Thieme

Essential Step-by-Step Techniques for Minimally Invasive Spinal Surgery

Roger Härtl, MD
Hansen-MacDonald Professor of Neurological Surgery;
Director of Neurosurgery Spine;
Director of the Weill Cornell Medicine Center for Comprehensive Spine Care
Weill Cornell Medicine & New York Presbyterian Och Spine
New York, New York, USA

Rodrigo Navarro-Ramirez, MD, MS
Spine-Fellowship Trained Neurosurgeon
Department of Neurological Surgery
Weill Cornell Medicine & New York Presbyterian Och Spine
New York, New York, USA

928 illustrations

Thieme
New York • Stuttgart • Delhi • Rio de Janeiro

Library of Congress Cataloging-in-Publication Data is available from the publisher.

Important note: Medicine is an ever-changing science undergoing continual development. Research and clinical experience are continually expanding our knowledge, in particular our knowledge of proper treatment and drug therapy. Insofar as this book mentions any dosage or application, readers may rest assured that the authors, editors, and publishers have made every effort to ensure that such references are in accordance with **the state of knowledge at the time of production of the book.**

Nevertheless, this does not involve, imply, or express any guarantee or responsibility on the part of the publishers in respect to any dosage instructions and forms of applications stated in the book. **Every user is requested to examine carefully** the manufacturers' leaflets accompanying each drug and to check, if necessary in consultation with a physician or specialist, whether the dosage schedules mentioned therein or the contraindications stated by the manufacturers differ from the statements made in the present book. Such examination is particularly important with drugs that are either rarely used or have been newly released on the market. Every dosage schedule or every form of application used is entirely at the user's own risk and responsibility. The authors and publishers request every user to report to the publishers any discrepancies or inaccuracies noticed. If errors in this work are found after publication, errata will be posted at www.thieme.com on the product description page.

Some of the product names, patents, and registered designs referred to in this book are in fact registered trademarks or proprietary names even though specific reference to this fact is not always made in the text. Therefore, the appearance of a name without designation as proprietary is not to be construed as a representation by the publisher that it is in the public domain.

Thieme addresses people of all gender identities equally. We encourage our authors to use gender-neutral or gender-equal expressions wherever the context allows.

Thieme Medical Publishers, Inc.
333 Seventh Avenue, 18th Floor,
New York, NY 10001, USA
www.thieme.com
+1 800 782 3488, customerservice@thieme.com

Cover design: © Thieme
Cover images source: © Thieme/Thom Graves
Typesetting by DiTech Process Solutions, India

Printed in India by Replika Press Pvt. Ltd. 5 4 3 2

ISBN: 978-1-68420-009-2

Also available as an e-book:
eISBN (PDF): 978-1-68420-010-8
eISBN (epub): 978-1-63853-623-9

To Alasha, Sebastian, and Julian. *Keep your eyes on the stars, and your feet on the ground. (Theodore Roosevelt)*

-Roger Härtl, MD

Dedicated to my parents.

To the students, residents, and fellows who inspired me to do this. This book was made thinking of you and I hope you find it useful.

To those role models who shaped my life and career inside and outside the operating room, I admire you and I will always be grateful: Roger H, Jean O, Peter J, Roberto DL, Max T, and Dr. Q.

Pablo L, Becky A, and AMSA, thanks for making dreams a reality through your cause.

-Rodrigo Navarro-Ramirez, MD, MS

In Memory of Khai Lam (1966-2021)

Contents

Videos ... xx

Foreword ... xxii

Preface ... xxiii

Contributors ... xxiv

Part I Introduction to MISS ... 1

1. Definition of MISS: The "6 Ts": Target/Technology/Technique/Teaching and Training/Testing/Talent ... 2

Roger Härtl, Sertac Kirnaz, Juan Del Castillo-Calcáneo, and Ibrahim Hussain

1.1 Definition of Minimally Invasive Spine Surgery ... 2

1.2 Potential of Minimally Invasive Spinal Surgery ... 3

1.3 The "6 Ts" to Success in MISS: Components for a Successful MISS Practice ... 4

1.4 Conclusion ... 12

2. Global MISS: Perspectives from Asia, Australia, Europe, Middle East, North America, and South America ... 14

2.1 Asia ... 14
Guang-Xun Lin, Jin-Sung Luke Kim, and Louis Chang

2.2 Australia ... 15
Tony Goldschlager

2.3 Europe ... 16
H. Michael Mayer

2.4 Middle East ... 17
Magdy Gamal AbdelKader Youssef

2.5 North America ... 18
Jason I. Liounakos and Michael Y. Wang

2.6 South America ... 19
Luiz Pimenta, Rodrigo Amaral, Leonardo Oliveira, and Luis Marchi

Part II MISS Target ... 21

3. Target Philosophy in Degenerative Spinal Disorders: Correlation of Clinical Presentation, Physical Examination, and Response to Interventional Procedures ... 22

Bridget T. Carey, Jaspal Ricky Singh, Neel Mehta, Taylor Wong, Sertac Kirnaz, Michael Sein, and Roger Härtl

3.1 Introduction ... 22

3.2 Cervical Segment ... 22

3.3 Thoracic Segment ... 27

3.4 Lumbar Segment ... 28

3.5 Conclusion ... 33

4. Deformity and MIS: Limitation or Opportunity? ... 41

Catherine Miller, Ibrahim Hussain, Juan S. Uribe, Kai-Ming Fu, and Praveen Mummaneni

4.1 Introduction ... 41

4.2 Spinopelvic Parameters ... 41

4.3 Opportunity for MIS Deformity Correction ... 41

4.4 Limitations of MIS ... 42

4.5 Patient Selection ... 43

4.6 MISDEF Algorithm ... 43

4.7 Example Cases ... 44

4.8 Conclusion ... 46

5. Target: The Muscle as a Pain Generator and Key Element to Protect during MIS Surgery ... 49

Norman Marcus and Roger Härtl

5.1 The Role of Muscles in Back and Neck Pain—before, during, and after Minimally Invasive Surgery ... 49

5.2 Introduction ... 49

5.3 Background ... 49

5.4 Clinical Presentation of Muscle Pain ... 49

5.5 Neuroanatomy and Neurophysiology of Muscle Pain: Myogenic (MGP) versus Neurogenic Inflammation ... 49

5.6 Clinical Examination ... 50

5.7 Muscle Generated Pain and Spinal Surgery ... 51

5.8 Operative Considerations ... 51

5.9 Conclusion ... 51

Part III MISS Technology ... 55

6. Tubular and Specular Retractors in MISS ... 56

Christoph Wipplinger, Sara Lener, Sertac Kirnaz, Ahmed Abdelsalam, Roger Härtl, and Claudius Thomé

6.1 Introduction ... 56

6.2 Tubular Retractor ... 56

6.3 Specular Retractor ... 57

6.4 Conclusion ... 59

6.5 Future Perspective ... 59

7. Navigation in MISS ... 61

Rodrigo Navarro-Ramirez, Alisson R. Teles, Franziska Anna Schmidt, Sertac Kirnaz, and Roger Härtl

7.1 Introduction ... 61

7.2 Technology ... 62

7.3 Image Acquisition ... 63

7.4 Registration System ... 63

7.5 Tracking System ... 63

7.6 Types of Navigation Systems ... 64

7.7 Teaching and Training ... 76

7.8 Conclusion ... 76

8. Robotics: Background and Current Role ... 79

Sean M. Barber, Meng Huang, Paul Holman, and Isador H. Lieberman

8.1 Introduction ... 79

8.2 Benefits and Limitations of Robotics in Spine Surgery ... 79

8.3 Early Evolution of Spinal Robotics 81

8.4 Robot-Assistance and Integrated Navigation 81

8.5 Basic Technique and Workflow 82

8.6 Learning Curve 83

8.7 Pearls and Pitfalls 84

8.8 Future Directions 84

9. Microscope in MISS 87

Avelino Parajón, Robert Nicholas Hernandez, Sertac Kirnaz, and Andreas Korge

9.1 Introduction 87

9.2 Historical Overview 87

9.3 Advantages of Using the Microscope in MISS 88

9.4 Disadvantages of the Microscope 89

9.5 Characteristics of Modern Spine/MISS Microscopes 91

9.6 Differences between Microscopes and Loupes 91

9.7 Operating Room Setup and Handling of Microscopes 91

9.8 Future 92

9.9 Training 92

10. Endoscope in MISS: How to Adopt and Change 95

Albert E. Telfeian

10.1 Introduction 95

10.2 Target 95

10.3 Pathologies Treated 96

10.4 Technology 96

10.5 Technique: Step-by-Step 96

10.6 Expanding Indications 97

10.7 Teaching and Training 100

10.8 Conclusion 100

Part IV MISS Techniques 102

11. Three Surgical Principles of MISS: Contralateral Decompression, Minimize Instability, and Indirect Decompression 103

Ibrahim Hussain, Rodrigo Navarro-Ramirez, Sertac Kirnaz, and Roger Härtl

11.1 Introduction 103

11.2 Contralateral Decompression 103

11.3 Minimizing Instability 106

11.4 Indirect Decompression 107

11.5 Conclusion 109

12. Surgical Techniques and Instrumentation in MISS 110

Robert Nicholas Hernandez, Sertac Kirnaz, and Michael S. Virk

12.1 Introduction 110

12.2 Bayoneted or Curved Instrumentation 110

12.3 Retractors 110

12.4 Drills 111

12.5 Visualization ... 111

12.6 Endoscopic Spine Surgery ... 112

12.7 Cerebral Spinal Fluid Leak Repair ... 112

12.8 Conclusion ... 113

13. Dural Repair in MISS and CSF Leak Management ... 114

Ramin A. Morshed, Young M. Lee, and Dean Chou

13.1 Introduction ... 114

13.2 Techniques for Repair ... 114

13.3 Conclusion ... 116

14. How to Achieve a Successful Fusion with MIS Techniques ... 118

Nickul S. Jain and Jeffrey C. Wang

14.1 Introduction ... 118

14.2 Host Factors ... 118

14.3 Interbody Fusion ... 121

14.4 Author's Preferred Technique for MIS TLIF ... 121

14.5 Discussion ... 123

15. Surgical Tips, Tricks, and Techniques to Minimize Invasiveness; General Advice on How to Handle Fluoroscopy, Blood Loss, and Infection Rates ... 126

Eric H. Elowitz

15.1 Introduction ... 126

15.2 Patient Evaluation and Selection ... 126

15.3 Preoperative Planning ... 127

15.4 Incision Planning and Tubular Considerations ... 127

15.5 Incision Planning for Lumbar Fusions ... 128

15.6 Fluoroscopy/Radiation Exposure ... 128

15.7 Navigation and Robotics ... 128

15.8 Blood Loss Minimization ... 128

15.9 Infection Rates ... 129

15.10 Conclusion ... 130

16. Perioperative Management; ERAS ... 132

G. Damian Brusko, Karthik Madhavan, and Michael Y. Wang

16.1 Introduction ... 132

16.2 Basic Principles of Enhanced Recovery ... 132

16.3 Incorporating ERAS into Minimally Invasive Spine Surgery ... 132

16.4 Implementation of ERAS in Spine Surgery ... 134

16.5 Conclusion ... 134

17. Key Elements to Safely Transition from Inpatient to Outpatient Spine Surgery ... 136

Richard Wohns

17.1 Proper Procedure Choices ... 136

17.2 Lumbar Spine ... 136

17.3 Cervical Spine ... 138

18. Posterior Cervical Foraminotomy/Discectomy 141
Luca Papavero

18.1 Introduction 141
18.2 Patient Selection: Indications, Contraindications 141
18.3 Preoperative Planning 141
18.4 Patient Positioning and Labeling of the Disc Space 142
18.5 Surgical Technique 142
18.6 Postoperative Care 143
18.7 Complications and Avoidance 143
18.8 Tips and Tricks 143

19. Unilateral Tubular Over-the-Top Cervical Laminectomy for Cervical Stenosis 149
Robert Nicholas Hernandez, Sergio Soriano-Solis, and José-Antonio Soriano-Sánchez

19.1 Introduction 149
19.2 Indications 149
19.3 Contraindications 149
19.4 Preoperative Planning 149
19.5 Surgical Steps 150
19.6 Postoperative Care 154
19.7 Complication Avoidance 154
19.8 Tips and Tricks 155
19.9 Conclusion 156

20. Posterior Cervical Facet Cages DTRAX 157
Melissa Meyer, John B. Ferraro, and Rahul V. Shah

20.1 Introduction 157
20.2 Indications 157
20.3 Contraindications 157
20.4 Preoperative Planning 157
20.5 Patient Positioning 157
20.6 Surgical Technique 158
20.7 Postoperative Care 161
20.8 Complications and Avoidance 162
20.9 Tips and Tricks 162

21. MIS Endoscopic Approaches for OC–C1–C2 Pathology 163
Rafael Uribe, Sertac Kirnaz, and Theodore H. Schwartz

21.1 Introduction 163
21.2 Indications 163
21.3 Techniques 163
21.4 Complication Avoidance and Management 167
21.5 Postoperative Care 168
21.6 Case Examples 168
21.7 Conclusion 169

22. Posterior Muscle Sparing Approaches for Decompression, Laminoplasty, and Laminectomy 171
Lionel N. Metz, Martin H. Pham, Kevin M. Hwang, and K. Daniel Riew

22.1 Introduction 171
22.2 Patient Selection: Indications, Contraindications 171
22.3 Preoperative Planning 172
22.4 Patient Positioning 173
22.5 Surgical Technique 174
22.6 Tips and Tricks 180

23. Minimally Invasive C1/C2 Fusion 182
Marcus Richter

23.1 Introduction 182
23.2 Indications 182
23.3 Contraindications 183
23.4 Preoperative Planning 183
23.5 Patient Positioning 183
23.6 Surgical Steps 184
23.7 Postoperative Care 187
23.8 Complication Avoidance 187
23.9 Tips and Tricks 190
23.10 Conclusion 190

24. Cervical Three-Dimensional Navigation to Facilitate Minimally Invasive Spine Surgery 191
Maziyar A. Kalani, Iain H. Kalfas, and Michael P. Steinmetz

24.1 Introduction 191
24.2 Indications 191
24.3 Contraindications 192
24.4 Preoperative Planning 192
24.5 Patient Positioning 192
24.6 Surgical Steps 192
24.7 Postoperative Care 194
24.8 Complication Avoidance 194
24.9 Tips and Tricks 195

25. Thoracic Vertebroplasty and Kyphoplasty 197
Justin Schwarz, Srikanth Boddu, Ibrahim Hussain, Alejandro Santillan, and Athos Patsalides

25.1 Introduction 197
25.2 Indications 197
25.3 Contraindications 197
25.4 Preoperative Planning 198
25.5 Patient Positioning 198
25.6 Surgical Steps 198
25.7 Postoperative Care 201
25.8 Complication Avoidance 201
25.9 Tips and Tricks 202
25.10 Conclusion 202

26. Thoracic Discectomy: Posterior Transpedicular Tubular Approach 203
Christopher D. Witiw, Brian T. David, and Richard G. Fessler

26.1 Introduction 203
26.2 Indications 203
26.3 Contraindications 203
26.4 Preoperative Planning 203
26.5 Patient Positioning 204
26.6 Surgical Steps 204
26.7 Postoperative Care 205
26.8 Complication Avoidance 205
26.9 Tips and Tricks 205
26.10 Conclusion 206

27. Lateral Retropleural Thoracic Discectomy and Corpectomy 207
David S. Xu, Jakub Godzik, S. Harrison Farber, Shashank V. Gandhi, Ernest J. Wright, Courtney Hemphill, Sebastian Uribe, and Juan S. Uribe

27.1 Introduction 207
27.2 Indications 207
27.3 Contraindications 207
27.4 Preoperative Planning 207
27.5 Patient Positioning 207
27.6 Step-by-Step Surgical Technique with Example 208
27.7 Postoperative Care 211
27.8 Complications and Avoidance 211
27.9 Tips and Tricks 213
27.10 Conclusion 213

28. Mini-Open Pedicle Subtraction Osteotomy for Deformity Correction 214
Cory Hartman, Jakub Godzik, Esteban Quiceno, and Juan S. Uribe

28.1 Introduction 214
28.2 Indications 215
28.3 Contraindications 215
28.4 Preoperative Planning 215
28.5 Patient Positioning 216
28.6 Surgical Steps 216
28.7 Postoperative Care 217
28.8 Complication Avoidance 218
28.9 Tips and Tricks 218
28.10 Conclusion 218

29. Posterior Paramedian Endoscopic Thoracic Discectomy 220
Raj Nangunoori, Diana H. Jho, David H. Jho, and Hae-Dong Jho

29.1 Introduction 220
29.2 Evolution of the Paramedian Approach 220
29.3 Patient Selection 221
29.4 Preoperative Planning and Patient Positioning 221
29.5 Surgical Technique 222
29.6 Postoperative Care 224

29.7 Complications and Avoidance ... 224
29.8 Tips and Tricks ... 224

30. Transpedicular Corpectomy and Fusion for Metastatic Tumor or Infection ... 226
Young M. Lee, Ramin A. Morshed, and Dean Chou

30.1 Introduction ... 226
30.2 Patient Selection: Indications and Contraindications ... 226
30.3 Preoperative Planning ... 226
30.4 Patient Positioning ... 226
30.5 Surgical Technique with Illustration/ Example ... 226
30.6 Postoperative Care ... 228
30.7 Complications and Avoidance ... 229

31. Techniques to Decrease the Invasiveness of Thoracic Deformity Correction ... 231
Brenton Pennicooke, Robert Nicholas Hernandez, and Michael S. Virk

31.1 Introduction ... 231
31.2 Computer-Assisted Navigation/Robotics/ Planning Software ... 231
31.3 Minimally Invasive Approaches to Three-Column Osteotomies and Expandable Cages ... 232
31.4 Percutaneous/Transfascial Instrumentation ... 233
31.5 Facet Joint Fusion and Arthrodesis ... 233
31.6 Optical Adjuncts and Visualization ... 234
31.7 Limitations ... 235
31.8 Conclusion ... 235

32. Unilateral Lumbar Approach for Over-the-Top Bilateral Decompression ... 238
Franziska C. Heider, Andreas Korge, and H. Michael Mayer

32.1 Introduction ... 238
32.2 Indications ... 238
32.3 Contraindications ... 238
32.4 Preoperative Planning ... 239
32.5 Patient Positioning ... 239
32.6 Surgical Steps ... 240
32.7 Postoperative Care ... 242
32.8 Complication Avoidance ... 243
32.9 Tips and Tricks ... 243
32.10 Conclusion ... 243

33. Far-Lateral Lumbar Discectomies ... 245
Eric H. Elowitz

33.1 Introduction ... 245
33.2 Indications ... 245
33.3 Contraindications ... 246
33.4 Preoperative Planning ... 246
33.5 Patient Positioning ... 246
33.6 Surgical Steps ... 247
33.7 Postoperative Care ... 249
33.8 Complication Avoidance ... 249

33.9 Tips and Tricks ... 250
33.10 Conclusion ... 250

34. Percutaneous Full-Endoscopic Interlaminar Approach for Lumbar Pathologies: Disc Herniation and Lumbar Spinal Stenosis ... 253
Javier Quillo-Olvera and Jin-Sung Luke Kim

34.1 Introduction ... 253
34.2 Indications ... 253
34.3 Contraindications ... 254
34.4 Preoperative Planning ... 254
34.5 Patient Positioning ... 254
34.6 Surgical Steps ... 254
34.7 Postoperative Care ... 258
34.8 Complication Avoidance ... 260
34.9 Tips and Tricks ... 260
34.10 Conclusion ... 260

35. Transforaminal Approach for Endoscopic Decompression ... 262
Ralf Wagner

35.1 Introduction ... 262
35.2 Indications ... 263
35.3 Contraindications ... 263
35.4 Preoperative Planning ... 263
35.5 Patient Positioning ... 264
35.6 Surgical Technique ... 264
35.7 Postoperative Care ... 270
35.8 Complication Avoidance ... 270
35.9 Tips and Tricks ... 270
35.10 Conclusion ... 271

36. Endoscopic Interlaminar Lumbar Laminectomy ... 273
Christoph Hofstetter

36.1 Introduction ... 273
36.2 Patient Selection ... 273
36.3 Indications ... 273
36.4 Surgical Technique ... 273
36.5 Tips and Tricks ... 278
36.6 Complications and Avoidance ... 278

37. LLIF T12/L1-L2 ... 279
Cristiano Magalhães Menezes and Érica Godinho Menezes

37.1 Introduction ... 279
37.2 Indications ... 279
37.3 Contraindications ... 279
37.4 Preoperative Planning ... 280
37.5 Patient Positioning ... 280
37.6 Surgical Steps ... 281
37.7 Postoperative Care ... 283
37.8 Complication Avoidance ... 283
37.9 Tips and Tricks ... 284
37.10 Conclusion ... 284

38. LLIF L2/3/4/5 ... 286
Frank M. Phillips and Sravisht Iyer

38.1 Introduction ... 286
38.2 Indications ... 286
38.3 Contraindications ... 286
38.4 Preoperative Planning ... 286
38.5 Patient Positioning ... 287
38.6 Surgical Steps ... 290
38.7 Postoperative Care ... 291
38.8 Complications and Avoidance ... 291
38.9 Tips and Tricks ... 291
38.10 Conclusion ... 292

39. Translumbar Surgery Comparison: Four Surgeons and Regions ... 293
Luiz Pimenta, Khai Lam†, Massimo Balsano, and Masato Tanaka

39.1 How I Do It ... 293

40. Minimally Invasive Oblique Anterior Lumbar Interbody Fusion ... 308
H. Michael Mayer, Andreas Korge, Frizzi Mayer, Franziska C. Heider, and Christoph Mehren

40.1 Introduction ... 308
40.2 Indications ... 308
40.3 Contraindications ... 308
40.4 Preoperative Planning ... 308
40.5 Patient Positioning ... 309
40.6 Surgical Steps ... 309
40.7 Postoperative Care ... 312
40.8 Complication Avoidance/Tips and Tricks ... 312
40.9 Conclusion ... 313

41. Maximum Access Surgery Posterior Lumbar Interbody Fusion ... 314
Joel Martin, Laura Hein, Pavan S. Upadhyayula, Vincent Cheung, and William Taylor

41.1 Introduction ... 314
41.2 Indications ... 314
41.3 Contraindications ... 314
41.4 Preoperative Planning ... 314
41.5 Patient Positioning ... 314
41.6 Surgical Technique ... 315
41.7 Postoperative Care ... 317
41.8 Complications and Avoidance ... 318
41.9 Tips and Tricks ... 320
41.10 Conclusions ... 320

42. MIS-TLIF with Total Navigation and Expandable Interbody Cages ... 322
Rodrigo Navarro-Ramirez, Sertac Kirnaz, and Roger Härtl

42.1 Introduction ... 322
42.2 Patient Selection: Indications and Contraindications ... 322
42.3 Preoperative Planning ... 322
42.4 Patient Positioning ... 323
42.5 Surgical Technique ... 324

42.6 Postoperative Care 326
42.7 Complications and Avoidance 329
42.8 Conclusion 329

43. MIS-TLIF Comparison: Four Surgeons and Regions 331
Seang-Beng Tan, Kevin Foley, Nestor Taboada, and Giuseppe Barbagallo

43.1 How I Do It 331

44. Percutaneous Pedicle Screw Fixation and MISS SI Joint Fusion 343
Greg Anderson

44.1 Introduction 343
44.2 Indications 343
44.3 Contraindications 343
44.4 Technique 343
44.5 Complication and Avoidance 346
44.6 Tips and Tricks 346
44.7 MIS SI Joint Fusion 347

45. Intradural Extramedullary Tumors 350
Hani Malone, Richard G. Fessler, and John E. O'Toole

45.1 Introduction 350
45.2 Patient Selection: Indications and Contraindications 350
45.3 Preoperative Planning 351
45.4 Technique 352
45.5 Postoperative Care 354
45.6 Complications and Avoidance 354
45.7 Tips and Tricks 354
45.8 Conclusion 355

46. Three-Dimensional Navigation in Lumbar Spine to Facilitate Minimally Invasive Spine Surgery 356
Jang W. Yoon, Gaetano De Biase, and Eric W. Nottmeier

46.1 Introduction 356
46.2 Preoperative Planning 356
46.3 Patient Selection: Indications and Contraindications 356
46.4 Patient Positioning 356
46.5 Surgical Technique 357
46.6 Use of Robotics and Augmented Reality in Spine Surgery: Future Implications 358

47. Strategies to Minimize Invasiveness and Optimize Success: OC Fusion 360
Bernhard Meyer and Sandro M. Krieg

47.1 Introduction 360
47.2 Indications for OC Fusion 360
47.3 Risks 360
47.4 Outcomes 360
47.5 Options for Reducing Invasiveness 361
47.6 Case 1 361

47.7 Case 2 ... 363
47.8 Discussion ... 365
47.9 Conclusion ... 365

48. Strategies to Minimize Invasiveness and Optimize Success: Cervical Front/Back Surgery for Deformity Correction ... 367
Lee A. Tan and K. Daniel Riew

48.1 Introduction ... 367
48.2 Surgical Planning for Cervical Spine Deformity ... 367
48.3 Surgical Technique to Minimize Invasiveness ... 368
48.4 Case Illustration ... 368
48.5 Conclusion ... 372

49. MIS Cervical Pedicle Screws—Percutaneous-Assisted Technique ... 373
Marcus Richter and Philipp Hartung

49.1 Introduction ... 373
49.2 Indications ... 374
49.3 Contraindications ... 374
49.4 Preoperative Planning ... 374
49.5 Patient Positioning ... 374
49.6 Surgical Steps ... 375
49.7 Postoperative Care ... 379
49.8 Complication Avoidance ... 380
49.9 Tips and Tricks ... 381
49.10 Conclusion ... 381

50. Treatment of Degenerative Lumbar Scoliosis with Minimally Invasive Multilevel LLIF in Combination with Lateral ALIF ... 382
James E. Dowdell, Giuseppe Barbagallo, and Sheeraz Qureshi

50.1 Introduction ... 382
50.2 Preoperative Presentation ... 382
50.3 Imaging Studies ... 382
50.4 Indications for Surgery ... 382
50.5 Case Presentation ... 383
50.6 Applied Anatomy of the Lateral Approach to the Spine ... 384
50.7 Surgical Procedure ... 385
50.8 Surgical Steps ... 386
50.9 Postoperative Course ... 391
50.10 Back to Case ... 392
50.11 Tips and Pearls for Treating ADLS with Minimally Invasive Surgery ... 393

51. Strategies to Minimize Invasiveness and Optimize Success: T10-Pelvis ... 395
Neel Anand, Alisa Alayan, and Sheila Kahwaty

51.1 Preoperative Presentation ... 395
51.2 Imaging Studies ... 395
51.3 Decision-Making for MIS ... 395
51.4 Factors Favoring Open Surgery ... 395

51.5 Details of Surgery 395

51.6 Trips and Tricks 402

52. Lifestyle Medicine: Optimizing Recovery Following MIS of the Spine 403

Jaspal Ricky Singh and Kyle F. Worell

52.1 Benefits of Minimally Invasive Spine Surgery 403

52.2 Exercise and Spine Therapy 403

52.3 Smoking Effects in Spine Surgery 407

52.4 Health and Wellness Coaching 408

53. Three-Dimensional Navigation in MISS 410

Bernhard Meyer and Yu-Mi Ryang

53.1 Introduction 410

53.2 State-of-the-Art—Where Are We Heading? 410

53.3 Future Perspectives 410

53.4 Conclusion 411

Part V Teaching and Training/Future 413

54. Surgical Training and Simulation in MISS 414

Carolin Melcher, Thana Theofanis, Yusef Mosley, Geoffrey Stricsek, Sertac Kirnaz, and James S. Harrop

54.1 Introduction 414

54.2 Methods 414

55. The Role of Biologics in Minimally Invasive Spine Surgery 420

Howard An

55.1 Introduction 420

55.2 Biologics for Spinal Arthrodesis 420

55.3 Conclusion 421

56. Summary and Outlook—Future of Lumbar Minimally Invasive Surgery 423

Joel Martin, Laura Hein, Vincent Cheung, and William Taylor

56.1 Adoption and Diffusion 423

56.2 Patient Care and Procedures 423

57. Achieving MISS on a Global Level 427

Roger Härtl, Franziska Anna Schmidt, Taylor Wong, and Sertac Kirnaz

57.1 Introduction 427

57.2 MISS and Leapfrogging 428

57.3 Economic Impact of MISS on Health Care in Health Care Systems Worldwide 428

Index 430

Videos

Video 11.1 MIS tubular decompression.

Video 13.1 CSF-leak MIS dural repair.

Video 18.1 Posterior cervical foraminotomy.

Video 19.1 MIS tubular cervical laminectomy.

Video 20.1 This video demonstrates steps for the DTRAX procedure, beginning with room setup. Patient positioning and C-arm set up is shown. The step-by-step procedure for DTRAX placement is then reviewed.

Video 24.1 Cervical 3D navigation to facilitate MISS.

Video 25.1 Thoracic vertebroplasty and kyphoplasty.

Video 26.1 Decompression of a symptomatic T7/8 disc herniation via a right-sided posterior transpedicular tubular approach.

Video 27.1 Minimally invasive lateral retropleural thoracic discectomy.

Video 30.1 Mini-open transpedicular corpectomy.

Video 32.1 Unilateral lumbar approach.

Video 34.1 Full-endoscopic lumbar interlaminar discectomy.

Video 34.2 Full-endoscopic interlaminar decompression for lumbar spinal stenosis.

Video 35.1 First steps for the endoscopic approach with TESSYS.

Video 35.2 First steps for the intradiscal endoscopic approach.

Video 35.3 First steps for the far lateral endoscopic approach.

Video 35.4 First steps for the transpedicular endoscopic approach.

Video 35.5 First steps for the contralateral endoscopic approach.

Video 35.6 First steps for the dorsolateral endoscopic approach.

Video 37.1 LLIF step-by-step technique.

Video 38.1 Lateral lumbar interbody fusion L2/L3/L4/L5.

Video 42.1 Total navigation MIS TLIF.

Video 43.1 MIS TLIF cage insertion with K-wire through the retractor.

Video 45.1 Intradural extramedullary tumors.

Video 49.1 Pedicle screws cervical MIS.

Foreword

Why is a spinal deformity surgeon with 30 years' experience who treats pediatric and adult patients via open posterior approaches writing the foreword for the most authoritative, complete, and detailed minimally invasive spine surgery (MISS) textbook ever written?

My answer comes from the first chapter of this incredibly valuable and timely book: Definition of MISS: The "6Ts": Target/Technology/Technique/Teaching and Training/Testing/Talent. In my vast experience of treating the entire spectrum of the most straightforward as well as the most complex spinal deformities, these "6Ts" are not only the hallmarks of perfecting MISS, but also open deformity surgery, and in reality, any type of successful spinal surgery. Behind the 6Ts is the mastery of spinal, neural, and perivertebral anatomy, as well as the optimization of surgical instruments, implants, and techniques that require proper training and talent, and then the performance of critical review of outcomes. This defines the profession of spinal surgery whether performing an endoscopic discectomy at L4–L5 for a posterolateral herniated nucleus pulposus (HNP), or a C2-sacrum/ilium total spinal reconstruction for a severe kyphotic osteoporotic spinal column collapse. That is why I agreed to write this foreword as someone who does not practice MISS on a daily basis, but nonetheless understands, respects, and appreciates those spinal surgeons who have revolutionized the quickly advancing field of MISS.

The entire tone of this monumental treatise on the state-of-the-art MISS begins with the first chapter by providing the definition of MISS as developed by a recent consensus by AOSpine: "A suite of technology-dependent techniques and procedures that reduces local operative tissue damage and systemic surgical stress, enabling earlier return to function and striving for better outcomes than traditional techniques." This initial and the following 56 chapters in this incredibly comprehensive work go on to describe, in great detail, how MISS can be applied to nearly any spinal operation. In painstaking detail, the appropriate indications, pathoanatomy, specific techniques, and equipment, along with valuable pearls and pitfalls, are provided to ensure the reader is versed in all aspects of MISS treatment of various spinal pathologies. Two of the highlights of this book include the reliance on plentiful images, figures, anatomic drawings, and imaging studies to illustrate the relevant anatomic approaches and corridors, and the emphasis on how anatomic mastery is critical to MISS. Additionally, it is recognized throughout the book that there are numerous idiosyncratic techniques used by the various surgeon contributors to accomplish their MISS goals—not a one-size-fits-all approach. This is highlighted nicely in the outstanding Chapter 43 on MIS-TLIF Comparison: Four Surgeons and Regions where one of the most commonly performed MISS surgeries is detailed step by step by four surgeons from various parts of the world: Asia, Dr. Seang-Beng Tan; Europe, Dr. Guiseppe Barbagallo; Latin America, Dr. Nestor Taboada; and North America, Dr. Kevin Foley. To me, this unique chapter epitomizes the global coverage of this topic in such a comparative and detailed manner that I personally have never seen before in any textbook chapter—truly incredible work!

Obviously, I am unable to comment on all of the chapters included, but do want to emphasize that every operative spinal pathology, along with specific MISS technique and specialized equipment needs, is covered in this exhaustive review. From Chapter 6 "Tubular and Specular Retractors in MISS" to Chapter 12 "Surgical Techniques and Instrumentation in MISS" to Chapter 14 "How to Achieve a Successful Fusion with MIS Techniques," to the final Chapter 57 "Achieving MISS on a Global Level," no stone is left unturned to provide the reader with the most complete and practical guide on MISS. The direction and groundwork for the entire array of chapters are really set by the illustrative cover: understanding relevant spinal anatomy, corridors, and targets to get to the relevant pathology as directly and with the least invasive method possible to accomplish the operative goals—this book cover illustration truly does speak a thousand words!

Having experienced putting chapters together as an editor of several spinal surgery textbooks, I truly understand the unbelievable commitment and effort needed to see this type of book to completion. Thus, I want to personally congratulate Dr. Roger Härtl and Dr. Rodrigo Navarro-Ramirez, the forces behind this seminal textbook, for their vision, leadership, and passion for MISS. They, along with all of the contributing surgeon authors, have created the current "Bible" of MISS that will help so many trainees and practicing spinal surgeons who will benefit from the expertise presented. This will then be translated into exponentially positive outcomes for many future patients afflicted with various spinal conditions who will be treated by MISS around the world, so thanks to all of you involved in this book. Because of you, the profession of spinal surgery, and specifically the subspeciality of MISS, has become better understood, much more global, and extremely successful. Congratulations!

Larry Lenke, MD
Surgeon-in-chief
New York Presbyterian Och Spine
New York, New York, USA

Preface

We are pleased to present our first edition of the *Essential Step-by-Step Techniques for Minimally Invasive Spinal Surgery*. Our goal is to gather MISS techniques in a comprehensive way and make them accessible for all spine surgeons regardless of their level of training. We understand that MISS is global and constantly evolving. However, appropriate patient selection (Target), access to hardware/software (Technology), special surgical technique (Technique), adequate education (Training), critical thinking, outcome evaluation (Testing), and surgical excellence (Talent) remain critical and represent the core elements that interact and determine the success of *any* surgery but MISS in particular.

In this book, we asked operative and nonoperative experts from around the world to contribute their experience and pearls surrounding the operative and perioperative management of MISS. We asked MISS expert surgeons to describe not only the indications and contraindications of the procedures, but also their step-by-step techniques, tips/tricks, complication avoidance, and postoperative care.

Essential Step-by-Step Techniques for Minimally Invasive Spinal Surgery is generously equipped with media (illustrations, pictures, figures, tables, comparative chapters, and videos) in an effort to share with the reader the "experience" of the experts/contributors. We are confident that the readers will find in this book a new reference to learn, review, and implement the core elements of MISS into their own practice.

We are certain that this book will become part of the basic armamentarium for all of those interested in spine surgery and minimally invasive techniques as we all aim for excellence and better patient surgical outcomes.

Roger Härtl, MD
Rodrigo Navarro-Ramirez, MD, MS

Contributors

Ahmed Abdelsalam, MD
Neurovascular Clinical Research Fellow
Department of Neurological Surgery
University of Miami
Miller School of Medicine
Miami, Florida, USA

Alisa Alayan, MD
Spine Surgeon
Spine Center
Cedars-Sinai Medical Center
Los Angeles, California, USA

Rodrigo Amaral, MD
Orthopaedic Spine Surgeon
São Paulo, São Paulo, Brazil

Howard An, MD
Professor and Director
Spine Surgery
Rush University Medical Center
Chicago, Illinois, USA

Neel Anand, MD, FAAOS
Professor of Orthopaedic Surgery
Department of Orthopaedic Surgery
Minimally Invasive Spine Surgery Spine Center
Cedars-Sinai Medical Center
Los Angeles, California, USA

Greg Anderson, MD
Orthopedic and Spine Surgeon
Rothman Orthopaedic Institute
Philadelphia, Pennsylvania, USA

Massimo Balsano, MD
Direttore UOC Ortopedia e Chirurgia Vertebrale
Centro Regionale Hub per la Chirurgia Vertebrale
Azienda Ospedaliera Universitaria
Head of Spinal Regional Department
University and Hospital Trust of Verona
Verona, Italy

Giuseppe Barbagallo, MD
Full Professor and Chairman
Department of Neurosurgery
Policlinico "G. Rodolico - San Marco" University Hospital
Catania, Italy

Sean M. Barber, MD
Neurosurgeon
Department of Neurosurgery
Houston Methodist Neurological Institute
Houston Methodist Hospital
Houston, Texas, USA

Srikanth Boddu, MD
Interventional Neuroradiologist
New York Presbyterian Hospital
Weill Cornell Medical College
New York, New York, USA

G. Damian Brusko, MD
Department of Neurological Surgery
University of Miami Miller School of Medicine
Miami, Florida, USA

Bridget T. Carey, MD
Assistant Professor of Clinical Neurology
Weill Cornell Medical College;
Assistant Attending Neurologist
Hospital for Special Surgery
New York, New York, USA

Juan Del Castillo-Calcáneo, MD
Neurosurgeon
American British Cowdray Medical Center
Mexico City, Mexico

Louis Chang, MD, FAANS, FACS
Assistant Professor
Department of Neurosurgery
New York Presbyterian Hospital
Weill Cornell Medical College
New York, New York, USA

Vincent Cheung, MD
Neurosurgeon
Anaheim Medical Center
Anaheim, California, USA

Dean Chou, MD
Professor of Neurosurgery
Department of Neurological Surgery
University of California at San Francisco
San Francisco, California, USA

Brian T. David, PhD
Assistant Professor
Department of Neurosurgery
Rush University Medical College
Chicago, Illinois, USA

Gaetano De Biase, MD
Research Fellow
Department of Neurosurgery
Mayo Clinic
Jacksonville, Florida, USA

James E. Dowdell, MD
Assistant Professor of Spine Surgery
Hospital for Special Surgery
Weill Cornell Medical College
New York, New York, USA

Eric H. Elowitz, MD
Associate Professor
Department of Neurosurgery
New York-Presbyterian Hospital
Weill-Cornell Medicine Brain and Spine Center
New York, New York, USA

S. Harrison Farber, MD
Department of Neurosurgery
Barrow Neurological Institute
Phoenix, Arizona, USA

John B. Ferraro, MHS, PA-C
Physician Assistant
Inspira Health Network
Vineland, New Jersey, USA

Richard G. Fessler, MD, PhD
Professor of Neurosurgery
Department of Neurosurgery
Rush University Medical Center
Chicago, Illinois, USA

Kevin Foley, MD
Professor of Neurosurgery
Department of Neurosurgery
University of Tennessee
Knoxville, Tennessee, USA

Kai-Ming Fu, MD
Associate Professor of Neurological and Spinal Surgery
Department of Neurological Surgery
Weill Cornell Medical College
New York, New York, USA

Shashank V. Gandhi, MD
Neurosurgeon
Department of Neurological Surgery
Texas Back Institute
Plano, Texas, USA

Jakub Godzik, MD
Department of Neurosurgery
Barrow Neurological Institute
St Joseph's Hospital and Medical Center
Phoenix, Arizona, USA

Tony Goldschlager, MBBS, DCH (London), PhD, FRACS
Neurosurgeon
Head of Endoscopic Skull Base Surgery and Minimally Invasive Spine Surgery
Monash University
Melbourne, Victoria, Australia

James S. Harrop, MD, MSHQS, FACS
Professor
Departments of Neurological and Orthopedic Surgery;
Director
Division of Spine and Peripheral Nerve Surgery;
Co-Director Neurologic Surgery Quality and Safety;
Neurosurgery Director
Delaware Valley SCI Center
Thomas Jefferson University
Philadelphia, Pennsylvania, USA

Roger Härtl, MD
Hansen-MacDonald Professor of Neurological Surgery;
Director of Neurosurgery Spine;
Director of the Weill Cornell Medicine Center for Comprehensive Spine Care
Weill Cornell Medicine & New York Presbyterian Och Spine
New York, New York, USA

Cory Hartman, MD
Neurosurgeon
Department of Neurosurgery
Barrow Neurological institute
St Joseph's Hospital and Medical Center
Phoenix, Arizona, USA

Philipp Hartung, MD
Spine Center
St. Josefs-Hospital
Wiesbaden, Germany

Franziska C. Heider, MD
Schön Klinik Munich Harlaching
Spine Center
Academic Teaching Hospital of the Paracelsus Medical University Salzburg (AU)
Harlachinger, Munich, Germany

Laura Hein, MSc
Tulane University
New Orleans, Louisiana, USA

Courtney Hemphill
Department of Neurosurgery
Barrow Neurological Institute
St. Joseph's Hospital and Medical Center
Phoenix, Arizona, USA

Robert Nicholas Hernandez, MD
Penn Medicine – Lancaster General Health Physicians
Lancaster General Health Crooked Oak
Lancaster, Pennsylvania, USA

Christoph Hofstetter, MD, PhD
Associate Professor
Department of Neurological Surgery
University of Washington
Seattle, Washington, USA

Paul Holman, MD
Neurosurgeon
Department of Neurosurgery
Houston Methodist Neurological Institute
Houston Methodist Hospital
Houston, Texas, USA

Meng Huang, MD
Neurological Spine Surgery Specialist
Department of Neurosurgery
Houston Methodist Neurological Institute
Houston Methodist Hospital
Houston, Texas, USA

Ibrahim Hussain, MD
Associate Professor of Neurological Surgery, Spinal Surgery
Department of Neurological Surgery
Weill Cornell Medical College
New York, New York, USA

Kevin M. Hwang, MD
Spine Surgery Fellow
Department of Orthopaedic Surgery
Massachusetts General Hospital
Boston, Massachusetts, USA

Sravisht Iyer, MD
Assistant Attending Orthopedic Surgeon
Hospital for Special Surgery;
Assistant Professor in Orthopedic Surgery
Weill Cornell Medical College
New York, New York, USA

Nickul S. Jain, MD
Orthopaedic Surgeon
Southern California Orthopedic Institute
Bakersfield, California, USA

David H. Jho, MD, PhD
Associate Professor
Department of Neurosurgery
Drexel University College of Medicine
Philadelphia, Pennsylvania, USA

Diana H. Jho, MD
Assistant Professor
Department of Neurological Surgery
Penn State Health
Hershey, Pennsylvania, USA

Hae-Dong Jho, MD, PhD
Professor and Chair
Department of Neuroendoscopy
Allegheny General Hospital
Drexel University College of Medicine
Philadelphia, Pennsylvania, USA

Sheila Kahwaty, PA-C, MPAS
Spine Center
Cedars-Sinai Medical Center
Los Angeles, California, USA

Maziyar A. Kalani, MD
Neurosurgeon
Department of Neurological Surgery
Mayo Clinic
Phoenix, Arizona, USA

Iain H. Kalfas, MD
Neurosurgeon
Cleveland Clinic Center for Spine Health
Neurological Institute
Cleveland Clinic Foundation
Cleveland, Ohio, USA

Jin-Sung Luke Kim, MD, PhD
Professor
Spine Center
Department of Neurosurgery
Seoul St. Mary's Hospital
College of Medicine
The Catholic University of Korea
Seoul, Korea

Sertac Kirnaz, MD
Spine Research Fellow
Department of Neurological Surgery
Weill Cornell Medicine
New York, New York, USA

Andreas Korge, MD
Schön Klinik Munich Harlaching
Spine Center
Academic Teaching Hospital of the Paracelsus Medical University Salzburg (AU)
Harlachinger, Munich, Germany

Sandro M. Krieg, MD
Senior Attending Neurosurgeon
Department of Neurosurgery
Klinikum rechts der Isar
School of Medicine
Technische Universität München
Munich, Germany

Khai Lam†, FRCS
King Edward VII's Hospital
The London Clinic
London, UK

Young M. Lee, MD
Neurosurgeon
Department of Neurological Surgery
University of California
San Francisco, California, USA

Sara Lener, MD
Spine Research Fellow
New York Presbyterian Hospital
Weill Cornell Medical College
New York, New York, USA

Isador H. Lieberman, MD
Neurosurgeon and Orthopedic Surgeon
Departments of Neurological and Orthopedic Surgery
Texas Back Institute
Plano, Texas, USA

Guang-Xun Lin, PhD
Department of Orthopedics
The Catholic University of Korea
Seoul, South Korea

Jason I. Liounakos, MD
Neurosurgeon
University of Miami
Miami, Florida, USA

Karthik Madhavan, MD
Assistant Professor of Neurosurgery
Department of Neurological Surgery
University of North Dakota School of Medicine and Health Sciences
Fargo, North Dakota, USA

Hani Malone, MD
Scripps Clinic Neurosurgery
San Diego Spine Foundation
San Diego, California, USA

Luis Marchi, MS
Department of Minimally Invasive Surgery
Instituto de Patologia da Coluna
São Paulo, Brazil

Norman Marcus, MD
Director
Clinical Muscle Pain Research
New York Presbyterian Hospital
Weill Cornell Medical College
New York, New York, USA

Joel Martin, MD
Neurosurgery Spine Fellow
University of Miami
Miami, Florida, USA

Frizzi Mayer, BA
Ludwig-Maximilians University of Munich
Munich, Germany

H. Michael Mayer, MD, PhD
Schön Klinik Munich Harlaching
Spine Center
Academic Teaching Hospital of the Paracelsus Medical University Salzburg (AU)
Harlachinger, Munich, Germany

† Deceased

Christoph Mehren, MD
Head of Department
Spine Center
The Schoen Clinic
Harlachinger, Munich, Germany

Neel Mehta, MD
Division Chief of Pain Management
New York Presbyterian Hospital
Weill Cornell Medical College
New York, New York, USA

Carolin Melcher, MD
Consultant
Division of Spine Surgery
Department of Orthopedic Surgery (RKU)
University Hospital of Ulm
Ulm, Germany

Cristiano Magalhães Menezes, MD, PhD
Spine Surgeon
Instituto Columna
Belo Horizonte, Brazil

Érica Godinho Menezes, MD
Universidade Federal de Minas
Belo Horizonte, Brazil

Lionel N. Metz, MD
Orthopaedic Surgeon
Department of Orthopaedic Surgery
University of California
San Francisco, California, USA

Bernhard Meyer, MD
Department of Neurosurgery
Klinikum rechts der Isar, School of Medicine, Technische Universität München
Munich, Germany

Melissa Meyer, DO
Inspira Health Network
Vineland, New Jersey, USA

Catherine Miller, MD
Neurosurgeon
Department of Neurological Surgery
University of California
San Francisco, California, USA

Ramin A. Morshed, MD
Resident Physician
Department of Neurological Surgery
University of California
San Francisco, California, USA

Yusef Mosley, MD
Department of Neurological Surgery
Thomas Jefferson University Hospital
Philadelphia, Pennsylvania, USA

Praveen Mummaneni, MD
Department of Neurological Surgery
University of California
San Francisco, California, USA

Raj Nangunoori, MD
Department of Neurosurgery
New York Presbyterian Hospital
Weill Cornell Medical College
New York, New York, USA

Rodrigo Navarro-Ramirez, MD, MS
Spine-Fellowship Trained Neurosurgeon
Department of Neurological Surgery
Weill Cornell Medicine & New York Presbyterian Och Spine
New York, New York, USA

Eric W. Nottmeier, MD
Professor of Neurosurgery
Department of Neurosurgery
Mayo Clinic
Jacksonville, Florida, USA

Leonardo Oliveira, MD
Department of Sports Medicine
Cleveland Clinic
Weston, Florida, USA

John E. O'Toole, MD, MS
Professor of Neurosurgery
Co-Director, Coleman Foundation Comprehensive Spine Tumor Clinic
Rush University Medical Center
Chicago, Illinois, USA

Luca Papavero, MD, PhD
Spine Surgeon
Clinic for Spine Surgery – Schoen Clinic Hamburg Eilbek
Hamburg, Germany

Avelino Parajón, MD
Head of Neurosurgery
University Hospital Ramón y Cajal
Madrid, Spain

Athos Patsalides, MD
Department of Neurological Surgery
New York Presbyterian Hospital
Weill Cornell Medical College
New York, New York, USA

Brenton Pennicooke, MD
Resident Physician
New York Presbyterian Hospital
Weill Cornell Medical College
New York, New York, USA

Martin H. Pham, MD
Assistant Professor
Department of Neurological Surgery
UC San Diego School of Medicine
San Diego, California, USA

Frank M. Phillips, MD
Ronald DeWald, Endowed Professor of Spinal Deformities;
Director
Division of Spine Surgery;
Section Head
Minimally Invasive Spine Surgery;
Fellowship Co-Director
Spine Surgery
Rush University Medical Center
Chicago, Illinois, USA

Luiz Pimenta, MD, PhD
Instituto de Patologia da Coluna
R. Vergueiro, São Paulo, São Paulo, Brazil

Esteban Quiceno, MD
Neurosurgeon
Department of Neurosurgery
Universidad de Antioquia
Medellín, Colombia

Javier Quillo-Olvera, MD
Spinal Neurosurgeon
Hospital Star Medica Queretaro
Medical School
Anáhuac University
Queretaro City, Mexico

Sheeraz Qureshi, MD, MBA
Associate Professor of Spine Surgery
Hospital for Special Surgery
New York, New York, USA

Marcus Richter, MD
Professor
Spine Center
St. Josefs-Hospital
Wiesbaden, Germany

K. Daniel Riew, MD
Department of Orthopaedic and Neurological Surgery
Och Spine Hospital
Columbia University Medical Center
New York Presbyterian Hospital
Weill-Cornell Medical College
New York, New York, USA

Yu-Mi Ryang, MD
Head of the Department of Neurosurgery
Center for Spine Therapy
Helios Klinikum Berlin-Buch
Berlin, Germany

Alejandro Santillan, MD
Interventional Neuroradiologist
Department of Radiology and Medical Imaging
University of Virginia
Charlottesville, Virginia, USA

Franziska Anna Schmidt, MD
Department of Neurosurgery
Medical University of Innsbruck
Innsbruck, Austria

Theodore H. Schwartz, MD
Vice Chair for Clinical Research
David and Ursel Barnes Professor in Minimally Invasive Surgery;
Professor of Neurosurgery, Neurology, and Otolaryngology;
Director
Center for Epilepsy and Pituitary Surgery
Co-Director
Surgical Neuro-oncology
New York Presbyterian Hospital
Weill Cornell Medical College
New York, New York, USA

Justin Schwarz, MD
Assistant Professor
Department of Neurological Surgery
New York-Presbyterian Hospital
Weill Cornell Medical College
New York, New York, USA

Michael Sein, MD
Assistant Professor of Rehabilitation Medicine
New York Presbyterian Hospital
Weill Cornell Medical College
New York, New York, USA

Rahul V. Shah, MD
Adjunct Clinical Professor of Orthopedic Surgery
Rowan University School of Osteopathic Medicine
Inspira Health Network
Vineland, New Jersey, USA

Jaspal Ricky Singh, MD
Vice Chair and Associate Professor
Department of Rehabilitation Medicine
Weill Cornell Medicine
New York Presbyterian Och Spine Center
New York, New York, USA

José-Antonio Soriano-Sánchez, MD
Neurosurgeon
Centro Medico ABC
Mexico City, Mexico

Sergio Soriano-Solis, MD
Spine Surgeon
Centro Medico ABC
Mexico City, Mexico

Michael P. Steinmetz, MD
Chairman
Department of Neurosurgery
Cleveland Clinic Lerner College of Medicine;
Director
Center for Spine Health
Neurological Institute
Cleveland, Ohio, USA

Geoffrey Stricsek, MD
Assistant Professor
Department of Neurosurgery
Northwestern Medical Group
Chicago, Illinois, USA

Nestor Taboada, MD
Neurosurgeon
Clinica Bautista
Barranquilla, Colombia

Lee A. Tan, MD
Assistant Professor
Department of Neurological Surgery
UCSF Medical Center
San Francisco, California, USA

Seang-Beng Tan, MD
Orthopaedic Surgeon
Mount Elizabeth Medical Center
Singapore

Masato Tanaka, MD
Vice President
Okayama Rosai Hospital
Okayama, Japan

William Taylor, MD
Clinical Professor
Department of Neurological Surgery
University of California
San Diego, California, USA

Alisson R. Teles, MD
Neurociruugião
Cirugia de Coluna
Hospital Moinhos de Vento
Porto Alegre
Rio Grande do Sul, Brazil

Albert E. Telfeian, MD, PhD
Professor of Neurosurgery
Department of Neurosurgery
Rhode Island Hospital
The Warren Alpert Medical School of Brown University
Providence, Rhode Island, USA

Thana Theofanis, MD
Neurosurgeon
Department of Neurological Surgery
Thomas Jefferson University Hospital
Philadelphia, Pennsylvania, USA

Claudius Thomé
Professor and Chairman
Department of Neurosurgery
Medical University of Innsbruck
Innsbruck, Austria

Pavan S. Upadhyayula, MD
University of California
San Diego, California, USA

Juan S. Uribe, MD
Neurosurgeon
Department of Neurosurgery
Barrow Neurological Institute
St Joseph's Hospital and Medical Center
Phoenix, Arizona, USA

Rafael Uribe, MD, MHS
Department of Neurological Surgery
New York Presbyterian Hospital
Weill Cornell Medical College
New York, New York, USA

Sebastian Uribe
The Johns Hopkins University
Baltimore, Maryland, USA

Michael S. Virk, MD, PhD
Assistant Professor, Neurosurgeon, and Spine Surgeon
Department of Neurological Surgery
New York Presbyterian Hospital
Weill Cornell Medical College
New York, New York, USA

Ralf Wagner, MD
Orthopaedic and Spine Surgeon
Ligamenta Spine Surgery Clinic
Frankfurt, Germany

Jeffrey C. Wang, MD
Chief
Orthopaedic Spine Service;
Co-Director;
Professor of Orthopaedic Surgery and Neurosurgery
USC Spine Center
Los Angeles, California, USA

Michael Y. Wang, MD
Department of Neurological Surgery
University of Miami Miller School of Medicine
Miami, Florida, USA

Christoph Wipplinger, MD
Research Fellow
Weill Cornell Medical College
New York Presbyterian Hospital
New York, New York, USA

Christopher D. Witiw, MD
Neurosurgeon
Department of Neurosurgery
St. Michael's Hospital
University of Toronto
Toronto, Ontario, Canada

Richard Wohns, MD
Neurosurgeon
NeoSpine
Puyallup, Washington, USA

Taylor Wong, BA
Research Fellow
Department of Neurological Surgery
Weill Cornell Medicine
New York, New York, USA

Kyle F. Worell, DC, PSP DipACLM
Primary Spine Care, Sports & Lifestyle Medicine
Manhattan Sports Medicine
Manhattan Spine Care
New York, New York, USA

Ernest J. Wright, MD
Neurosurgeon
Department of Spine Surgery
Ascension Medical Group
Nashville, Tennessee, USA

David S. Xu, MD
Assistant Professor
Department of Neurosurgery
Baylor College of Medicine
Houston, Texas, USA

Jang W. Yoon, MD
Assistant Professor of Clinical Neurosurgery
Department of Neurosurgery
University of Pennsylvania
Philadelphia, Pennsylvania, USA

Magdy Gamal AbdelKader Youssef
Head of Spine Unit
International Medical Center IMC;
Professor of Spine Surgery
Ain-Shams University
Cairo, Egypt

Part I

Introduction to MISS

1 Definition of MISS: The “6 Ts”: Target/Technology/Technique/Teaching and Training/Testing/Talent *2*

2 Global MISS: Perspectives from Asia, Australia, Europe, Middle East, North America, and South America *14*

I

1 Definition of MISS: The "6 Ts": Target/Technology/Technique/Teaching and Training/Testing/Talent

Roger Härtl, Sertac Kirnaz, Juan Del Castillo-Calcáneo, and Ibrahim Hussain

Summary

This chapter provides the framework for success with minimally invasive spine surgery (MISS). To illustrate this, we developed the "6 Ts" to create a foundation for successful MISS procedures. The "6 Ts" are: target, tools, technique, training, testing, and talent. These six attributes inform one another as they develop, thus patient selection for MISS improves as mastery of the tools improves as well. MISS is an evolving field and using the "6 Ts" provides a method for reaching the main goal of MISS, which is to treat spinal pathologies with minimal invasion.

Keywords: minimally invasive spine surgery, tubular retractor, indirect decompression, navigation, muscle-sparing spine surgery, over-the-top decompression

1.1 Definition of Minimally Invasive Spine Surgery

Spinal surgery that attempts to reduce the invasiveness of traditional spinal procedures is attracting considerable and growing interest worldwide. This type of surgery has been called "less invasive," "minimal access," or "minimally destructive" spinal surgery. For the purpose of this book, we decided to stick with the most widely used term: "minimally invasive spine surgery" (MISS). We realize and acknowledge that there is not one perfect descriptive term, as this type of surgery is evolving and surgeons in different regions have variable access to MISS-enabling technology and training. Based on the recent consensus definition by AOSpine, MISS can be defined as a "suite of technology-dependent techniques and procedures that reduces local operative tissue damage and systemic surgical stress, enabling earlier return to function [and] striving for better outcomes than traditional techniques."[1,2]

This definition already implies what we call as the six principles that surgeons should consider when engaging in MISS, i.e., the "6 Ts" (▶ Fig. 1.1):

- Target: Appropriate patient and procedural selection.
- Technology: Specialized technology that enables or facilitates MISS.
- Technique: Surgical and perioperative techniques and procedures.
- Training: Adequate training and teaching of the surgeon, collaborating team, and trainees.
- Testing: Critical review and testing of surgical outcomes (research).
- Talent: Development of surgical talent.

The goal of MISS is to leave the smallest possible "surgical footprint" while achieving the goal of traditional open surgery. MISS emphasizes attaining the best functional outcome for the patient, free of unnecessary iatrogenic risk exposure.

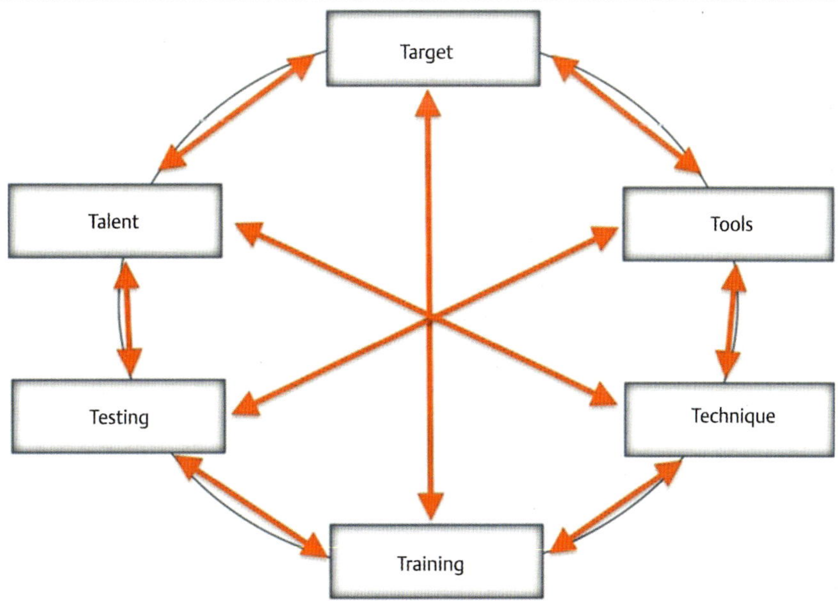

Fig. 1.1 The "6 Ts" to success in spinal minimally invasive spine surgery (MISS). These are all interactive. For example, the results of data collection, research and outcome assessment (testing) over time will refine our surgical decision-making process (target). The tools and techniques used will determine the surgical teaching and training required to master MISS. Training and teaching are central to all innovation and are used to develop talent.

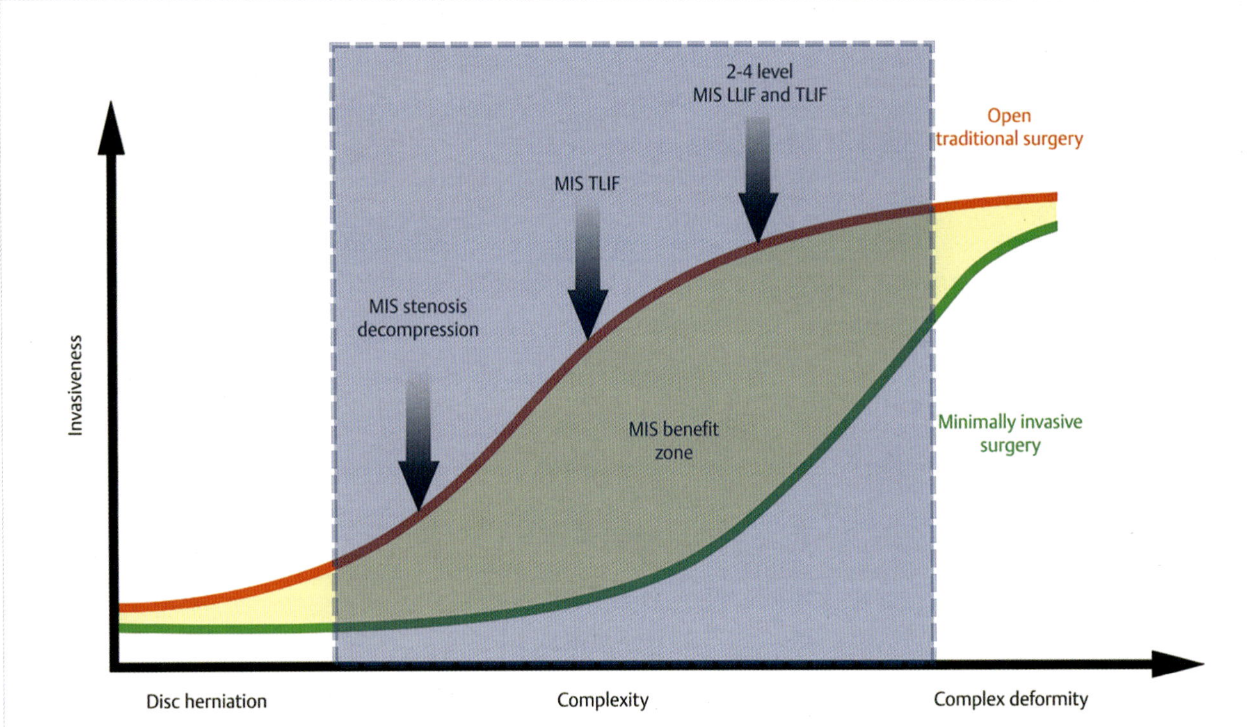

Fig. 1.2 Relating the complexity of the procedure to the invasiveness of the system used (see ▶ Table 1.1), complexity increases from a single-disc herniation to single-level lumbar stenosis, to multi-level instability and/or deformity requiring fusion.

1.2 Potential of Minimally Invasive Spinal Surgery

Approximately 1.6 million instrumented spinal procedures are done in the United States each year.[3] Most decompressions and approximately 50% of fusion procedures can be performed completely or partially using MISS. Therefore, an estimated 75% of all spinal surgeries could be performed completely or partially using MISS instead of conventional techniques, indicating that the full potential of MISS is yet to be recognized. The most challenging aspect for MISS is still the treatment of significant and multilevel deformities, but progress is being made in at least partially applying some of the benefits of MISS, such as percutaneous screw placement, navigation, lateral approaches, etc.

Which procedures and pathologies currently benefit most from MISS? Let us plot the complexity of thoracolumbar procedures against their invasiveness (▶ Fig. 1.2). This is a somewhat arbitrary and subjective approach, but it effectively demonstrates the current role of MISS compared with open traditional surgery. In terms of procedure complexity, the spectrum ranges from simple lumbar disc herniation on the left to single- and multilevel lumbar stenosis decompression, single-level spondylolisthesis cases treated with MIS transforaminal lumbar interbody fusion (TLIF), multilevel lateral and then combined lateral/TLIF, and possibly anterior lumbar interbody fusion procedures for moderate deformities. All the way on the right, we find complex deformities defined as fused or rigid spines requiring more than five levels of instrumentation. Invasiveness on the Y-axis can be assessed by looking at surgical parameters such as intraoperative blood loss, infection risk, length of stay, postoperative pain levels, etc. (▶ Table 1.1).

Table 1.1 Factors that determine invasiveness and complexity of spinal procedures

Invasiveness factors	Complexity factors
Length of procedure	Technical demands to surgeon and staff
Blood loss	Predictability of outcome
Infection risk	Use of technology
Incision length and size of tissue exposure	Number of stages and steps in a procedure
Associated fluid shifts	Use of implants
General vs. local anesthesia	Revision surgery
Postoperative pain levels	Intradural vs. extradural
Perioperative risks	Degree of deformity correction required

Literature and experience show that with the very-low-level complexity cases, there is no big difference between MISS and open traditional surgery when it comes to outcome and invasiveness (▶ Fig. 1.3). For example, patients with simple lumbar disc herniation for the most part will do equally well whether treated by a well-trained endoscopic spine surgeon, via tubular surgery, or by open microdiscectomy.[4,5] However, when we move to a slightly more complex operation, such as a decompression for severe lumbar spinal stenosis, there is already a clear advantage for MISS. Studies show that performing this decompression through tubes or specular retractors using a unilateral laminectomy for bilateral decompression (ULBD) is associated

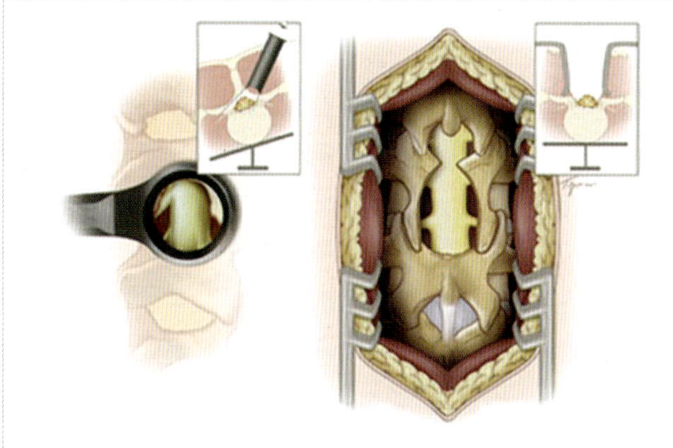

Fig. 1.3 Comparison of surgical approach and bony removal between minimally invasive spine surgery (*left*) and open spine surgery (*right*).

with multiple benefits to the patient, including earlier return to work, less pain, and lower risk of infection[6,7,8,9,10] when compared with traditional open surgery. When it comes to patients with lumbar stenosis and spondylolisthesis, the difference between MISS and traditional open surgery is even more pronounced because open surgery will frequently be performed by combining a decompression with fusion, whereas with MISS a fusion can be avoided if the spondylolisthesis is stable.[11] For patients with unstable spondylolisthesis, studies have shown that MIS TLIF is associated with benefits over open fusion and/or TLIF, including reduction in length of stay, decreased infection rates, and decreased costs.[11,12] Further to the right, we move toward mild and moderate deformity pathologies that can frequently be treated by taking advantage of less invasive lateral, oblique, or anterior indirect decompression and fusion procedures, all of which provide excellent clinical results while minimizing complications and invasiveness. As we move to the right, even the MISS treatment interventions become more complex and less "minimally invasive". This is mainly based on the increase in operative time, number of different access sites, and number of MISS procedures required to achieve the overall surgical goal. Finally, for rigid curves requiring more than 5-level surgery including L5/S1, rigid deformities requiring more than 10-level fusion, or previously instrumented multilevel fusions, the downsides of MISS currently outweigh the potential benefits. Based on the work by the International Spine Study Group, a recommendation was developed for the treatment of adult degenerative scoliosis[13] and recently updated. Compared to the previous algorithm from 2014,[13] the introduction of new technology, such as expandable cages, lateral techniques, anterior column release (ACR), and other technologies and procedures, has expanded the indications for MISS for deformity correction to now include patients with deformities and even with significant lumbar lordosis–pelvic incidence (LL-PI) mismatch.[14]

Based on these thoughts, it is our belief that the greatest benefits of MISS are currently for the treatment of pathologies ranging from lumbar disc herniation to moderate deformities up to approximately five levels, which can be considered as the "benefit zone" for MISS. However, this benefit zone for MISS is constantly being expanded with the expansion of MISS components into more complex surgical pathologies. Examples of this would include the use of lateral ACR procedures with hyperlordotic cages combined with more traditional and open osteotomy procedures performed posteriorly (Chapters 27 and 28). Other examples include the adoption of three-dimensional (3D) navigation and robotic surgery in multilevel deformity correction procedures and preoperative 3D planning and virtual augmentation in, for example, complex tumor resections, which may contribute to overall less invasive surgery.

These considerations demonstrate that MISS has already gained a significant role in spinal surgery that will become even more prominent as technology and techniques evolve. Indeed, a future of spinal surgery without an adoption of MISS techniques and principles does not seem to be possible.

1.3 The "6 Ts" to Success in MISS: Components for a Successful MISS Practice

The "6 Ts" of MISS represent a concept that references the key elements determining the success of MISS and the MISS surgeon over time, these are: target, technology, technique, teaching and training, testing, and talent. We will further describe each of the "Ts" in relation to MISS. It is important to realize that these are all interactive. For example, over time the results of data collection, research, and outcomes assessments (testing) will refine our surgical decision-making process (target) which in turn will influence the next generation of MISS surgeons (teaching and training). The tools and techniques used will determine the surgical teaching and training required to master MISS. As research shows, talent is highly dependent on the correct teaching and training methodology.

1.3.1 Target

"Target philosophy" is described as choosing the right operation for the appropriate patient and pathology. This decision-making process is one of the most complex problems in spinal surgery because there is very little science to guide the surgeon and patient. Spinal surgical decision-making is based to a large extent on the surgeon's experience and background, training level, and patient expectations and beliefs which are not always clear or measurable. By including the target philosophy in our "6 T" concept of the key elements for success, we try to shed some light on the difficult decision-making process in spinal surgery. The classic dilemma with spinal surgery is the poor correlation between patient's signs and symptoms, imaging findings, patient expectations, and ultimately patient outcome. If in doubt, a conservative approach may be sometimes the best option: *The "least invasive" MISS operation is the one not performed because of a lack of correlation between patient signs and symptoms, imaging findings, and expected outcome.* On the other hand, if there is a correlation, we struggle as MISS surgeons to balance treating only the patient's current signs and symptoms versus more extensive surgery that anticipates future deterioration as a result of the natural history, as a result of the surgical intervention, or both. This highlights the challenge we have with defining the natural history of untreated or minimally treated degenerative spinal disease; at what point should we treat abnormal imaging findings even though the patient may not be (yet) symptomatic?

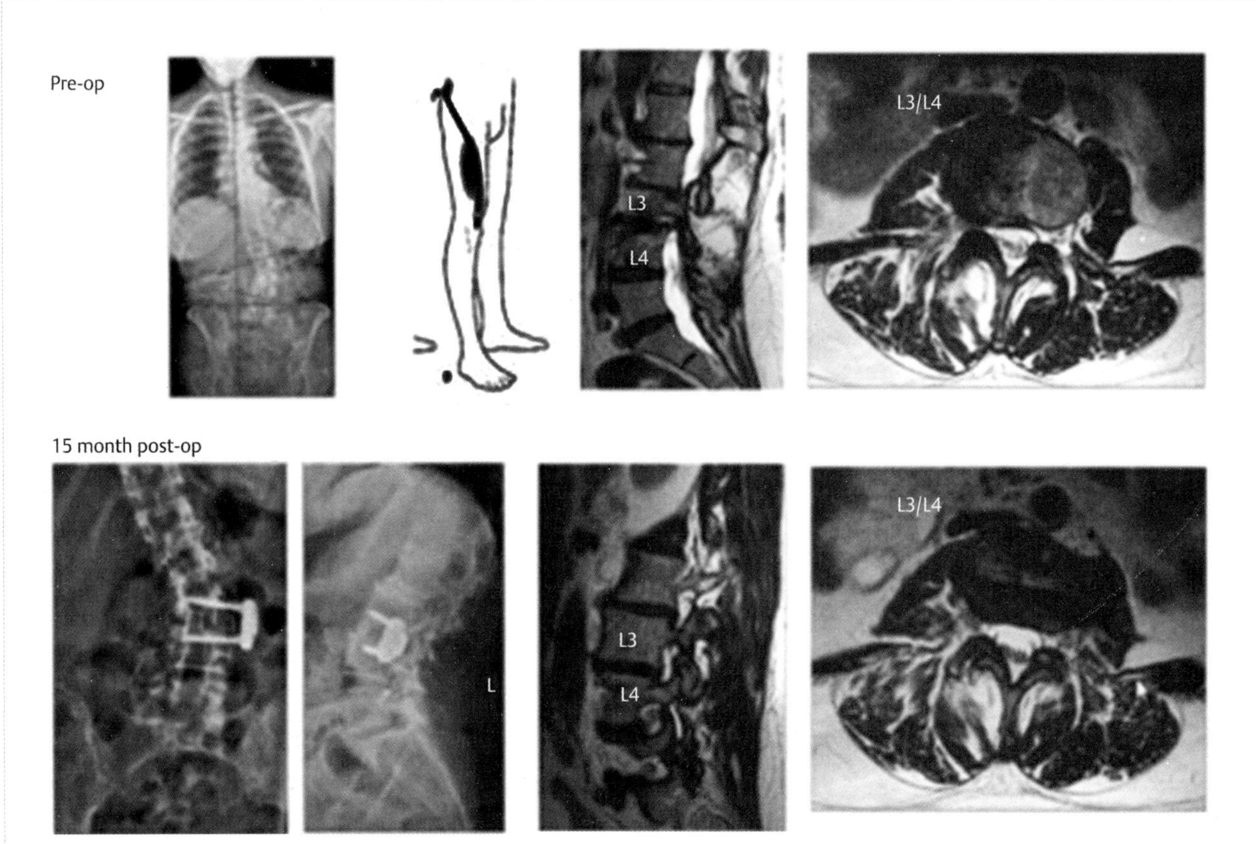

Fig. 1.4 Imaging of an elderly patient who presented with significant right-sided L3 radiculopathy without mechanical back pain. Imaging demonstrates significant degenerative scoliosis with single-level foraminal compression in the concavity of the curve. Patient had pain resolve 15 weeks post operation.

Take, for example, an elderly patient who presented without mechanical back pain but with a significant right-sided L3 radiculopathy. Imaging demonstrated a significant degenerative scoliosis with single-level foraminal compression in the concavity of the curve (▶ Fig. 1.4). This patient was treated successfully with an ambulatory single-level translumbar discectomy and fusion. However, several perioperative questions arise: Should this patient have undergone a bigger surgery that addresses the deformity? Will the one-level fusion accelerate the deformity progression above and below? A clear answer cannot be provided at this time, and surgical decision-making will therefore be guided by the patient's expectations, the surgeon's recommendation and experience, and a comprehensive discussion between both parties.

Because of the small exposure and limited access to the spine in MISS, it is of great importance to preoperatively diagnose the patient's underlying problem as accurately as possible. One goal of MISS is to minimize surgical overtreatment and iatrogenic morbidity due to unnecessary "prophylactic" surgery. Once the decision for an operation has been made, the surgeon has to be sure that the surgical approach chosen will allow effective treatment of the patient's problem. Most patients with degenerative disorders will present with pain-related symptoms that may be difficult to localize. Therefore, the well-trained MISS surgeon must be adept at taking a detailed clinical history, performing a thorough neurologic assessment, excluding other common musculoskeletal or other etiologies of symptom generation, and must be able to correlate the examination findings and patient's complaints to the imaging studies. Furthermore, the surgeon must understand the different types of pain encountered and their relationship to the anatomy (▶ Fig. 1.5). For more details, see Chapter 3.

Sound and targeted surgical decision-making in MISS for degenerative disorders will typically require following three steps (▶ Fig. 1.6):

1. Understanding and classification of the different types of pain patterns. Broad categories are radicular pain, neurogenic claudication-type pain, mechanical axial neck and back pain, and signs and symptoms due to spinal cord or cauda equina compression (Chapter 3). Muscle-generated pain is increasingly being recognized as an independent source of back and neck pain and will be covered separately in Chapter 5.
2. Next is accurate diagnosis of the patient's underlying pathology (▶ Fig. 1.7). In addition to step 1, this will require synthesis of a careful clinical examination and history taking, review of imaging studies, and sometimes additional testing such as electromyography, nerve conduction studies, or diagnostic injections. This is best accomplished using a team-based approach with other subspecialists such as pain anesthesiologists, physiatrists, and neurologists all involved in the workup. In more complex cases, careful review of imaging studies with a radiologist with advanced expertise in spinal pathology is also helpful.

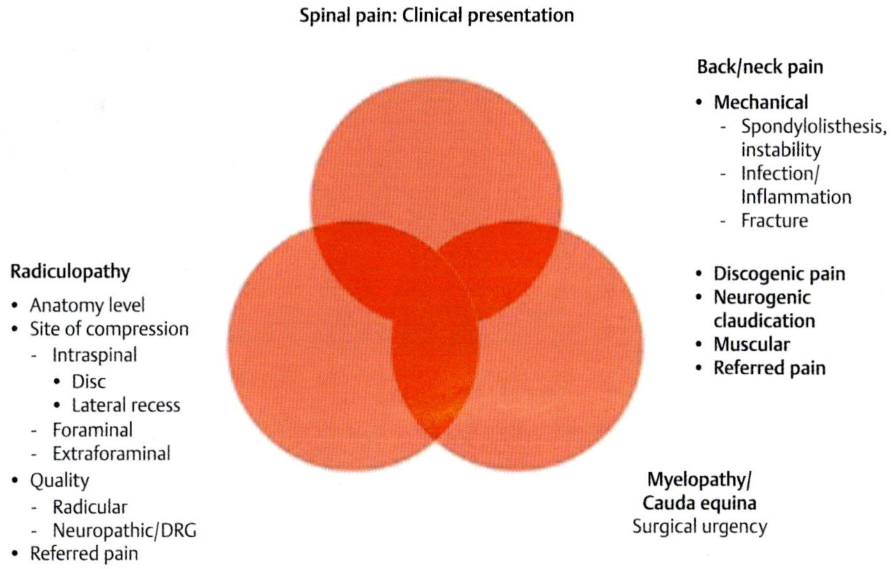

Fig. 1.5 Understanding the different types of pain patters and their correlation to the clinical examination and imaging.

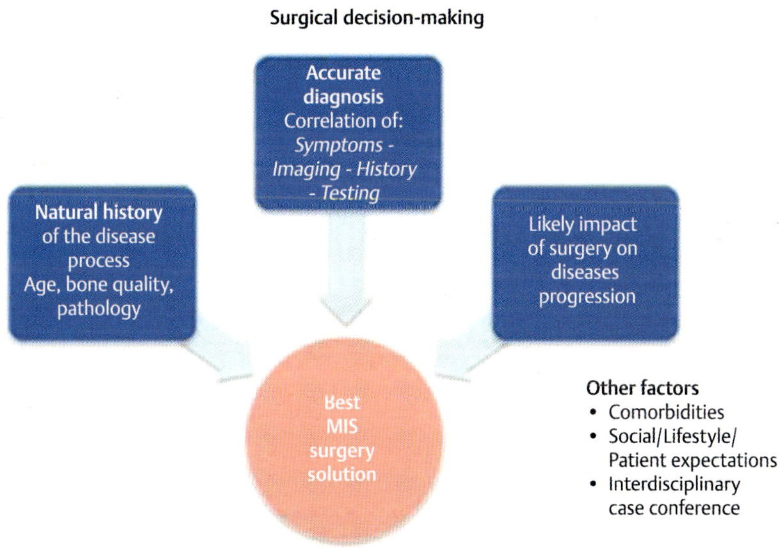

Fig. 1.6 Factors of surgical decision-making.

3. Surgical decision-making not only involves a careful consideration of steps 1 and 2, but also an understanding of the natural history of the underlying pathology and the likely impact of surgery on the disease process (▶ Fig. 1.8). For example, in the example mentioned above, it would be important to understand the natural history of degenerative scoliosis over time (which is poorly understood currently). How likely is the curve to worsen over time and require additional surgical treatment in 5, 10, or 20 years? On the other hand, what impact and unwanted side effects will surgical intervention have over time? Will surgery worsen the patient's current biomechanics and accelerate the disease process? Another common example is the patient with lumbar stenosis and spondylolisthesis; will a decompression alone cause instability that will worsen the slip and require a fusion later on?

Other factors that have to be considered in the surgical decision-making process include age, functional status, and comorbidities such as obesity, osteoporosis, and cardiac/pulmonary/vascular disease, and vascular disease among others. Finally, surgical decision-making in MISS must take into consideration the patient's expectations, lifestyle, and social factors, much more than in other surgical subspecialties. For example, if the patient is an avid athlete and wishes to return to an active

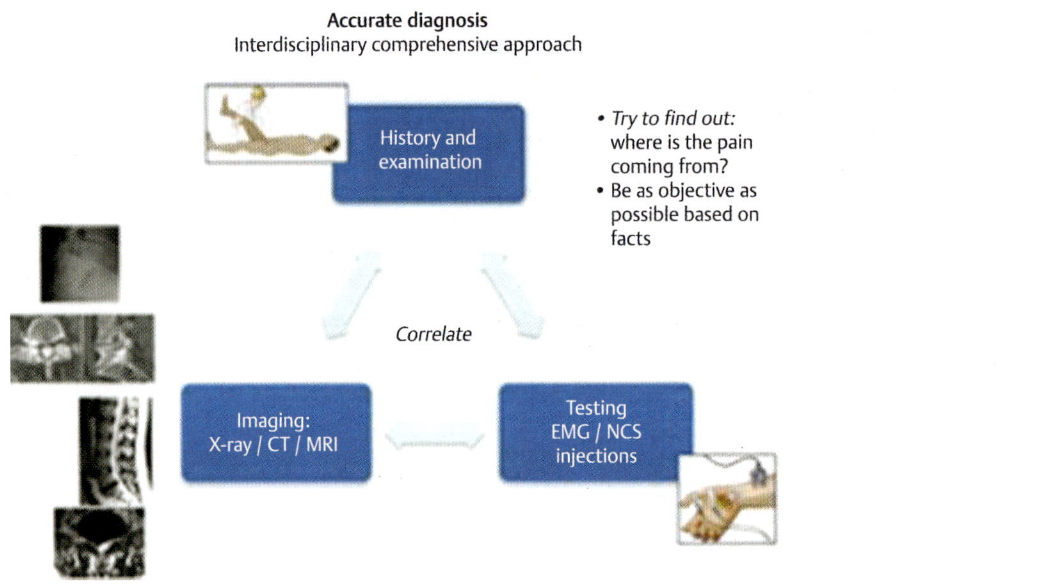

Fig. 1.7 Accurate diagnosis of the patient's underlying pathology.

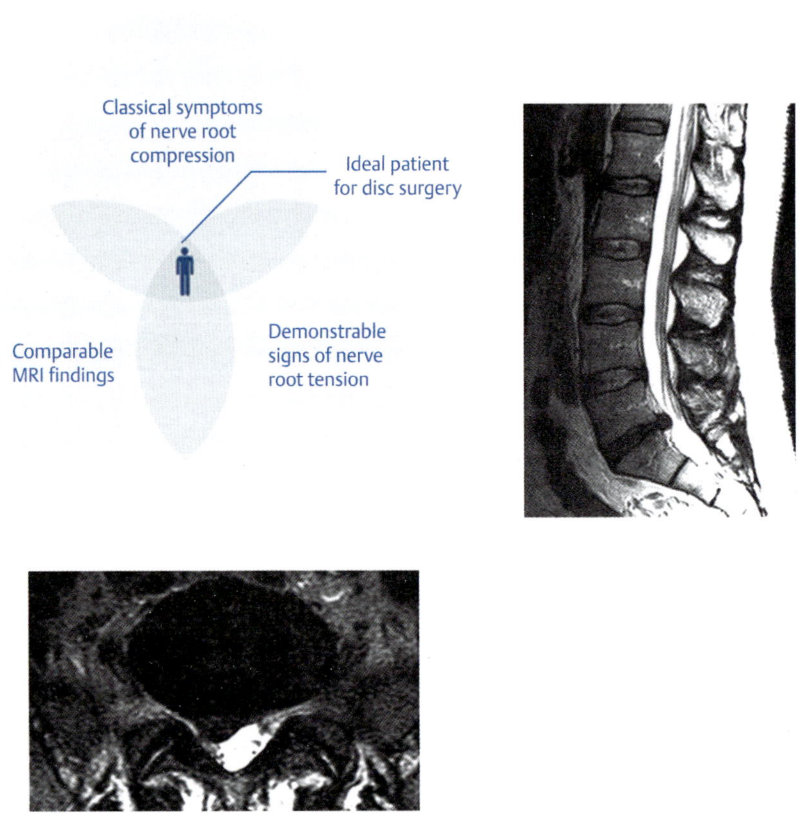

Fig. 1.8 Example from AO MIS book: Signs and symptoms and imaging findings have to come together and support the diagnosis before a surgical treatment decision should be made.

lifestyle, the surgical decision may be different than in a patient who lives a sedentary lifestyle and wishes for nothing more than to be able to carry out daily activities without issues. Social networks and support systems also play an important role, as these factors are significant in the postsurgical recovery process. For example, a patient with a strong support system might be able to handle a more complicated recovery than one who has limited support system. Patient expectations have to be

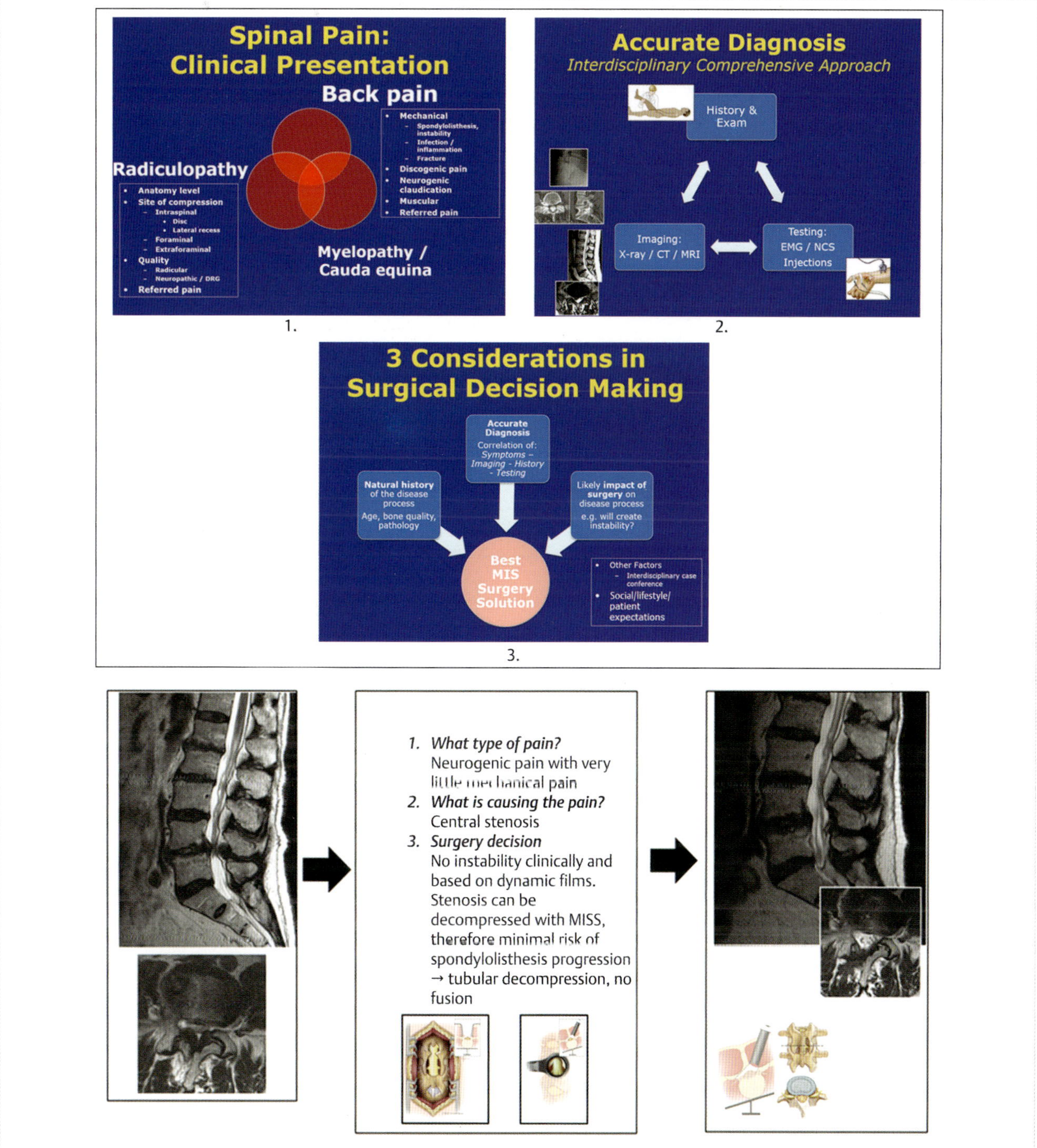

Fig. 1.9 Example of surgical decision-making using the three-step target philosophy as outlined. A 65-year-old patient with severe lumbar stenosis and grade I spondylolisthesis who had failed nonoperative treatment. His symptoms were inability to walk more than 100 meters which caused him pain in his buttocks bilaterally. This was relieved by sitting down (neurogenic claudication). On clinical examination, there was no mechanical low back pain and dynamic flexion–extension films did not show any instability. No radicular pain below the knees. Lower extremity pulses were normal and symmetric. Decision was a tubular approach for a unilateral laminectomy for bilateral decompression without stabilization.

considered and, if not realistic, need to be addressed before making a final decision. All of this is especially relevant and requires extra careful consideration in MISS because of the targeted nature of what we do in the operating room (OR). Since we frequently involve other spinal specialists in the initial workup, it can be very helpful to discuss the final surgical plan in an interdisciplinary setting. For this reason, we have included in this book chapters on accurate workup (Chapter 3) and lifestyle-related issues and expectations (Chapter 52). We have also included a separate chapter on the importance of muscle as a pain generator, which is increasingly being recognized as an independent source of back and neck pain (Chapter 5).

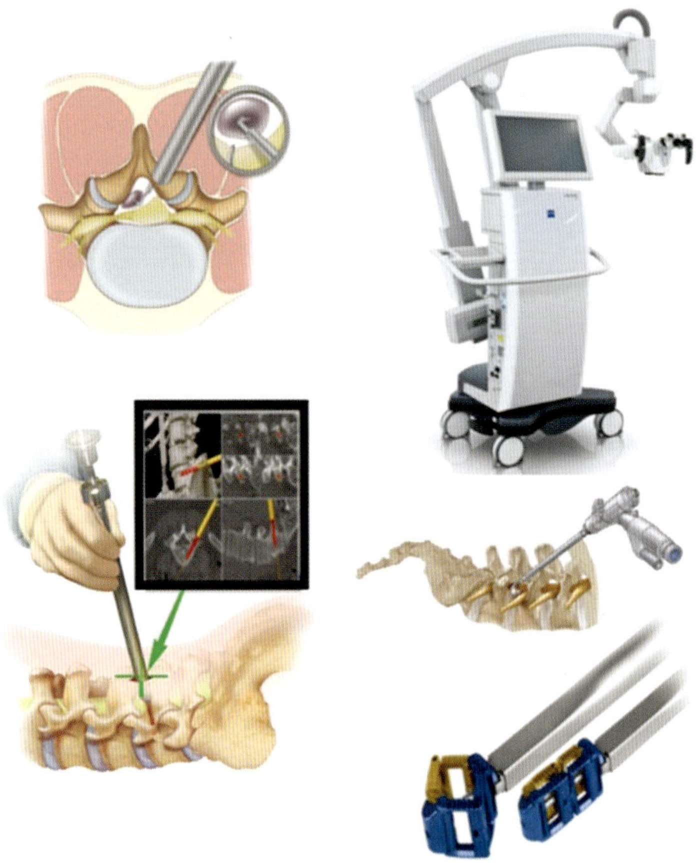

Fig. 1.10 Fundamental tools/technologies for performing minimally invasive spine surgery techniques.

In summary, the importance of the target philosophy in accurate surgical decision-making cannot be overemphasized and lies at the core of successful MISS. See ▶ Fig. 1.9 for a case-based example on surgical decision-making based on the three-step target philosophy.

1.3.2 Tools and Technology

This refers to surgical tools and instruments available in the OR to perform MISS. These are rapidly evolving, especially in terms of implant technology, imaging and navigation, and surgical planning software. In the absence of the tools necessary for MISS, conventional open surgery may be a safer alternative.

Some of the fundamental tools/technologies for performing MISS techniques are as follows (▶ Fig. 1.10):

- Access: tubular or specular retractors, endoscope.
- Visualization and illumination: microscope, exoscope, endoscope.
- Special implants (e.g., expandable cages, hyperlordotic cages, stand-alone cages, cannulated screws, percutaneous single-step pedicle screw system, etc.).
- Curved, bayoneted, and extended instruments.
- Intraoperative imaging system with two-dimensional (2D) and 3D navigation, robotic guidance systems.
- Surgical planning and augmented reality software.

Although not all of these tools are necessary for MISS, the broad categories should be covered in order to enable MISS: This includes access technologies such as tubular retractors or the endoscope; visualization, illumination, and magnification with a surgical microscope; fluoroscopy or computer navigation; and special implants including various interbody cages and cannulated pedicle screws. One particularly helpful tool for MISS is the surgical microscope, which gives the surgeon the depth resolution necessary to guide surgical decision-making when working in fields with limited exposure. Current surgical microscopes come equipped with integrated navigation technology and high-definition video documentation systems. They also allow for easy editing and transfer of videos to handheld devices. Imaging in spine surgery is essential for the accurate localization of the pathology to be treated, avoidance of wrong level surgery, and the proper insertion of implants. This is even more important in MISS procedures, which lack open visualization of anatomical reference points that can be used as a basis for orientation and implant placement. For example, the Airo® CT scanner (Brainlab AG, Feldkirchen, Germany) greatly expands navigation from a tool used solely for instrumentation navigation to one used for intraoperative planning and guidance throughout the entirety of MISS procedures. It has introduced an era of "total navigation," that is, the use of navigation for all steps of the procedure—from pathology localization and incision

planning, to screw placement, tubular decompression, cage placement, and rod measurement without the need for fluoroscopy.[15] The 3D navigation has improved the workflow of MISS by increasing accuracy of localization and hardware implantation and decreasing the amount of radiation the surgical staff is exposed to. Total navigation makes spine surgery safer, more accurate, and enhances efficient and reproducible workflows (Chapter 42). Robotic surgery is another evolving technology that holds great promise, as is augmented and virtual reality (Chapter 8).

The paradigm shift from open surgery to MISS was achieved gradually with the development of new technologies. Tools and technologies will be covered in most of the following chapters, and surgeons are naturally well-exposed to these at meetings and surgical courses.

1.3.3 Surgical Technique

Surgical technique is intimately related to the surgeon's operative background, mentorship, and training during residency and fellowship, as well as the current operative experience in MISS. There are at least three characteristic surgical techniques that are relevant for the vast majority of MISS procedures that are not generally taught in spinal programs. These include:

1. Spinal surgery via a tubular or specular retractor or via the endoscope to achieve a bilateral decompression and a contralateral foraminotomy through a unilateral, minimally invasive approach. This is also frequently called "over-the-top" decompression. For example, in lumbar spinal stenosis, the tubular decompression procedure has been named "unilateral laminotomy for bilateral decompression."[7]
2. The technique of minimizing iatrogenic instability using "over-the-top" type decompression approaches. This reduces the need for instrumentation and fusion surgery. We now routinely use this in patients with lumbar stenosis and stable grade I spondylolisthesis, for the contralateral approach for decompression of synovial cysts, contralateral approach for decompression of intraforaminal pathology, and for the treatment of two-level lumbar pathology where one level requires a fusion and the adjacent level with stenosis requires just a decompression.[7,16]
3. The lateral, oblique, or anterior technique of indirect decompression of central and foraminal stenosis. The challenge currently lies in the accurate prediction of successful indirect decompression and the determination of which patients should also undergo a direct decompression. In addition, these approaches also allow a certain degree of deformity correction depending on the type of implants and techniques used.

Other surgical technique-related topics include, for example, the effective and safe integration of 2D/3D navigation and robotic surgery into the surgical workflow. Moreover, the use of special anesthetic enhanced recovery after surgery (ERAS) approaches falls into this category and will be covered in Chapter 16.

1.3.4 Teaching/Training

As with all new techniques, the process of attaining surgical proficiency involves a learning curve.[5,17,18] As MISS continues to become more prominent in the field of spine surgery, residents are being exposed to MISS techniques earlier in their training. At institutions where MISS is performed frequently, residents may graduate competent in MISS techniques, thus eliminating the learning curve faced by spine surgeons who are new to MISS. Educating future generations of surgeons on MISS is crucial to the advancement of the field. However, the complexity of MISS is rapidly evolving and even MISS-trained surgeons have to find ways to effectively keep up with new developments. For surgeons who have not yet reached the plateau of the learning curve, it is crucial to understand how to maximize their ability to reach it safely and efficiently. Therefore, essentially all surgeons will face a time where they have to train. The best way to become proficient is to teach others, so teaching and training are intricately interwoven and go both ways—teaching yourself and teaching others.

For those who are already experts in MISS, they will have to train colleagues, residents, and fellows, so teaching and training will be equally important for them. Recently, surgical simulation using very realistic models has become available and allows surgeons to train in the basic skills and procedures in MISS.[19] In addition, attending courses aimed specifically at educating surgeons in MISS procedures can be immensely valuable as well as visiting and observing other expert surgeons. This will be covered further in Chapter 54.

1.3.5 Curriculum Development

It is important to develop a curriculum for the teaching and training of MISS (▸ Table 1.2).[1] For example, the approach taken by AOSpine breaks MISS up into nine basic skills and nine basic procedures which are expanded over time.[1] This includes a stepwise program using videos, surgical simulation, lectures, and online teaching material to minimize the learning curve for surgeons. Most of these will be also covered in this book.

Table 1.2 AOSpine MISS curriculum[1]

Basic MISS skills	Basic MISS procedure
Using a microscope	Microscopic interlaminar lumbar discectomy
Using an endoscope	Microscopic posterior cervical foraminotomy
Using a burr with an endoscope	Microscopic extraforaminal lumbar discectomy
Using a drill for MISS	Endoscopic interlaminar lumbar discectomy
Using 2D and 3D navigation and assistive technologies	Endoscopic transforaminal lumbar foraminotomy and discectomy
Managing a dural tear	Endoscopic ULBD (endoscopic "over-the-top" decompression or endoscopic ULBD)
Bleeding control	Microscopic ULBD ("over-the-top" decompression)
Maximizing arthrodesis	Percutaneous screw and rod placement
What to do when lost	TLIF

Abbreviations: 2D, two-dimension; 3D, three-dimension; MISS, minimally invasive spine surgery; TLIF, transforaminal lumbar interbody fusion; ULBD, unilateral laminectomy for bilateral decompression.

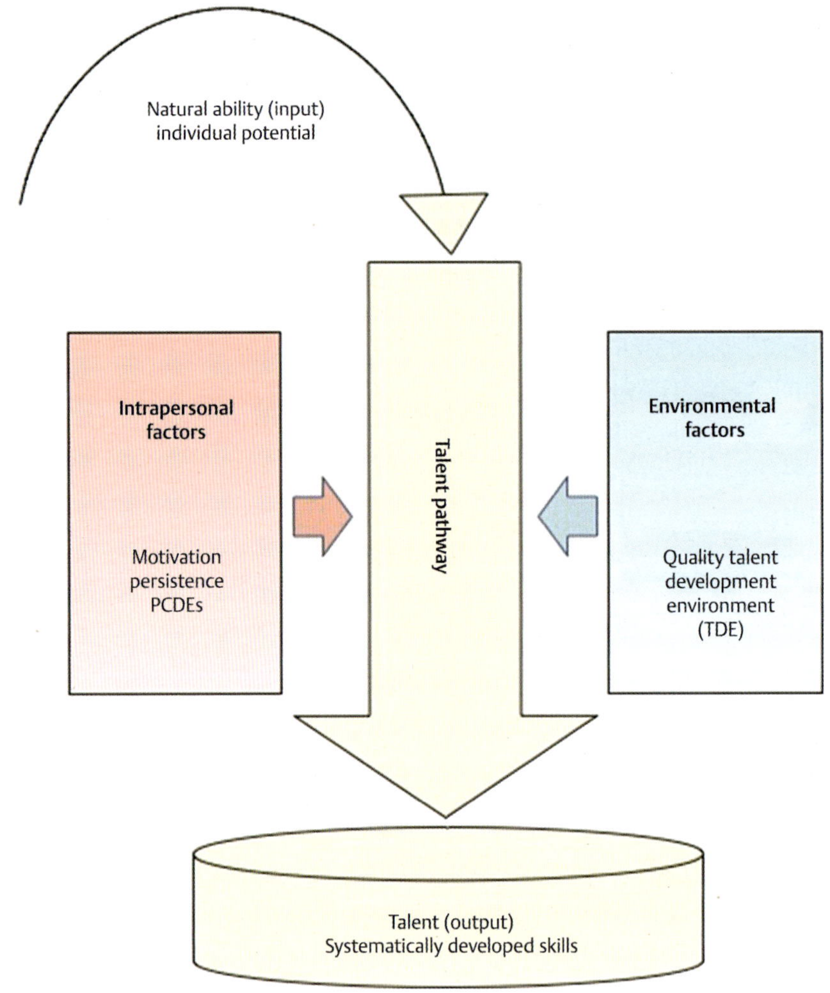

Fig. 1.11 Talent is developed by one's natural ability, intrapersonal factors, and environmental factors.

1.3.6 Testing: Research and Outcomes

Continuous outcome tracking and research are essential, especially for novice MISS surgeons. Following your outcomes closely will allow you to identify deficiencies and strengths, and will allow you to focus your time and attention on areas that may need improvement. It will also affect all other aspects of the "6 Ts." It may affect over time your surgical decision-making process or whether you decide to invest in a certain technology. For example, if you are not happy with screw accuracy or radiation exposure, you may decide to invest in 3D navigation. These decisions are best made using objective data. Outcome tracking will also help in the counseling of patients. MISS is an evolving field, so input from a broad pool of surgeons who practice it is vital for evolving techniques. As a surgeon, you may decide to join one of the larger organizations and get engaged in research and clinical studies in order to advance the field of MISS.

1.3.7 Talent and Aptitude

The question has been posed whether some surgeons possess preexisting nonsurgical competence that gives them an advantage over other surgeons who come without these skills or attributes. Examples for these competences are innate handiness, regular eating with chopsticks, experience with computer games, playing a musical instrument, etc.[20,21,22,23,24,25,26,27] In the aviation industry, for example, aspiring pilots have to prove their aptitude in a selection process. Talent or aptitude is usually viewed as an individual's ability without consideration of the process of development that led to this ability.

The concept of talent in surgery appears to be more complex. Although excellent surgical skills are important, a truly successful surgeon is also characterized by attributes such as enthusiasm, resilience, caring attitude toward her or his patients, self-discipline and criticism, physical fitness, and commitment.[28] From sports we know that some of the most successful athletes were able to compensate for physical disadvantages with strengths in another area (commitment, determination, hard work).[29] Therefore, testing manual dexterity in students will not be sufficient to assess surgical talent or aptitude. Significant insight comes from talent development research in sports. Gagne argued that innate natural abilities exist but they need to be actualized and appreciated by a context in order to flourish.[30] He developed a "Differentiated Model of Giftedness and Talent" that describes

how coaching or training can transform skills or natural abilities into true excellence and talent (▶ Fig. 1.11).[31]

Ericcson, Nandagopal, and Roring introduced the concept of "deliberate practice" for how expertise, expert performance, and experts develop. Deliberate practice is "when individuals engage in practice activities (which are, at least initially, designed by teachers and coaches) with full concentration on improving some specific aspect of performance."[32] They studied deliberate practice in expert musicians, which led to the theory that 10,000 hours of practice is needed to achieve expert performance.[33]

Similar ideas have also been taken up in the popular press by Daniel Coyle who published the book *The Talent Code: Greatness Isn't Born. It's Grown.*[34] Research shows that surgical skills can be improved significantly when using appropriate teaching and learning techniques, independent from a preexisting skill level.[35] The environment, including adequate teaching and training, has an important impact on whether talent can be developed and optimized. As summarized in a study by Jensen et al., "Individual skills make good surgeons, the mixture of skills provide the potential to become talented, while the person-environment fit is what determines if the talent potential can be realized."[36]

1.4 Conclusion

MISS is an advancing field which has rapidly progressed in the past decade and will continue to expand its role in treating complex spinal pathology. The "6 Ts" outline the basic principles for successful MISS. MISS is a dynamic field that develops in parallel with technology, especially as new technologies impact imaging and surgical implementation. The ultimate goal of MISS is to accomplish spinal health in the least invasive manner while avoiding complications and overtreatment. Of the six principles covered, the "target philosophy" is the one least covered in publications, books, or at meetings and should therefore be considered carefully.

References

[1] Schmidt FA, Wong T, Kirnaz S, et al. Development of a curriculum for minimally invasive spine surgery (MISS) 122S. Global Spine J. 2020; 10 Suppl 2:122S–125S

[2] McAfee PC, Phillips FM, Andersson G, et al. Minimally invasive spine surgery. Spine. 2010; 35 Suppl 26:S271–S273

[3] Dyrda, L. Surgeons perform 1.62M instrumented spinal fusions per year in the US: 5 things to know. [online] Beckersspine.com. Accessed 22 July 2021

[4] Arts MP, Brand R, van den Akker ME, Koes BW, Bartels RH, Peul WC, Leiden-The Hague Spine Intervention Prognostic Study Group (SIPS). Tubular diskectomy vs conventional microdiskectomy for sciatica: a randomized controlled trial. JAMA. 2009; 302(2):149–158

[5] Parikh K, Tomasino A, Knopman J, Boockvar J, Härtl R. Operative results and learning curve: microscope-assisted tubular microsurgery for 1- and 2-level discectomies and laminectomies. Neurosurg Focus. 2008; 25(2):E14

[6] Härtl R, Korge A. Minimally invasive spine surgery: techniques, evidence, and controversies. Thieme; 2012

[7] Boukebir MA, Berlin CD, Navarro-Ramirez R, et al. Ten-Step minimally invasive spine lumbar decompression and dural repair through tubular retractors. Oper Neurosurg (Hagerstown). 2017; 13(2):232–245

[8] Guiot BH, Khoo LT, Fessler RG. A minimally invasive technique for decompression of the lumbar spine. Spine. 2002; 27(4):432–438

[9] Khoo LT, Fessler RG. Microendoscopic decompressive laminotomy for the treatment of lumbar stenosis. Neurosurgery. 2002; 51 Suppl 5:S146–S154

[10] Palmer S, Turner R, Palmer R. Bilateral decompressive surgery in lumbar spinal stenosis associated with spondylolisthesis: unilateral approach and use of a microscope and tubular retractor system. Neurosurg Focus. 2002; 13(1):E4

[11] Schöller K, Alimi M, Cong GT, Christos P, Härtl R. Lumbar spinal stenosis associated with degenerative lumbar spondylolisthesis: a systematic review and meta-analysis of secondary fusion rates following open vs minimally invasive decompression. Neurosurgery. 2017; 80(3):355–367

[12] Ge DH, Stekas ND, Varlotta CG, et al. Comparative analysis of two transforaminal lumbar interbody fusion techniques: open TLIF versus Wiltse MIS TLIF. Spine. 2019; 44(9):E555–E560

[13] Mummaneni PV, Shaffrey CI, Lenke LG, et al. Minimally Invasive Surgery Section of the International Spine Study Group. The minimally invasive spinal deformity surgery algorithm: a reproducible rational framework for decision making in minimally invasive spinal deformity surgery. Neurosurg Focus. 2014; 36(5):E6

[14] Mummaneni PV, Park P, Shaffrey CI, et al. International Spine Study Group (ISSG). The MISDEF2 algorithm: an updated algorithm for patient selection in minimally invasive deformity surgery. J Neurosurg Spine. 2019; 32(2):221–228

[15] Navarro-Ramirez R, Lang G, Lian X, et al. Total navigation in spine surgery: a concise guide to eliminate fluoroscopy using a portable intraoperative computed tomography 3-dimensional navigation system. World Neurosurg. 2017; 100:325–335

[16] Wipplinger C, Melcher C, Hernandez RN, et al. "One and a half" minimally invasive transforaminal lumbar interbody fusion: single level transforaminal lumbar interbody fusion with adjacent segment unilateral laminotomy for bilateral decompression for spondylolisthesis with bisegmental stenosis. J Spine Surg. 2018; 4(4):780–786

[17] Lau D, Lee JG, Han SJ, Lu DC, Chou D. Complications and perioperative factors associated with learning the technique of minimally invasive transforaminal lumbar interbody fusion (TLIF). J Clin Neurosci. 2011; 18(5):624–627

[18] Son-Hing JP, Blakemore LC, Poe-Kochert C, Thompson GH. Video-assisted thoracoscopic surgery in idiopathic scoliosis: evaluation of the learning curve. Spine. 2007; 32(6):703–707

[19] Pfandler M, Lazarovici M, Stefan P, Wucherer P, Weigl M. Virtual reality-based simulators for spine surgery: a systematic review. Spine J. 2017; 17(9):1352–1363

[20] Buckley CE, Kavanagh DO, Gallagher TK, Conroy RM, Traynor OJ, Neary PC. Does aptitude influence the rate at which proficiency is achieved for laparoscopic appendectomy? J Am Coll Surg. 2013; 217(6):1020–1027

[21] Grantcharov TP, Bardram L, Funch-Jensen P, Rosenberg J. Impact of hand dominance, gender, and experience with computer games on performance in virtual reality laparoscopy. Surg Endosc. 2003; 17(7):1082–1085

[22] Boyd T, Jung I, Van Sickle K, Schwesinger W, Michalek J, Bingener J. Music experience influences laparoscopic skills performance. JSLS. 2008; 12 (3):292–294

[23] Donnon T, DesCôteaux JG, Violato C. Impact of cognitive imaging and sex differences on the development of laparoscopic suturing skills. Can J Surg. 2005; 48(5):387–393

[24] White MT, Welch K. Does gender predict performance of novices undergoing Fundamentals of Laparoscopic Surgery (FLS) training? Am J Surg. 2012; 203 (3):397–400, discussion 400

[25] Thorson CM, Kelly JP, Forse RA, Turaga KK. Can we continue to ignore gender differences in performance on simulation trainers? J Laparoendosc Adv Surg Tech A. 2011; 21(4):329–333

[26] Rosenberg BH, Landsittel D, Averch TD. Can video games be used to predict or improve laparoscopic skills? J Endourol. 2005; 19(3):372–376

[27] Rosser JC, Jr, Lynch PJ, Cuddihy L, Gentile DA, Klonsky J, Merrell R. The impact of video games on training surgeons in the 21st century. Arch Surg. 2007; 142(2):181–186, 186

[28] Schmidt-Tintemann U. [Women in surgery]. Zeitschrift fur alle Gebiete der operativen Medizen. Chirurg. 1997; 68(6):583–585

[29] Abbott A, Collins D. A theoretical and empirical analysis of a 'state of the art' talent identification model. High Abil Stud. 2002; 13(2):157–178

[30] Gagné F. From genes to talent: the DMGT/CMTD perspective. Rev Educ. 2015; 368:12–37

[31] Gagné F. Nature or nurture? A re-examination of Sloboda and Howe's (1991) interview study on talent development in music. Psychol Music. 1999; 27 (1):38–51

[32] Ericsson KA, Nandagopal K, Roring RW. Toward a science of exceptional achievement: attaining superior performance through deliberate practice. Ann N Y Acad Sci. 2009; 1172(1):199–217

[33] Ericsson KA. Deliberate practice and the acquisition and maintenance of expert performance in medicine and related domains. Acad Med. 2004; 79 (10) Suppl:S70–S81

[34] Coyle D. The Talent Code: Greatness Isn't Born. It's Grown. New York: Random House Publishing Group; 2009

[35] Lindlohr C, Lefering R, Saad S, Heiss MM, Pape-Köhler C. Training or non-surgical factors-what determines a good surgical performance? A randomised controlled trial. Langenbecks Arch Surg. 2017; 402(4):645–653

[36] Jensen RD, Christensen MK, LaDonna KA, Seyer-Hansen M, Cristancho S. How surgeons conceptualize talent: a qualitative study using sport science as a lens. J Surg Educ. 2017; 74(6):992–1000

2 Global MISS: Perspectives from Asia, Australia, Europe, Middle East, North America, and South America

Summary
Spine surgical techniques including MIS are described to be uniform and reproducible. However, adaptation to the techniques is encountered around the world depending on multiple factors: regulatory organisms, government regulations, technology access, cultural practices among others. These differences sometimes promote change, innovation, and improvement of clinical practice. This chapter represents a unique opportunity for the reader to experience and learn the MIS perspective of spine surgeons from six different geographical regions around the world.

Keywords: global surgery, global spine surgery, international spine surgery, international MIS surgery, Asian spine surgery, European spine surgery, Latin American spine surgery, Middle Eastern spine surgery

2.1 Asia

Guang-Xun Lin, Jin-Sung Luke Kim, and Louis Chang

Over the past decade, minimally invasive spine surgery (MISS) has gained rapid popularity around the world. With available technologies, MISS can now be performed using advanced surgical tools and background knowledge to treat a myriad of spinal pathologies, including lumbar disc herniation, spinal stenosis, and use in fusion surgery.[1,2,3]

Surveying the current state of MISS in the Asian region, we can roughly divide its application into five categories: (1) microendoscopic discectomy (MED); (2) full-endoscopic lumbar discectomy (FELD); (3) percutaneous endoscopic lumbar discectomy (PELD); (4) MISS fusion (transforaminal/lateral/oblique-lumbar interbody fusion [TLIF/LLIF/OLIF]), with or without navigation (i.e., O-arm); and (5) miscellaneous percutaneous procedures such as percutaneous vertebroplasty (PVP) or percutaneous kyphoplasty (PKP), etc.

The technique for percutaneous arthroscopic nucleotomy through a posterolateral approach was introduced by Kambin in 1973[4] and Hijikata et al in 1975.[5] The first documented microdiscectomy procedures were reported by Yasargil[6] and Caspar[7] in 1977. The MED technique was later developed in 1999 by Foley et al.[8] Since 2002, Foley's introduction of MISS fusion has shown significant progress and has been widely used for the treatment of lumbar degenerative disease.[9] The minimally invasive LLIF technique was first described by Ozgur et al in 2006.[10] The minimally invasive retroperitoneal lumbar approach was then introduced by M. Mayer in 1997, but the term OLIF was coined in 2012.[11] Image-guidance techniques in spinal surgery procedures have been implemented since 1995.[12] In addition, PVP was performed initially in 1984 by Galibert et al[13] and PKP was then developed in the mid-1990s by Garfin et al.[14]

Several factors that characterize the region-specific strengths, weaknesses, opportunities, and threats can be identified.

2.1.1 Strengths

The development of MISS in Asia is mainly concentrated in East Asia and India. Since 2000, five countries in Asia have published the largest number of articles in the field of MISS each year.[15] Academic activities such as conferences and courses are also the most active in this geographic region. ▶ Table 2.1 summarizes the timeline of development of MISS techniques in the top five Asian countries.

The strong support of MISS associations also played an important role in the growth of MISS in Asia. As early as 2002, South Korea established a MISS association, named Korean Minimally Invasive Spine Surgery Society (KOMISS), to promote and develop the MISS field led by C. K. Park. In 2003, the COA-CMISS and CSSA-CMISS were established in China. Subsequently, Japanese Society of Minimally Invasive Spine Surgery (JASMISS), Taiwan Society of Minimally Invasive Spine Surgery (TSMISS), and Minimally Invasive Spine Surgeons of India (MISSICON) also established their respective MISS associations. These societies have made significant contributions to the development of MISS in the Asian countries.

Of the major countries in Asia, the role of South Korea in MISS was most prominent and most of the minimally invasive

Table 2.1 MISS development timeline in the top five Asian countries

Country	MED	FELD or PELD	MISS fusion (MISS-TLIF/DLIF/OLIF)	Navigation (O-arm)	Others
China	1998	2005	MISS-TLIF from 2006 DLIF from 2012 OLIF from 2014	2013	PKP from 2002
India	2000s	2000	OLIF from 2016	2015	PVP from 2000
Japan	1998	2003	OLIF from 2012	2000s	2011
South Korea	1990s	1992	DLIF from 2011 OLIF from 2012	2009	PVP from 1999 PKP from 2001
Taiwan	2001	1997	2010s	2000s	2000s

Abbreviations: DLIF, direct lumbar interbody fusion; FESS, full-endoscopic spinal surgery; MED, microendoscopic discectomy; MISS, minimally invasive spine surgery; OLIF, oblique lumbar interbody fusion; PELD, percutaneous endoscopic lumbar discectomy; PKP, percutaneous kyphoplasty; PVP, percutaneous vertebroplasty; TLIF, transforaminal lumbar interbody fusion.

surgeries were first performed in South Korea (PVP by C. K. Park in 1999, PELD by S. H. Lee in 2002, DLIF/OLIF by J. S. Kim).

The accelerated development of MISS in Asia may be, in part, due to cultural factors and the reluctance of many Asians, especially East Asians, to accept major surgery. Today, endoscopic spinal surgery in Asia has become one of the mainstream approaches to spine surgery unlike in the United States or Europe. This is reflected by the establishment of International Society of Endoscopic Spine Surgery (ISESS) in 2017 for the advancement of endoscopic surgical techniques in spine and the overall development of global MISS. The contributions of ISESS have propelled Asia's position in the field of endoscopic spinal surgery.

2.1.2 Weaknesses

The significant differences between geographic regions in Asia when it comes to economic status and medical infrastructure could be considered among overall weakness of this region. The abovementioned countries clearly spearhead MISS, while many of the other countries are still far behind.

2.1.3 Opportunities

As technology continues to advance and the indications for surgery expand over the years, we have found that endoscopic spinal surgery can not only be used to treat the simple disc herniation but also effectively address lumbar stenosis.[2,16,17] Moreover, there have been a few reports on endoscopy-assisted interbody fusion procedure[3] and other applications of endoscopic spine surgery, such as unilateral biportal endoscopic (UBE) technique, which is considered endoscopic-assisted rather than full endoscopic spine surgery.[18,19,20]

The improvements in surgical techniques, technologies, and instruments, along with the cultural differences in Asia, have allowed MISS to gain popularity over traditional spinal surgeries in Asia.

2.1.4 Threats

The focus on endoscopic surgery has led to a slower development in other areas of MISS in this region, as seen in ▶ Table 2.1. Although percutaneous technologies were described as early as the early 1990s, other very well accepted MISS procedures and technologies such as fusion and navigation were published later, when compared to other regions. This may be a challenge going forward.

References

[1] Ruetten S, Komp M, Merk H, Godolias G. Full-endoscopic interlaminar and transforaminal lumbar discectomy versus conventional microsurgical technique: a prospective, randomized, controlled study. Spine. 2008; 33(9):931–939

[2] Komp M, Hahn P, Oezdemir S, et al. Bilateral spinal decompression of lumbar central stenosis with the full-endoscopic interlaminar versus microsurgical laminotomy technique: a prospective, randomized, controlled study. Pain Physician. 2015; 18(1):61–70

[3] Youn MS, Shin JK, Goh TS, Lee JS. Full endoscopic lumbar interbody fusion (FELIF): technical note. Eur Spine J. 2018; 27(8):1949–1955

[4] Kambin P, ed. Arthroscopic Microdiscectomy: Minimal Intervention Spinal Surgery. Baltimore, MD: Urban & Schwarzenberg; 1990

[5] Hijikata S, Yamagishi M, Nakayama T, Oomori K. Percutaneous discectomy: a new treatment method for lumbar disc herniation. J Toden Hosp. 1975; 5:5–13

[6] Yasargil MG. Microsurgical operations of herniated lumbar disc. Adv Neurosurg. 1977; 4:81–82

[7] Caspar W. A new surgical procedure for lumbar disc herniation causing less tissue damage through a microsurgical approach. Adv Neurosurgs. 1977; 4:74–80

[8] Foley KT, Smith MM, Rampersaud YR. Microendoscopic approach to far-lateral lumbar disc herniation. Neurosurg Focus. 1999; 7(5):e5

[9] Foley KT, Holly LT, Schwender JD. Minimally invasive lumbar fusion. Spine. 2003; 28(15) Suppl:S26–S35

[10] Ozgur BM, Aryan HE, Pimenta L, Taylor WR. Extreme Lateral Interbody Fusion (XLIF): a novel surgical technique for anterior lumbar interbody fusion. Spine J. 2006; 6(4):435–443

[11] Silvestre C, Mac-Thiong J-M, Hilmi R, Roussouly P. Complications and morbidities of mini-open anterior retroperitoneal lumbar interbody fusion: oblique lumbar interbody fusion in 179 patients. Asian Spine J. 2012; 6(2):89–97

[12] Amiot LP, Labelle H, DeGuise JA, Sati M, Brodeur P, Rivard CH. Computer-assisted pedicle screw fixation. A feasibility study. Spine. 1995; 20(10):1208–1212

[13] Galibert P, Deramond H, Rosat P, Le Gars D. [Preliminary note on the treatment of vertebral angioma by percutaneous acrylic vertebroplasty]. Neurochirurgie. 1987; 33(2):166–168

[14] Garfin SR, Yuan HA, Reiley MA. New technologies in spine: kyphoplasty and vertebroplasty for the treatment of painful osteoporotic compression fractures. Spine. 2001; 26(14):1511–1515

[15] Fan G, Han R, Zhang H, He S, Chen Z. Worldwide research productivity in the field of minimally invasive spine surgery: a 20-year survey of publication activities. Spine. 2017; 42(22):1717–1722

[16] Ruetten S, Komp M, Merk H, Godolias G. Surgical treatment for lumbar lateral recess stenosis with the full-endoscopic interlaminar approach versus conventional microsurgical technique: a prospective, randomized, controlled study. J Neurosurg Spine. 2009; 10(5):476–485

[17] Komp M, Hahn P, Merk H, Godolias G, Ruetten S. Bilateral operation of lumbar degenerative central spinal stenosis in full-endoscopic interlaminar technique with unilateral approach: prospective 2-year results of 74 patients. J Spinal Disord Tech. 2011; 24(5):281–287

[18] He EX, Guo J, Ling QJ, Yin ZX, Wang Y, Li M. Application of a narrow-surface cage in full endoscopic minimally invasive transforaminal lumbar interbody fusion. Int J Surg. 2017; 42:83–89

[19] Hwa Eum J, Hwa Heo D, Son SK, Park CK. Percutaneous biportal endoscopic decompression for lumbar spinal stenosis: a technical note and preliminary clinical results. J Neurosurg Spine. 2016; 24(4):602–607

[20] Heo DH, Son SK, Eum JH, Park CK. Fully endoscopic lumbar interbody fusion using a percutaneous unilateral biportal endoscopic technique: technical note and preliminary clinical results. Neurosurg Focus. 2017; 43(2):E8

2.2 Australia

Tony Goldschlager

Like most of the world, spine surgery in Australasia is performed by both orthopaedic surgeons and neurosurgeons. The training, however, is managed and regulated by a central body, the Royal Australasian College of Surgeons (RACS). This body is responsible for resident placements, which are rotated among accredited hospitals to provide trainees with a breadth of experience. This means that exposure to MISS during residency is dependent on the supervising surgeons encountered on these rotations, which is generally limited to a duration of no more than 2 years in a given hospital. It is fair to say that in Australasia MISS is generally a skill developed during post-fellowship training; however, this is changing.

The health care system in Australia is divided between the public and the private sector and this provides specific

opportunities. Teaching and training typically occur in the public sector, which is generally of high standard but less efficient than the private sector. High-volume, single-surgeon surgery is performed in the private sector, which enables outcome research on specific MISS techniques. This is reflected in the Australasian MISS publications. A search of PubMed on "minimally invasive spine surgery" and "Australia" since 2010 has revealed 62 publications. Many of these publications are single-surgeon consecutive series, while some are descriptions of new techniques.

It is difficult to know the true extent of MISS is Australasia but it certainly appears to be increasing. We recently conducted a survey of Australasian neurosurgeons on their practice of microdiscectomy. This survey sheds some light on current Australasian neurosurgical practice. The majority of responders use microscopic (76.5%) or loupe (20.6%) magnification, but 2.9% use no magnification. The majority of surgeons (77%) perform unilateral muscle dissection; 21% use tubular retractors but almost 3% utilize a bilateral muscle dissection exposure.[1] There is a significant number of neurosurgeons who perform "simple spine surgery" only, such as microdiscectomy and laminectomy. These surgeons typically do not perform instrumented operations. For those that do, navigation and robotic technologies are being acquired and utilized by an increasing number of Australasian hospitals. Surgeons are tending to adopt MISS techniques and technologies. However, the challenges are that comparatively, the Australasian market is small and a separate regulatory pathway, through the Therapeutic Goods Administration (TGA), exists. This means that Australasian spine surgeons have lesser and later exposure to new technologies.

In summary, MISS in Australasia is increasing. Many Australasian spine surgeons undertake fellowships overseas where new skills and linkages are developed. The Australasian health landscape provides unique opportunities to develop and study MISS technology and techniques.

2.2.1 Strengths

- Highly trained surgeons.
- Latest techniques readily adopted.
- Regional regulatory body.
- Shorter hospital stay.

2.2.2 Weaknesses

- Regional regulatory body.
- Variable availability of imaging modalities.
- Reliant on consumables which increases hospital costs.

2.2.3 Threats

- Prosthesis costs.
- Insurance bodies may limit access to some procedures.

2.2.4 Opportunities

- Global adoption of locally invented technologies.
- Great training ground for fellowships.

Reference

[1] Daly CD, Lim K-Z, Ghosh P, Goldschlager T. Perioperative care for lumbar microdiscectomy: a survey of Australasian neurosurgeons. J Spine Surg. 2018; 4(1):1–8

2.3 Europe

H. Michael Mayer

2.3.1 Introduction

The history of MISS in Europe dates back to the late 1970s of the last century when Yasargil and Caspar independently published their papers on the first microsurgical discectomy.[1,2] Since then, a variety of different minimally invasive techniques have been inaugurated by European spine surgeons: such as microsurgical anterior cervical discectomy and fusion (ACDF)[3] or disc replacement,[4,5] endoscopic discectomies,[6,7,8] thoracoscopic approaches for disc herniations or fractures,[9,10] microsurgical and endoscopic lumbar decompression techniques,[11,12,13] mini-open anterior lumbar interbody fusion (ALIF), oblique lumbar interbody fusion (OLIF),[14] vertebroplasty, kyphoplasty, or vertebral body stenting[15] etc. just to mention a few which have become "standard techniques" in high-level spine centers in Europe.

If we look at the surgical spectrum of spine centers in Europe, minimally invasive techniques are applied more or less in 50 to 70% of all spine operations. Either the complete operation is performed in an MISS technique (e.g., endoscopic discectomy) or parts of the operation are performed in an MISS technique (e.g., MISS-TLIF).

Independent of the discussion about the benefits and risks of MISS techniques is the fact that such techniques are nothing else than the normal evolution of surgical techniques according to the Hippocratic principle of: "First do no harm" to the patient.

I have tried to summarize the current situation of MISS in Europe with a simple personal SWOT (Strengths, Weaknesses, Opportunities, Threats) analysis.

2.3.2 Strengths

Due to very strong and dynamic research and development activities of European Medtech companies in the 1980s, 1990s of the last, and the first 5 years of the current century, a number of MISS techniques have been refined technically and have become standard in nearly every spine center in Europe. Examples are: microsurgical lumbar discectomies, microsurgical decompression techniques for spinal stenosis, microsurgical cervical foraminotomies and ACDF, percutaneous pedicle screw placement with or without navigation, mini-open approaches to the anterior lumbar spine (ALIF, OLIF), thoracoscopic or mini-open approaches for fracture treatment and thoracic discectomies, vertebroplasty, kyphoplasty, and vertebral body stenting. All these techniques have demonstrated the strengths of MISS, which is the reduction of surgical trauma and collateral tissue damage. The resulting clinical effects and benefits are less blood loss, less perioperative and postoperative morbidity, shorter hospitalization times, and faster rehabilitation. These are the

main strengths of MISS in spine surgery and it has been demonstrated in a number of clinical studies that the mid- and long-term outcomes are the same or even better as compared to non-MISS techniques.

2.3.3 Weaknesses

It seems to be clear that the primary goals of any new surgical technique should be beneficial for the patient. This can only be realized if the goal of surgery can be achieved in the same way as with conventional techniques, that is, the technical and clinical outcome should be the same but with less invasiveness. This, on the other hand, requires an adequate technology and surgical training. Whereas technology is not a problem, the training of innovative MISS techniques is. The opportunities to learn are focused on lab training with simple sawbone models or wet labs where approaches and tissue handling can be learned best. However, experience still has to be gained on operating patients. The more complex the procedure is, the longer are the "learning curves." A learning curve is nearly always associated with higher perioperative morbidity, higher complication rates as well as inferior clinical outcomes. This implies that the surgeon exposes earlier patients to a higher risk so that later patients can benefit from a new technique. This is immanent to all learning processes in medicine as long as we don't have other training tools.

2.3.4 Opportunities

The research and development of teaching and training tools for young surgeons are great opportunities which new technologies provide. The use of virtual or augmented reality and the creation of surgical simulators might enable us to shift parts of our learning curves from the operating theater to the lab. "Serious games" or apps might help to assess and practice typical basic MISS skills such as three-dimensional orientation, fine-motor skills, hand-eye coordination etc. before we enter the operating theater. The affinity of the younger surgeon generation to such technologies will help.

We are still in a comfortable position in Europe to be able to use the "latest" technology (e.g., fourth-generation cervical disc replacement, stand-alone ACDF, all kinds of lumbar fusion techniques etc.). However, "European ideas" in MISS become more difficult to realize with US market-driven Medtech companies because of regulatory issues (see "Threats" below). The window of opportunities opens in Asia. Asian countries have taken the lead in a variety of innovative MISS techniques such as endoscopic surgery, 3D-printed (individual) implant technology, electromagnetic navigation, and intraoperative robotics. Thus, the opportunities for European MISS surgeons are growing with closer cooperation with our Asian colleagues or Asian companies. The growing number of Asian fellows in European spine centers and closer cooperation between Asian and European spine centers underline this development.

2.3.5 Threats

There are a number of threats, which might slow down the further development of MISS techniques in spine surgery. The call for evidence-based data and cost efficiency by insurance companies and health care politics is increasingly challenging. Stricter regulatory requirements make it more difficult, costly, and finally unattractive to develop new techniques even if new implants can be sold with such techniques. With a look at the global market situation, the fact that the US market is still the most important one has slowed down innovation in spine surgery tremendously. Although the number of 510,000 approvals of spine products through the FDA has remained more or less constant in the last years, the number of true FDA IDE approvals in spine products has dropped dramatically. Many innovative technologies are simply not realized by manufacturers, because they don't see a chance to get FDA approval in an acceptable time span. If European health care politics, payers, and Medtech companies continue to adopt the FDA regulatory "philosophy" we may not only see a stagnancy but probably a decline of MISS applications in European spine surgery.

References

[1] Caspar W. A new surgical procedure for lumbar disc herniation causing less tissue damage due to a microsurgical approach. Adv Neurosurg. 1977; 4:74–80

[2] Yasargil MG. Microsurgical operation of the herniated lumbar disc. In: Wüllenweber R, Brock M, Hamer J, Klinger M, Spoerri O, eds. Lumbar Disc Adult Hydrocephalus. Advances in Neurosurgery. 4th ed. Berlin, Heidelberg; New York: Springer; 1977:81–82

[3] Caspar W, Barbier DD, Klara PM. Anterior cervical fusion and Caspar plate stabilization for cervical trauma. Neurosurgery. 1989; 25(4):491–502

[4] Mayer HM, Wiechert K, Korge A, Qose I. Minimally invasive total disc replacement: surgical technique and preliminary clinical results. Eur Spine J. 2002; 11 Suppl 2:S124–S130

[5] Bertagnoli R, Kumar S. Indications for full prosthetic disc arthroplasty: a correlation of clinical outcome against a variety of indications. Eur Spine J. 2002; 11 Suppl 2:S131–S136

[6] Schreiber A, Suezawa Y, Leu H. Does percutaneous nucleotomy with discoscopy replace conventional discectomy? Eight years of experience and results in treatment of herniated lumbar disc. Clin Orthop Relat Res. 1989(238):35–42

[7] Mayer HM, Brock M. Percutaneous endoscopic discectomy: surgical technique and preliminary results compared to microsurgical discectomy. J Neurosurg. 1993; 78(2):216–225

[8] Ruetten S, Komp M, Godolias G. A new full-endoscopic technique for the interlaminar operation of lumbar disc herniations using 6-mm endoscopes: prospective 2-year results of 331 patients. Minim Invasive Neurosurg. 2006; 49(2):80–87

[9] Rosenthal D, Dickman CA. Thoracoscopic microsurgical excision of herniated thoracic discs. J Neurosurg. 1998; 89(2):224–235

[10] Potulski M, Beisse R, Bühren V. Thorascopically guided therapy of the "anterior column". Technique and results. Orthopade. 1999; 28(8):723–730

[11] Spetzger U, Bertalanffy H, Reinges MH, Gilsbach JM. Unilateral laminotomy for bilateral decompression of lumbar spinal stenosis. Part II: Clinical experiences. Acta Neurochir (Wien). 1997; 139(5):397–403

[12] Ruetten S, Komp M, Merk H, Godolias G. Surgical treatment for lumbar lateral recess stenosis with the full-endoscopic interlaminar approach versus conventional microsurgical technique: a prospective, randomized, controlled study. J Neurosurg Spine. 2009; 10(5):476–485

[13] Mayer HM, Heider F. "Slalom": microsurgical cross-over decompression for multilevel degenerative lumbar stenosis. BioMed Res Int. 2016; 2016:9074257

[14] Mayer HM. A new microsurgical technique for minimally invasive anterior lumbar interbody fusion. Spine. 1997; 22(6):691–699, discussion 700

[15] Heini PF, Orler R. Kyphoplasty for treatment of osteoporotic vertebral fractures. Eur Spine J. 2004; 13(3):184–192

2.4 Middle East

Magdy Gamal AbdelKader Youssef

2.4.1 Introduction

The Middle East is home to some of the oldest civilizations. Science, medicine, and surgery were explored early with many

advances made hundreds of years before they were described in the western world. Minimally invasive surgery was not an exception, and it was first mentioned in early Egyptian civilization and was drawn in papyrus for many surgical fields with instruments that mimicked many recent tools.

2.4.2 Strengths

Individual surgeons in our region show great interest and enthusiasm in MISS and it has been focally adopted very successfully with limited penetration.

2.4.3 Weaknesses

Although MISS started years ago in a revolutionary way in Europe and North America targeting less morbidity and early return to work, it did not get that attention in the Middle East. It showed a delayed start due to many factors, including reluctance on the part of surgeons, health insurance system, patient's compliance and needs, and lack of proper companies and media support. Most patients are treated by government health insurance facilities as well as private health insurance companies, and for these facilities, MISS is not their top priority to optimize cost effectiveness from their point of view.

Meanwhile, foreign companies are not always ready to lower the cost for the Middle East region and, even more important, are not offering much training for surgeons to bridge the relatively long MISS learning curve. This leaves surgeons hesitant to do MISS and they tend to stick to open surgery, aiming for safety and predictable results and avoiding complications. As a result, surgeons who do not have access to technology and training will sometimes turn against such progress in their facilities especially when they are heading their departments and see no possible way to participate in what they consider as "fashionable" surgery.

Hospitals in the Middle East are also looking for the best deals from their point of view before paying for very expensive MISS tools; costly navigation and endoscopic instruments mean lower profit for them, thus ignoring the benefits in the long term.

2.4.4 Opportunities

Recently, some progress has been made regarding MISS based on personal interest of some enthusiastic surgeons, mainly in academia, who started on their own to buy affordable tools to enter this field despite the financial barriers. Such personal efforts started to spread the spirit to others and obliged companies to help in providing tools and share training and ask expert surgeons to visit Middle East countries. This spirit was reflected positively in the media and started to spread the message to many others, explaining the benefits of MISS to patients who started seeking such appealing way of management which gained promising popularity in past few years.

For the MISS revolution to spread in this region, it will be necessary to have a real interest and appreciation of hospitals and government institutions regarding the benefits of MISS, which will lower the cost and hospital stay in the long term, especially endoscopic and tube assisted microscopic surgeries that might replace traditional open surgery to be the new gold standard in lumbar discectomies, percutaneous fixation to take bigger share in fracture stabilization, and vertebroplasty to help more osteoporotic cases. From these categories, MISS can extend to other indications in many other pathologies based on advances in radiology and technical support from companies. Industry should offer more professional training for the whole surgical team to take MISS to a higher level. Training is the key factor in MISS progression even in low resource settings if the available basic tools can be properly used by properly trained spine surgeons.

2.4.5 Threats

The costs of providing MISS technology and implants from companies abroad are prohibitively high. Importing tools by foreign currency is not cost effective, especially when patients at present can hardly share some of the medical costs. On the other hand, some equipment and tools such as tubular retractor and endoscopes could be purchased at relatively low prices and, with proper training, may allow the introduction of MISS technology without necessarily having to invest in very expensive navigation systems, robotics, and the whole spectrum of MISS implants.

2.5 North America

Jason I. Liounakos and Michael Y. Wang

2.5.1 Introduction

Techniques in MISS are rapidly changing the way spine care is delivered is North America. The needs of the patient, surgeon, and economy are responsible for such widespread interest, translating to an increased rate of adoption and technological advancement over recent years. Together, these factors provide the optimal environment for the proliferation of MISS, as evidenced by trends in the literature with almost half of all peer-reviewed articles relating to MISS originating from the USA.[1] This section provides an overview of the driving forces behind increased utilization and advancement using a strengths, weaknesses, opportunities, and threats (SWOT) analysis.

2.5.2 Strengths

MISS for the appropriate indications appears to deliver at least equivalent clinical outcomes compared to conventional open surgery, while decreasing morbidity and recovery time.[2,3,4] Patients in North America are sensitive to this and many actively seek out minimally invasive options for their ailments. Moreover, degenerative disc disease and associated pathologies leading to pain and disability are more prevalent with age. Due to declining birth rates and rapidly increasing life expectancy, a dramatic upward shift in the global age structure is occurring. This will almost certainly lead to an increased number of spine surgeries being performed on an increasingly aged population with more medical comorbidities.[5] This fact, coupled with hospital and physician reimbursement shifting to a more outcome-focused model, has resulted in an emphasis on minimally invasive alternatives and enhanced recovery after surgery (ERAS)®

programs. All of these factors, combined with the almost universal availability of MISS equipment in the USA and a strong academic culture, result in the ideal environment for MISS to thrive and evolve.

2.5.3 Weaknesses

The learning curve associated with MISS techniques likely represents its most significant weakness, particularly for established surgeons. Fortunately, this may all but disappear as the current generation of trainees advance into practice, as residency and fellowship programs are now demanding mastery of techniques such as LLIF, MISS-TLIF, ALIF, and percutaneous placement of instrumentation. Spinal endoscopy remains less widely adopted likely owing to an even steeper learning curve as reported in multiple studies.[6,7] As exposure to endoscopy continues to increase in residency and the potential long-term benefits and cost-savings are fully realized, this too will be minimized. In addition, countless organized courses are now available to increase exposure to all these techniques for both residents and practicing surgeons alike.

2.5.4 Opportunities

The United States' health care system is heavily influenced by private and public economic interests. As such, it is through healthy competition that North America has remained the leader in spinal technology and innovation over the past 20 years. As value and cost-effectiveness become increasingly important in health care economics, numerous studies have begun to evaluate the economic impact of MISS. The greatest benefits appear to come from decreasing hospital length of stay, postoperative medical complications, narcotic reliance, and the rate of discharge to rehabilitation facilities.[8,9,10] Moreover, MISS may be readily performed in ambulatory surgical centers, resulting in significant cost reductions compared to tertiary medical centers.[11] As surgeons in the USA continue to push the boundary of what is capable of being performed in the outpatient setting, the opportunities for advancement of MISS will only grow.

2.5.5 Threats

As discussed, one area of MISS that has not seen much widespread adoption in the USA is spinal endoscopy. The primary reasons for this include high initial perceived cost of establishing an endoscopic program, steep learning curve, and poor reimbursement. The result is limited adoption outside of boutique, privately owned, ambulatory surgery practices. As the potential for long-term savings is realized, this should lead to a paradigm shift toward increased endoscopic utilization. In our own center, utilizing a novel awake endoscopic-assisted TLIF procedure, coupled with an ERAS protocol, we have shown a 15.2% reduction in acute care costs compared to standard MISS-TLIF.[12]

2.5.6 Conclusions

MISS in North America has seen widespread adoption and advancement at a break-neck pace over the past 20 years. The promise of equivalent or better outcomes, coupled with reduced soft tissue trauma, minimal blood loss, shorter hospital length of stay (or even outpatient surgery), reduced narcotic reliance, and faster postoperative recovery, is highly desirable to both patients and surgeons alike. Bountiful resources and incentives for progress have made North America, and particularly the USA, a leader in furthering MISS.

References

[1] Fan G, Han R, Zhang H, He S, Chen Z. Worldwide research productivity in the field of minimally invasive spine surgery: a 20-year survey of publication activities. Spine. 2017; 42(22):1717–1722

[2] Wang X, Borgman B, Vertuani S, Nilsson J. A systematic literature review of time to return to work and narcotic use after lumbar spinal fusion using minimal invasive and open surgery techniques. BMC Health Serv Res. 2017; 17 (1):446

[3] Patel AA, Zfass-Mendez M, Lebwohl NH, et al. Minimally invasive versus open lumbar fusion: a comparison of blood loss, surgical complications, and hospital course. Iowa Orthop J. 2015; 35:130–134

[4] Goldstein CL, Macwan K, Sundararajan K, Rampersaud YR. Perioperative outcomes and adverse events of minimally invasive versus open posterior lumbar fusion: meta-analysis and systematic review. J Neurosurg Spine. 2016; 24 (3):416–427

[5] Fehlings MG, Tetreault L, Nater A, et al. The aging of the global population: the changing epidemiology of disease and spinal disorders. Neurosurgery. 2015; 77 Suppl 4:S1–S5

[6] Hsu HT, Chang SJ, Yang SS, Chai CL. Learning curve of full-endoscopic lumbar discectomy. Eur Spine J. 2013; 22(4):727–733

[7] Morgenstern R, Morgenstern C, Yeung AT. The learning curve in foraminal endoscopic discectomy: experience needed to achieve a 90% success rate. SAS J. 2007; 1(3):100–107

[8] Hofstetter CP, Hofer AS, Wang MY. Economic impact of minimally invasive lumbar surgery. World J Orthop. 2015; 6(2):190–201

[9] Hopkins B, Mazmudar A, Kesavabhotla K, Patel AA. Economic Value in Minimally Invasive Spine Surgery. Curr Rev Musculoskelet Med. 2019; 12(3):300–304

[10] Parker SL, Adogwa O, Bydon A, Cheng J, McGirt MJ. Cost-effectiveness of minimally invasive versus open transforaminal lumbar interbody fusion for degenerative spondylolisthesis associated low-back and leg pain over two years. World Neurosurg. 2012; 78(1–2):178–184

[11] Mok JK, Gang CH, Qureshi S, McAnany SJ. Using minimally invasive techniques adds to the value equation for select patients. J Spine Surg. 2019; 5 Suppl 1:S101–S107

[12] Wang MY, Chang HK, Grossman J. Reduced acute care costs with the ERAS® minimally invasive transforaminal lumbar interbody fusion compared with conventional minimally invasive transforaminal lumbar interbody fusion. Neurosurgery. 2018; 83(4):827–834

2.6 South America

Luiz Pimenta, Rodrigo Amaral, Leonardo Oliveira, and Luis Marchi

2.6.1 Introduction

The aim of MISS is to provide the patient with the same or better results compared to traditional open procedures, with the difference that it causes less collateral tissue damage; decreases morbidity, blood loss, and length of hospital stay; and gives the patient a more rapid recovery and return to daily activities, with clinical and socioeconomic positive effects.[1] Research and clinical trials resulting in a critical evaluation, publications, and finally education and training of surgeons are important mechanisms by which MISS can and should be analyzed and promoted. In this regard, we can identify a number of different strengths, weaknesses, opportunities, and threats (SWOT) that are characteristic for our region.[2]

Table 2.2 Summary of strengths, weaknesses, opportunities, and threats of MISS from experts around the world

Strengths (+)	Weaknesses (–)
• Reduced surgical trauma and collateral tissue damage • Decreased morbidity and recovery time than open surgery • Strong support and involvement in academic activities (i.e., MISS publications), increasing worldwide visibility for countries • Shift to a more outcome-focused model as life expectancy increases and individuals with more medical comorbidities are in need of spine surgery	• Difficult learning curve • High initial costs and lack of financial support and investment for surgeon training and research • Significant differences in economic status and medical infrastructure between different geographic regions • Reluctance due to surgeons, health insurance systems, patient compliance, and lack proper company and media support • Lack of interest to focus on long-term benefits by hospitals
Opportunities (+)	**Threats (–)**

• Significant cost reductions due to decreased length hospital of stay, postoperative medical complications, narcotic reliance, and rate of discharge to rehabilitation facilities
• Better integration and exchange of expertise and knowledge
• Provides a training ground for fellowships
• Development of teaching and training tools (i.e., virtual or augmented reality, apps, simulators)
• Technology advancement has expanded the use of MISS (i.e., endoscopic spinal surgery) to treat other pathologies that were otherwise not regularly treated by MISS
• Global adoption of locally invented technologies
	• Regulatory bodies/entities
	  ◦ Prevent new technologies from entering the market
	  ◦ Create strict regulatory requirements that make it more difficult and costly to develop new techniques
	  ◦ Demand for more evidence-based data and cost efficiency to support MISS
	• High cost to provide MISS technology and implants from foreign companies in countries that do not have locally available technologies
	• Endoscopy
	  ◦ Lack of widespread adoption due to cost, difficult learning curve, and poor reimbursement
	  ◦ High focus on endoscopic surgery slows the development of other areas in MISS

2.6.2 Strengths

To achieve worldwide visibility, papers must be published in high-quality journals.[3] Federal and state research agencies have allowed an increased number of spine publications over the past 10 years, contributing to the change of Brazil in the worldwide ranking index from the 22nd position in 1998 to 13th in 2008.[4] There is also an increasing number of publications in the last few years, of mainly clinical studies and case reports, mostly regarding spinal cord injury and minimally invasive surgical techniques. However, the number of citations per year did not change, despite higher level of evidence produced by publications.

2.6.3 Weaknesses

There are many factors that hinder scientific production in South America, namely, difficulty with language, lack of interest in research, absence of economic resources, and lower quality of publications.[5] The main challenges to perform valid science are lack of financial support and investment for training researchers to conduct high-level research, providing conditions for exchanging knowledge, promoting multicenter research projects, and obtaining funds from governmental and private entities to increase not only the number but also quality of publications.

2.6.4 Opportunities

Latin American surgeons must seek better integration and exchange of expertise, using the strengths of each research center to generate scientific works of excellence despite all the difficulties faced in our region.

2.6.5 Threats

As for the adoption of MISS techniques in Latin America, particularly in Brazil, we still face some barriers that slows a wider adoption of MISS. The first one is to obtain the Brazilian Health Regulatory Agency (ANVISA) approval and registry, which may take several years and it is a very expensive process. Additionally, our public health system and some of our particular practices still use old guidelines developed before the MISS expansion. Thus, the entry of new products in the market, mainly public hospitals, is difficult. In order to break these barriers, new codification manuals are being employed by Sociedade Brasileira de Coluna (SBC), and other societies, in which they include the new technologies. Despite these difficulties, several market research groups point out that the MISS will lead the advance of spinal surgery in Latin America, with a key role for MISS interbody fusion implants.

Specifically in Brazil, we do have some delays in clinical trial due to the ANVISA and CONEP bureaucracy, which makes it difficult to initiate trials. However, we have one of the most heterogeneous populations in the world, making Brazil a good candidate for any clinical trial. Currently, based on clinicaltrial.gov, only two MISS-related studies are being carried out in the South American region.

Summary of strengths, weaknesses, opportunities, and threats of MISS from experts around the world have been listed in ▸ Table 2.2.

References

[1] McAfee PC, Phillips FM, Andersson G, et al. Minimally invasive spine surgery. Spine. dezembro de. 2010; 35(26) Suppl:S271–S273

[2] Veiga de Cabo J. [Visibility of scientific journals and initiatives to improve the diffusion of Spanish publications]. Nutr Hosp. agosto de. 2003; 18(4):177–180

[3] Sánchez-Tarragó N, Caballero-Rivero A, Trzesniak P, et al. Scientific journals in Latin America on their way towards open access: a diagnosis on policies and editorial strategies. Transinformacao. agosto de. 2016; 28(2):159–172

[4] Falavigna A, Botelho RV, Teles AR, et al. Twelve Years of Scientific Production on Medline by Latin American Spine Surgeons. PLoS ONE [Internet]. 5 de fevereiro de 2014 [citado 27 de janeiro de 2018];9(2). Disponível em: https://www.ncbi.nlm.nih.gov/pmc/articles/PMC3914870/

[5] Cristina Pabón Escobar S, Costa, C M. Visibility of Latin American scientific publications: the example of Bolivia. J Sci Commun. 2006; 5(2):A01

Part II

MISS Target

3 Target Philosophy in Degenerative Spinal Disorders: Correlation of Clinical Presentation, Physical Examination, and Response to Interventional Procedures *22*

4 Deformity and MIS: Limitation or Opportunity? *41*

5 Target: The Muscle as a Pain Generator and Key Element to Protect during MIS Surgery *49*

II

3 Target Philosophy in Degenerative Spinal Disorders: Correlation of Clinical Presentation, Physical Examination, and Response to Interventional Procedures

Bridget T. Carey, Jaspal Ricky Singh, Neel Mehta, Taylor Wong, Sertac Kirnaz, Michael Sein, and Roger Härtl

Summary

The success of MISS in this setting relies upon identifying a clear surgical target, so as to minimize surgical overtreatment and optimize subjective and objective patient outcomes. It is critical to note that not all radiographic evidence of "wear and tear" is necessarily pathological or problematic. This chapter will cover the typical patient presentations for common degenerative spinal conditions, along with the neurologic and musculoskeletal examination maneuvers, electrodiagnostic studies, and diagnostic injections that the minimally invasive spine surgeon must be aware of in order to determine the proper diagnosis.

Keywords: diagnostic injections, EMG, minimally invasive spine surgery, musculoskeletal examination, spinal imaging, spinal pathologies

3.1 Introduction

Precise diagnosis is of utmost importance for the decision-making process in minimally invasive spine surgery (MISS) for degenerative spine conditions. The success of MISS in this setting relies upon identifying a clear surgical target, so as to minimize surgical overtreatment and optimize subjective and objective patient outcomes.

Several questions are crucial in this context: How can we accurately describe and diagnose pain? How can we use the clinical examination, imaging studies, electrophysiological testing, injections, and other tests to precisely and accurately localize the pain generator? For example, many patients have complex, multilevel spinal pathology on imaging: how can we determine the most appropriate site to target with a successful surgical intervention?

The majority of patients with degenerative disorders who are at the point where surgical intervention is being considered present with pain as a dominant symptom. A careful pain history will allow the surgeon to elucidate the probable predominant pain generator. Pain resulting from degenerative spine disease can be characterized based on its quality, location, radiation, and provoking and palliating factors. The pattern of these pain characteristics often suggests the responsible focal etiology. Therefore, an accurate understanding of the type of pain a patient is experiencing is of great importance in the diagnosis and identification of the underlying pathology that may or may not be surgically treatable.

At our interdisciplinary spine center, we use thorough history and physical examination as the basis of diagnosis, and then, as needed, utilize electrodiagnostic studies, diagnostic injections, and imaging studies to confirm, refute, and/or more precisely localize the site of pathology responsible for the patient's most problematic pain symptoms. Once a diagnosis has been reached, the surgeon may determine whether this site is amenable to surgical intervention.

In this chapter, we review typical patient presentations for common degenerative spinal conditions, along with the neurologic and musculoskeletal examination maneuvers, electrodiagnostic studies, and diagnostic injections that the minimally invasive spine surgeon must be aware of in order to determine the proper diagnosis. We will also discuss some of the extraspinal musculoskeletal pathology that may masquerade as a spinal condition and confound the diagnostician. Based on clinical experience and literature, we describe the most frequently encountered pain patterns affecting each anatomical spinal segment, and how their recognition can guide in the diagnosis and accurate surgical decision-making.

> The goal of MISS in degenerative spinal disorders is to precisely *target* the pain generator and decompress/stabilize the spinal anatomy if needed, without overtreating the patient.

3.2 Cervical Segment

a) **Introduction:** In anatomical terms the cervical spine can be divided into three units: the C1 atlas, the C2 axis, and the remaining C3–C7 typical cervical vertebrae. In functional terms these units can be regarded as the cradle, the axis, and the column.[1]

b) **Cervical central canal stenosis:**

1. **Clinical presentation:** Central stenosis of the cervical spine may clinically manifest in a number of ways, depending on the degree and precise location of degenerative change. Neck pain may or may not be a significant presenting symptom. More commonly, the presentation involves neurological signs and symptoms. Gait instability, hand clumsiness, and proximal lower extremity weakness may all be presenting symptoms, along with overt upper extremity weakness.
2. **Physical examination:**
    i) **Neurologic examination:** The primary neuropathic pathology in central canal stenosis involves the spinal cord. Compression of the cervical spinal cord results in disruption of white matter tracts, the clinical correlate of which is myelopathy. Muscle tone may be increased in the upper and lower extremities. Deep tendon reflexes (DTRs) become abnormally brisk. Weakness of the arms and proximal lower extremities may occur, and there may be impairment of manual dexterity out of proportion to weakness, reflecting compression on

the corticospinal tracts. Pathological reflexes may be present, such as positive Babinski's and Hoffman's signs.

ii) **Provocative maneuvers:** Lhermitte's sign is characterized by the development of paresthesias and/or burning pain down the back and into the extremities upon neck flexion. The absence of this sign does not rule out cervical spinal cord impingement; however, its presence will generally rule it in.

3. **Electrodiagnostics:** If concomitant neural foraminal stenosis is not present, nerve conduction studies (NCS)/ electromyography (EMG) will be normal (see Section 3.2c, point 3). In patients with cervical spinal cord compression who have a normal clinical examination, abnormal EMG findings may be helpful in determining whether a decompression should be considered.
4. **Diagnostic injections:** In patients with cervical spinal stenosis and cord compression, injections are usually not helpful since these patients typically do not present with pain as a dominant symptom. Other symptoms such as numbness or tingling do not respond to injections. In patients with severe spinal cord compression, injections may actually be contraindicated.

c) **Cervical radiculopathy and neural foraminal stenosis:**

1. **Clinical presentation:** Patients suffering from cervical radiculopathy most commonly experience a sense of pain radiating from the neck or upper back region into one or both upper extremities. They may complain of pain, numbness, or paresthesias in the sensory distribution of the affected nerve root or roots (▶ Fig. 3.1). Of note, C7 nerve root compression can be associated with pain between the shoulder blades, with or without classic C8 dermatomal pattern pain. Patients may also note arm weakness or muscle atrophy. Typically, the symptoms are unilateral. Root tension signs are typically present. As a consequence, patients with cervical radiculopathy may be noted to place the hand of the affected extremity on top of their head: this reduces tension along the nerve and leads to symptom relief. Flexion typically relieves the pain while extension and/or tilting toward the side of the pain exacerbates it.
2. **Physical examination:**

i) **Neurologic examination:** Motor examination includes the visual inspection of muscle for atrophy or fasciculations, which occur in the setting of loss of neural connection between the anterior horn cells and the peripheral motor nerve. Muscle tone should be normal or decreased: if increased, suspicion for myelopathy arises, indicating spinal cord involvement either as an alternative or in addition to root pathology. Muscle strength is assessed with resistance testing of individual muscle groups to include the C5–T1 myotomes, which innervate the musculature of the upper extremities via the brachial plexus (▶ Fig. 3.2). Sensory examination may elicit hypesthesia, hyperesthesia, induced paresthesia, or a combination of sensory derangements in the affected dermatome. If sensory changes are diffuse or bilateral, this argues against radicular etiology. DTRs of the upper extremities should be decreased or absent, specifically the biceps tendon DTR for C5/C6 radiculopathy and the triceps tendon DTR for C7/C8 radiculopathy.

Compression of the C4 nerve at the C3/C4 level is a frequently overlooked diagnosis and can be associated with pain radiating into the tip of the shoulder. The C4 root may in part be assessed by examination of the rhomboid muscle group, which this root innervates along with C5, via the dorsal scapular nerve. Assessment of the cervical roots superior to C4 (i.e., superior to the brachial plexus) is generally based on

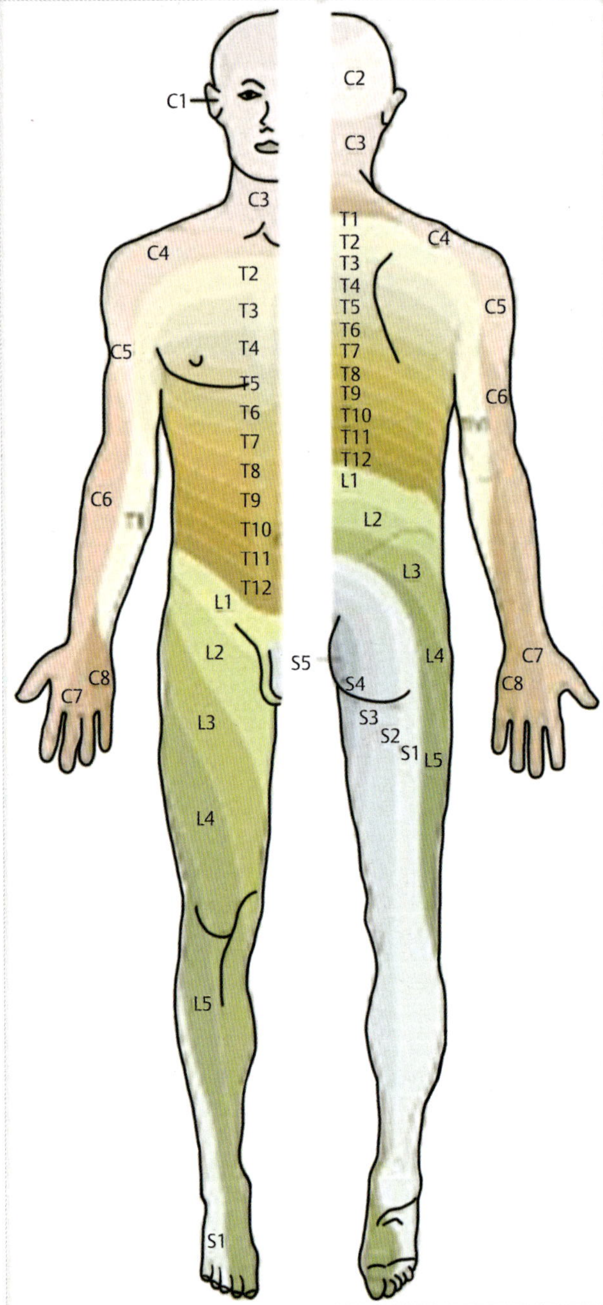

Fig. 3.1 Dermatomes. (Reproduced from Alignment Examination. In: Vialle L, Vialle L, ed. AOSpine Masters Series, Volume 8: Back Pain. 1st Edition. New York: Thieme; 2016.)

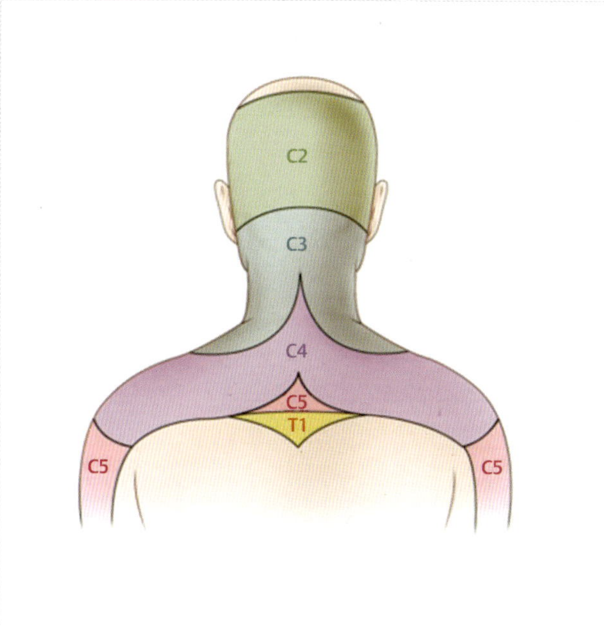

Fig. 3.2 Upper posterior dermatomal distribution of C2–T1. (Reproduced from Motor. In: Albert T, Vaccaro A, ed. Physical Examination of the Spine. 2nd Edition. New York: Thieme; 2016.)

symptoms. C2 and/or C3 radiculopathy often presents as posterior lateralized headache, which is actually radicular cephalgia along the dermatomal distribution.

3. **Electrodiagnostics:** NCS and needle EMG can be useful diagnostic tools in the localization and prognosis of radicular nerve injury. The goal of NCS/EMG for cervical radicular disease is to perform an electrophysiologic interrogation of the cervical nerve roots. Conventional NCS/EMG testing for cervical radiculopathy is easily performed in the outpatient setting and is generally well tolerated by patients. A typical study allows for the thorough assessment of C4–T1 nerve roots through the electrodiagnostic study of the upper extremities, shoulder girdle, and the cervical paraspinal musculature. It is important to note that needle EMG will be normal in patients with low grade compression injury to the nerve root, that is, a demyelinating injury with axonal sparing. Significant axonal dropout must occur prior to the development of electrophysiological evidence of denervation of muscles sharing the affected myotome. Thus, a normal EMG does not rule out radiculopathy. An abnormal study, however, can confirm it. Further, the degree of denervation occurring within a muscle can define the severity of neurological injury, and therefore generally speaking indicate the urgency for surgical intervention.
   The sensitivity of needle EMG is dependent on the timing of the study. Spontaneous electrical activity of muscle fibers in the form of positive sharp waves and/or fibrillation potentials begins to be observed 10 to 14 days after interference of axonal innervation to the motor end plates. This finding indicates axonal injury and resultant muscle fiber denervation. In the case of radiculopathy, this finding confirms significant neurological damage to the nerve root. A study performed prior to 14 days following injury may precede the development of this electrophysiologic finding, and therefore appear spuriously normal.
   Findings of denervation on needle EMG are concerning because by definition they confirm axonal injury. Prognostication for recovery of neurological function following injury to peripheral nerve is directly related to the degree of injury. An abnormal EMG, therefore, indicates an injury beyond neuropraxia and, hence, a risk of permanent neurological deficit. If little or no findings of reinnervation are observed by 12 weeks after onset of an axonal injury, this indicates a higher lever injury and is a poor prognostic sign. From the neurological perspective, the identification of axonal injury on the basis of denervation on needle EMG indicates risk of neurological deficit with incomplete recovery. Surgical decompression is indicated to protect neurological function in these cases, with the most favorable prognosis occurring with prompt surgical intervention. The rationale is that compression injury occurs over time, and if left alone, a low-level injury with prognosis for good recovery evolves into a higher level injury with increasingly poorer prognosis for recovery.
4. **Diagnostic injections:** Epidural steroid injections are useful for short-term relief from neuropathic symptoms. Diagnostic epidural injection using a local anesthetic alone or with steroid can be used to confirm that radicular pain is due to neural foraminal stenosis at a specific vertebral level. If the patient's symptoms are temporarily relieved with a targeted injection to the suspected clinically correlated level, this is considered a positive diagnostic test. For this purpose, interlaminar injections can be performed more easily; however, this technique may be less selective. Transforaminal epidural steroid injections with ultrasound or CT guidance can be performed, but caution should be taken to avoid intravascular injection that may be more difficult to see with fluoroscopic guidance.[2,3,4,5,6]

d) **Cervical facet joint arthropathy:**

1. **Clinical presentation:** The facet joints are true synovial joints. A patient with spinal arthritis will often find that periods of inactivity lead to stiffness and reduced spinal range of motion. Symptoms are typically prominent upon getting out of bed in the morning, or rising from a chair following prolonged sitting. Often times, these symptoms will dissipate following commencement of physical activity or by application of heat to the affected area, only to recur following the next period of inactivity.
   In addition, advanced arthropathy of the upper cervical spine may lead to cervicogenic headaches. Irritation of the C2/C3 roots may occur on the basis of neural foraminal stenosis through joint hypertrophy. These roots give rise to the greater and lesser occipital nerves which innervate the head (▶ Fig. 3.3).
2. **Physical examination:**
   i) **Neurologic examination:** In general, the neurologic examination should be normal in patients with facet mediated symptoms. Neuromuscular examination may reveal decreased cervical range of motion. Paraspinal muscle spasm may be present.

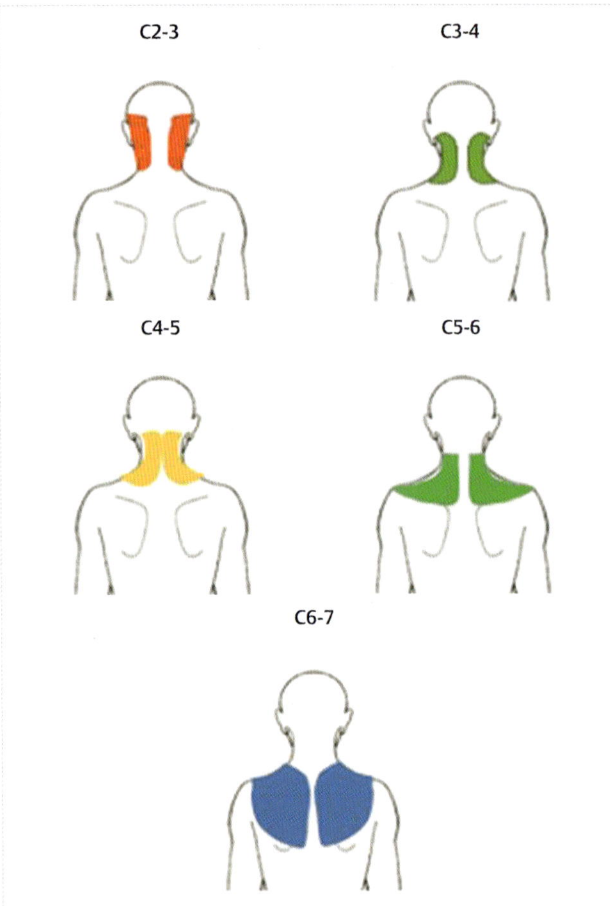

Fig. 3.3 Projection of facet-related pain. (Image used with permission from Dr. Jaspal Ricky Singh.)

ii) **Provocative maneuvers:** Facet loading is used to elicit pain in the affected joint. This maneuver is performed by having the patient rotate and extend the cervical spine toward the symptomatic side. Diminished range of motion, audible crepitus, or increased discomfort are suggestive of facet mediated symptoms. A similar maneuver is the Spurling's maneuver used for the workup of patients with suspected foraminal nerve root compression. However, in these patients radiating radicular pain is elucidated. In patients with facet joint pathology the pain will be more localized and not radiating.

3. **Electrodiagnostics**: Normal.
4. **Diagnostic injections**: Diagnostic facet joint blocks may be performed on the clinically suspected symptomatic level. It is important to note that over a third of diagnostic facet joint blocks yield false positive results. Therefore, repeated blocks with two distinct anesthetic agents are recommended to improve diagnostic value.[7,8,9]

e) **Myofascial neck pain or muscle generated pain**

1. **Clinical presentation:** Pain attributed to muscle and its surrounding fascia is termed myofascial pain. The quality of pain is usually described as a dull aching sensation, made worse with aggressive activity and prolonged positioning. Cervical myofascial pain is believed to result from overuse of or trauma to the muscles that support the shoulders and neck. It can also result from compensation for underlying spinal pathology, such as the conditions discussed above. In the cervical spine, the muscles most often implicated in myofascial pain are the trapezius, levator scapulae, rhomboids, and paraspinals (▶ Fig. 3.4). Chapter 5 covers muscular generated pain in detail.
2. **Physical examination**: The hallmark of myofascial pain is the presence of trigger points: discrete, focal, hyperirritable areas located in a taut band of skeletal muscle. Trigger points produce pain locally and in a referred pattern when palpated:
   i) **Neurologic examination**: Normal
   ii) **Provocative maneuvers**: Trigger point palpation should elicit the patient's index pain and referred pain patterns. On deep palpation, a muscle twitch response may be seen as well.
3. **Electrodiagnostics**: Normal.
4. **Diagnostic injections**: Injection for the treatment of symptomatic trigger points is both therapeutic and diagnostic. Trigger points are diagnosed by examining signs, symptoms, pain patterns, and manual palpation. Using a 25-gauge needle, the muscle is injected either with saline, local anesthetic, or steroid or a combination of the above. Ultrasound guidance can be used for muscle specificity and avoiding lung or nerve injury. Care should be taken to avoid infection, nerve injection, pneumothorax, and intrathecal injection.[10,11,12,13,14,15] Also refer to Chapter 5.

f) **Primary shoulder pathology**

1. **Clinical presentation:** Overuse injuries of the shoulder are common and can be due to issues involving soft tissue derangements such as rotator cuff tendinopathy, as well as arthropathy of the glenohumeral, sternoclavicular, or acromioclavicular joints. Patients with these conditions may report that pain localizes to the shoulder but may also have referred pain into the neck or upper arm, which can mimic radicular pain. Symptoms tend to be brought on by overhead activities such as reaching to a high shelf or washing one's hair.
2. **Physical examination:**
   i) **Neurologic examination:** Normal. However, pain may limit isolated muscle testing of shoulder girdle and/or rotator cuff musculature which may be confounding.
   ii) **Provocative maneuvers:** The two most commonly performed tests for shoulder impingement are the Neer test and the Hawkins test. In the Neer test, the examiner stabilizes the scapula while passively elevating the shoulder, in effect compressing the humeral head into the acromion.
   iii) In the Hawkins test, the examiner elevates the arm to 90 degrees of abduction and applies an internal rotation force, sandwiching the tendons of the rotator cuff under the acromion.
   iv) Both tests attempt to reduce the acromiohumeral interval to "impinge" the soft tissues in between these bony surfaces.
3. **Electrodiagnostics**: Normal.
4. **Diagnostic injections**: Diagnostic intra-articular shoulder injection can assist to rule in or rule out the shoulder joint as the underlying pain source. These can be performed with ultrasound or fluoroscopic guidance for precise placement.

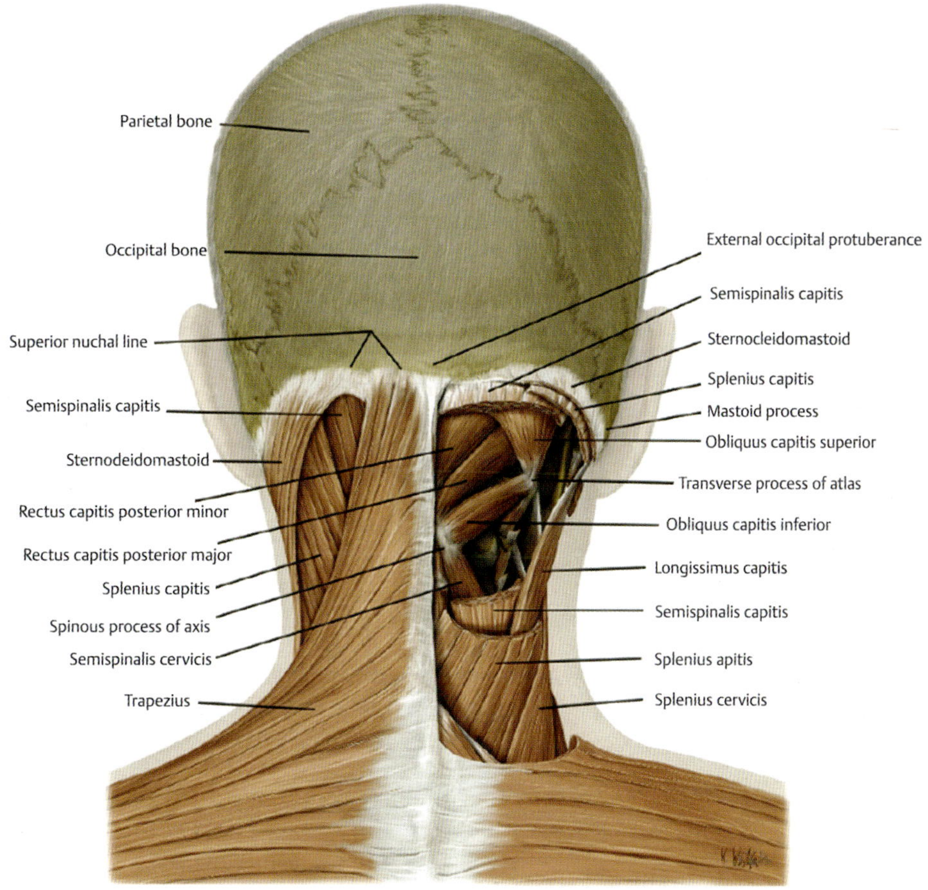

Fig. 3.4 Posterior cervical superficial and deep musculature. (Reproduced from Schuenke M, Schulte E, Schumacher U, eds. Thieme Atlas of Anatomy. General Anatomy and Musculoskeletal System. New York: Thieme; 2006. © Thieme, 2005. Illustration by Karl Wesker.)

Further injections can be considered for isolating the suprascapular nerve using ultrasound, to determine if entrapment is the cause of shoulder versus neck pain.[16,17,18]

g) **Brachial plexopathy:**

1. **Clinical presentation:** Brachial plexopathy may occur due to trauma, physiological compression (thoracic outlet syndrome, discussed in Section 3.3b), or due to an idiopathic inflammatory event (Parsonage-Turner syndrome). The typical manifestation of brachial plexopathy is pain, which can occur in the anterior neck region and clavicular region, and radiate distally along affected peripheral nerve courses (▶ Fig. 3.5). Sensory and motor deficits may be present as well, affecting the territory of the regional plexus involvement.
   The diagnosis of idiopathic brachial plexopathy, or Parsonage-Turner syndrome, is made on the basis of clinical history, radiographic exclusion of cervical root pathology, and confirmatory electrodiagnostic studies. The classic presentation consists of the development of severe unilateral pain of the neck and shoulder region, which lasts for several days, and then subsequently subsides. The pain is not mechanical, and thus cannot be alleviated by body movement or positioning. Classically, as the pain subsides, weakness develops, with varying degrees of associated sensory deficit.
2. **Physical examination:** Neurologic examination will identify motor and sensory deficits in a peripheral pattern, which localizes to the plexus as opposed to isolated peripheral nerve or dermatome/myotome pattern. If the upper plexus is involved, the biceps and brachioradialis DTRs will be decreased or absent. If the lower plexus is involved, the triceps DTR will be decreased or absent.
3. **Electrodiagnostics**: NCS/EMG will reveal abnormal sensory and motor NCS of affected plexus branches.
4. **Diagnostic injections:** A brachial plexus block of local anesthetic (at the interscalene groove, supraclavicular, or infraclavicular areas) can be considered. Ultrasound guidance or nerve stimulation is strongly suggested for accuracy, and steroid can be added for potentially therapeutic relief.[19] Imaging studies including a brachial plexus MRI can also be helpful.

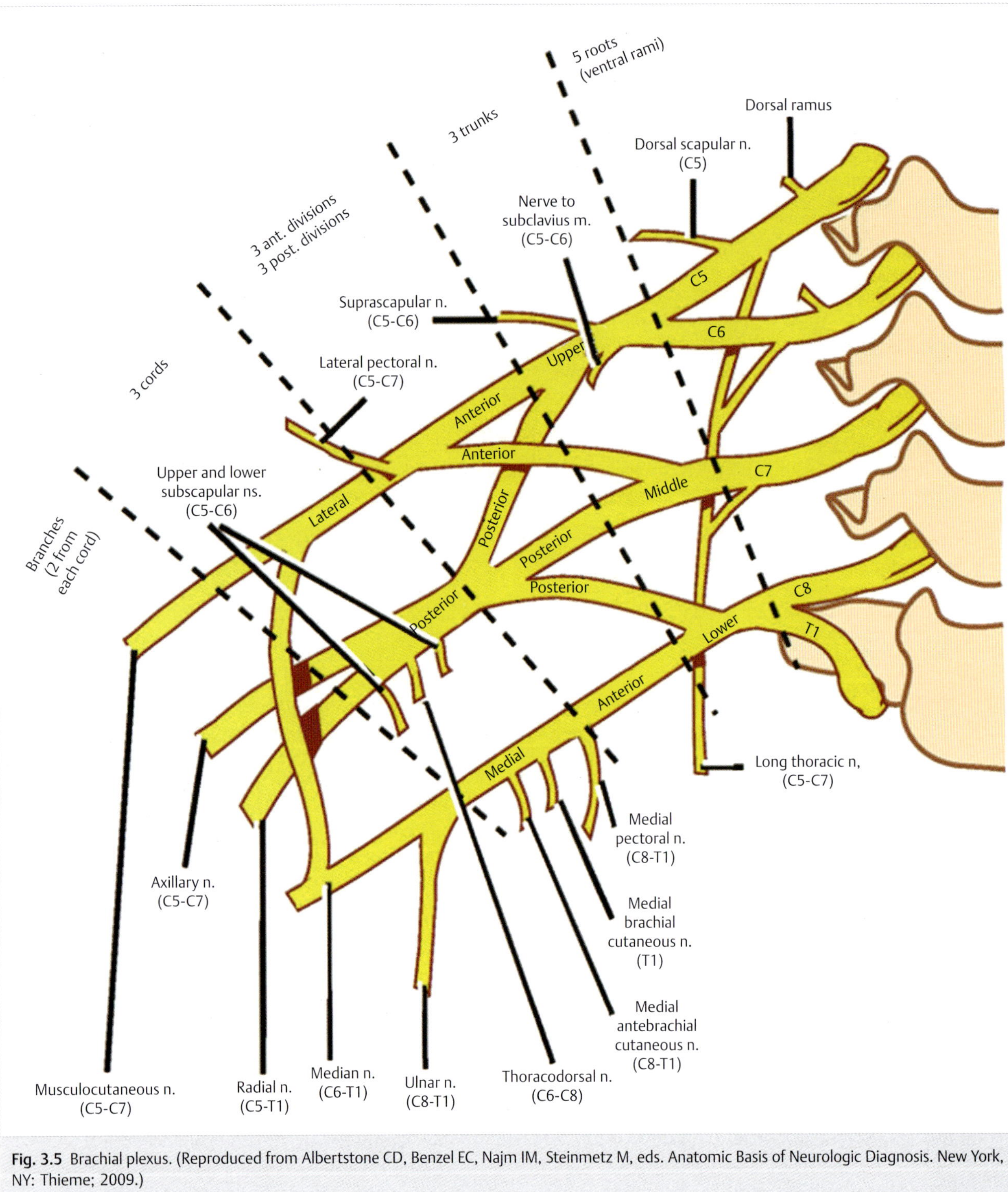

Fig. 3.5 Brachial plexus. (Reproduced from Albertstone CD, Benzel EC, Najm IM, Steinmetz M, eds. Anatomic Basis of Neurologic Diagnosis. New York, NY: Thieme; 2009.)

3.3 Thoracic Segment

a) **Thoracic radiculopathy and neural foraminal stenosis:**

1. **Clinical presentation:** Patients suffering from thoracic radiculopathy complain of pain, numbness, tingling, and/or paresthesias in the dermatomal distribution of the affected nerve root or roots, typically radiating from the axial back along the ribs ipsilateral to the stenosis. A thorough skin examination is especially important in this region to rule out acute herpes zoster reactivation, or shingles. Patients should also be asked about past episodes of shingles, as postherpetic neuralgia can be easily confused with a thoracic radiculopathy.

2. **Physical examination:**
   i) **Neurologic examination:** On neurological examination, sensory disturbances may be present in the affected thoracic dermatome. These may manifest as hypesthesia, paresthesias, or hyperesthesia. Because the nerve roots exiting the thoracic spine do not form plexuses, the motor branches of the thoracic spinal roots innervate segmental myotomes corresponding to the dermatomal pattern, supplying local intercostal and paraspinal muscles. Due to overlapping innervation of these territories, clinical weakness of the trunk musculature is seldom elicited. There are no DTR arcs involving the thoracic roots; thus, DTRs of the limbs are normal in thoracic radicular lesions.
   ii) **Provocative maneuvers:** No specific provocative maneuvers have been established for thoracic disc herniations.
3. **Electrodiagnostics:** Needle EMG of the thoracic paraspinal musculature can reveal findings of denervation due to radicular pathology. Although this finding would support thoracic radiculopathy, localization to a precise level cannot be confirmed due to overlapping myotomal innervation with the levels above and below a particular numbered vertebral segment.
4. **Diagnostic injections:** See cervical epidural injections for similar application to thoracic disc pathology (Section 3.2c, point 4).

b) **Thoracic outlet syndrome:**
1. **Clinical presentation:** Thoracic outlet syndrome (TOS) consists of a constellation of signs and symptoms, including paresthesias and aching pain in the neck, shoulder, and arm. The cause is thought to be compression of the brachial plexus and/or the subclavian artery and vein as they exit the space between the shoulder girdle and the first rib, or compression from congenitally abnormal structures such as cervical ribs. One or many of the structures may be compressed, thus giving the syndrome a varied clinical expression. TOS is seen most commonly in women between 25 and 50 years of age. Although the symptoms of TOS vary, compression or ischemia due to vascular compression of neural structures accounts for most cases.
2. **Physical examination:**
   i) **Neurologic examination:** The neurological examination is usually nonfocal in TOS; however, patchy mild deficits corresponding to brachial plexus dysfunction may be observed. Relative hyporeflexia of the DTRs of the affected limb may be present.
   ii) **Provocative maneuvers:** The symptoms of TOS may be elicited by various maneuvers, including the Adson test and the elevated arm stress test. The Adson test is carried out by palpating the radial pulse on the affected side with the patient's neck extended and the head turned toward the affected side. A diminished pulse suggests TOS. The elevated arm stress test, also called Roos test, is performed by having the patient hold his or her arms over the head while opening and closing the hands. Normally, patients without TOS can perform this maneuver for approximately 3 minutes prior to fatigue, whereas those suffering from TOS experience the onset of symptoms within 30 seconds.[20]
3. **Electrodiagnostics:** TOS due to a cervical rib generally results in compression of the lower trunks and division of the brachial plexus. Abnormal electrodiagnostic studies involving predominantly ulnar and radial nerves with sparing of axillary and musculocutaneous nerves is the most frequently observed pattern. TOS due to vascular or other causes may result in patchy abnormalities.
4. **Diagnostic injections:** Injections of local anesthetic with or without steroid to the regional musculature such as the scalene muscles have been performed but are nonspecific in the diagnosis. Ultrasound guidance is generally used for accuracy.[21,22]

3.4 Lumbar Segment

a) **Introduction:** The lumbar spine is the base of support for the upper back and limbs, and any loads that they carry. The lumbar spine serves to transmit these loads to the pelvis and lower limbs.[23] A moderate amount of range of motion is permitted in flexion/extension, lateral bending, and rotation planes. There are several anatomical zones and levels that guide surgeons in devising a targeted treatment plan for spinal pathologies (▶ Fig. 3.6 and ▶ Fig. 3.7).

b) **Lumbar central canal stenosis:**
1. **Clinical presentation:** Neurogenic claudication is the sine qua non of lumbar central canal stenosis and manifests in a characteristic manner as pain and weakness in the legs while walking that disappears with lumbar spine flexion or by assuming a seated position. In addition, patients with lumbar spinal stenosis may experience lower extremity numbness and paresthesias in the distribution of the affected nerve roots. It can also present as painless fatigue when walking.
   The causes of spinal stenosis include bulging or herniated discs, facet arthropathy, and thickening of the epidural fat or ligamentum flavum, which encroach upon the spinal canal. Lumbar extension increases this crowding while flexion reduces it. On the basis of these mechanics, some stenotic individuals find walking downhill particularly uncomfortable, while bicycling may be no problem. This may be a useful discriminator between neurogenic claudication versus intermittent claudication due to peripheral vascular disease. The factors that incite central lumbar canal stenosis tend to worsen with age. Therefore, central canal stenosis is rarely seen in patients younger than 60 years of age.[26]
   In cases of severe neurological compression due to central lumbar canal stenosis, disturbance of bladder and/or bowel function may ensue as part of the clinical cauda equina syndrome, which is a surgical emergency.
2. **Physical examination:**
   i) **Neurologic examination:** The neurologic examination of the lower extremities varies dependent on the severity of compression, and the level of compression. In mildly symptomatic patients, the examination may be normal; however, at least subtle abnormalities such as hypoactive lower extremity DTRs are present in most individuals.

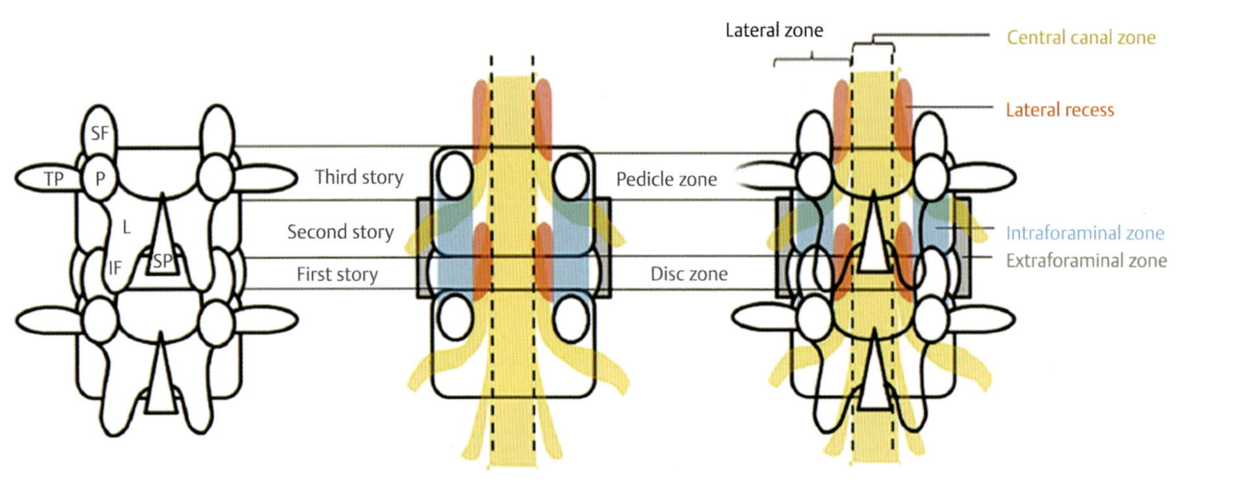

Fig. 3.6 This diagram summarizes the potential zones and levels (stories) of disc fragments and other spinal pathologies based on anatomical boundaries familiar to surgeons. (Based on Wiltse et al's work.[24])

If compression occurs below the conus medullaris, any or all of the roots of the cauda equina may be involved to varying extents, resulting in patchy bilateral sensory and motor deficits in the legs, with decreased patellar and Achilles DTRs.

If compression occurs involving the conus medullaris, hyperreflexia and increased tone may occur.

Bowel and bladder function should always be considered.

ii) **Provocative maneuvers:** Patients often have a positive stoop test: when walking, the patient stoops forward, gradually reduces walking speed, and sometimes will stoop forward until he or she finally stops.[27]

3. **Electrodiagnostics:**
   An unfortunate limitation of electrodiagnostics in the study of lumbar stenosis occurs due to the fact that the nerves in the cauda equina are peripheralized in histology, despite their intrathecal location. Central canal stenosis resulting in cauda equina compression will generally manifest on NCS/EMG as polyradiculopathy, which by definition, is what it is. An electrophysiologically abnormal L5 nerve root, for example, will result in the same NCS/EMG findings whether the site of compression is within the neural foramen or in the central canal. In this case, NCS/EMG is therefore useful to rule out additional or alternative etiologies for pain and weakness, but is limited in localizing foraminal versus central canal compression.
4. **Diagnostic injections:** Epidural steroid injections are useful for short-term relief of neuropathic symptoms. Diagnostic epidural injection using a local anesthetic with steroid alone can be used to confirm radicular pain, since it generates from a specific spinal level. If the patient's symptoms are temporarily relieved with localized injection, the local origin of radicular pain is confirmed (also see Section 3.2b, point 4).
   Understanding the anatomy and the different potential nerve compression sites in the lumbar spine and correlating them with the patient's symptoms and imaging findings are key in designing a successful minimally invasive procedure. Clinical examination, electrophysiology, and provocative testing as discussed in this chapter can be crucial in identifying the correct surgical "target."

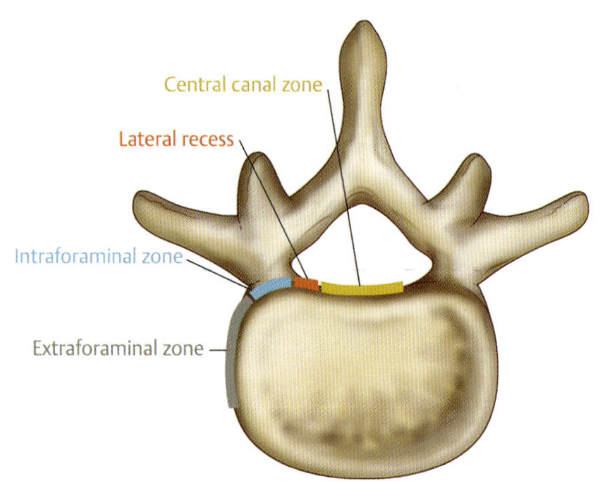

Fig. 3.7 Diagram representing the anatomic zone based on axial imaging.[24] Understanding the exact location of the pathology guides the surgeon in devising a targeted treatment plan. For example, the editors recommend treating a lumbar disc herniation via tubular surgery with the following access strategies[25]: Central canal—ipsilateral approach; lateral recess—ipsilateral approach at L4/5/S1, consider contralateral approach higher up in order to protect the pars; foraminal zone—contralateral over the top approach or far-lateral approach, depending on how medial/lateral the disc is located; extraforaminal zone—far-lateral approach.

c) **Lateral recess stenosis:**
1. **Clinical presentation:** The lumbar spinal nerve roots lie in the lateral recess and extend to the medial border of the superior articular facet at the lower portion of the vertebral foramen of the level above.[28] Diagnosis of lateral recess stenosis and the determination of the specific nerve root or roots involved can be challenging, owing to the intermediate location of the lateral recess between the

central canal and the neural foramen. Patients may present with variable symptoms of neurogenic claudication to focal radiculopathy based on the degree and region of the lateral recess affected. Because of this, no common presenting symptom is specific to lateral recess stenosis. However, the radicular pain from lateral recess stenosis will be different from the pain caused by foraminal or extraforaminal dorsal root ganglion (DRG) compression—sharp and shooting versus burning and dysesthetic.

2. **Physical examination:**
   i) **Neurologic examination:** The detailed motor examination should be performed. Sensory examination may elicit hypesthesia, hyperesthesia, induced paresthesia, or a combination of sensory derangements in the affected dermatome. DTRs of the lower extremities may be decreased or absent, specifically the patellar DTR in L4 radiculopathy and the Achilles DTR in S1 radiculopathy.
   ii) **Provocative maneuvers:** No specific provocative maneuvers exist for lateral recess stenosis.
3. **Electrodiagnostics:** A typical NCS/EMG study performed for the evaluation of lumbar radiculopathy includes NCS of the lower extremities, and needle EMG of select lower limb, hip, and lumbar paraspinal muscles so as to include evaluation of L1–S1 myotomes. NCS will reveal prolonged peroneal late responses in L5 radiculopathy, and prolonged tibial late responses in S1 radiculopathy.
   The same principles of timing and analysis apply as discussed in Section 3.2c, point 3.
4. **Diagnostic injections:** Epidural injections as described in Section 3.2b, point 4, apply here, but can be more targeted for laterality. However, in differentiating lateral recess from other causes of stenosis, placement of the needle in the lateral recess may aid in diagnosis, but is limited by unpredictable spread of the injectate.

d) **Central/posterolateral disc herniation**

1. **Clinical presentation:** Radicular shooting, sciatica-type pain from compression of the traversing nerve root. Straight leg sign will be positive. Weakness and sensory deficits in a dermatomal distribution. Note that while posterolateral disc herniation is the most common reason for radicular shooting pain, there are multiple compression sites that can cause similar pain distribution, especially in the case of L5 pain (▶ Fig. 3.8).
2. **Physical examination:**
   i) **Neurologic examination:** The detailed motor examination should be performed. Sensory examination may elicit hypesthesia, hyperesthesia, induced paresthesia, or a combination of sensory derangements in the affected dermatome. DTRs of the lower extremities may be decreased or absent, specifically the patellar DTR in L4 radiculopathy and the Achilles DTR in S1 radiculopathy.
   ii) **Provocative maneuvers:** Straight leg sign or slump sit test
3. **Electrodiagnostics:** A typical NCS/EMG study performed for the evaluation of lumbar radiculopathy includes NCS of the lower extremities, and needle EMG of select lower limb, hip, and lumbar paraspinal muscles so as to include evaluation of L1–S1 myotomes. NCS will reveal prolonged peroneal late responses in L5 radiculopathy, and

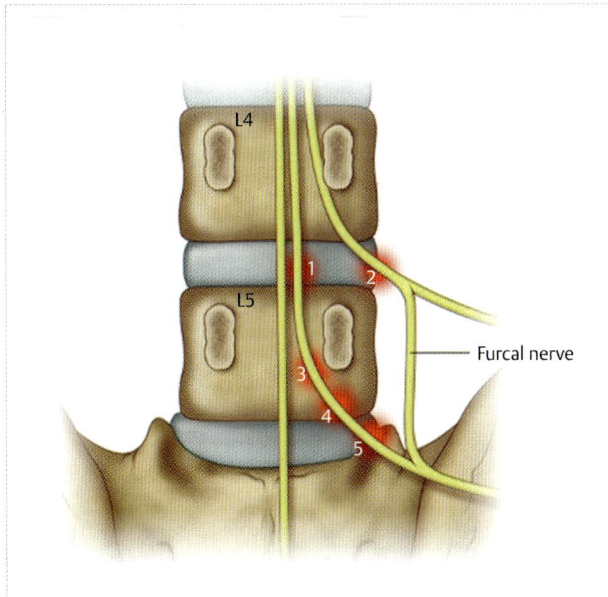

Fig. 3.8 Diagram demonstrating the five points of nerve compression of the L5 nerve that can result in L5 radiculopathy: (1) Posterolateral disc herniation, L4/5 compressing the L5 nerve; (2) foraminal disc L4/5 compressing the furcal nerve.[29] The furcal nerve is an independent nerve in the L4 foramen that links up to the L5 nerve. (3) Disc medial to L5 pedicle; (4) foraminal disc L5/S1; (5) extraforaminal disc L5/S1. (4) and (5) can result in compression of the dorsal root ganglion (DRG) which can be associated with burning pain and sensory dysesthesia. This diagram was modified from Chapter 26 in Young and McCullough.[30]

   prolonged tibial late responses in S1 radiculopathy.
   The same principles of timing and analysis apply as discussed in Section 3.2c, point 3.
4. **Diagnostic injections:** Epidural injections as described in Section 3.2b, point 4, apply here, but can be more targeted for laterality.

e) **Lumbar neural foraminal or extraforaminal stenosis:**

1. **Clinical presentation:** Patients suffering from foraminal or extraforaminal bony stenosis most commonly experience pain and dysesthesias of a single dermatome, radiating from the back or buttock region into one of the lower extremities. Similarly, weakness is typically seen involving a specific myotome. Symptoms are usually unilateral, but bilateral foraminal narrowing can be seen in the setting of spondylolisthesis or diffuse lumbar disc bulging. The pain is frequently characterized by a burning and on fire type character associated with sensory dysesthesia from compression of sensory DRG.
2. **Physical examination:**
   i) **Neurologic examination:** Muscle strength is assessed with resistance testing of individual muscle groups to include the L1–S1 myotomes. Sensory examination may elicit hypesthesia, hyperesthesia, induced paresthesia, or a combination of sensory derangements in the affected dermatome. DTRs of the lower extremities may be decreased or absent, specifically the patellar DTR in L4 radiculopathy and the Achilles DTR in S1 radiculopathy.

ii) **Provocative maneuvers:** The lumbar foraminal compression test or modified Kemp's test is the corollary for lumbar foraminal stenosis as the Spurling's maneuver is to cervical foraminal stenosis. The patient's arms are on the side of the body or on the hips. The examiner places the lumbar spine in hyperextension, along with combined ipsilateral lateral flexion and rotation to end range toward the symptomatic side, sustained for up to 30 seconds. Similar to the Spurling's maneuver, a positive test should recreate the patient's index radicular symptoms. A reproduction of nonradicular paraspinal back pain would indicate facet joint pathology.

3. **Electrodiagnostics:** NCS/EMG is useful in the evaluation of neurological injury due to lumbar disease for a number of reasons. First, NCS/EMG can confirm the diagnosis of radicular injury, localize the affected lumbar root or roots, and assess the severity of injury. Equally important, NCS/EMG can identify alternative distal nerve pathology, such as generalized sensorimotor polyneuropathy, focal neuropathies, and other disorders such as motor neuron disease or primary myopathy. Any of these pathological processes, for example, can result in a foot drop.
A typical NCS/EMG study performed for the evaluation of lumbar radiculopathy includes NCS of the lower extremities, and needle EMG of selected lower limb, hip, and lumbar paraspinal muscles so as to include evaluation of L1–S1 myotomes. The same principles of timing and analysis apply as discussed in Section 3.2c.
4. **Diagnostic injections:** Transforaminal epidural injections, with or without steroids, can be useful for short-term relief from neuropathic symptoms. Whether symptoms are related to mechanical compression of the nerve or to an inflammatory radiculitis, the injection can be used to confirm that radicular pain is due to neural foraminal stenosis at a specific vertebral level. If the patient's symptoms are temporarily relieved with a targeted injection to the suspected clinically correlated level, this is considered a positive diagnostic test.

f) **Lumbar facet joint arthropathy:**

1. **Clinical presentation:** Lumbar facet joint osteoarthritis leads to localized unilateral or bilateral lumbar region pain, which may radiate to the buttocks, groin, and thighs. Symptoms are generally worse in the morning after arising from bed, and during periods of inactivity. An associated sense of stiffness is generally present. The discomfort may improve with activity or the application of heat.[31]
2. **Physical examination:**
   i) **Neurologic examination:** Normal. Neuromuscular examination may reveal decreased lumbar range of motion, or palpable paraspinal muscle spasm.
   ii) **Provocative maneuvers:** Kemp's test, also called facet loading, requires the patient to perform extension combined with rotation of the spinal region of interest, with a positive test defined as a reproduction of the patient's axial back pain (▶ Fig. 3.9). If radicular symptoms are elicited, foraminal stenosis should be considered instead.
3. **Electrodiagnostics**: Normal.
4. **Diagnostic injections**: Diagnostic facet joint blocks may be performed on the clinically suspected symptomatic level. It is important to note that over a third of diagnostic facet joint blocks yield false positive results. Therefore, repeated blocks with two distinct local anesthetic agents are recommended to improve diagnostic value.[7,8,9]

g) **Sacroiliac joint pain:**

1. **Clinical presentation:** The sacroiliac joint (SIJ) is a diarthrodial joint encapsulated by strong fibrous ligaments. SIJ innervation is typically supplied by the sensory nerves of S1–S3 with additional L4 and L5 contribution in some individuals. SIJ arthropathy has been identified as the pain generator in up to 30% of all presenting low back pain.
Patients often present with unilateral, medial buttock discomfort and pain in sacral sulcus. The distinguishing feature of SIJ pain is lack of pain superior to the L5/S1 level. Pain may be referred to the hip or groin. Muscle imbalance may occur, leading to weakness of the gluteus medius muscle with reactive tightening of the piriformis and quadratus lumborum muscles. Given the distribution of symptoms, discogenic, facetogenic, and myofascial pain generators must be ruled out. Bilateral SIJ pathology may be indicative of a primary inflammatory arthropathy, such as ankylosing spondylitis.
2. **Physical examination**:
   i) **Neurologic examination:** Normal. Nerve root tension signs should be absent.
   ii) **Provocative maneuvers:** Patrick's test: One of the most commonly used provocative maneuvers for diagnostic SIJ pain. It is also called the **FABER** maneuver after the acronym for the passive positioning of the ipsilateral hip in **F**lexion, **AB**duction, and **E**xternal **R**otation. With the patient lying supine, the ankle of the affected extremity is placed on the contralateral knee to create a figure-4 position. The examiner places his or her hand along the medial aspect of the knee of the tested extremity and applies downward pressure toward the examination table, while simultaneously providing counterpressure with the other hand on the contralateral anterior superior iliac spine (ASIS). A positive test reproduces back or buttock pain, whereas groin pain is more indicative of hip joint pathology.
   Gaenslen's test: With the patient supine, the hip is maximally flexed on the affected side, and the opposite hip is extended. This may require the patient to hang the extended leg off the examination table. A positive test reproduces ipsilateral buttock or SIJ pain on the side where the hip is flexed.
   Fortin's finger test is a simple and reliable diagnostic aid. The patient points to the area of pain with one finger (▶ Fig. 3.10). The result is positive if the site is within 1 cm of the posterior superior iliac spine.[32] Palpation in that area reproduces the typical pain.
3. **Electrodiagnostics**: Normal.
4. **Diagnostic injections**: Other than inflammatory sacroiliitis, SIJ dysfunction is extremely difficult to identify on imaging. Therefore, SIJ diagnostic block is a method to distinguish SIJ mediated symptoms from other potential pain generators in the surrounding region. SIJ block can be performed under fluoroscopy or ultrasound guidance in an

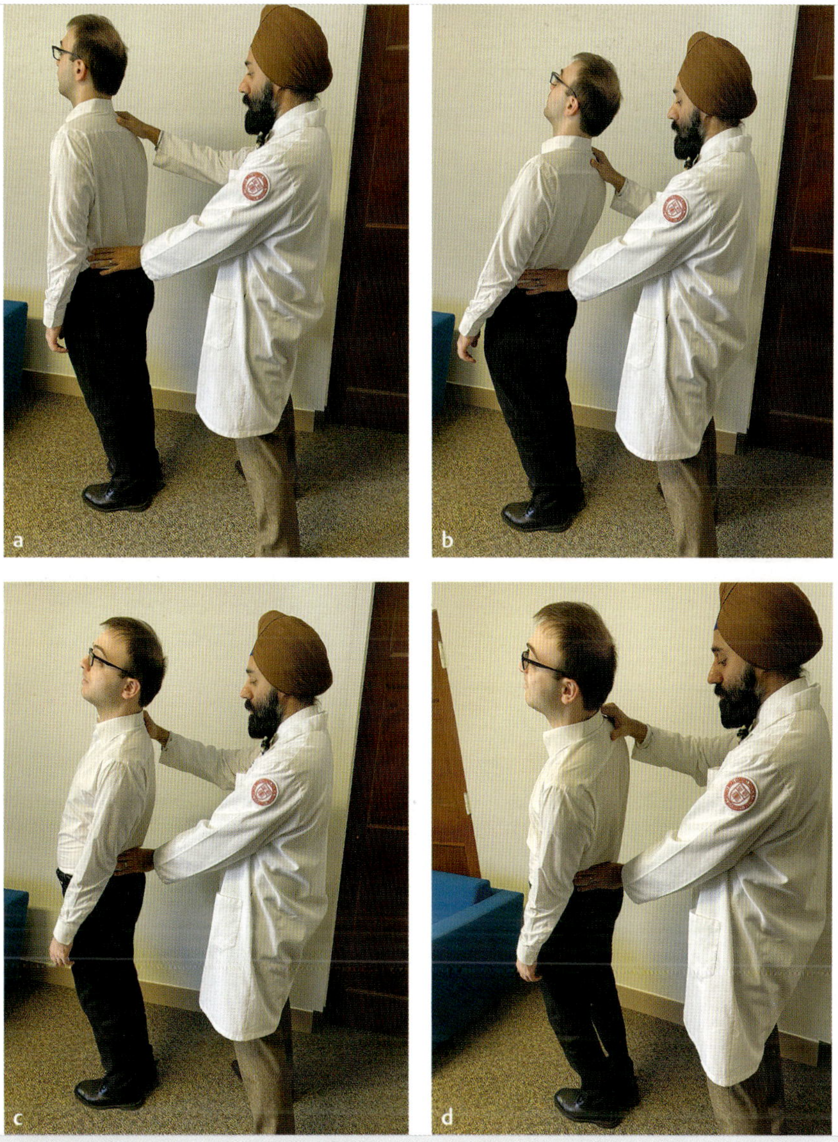

Fig. 3.9 The purpose of the Kemp's test and modified Kemp's test is to assess the lumbar spine facet joints and the neural foramen, respectively. Kemp's test uses the patient's trunk both as a lever to induce tension and as a compressive force. This is a provocation test to detect pain. Local pain suggests a facet cause, while radiating pain into the leg is more suggestive of nerve root irritation in the foramen, especially if the pain is below the knee. **(a)** Neutral standing position, **(b)** the examiner places the lumbar spine in hyperextension, **(c)** the examiner places the lumbar spine in ipsilateral lateral flexion, **(d)** the examiner rotates the lumbar spine to end range toward the symptomatic side, sustained for up to 30 seconds.

outpatient setting. The standard method is the inferior approach. However, due to SIJ fusion or osteoarthritic changes, a superior approach may be useful. In a systematic review consisting 11 diagnostic accuracy and 14 therapeutic studies, Simopoulos and colleagues found levels II and III evidence supporting a series of two injections that resulted in 70% pain relief in each or 75% pain improvement after a single block respectively as the procedure standard. Intra- and periarticular SIJ injections have shown to be equally efficacious.[33,34]

h) **Piriformis syndrome:**

1. **Clinical presentation:** Piriformis syndrome is an entrapment neuropathy caused by compression of the sciatic nerve by the piriformis muscle as it passes through the sciatic notch. Patients will present with pain, numbness, paresthesias, and weakness in the distribution of the sciatic nerve.
Variant anatomy of the piriformis exists. In one variation, the fibular branch of the sciatic nerve passes through the belly of the piriformis muscle, placing these nerve fibers at greater risk of being entrapped with piriformis activation. This variant is thought to be seen in approximately 9% of individuals.[35]
2. **Physical examination:**
   i) **Neurologic examination:** The motor and sensory changes of piriformis syndrome may reveal sensory and/or motor deficits limited to the distribution of the sciatic nerve below the sciatic notch.
   ii) **Provocative maneuvers:** The corollary of the FABER test for SIJ pain is the **FADIR** test for piriformis pain. In this maneuver, the examiner attempts to stretch the piriformis muscle taut to aggravate sciatic nerve

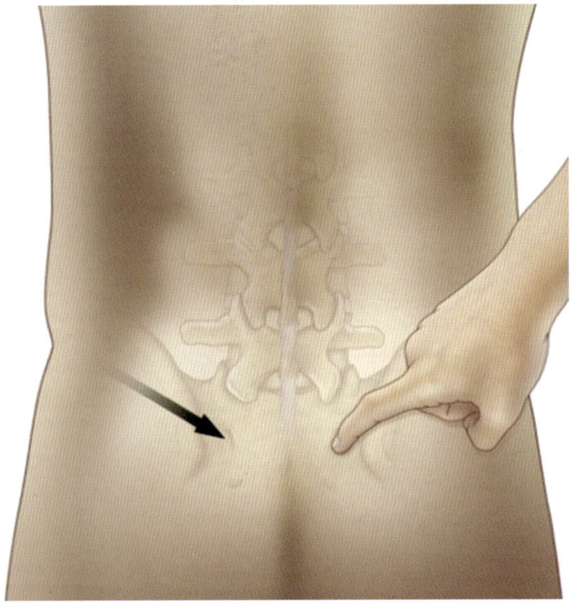

Fig. 3.10 Fortin's finger test.

entrapment. To accomplish this, the examiner passively ranges the hip of the symptomatic side of the supine patient in **F**lexion, **AD**duction, and **I**nternal **R**otation. This distracts the attachment sites of the piriformis, the sacrum, and the greater trochanter.

3. **Electrodiagnostics:** NCS/EMG of the lower extremities may reveal findings of sciatic neuropathy. Electrodiagnostic abnormalities may be subtle. A delayed H-reflex response on the affected side is perhaps the most sensitive finding. The yield for this may be increased by performing the study with the leg in an abducted, flexed, and internally rotated position, which induces increased pressure from the piriformis muscle onto the sciatic nerve.[36]
4. **Diagnostic injections:** Injection of local anesthetic in the region of the sciatic nerve and piriformis muscle at this level serves as a diagnosis. Steroid can be added for possible therapeutic benefit. Fluoroscopic guidance with nerve stimulator technique has been used, but more commonly ultrasound localization of the muscle is more acceptable.[37]

i) **Hip osteoarthritis:**

1. **Clinical presentation:** Hip osteoarthritis (OA) is extremely common. A population-based study from the US showed an incidence rate of 0.5 per 1,000 cases per year.[38] Patients present with aching pain and stiffness usually felt deep in the anterior groin but may refer to the anteromedial or lateral thigh and occasionally the buttocks. This can mimic an L2, L3, or L4 lumbar radiculopathy. Pain is exacerbated particularly by rising from a seated position and during the initial phases of ambulation.[39] Morning stiffness is a hallmark of hip OA, much like facet joint arthropathy.
2. **Physical examination:**
   i) **Neurologic examination:** Normal. However pain may limit hip flexion and abduction strength.
   ii) **Provocative maneuvers:** Passive range of motion testing looks for pain emanating from the hip joint as the femoroacetabular ball-and-socket joint is activated. To test internal and external rotation, the examiner flexes both hip and knee at 90 degrees, then rotating back and forth, both internally and externally. Pain is often elicited at the end ranges, particular on internal rotation.
3. **Electrodiagnostics**: Normal.
4. **Diagnostic injections**: Diagnostic intra-articular hip injection can assist to rule in or rule out the hip joint as the underlying pain source. The hip injection may be performed under either fluoroscopy or ultrasound guidance to help reduce accidental needle injury. Injection of local anesthetic alone can be used for diagnostic purposes, but steroid is often added for therapeutic benefit.

j) **Myofascial back pain or muscle generated pain**:

1. **Clinical presentation:** As previously described in Section 3.2e, pain attributed to muscle and its surrounding fascia is termed myofascial pain. The quality of pain is usually described as a dull aching sensation, made worse with aggressive activity and prolonged positioning. Lumbar myofascial pain is believed to result from overuse of or trauma to the muscles that support posture. It can also result from compensation for underlying spinal pathology, such as the conditions discussed above.
   An alternative diagnostic approach to myofascial pain was described by Marcus et al.[10] Instead of locating trigger points, muscle pain amenable to injection (MPAI) was identified using a hand-held muscle pain detection device (MPDD). MPDD establishes the pathological muscle–tendon junction and muscle belly by provoking a targeted contraction in the painful area that in turn stimulates the pain generating nociceptors in the sore muscle. Unlike trigger point injections, MPAI diagnostic/therapeutic approach includes mechanical stimulation with the needle tip and injection to the entheses and along the entire tissue where the sensitized nociceptors are found. This approach was shown to be effective in identifying and treating back pain that was once thought to be caused by structural pathology in the spine, needing surgical intervention, as well as post-laminectomy syndrome (see Chapter 5).

3.5 Conclusion

The human spine is unique in its longitudinal orientation, and structural adaptations have evolved for the management of axial loading and the mechanical stresses of a longitudinal plane of gravity. It is critical to note that not all radiographic evidence of "wear and tear" is necessarily pathological or problematic. The development of pain and/or neurological deficits may be based on a small focus of injury among a field of nonsymptomatic radiographic abnormalities. The accurate identification of these foci allows MISS to be precisely targeted and extremely effective in appropriately selected patients (▶ Table 3.1).

Table 3.1 Correlation of pain symptoms, clinical examination, and anatomical localization of pathology in degenerative spinal disorders

Most commonly used descriptive term	Symptoms	Examination	Imaging findings
Neurogenic claudication	Intermittent unilateral or bilateral leg and buttock pain worse with standing and walking, relieved with sitting or leaning forward	Positive stoop test	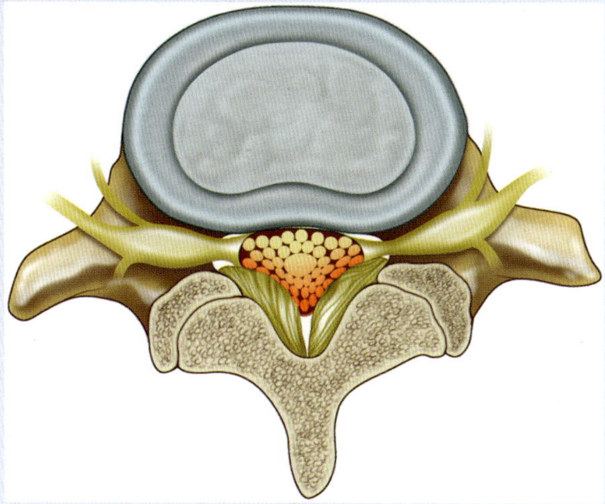
Radicular pain—posterolateral disc herniation	Sciatica, myotomal/dermatomal pain Sharp, electric shock Starts proximal and radiates distal Not affected by palpation Sitting worse than standing	Positive straight leg sign Positive slump sit test	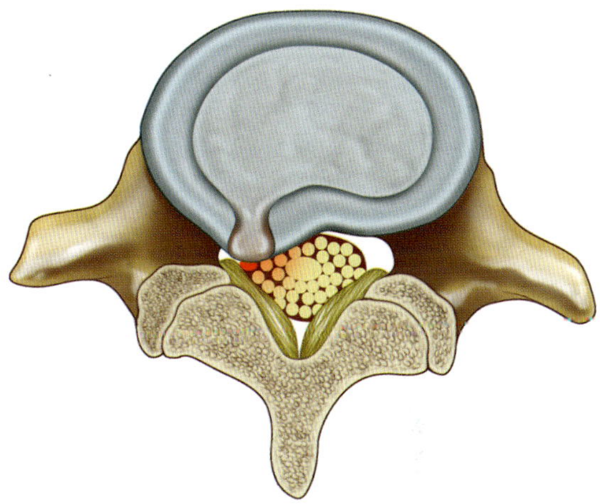

(Continued)

Table 3.1 *(Continued)* Correlation of pain symptoms, clinical examination, and anatomical localization of pathology in degenerative spinal disorders

Most commonly used descriptive term	Symptoms	Examination	Imaging findings
Radicular pain—lateral recess stenosis	Sciatica, myotomal/dermatomal pain Sharp, electric shock Starts proximal and radiates distal Not affected by palpation	Positive straight leg sign Positive slump sit test	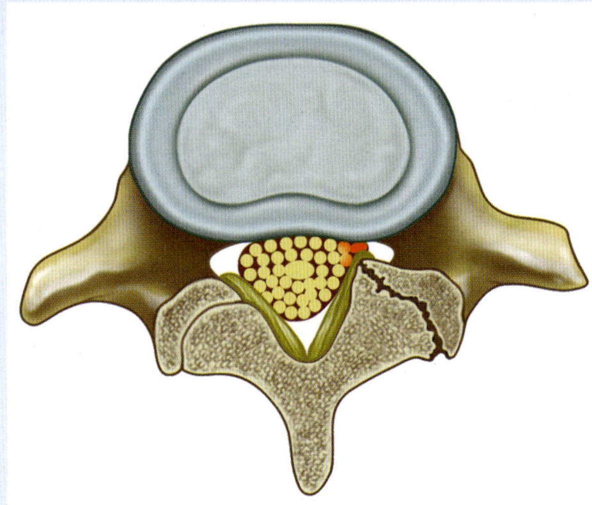
Radicular pain Foraminal/extraforaminal soft disc	Leg pain, burning, on fire, sensory dysesthesia from compression of sensory DRG	Positive straight leg sign Positive slump sit test Positive Kemp's loading test—reproduces radicular pain in cervical spine: Positive Spurling's sign	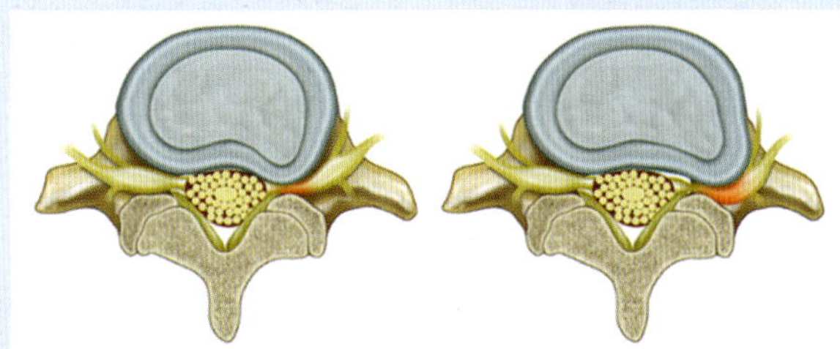 Foraminal (*left*), extraforaminal (*right*)
Radicular pain—foraminal bony compression ("vertical compression")	Sciatica, myotomal/dermatomal pain Standing and walking worse	Positive Kemp's loading test—reproduces radicular pain	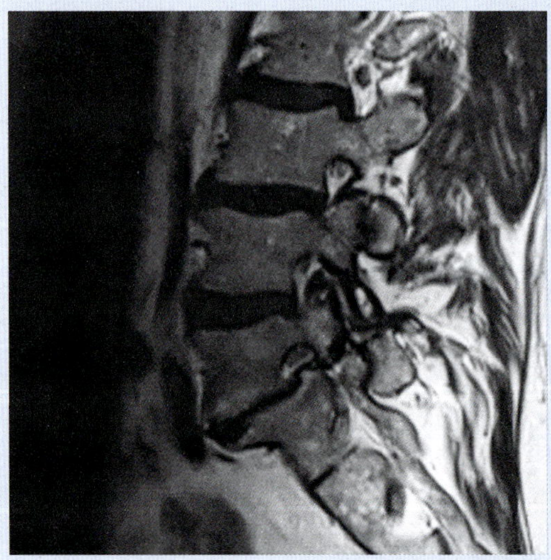

(Continued)

Table 3.1 *(Continued)* Correlation of pain symptoms, clinical examination, and anatomical localization of pathology in degenerative spinal disorders

Most commonly used descriptive term	Symptoms	Examination	Imaging findings
Mechanical low-back pain	Deep and agonizing nonradicular pain that is worsened by spinal loading (i.e., standing, walking, lifting); improved by spinal unloading (i.e., sitting, lying in bed) Worse later in day		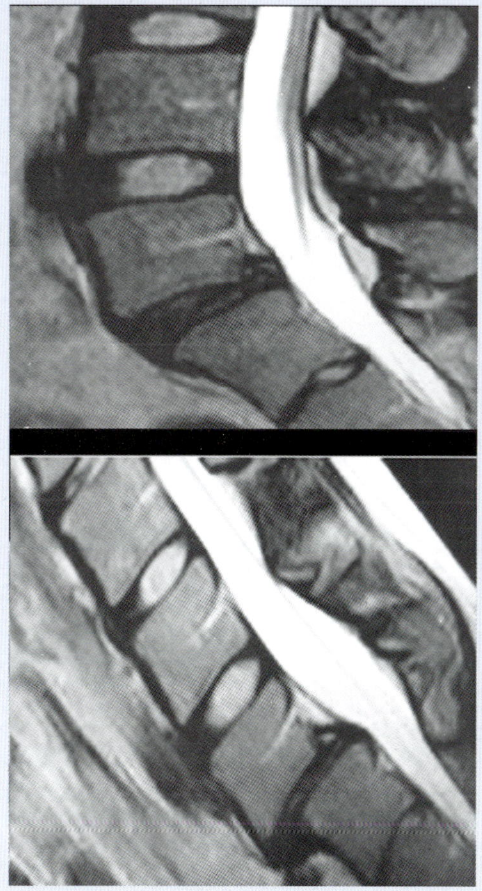 L5/S1 instability on dynamic MRI Extension (*top*), flexion (*bottom*)
Facet joint pain	Extension pain	Positive Kemp's loading test—reproduces nonradicular back pain	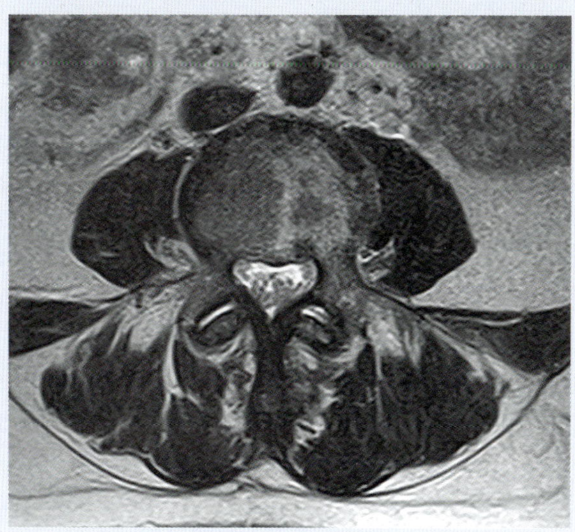

(Continued)

Table 3.1 *(Continued)* Correlation of pain symptoms, clinical examination, and anatomical localization of pathology in degenerative spinal disorders

Most commonly used descriptive term	Symptoms	Examination	Imaging findings
Discogenic pain	Similar to mechanical back pain Nonradicular	Discogram	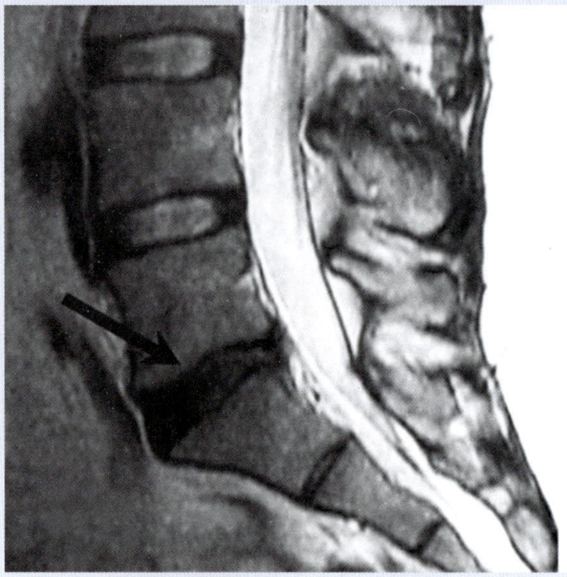
Myogenic/Muscle generated pain (MGP)	Dull aching sensation, made worse with aggressive activity and prolonged positioning	Palpation, also see Chapter 5	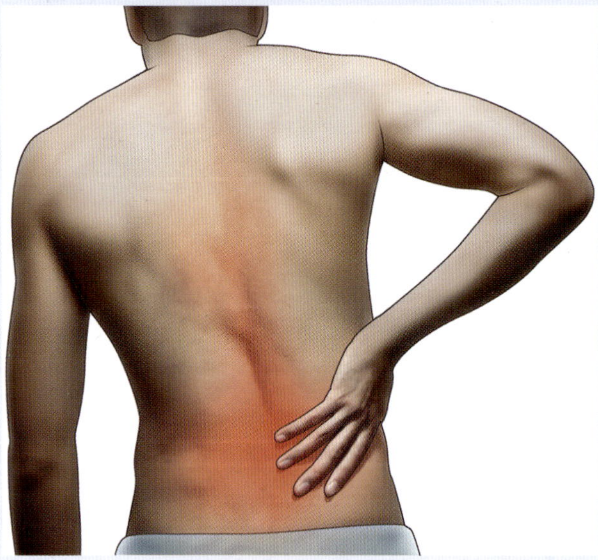 Imaging is normal

(Continued)

Table 3.1 *(Continued)* Correlation of pain symptoms, clinical examination, and anatomical localization of pathology in degenerative spinal disorders

Most commonly used descriptive term	Symptoms	Examination	Imaging findings
SIJ pain	Localized pain and tenderness over SIJ	Fortin's finger test	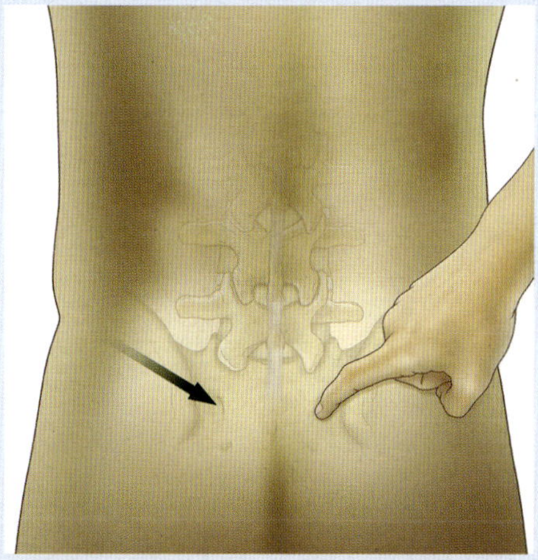
Trochanter bursa and IT band	Tenderness to palpation over the lateral hip, greater trochanter, and down the IT band	Positive Ober's test	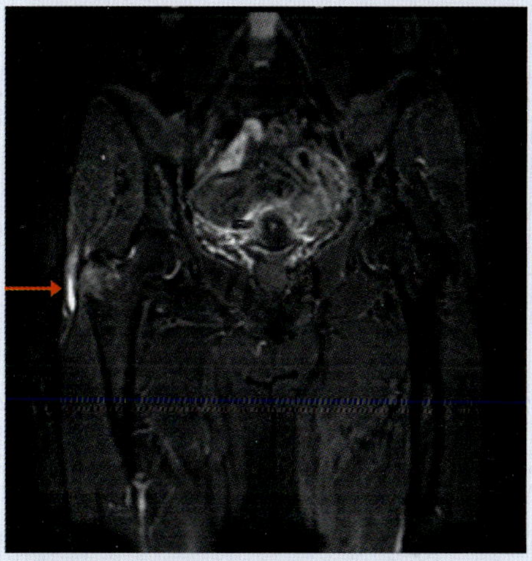 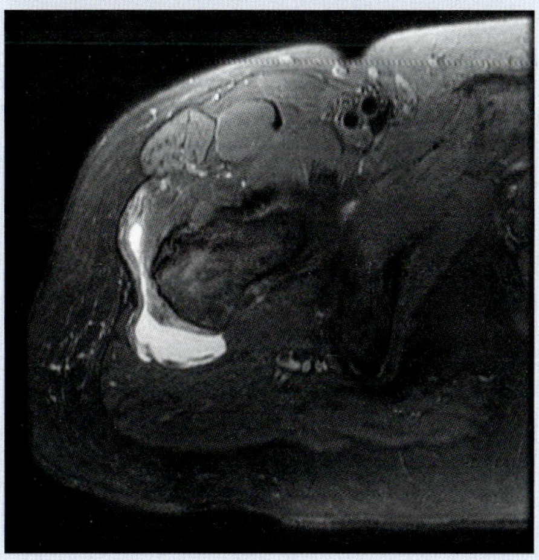

(Continued)

Table 3.1 *(Continued)* Correlation of pain symptoms, clinical examination, and anatomical localization of pathology in degenerative spinal disorders

Most commonly used descriptive term	Symptoms	Examination	Imaging findings
Piriformis	Tenderness to palpation over the inferolateral quadrant of the buttock, sometimes radiating down to the posterior thigh into the calf if there is compression of the sciatic nerve as it transverses by piriformis muscle	Buttock pain that occurs not over the SIJ, but into the gluteal crease	Imaging is normal
Hip	Almost universal pain radiating into the ipsilateral groin and thigh, rarely buttock pain	Internal rotation deficits; positive IROP	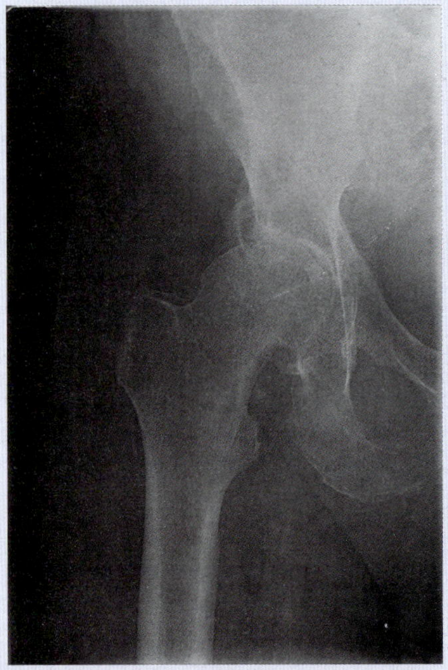 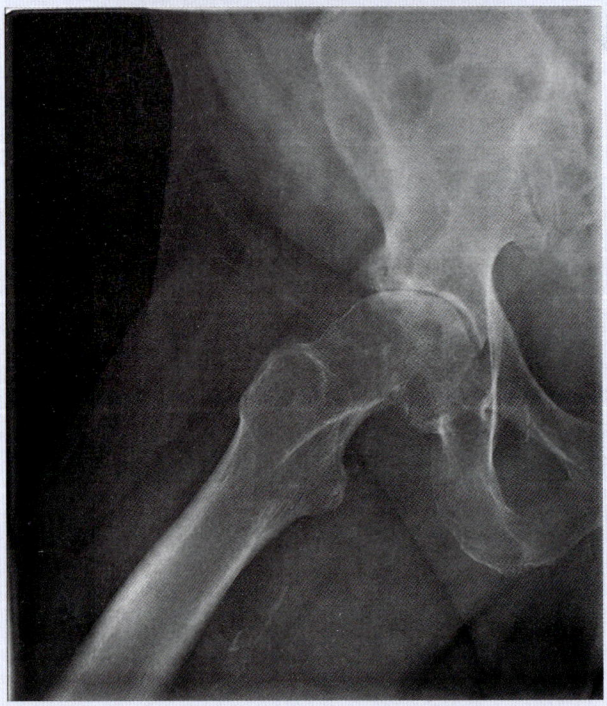

Abbreviations: DRG, dorsal root ganglion; IROP, internal rotation over pressure; IT, iliotibial; MRI, magnetic resonance imaging; SIJ, sacroiliac joint.

References

[1] Bogduk N, Mercer S. Biomechanics of the cervical spine. I: Normal kinematics. Clin Biomech (Bristol, Avon). 2000; 15(9):633–648

[2] Kawakami M, Weinstein JN, Chatani K, Spratt KF, Meller ST, Gebhart GF. Experimental lumbar radiculopathy. Behavioral and histologic changes in a model of radicular pain after spinal nerve root irritation with chromic gut ligatures in the rat. Spine. 1994; 19(16):1795–1802

[3] Quraishi NA. Transforaminal injection of corticosteroids for lumbar radiculopathy: systematic review and meta-analysis. Eur Spine J. 2012; 21(2):214–219

[4] Sasso RC, Macadaeg K, Nordmann D, Smith M. Selective nerve root injections can predict surgical outcome for lumbar and cervical radiculopathy: comparison to magnetic resonance imaging. J Spinal Disord Tech. 2005; 18(6):471–478

[5] Wallace MA, Fukui MB, Williams RL, Ku A, Baghai P. Complications of cervical selective nerve root blocks performed with fluoroscopic guidance. AJR Am J Roentgenol. 2007; 188(5):1218–1221

[6] Huston CW, Slipman CW, Garvin C. Complications and side effects of cervical and lumbosacral selective nerve root injections. Arch Phys Med Rehabil. 2005; 86(2):277–283

[7] Jackson RP, Jacobs RR, Montesano PX. 1988 Volvo award in clinical sciences. Facet joint injection in low-back pain. A prospective statistical study. Spine. 1988; 13(9):966–971

[8] Manchukonda R, Manchikanti KN, Cash KA, Pampati V, Manchikanti L. Facet joint pain in chronic spinal pain: an evaluation of prevalence and false-positive rate of diagnostic blocks. J Spinal Disord Tech. 2007; 20(7):539–545

[9] Stanley D, McLaren MI, Euinton HA, Getty CJ. A prospective study of nerve root infiltration in the diagnosis of sciatica. A comparison with radiculography, computed tomography, and operative findings. Spine. 1990; 15(6):540–543

[10] Marcus NJ, Gracely EJ, Keefe KO. A comprehensive protocol to diagnose and treat pain of muscular origin may successfully and reliably decrease or eliminate pain in a chronic pain population. Pain Med. 2010; 11(1):25–34

[11] Marcus NJ, Shrikhande AA, McCarberg B, Gracely E. A preliminary study to determine if a muscle pain protocol can produce long-term relief in chronic back pain patients. Pain Med. 2013; 14(8):1212–1221

[12] Shafer N. Pneumothorax following "trigger point" injection. JAMA. 1970; 213 (7):1193–1193

[13] Nelson LS, Hoffman RS. Intrathecal injection: unusual complication of trigger-point injection therapy. Ann Emerg Med. 1998; 32(4):506–508

[14] Elias M. Cervical epidural abscess following trigger point injection. J Pain Symptom Manage. 1994; 9(2):71–72

[15] Zink W, Graf BM. Local anesthetic myotoxicity. Reg Anesth Pain Med. 2004; 29(4):333–340

[16] Gorski JM, Schwartz LH. Shoulder impingement presenting as neck pain. J Bone Joint Surg Am. 2003; 85(4):635–638

[17] Hawkins RJ, Bilco T, Bonutti P. Cervical spine and shoulder pain. Clin Orthop Relat Res. 1990(258):142–146

[18] Manifold SG, McCann PD. Cervical radiculitis and shoulder disorders. Clin Orthop Relat Res. 1999(368):105–113

[19] Cormick W. Ultrasound guided therapeutic injections of the cervical spine and brachial plexus. Australas J Ultrasound Med. 2014; 17(1):11–19

[20] Roos DB. The place for scalenectomy and first-rib resection in thoracic outlet syndrome. Surgery. 1982; 92(6):1077–1085

[21] Bottros MM, AuBuchon JD, McLaughlin LN, Altchek DW, Illig KA, Thompson RW. Exercise-enhanced, ultrasound-guided anterior scalene muscle/pectoralis minor muscle blocks can facilitate the diagnosis of neurogenic thoracic outlet syndrome in the high-performance overhead athlete. Am J Sports Med. 2017; 45(1):189–194

[22] Braun RM, Shah KN, Rechnic M, Doehr S, Woods N. Quantitative assessment of scalene muscle block for the diagnosis of suspected thoracic outlet syndrome. J Hand Surg Am. 2015; 40(11):2255–2261

[23] Bogduk N, Baker RM. Clinical and Radiological Anatomy of the Lumbar Spine. Elsevier/Churchill Livingstone; 2012

[24] Wiltse LL, Berger PE, McCulloch JA. A system for reporting the size and location of lesions in the spine. Spine. 1997; 22(13):1534–1537

[25] Boukebir MA, Berlin CD, Navarro-Ramirez R, et al. Ten-step minimally invasive spine lumbar decompression and dural repair through tubular retractors. Oper Neurosurg (Hagerstown). 2017; 13(2):232–245

[26] Porter RW. Spinal stenosis and neurogenic claudication. Spine. 1996; 21 (17):2046–2052

[27] Dyck P. The stoop-test in lumbar entrapment radiculopathy. Spine. 1979; 4 (1):89–92

[28] Kim DH. Minimally Invasive Percutaneous Spinal Techniques E-Book. Elsevier Health Sciences; 2010

[29] Kikuchi S, Hasue M, Nishiyama K, Ito T. Anatomic and clinical studies of radicular symptoms. Spine. 1984; 9(1):23–30

[30] Young PH, McCulloch JA. Essentials of Spinal Microsurgery. Lippincott-Raven; 1998

[31] Kalichman L, Hunter DJ. Lumbar facet joint osteoarthritis: a review. Paper presented at: Seminars in arthritis and rheumatism 2007

[32] Fortin JD, Falco FJ. The Fortin finger test: an indicator of sacroiliac pain. Am J Orthop. 1997; 26(7):477–480

[33] Simopoulos TT, Manchikanti L, Gupta S, et al. Systematic review of the diagnostic accuracy and therapeutic effectiveness of sacroiliac joint interventions. Pain Physician. 2015; 18(5):E713–E756

[34] Nacey NC, Patrie JT, Fox MG. Fluoroscopically guided sacroiliac joint injections: comparison of the effects of intraarticular and periarticular injections on immediate and short-term pain relief. AJR Am J Roentgenol. 2016; 207 (5):1055–1061

[35] Lewis S, Jurak J, Lee C, Lewis R, Gest T. Anatomical variations of the sciatic nerve, in relation to the piriformis muscle. Translational Research in Anatomy.. 2016; 5:15–19

[36] Fishman LM, Zybert PA. Electrophysiologic evidence of piriformis syndrome. Arch Phys Med Rehabil. 1992; 73(4):359–364

[37] Benzon HT, Katz JA, Benzon HA, Iqbal MS. Piriformis syndrome: anatomic considerations, a new injection technique, and a review of the literature. Anesthesiology. 2003; 98(6):1442–1448

[38] Wilson MG, Michet CJ Jr, Ilstrup DM, Melton LJ III. Idiopathic symptomatic osteoarthritis of the hip and knee: a population based incidence study. Paper presented at: Mayo Clinic Proceedings 1990

[39] Altman R, Alarcón G, Appelrouth D, et al. The American College of Rheumatology criteria for the classification and reporting of osteoarthritis of the hip. Arthritis Rheum. 1991; 34(5):505–514

4 Deformity and MIS: Limitation or Opportunity?

Catherine Miller, Ibrahim Hussain, Juan S. Uribe, Kai-Ming Fu, and Praveen Mummaneni

Summary
Adult spinal deformity comprises a complex and wide spectrum of spinal disease. Sagittal balance and spinopelvic parameters have been shown to correlate with disability and patient reported outcomes. Adult deformity correction has traditionally been treated with open surgical correction but is associated with high complication rates. Minimally invasive surgery (MIS) techniques were developed as alternative corrective strategies in an effort to decrease the perioperative complications and morbidity associated with open deformity correction surgery. Proper patient selection is critical to ensure adequate deformity correction using MIS techniques and depends on the patients, their symptoms, the deformity, and the spinopelvic parameters.

Keywords: minimally invasive, adult spinal deformity, spinopelvic parameters, sagittal balance, pelvic incidence, lumbar lordosis, MISDEF2 algorithm

4.1 Introduction

Adult spinal deformity comprises a complex and wide spectrum of spinal disease ranging from progression of adolescent idiopathic scoliosis to degenerative scoliosis from asymmetric degeneration of the spine.[1] Depending on the type and severity of the spinal deformity, patients often have significant disability. They can present with obvious abnormalities in posture, deformity of the body, and pain and neurologic dysfunction as a result of structural changes and/or impingement of neural elements.

Adult spinal deformity continues to be a challenging disease faced by spine surgeons. In 2016, elderly patients (age > 65 years) made up 14.5% of the United States population.[2] The prevalence of scoliosis in this age group has been reported to be as high as 68%.[3] With the increasing elderly population, there is a rising number of patients being evaluated for possible deformity correction. Significant investigation is underway to determine which of these patients will benefit from correction of their deformity and through which surgical approach (traditional open surgery versus minimally invasive techniques).

4.2 Spinopelvic Parameters

The extent of spinal deformity is determined through radiographic evaluation of the spine. Sagittal balance is influenced by the relationship between the pelvis and the spine. Ideal balance maintains the head over the center of the pelvis. If sagittal imbalance is present, a person can use compensatory measures (hip extension, pelvic retroversion) to bring the spine toward normal alignment, but this compensation has limits. Spinopelvic parameters are used in the assessment of deformity to determine the degree of sagittal imbalance and its relationship to the pelvis (▶ Fig. 4.1). These parameters have been shown to correlate with health-related quality of life scores and disability, both prior to and after deformity correction.

Sagittal balance is measured by the sagittal vertebral axis (SVA) from 36 inch standing X-rays. SVA is the distance from a plumb line drawn down from the midpoint of the C7 vertebral body to the dorsal corner of the end plate of S1. The SVA is positive if the plumb line falls ventral to the dorsal corner of the end plate of S1 and negative if the plumb lines fall dorsal to this point. Normal SVA is 0 to 5 cm.

Pelvic incidence (PI) is the angle between a line drawn perpendicular to the midpoint of the sacral end plate and a line from this point to the center of the femoral heads. PI is a constant value that is not affected by body posture and is the sum of the sacral slope (SS) and pelvic tilt (PT). SS is the angle between the horizontal and a line along the sacral end plate. Pelvic compensation is measured by the PT. PT is the angle between a vertical line drawn upwards from the center of the femoral heads and a line drawn from the center of the femoral heads to the midpoint of the sacral end plate.

Lumbar lordosis (LL) is the angle between the lines drawn parallel to the superior end plate of L1 and the sacral end plate. It has been shown that there is a relationship between LL and PI with the ideal difference less than 10 degrees (PI-LL ≤ 10 degrees).

Glassman et al reviewed 752 patients with adult spinal deformity from a multicenter prospective database and found that increasing SVA was associated with a linear worsening of health-reported quality of life scores (Scoliosis Research Society patient questionnaire [SRS-29], Oswestry Disability Index [ODI], and Medical Outcomes Study Short Form [SF-12]).[4] Schwab et al evaluated disability in 492 adult spinal deformity patients from a multicenter database. They found that SVA, PT, and PI-LL mismatch were key factors to impact disability in deformity patients.[5] In a study reviewing 125 adult patients with flatback deformity (PI-LL mismatch > 10 degrees), with and without normal SVA, Smith et al found that a PI-LL mismatch was associated with significant disability.[6]

4.3 Opportunity for MIS Deformity Correction

Degenerative adult scoliosis is a progressive disease which worsens significantly over time. Curves tend to increase 1 to 2 degrees per year, with lateral listhesis being a documented risk factor for progression. Patients with lumbar stenosis who have concomitant scoliosis often demonstrate a significant increase in deformity 1 year after decompression surgery.[7,8,9] The operative treatment of patients with deformity takes this into account by relieving compression of neural structures, realigning the spine to achieve global spinal balance, and promoting arthrodesis. This has traditionally been accomplished with open surgical techniques, which require extensive spinal

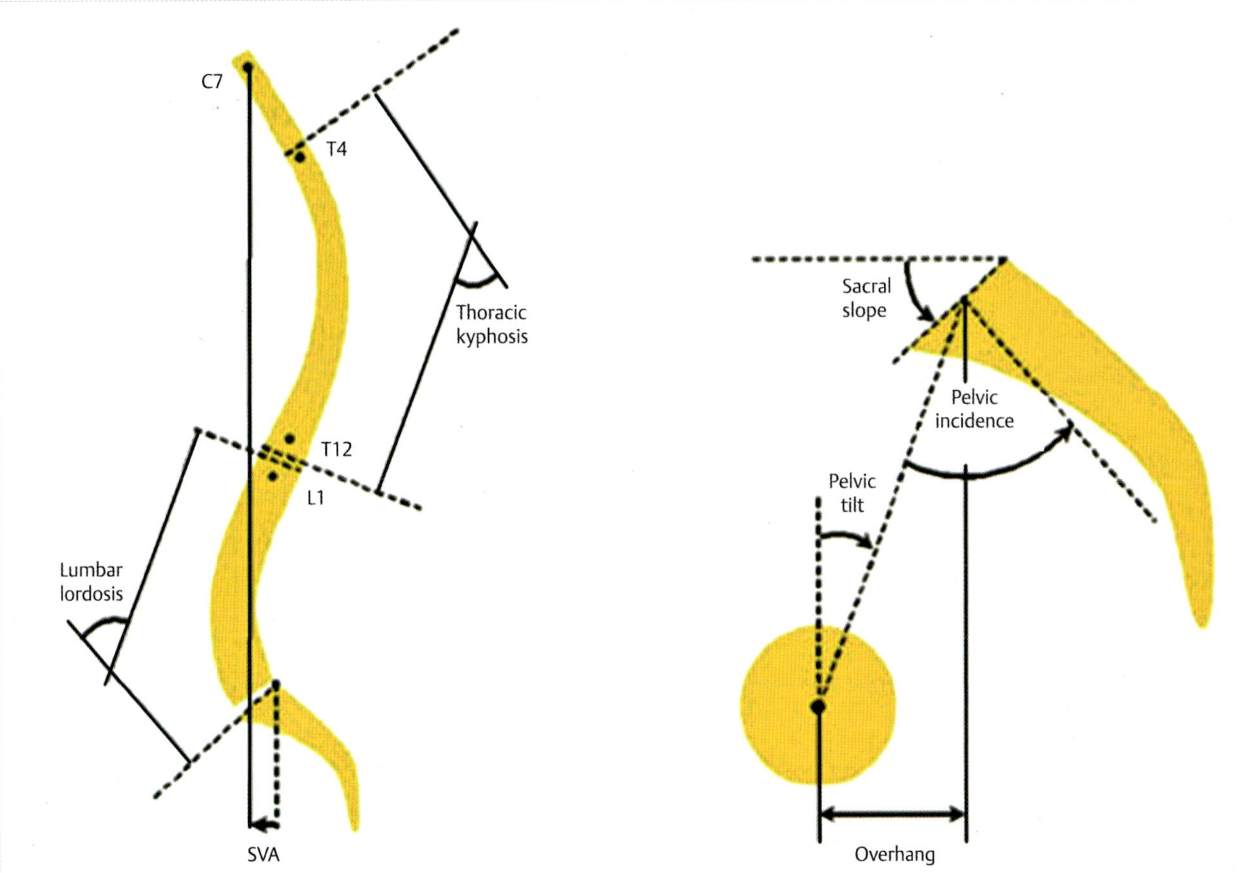

Fig. 4.1 Spinopelvic parameters: Lumbar lordosis, pelvic incidence, pelvic tilt, and sacral slope.

exposure with muscle retraction, long operative times, and significant blood loss. Deformity correction surgery has been associated with high perioperative morbidity, with historical reports citing complications rates ranging from 20 to 80%.[10,11,12] The International Spine Study Group (ISSG) performed a multicenter study in which they reviewed 953 adult spinal deformity patients who underwent surgical correction. They reported a 7.6% rate of major complications, with the most common complications being excessive blood loss, pulmonary embolism, and wound infection requiring reoperation.[13] Another study performed a retrospective review of 206 patients who underwent deformity correction from a multicenter database. They found major complication rates varied from 6 to 29%, with complications occurring more frequently in older patients.[14] In a study examining 407 deformity corrective procedures, Pateder et al found a 30-day mortality rate of 2.4%.[15]

In an effort to decrease the perioperative complications and morbidity associated with open deformity correction surgery, minimally invasive surgery (MIS) techniques were developed as alternative corrective strategies. These techniques allow for less disruption to the paraspinal musculature through the utilization of various MIS retractor systems while achieving the same goals as open deformity correction surgery. Several studies have shown that MIS for deformity can result in less blood loss, shorter hospital stays, and earlier postoperative recovery for appropriately selected patients with moderate deformities.[16,17,18,19,20]

MIS techniques were developed as alternative corrective strategies in an effort to decrease the perioperative complications and morbidity associated with open deformity correction surgery. Proper patient selection is critical to ensure adequate deformity correction using MIS techniques.

4.4 Limitations of MIS

As MIS techniques gained popularity for deformity correction, additional research has been published which identify some of the limitations of MIS. Early studies of MIS techniques showed improved coronal balance; however some patients did not achieve optimal sagittal correction.[21,22] Dakwar et al published a series of 25 adult patients who underwent MIS for deformity correction using the minimally invasive lateral transpsoas approach. Perioperative complications occurred in 12% of the patients. Although they had improvement in clinical outcomes and coronal balance, one-third of the patients in this early study did not have restoration of their sagittal balance.[23]

Because of limited bony exposure for a fusion surface, pseudarthrosis has been reported in MIS for deformity, especially at levels where an interbody fusion is not used. Wang and Mummaneni reviewed 23 patients who underwent MIS for

deformity correction. There was improvement in both clinical and radiographic results; however, 28.6% of patients who underwent posterolateral (without interbody) fusion had pseudarthrosis.[24]

Over time, MIS techniques have advanced with the use of hyperlordotic grafts and anterior column reconstructions with practices involving anterolateral stand-alone instrumentation, circumferential MIS (cMIS), and hybrid surgery (MIS + open). The ISSG studied 85 consecutive patents undergoing deformity correction from a multicenter database and compared the results of stand-alone fusion, cMIS, and hybrid surgeries. They found similar clinical outcomes between the three groups; however the hybrid group achieved greater coronal and sagittal correction, albeit with high complication rates. For coronal curve correction, they found a ceiling effect of typical lordosis corrections of 23, 34, and 55 degrees for stand-alone, cMIS, and hybrid, respectively. Only the hybrid approach allowed for statistically significant improvements in sagittal plane correction and also markedly greater improvement in LL.[25]

4.5 Patient Selection

Despite the advancements in MIS for deformity correction and its reported advantages, not every patient is a suitable candidate to undergo deformity correction through a minimally invasive approach. Literature has shown that several factors can help determine this, such as flexibility of the curve, spinopelvic alignment, and the degree of the sagittal deformity. Mundis et al investigated 63 deformity patients who underwent cMIS or posterior MIS correction and divided the patients into groups based on their baseline SRS-Schwab global alignment modifier. They found that those with less sagittal imbalance had greater improvement in ODI and numeric rating scale (NRS) in back and leg scores. The group with severe sagittal imbalance was not adequately treated with an MIS approach and similar deformities may be better suited for traditional open correction.[26]

Eastlack et al and the ISSG evaluated baseline characteristics of 350 patients who underwent either open or MIS for deformity correction from two multicenter databases. The approach was determined by surgeon's preference. The MIS group was slightly older with worse preoperative ODI scores. They had smaller coronal deformities but similar sagittal malalignment. MIS was more often used in patients with SVA < 6 cm and PI-LL mismatch < 30 degrees.[27]

4.6 MISDEF Algorithm

Given the complexity of adult spinal deformity and the numerous available surgical techniques, the Minimally Invasive Spinal Deformity (MISDEF) algorithm was developed to help guide surgeons in selecting the optimal surgical approach for their deformity patients who had failed nonoperative management.[28] This algorithm was established using the Delphi approach to ensure agreement from experts in the field. The initial iteration of the algorithm divided patients into three classes based on various radiographic parameters. As MIS techniques and instrumentation evolved, an updated MISDEF2 algorithm was developed. The MISDEF2 algorithm included a new class in which newer circumferential MIS and hybrid strategies could be utilized resulting in four total classes (▶ Fig. 4.2).[28]

Clinical symptoms and radiographic parameters were considered in the development of the algorithm, culminating into four general classes of deformities, which guide the surgical approaches. Radiographic parameters, which have been shown to influence disability and outcomes, such as v SVA, PT, PI-LL, lateral listhesis, and coronal Cobb angle, were utilized in the algorithm.

4.6.1 Class 1

A Class 1 deformity is mild and causes symptoms of neurogenic claudication or radiculopathy from central, lateral recess, or foraminal stenosis. There should be minimal back pain attributable to the deformity. These deformities are flexible curves with an SVA < 6 cm, PT < 25 degrees, PI-LL mismatch < 10 degrees, lateral listhesis < 6 mm, and coronal Cobb angle < 20 degrees. These patients, at most, have a Meyerding Grade 1 spondylolisthesis.

The goal of treatment in these patients is decompression of the neural elements and not correction of the mild spinal deformity. Appropriate surgical approach is an MIS or mini-open (muscle sparing) decompression or single level fusion. Using fixed tubular retractors or small expandable retractors through muscle sparing approach, one can perform an ipsilateral hemilaminotomy and foraminotomy, as well as a contralateral decompression by angling the retractor medially. MIS decompression can be performed at one or two levels through the same incision. If a mobile Grade 1 spondylolisthesis is present, minimally invasive fusion can also be performed via transforaminal interbody fusion (TLIF) or lateral interbody fusion (LIF).

4.6.2 Class 2

Patients with a Class 2 deformity have symptoms related to stenosis, similar to Class 1; however they have back pain as their dominant symptom. These patients have SVA < 6 cm, PT < 25 degrees, PI-LL mismatch of 10 to 30 degrees, thoracic kyphosis < 60 degrees, and coronal Cobb angle > 20 degrees. Patients with SVA > 6 cm but having curves that partially correct while supine also belong to Class 2.

For this class, the goals of treatment are both decompression with some deformity correction. Decompression of single or multiple levels is obtained via similar minimally invasive techniques as described for Class 1. Unlike Class 1, these patients require multiple levels of fusion, extending across the apex of their curve. Instrumentation and interbody fusion are accomplished via minimally invasive techniques to achieve correction of the deformity with or without concomitant decompression.

4.6.3 Class 3

Patients in Class 3 are different from those initially described in the first MISDEF algorithm. Preoperatively, the curve may be rigid with SVA > 6 cm, PT > 25 degrees, PI-LL mismatch > 30 degrees, thoracic kyphosis > 60 degrees, and thoracolumbar kyphosis > 10 degrees. These patients can be adequately treated with minimally invasive techniques; however, they should only

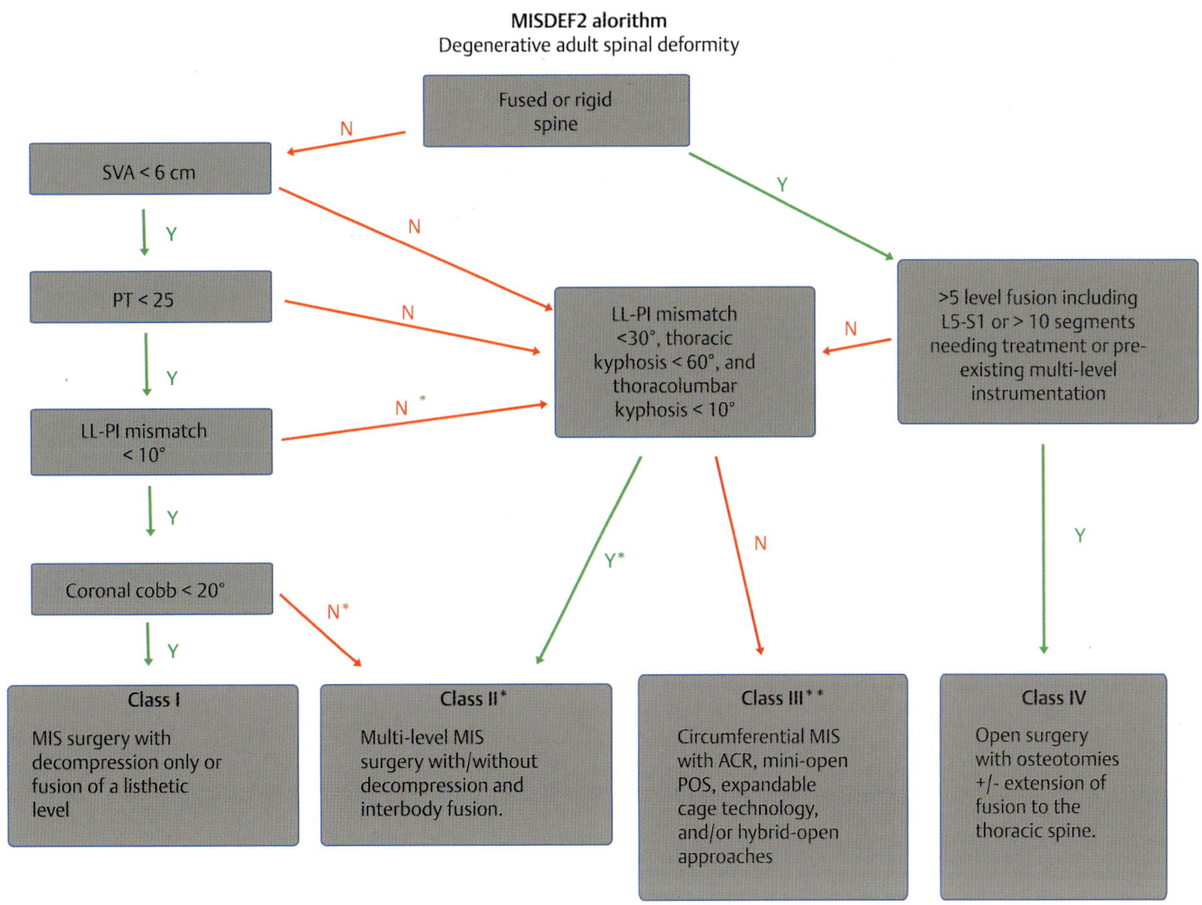

Fig. 4.2 Minimally Invasive Spinal Deformity (MISDEF2) algorithm is a guide to assist with decision-making on which adult spinal deformity patients are candidates for minimally invasive surgical approaches. (Reprinted with permission from Mummaneni PV, Park P, Shaffrey CI, et al. The minimally invasive interbody selection algorithm for spinal deformity. J Neurosurg Spine 2021; 34(5): 741–748.)

be performed by experienced MIS surgeons. Sagittal correction can be achieved through anterior longitudinal ligament (ALL) release, hyperlordotic cages, and mini-open pedicle subtraction osteotomy (PSO).[29,30,31,32] Hybrid procedures can also be utilized here, where MIS techniques are used for anterior reconstruction/interbody placement and pedicle screw instrumentation/osteotomies are performed through open posterior approaches to achieve the greatest degree of correction.

4.6.4 Class 4

Patients in Class 4 present with back and leg pain with significant coronal and/or sagittal imbalance. Preoperatively, the curve is rigid with SVA > 6 cm. These patients have fixed deformities and the goal of their treatment is correction of the deformity in both the coronal and sagittal planes. Correction often requires fusion of more than five levels, including L5–S1, or instrumentation of more than 10 segments. These patients may also have pre-existing multilevel instrumentation and require three column osteotomies or extension to the thoracic spine, given the severity of the deformity. MIS techniques are not suitable for these large deformities as they cannot achieve similar realignment compared to traditional open surgery.

The reliability of the algorithm was tested using 24 representative spinal deformity cases provided to 14 fellowship-trained spinal surgeons at two separate time points. A short history of symptoms, imaging (X-rays, magnetic resonance imaging [MRI] images), and measured radiographic parameters were included for each case. Interobserver kappa was 0.85 and 0.82 for separate assessments and intraobserver kappa was 0.8, demonstrating substantial agreement.[28]

4.7 Example Cases

4.7.1 Class 1 (▶ Fig. 4.3)

A 68-year-old woman presented with severe left leg radiculopathy and mild low back pain. Her MRI revealed a Grade 1 L4–L5 spondylolisthesis and a left L4–L5 facet cyst causing foraminal stenosis. Flexion/extension X-rays showed dynamic instability at the L4–L5 level. Preoperative 36-inch standing X-rays showed degenerative lumbar scoliosis with an SVA of 0 cm, LL of 53 degrees, PI of 52 degrees, PI-LL mismatch of 1 degree, PT of 14 degrees, and coronal cobb angle of 21 degrees. Despite her lumbar scoliosis, her clinical symptoms correlated with her L4–L5 spondylolisthesis. She failed conservative measures and

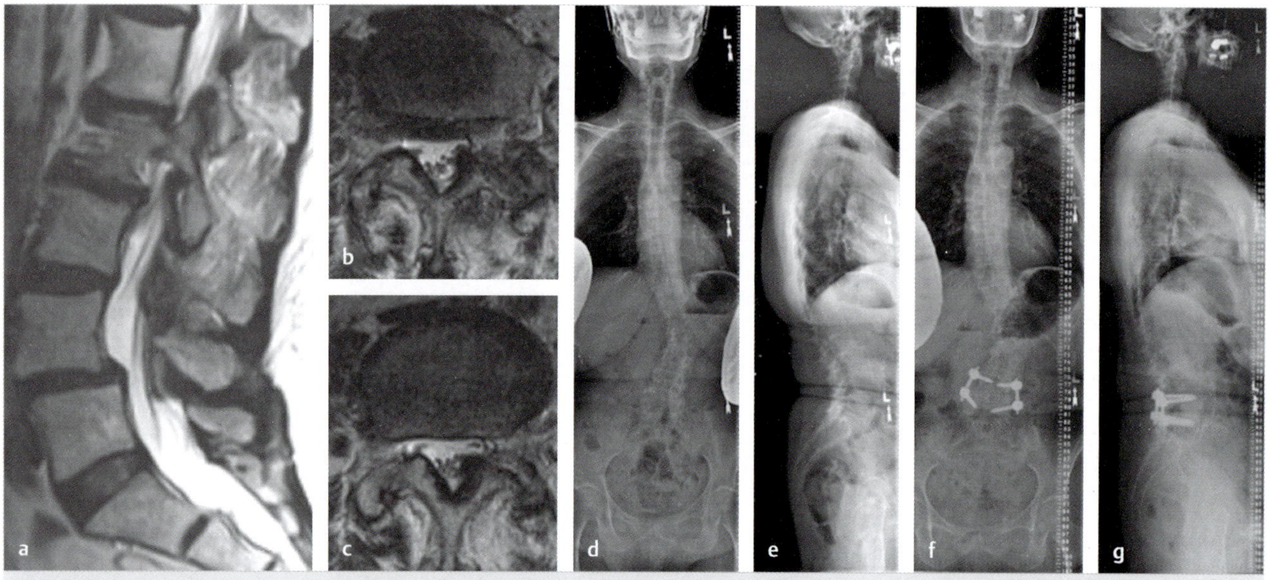

Fig. 4.3 Class 1 example: A 68-year-old woman with left leg radiculopathy and mild back pain. T2-weighted sagittal **(a)** and axial **(b, c)** magnetic resonance imaging (MRI) shows the Grade 1 L4–L5 spondylolisthesis and facet cyst causing foraminal stenosis. Preoperative 36-inch standing X-rays **(d, e)** demonstrate a lumbar degenerative scoliosis but overall normal coronal and sagittal balance. Postoperative 36-inch standing X-rays **(f, g)** illustrate maintenance of her coronal and sagittal balance after a minimally invasive surgery (MIS) of L4–L5 via transforaminal interbody fusion (TLIF).

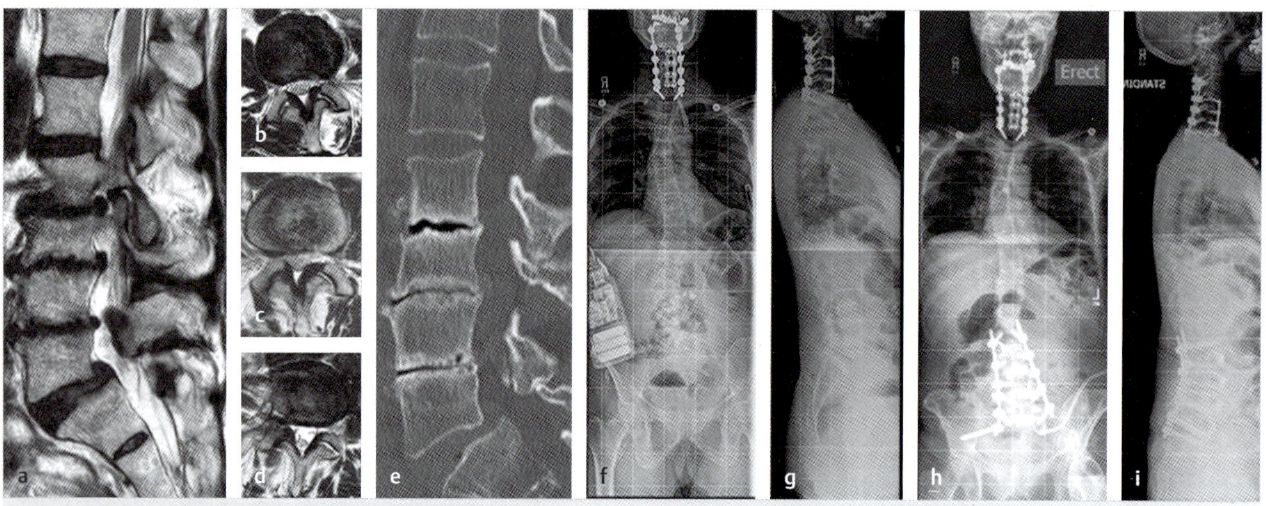

Fig. 4.4 Class 2 example: A 62-year-old female presented with chronic low back pain and right leg pain and weakness. T2-weighted axial **(a)** and sagittal **(b–d)** magnetic resonance imaging (MRI) showing multilevel degenerative disease with central and foraminal stenosis. Sagittal computed tomography (CT) scan **(e)** displays a rigid curve with anterior lipping osteophytes at L2-3-4 and spondylolisthesis at L5–S1. Preoperative 36-inch standing X-rays **(f, g)** showing thoracolumbar scoliosis. She underwent L2–S1 anterior lumbar interbody fusion (ALIF), followed by L2-pelvic minimally invasive surgery (MIS) instrumentation. Postoperative 36-inch standing X-rays **(h, i)** show straightening of the lumbar scoliosis and maintenance of coronal and sagittal balance.

underwent an MIS L4–L5 TLIF with complete resolution of her symptoms. Her postoperative X-rays showed SVA of 0 cm, LL of 50 degrees, PI of 52 degrees, PI-LL mismatch of 2 degrees, PT of 18 degrees, and coronal Cobb angle of 21 degrees.

4.7.2 Class 2 (▸ Fig. 4.4)

A 62-year-old woman presented with chronic low back pain and right leg pain and weakness. She had tried and failed several conservative measures. Her MRI showed multilevel degenerative disc disease causing central and foraminal stenosis, as well as a Grade 1 L5–S1 spondylolisthesis. Preoperative 36-inch standing X-rays displayed thoracolumbar scoliosis with SVA of −1.5 cm, LL of 60 degrees, PI of 65 degrees, PI-LL of mismatch 5 degrees, PT of 25 degrees, and lumbar coronal Cobb angle of 31 degrees. Postoperatively, her imaging shows SVA of 1 cm, LL of 58 degrees, PI of 65 degrees, PI-LL mismatch of 7 degrees, PT of 17 degrees, and coronal Cobb angle of 2 degrees.

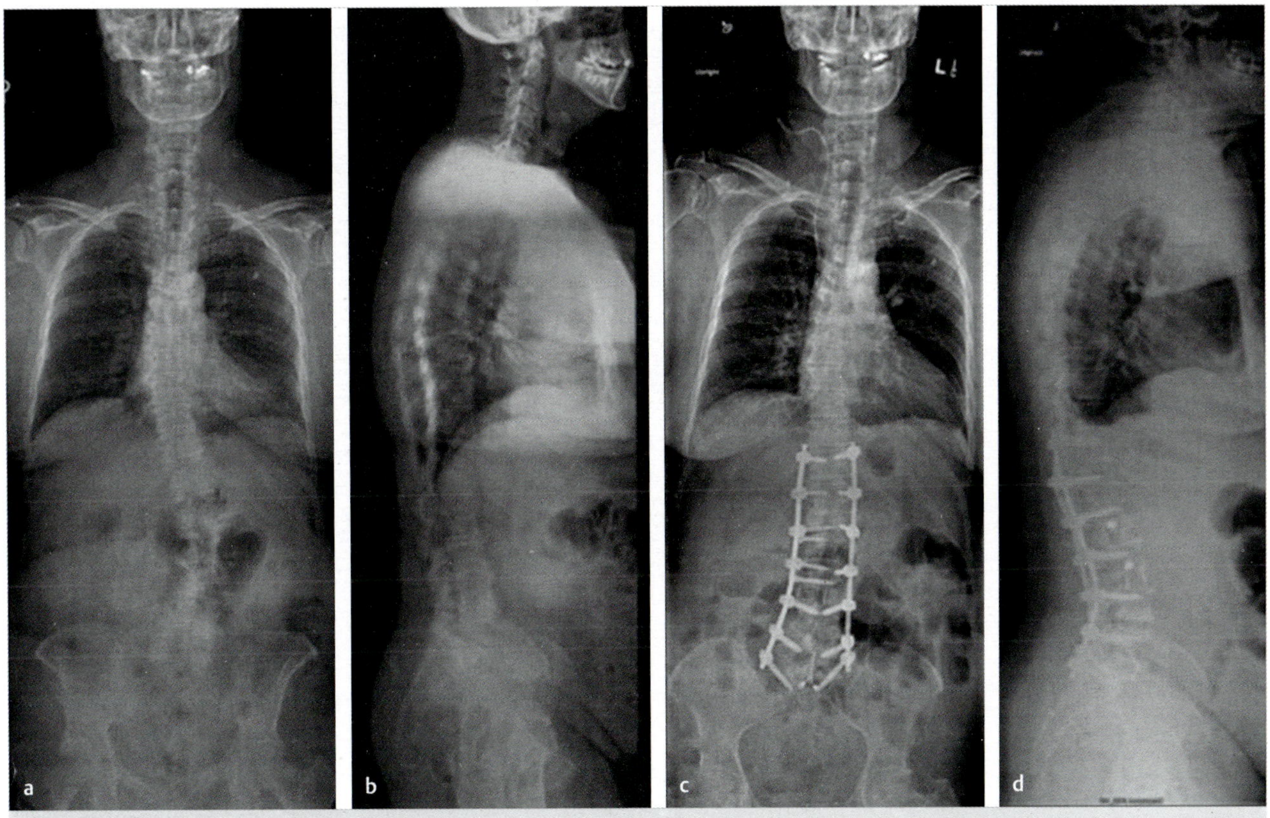

Fig. 4.5 Class 3 example: Preoperative 36-inch standing X-rays **(a, b)** showing thoracolumbar scoliosis and coronal levoscoliosis and flattening of the lumbar spine. There is a preoperative PI-LL mismatch of 33 degrees (PI = 57 degrees and LL = 24 degrees). The patient underwent circumferential minimally invasive surgery (cMIS) with single level anterior lumbar interbody fusion (ALIF), multi-level lateral lumbar interbody fusion (LLIF), anterior column realignment (ACR) at L3–L4 with hyperlordotic cage placement, and percutaneous pedicle screw instrumentation. Postoperative 36-inch standing X-rays **(c, d)** show that LL was increased to 56 degrees, with a new PI-LL mismatch of 1 degree while preserving sagittal vertebral axis (SVA) at around 7 cm.

4.7.3 Class 3 (▶ Fig. 4.5)

A 68-year-old male presented with low back pain and multilevel radicular pain. His preoperative X-rays demonstrated a coronal levoscoliosis, flatback morphology, SVA of 7.5 cm, PI of 57 degrees, LL of 24 degrees, PI-LL of mismatch 33 degrees, and PT of 27 degrees. The patient underwent cMIS with single level anterior lumbar interbody fusion (ALIF), multilevel lateral lumbar interbody fusion (LLIF), anterior column realignment (ACR) at L3–L4 with hyperlordotic cage placement, and T12–S1 percutaneous pedicle screw instrumentation. Postoperatively, PT was 19 degrees and LL was increased to 56 degrees with a new PI-LL mismatch of 1 degrees. SVA was preserved at 7 cm.

4.7.4 Class 4 (▶ Fig. 4.6)

A 72-year-old man presented with bilateral leg pain and numbness. He had a history of prior placement of interspinous distraction and L1–L2 fusion. His imaging showed a fixed sagittal plane deformity with L1–L2 spondylolisthesis and advanced arthropathy at L3–S1, causing severe stenosis from L1 to S1. His preoperative X-rays exhibited SVA of + 17 cm, LL of 7 degrees, PI of 54 degrees, PI-LL mismatch of 47 degrees, and PT of 28 degrees. He underwent removal of prior hardware, T10 pelvis instrumentation, L1–S1 decompressive laminectomies, L2 pedicle subtraction osteotomy, and L5–S1 TLIF. He had complete resolution of his pain with minimal residual numbness. His postoperative X-rays showed SVA of 3 cm, LL of 45 degrees, PI of 54 degrees, PI-LL mismatch of 9 degrees, and PT of 26 degrees.

4.8 Conclusion

Adult spinal deformity comprises a complex and wide spectrum of spinal disease. Sagittal balance and spinopelvic parameters have shown to correlate with disability and patient reported outcomes. Deformity correction has traditionally been treated with open surgical correction but is associated with high complication rates. MIS techniques were developed as alternative corrective strategies in an effort to decrease the perioperative complications and morbidity associated with open deformity correction surgery. Proper patient selection is critical to ensure adequate deformity correction and depends on the patients, their symptoms, the deformity, and the spinopelvic parameters. The MISDEF algorithm presents a guideline for surgeons to decide which of their patients are suitable candidates for MIS deformity correction.

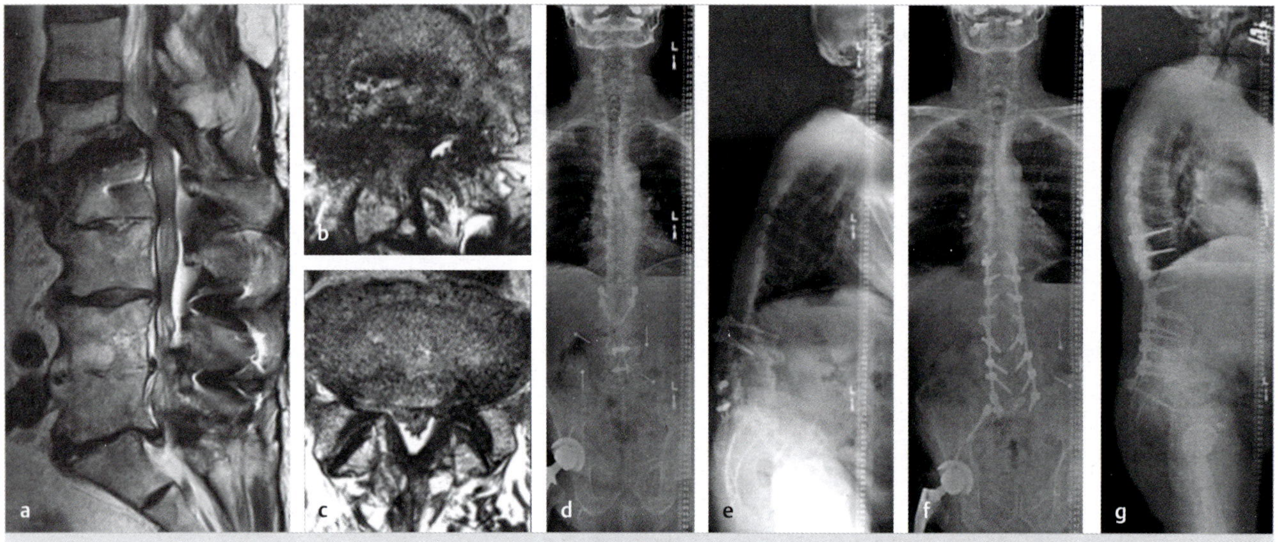

Fig. 4.6 Class 4 example: A 72-year-old man presented with progressive bilateral leg pain and numbness. T2-weighted sagittal **(a)** and axial magnetic resonance imaging (MRI) at L1–L2 **(b)** and L5–S1 **(c)** shows severe multilevel stenosis from L1 to S1, L1–L2 spondylolisthesis, and L5 retrolisthesis. Preoperative 36-inch standing X-rays **(d, e)** display the fixed sagittal plane deformity with focal kyphosis at L1–L2. The patient underwent an open T10 pelvis instrumentation and decompression, L2 pedicle subtraction osteotomy, and L5–S1 transforaminal interbody fusion (TLIF). Postoperative 36-inch standing X-rays **(f, g)** show restoration of sagittal balance.

References

[1] Birknes JK, White AP, Albert TJ, Shaffrey CI, Harrop JS. Adult degenerative scoliosis: a review. Neurosurgery. 2008; 63(3) Suppl:94–103

[2] The United States Census Bureau Statistics. 2016. (Accessed from: https://data.census.gov/cedsci/table?d=ACS%205-Year%20Estimates%20Data%20Profiles&tid=ACSDP5Y2016.DP05)

[3] Schwab F, Dubey A, Gamez L, et al. Adult scoliosis: prevalence, SF-36, and nutritional parameters in an elderly volunteer population. Spine. 2005; 30 (9):1082–1085

[4] Glassman SD, Bridwell K, Dimar JR, Horton W, Berven S, Schwab F. The impact of positive sagittal balance in adult spinal deformity. Spine. 2005; 30 (18):2024–2029

[5] Schwab FJ, Blondel B, Bess S, et al. International Spine Study Group (ISSG). Radiographical spinopelvic parameters and disability in the setting of adult spinal deformity: a prospective multicenter analysis. Spine. 2013; 38(13): E803–E812

[6] Smith JS, Singh M, Klineberg E, et al. International Spine Study Group. Surgical treatment of pathological loss of lumbar lordosis (flatback) in patients with normal sagittal vertical axis achieves similar clinical improvement as surgical treatment of elevated sagittal vertical axis: clinical article. J Neurosurg Spine. 2014; 21(2):160–170

[7] Chin KR, Furey C, Bohlman HH. Risk of progression in de novo low-magnitude degenerative lumbar curves: natural history and literature review. Am J Orthop. 2009; 38(8):404–409

[8] Tsutsui S, Yoshimura N, Watanuki A, et al. Risk factors and natural history of de novo degenerative lumbar scoliosis in a community-based cohort: the Miyama study. Spine Deform. 2013; 1(4):287–292

[9] Hosogane N, Watanabe K, Kono H, Saito M, Toyama Y, Matsumoto M. Curve progression after decompression surgery in patients with mild degenerative scoliosis. J Neurosurg Spine. 2013; 18(4):321–326

[10] Aebi M. The adult scoliosis. Eur Spine J. 2005; 14(10):925–948

[11] Carreon LY, Puno RM, Dimar JR, II, Glassman SD, Johnson JR. Perioperative complications of posterior lumbar decompression and arthrodesis in older adults. J Bone Joint Surg Am. 2003; 85(11):2089–2092

[12] Zurbriggen C, Markwalder TM, Wyss S. Long-term results in patients treated with posterior instrumentation and fusion for degenerative scoliosis of the lumbar spine. Acta Neurochir (Wien). 1999; 141(1):21–26

[13] Schwab FJ, Hawkinson N, Lafage V, et al. International Spine Study Group. Risk factors for major peri-operative complications in adult spinal deformity surgery: a multi-center review of 953 consecutive patients. Eur Spine J. 2012; 21(12):2603–2610

[14] Smith JS, Shaffrey CI, Glassman SD, et al. Spinal Deformity Study Group. Risk-benefit assessment of surgery for adult scoliosis: an analysis based on patient age. Spine. 2011; 36(10):817–824

[15] Pateder DB, Gonzales RA, Kebaish KM, Cohen DB, Chang JY, Kostuik JP. Short-term mortality and its association with independent risk factors in adult spinal deformity surgery. Spine. 2008; 33(11):1224–1228

[16] Dhall SS, Wang MY, Mummaneni PV. Clinical and radiographic comparison of mini-open transforaminal lumbar interbody fusion with open transforaminal lumbar interbody fusion in 42 patients with long-term follow-up. J Neurosurg Spine. 2008; 9(6):560–565

[17] Foley KT, Gupta SK. Percutaneous pedicle screw fixation of the lumbar spine: preliminary clinical results. J Neurosurg. 2002; 97(1) Suppl:7–12

[18] Guiot BH, Khoo LT, Fessler RG. A minimally invasive technique for decompression of the lumbar spine. Spine. 2002; 27(4):432–438

[19] Khoo LT, Palmer S, Laich DT, Fessler RG. Minimally invasive percutaneous posterior lumbar interbody fusion. Neurosurgery. 2002; 51(5) Suppl:S166–S181

[20] Park Y, Ha JW. Comparison of one-level posterior lumbar interbody fusion performed with a minimally invasive approach or a traditional open approach. Spine. 2007; 32(5):537–543

[21] Anand N, Rosemann R, Khalsa B, Baron EM. Mid-term to long-term clinical and functional outcomes of minimally invasive correction and fusion for adults with scoliosis. Neurosurg Focus. 2010; 28(3):E6

[22] Tormenti MJ, Maserati MB, Bonfield CM, Okonkwo DO, Kanter AS. Complications and radiographic correction in adult scoliosis following combined transpsoas extreme lateral interbody fusion and posterior pedicle screw instrumentation. Neurosurg Focus. 2010; 28(3):E7

[23] Dakwar E, Cardona RF, Smith DA, Uribe JS. Early outcomes and safety of the minimally invasive, lateral retroperitoneal transpsoas approach for adult degenerative scoliosis. Neurosurg Focus. 2010; 28(3):E8

[24] Wang MY, Mummaneni PV. Minimally invasive surgery for thoracolumbar spinal deformity: initial clinical experience with clinical and radiographic outcomes. Neurosurg Focus. 2010; 28(3):E9
[25] Wang MY, Mummaneni PV, Fu KM, et al. Minimally Invasive Surgery Section of the International Spine Study Group. Less invasive surgery for treating adult spinal deformities: ceiling effects for deformity correction with 3 different techniques. Neurosurg Focus. 2014; 36(5):E12
[26] Mundis GM, Jr, Turner JD, Deverin V, et al. International Spine Study Group. A critical analysis of sagittal plane deformity correction with minimally invasive adult spinal deformity surgery: a 2-year follow-up study. Spine Deform. 2017; 5(4):265–271
[27] Eastlack RK, Mundis GM, Jr, Wang M, et al. International Spine Study Group. Is there a patient profile that characterizes a patient with adult spinal deformity as a candidate for minimally invasive surgery? Global Spine J. 2017; 7(7):703–708
[28] Mummaneni PV, Park P, Shaffrey CI, et al. International Spine Study Group (ISSG). The MISDEF2 algorithm: an updated algorithm for patient selection in minimally invasive deformity surgery. J Neurosurg Spine. 2019; 32(2):221–228
[29] Akbarnia BA, Mundis GM, Jr, Moazzaz P, et al. Anterior column realignment (ACR) for focal kyphotic spinal deformity using a lateral transpsoas approach and ALL release. J Spinal Disord Tech. 2014; 27(1):29–39
[30] Turner JD, Akbarnia BA, Eastlack RK, et al. Radiographic outcomes of anterior column realignment for adult sagittal plane deformity: a multicenter analysis. Eur Spine J. 2015; 24 Suppl 3:427–432
[31] Wang MY, Bordon G. Mini-open pedicle subtraction osteotomy as a treatment for severe adult spinal deformities: case series with initial clinical and radiographic outcomes. J Neurosurg Spine. 2016; 24(5):769–776
[32] Wang MY, Madhavan K. Mini-open pedicle subtraction osteotomy: surgical technique. World Neurosurg. 2014; 81(5–6):843.e11–843.e14

5 Target: The Muscle as a Pain Generator and Key Element to Protect during MIS Surgery

Norman Marcus and Roger Härtl

Summary

Dr. Normam Marcus is a skilled clinician who has dedicated part of his career to the study of muscle physiopathology and its role as "back pain" generator. His approach has proven to be an effective tool in those patients where pain diagnosis/treatment is challenging. In this chapter, Dr. Marcus guides the reader through the rationale of his approach and how to implement this approach into a multidisciplinary practice.

Keywords: Ehlers Danlos, ED, muscle pain, back pain, low back pain, discogenic pain, mechanical back pain, radicular pain, myogenic pain

5.1 The Role of Muscles in Back and Neck Pain—before, during, and after Minimally Invasive Surgery

Soft tissue includes ligaments, fascia, and muscle/tendon. For simplicity, muscles will be used in this chapter to represent soft tissue, acknowledging that the other soft tissue representatives are important pain generators as well. Appreciation of the pathophysiologic and functional causes of muscle pain may improve spine surgery outcomes.

5.2 Introduction

Muscles constitute approximately 40% of the body by weight and are thought to be an important cause of nonspecific/idiopathic low back pain in as many as 85% of patients presenting with nonradiating back pain.[1] The overriding concept of this chapter is that muscle is an important primary source of back pain. It is then reasonable to assume that persistent low back pain, often encountered as a common symptom in failed back surgery syndrome (FBSS), can be a function of muscle generated pain, and may be present before as well as after spine surgery. Therefore, careful preoperative evaluation for muscle generated pain is crucial in avoiding FBSS. This requires a thorough musculoskeletal evaluation and emphasis on muscle strengthening and flexibility training in order to avoid mistakenly operating on a patient who suffers from muscle related pain.

With the increasing rates of spine surgery, there is an increased incidence of FBSS.[2] Newer soft tissue sparing procedures (minimally invasive surgery [MIS]) hold the promise of diminished trauma and subsequent incidence of FBSS, but even though postoperative pain is less in MIS compared to open procedures for the first 6 months, a significant number of patients still experience mild-to-moderate pain and disability 5 years after surgery.[3] This raises the concern that, regardless of the surgery, some of this pain may have been present before as "muscle generated pain" (MGP). Muscle-related back or neck pain may exist even after a perfectly performed MIS procedure. The surgical team that anticipates this possibility will have a greater degree of success in appropriately selecting patients for surgery and managing postoperative pain.

5.3 Background

Since the seminal report of Mixter and Barr in 1934[4] of a disc herniation causing sciatic pain and a second paper in 1935,[5] suggesting that nonradiating back pain was disc related, the field of spine surgery has looked to the neuraxis as the source of the back pain and surgery as often inevitable. Faculty at the Weill Cornell Center for Comprehensive Spine Care, believing that ignored MGP may be a contributing etiology for FBSS in technically successful spine surgery, have begun to examine the role of muscles in clinical back pain presentations. Fishbain et al[6] pointed out that it is difficult to distinguish neuropathic pain from soft tissue generated pain: Without knowledge of the pathophysiologic mechanisms causing muscle pain, in a patient presenting with regional pain, the putative diagnosis will usually be neuraxial. For example, a patient complaining of pain in the low back, buttock, and thigh with magnetic resonance imaging (MRI) evidence of an L4/L5 disc will most often be assessed as having pain that reflects root compression and not be assessed for muscles in the low back and buttock as a possible source of the pain. A 2011 study[7] described variables contributing to the incidence of FBSS: (1) preoperatively, (2) perioperatively, and (3) postoperatively. MGP as a putative source of back and/or leg pain was not mentioned.

5.4 Clinical Presentation of Muscle Pain

Muscle pain is typically described as a dull aching sensation, made worse with aggressive activity and prolonged positioning. A muscle that is a source of pain is found to have *inhibition of* electrical activity with associated problems in coordination and flexibility related to *increased* activity in antagonist groups.[8] This phenomenon is known as the "pain-adaptation model."

Sensitized muscles and muscles that are painful due to referred pain patterns (see below) may present with increased muscle tone.[9] Nerves traveling through or adjacent to stiffened muscles may become compressed, suggesting a neuropathic problem of which the piriformis syndrome is only one example.[10]

5.5 Neuroanatomy and Neurophysiology of Muscle Pain[11]: Myogenic (MGP) versus Neurogenic Inflammation

The nociceptive signal is transmitted to the central nervous system where it may be ultimately experienced in the cerebral cortex as pain. The nociceptor may be stimulated by compression

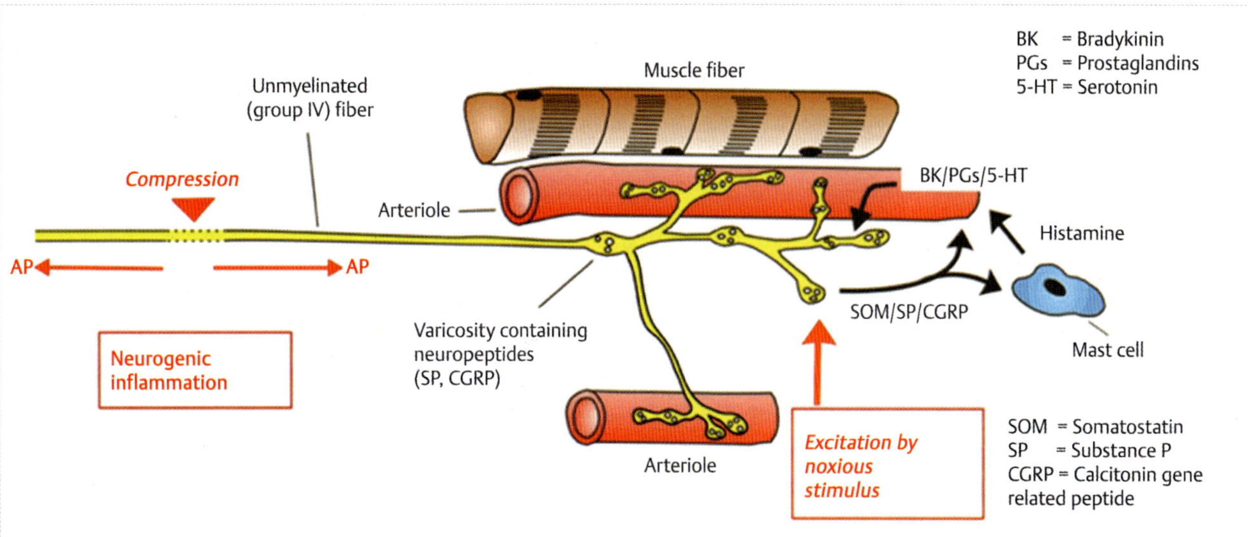

Fig. 5.1 Schematic of group IV muscle nociceptor. Neurogenic and myogenic pain. Pathoanatomical changes in the neuraxis may produce compression of the afferent group IV fibers close to the spine producing neurogenic inflammation consisting of a retrograde impulse distally to the muscle causing release of neuroexcitatory and vasoactive substances from varicosities on the nerve, arteriolar endothelium, mast cells, and platelets and an anterograde stimulation to synapse with a dorsal horn neuron (DHN). Myogenic excitation results from noxious stimuli to the muscle tissue strong enough to depolarize high threshold mechano/chemo receptors causing an action potential and release of glutamate into the synapse with the DHN and peripheral release of the same neuroexcitatory substances above.

Table 5.1 Kraus-Weber test for trunk muscle strength and flexibility: exercises and measurements

Test	Measurement
Floor touch—knees extended, feet together	Flexibility of low back muscles, hamstrings, and calves
Leg lift supine	Strength of abdominals and hip flexors
Sit up with legs extended	Strength of abdominals and hip flexors
Sit up with knees bent	Eliminating hip flexors, testing abdominal muscle strength
Lifting lower body and then upper body from the mat while prone	Back muscle extensor strength

of the afferent neuron close to the spinal cord (see ▶ Fig. 5.1, for example, from a herniated lumbar or cervical disc, severe lateral recess stenosis, or spondylolisthesis causing compression of an exiting nerve root in the foramen). In this case, the neural compression elicits an action potential that can travel back to the spinal cord producing neuropathic pain. At the same time, however, an action potential can also travel peripherally to the muscle tissue with release of neuropeptides resulting in neurogenic inflammation. Clinically, the patient with afferent nerve compression could then have neurogenic induced muscle inflammation complicating the neuropathic presentation.

A microsurgical discectomy or decompression and fusion to treat the nerve compression may eliminate or diminish the anterograde stimulation travelling to the spinal cord and retrograde stimulation peripherally toward the muscle. Although the neuropathic pain component will decrease, immediately or over time, the significant muscle changes induced by the neurogenic inflammation may persist for a variable period and can result in significant persistent postoperative MGP, which, if not considered, will be difficult to treat. The patient may then be pessimistically diagnosed as suffering from FBSS.

If noxious stimuli are persistent or recur repeatedly, the peripheral nerve may become sensitized with accompanying persistent tenderness and local spread of hypersensitivity as a reflection of retrograde stimulation to uninvolved branches of the free nerve ending, and concomitant sensitization of dorsal horn neurons (DHNs), which may result in the opening of ineffective channels to DHN at different levels in the spinal cord, producing referred pain patterns to muscles that are not the direct source of pain. For example, a sensitized serratus anterior may refer pain to cervical paraspinal muscles causing pain in the lateral neck that may mistakenly be attributed to degenerative changes in the cervical spine.

5.6 Clinical Examination

The possible sources of pain may be identified with a soft tissue assessment for muscle dysfunction. The examination includes the following steps:

a) Observation of asymmetric muscle stiffness and/or spasm. Asymmetry of:
   1. Hip height with associated equal leg length (from anterior superior iliac spine [ASIS] to medial malleolus).
   2. Asymmetry of resting ankle rotation while lying supine with legs extended.

b) Kraus-Weber test for trunk muscle strength and flexibility (▶ Table 5.1).

c) Palpation of muscles and fascia in lower body most often involved as pain generators, demonstrating increased tenderness to pressure relative to a muscle in an uninvolved nonpainful region. (A pressure algometer may provide greater accuracy in determining how much pressure is perceived as uncomfortable.)[12]

The back or neck examination is done in prone position with pillows under hips and ankles (chest and head), which is a stressless position. The supine examination is done lying flat.

In order to apply consistent pressure, the examiners should have an idea of how much pressure they are applying with their fingers (thumb or fingers two to four). Normal muscle in an otherwise healthy adult is generally not tender with pressures below approximately 3.5 kg/cm^2.

The pressure should be applied to all putative pain generating muscles in the region of the pain complaint including putative antagonists. Muscles identified as tender (causing tenderness at lower pressures) should also prompt an examination of the contralateral muscle for comparison.

5.7 Muscle Generated Pain and Spinal Surgery

A pilot study in the Orthopedic Spine Surgery Division of Kaiser Permanente in San Diego to identify and treat specific muscles causing back and leg pain in patients scheduled for spine surgery resulted in four of seven patients' surgeries being cancelled with three still having reported relief 77 weeks after treatment.[13]

If all patients being considered for spine surgery were screened for the presence of MGP, and if identified muscles were treated, it is suggested that successful surgical outcome rates would be higher because prior recognition and treatment of soft tissue pain will decrease unnecessary surgeries.

In the same paper, 97 patients presenting with persistent pain, who had failed typical pain medicine interventions such as epidural steroid injections, facet blocks, radiofrequency ablation, spinal cord stimulation, and spine surgery, were also assessed with the same protocol to identify and treat sensitized muscles. At 77 weeks post treatment, successful reduction in pain and improvement in activities of daily living (ADLs) were sustained, suggesting that soft tissue evaluation should be a standard element of care in FBSS.

5.8 Operative Considerations

Surgeons performing MIS have always understood that muscles are important in postoperative recovery. Indeed, surgical approaches often emphasize muscle sparing in an attempt to improve both the speed of postoperative recovery and functional outcome.

The traditional subperiosteal midline approach sacrifices large portions of the posterior stabilizing elements, including ligaments, tendons, and bony structures. It may also lead to denervation and devascularization of the adjacent muscles. The use of self-retaining retractors may also result in muscle atrophy,[14,15,16] which in turn can lead to decreased force production capacity.[17] Mayer et al[18] evaluated trunk muscle strength in patients who had undergone lumbar surgery and found diminished strength in subjects who had undergone open fusion procedures compared to those who had undergone discectomy. Muscle denervation due to extensive exposure, especially over the facet joint and pars interarticularis, is another source of muscle atrophy. These factors conceptually impact patient recovery and long-term effects of surgery, both at the index level and adjacent segments.[19,20] This topic has been recently reviewed by Kim et al.[21,22]

Stevens et al[20] assessed the appearance of the multifidus muscle via MRI in patients treated by open versus MISS lumbar interbody fusion techniques, and found marked intermuscular edema on MRI at 6 months postsurgery in the open surgery group. In contrast, normal muscle appearance was observed on MRI in patients in the MISS group (▶ Fig. 5.2).

However, it is important to understand that patients after MISS procedures can still suffer from significant MGP, especially if it was present before surgery and was not accurately diagnosed.

The emerging observations concerning suspected MGP as explained above and its treatment, as shown in ▶ Fig. 5.3, can therefore significantly impact the assessment and treatment of patients with spinal disorders. Failure to consider MGP may result in suboptimal outcomes even after the least invasive "technically successful" MIS.

Key Points

- Muscle can be an independent source of pain in patients with degenerative spinal disease (▶ Fig. 5.4).
- Understanding the pathophysiological mechanisms of muscle pain will enhance the capacity of the surgeon to identify muscles as a pre-existing or complicating postsurgical source of pain. Physical therapy and healthy exercise are key to treating muscle generated low back pain (see Chapter 54, ▶ Fig. 5.1).
- Even the least invasive MIS procedure may be compromised by MGP, especially if it was present before surgery.
- Educating patients about MGP can help in reassuring them concerning postoperative discomfort.
- An interdisciplinary approach, consisting of pain management, physiatry, physical therapy, and, when indicated, psychiatry/psychology, improves the ability to diagnose and treat MGP, ideally before considering surgery, and when it occurs after an otherwise successful MIS procedure.

5.9 Conclusion

Muscles as a source of common pain presentations should be included in the pre- and postgraduate curriculum of physicians. Reimbursement coding should be created to encourage a detailed and time-consuming methodology necessary for appropriate soft tissue assessment and treatment in patients being considered for spine surgery and in those with persistent pain following apparently successful surgeries.

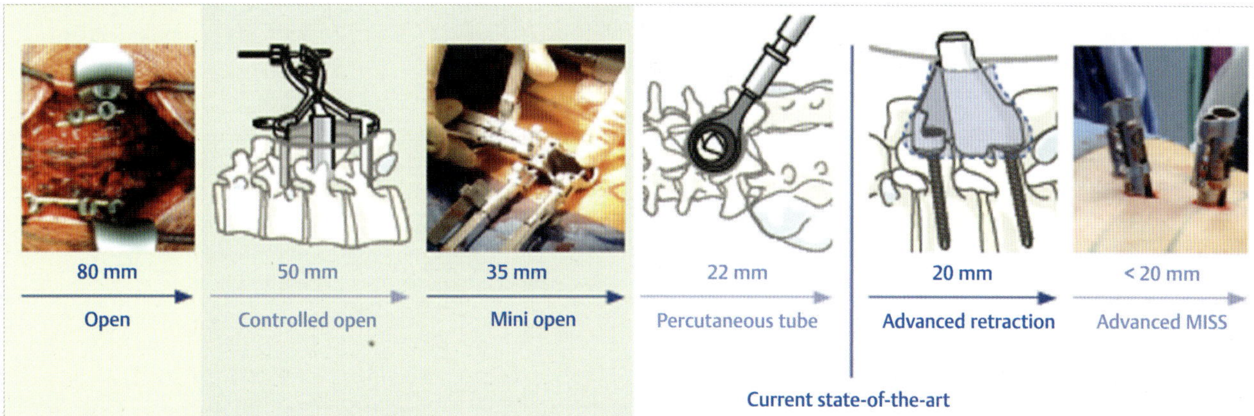

Fig. 5.2 Access progression for posterior fusion surgery of the lumbar spine. More than 90% of surgeries are currently performed by either open macrosurgical approaches or with an only slightly reduced approach extent (i.e., within the range "open" to "mini-open"). Minimally invasive spinal surgery (MISS) includes a variety of approach modifications ranging from "controlled open" to finger-size incisions.

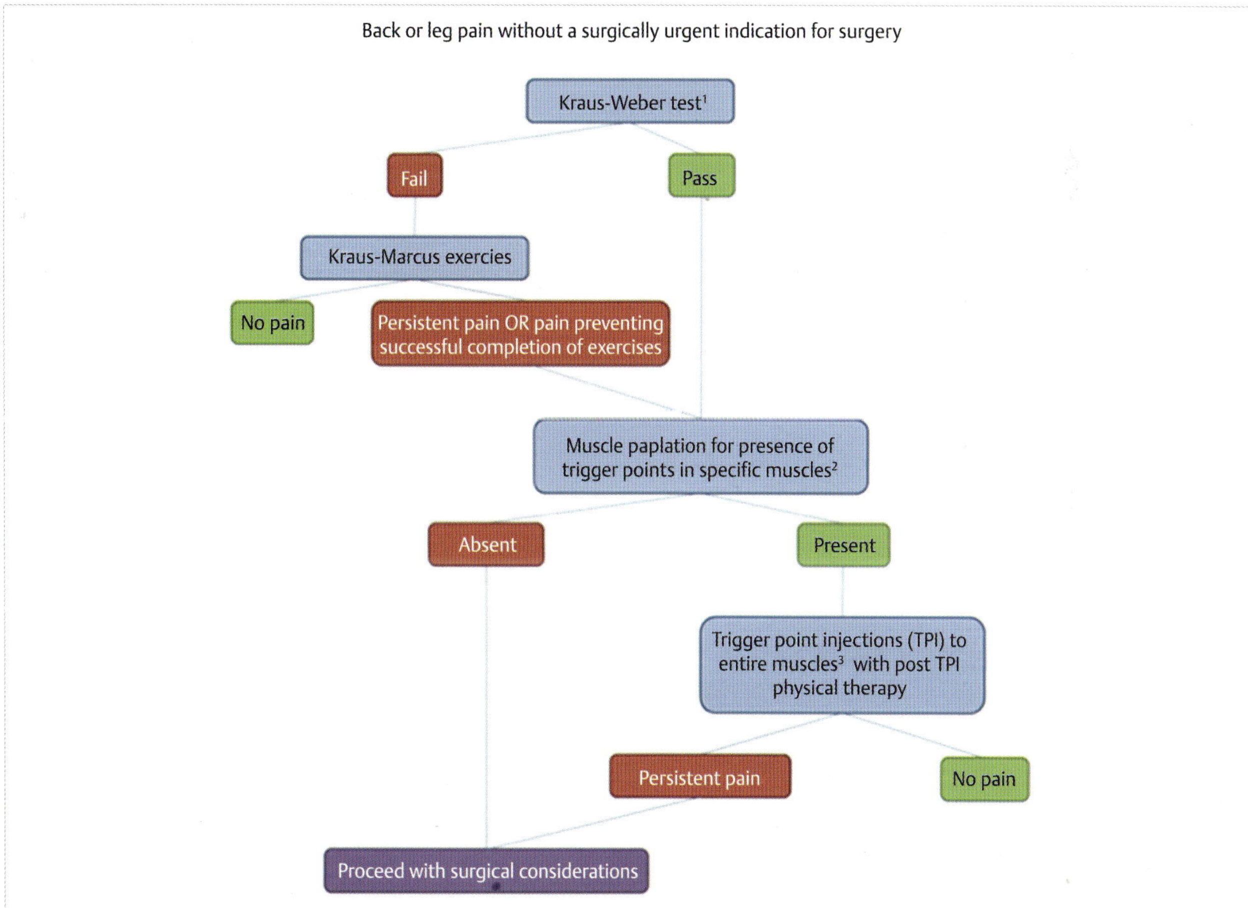

Fig. 5.3 We present a comprehensive approach to evaluate and treat muscle generated pain.[23] We acknowledge that other protocols exist and encourage comparative clinical outcome research. 1. Kraus-Weber test/exercises for key postural muscle strength and flexibility[24,25] for low back pain (and test for range of motion of cervical spine and shoulders). When tension is identified, it may be addressed with psychological/psychiatric interventions. 2. Identification of a specific muscle, not a tender spot in a region, is important because the highest density of nociceptors is in the attachments of the muscle tissue. 3. Specific muscle attachment sites need to be injected in order to produce optimal pain relief.[13]

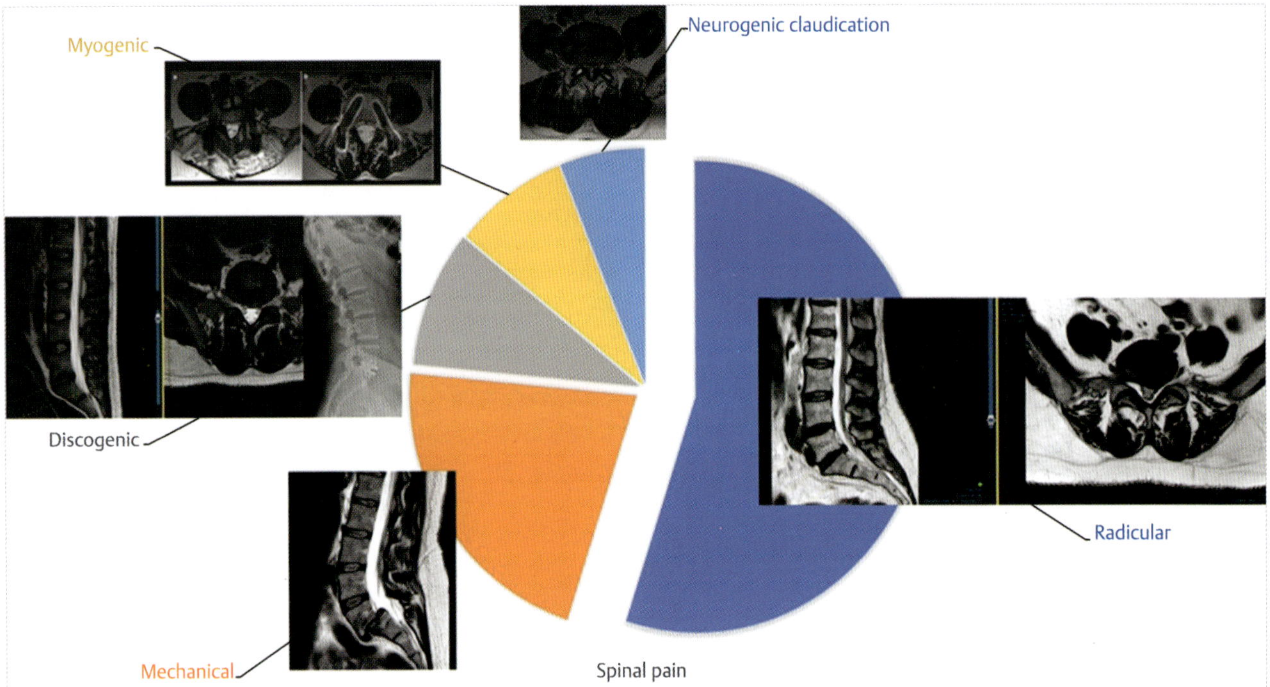

Fig. 5.4 Current concept of putative sources of spinal pain (future studies are needed to determine the incidence of MGP in FBSS): Clockwise from the right: Radicular is the most common (*dark blue*); as we can see, it may be present in the classic scenario of a lumbar disc herniation. Mechanical pain is the second most common where vertebral movement and displacement are the source of pain. Discogenic pain is present in some young patients like in this example of a patient with isolated disc degeneration of L5–S1. Myogenic pain or muscle generated pain (MGP) could be seen in patients with otherwise normal magnetic resonance imaging (MRI) scans or sometimes in patients such as this one who underwent corrective fusion surgery and now shows postoperative MRI findings consistent with muscle fat infiltration and is being diagnosed as suffering from failed back surgery syndrome (FBSS). Neurogenic claudication is mostly present in severe degenerative central stenosis.

References

[1] van Tulder M, Koes B. Chronic low back pain. Am Fam Physician. 2006; 74 (9):1577–1579

[2] Keller RB, Atlas SJ, Soule DN, Singer DE, Deyo RA. Relationship between rates and outcomes of operative treatment for lumbar disc herniation and spinal stenosis. J Bone Joint Surg Am. 1999; 81(6):752–762

[3] Machado GC, Witzleb AJ, Fritsch C, Maher CG, Ferreira PH, Ferreira ML. Patients with sciatica still experience pain and disability 5 years after surgery: a systematic review with meta-analysis of cohort studies. Eur J Pain. 2016; 20(10):1700–1709

[4] Mixter WJ, Barr JS. Rupture of the intervertebral disc with involvement of the spinal canal. N Engl J Med. 1934; 211(5):210–215

[5] Mixter WJ, Ayer JB. Herniation or rupture of the intervertebral disc into the spinal canal: report of thirty-four cases. N Engl J Med. 1935; 213(9):385–393

[6] Fishbain DA, Cole B, Lewis JE, Gao J. What is the evidence that neuropathic pain is present in chronic low back pain and soft tissue syndromes? An evidence-based structured review. Pain Med. 2014; 15(1):4–15

[7] Chan CW, Peng P. Failed back surgery syndrome. Pain Med. 2011; 12(4):577–606

[8] Graven-Nielsen T, Arendt-Nielsen L. Sensory and motor manifestations of muscle pain. J Musculoskeletal Pain. 2008; 16(1–2):93–105

[9] Mense S, Simons DG, Russell IJ. Muscle Pain: Understanding Its Nature, Diagnosis, and Treatment. Lippincott Williams & Wilkins; 2001

[10] Kopell HP, Thompson W. Peripheral Entrapment Neuropathies. Baltimore: Williams & Wilkins; 1963

[11] Marcus NJ, Mense S. Muscle pain: pathophysiology, evaluation, and treatment. In: Bajwa ZH, Wootton RJ, Warfield CA, eds. Principles and Practice of Pain Medicine. 3rd ed. McGraw-Hill Education Medical; 2016

[12] Walton DM, Macdermid JC, Nielson W, Teasell RW, Chiasson M, Brown L. Reliability, standard error, and minimum detectable change of clinical pressure pain threshold testing in people with and without acute neck pain. J Orthop Sports Phys Ther. 2011; 41(9):644–650

[13] Marcus NJ, Shrikhande AA, McCarberg B, Gracely E. A preliminary study to determine if a muscle pain protocol can produce long-term relief in chronic back pain patients. Pain Med. 2013; 14(8):1212–1221

[14] Datta G, Gnanalingham KK, Peterson D, et al. Back pain and disability after lumbar laminectomy: is there a relationship to muscle retraction? Neurosurgery. 2004; 54(6):1413–1420, discussion 1420

[15] Gejo R, Matsui H, Kawaguchi Y, Ishihara H, Tsuji H. Serial changes in trunk muscle performance after posterior lumbar surgery. Spine. 1999; 24 (10):1023–1028

[16] Gille O, Jolivet E, Dousset V, et al. Erector spinae muscle changes on magnetic resonance imaging following lumbar surgery through a posterior approach. Spine. 2007; 32(11):1236–1241

[17] Marras WS, Davis KG, Granata KP. Trunk muscle activities during asymmetric twisting motions. J Electromyogr Kinesiol. 1998; 8(4):247–256

[18] Mayer TG, Vanharanta H, Gatchel RJ, et al. Comparison of CT scan muscle measurements and isokinetic trunk strength in postoperative patients. Spine. 1989; 14(1):33–36

[19] Kim D-Y, Lee S-H, Chung SK, Lee H-Y. Comparison of multifidus muscle atrophy and trunk extension muscle strength: percutaneous versus open pedicle screw fixation. Spine. 2005; 30(1):123–129

[20] Stevens KJ, Spenciner DB, Griffiths KL, et al. Comparison of minimally invasive and conventional open posterolateral lumbar fusion using magnetic resonance imaging and retraction pressure studies. J Spinal Disord Tech. 2006; 19 (2):77–86

[21] Kim CW. Scientific basis of minimally invasive spine surgery: prevention of multifidus muscle injury during posterior lumbar surgery. Spine. 2010; 35 (26) Suppl:S281–S286
[22] Kim CW, Siemionow K, Anderson DG, Phillips FM. The current state of minimally invasive spine surgery. J Bone Joint Surg Am. 2011; 93(6):582–596
[23] Marcus NJ, Gracely EJ, Keefe KO. A comprehensive protocol to diagnose and treat pain of muscular origin may successfully and reliably decrease or eliminate pain in a chronic pain population. Pain Med. 2010; 11(1):25–34
[24] Kraus H, Marcus NJ. The reintroduction of an exercise program to directly treat low back pain of muscular origin. J Back Musculoskeletal Rehabil. 1997; 8(2):95–107
[25] Kraus H, Nagler W, Melleby A. Evaluation of an exercise program for back pain. Am Fam Physician. 1983; 28(3):153–158

Part III

MISS Technology

6 Tubular and Specular Retractors in MISS 56
7 Navigation in MISS 61
8 Robotics: Background and Current Role 79
9 Microscope in MISS 87
10 Endoscope in MISS: How to Adopt and Change 95

III

6 Tubular and Specular Retractors in MISS

Christoph Wipplinger, Sara Lener, Sertac Kirnaz, Ahmed Abdelsalam, Roger Härtl, and Claudius Thomé

Summary

The choice of the retractor system has been controversial since the introduction of minimally invasive spinal surgery (MISS). The great variety of available retractor systems can be categorized into tubular and specular retractors. Both retractor systems have various advantages and shortcomings. The main differences between them are the extent of dissection required in order to insert the retractor and the surgeon's visual field provided by the retractor.

While specular retractors require more extensive dissection than tubular retractors, the visual field is wider and expandable. However, tubular retractors cause far less soft-tissue damage and provide a more targeted approach. The choice of the retractor should, therefore, be based on the surgeon's experience as well as on the spine pathology that needs to be addressed.

Keywords: tubular retractor, specular retractor, minimally invasive spine surgery, lumbar decompression, lumbar disc herniation

6.1 Introduction

Since minimally invasive spinal surgery (MISS) was introduced, the choice of the retractor system has been a controversial topic. One of the main goals of MISS is to reduce trauma to the paraspinal tissues and muscle groups.[1] To achieve this, the retractor should be chosen carefully and adapted to the patient's and surgeon's needs.

Among the most frequently used systems, specular and tubular retractors are the most acclaimed. In 1991, Caspar et al implemented the use of a specular retractor for MISS discectomy procedures.[2] Later, in 1996, Smith and Foley performed the first microendoscopic lumbar discectomy through the so-called microendoscopic discectomy (MED) tubular retractor.[3] Within the past few years, retractor systems have progressively developed in parallel with the increase and advancement of MISS procedures. For example, the Minimal Exposure Tubular Retractor (METRx; Medtronic Sofamor Danek, Memphis, TN) MD tubular retractor system, which was a modified version of the original MED tube, was developed and first described in 2002 and allowed the use of a surgical microscope.[4] Since then, many different MISS retractor systems have emerged, involving both tubular and specular retractors.

The purpose of this chapter is to highlight the different features of tubular and specular retractor systems in MISS.

6.2 Tubular Retractor

The tubular retractor has revolutionized the practice of spinal surgery. While initially developed for endoscopically assisted surgery,[3] it has now become an indispensable tool for MISS surgery. The tubular retractor allows the treatment of focal lesions in a targeted manner without significantly distorting the normal anatomy. Although the initial indication for tubular microsurgery was lumbar microdiscectomy, the versatility of the technique has enabled a large variety of procedures. Today, tubes are used not only for lumbar, but also for cervical and thoracic spine surgery, spinal fusion, and even complex deformity corrections.[5]

Multilevel pathologies can be treated through small incisions and ports, resulting in minimal tissue trauma. Recently, tubular anterior cervical spine approaches have emerged and may replace wide anterior exposures, which have been associated with considerable morbidity such as dysphagia and poor cosmetic results.[6]

There are multiple commercially available tubular retractor systems (▶ Fig. 6.1) consisting of sequential dilators in diameter, all of which are marked in length to select the final appropriate retractor size for the case, several tubular retractors in lengths and diameters, a table clamp, and a holding arm. In practice, the diameter of the tube is dependent on pathology being treated. For example, microdiscectomies or cervical foraminotomies can be accomplished with 14-mm tubes, whereas fusion procedures may require tubes with diameters of up to 22 mm.

Sequential transmuscular dilation minimizes collateral tissue trauma and can better target the site of the pathology in comparison to open approaches. The insertion of a tubular retractor will merely split the paraspinal muscles, minimizing muscle trauma and facilitating rapid recovery after surgery. Tubular retractors are also less prone to cause a crush injury than self-retaining retractors. Furthermore, subperiosteal approaches are also more likely to lead to irreversible denervation of multifidus muscle during dissection.[7]

Pivoting of the tube allows for a larger exposure of the spine with minimal additional muscle dissection. The small size of the approach and the reduced tissue trauma have shown to minimize infection rates, especially in obese patients.[8,9] Subsequently, the reduced complication rates enable patients to recover faster, shortening hospital stays.[10] Apart from the obvious benefits such as less tissue damage, benefits also include socioeconomic advantages, decreasing the economic burden.[11]

The transmuscular approach minimizes dead space at the surgical site created by muscle detachment and extensive soft tissue retraction; thereby, reducing the risk of postoperative fluid collections such as seromas. The close approximation of tissues immediately after removal of the tube without a dead space also reduces the risk of cerebrospinal fluid (CSF) leaks. Small incidental durotomies may not require closure in tubular approaches; however, it is recommended.[12] Despite that, primary dural closure using a standard technique and surgical instruments can be challenging in this setting due to the limited surgical corridor through tubular retractor systems. If a watertight dural closure cannot be achieved, this may predispose patients to complications such as CSF fistula, pseudomeningocele, or wound infection.[13]

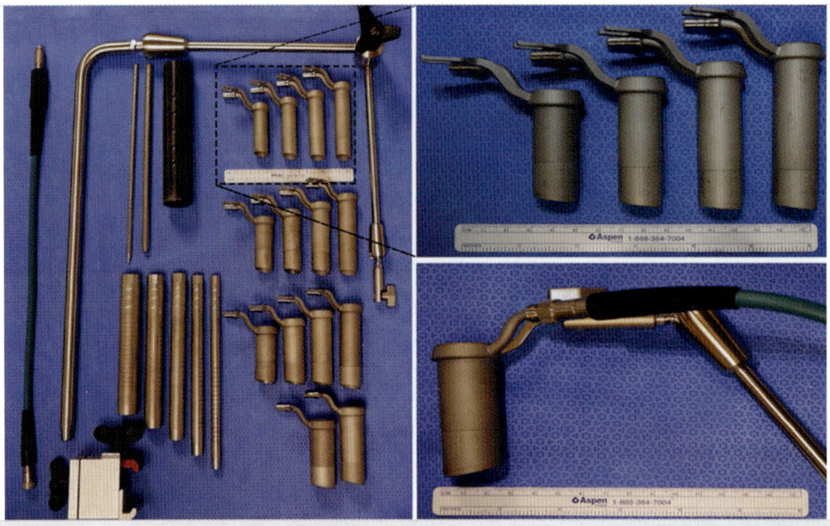

Fig. 6.1 Tubular retractors and sequential dilators (*left* image).

Tubular microsurgery has a more challenging learning curve than many open spinal techniques.[10] Three-dimensional orientation in a deep narrow field can be cumbersome due to the limited exposure of the anatomy, which may even be distorted as a result of the underlying pathology. Therefore, meticulous knowledge of the anatomy and preparation are required in order to be able to target the site of the spinal pathology precisely. As a result, tubular procedures may require extensive radiation that is dependent on the surgeon's experience, but can be overcome by using intraoperative navigation. A main advantage of tubular surgery compared with open or mini-open approaches is that no subperiostal muscle detachment is necessary. Furthermore, the use of tubular techniques in oblique lateral approaches, such as extraforaminal disc herniations or costotransversectomy trajectories, is advantageous as other approaches would require extensive open dissections.[7,14]

6.2.1 Example: Tubular Lumbar Microdiscectomy Approach

A small incision is made approximately 1 to 1.5 cm from the midline over the corresponding herniated disc space and facet joint. A blunt probe is then passed perpendicularly through the incision until the bony surface of the inferior edge of the lamina is encountered. Then a lateral fluoroscopy image should be taken to confirm the dilator position over the lamina/medial facet joint. Once the position is satisfactory, dilators of increasing diameter are inserted with a twisting motion to avoid undue pressure and plunging (special attention should be taken when using plastic sterile covers to not introduce the wrap inside of the wound). The tubular size necessary for a discectomy is approximately 16 mm, depending on the surgeon's experience. Fluoroscopy is then used to confirm that the dilator is positioned directly on the bone at the inferior edge of the lamina with no or minimal intervening soft tissue. The working channel is then secured with a rigid holding arm and directed slightly medially toward the lamina and spinous process (▶ Fig. 6.2). At this point, a muscle layer remaining on the bone often has to be removed using the monopolar. The subsequent steps are carried in a similar fashion as a standard microdiscectomy.

6.3 Specular Retractor

Specular retractors were introduced in order to minimize traditional macroscopic approaches to the spine. In 1991, Caspar utilized spreadable speculae for a less invasive lumbar microdiscectomy[2]. In a subperiostal midline approach, specular retractors are frequently used and offer some advantages. These advantages are predominantly applicable to surgeons who are less experienced with MISS and use the traditional open approach in a minimized fashion.

Except for minor changes, the basic design and mechanism for separating two or more retractor blades have remained relatively unchanged since its introduction. The fundamental structure of most specular retractors includes an elongated rack bar and two retracting arms: one fixed and one movable (▶ Fig. 6.3). Both arms normally extend in a direction perpendicular to the rack bar and the movable arm can be displaced along the rack bar. This is done using a crank, which also acts as a torque lever to activate a pinion mechanism when needed. Below the retractor arms, two blades are provided. The available blades vary in size, length, and design as different indications may require different mechanisms of retraction.[15]

The learning curve for the safe performance of surgeries through specular retractors is known to be steep. A major advantage of this approach is the relatively wide exposure of anatomical structures, which can be more extended at the depth than on the surface. A specular retractor provides a full view over the lamina, ligamentum flavum, and the spinous process, and thereby helps with orientation and eliminates the need to move the retractor cranially or caudally throughout the procedure. Other than tubular approaches, no table bar is needed to hold the retractor in place. Furthermore, this approach can be achieved without the aid of fluoroscopy and is solely based on anatomical landmarks if performed by an experienced spine surgeon. Nevertheless, one fluoroscopic shot is recommended after the final positioning of the retractor. This

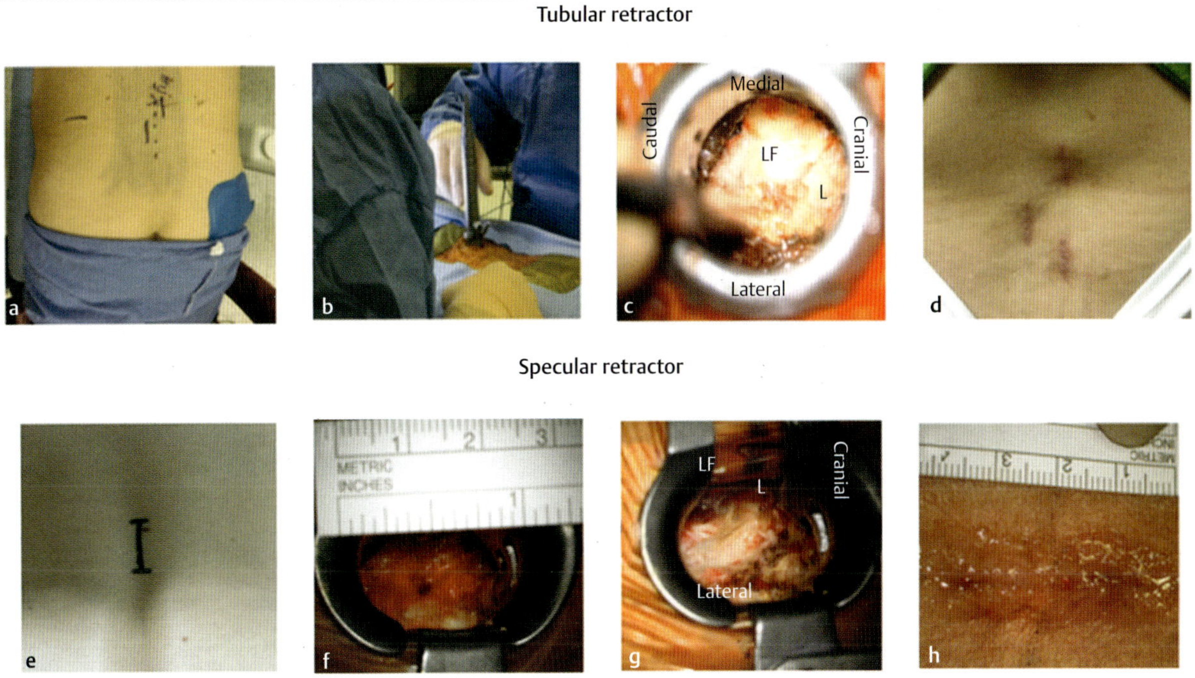

Fig. 6.2 Utilization of tubular and specular retractors, **(a)** paramedian skin marks, **(b)** serial dilation left, **(c)** overview of the operative field through an 18-mm tubular retractor, **(d)** healed scars after multilevel tubular surgery, **(e)** midline skin mark, **(f)** size of the operative field through a specular retractor, **(g)** overview of the operative field through a specular retractor, and **(h)** closed wound after specular surgery.

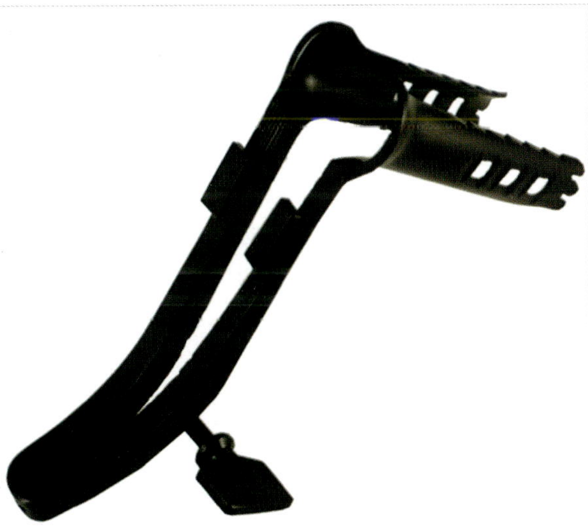

Fig. 6.3 Specular retractor for lumbar discectomy. (© Precision Surgical Instruments Ltd.)

leads to reduced radiation exposure for the surgeon and the patient. When operating with specular retractors, conventional surgical instruments can be used instead of bayoneted instruments necessary for tubular surgery. This may also facilitate the learning curve in MISS.

Mini-open procedures using specular retractors can be performed more easily and under direct vision, yet through small incisions.[16] The view of the operative field is seen in a tridimensional way and the anatomical landmarks can be easily identified. The real perception of depth is only given when using specular retractors. Therefore, the estimation of structures and the real distance handling of instruments is correlated with a lower incidence of dural tears when using a specular retractor as an untrained surgeon.[17] Furthermore, costs regarding the usage of specular retractors are low. They are widely available and the surgical instruments used are the same whether performing the open or mini-open procedure.[17] Furthermore, specular retractors can be used under fluoroscopic guidance as well as under computed tomography navigation.

The prolonged use of self-retaining retractors may cause a reduction in muscle function and has been suspected to increase scar tissue formation. The insertion of open retractors via a subperiosteal approach has been compared with the transmuscular insertion of tubular retractors in the lumbar paraspinal muscles. It was shown that the tubular type resulted in less muscle edema and a lower increase in intramuscular pressure, which is known to correlate with reduced intramuscular blood flow and the potential development of low back pain.[18]

6.3.1 Example: Mini-Open Lumbar Discectomy

The patient is positioned prone and the level of interest is localized under fluoroscopic guidance. The surgeon should stand on the side of the pathology with the assistant standing on the contralateral side. After sterile washing and covering, a 30-mm midline skin incision is made and subcutaneous tissue and fascia are dissected utilizing electrocautery. Muscle insertions at the spinous process are separated by electrocautery and then

Table 6.1 Overview about individual properties, advantages, and limitations

	Tubular retractor	Specular retractor
First description for spine MISS	1996	1991
Approach	Transmuscular	Subperiostal
Visual field	Narrow and fixed, can be extended by wanding the tube	Wide, expandable
Procedures	• Discectomy • Decompression • Foraminotomy • TLIF	• Discectomy • Decompression
Incision	Paramedian	Midline
Navigation/X-ray	Mandatory	Helpful
Visualization	Microscope	Microscope/loupes/headlight
Advantages	• Targeted • Minimized tissue trauma • Visual field extendable by wanding (contralateral side) • Feasible for revision surgery	• Expandable visual field • Little radiation needed • Feasible for revision surgeries • Visual field extendable by wanding (contralateral side)
Limitations	• Fluoroscopy/navigation required • Rigid/narrow visual field	• Increased soft tissue trauma • More limited view to contralateral side • Less targeted approach

Abbreviations: MISS, minimally invasive spine surgery; TLIF, transforaminal lumbar interbody fusion.

bluntly detached using a Cobb elevator. Once the muscles are properly detached and the bony landmarks are exposed, the expandable retractor and counter retractor are inserted, providing a wide overview over the lamina, ligamentum flavum, and spinous process (▶ Fig. 6.2). The subsequent steps are identical to those of a conventional microdiscectomy.

6.4 Conclusion

The type of retractor influences the surgical technique and is dependent on several intraoperative factors (▶ Table 6.1). Nevertheless, a comparison of the conventional lumbar microsurgical subperiosteal and the more recent tubular transmuscular approach showed that the early postoperative outcome after disc surgery (assessed via Visual Analog Scale and Oswestry Disability Index) was equivalent in both groups.[19,20] Therefore, the choice of the retractor should be made reasonably and adjusted to the type of patient and pathology while also taking into consideration the surgeon's skills and training level.

6.5 Future Perspective

A recently published review of the literature indicated that efforts are being made to address tissue ischemia as it pertains to specular retraction—experimental surgical retractors using integrated force and oxygenation sensors monitor[21] as well as "perfusion-stimulating retractors" are still under development.[15]

References

[1] Foley KT, Smith MM, Rampersaud YR. Microendoscopic approach to far-lateral lumbar disc herniation. Neurosurg Focus. 1999; 7(5):e5

[2] Caspar W, Campbell B, Barbier DD, Kretschmmer R, Gotfried Y. The Caspar microsurgical discectomy and comparison with a conventional standard lumbar disc procedure. Neurosurgery. 1991; 28(1):78–86, discussion 86–87

[3] Smith MM, Foley KT. Microendoscopic discectomy (MED): the first 100 cases. Neurosurgery. 1998; 43(3):702

[4] Palmer S. Use of a tubular retractor system in microscopic lumbar discectomy: 1 year prospective results in 135 patients. Neurosurg Focus. 2002; 13(2):E5

[5] Parikh K, Tomasino A, Knopman J, et al. Operative results and learning curve: microscope-assisted tubular microsurgery for 1- and 2-level discectomies and laminectomies. Neurosurg Focus. 2008; 25(2):E14

[6] Kulkarni AG, Patel A, Ankith N. A technical case report on use of tubular retractors for anterior cervical spine surgery. Eur Spine J. 201 8; 27:1:454

[7] Kim CW. Scientific basis of minimally invasive spine surgery: prevention of multifidus muscle injury during posterior lumbar surgery. Spine. 2010; 35 (26):S281–S286

[8] Senker W, Meznik C, Avian A, Berghold A. Perioperative morbidity and complications in minimal access surgery techniques in obese patients with degenerative lumbar disease. Eur Spine J. 2011; 20(7):1182–1187

[9] Shousha M, Cirovic D, Boehm H. Infection rate after minimally invasive noninstrumented spinal surgery based on 4350 procedures. Spine. 2015; 40 (3):201–205

[10] Alimi M, Hofstetter CP, Pyo SY, Paulo D, Härtl R. Minimally invasive laminectomy for lumbar spinal stenosis in patients with and without preoperative spondylolisthesis: clinical outcome and reoperation rates. J Neurosurg Spine. 2015; 22(4):339–352

[11] Oppenheimer JH, DeCastro I, McDonnell DE. Minimally invasive spine technology and minimally invasive spine surgery: a historical review. Neurosurg Focus. 2009; 27(3):E9

[12] Ruban D, O'Toole JE. Management of incidental durotomy in minimally invasive spine surgery. Neurosurg Focus. 2011; 31(4):E15

[13] Tan LA, Takagi I, Straus D, O'Toole JE. Management of intended durotomy in minimally invasive intradural spine surgery: clinical article. J Neurosurg Spine. 2014; 21(2):279–285

[14] Härtl R. The four pillars of minimally invasive spine surgery. In: Härtl R, Korge A, eds. Minimally Invasive Spine Surgery. Stuttgart: Georg Thieme Verlag; 2012

[15] Papavero L. Spinal Retractors, in Manual of Spine Surgery. Springer: Berlin; 2012:27–33

[16] Uehara M, Takahashi J, Kuraishi S, et al. Mini open foraminotomy for cervical radiculopathy: a comparison of large tubular and trimline retractors. Asian Spine J. 2015; 9(4):548–552

[17] Teli M, Lovi A, Brayda-Bruno M, et al. Higher risk of dural tears and recurrent herniation with lumbar micro-endoscopic discectomy. Eur Spine J. 2010; 19 (3):443–450

[18] Kobayashi Y, Sekiguchi M, Konno S, Kikuchi S. Increased intramuscular pressure in lumbar paraspinal muscles and low back pain: model development and expression of substance P in the dorsal root ganglion. Spine. 2010; 35 (15):1423–1428

[19] Brock M, Kunkel P, Papavero L. Lumbar microdiscectomy: subperiosteal versus transmuscular approach and influence on the early postoperative analgesic consumption. Eur Spine J. 2008; 17(4):518–522

[20] Schizas C, Tzinieris N, Tsiridis E, Kosmopoulos V. Minimally invasive versus open transforaminal lumbar interbody fusion: evaluating initial experience. Int Orthop. 2009; 33(6):1683–1688

[21] Fischer G, Talamini M, Marohn M, Kazanzides, et al. Intraoperative ischemia sensing surgical instruments. In: Conference Paper at the First International Conference on Complex Medical Engineering (CME) 2005: May 15-18. Kagawa International Conference Hall, Takamatsu, Japan. 2005

7 Navigation in MISS

Rodrigo Navarro-Ramirez, Alisson R. Teles, Franziska Anna Schmidt, Sertac Kirnaz, and Roger Härtl

Summary

Three-dimensional navigation options offer new opportunities for more precise navigation in minimally invasive spinal surgery (MISS), reduce radiation exposure for the surgical team, and accelerate surgical workflow. Recently, the concept of "total navigation" using intraoperative computed tomography (iCT) navigation (NAV) in spinal surgery has been introduced. Total navigation makes MISS safer and more accurate, and enhances efficient and reproducible workflows. Fluoroscopy and radiation exposure for the surgical staff can be eliminated in the majority of cases.

Keywords: navigation, neuronavigation, spine surgery imaging, intraoperative imaging, localization

7.1 Introduction

Spine surgery and spine instrumentation have been influenced by technological development, allowing treatment of more complex spinal pathology, while maintaining or restoring spinal stability and alignment.[1,2,3] Nowadays, spinal procedures have become more complex, and it is crucial to minimize complications like spinal cord injury, nerve root injury, and vascular injuries as well as dural tears and subsequent cerebrospinal fluid (CSF) leakage .[2,3] Minimizing complications requires surgeon's expertise and familiarity with surgical anatomy that in some cases is greatly facilitated through intraoperative imaging. This allows the surgeon to be precisely oriented despite the real-time anatomical shifting during surgery or when the patient's surgical field is reduced especially in MISS. When using MISS procedures, direct visualization of anatomical landmarks may be compromised and may make it necessary to count on the state-of-the-art imaging technology to reduce the risk of complications.[2,4]

The technology used to acquire intraoperative imaging has evolved from the discovery of X-rays in the late 19th century to the highly sophisticated intraoperative computed tomography (iCT) based navigation tools used today. In this chapter, we will describe the two main modalities of iCT available today, namely, Airo and O-arm.[2,3,5]

Computer-assisted spine surgery (CAS) is a computer-based technology that links spine image, acquired by conventional techniques, such as fluoroscopy and intraoperative cone beam computed tomography (iCBCT), with an accurate representation of intraoperative anatomy.[6,7] This gives the surgeon the ability to manipulate multiplanar CT or fluoroscopic images obtained during the surgical procedure in order to gain orientation intraoperatively and, therefore, enhance the accuracy of spine surgery, which are of upmost importance during spinal instrumentations. CAS can also help to minimize the surgical team's radiation exposure.

Accuracy of navigation systems for pedicle screw placement has been studied extensively in recent years. In summary, CAS has shown to increase screw placement accuracy and decrease the rate of malpositioned screw-related complications (> 95–99%)[8,9,10,11,12,13,14,15,16,17,18] when compared with free-hand and/or fluoroscopy-based techniques.[10,11] In addition, the use of three-dimensional iCT for intraoperative confirmation has the potential to eliminate reoperation for screw malposition.[19] Furthermore, the navigation techniques like iCT (fan beam) may eliminate radiation exposure of the surgical staff. However, the dose received by the patient may be still high. For example, the amount of radiation received from a chest X-ray (two views) is 0.1 mSv, for an upper GI fluoroscopic study, it is 6 mSv, and the mean of an iCT (fan beam) spine procedure is 13 mSv.[14,20]

Here, we present the tips, pearls, and workflow that we have used to perform three-dimensional iCT navigation using the two most common iCT systems available, Airo (Brainlab) and O-arm (Medtronic).

The increasing popularity of MISS has led to dependence upon image guidance, primarily intraoperative fluoroscopy, mainly because limited muscle dissection may prevent adequate exposure of the anatomical landmarks used for traditional free-hand techniques.[21] Although three-dimensional navigation increases instrumentation accuracy and reduces surgeon's exposure to radiation,[22] its implementation into the clinical practice has been challenged by its costs, and by surgeon's concerns about increased operative times, ease of use, integration into the surgical flow, and safety.[14]

In 2013, Härtl et al[23] published a global survey on the use of computer-aided spine surgery that provided interesting data on the use of spinal navigation. In this survey, approximately 80% of the respondents were favorable to the use of spinal navigation. However, despite its widespread availability, only 11% of spine surgeons in North America and Europe used navigation. The routine users of navigation mentioned following advantages: its accuracy, the potential of making complex surgery safer, and minimizing radiation exposure. The nonusers not only indicated lack of equipment and high costs as the most important reasons not to use navigation, but also inadequate training and increasing operative time.

It has been proposed that navigation systems might prolong overall operative time due to the time used for operating room (OR) setup and navigation workflow, as well as the time required to scan and register the patient intraoperatively. In fact, it has been shown that even when the overall operative time is prolonged, the time per screw insertion is shorter due to quicker identification of bony anatomy.[24,25] Of note, the new generation navigation settings require less scanning and registration time.

Hence, application of step-by-step guidelines might overcome potential delays related with the setup and workflow with intraoperative image-guided navigation, making it more efficient, reproducible, and diminishing the overall operative time.[26]

Every navigation system has its own characteristics and, consequently, the workflow, pearls, and pitfalls vary according to the navigation system being used.

We personally have used different systems over time, a journey of transition from conventional fluoroscopy to cone beam

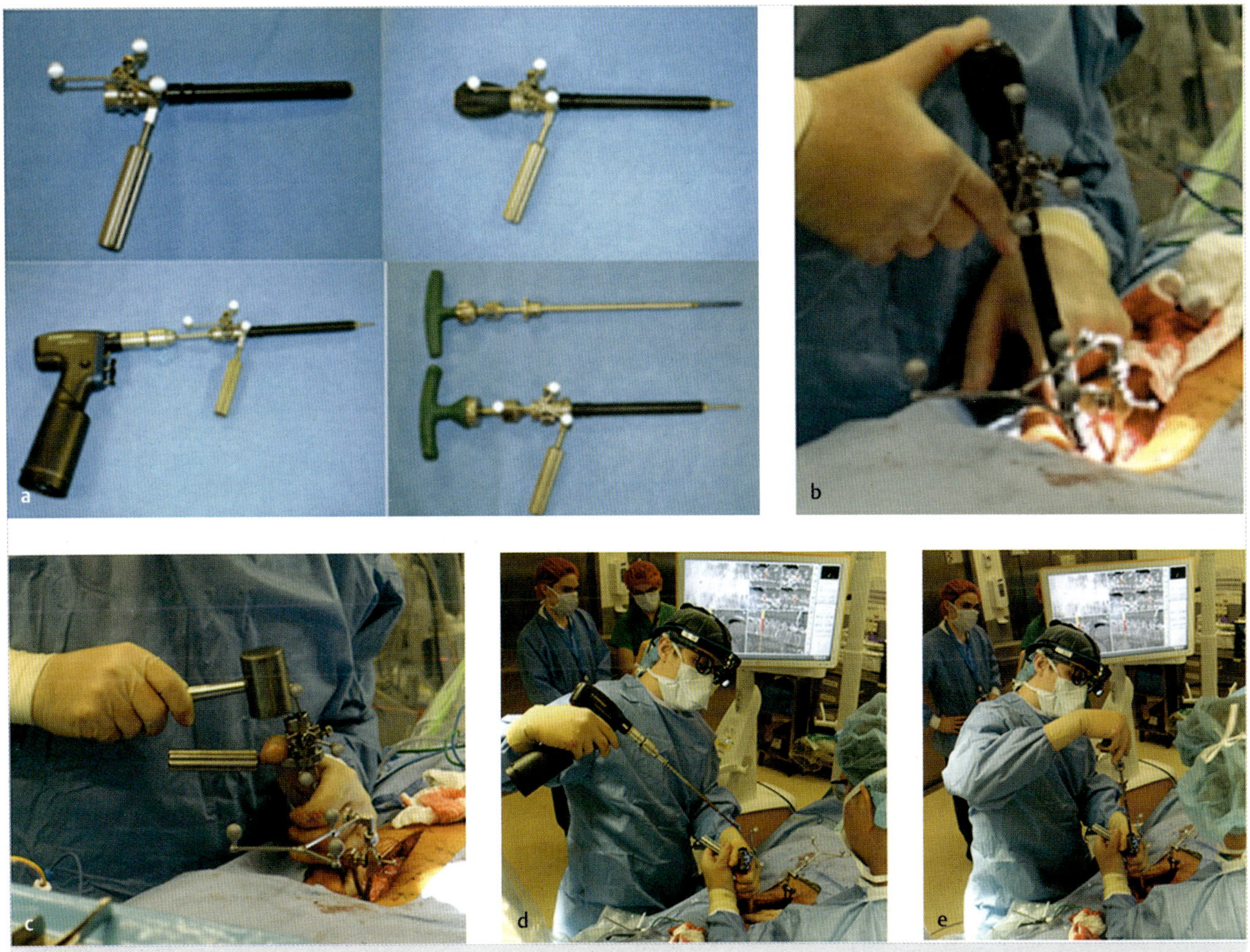

Fig. 7.1 (a) The navigated guide tube comprises a 170-mm-long tube with a 10-mm outer diameter and 8.3-mm cannulation and handle. A tissue protection sleeve and a trocar are made of polyetheretherketone (PEEK) material which facilitate percutaneous placement of the guide tube. An interface for attachment to an infrared reference array is positioned on a 270-degree rotatable collar on the proximal end to allow flexible positioning of the guide tube with respect to the navigation camera. **(b–e)** A drill, tap, and finally a pedicle screw without screw head can be inserted through this guide tube.

three-dimensional navigation, and lastly to three-dimensional iCT navigation in a process that has proven to be effective and perfectly applicable to any clinical practice. Also, we have introduced the concept of "Total Navigation," implying the use of iCT navigation in the steps of surgery, as an attempt to eliminate the radiation exposure for the surgical staff, elimination of K-wires for instrumentation,[27] and elimination of pedicle probe.

The elimination of K-wires represents a major improvement in this setting. Usually, the systems that use three-dimensional navigation for percutaneous screw placement work via K-wires and require a separate navigation of multiple instruments, such as the drill guide, awl, tap, and, finally, the screw. The idea behind the creation of a navigated guide tube was to reduce the number of instruments that need to be navigated and the potential risks associated with the K-wires (i.e., they can break or bend during the procedure and pose risk of visceral or vascular injuries). This navigated tube is attached to a reference array and is used to determine the ideal pedicle trajectory; an appropriately sized pedicle screw is simulated using the navigation software, and the navigated tube is gently impacted so that the teeth would hold on to the bony anatomy. A drill, tap, and finally a pedicle screw without screw head can be inserted through this guide tube[27] (▶ Fig. 7.1).

> Total three-dimensional navigation makes MISS safer and more accurate, eliminates fluoroscopy, and enhances efficient and reproducible workflows.

7.2 Technology

The initial step in integrating CAS with any type of spinal procedure is the acquisition of multiple successive images of the region of interest, a process that can be accomplished with either fluoroscopy or computed tomography (CT).[28] The CAS or image guidance technology (IGT) is available in a variety of setups, which may be differentiated according to the manner in which these images are captured, processed, and presented to the surgeon.[28] Usually, the elements that compose a navigation system

are: (1) a system for image acquisition that allows for the tracking of specialized instruments in relation to a single or multiple reference points attached to suitable anatomic landmarks and (2) a computer workstation that reconfigures this data set into a series of multiplanar images that are displayed on a monitor along with the relative position of any instrumentation within the operative field.[28]

7.3 Image Acquisition

Usually, the elements that allow for image acquisition consist of a camera optical localizer that interfaces with the image-processing computer workstation through emission of infrared light to the operative field or an electromagnetic (EM) registration system. Passive reflective spheres placed in a handheld navigational tool serve as the connection between the surgeon and the computer workstation. These passive reflectors can be also attached to the traditional surgical instruments like the drill guide, a tap, or a pedicle screwdriver. In order to calculate accurately the position of the instruments in the surgical field and the anatomic points where the tip of the instruments is resting, the spacing and positioning of the passive reflectors on each navigational probe or customized trackable surgical instrument are programmed into the computer workstation. In fact, after the infrared light is transmitted toward the operative field and reflected back to the optical localizer by the passive reflectors, the information is conveyed to the computer workstation allowing calculation of the spatial location, through matching spinal image data (CT or fluoroscopic images) to its corresponding surgical anatomy.[2,3]

7.4 Registration System

The accurate translation of spatial information into detailed renderings of spinal anatomy necessitates a stable frame of reference that enables the computer assisted system to calculate the relative positioning of instruments within the surgical field in all three dimensions. This process of establishing a relation between the "real" coordinate system, as defined by the patient's array, and the "virtual" coordinate system of the imaging data is called registration. Different registration techniques can be applied.[2,5]

7.4.1 Point-Matching Registration Technique

Several anatomical points are selected in CT and magnetic resonance imaging (MRI) data set and in the corresponding anatomy. These points have to be selected for each spinal level to be instrumented. Any anatomical landmark that can be identified, both preoperatively and intraoperatively, can be used as a reference point. Examples of some common points are: the tip of a spinous or transverse process or the apex of a facet joint. After selecting one of these points in the CT image data, the tip of the navigation tool is placed on the corresponding point in the surgical field, with the reflective spheres on the tool handle aimed toward the camera. Infrared light from the camera is reflected off the spheres, back toward the camera, and into the computer, which calculates the spatial position of the probe's tip and the anatomic structure it is resting on. This effectively "links" the point selected in the image data with the point selected in the surgical field. If a minimum of three points are registered, when the probe is placed on any other point in the surgical field, the corresponding point in the image data set will be identified on the computer workstation. The disadvantage of this technique is that any error on the part of the surgeon in selecting the specific anatomic points in the surgical field will result in varying degrees of navigational inaccuracy. This paired point protocol can also be performed in conjunction with surface matching.[2]

Another method of registration is CT-fluoro matching. This technique is used sometimes when the navigation system is preoperative CT based. When using this technique, the preoperative CT is matched to intraoperative two-dimensional fluro images of the spine, taken from different angles of the patient.[29]

7.4.2 Surface-Matching Registration Technique

Surface matching is a supplementary registration technique in which the surgeon randomly selects multiple anatomical points on the exposed posterior elements to provide supplementary topographic data. This technique does not preclude prior selection of the points in the image set, although several discrete points in both the image data set and in the surgical field are frequently needed to improve the accuracy of surface mapping. The positional information of these points is transferred to the workstation, and a topographic map of the selected anatomy is created and "matched" to the patient's image set. The concomitant use of the point-to-point and surface-matching approaches was shown to result in a significantly lower mean registration error compared with that of paired point matching alone for the insertion of pedicle screws.[2]

7.4.3 Automated Registration

Automated registration is performed without any input from the surgeon and with less potential for registration error. It can be performed only when the image data is acquired intraoperatively. This technique involves attaching a reference frame with reflective spheres to some site in the exposed spinal anatomy or, in lumbar surgery, to the iliac crest. A second reference frame is built into the intraoperative CT imaging scanner or fluoroscope. As the intraoperative images are acquired, the two reference frames allow for registration to occur without the need for the surgeon's input. The CT scanner or fluoroscope can then be removed, and real-time navigation of up to five separate spinal levels can be performed.[2,28,30]

7.5 Tracking System

The image guided navigation systems utilize either optical or EM tracking systems.[28]

7.5.1 Optical Tracking

As previously mentioned with the optical systems, a source produces a series of pulsed beam infrared light that are passively

reflected off the spheres on the surgical instruments and afterwards captured by a specialized camera or, alternatively, the camera may detect the infrared light that is actively emitted by an array of diodes that are fixed to the instruments and any number of reference points. The positional information obtained with these infrared signals is merged with the reference data that was previously acquired during the anatomic registration process, allowing specific location of the instrument to be identified in space and displayed on multiplanar images of the spine. The use of infrared wavelengths minimizes the distortion that may be caused by any surrounding metal or electrical fields present within the OR. The successful functioning of the optical system depends on a clear "line-of-sight" between the tracking device and the surgical field. The reflective array integral to all optical tracking systems increases the size and weight of these specialized instruments, which may make them more unwieldy for the surgeon to handle. It has also been suggested in the anesthesia literature that this infrared technology may interfere with pulse oximetry monitoring during anesthesia.

7.5.2 Electromagnetic Registration Systems

These systems have been developed as another method for tracking the location of instruments during surgical navigation to address the disadvantages of optical devices, namely, the need of a clear "line-of-sight" between the tracking device and the passive signal emitters (reflective spheres) in the surgical field.[31] This may restrict the operator's normal range of movement and thus limit the intuitive handling of the instruments. Moreover, the trackers needed for optical systems with active and passive reflectors are attached to the instruments and to the operation areas to be referenced and have anatomical and ergonomic disadvantages. For one thing, the instruments used are significantly larger and heavier, resulting in poorer ergonomics and handling for the operator.

In the EM systems, three orthogonal EM fields are generated by a transmitter attached to a fixed anatomic reference point, such as a spinous process. The positional data of these instruments are collected by a receiver and integrated to facilitate navigation. Since a line of sight is not required, the surgeon and nursing staff are able to work freely within the operative field. However, EM image guidance may be compromised by metal artifacts, including surgical implants, as well as by any EM fields originating from other equipment in the OR such as monopolar electrocautery, electrocardiogram monitoring, and cell phones. Given the limited area of these EM fields, the transmitter may also need to be repeatedly transferred to additional anatomic structures to obtain sufficient tracking information for multilevel procedures.[28,32]

7.6 Types of Navigation Systems

The two primary options for intraoperative imaging of the spine are still radiography and fluoroscopy. C-arm fluoroscopy remains a low cost and widely available mode of intraoperative image acquisition, which allows for the rapid and serial visualization of two-dimensional images in real time.[33]

Nonetheless, the past three decades of image-guided spine surgery have witnessed the development of multiple modalities for intraoperative imaging and navigation. The ultimate utility of these technologies depends on a critical appraisal of the unique advantages and disadvantages of each system (▶ Fig. 7.2).[2,34]

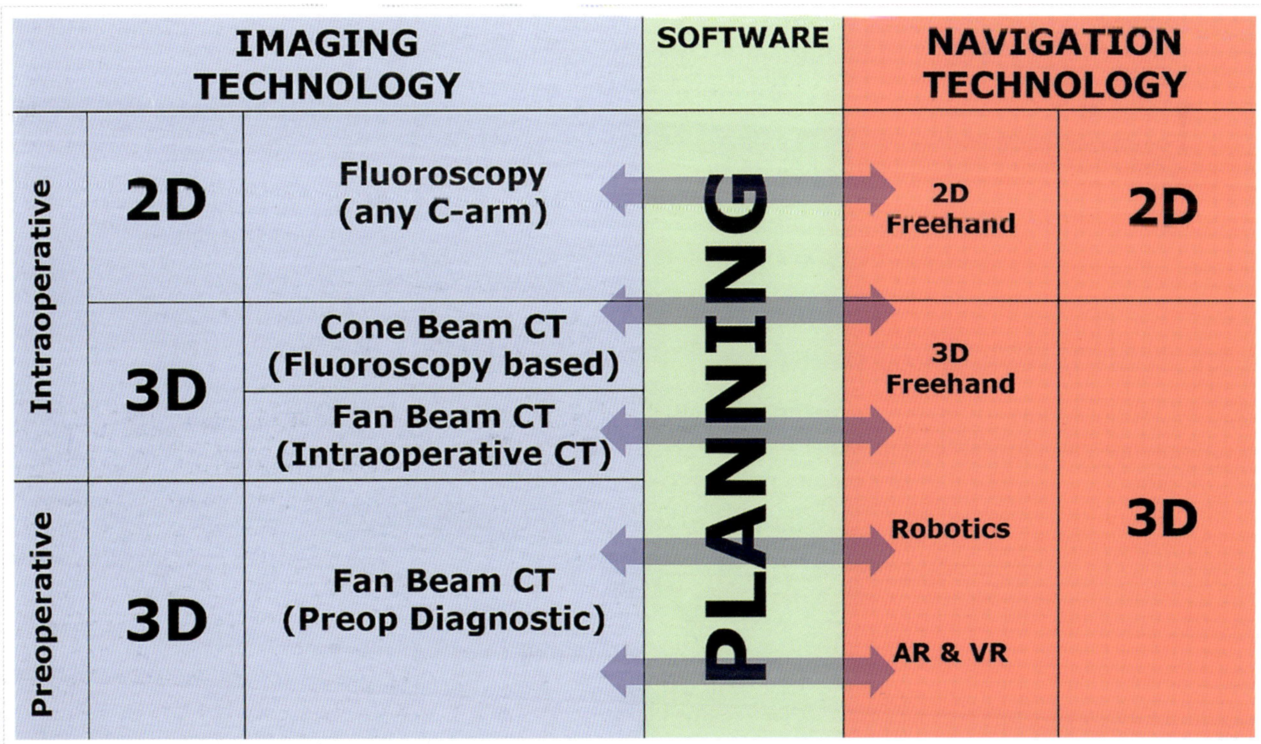

Fig. 7.2 Types of navigational systems.

7.6.1 Preoperative CT-Based Navigation/ Computer-Based Tomography

The first available mode of intraoperative navigation was this modality. This technique utilizes preoperative thin-slice scans and one of several registration processes to create a data set, which forms the basis for intraoperative navigation. In fact, prior to the surgery, a two-dimensional thin-cut CT through the region of interest is obtained and uploaded to a workstation where it creates a virtual three-dimensional reconstruction that can be used for planning the surgery, simulating the implants, etc. On this preoperative reconstruction, anatomical landmarks are selected for intraoperative registration.[29,34]

However, preoperative CT scans are acquired with the patient in a supine position, while during surgery patients are usually in the prone position. The resulting vertebral shift and realignment creates a risk for navigation errors. Therefore, to account for shifting anatomy during surgery, each level must be registered separately to accurately plan and perform the surgery.[33,35] One significant disadvantage of CT-based guidance systems is the need for surgeon-dependent registration of anatomic landmarks on preoperative CT images and the corresponding anatomy of the patient intraoperatively. In addition, extensive bony exposure is required for adequate registration and it may be difficult to identify landmarks for registration in patients with prior laminectomies.[33,34]

During navigation, the surgeon is presented reformatted CT images, on virtual three-dimensional multiplanar image reconstructions, with the selected screw entry point and trajectory superimposed on the images. This information is updated in real time as adjustments are made to the selected trajectory in the surgical field.[36]

One of the disadvantages of this technology was increased radiation exposure to the patient preoperatively.[33]

7.6.2 Intraoperative Image-Based Navigation

Intraoperative image-based navigation systems eliminate the need for surgeon-dependent registration step because the system is automatically registered through the acquisition of images intraoperatively. Thus, the need for spinal exposure for point matching is obviated. Furthermore, in this setting, as images are obtained after patient positioning, they are an accurate representation of vertebral anatomy at the time of surgery.[30]

Two-Dimensional Navigation—Fluoroscopy Based

"Virtual fluoroscopy" or two-dimensional fluoroscopy-based navigation is a strategy that combines a standard two-dimensional C-arm with a computer navigation system. It uses standard anteroposterior (AP) and lateral images of the spine acquired immediately before the start of the procedure.[36] Registration is performed automatically with a reference frame attached to the C-arm.[34] A series of fluoroscopy images in AP, lateral, and sometimes the pedicle oblique views are acquired with a reference frame attached to a stable anatomical landmark, often a spinous process in the vicinity of the vertebrae that will be operated. These images are transferred to the navigation workstation, and this data set is used to navigate implants on the virtual anatomy viewed on the screen (▶ Fig. 7.3). An infrared camera aimed at the reference arc and navigation tools allows continuous recognition of the navigation tools in relation to the relevant anatomy. A continuous "line of sight" must be kept between the infrared camera, the reference arc, and the navigation tools. The accuracy of the system will be maintained as long as the stability of the reference arc is maintained, motion segments do not change their position compared to acquired images, and the navigation tools are kept in line with the desired trajectory. Therefore, fluoro-based navigation allows a completely automatic registration of the spine, correction of image distortion, and reduction of radiation exposure to the staff; however, it is limited to two-dimensional projection images. As it does not provide three-dimensional visualization of the spinal anatomy during navigation, the risk of navigation errors is increased and abnormal axial anatomy is more likely to remain unrecognized. Errors may also be greater in cases of: poor bone quality, excess intra-abdominal gas, morbid obesity, spinal deformity, prior surgery, and congenital anomalies. Furthermore, image resolution is typically best in the center of the field and any structures around the periphery may appear distorted secondary to parallax, so to maintain the accuracy of navigation across several spinal segments, the process of data acquisition and anatomic registration may need to be repeated several times.[30,33,34]

In summary, two-dimensional navigation provides an easier learning curve for surgeons who are familiar and very comfortable with conventional anterior-posterior-lateral fluoroscopy. It is readily available and is easily incorporated into the workflow when using devices or techniques that require real-time X-ray control and require that fluoroscopy be brought into surgery. Such procedures include: cement injection in vertebroplasty procedures, kyphoplasty procedures, and the use of K-wires. Two-dimensional navigation can also be applied in situations that require frequent radiographic updates because of anatomy changes during surgery, such as translumbar discectomy and fusion procedures like extraforaminal lumbar interbody fusion, where the cage placement and its relationship between vertebrae require X-ray exposure. In these situations, 2DNAV will not eliminate the need for fluoroscopy, but can significantly reduce the need of continuous X-ray and will help to improve the workflow. For example, 2DNAV reduces the operative time and the risk of intraoperative contamination because the C-arm does not need to be continually repositioned during the case. This strategy is also preferable to preoperative CT-based navigation, which necessitates a suitable preoperative CT that must be matched to the corresponding anatomic structures by a manual registration process before navigation may proceed.

This navigational system is a relatively inexpensive navigational system (compared to three-dimensional navigation) that combines the benefits of navigation with affordable purchasing and maintenance costs, which can be of upmost importance when there are economic and infrastructural challenges. We have encouraged the use of navigation technologies whenever possible. We advocated the use of navigation whenever possible. During our annual mission in Tanzania, we effectively helped to implement potable hardware and two-dimensional navigation system in a hospital that had no prior experiences with such equipment.[37]

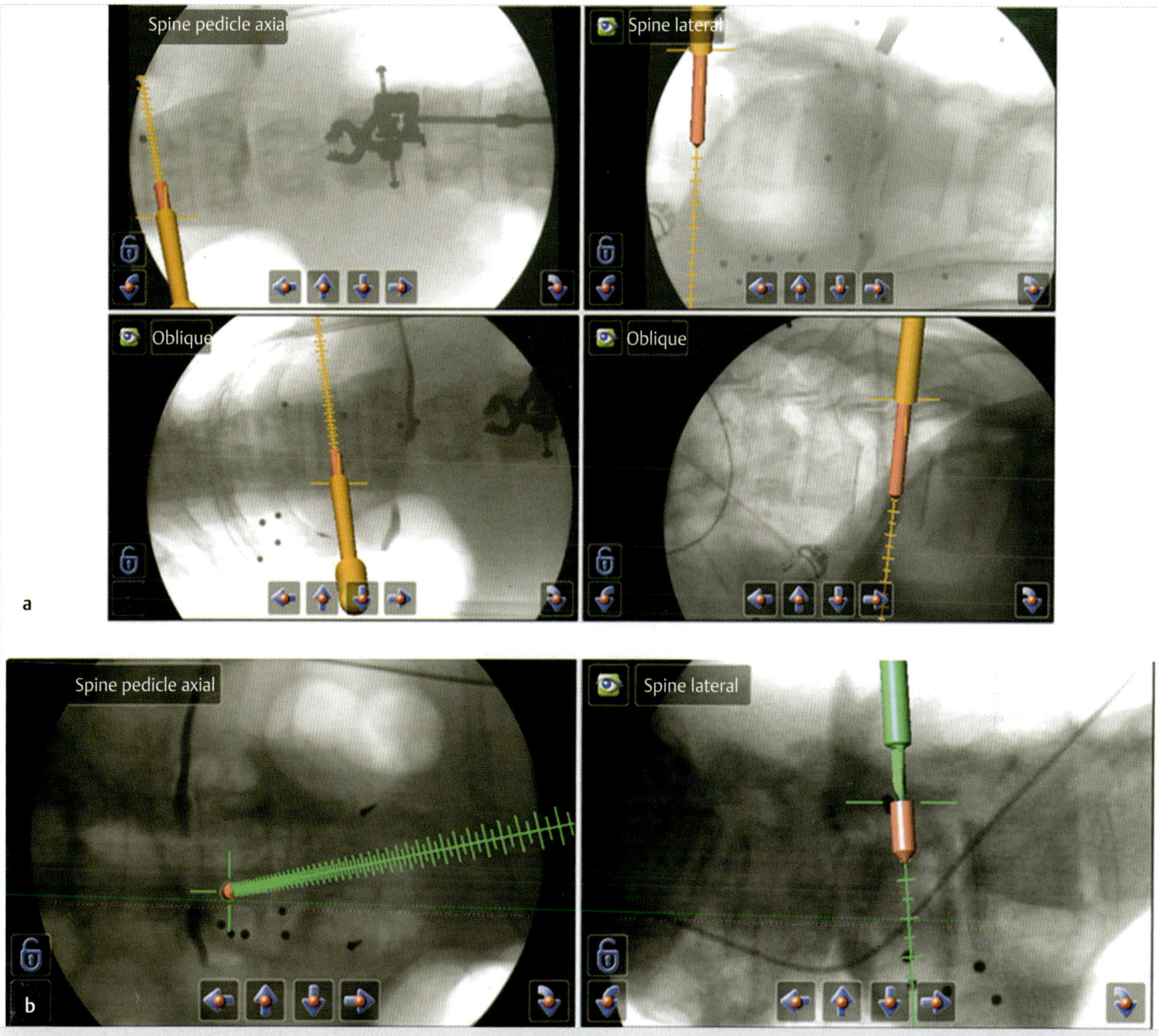

Fig. 7.3 Workstation screen demonstrating a fluoroscopic navigational system. **(a)** Standard anteroposterior (AP) and lateral views are provided with superimposed simulation to determine the ideal pedicle entry point, trajectory, and the appropriate pedicle screw size. **(b)** Simulation to determine the ideal medial/lateral trajectory—to avoid medial pedicle violation, initially a pedicle screw is simulated that is no longer than the pedicle. If this short, simulated screw does not breach the medial border of the pedicle on the AP view and seems to be in perfect medial/lateral position, simulation is lengthened until the desired screw length is achieved. (Used with permission from Njoku et al.[37])

Three-Dimensional Navigation—Fluoroscopy Based

The first system to appear was the three-dimensional fluoroscopy. It uses an isocentric C-arm fluoroscope or an enclosed fluoroscopy-based technology called cone beam CT (iCBCT) to generate a three-dimensional data set intraoperatively that can be used for surgical navigation when combined with an image guided system. The fluoroscope obtains multiple images during an automated 190 degrees rotation around the patient and these images are automatically reconstructed into multiplanar axial, coronal, and sagittal anatomic views.[38]

The iCBCT technology is a modality where a high-resolution three-dimensional view is acquired from the "spin" of a cone-shaped X-ray beam around the patient to a flat panel detector.[34,39] Embodiments of iCBCT include fixed-room C-arms, mobile C-arms, mobile U-arms, and mobile O-arms.[40] The multiple images generated by the spin are processed into a three-dimensional volumetric data set (axial, sagittal, and coronal anatomic CT-like views).[26,34] These reformatted images have less quality than the conventional CT imaging but are superior to isocentric C-arm imaging.

Like two-dimensional fluoroscopy-based navigation, iCBCT-based navigation systems perform automatic registration and eliminate the error caused by anatomic shift by scanning the patient in the surgical position.[41] The main disadvantage of iCBCT compared to intraoperative CT-based navigation, apart from the quality of the image, is that only several levels can be visualized at a time, depending on the scan volume per "spin." This is particularly relevant for large deformity surgeries where the entire surgical site cannot be included within one "spin," and the iCBCT device must be re-centered.[34]

At the end of the surgery, if the accuracy of the hardware needs to be checked, the axial reconstituted can be obtained right away to confirm the accurate placement of the hardware in all three planes (axial, coronal, and sagittal).[34]

Intraoperative exposure to radiation is of concern to both patients and the surgical team. When using these navigational systems, the acquisition of three-dimensional images of the surgical field is done while the surgical team and OR staff leave the room or stand behind a lead shield, and thus are removed from radiation exposure. However, this technique implies higher radiation for the patient.[42,43]

Intraoperative CT (iCT) Scan Navigation

The iCT navigation technology uses a portable CT scanner that translates in the rostral to caudal axis over the patient. The iCT navigation workstation registers the patient's anatomy and creates three-dimensional images using a fan beam CT scanner for image acquisition (▶ Fig. 7.4). These images allow for navigated instrumentation and for intraoperative planning throughout the procedure (e.g., one can plan the accurate measurement of the implants).[34]

The iCT computer-guided navigation technique affords immediate survey of screw/implants position and intraoperative revision.[44] Some advantages are the quality of the image that can be very similar to a diagnostic CT scanner for bone and soft tissue and much better than its previous generation of iCBCT machines.

Another advantage of iCT is that it has an extended scan volume capacity, which eliminates the need to re-center the device even in large deformity cases. Disadvantages include high cost, inferior ergonomics compared to two-dimensional navigation and some of the three-dimensional fluoroscopy-based navigation devices, increased preparation time, and less flexibility due to requirements for specialized operating tables.[34]

The latest generation of iCT overcame some of the limitations, such as flexibility and bigger size of the gantry.[14] Similar to the iCBCT, OR staff is not exposed to radiation, but the technique entails a higher radiation exposure for the patient.[34]

7.6.3 Robotic Navigation

Robotic navigation is the one of the most recent developments in spinal navigation.

On a specially designed graphic user interface with specific software, the surgeon uses preoperatively acquired CT images to plan the trajectory of the screws.

Intraoperatively fluoroscopic images (AP and lateral views) are obtained in order to facilitate automated registration. During navigation, the robotic arm moves into the appropriate position to guide screw insertion accurately along the appropriate trajectory.[2] Intraoperative image intensifier X-rays with targeting devices are then matched with the CT-based virtual images, as well as the surgeon's plan. A clamp is attached to the spinous process, or a minimally invasive frame is mounted on the iliac crest and on a spinous process. A miniature robot is then attached to the clamp and/or frame. On the basis of combined CT scan and image intensifier data, the robot aligns itself to the desired entry point and trajectory, as dictated by the surgeon's preoperative plan.[4]

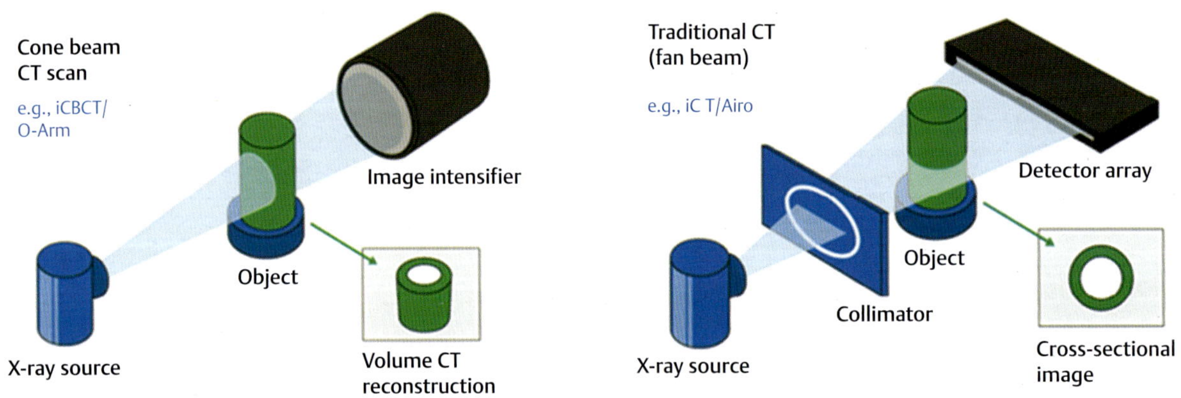

- Emits a "cone type" X-ray and is detected by a flat panel sensor
- Lower radiation dosage
- Lower cost
- Less artifacts with metallic objects
- No soft tissue definition
- Available for mobile 3D C-arm
- Possible to operate by nonradiologists

- Emits a "fan type" X-ray and is detected by a linear detector array
- Greater soft tissue definition
- Greater bone resolution
- Available for mobile and intraoperative utilization

Fig. 7.4 Differences between intraoperative computed tomography (iCT) (fan beam) and intraoperative cone beam computed tomography (iCBCT) (cone beam). Workstation screen demonstrating a fluoroscopic navigational system. Although iCT and iCBCT bear some similarities in the nature of the images they produce, they are inherently different imaging modalities. iCBCT is classified as a mobile X-ray system and uses a cone beam configuration, whereas iCT is classified as a true or conventional computed tomography (CT) scanner that uses a fan beam configuration.

Table 7.1 Advantages and disadvantages of the different navigational systems[5]

	Fluoroscopy	2D fluoro NAV	3D cbCT	3D iCT	3D preoperative CT
Major advantage	Only true real-time imaging modality	Navigation may be performed using images acquired intraoperatively in the surgical position. Automatic registration is possible	Three-dimensional images may be acquired during surgery and used for navigation	Higher resolution imaging and extended scan volume when compared to cbCT	Preoperative CT may be coupled to intraoperative navigation system
Need for intraoperative image acquisition?	Yes	Yes	Yes	Yes	No
Requires additional preoperative imaging?	No	No	No	No	Yes
Need for reregistration for multiple level surgeries?	No	No	No	No	Yes
Real-time image?	Yes	Yes (if needed)	Yes (if needed)	No	No
Screw accuracy	♦♦	♦♦	♦♦♦♦	♦♦♦♦	♦♦♦
Bone quality image	♦♦	♦♦	♦♦♦♦	♦♦♦♦	♦♦♦♦
Soft tissue quality image	–	–	♦	♦♦♦	♦♦♦♦
Surgical team's radiation exposure	♦♦♦♦	♦♦♦	–	–	–
Patient's radiation exposure	♦♦	♦	♦♦♦	♦♦♦♦	♦♦♦♦ (pre- + /– post-op)
Cost	♦	♦♦	♦♦♦♦	♦♦♦♦	♦♦♦
Level of expertise	♦	♦♦♦	♦♦♦♦	♦♦♦♦	♦♦♦
Hardware limitations (special calibrated tools)	No	No	Yes	Yes	Yes

Abbreviations: 3D cbCT, intraoperative cone beam computed tomography; 3D iCT, three-dimensional intraoperative computed tomography; CT, computed tomography.

Studies reporting procedures using robotic surgery have found high levels of accuracy for implant placements. The downsides of robotic surgery include the fact that active tracking is not possible, and that implant accuracy can only be checked after surgery via CT scan (▶ Table 7.1).[4]

7.6.4 Technique

Although iCT and iCBCT bear some similarities in the nature of the images they produce, they are inherently different imaging modalities. iCBCT is classified as a mobile X-ray system and uses a cone beam configuration, whereas iCT is classified as a true or conventional CT scanner that uses a fan beam configuration. In the interest of reflecting our experience with the navigation systems, we will describe the workflows for the two most common iCT navigation systems, Airo® and O-arm®. However, we acknowledge the navigation modalities presented are not limited to these two brands and analogous brands are referenced under the above classification.

Airo-iCT Operating Room Setup

The iCT-guided NAV included the CT scanner, an image-guidance system, an infrared tracking camera navigation system (Brainlab CurveTM, Brainlab AG, Feldkirchen, Germany), and a patient reference array (RA) (Brainlab AG, Feldkirchen, Germany). The design of the iCT scanner combined a large gantry opening (107 cm) with a slim gantry (30.5 × 38 cm) and a small footprint (1.5 m^2). Scan capacity (length of the image acquired) is approximately 60 cm. The suspension-controlled electrical drive system allowed the machinery to be moved around the OR. A mobile, radiolucent carbon fiber table (Trumpf TruSystem 7500, TRUMPF Inc., Farmington, Connecticut, USA) was attached to the gantry during surgery. iCT and CurveTM systems were connected to an automatic image-transfer device and an image patient co-registration that assisted in navigation. Precalibrated or manually calibrated instruments could be used with navigation for enhanced workflow[14] (▶ Table 7.2 and ▶ Fig. 7.5).

Airo Setup of the iCT NAV for "Total Navigation"

a) Before surgery, the iCT NAV is positioned parallel to the rail system and the gantry, facing anesthesia (▶ Fig. 7.5a).
b) After the patient is anesthetized on a transport bed parallel to the gantry, the gantry of the portable iCT system is rotated perpendicular to the rails into the scan position (▶ Fig. 7.5b).
c) Hereafter, a Trumpf carbon fiber tabletop with a T3 frame is connected to the Trumpf column on the integrated rail system.
d) Intubation and insertion of the needle electrodes for EMG monitoring is conducted, followed by flipping the patient onto the T3 frame.
e) Next, the patient is positioned on and taped to the table. Adequate taping is important since it minimizes anatomical displacement, especially in obese patients. Care has to be taken not to tape too tightly in order to avoid skin necrosis or pressure points.

Table 7.2 Tips to improve accuracy in intraoperative computed tomography guided navigation[14]

Draping	• Securing the patient with tape to the OR table minimizes tissue movement • Tape across the chest and hips and laterally from the patient's side downwards
Intraoperative scan	• Include anatomic landmarks (e.g., lumbar spine: sacrum and/or the lowest and/or the first rib), allowing accurate determination of the index level/pathology • Obtain intraoperative CT immediately before it is actually needed (sometimes after the anatomic structures have been exposed, e.g., posterior cervical cases, this minimizes the chances of shift and inaccuracies caused by surgical manipulation)
Verification of accuracy	• Verify anatomical landmarks with navigation at every crucial step (e.g., screw placement and drill utilization), especially in MISS where landmarks are limited (e.g., in MISS lumbar cases, point out the tip of the transverse process after skin incision) • Constantly compare the position and tactile feedback of the navigated instrument during surgery • Reflective markers should not be contaminated
Master the anatomy	• Intraoperative navigation does not substitute the need to know the anatomy
Prevent excessive movement	• Throughout the procedure confirm stable placement and avoid hitting the array during surgery • Avoid pressure, mechanical impact (with hammers or mallet), or movements • Use a battery-driven drill to prepare screw holes and avoid Jamshidi needles (too much pressure, can move the patient)
"Hands-off test"	• After full insertion of the tap into the pedicle, let go of the instrument • If the screw simulation on the navigation screen demonstrates an adequately positioned screw in the pedicle without breach, this is usually confirmation of a well-placed screw trajectory (this test should be avoided in patients with poor bone quality and in the cervical spine)
Neuromonitoring	• Intraoperative neuromonitoring and screw stimulation with a cutoff of approximately 9 mAmp
Verification of position	• iCT scan after implantation of instrumentation/implants to verify desired position and accuracy

Abbreviations: CT, computed tomography; iCT, intraoperative computed tomography; MISS, minimally invasive spinal surgery; OR, operating room.

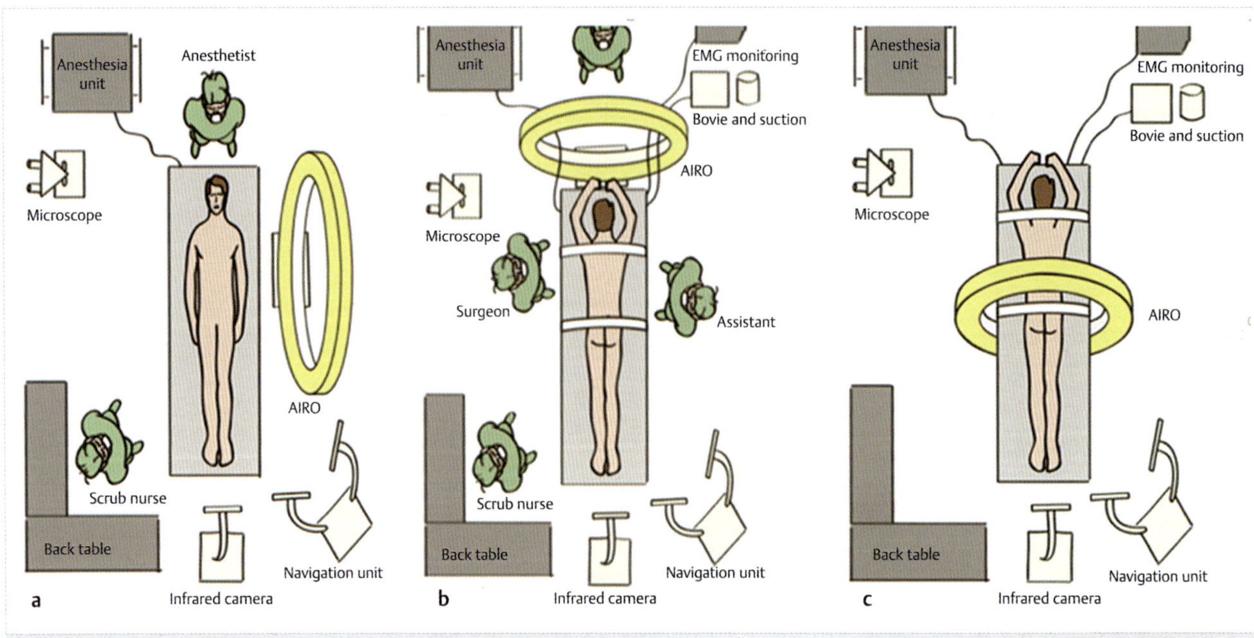

Fig. 7.5 Intraoperative computed tomography (iCT) operating room (OR) setup. From *left*: **(a)** Before surgery, the iCT is parallel to the rail system. **(b)** Intraoperative OR suite setup. The patient is face down with arms up for a lumbar procedure (note: arms should be placed down at the side for cervical surgery). It is important to lead all anesthesia, electromyography, Bovie, and suction cords through the gantry of the iCT. Cloth tape is applied across the chest and hips and laterally from the patient's side downwards in order to minimize tissue movement and shifting during surgery. **(c)** OR suite setup when taking iCT scans of the patient. All personnel leave the room while the iCT is in use.[14]

f) The gantry is located on the cranial side of the patient and all the cables (Bovie, suction, and EMG monitoring, etc.) are let through the gantry.

g) While the iCT-scanner is running, the surgical staff leaves the room, and thus avoid unnecessary radiation exposure (▶ Fig. 7.5c).

h) For MISS cases, a drill guide tube is calibrated and connected above the desired entry point through a small skin and fascial incision. The use of a navigated guide tube streamlines the workflow by eliminating K-wires and the need to navigate multiple instruments (point, drill, tap, screw). The navigated guide tube is used for drilling, tapping, and screw placement[27] (▶ Fig. 7.6a, b).

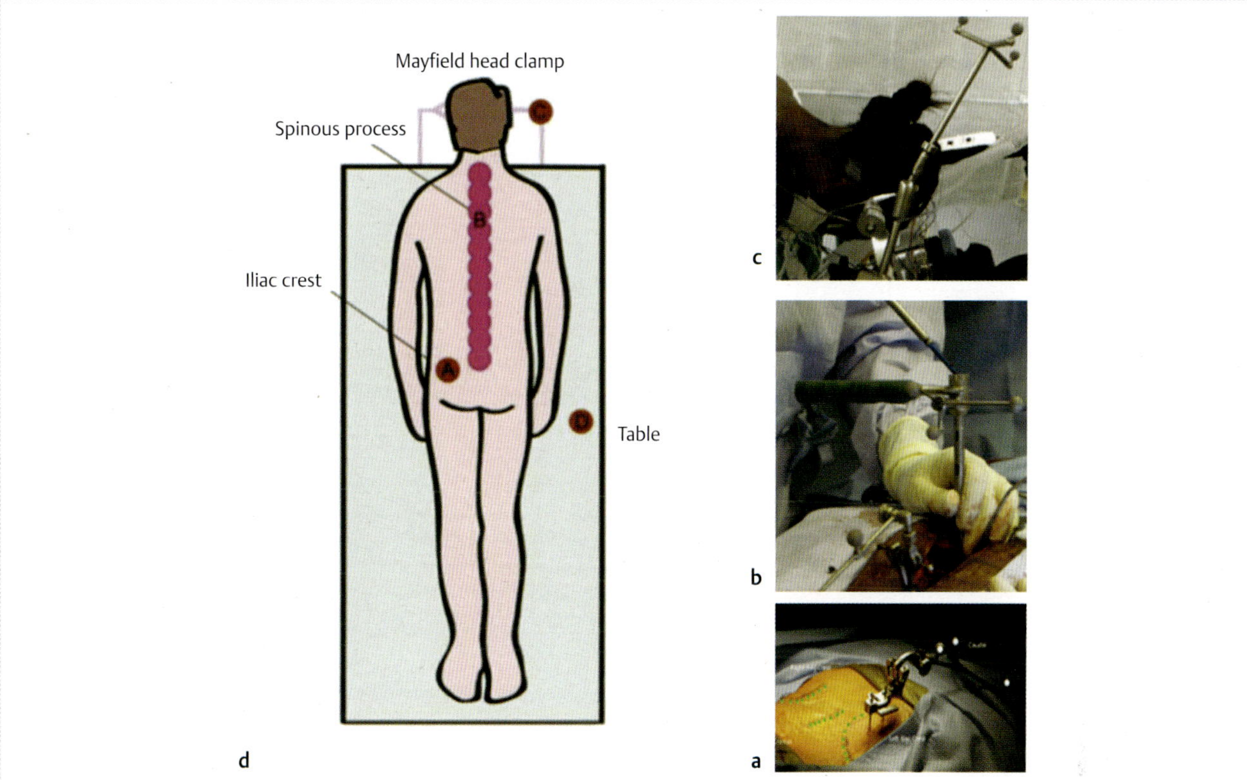

Fig. 7.6 Reference array. **(a)** For pathology of pelvic T12, the reference array (RA) is placed in posterior iliac crest via a two-pin fixator (*lower right*). **(b)** For pathology of C3–T11, the RA is placed on a spinous process (*mid right*). **(c)** For pathology of C0–C3, the RA is docked in the Mayfield head clamp (*top right*). **(d)** For localization (e.g., intradural tumor, thoracic disc herniation) from occiput to pelvic, the RA is attached to the table with the patient adequately immobilized with tape (not shown).[14]

i) In cases that require additional decompression and placement of a cage, the following steps are followed: Bone graft can be harvested from the iliac crest and the pointer can be used for best localization of appropriate iliac crest bone. In cases where a tubular retractor is placed for decompression and facetectomy, the fascial incision for the tubular retractor is determined with navigation. The fascial incision is typically 2 to 3 cm medial to the fascial incision required for screw placement. The pointer identifies the inferior edge of the lamina and the facet joint. Over a series of tubular dilators, the retractor is then placed and adequate exposure of the anatomy is again confirmed with the navigated pointer. The decompression and facetectomy is performed under the microscope and can also be done with the assistance of navigation. Navigation at this point will also be helpful to determine, for example, the localization of the pedicle, the disc space, and the trajectory of the disc space. We then use navigation to determine the trajectory of the discectomy and cage placement.
j) After placement of the cage, a control CT scan is obtained. Based on this CT scan the length of the rods can be determined either with navigation or directly from the computer screen.

Airo-iCT Workflow for Localization of Spinal Pathology

This workflow is useful for spine tumors and cervical instrumentation cases:

a) The patient is placed either prone or supine and secured to the table using cloth tape as described in the lumbar total navigation workflow.
b) The RA is placed and secured either to the table or to a Mayfield head-holder (▶ Fig. 7.6c) depending on the anatomical region of interest.
c) For the preoperative scan, two half sheets are draped around the incision site and the region of interest is marked on the drape.
d) An infrared camera is positioned toward the RA and the reflective markers on the gantry.
e) All personnel leave the OR before a radiology technician initializes the scan via a remote control. This eliminates X-ray exposure of the surgical staff.
f) After the scan, the images are automatically transferred to the NAV.
g) The site of incision and its proper trajectory are identified with a pointer. In open cases, accuracy could be confirmed by palpation of anatomical landmarks (i.e., spinous transverse process at several levels). In MISS, the tip of a transverse process is used to verify accuracy.
h) Displacement of anatomical structures must be taken into consideration and rescanning or anatomical landmark confirmation may be necessary, especially when treating intradural spine tumors.
i) A final CT is obtained in those cases where permanent hardware is implanted, especially in thoracic and/or occipitocervical instrumentations (▶ Fig. 7.7, ▶ Fig. 7.8, ▶ Fig. 7.9, ▶ Fig. 7.10, and ▶ Fig. 7.11).

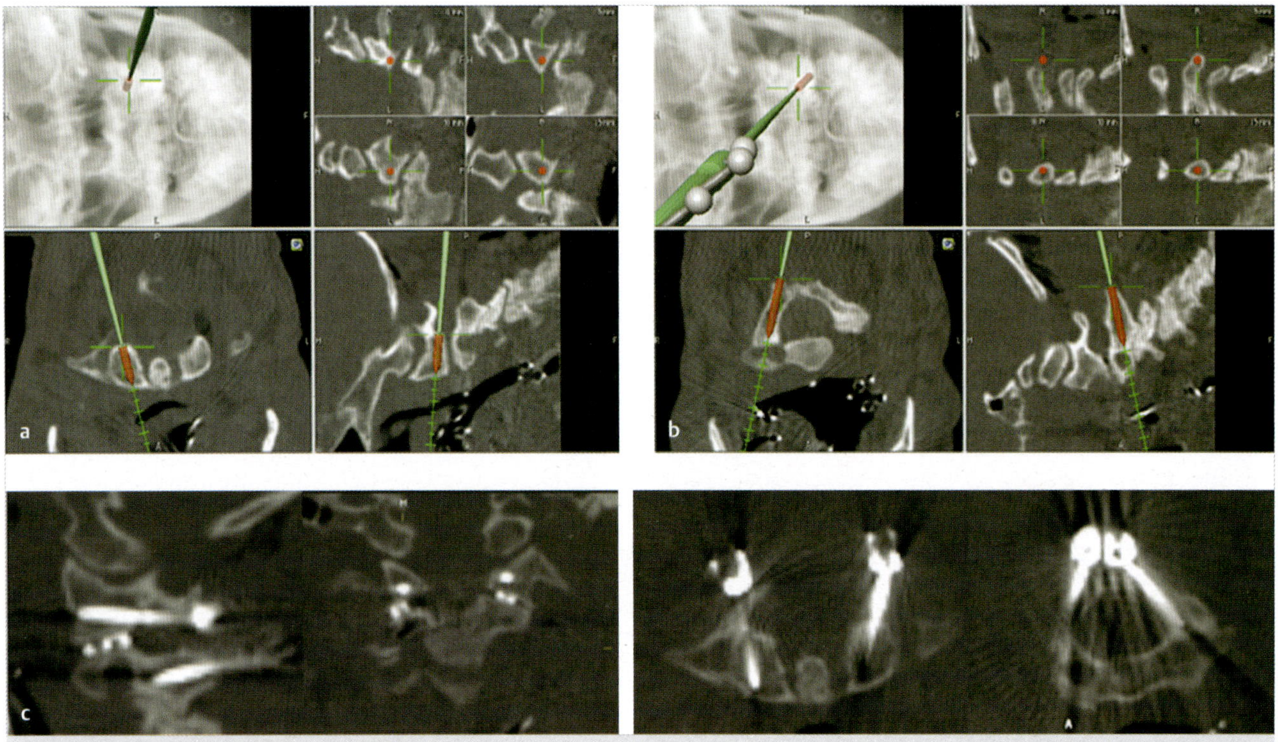

Fig. 7.7 **(a)** Planning of C1 lateral mass screw (size and screw position). **(b)** Planning for C2 laminar screws. **(c)** Survey of pedicle screw and C1–C2 lateral cage bilateral.

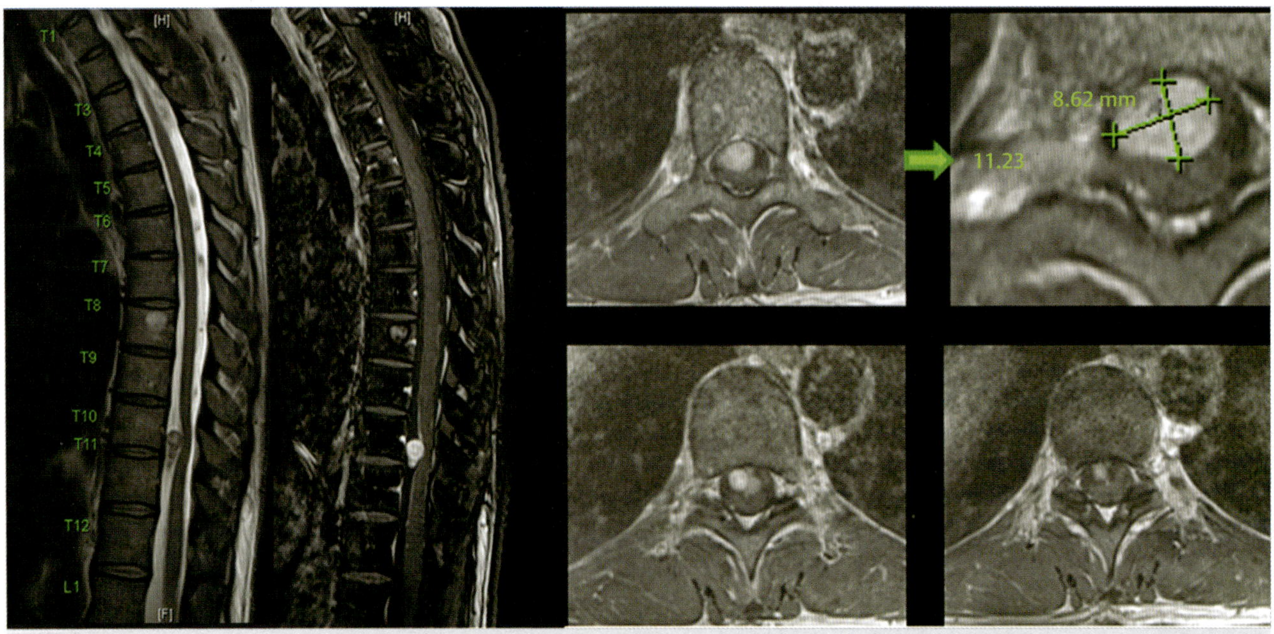

Fig. 7.8 Magnetic resonance imaging (MRI) of the thoracic spine (T2 sagittal, T1 sagittal, and axial with gadolinium) showing an enhancing intradural extramedullary lesion extending from mid T10 to T11 level with mass effect and flattening of the ventral cord with displacement of the cord posterior, without abnormal cord signal.

Airo-iCT Workflow for Single-Step Pedicle Screw System (SSPSS)

Traditional MIS pedicle screw systems are cumbersome, requiring multiple steps and instruments, including placement of Jamshidi needles, K-wires, power drill, tap, and finally, screw placement. Multiple companies have introduced navigable single-step pedicle screw systems (SSPSSs) for percutaneous and mini-open placement. Compared to conventional pedicle screw systems, this technology eliminates the need for K-wires. It

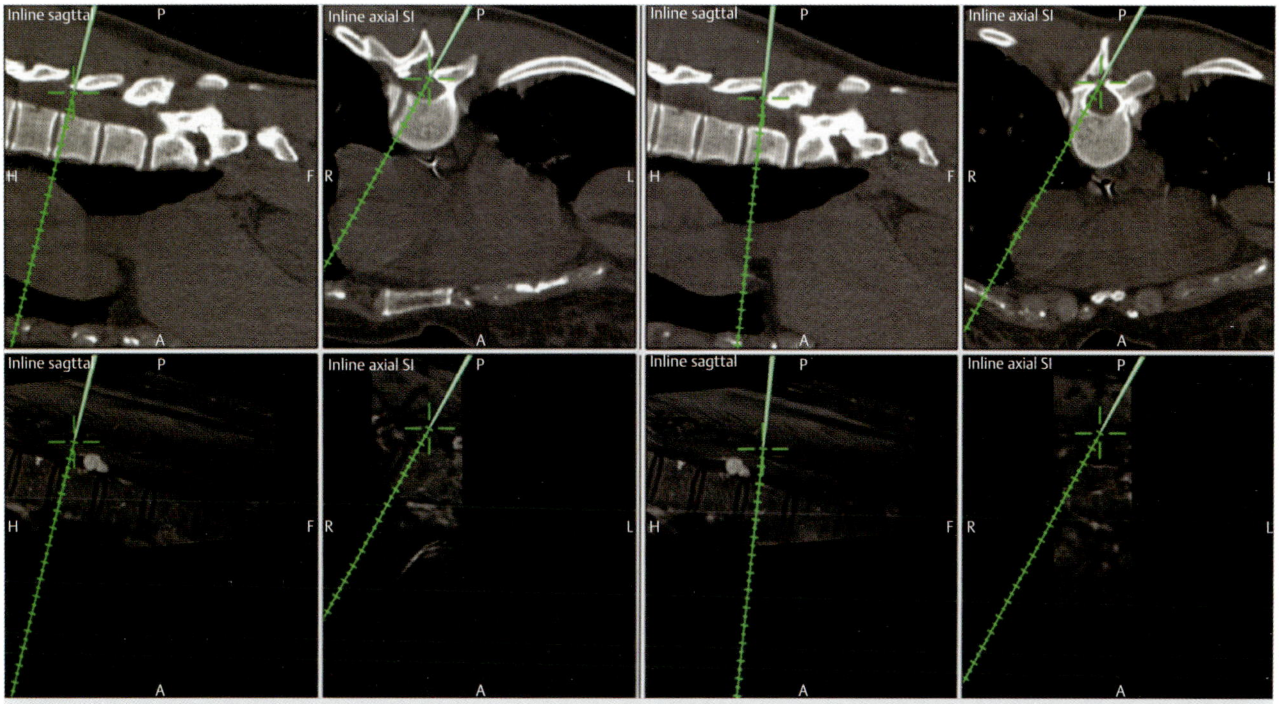

Fig. 7.9 Preoperative magnetic resonance imaging (MRI) merged with intraoperative computed tomography (iCT) image for location purposes.

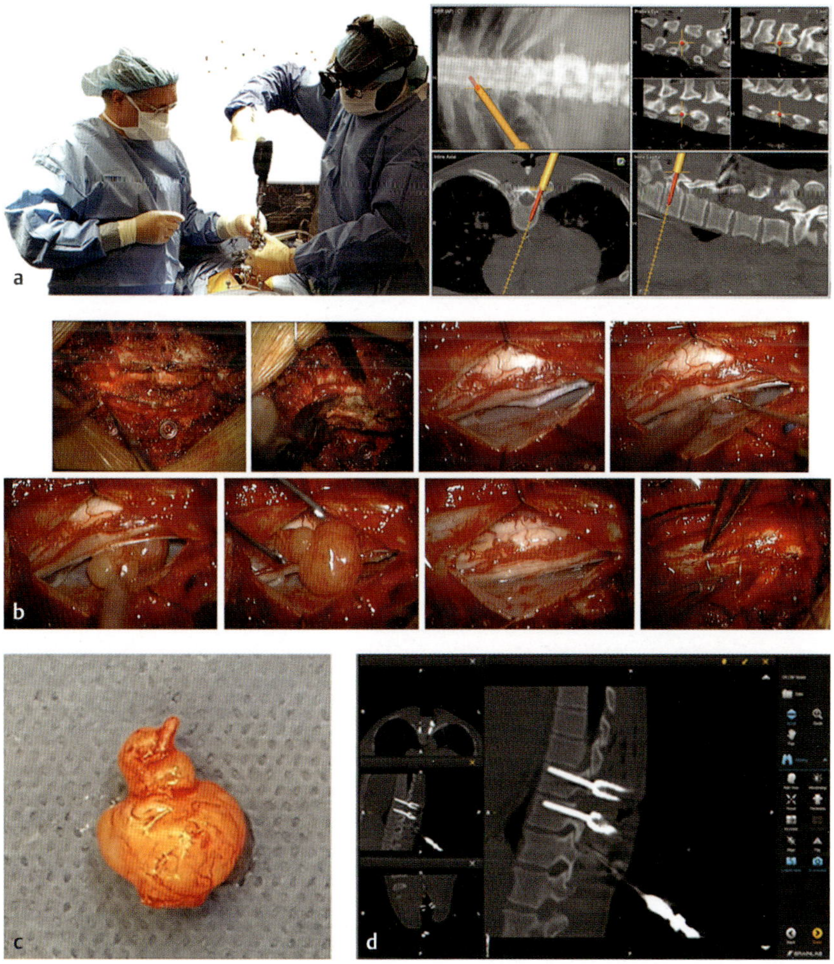

Fig. 7.10 **(a)** Introduction of transpedicular screws in T10 and T11 with the navigated guide tube. **(b)** Intraoperative images. **(c)** Tumor. **(d)** Intraoperative computed tomography (iCT) after pedicle screws insertion and resection of the tumor.

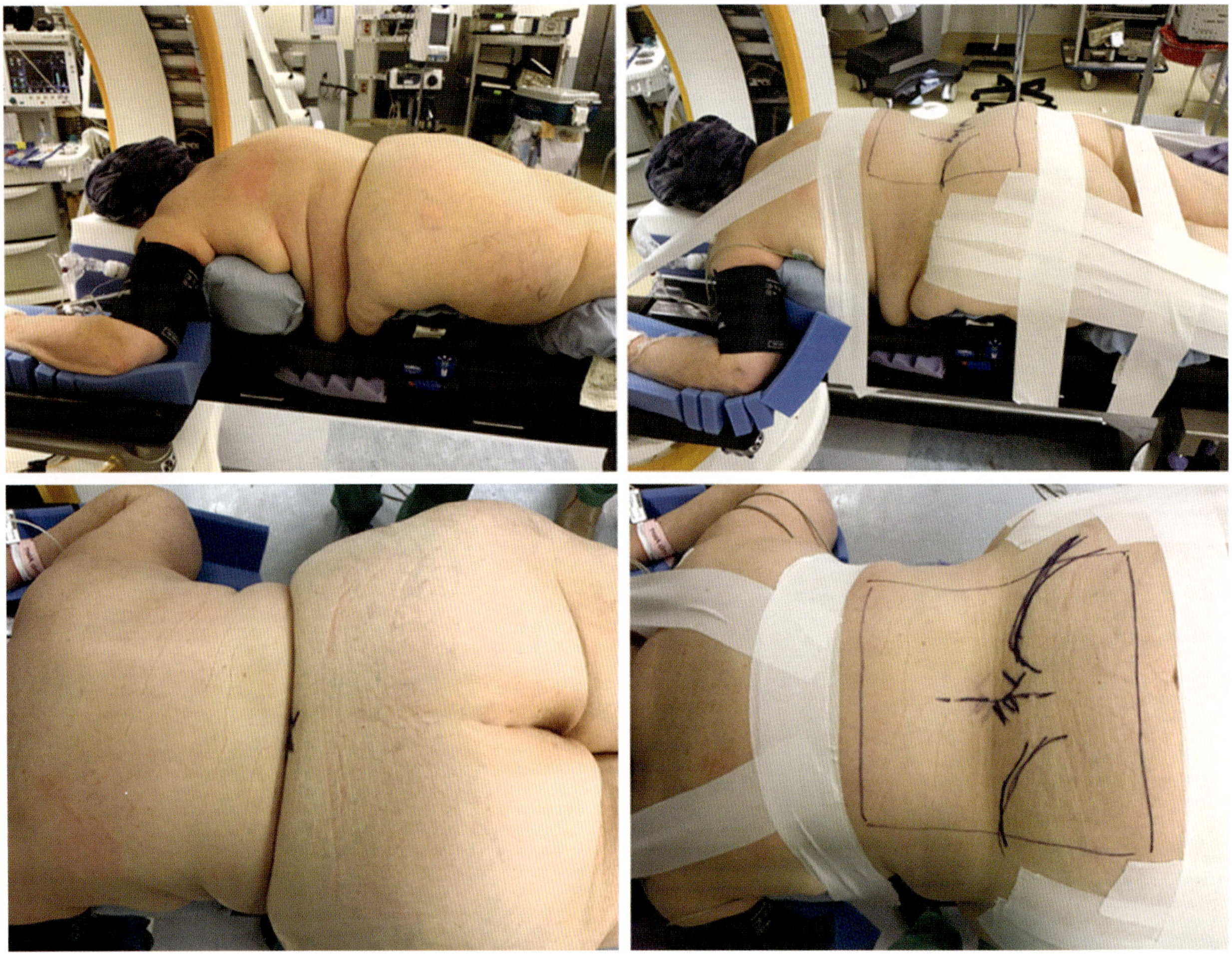

Fig. 7.11 Pictures showing the patient positioning and fixation with tape before the first scan.

combines docking, tapping, and screw placement into one step with a single device that needs to be registered only once for intraoperative navigation (▶ Fig. 7.12).

A case series revealed that with the use of SSPSS the accuracy rate is 93%. This result is comparable to the literature, for example, to a previous meta-analysis which described a median accuracy rate of 95.2% in navigated pedicle screw placement.[45,46,47,48] Furthermore, it was seen that SSPSS is more time saving. The time per screw was 2.45 minutes, which is less than what the literature describes.[14,45,49,50] A downside of SSPSS is the sharp stylet, which can potentially harm surrounding tissue. However, SSPSS is a promising technique and can improve the efficiency of pedicle screw insertion while reducing radiation exposure to the OR staff.

a) The navigation wand is used to identify the optimal trajectory for pedicle screw insertion at each level on each side. The skin is marked over these areas. Usually, one skin incision can be made on each side with separate fascial openings per level.
b) Manual verification is done using the Brainlab pointer by identifying and palpating a transverse process at a distance from the reference array.
c) The SSPSS device with navigation star is registered and calibrated (▶ Fig. 7.13). This eliminates the need for K-wires. A short stylet is exposed at the tip of the screw and used to dock on the lateral aspect of the superior articulating facet of the level to be instrumented (▶ Fig. 7.14). To ensure that the stylet is engaged in bone, gentle malleting is necessary. The required trajectory is aligned; then the self-tapping screw is inserted. To maintain the ideal trajectory, it is essential to hold the SSPSS device in a manner that allows the navigation to be facing the camera of the navigation station (▶ Fig. 7.15).
d) Once the pedicle screw enters the vertebral body, the stylet is retracted. With this single-step technique, there is no need for extra drilling or taping.
e) A final CT is done while leaving the navigation reference in place in case further adjustment of the instruments or decompression is needed.
f) The wound is generously irrigated and washed after meticulous hemostasis is performed. Osteostimulative bone graft is packed under the rod. Local anesthesia is used to infiltrate the muscle and the wound is closed.

O-Arm iCT Operating Room Setup and Navigation

The O-arm™ navigation system includes the cone-beam mobile CT scanner (O-arm™ imaging system, Medtronic), the LED

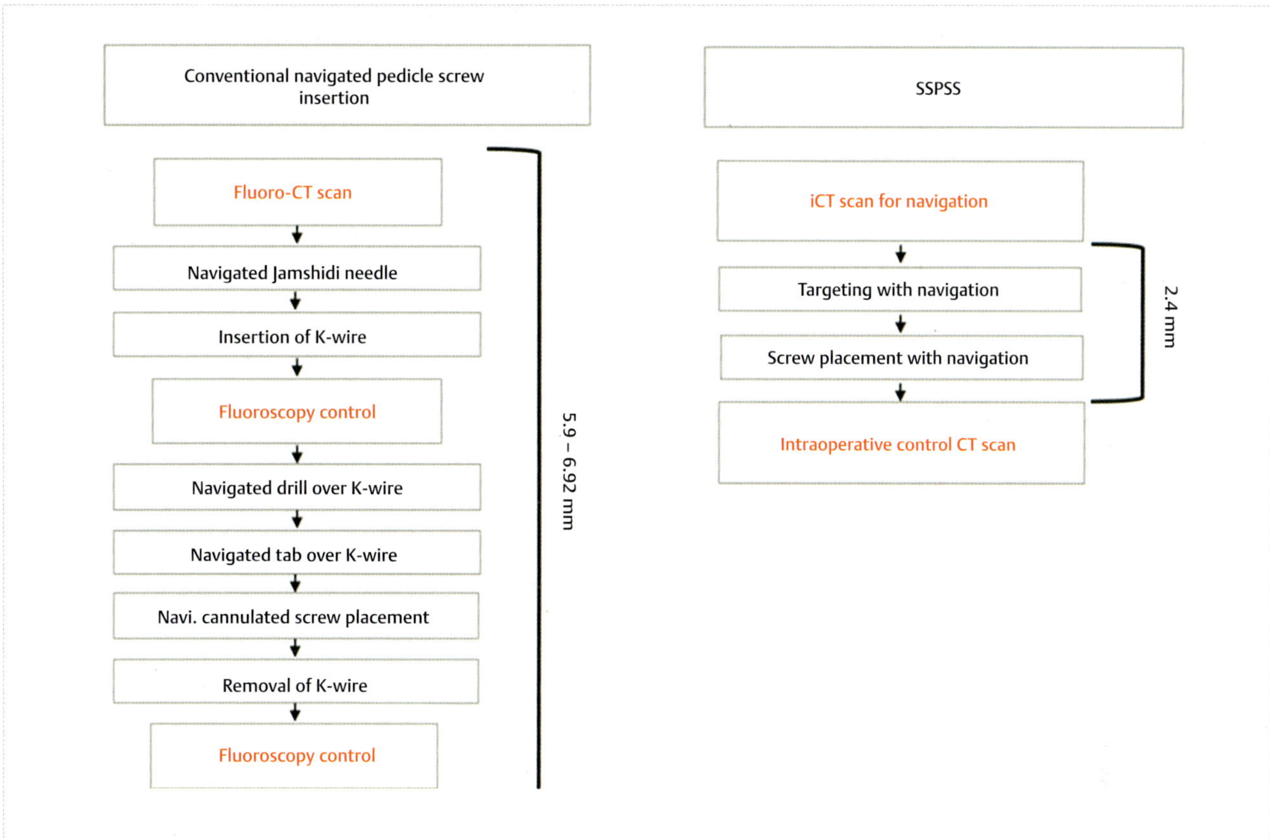

Fig. 7.12 Flowchart illustrating the different workflow among conventional navigated pedicle screw insertion versus the single-step pedicle screw system.

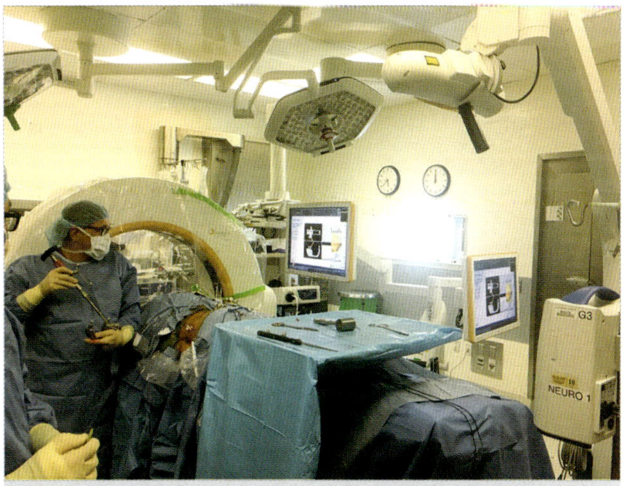

Fig. 7.13 The SSPSS device with navigation star is registered and calibrated.

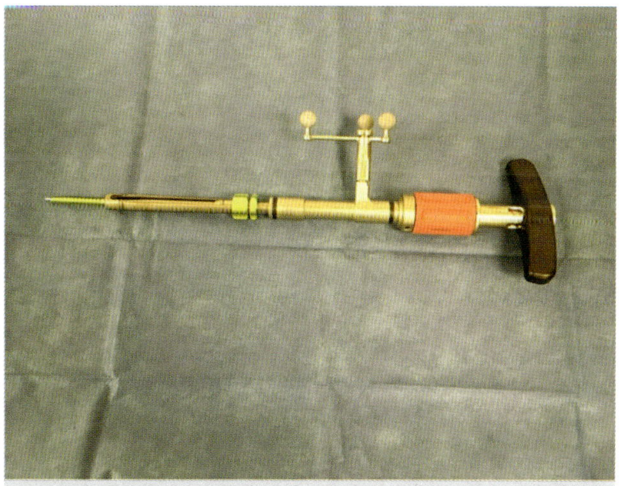

Fig. 7.14 Picture showing an SSPSS navigated screw inserter and the navigated stylet that can be extended to a maximum of 5 mm beyond the tip of the screw.

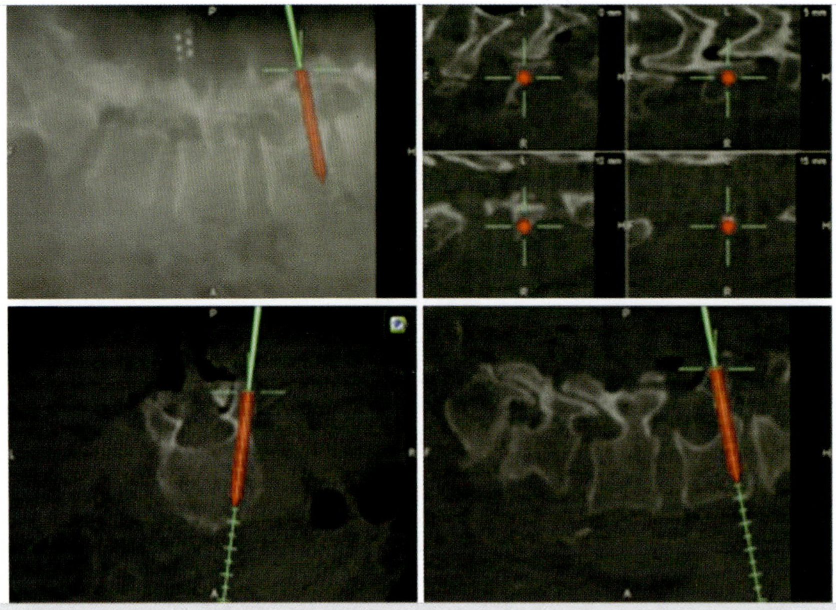

Fig. 7.15 Intraoperative computed tomography (CT) scan of a 66-year-old female patient showing the L3 screw insertion.

detector camera, and the computer-assisted surgical navigation workstation (Medtronic Stealth Station™, Medtronic, Minneapolis, MN, USA). The O-arm measures 280.6 and 202.2 cm with the gantry closed and opened, respectively; the gantry opening is 69.9 cm and the bore diameter is 96.5 cm. Scan capacity (length of the image acquired) is approximately 30 cm.

General patient positioning for spine navigation is not different from standard spine positioning. However, the appropriate selection of an OR surgical table for image guidance is very important:

a) The design of the O-arm™ works ideally with the Jackson radiolucent spinal table, which presents a core structure with minimal radiodense metal resulting in minimal radiographic artifact and enables the mobile CT scanner to be positioned along any level of the spinal axis. Any table that has a base can obstruct movement along the axis of the patient and table. The CT scanner can be left outside the OR until image acquisition is required (i.e., after patient positioning, approach, and registration process).

b) Before image acquisition, sterile draping of the CT scanner is a consideration. The O-arm can be either covered with its sterile cover (▶ Fig. 7.16a), or an alternative drape can cover the patient until the mobile scanner acquires the images (▶ Fig. 7.16b). In our opinion, the use of an extra drape on the patient avoids possible problems of the O-arm cover (i.e., getting caught between the shields, increasing surgical time) while being safe and faster.

c) The surgical area should be sterilely prepped and the draping should be as wide as possible as this allows for skin surface anatomy identification and gives orientation during the entire procedure, particularly in MISS cases. Different options for navigated reference frame exist depending on the region of interest. For posterior cervical cases, navigated reference frame options include the spinous process clamp and the Mayfield reference frame. For thoracic and lumbar spine, a spinous process clamp or pedicle screw-based reference frame can be used. In addition, the reference pin into the ilium is an option for lumbar cases. The camera can be placed either at the foot or at the head of the table. Consideration to the "line-of-sight" issues for the navigated reference frame and the LED camera should determine the location. These issues can cause some workflow disruption during the procedure, so care should be taken to make sure the line of sight is clear of any obstructions and the reflective surfaces are free of bloodstains. During the entire procedure, careful attention to not move the reference frame is key for navigation accuracy.

d) The image acquisition starts with localizing X-rays in both AP and lateral views, and the CT scanner is positioned to maximize the working area. In this step, the LED camera is adjusted to make sure the reference frame and iCT are visible. While the CT is running, operative personnel should temporarily leave the OR in order to avoid radiation exposure. After image acquisition, the surgeon checks the navigation workstation and review for image quality. The O-arm can be removed from the OR. In deformity cases, usually more than one spin is necessary; for regular T10-pelvis instrumentation, the usual number of spins is two or three. The next step is the calibration of the navigated instruments followed by a final check of navigation accuracy with known spinal anatomical landmarks; normally following the lamina along the border is enough, although TP's are always another option if lateral dissection is not a problem. Check of navigation accuracy is a critical step and it should be performed as many times as needed to ensure system accuracy and prevent potential complications.

e) The navigated instruments are then used for spinal instrumentation. Ideal trajectory is visualized and confirmed in real time on the navigation workstation (▶ Fig. 7.17a). Spinal measurements can be done at the workstation in order to select the appropriate screw size.

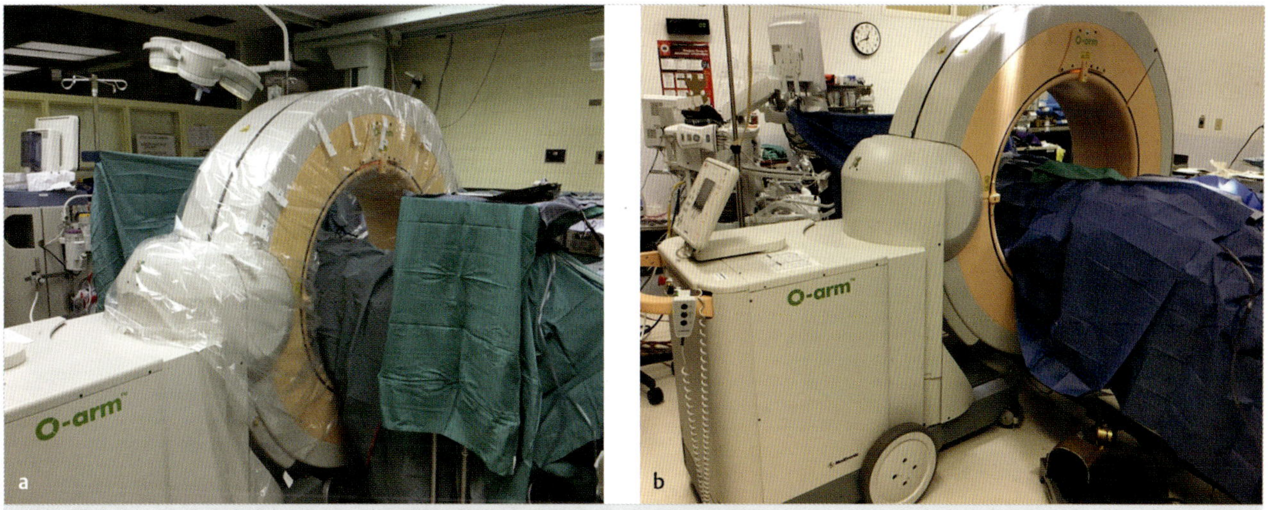

Fig. 7.16 **(a)** O-arm setup with a cover. **(b)** O-arm setup with two extra sterile half sheets.

f) For percutaneous screw placement, skin incision is planned using the navigation. After fascial incision, the navigated drill is used to make the initial hole. This is followed by the power-drilling of the tract using a predefined length (▶ Fig. 7.17b) (i.e., 30 mm for lumbar pedicle screws).
g) The power-drilling technique is preferred by the authors mainly because it minimizes manipulation of the patient, reducing the risk of spine shift and inaccuracy during the procedure. After the tract is made into the pedicle, a guide wire is inserted through the tract to maintain pedicle trajectory and position. Careful attention should be paid when managing the guide wires in MISS as the tip is not navigated in real time. The authors measure the wire about 1 cm longer than the initial length of drilling and penetrate the wire into the vertebral body, protecting the wire from movement while not perforating the anterior cortex of the vertebral body.
h) After tapping (▶ Fig. 7.17c), the pedicle screw is inserted using the navigated screw-driver. We recommend removing the guide wire during the insertion of the pedicle screw (i.e., when the screw crosses the junction of the pedicle to the vertebral body) in order to avoid inadvertent guide wire advancement. For open surgical approaches, the guide wires are not necessary.
i) Navigation accuracy must be constantly maintained and monitored throughout the surgery. Avoiding excess force and torque on the spine is extremely important in navigated cases. In addition, confirmation of navigation accuracy should always be done before any pedicle cannulation by touching identified spine anatomy and confirming on the image-guided system.

7.7 Teaching and Training

7.7.1 Learning Curve

As the concerns with learning curve and deceleration of the surgical workflow appear to be the major drawbacks, limiting its applicability, mastering the workflow before surgery is suggested. The main goal of navigation has to be to enhance safety, accuracy, and diminish (almost eliminate) radiation exposure to the staff and ultimately to the patient.[14]

The applications of navigation in spine surgery have been successfully expanding in the last years, from the classic usage in screw insertion (more and more in all segments of the spine) to interbody fusion (lateral lumbar interbody fusion,[51] transforaminal lumbar interbody fusion,[48] posterior lumbar interbody fusion)[52,53] and spinal tumor resections.[54,55]

7.7.2 Tips and Tricks

1. In real-time navigation, avoiding excessive pressure or spine manipulation is key to preventing affecting accuracy.
2. Navigation is a dynamic process. Calibrate and recalibrate as many times as needed and confirm the accuracy with anatomical landmarks before any critical step.
3. Be aware of radiation exposure and try to minimize the dose to the patient as much as possible.

7.8 Conclusion

The learning curve of navigation in spinal fusion procedures requires: mastering the anatomy, gently manipulating the spine, and decreasing the pressure applied over anatomical structures during the procedure to minimize anatomical shifting. Repetitive confirmation using anatomical landmarks must be used as frequently as needed to ensure the patient's safety. Thus, it is important to understand the technology, scope of action, pros and cons, and the workflow used by experts when treating surgical pathologies of different regions of the spine.

Using navigation for spinal fusion procedures optimizes pathology localization in challenging cases such as spinal tumors, spine surgery in obese patients, and deformity cases. It also helps to improve technical aspects of the surgery such as appropriate hardware selection (screws, rods, cages).

Nowadays, spinal navigation is used in spine centers all over the world and has proven to be safe, accurate, and efficient.

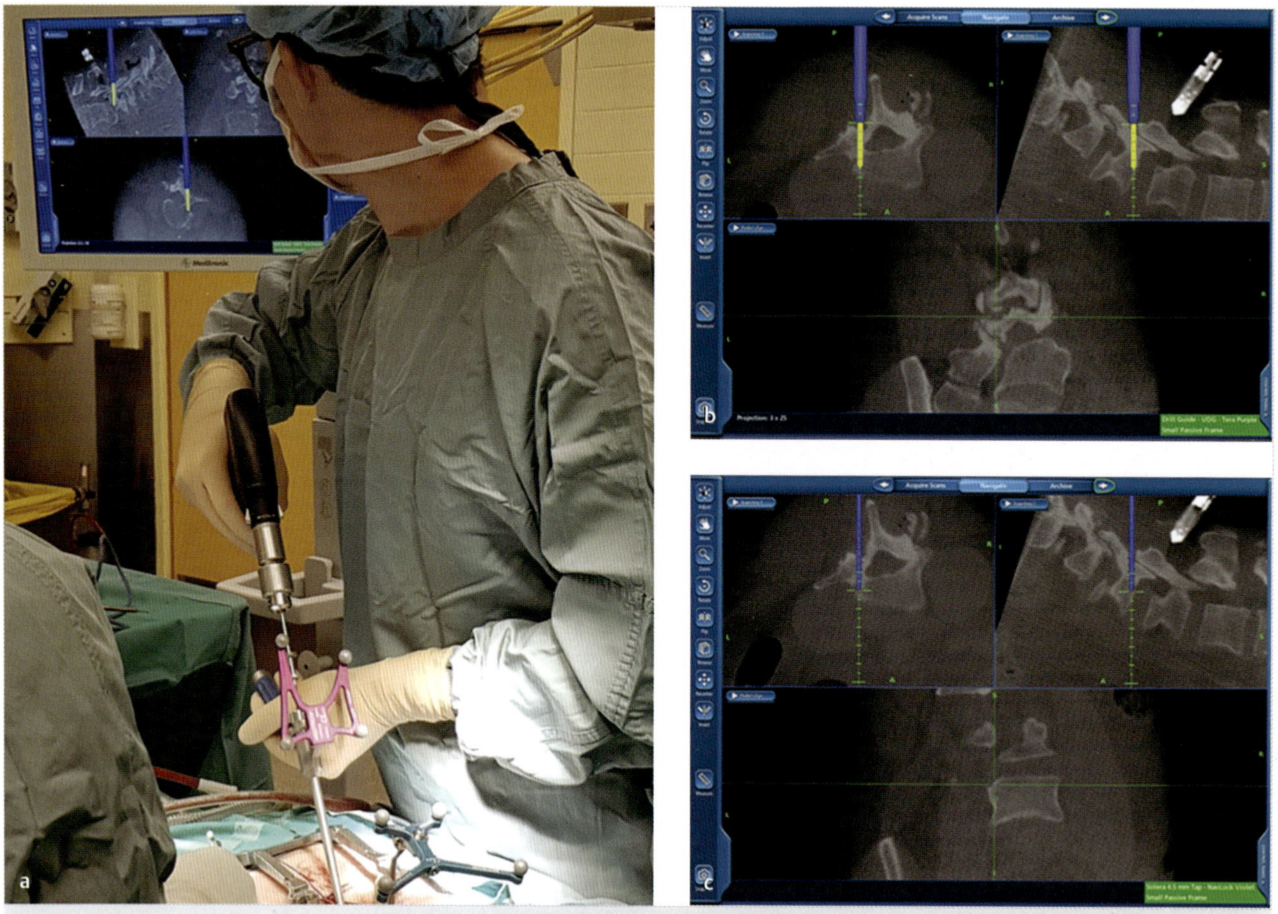

Fig. 7.17 **(a)** Navigation in a cortical screw trajectory case using the guide tube and the power drill showing the arrangement of the navigation tool and its relationship to the reference array. **(b)** Image showing the predicted trajectory for the cortical screws with a 35-mm offset. **(c)** Image of the navigated "Tap" tool as it goes into the previously drilled canal.

References

[1] Malhotra D, Kalb S, Rodriguez-Martinez N, et al. Instrumentation of the posterior thoracolumbar spine: from wires to pedicle screws. Neurosurgery. 2014; 10 Suppl 4:497–504, discussion 505

[2] Kalfas IH. Image-guided spinal navigation: application to spinal metastases. Neurosurg Focus. 2001; 11(6):e5

[3] Kalfas IH. Image-guided spinal navigation: principles and clinical applications. In: Ozgur B, Benzel E, Garfin S, eds. Minimally Invasive Spine Surgery: A Practical Guide to Anatomy and Techniques. 1st ed. Springer-Verlag New York; 2012

[4] Härtl R, Korge A. Minimally Invasive Spine Surgery: Techniques, Evidence, and Controversies. 1st ed. Thieme; 2012

[5] Mezger U, Jendrewski C, Bartels M. Navigation in surgery. Langenbecks Arch Surg. 2013; 398(4):501–514

[6] Kalfas IH, Kormos DW, Murphy MA, et al. Application of frameless stereotaxy to pedicle screw fixation of the spine. J Neurosurg. 1995; 83(4):641–647

[7] Murphy MA, McKenzie RL, Kormos DW, Kalfas IH. Frameless stereotaxis for the insertion of lumbar pedicle screws. J Clin Neurosci. 1994; 1(4):257–260

[8] Allam Y, Silbermann J, Riese F, Greiner-Perth R. Computer tomography assessment of pedicle screw placement in thoracic spine: comparison between free hand and a generic 3D-based navigation techniques. Eur Spine J. 2013; 22(3):648–653

[9] Tian NF, Huang QS, Zhou P, et al. Pedicle screw insertion accuracy with different assisted methods: a systematic review and meta-analysis of comparative studies. Eur Spine J. 2011; 20(6):846–859

[10] Rivkin MA, Yocom SS. Thoracolumbar instrumentation with CT-guided navigation (O-arm) in 270 consecutive patients: accuracy rates and lessons learned. Neurosurg Focus. 2014; 36(3):E7

[11] Aoude AA, Fortin M, Figueiredo R, Jarzem P, Ouellet J, Weber MH. Methods to determine pedicle screw placement accuracy in spine surgery: a systematic review. Eur Spine J. 2015; 24(5):990–1004

[12] Kotani Y, Abumi K, Ito M, et al. Accuracy analysis of pedicle screw placement in posterior scoliosis surgery: comparison between conventional fluoroscopic and computer-assisted technique. Spine. 2007; 32(14):1543–1550

[13] Laine T, Lund T, Ylikoski M, Lohikoski J, Schlenzka D. Accuracy of pedicle screw insertion with and without computer assistance: a randomised controlled clinical study in 100 consecutive patients. Eur Spine J. 2000; 9 (3):235–240

[14] Navarro-Ramirez R, Lang G, Lian X, et al. Total navigation in spine surgery; a concise guide to eliminate fluoroscopy using a portable intraoperative computed tomography 3-dimensional navigation system. World Neurosurg. 2017; 100:325–335

[15] Gelalis ID, Paschos NK, Pakos EE, et al. Accuracy of pedicle screw placement: a systematic review of prospective in vivo studies comparing free hand, fluoroscopy guidance and navigation techniques. Eur Spine J. 2012; 21(2):247–255

[16] Shin MH, Ryu KS, Park CK. Accuracy and safety in pedicle screw placement in the thoracic and lumbar spines: comparison study between conventional C-arm fluoroscopy and navigation coupled with O-Arm® guided methods. J Korean Neurosurg Soc. 2012; 52(3):204–209

[17] Van de Kelft E, Costa F, Van der Planken D, Schils F. A prospective multicenter registry on the accuracy of pedicle screw placement in the thoracic, lumbar, and sacral levels with the use of the O-arm imaging system and StealthStation Navigation. Spine. 2012; 37(25):E1580–E1587

[18] Scheufler KM, Franke J, Eckardt A, Dohmen H. Accuracy of image-guided pedicle screw placement using intraoperative computed tomography-based navigation with automated referencing, part I: cervicothoracic spine. Neurosurgery. 2011; 69(4):782–795, discussion 795

[19] Santos ER, Sembrano JN, Yson SC, Polly DW, Jr. Comparison of open and percutaneous lumbar pedicle screw revision rate using 3-D image guidance and intraoperative CT. Orthopedics. 2015; 38(2):e129–e134

[20] American Society of Radiologic Technologists. X-ray risk calculator. 2016 [cited 2017 03302017]; Available from: http://www.xrayrisk.com/calculator/calculator-normal-studies.php?id=26

[21] Houten JK, Nasser R, Baxi N. Clinical assessment of percutaneous lumbar pedicle screw placement using the O-arm multidimensional surgical imaging system. Neurosurgery. 2012; 70(4):990–995

[22] Slomczykowski M, Roberto M, Schneeberger P, Ozdoba C, Vock P. Radiation dose for pedicle screw insertion: fluoroscopic method versus computer-assisted surgery. Spine. 1999; 24(10):975–982, discussion 983

[23] Härtl R, Lam KS, Wang J, Korge A, Kandziora F, Audigé L. Worldwide survey on the use of navigation in spine surgery. World Neurosurg. 2013; 79 (1):162–172

[24] Khanna AR, Yanamadala V, Coumans JV. Effect of intraoperative navigation on operative time in 1-level lumbar fusion surgery. J Clin Neurosci. 2016; 32:72–76

[25] Meng XT, Guan XF, Zhang HL, He SS. Computer navigation versus fluoroscopy-guided navigation for thoracic pedicle screw placement: a meta-analysis. Neurosurg Rev. 2016; 39(3):385–391

[26] Nottmeier EW. A review of image-guided spinal surgery. J Neurosurg Sci. 2012; 56(1):35–47

[27] Shin BJ, Njoku IU, Tsiouris AJ, Härtl R. Navigated guide tube for the placement of mini-open pedicle screws using stereotactic 3D navigation without the use of K-wires: technical note. J Neurosurg Spine. 2013; 18(2):178–183

[28] Patel AA, Whang PG, Vaccaro AR. Overview of computer-assisted image-guided surgery of the spine. Semin Spine Surg. 2008; 20(3):186–194

[29] Ringel F, Villard J, Ryang YM, Meyer B. Navigation, robotics, and intraoperative imaging in spinal surgery. In: Schramm J, ed. Advances and Technical Standards in Neurosurgery. Vol. 41. Springer International Publishing; 2014:3–22

[30] Acosta FL, Jr, Thompson TL, Campbell S, Weinstein PR, Ames CP. Use of intraoperative isocentric C-arm 3D fluoroscopy for sextant percutaneous pedicle screw placement: case report and review of the literature. Spine J. 2005; 5 (3):339–343

[31] Hedrick MH, Fraser JK. Processing Regenerative Cells from Adipose Tissue for Placement in Patient Suffering from e.g. Liver Disorder Involves Separating, Concentrating, and Manipulating Regenerative Cells for Enhancement of Therapeutic Effects. Cytori Therapeutics Inc.; 2008

[32] Hahn P, Oezdemir S, Komp M, et al. A new electromagnetic navigation system for pedicle screws placement: a human cadaver study at the lumbar spine. PLoS One. 2015; 10(7):e0133708

[33] Holly LT. Image-guided spinal surgery. Int J Med Robot. 2006; 2(1):7–15

[34] Karhade AV, Vasudeva VS, Pompeu YA, Lu Y. Image guided spine surgery: available technology and future potential. Austin Neurosurg Open Access. 2016; 3(1):1–5

[35] Papadopoulos EC, Girardi FP, Sama A, Sandhu HS, Cammisa FP, Jr Accuracy of single-time, multilevel registration in image-guided spinal surgery. Spine J. 2005; 5(3):263–267, discussion 268

[36] Kalfas IH. Benzel's Spine Surgery—193 Intraoperative Imaging of the Spine. 4th ed. Elsevier; 2017

[37] Njoku I, Wanin O, Assey A, et al. Minimally invasive 2D navigation-assisted treatment of thoracolumbar spinal fractures in East Africa: a case report. Cureus. 2016; 8(2):e507

[38] Holly LT, Foley KT. Three-dimensional fluoroscopy-guided percutaneous thoracolumbar pedicle screw placement. Technical note. J Neurosurg. 2003; 99(3) Suppl:324–329

[39] Scarfe WC, Farman AG. What is cone-beam CT and how does it work? Dent Clin North Am. 2008; 52(4):707–730, v

[40] Schafer S, Nithiananthan S, Mirota DJ, et al. Mobile C-arm cone-beam CT for guidance of spine surgery: image quality, radiation dose, and integration with interventional guidance. Med Phys. 2011; 38(8):4563–4574

[41] Tjardes T, Shafizadeh S, Rixen D, et al. Image-guided spine surgery: state of the art and future directions. Eur Spine J. 2010; 19(1):25–45

[42] Baaj AA, Beckman J, Smith DA. O-Arm-based image guidance in minimally invasive spine surgery: technical note. Clin Neurol Neurosurg. 2013; 115 (3):342–345

[43] Mendelsohn D, Strelzow J, Dea N, et al. Patient and surgeon radiation exposure during spinal instrumentation using intraoperative computed tomography-based navigation. Spine J. 2016; 16(3):343–354

[44] Lee M-H, Lin MH-C, Weng H-H, et al. Feasibility of intra-operative computed tomography navigation system for pedicle screw insertion of the thoracolumbar spine. J Spinal Disord Tech. 2013; 26(5):E183–E187

[45] Schmidt FA,, Lekuya H, Kirnaz S, et al. Novel MIS 3D NAV single step pedicle screw system (SSPSS): workflow, accuracy and initial clinical experience. Int J Spine Surg. 2020

[46] Fraser J, Gebhard H, Irie D, Parikh K, Härtl R. Iso-C/3-dimensional neuronavigation versus conventional fluoroscopy for minimally invasive pedicle screw placement in lumbar fusion. Minim Invasive Neurosurg. 2010; 53(4):184–190

[47] Kosmopoulos V, Schizas C. Pedicle screw placement accuracy: a meta-analysis. Spine. 2007; 32(3):E111–E120

[48] Lian X, Navarro-Ramirez R, Berlin C, et al. Total 3D Airo® navigation for minimally invasive transforaminal lumbar interbody fusion. BioMed Res Int. 2016; 2016:5027340

[49] Blizzard DJ, Thomas JA. MIS single-position lateral and oblique lateral lumbar interbody fusion and bilateral pedicle screw fixation: feasibility and perioperative results. Spine. 2018; 43(6):440–446

[50] Spitz SM, Sandhu FA, Voyadzis JM. Percutaneous "K-wireless" pedicle screw fixation technique: an evaluation of the initial experience of 100 screws with assessment of accuracy, radiation exposure, and procedure time. J Neurosurg Spine. 2015; 22(4):422–431

[51] Joseph JR, Smith BW, Patel RD, Park P. Use of 3D CT-based navigation in minimally invasive lateral lumbar interbody fusion. J Neurosurg Spine. 2016; 25 (3):339–344

[52] Wang Y, Liu H, Hu Y, Yi X, Li C. Navigated 2-level posterior lumbar fusion: a 5-cm-incision procedure. J Orthop Surg Res. 2016; 11:1

[53] Kim TT, Johnson JP, Pashman R, Drazin D. Minimally invasive spinal surgery with intraoperative image-guided navigation. BioMed Res Int. 2016; 2016:5716235

[54] Nasser R, Drazin D, Nakhla J, et al. Resection of spinal column tumors utilizing image-guided navigation: a multicenter analysis. Neurosurg Focus. 2016; 41 (2):E15

[55] Yang YK, Chan CM, Zhang Q, Xu HR, Niu XH. Computer navigation-aided resection of sacral chordomas. Chin Med J (Engl). 2016; 129(2):162–168

8 Robotics: Background and Current Role

Sean M. Barber, Meng Huang, Paul Holman, and Isador H. Lieberman

Summary

Early experience with spinal robotic systems have shown them to be a useful tool for assisting with pedicle screw placement, albeit with some limitations. Future improvements in robotic technology have the potential to expand the applications of these devices to involvement with more advanced spinal surgery tasks.

Keywords: spinal robotics, robotic surgery, pedicle screw, spinal navigation

8.1 Introduction

In the field of surgery, improvements in diagnostic and therapeutic capability are often driven by technological innovation. Advances in sterile technique (e.g., autoclave), hemostasis (e.g., bipolar electrocautery), diagnostic imaging (e.g., computed tomography [CT], magnetic resonance imaging), and surgical visualization (e.g., operating microscope, endoscopy) have each led to improvements in surgical potential and/or outcomes, together drastically altering the landscape of surgical practice as a whole. Not every advance in surgical technology, however, proves useful or cost-effective enough to warrant widespread adoption. Occasionally, technological progress arises without identifiable applications or with flaws that dilute its value and practicality to unacceptable levels. Rigorous and objective analysis of new surgical technology is paramount to ensuring that the benefits provided are not outweighed by the costs of implementation, and that technology for the sake of technology is rejected.

Over the past decade, stereotactic spinal navigation has slowly emerged as a widespread enabling technology in both complex and minimally invasive spinal surgery. Value has been demonstrated in improved accuracy of screw insertion, reduction in occupational radiation exposure, and facilitation of both minimally invasive and complex revision surgery. Robotic surgical systems designed specifically for spine surgery are now emerging as competitive or complementary tools for the use of spinal navigation. Although robotic surgery has proven to be a feasible alternative to open and endoscopic/laparoscopic techniques in other surgical specialties,[1,2,3,4,5,6,7] robotic-assisted spinal surgery has yet to achieve widespread adoption. The role of robotic devices in the everyday spine surgery practice remains ill-defined. What benefits do such devices confer? How can they be effectively incorporated into the operative workflow? How steep is the learning curve, and what potential risks are involved? The goal of this chapter is to address these concerns and provide an understanding of the current state and future directions of robotics in spine surgery.

8.2 Benefits and Limitations of Robotics in Spine Surgery

A wealth of potential opportunities exists for the incorporation of robotics into spine surgery, and the theoretical benefits associated with robotic surgical assistance in surgery in general—and spine surgery in particular—are numerous. The benefits of robotic surgical assistance can be divided into two broad categories: (1) reduction of human error, thus improving the safety and efficacy of current practice, and (2) augmenting human surgical capability such that procedures, approaches, and treatments, which were previously impractical are now feasible, reproducible, and safe.

Human error plays a role in a number of intraoperative complications in spine surgery. Humans are subject to fatigability, distraction, tremor, inconsistency and relative limitations in dexterity, memory, and an ability to detect and anticipate changes in the environment and surgical field, many of which may be improved upon with robotic assistance.

However, modern robotic technology also bears certain weaknesses including limited dexterity, high monetary cost, relatively large operating room space requirement, and poor independent decision-making capabilities, among others.

Spine surgery in particular seems well-suited to the use of robots, as many modern spinal procedures involve repeatedly performing similar mechanical tasks of relatively low complexity at multiple levels (e.g., laminectomy, discectomy, pedicle screw placement). Spinal robotic technology is still in its infancy, however, and the majority of objective evidence available regarding the benefits of robotic devices in spine surgery draws from the use of robots in a shared control model to assist with the placement of pedicle screws.

8.2.1 Pedicle Screw Accuracy

Currently available spinal robotic systems are passive and primarily assist with the localization and execution of a preplanned trajectory, lending themselves well to the placement of pedicle screws. There is little consensus, however, regarding how the accuracy of robot-assisted screws compare with screws placed via other methods. Several studies have shown significantly improved accuracy of pedicle screws placed with robotic assistance compared with conventional, fluoroscopy-guided or navigated techniques,[14,15,17] whereas others have shown statistically comparable[8,10,12,13,16,18] or inferior results[9] with robotic assistance. Many confounding variables exist when making such comparisons, however, including surgeon experience, the specific robotic device used, the method of intraoperative registration employed, whether the screws were placed percutaneously or open, and whether the robot was affixed directly to the bony anatomy (e.g., via a spinous process clamp or Schanz screw) or instead attached only to the operating table.

Roser et al evaluated 37 patients randomized to undergo pedicle screw instrumentation with freehand techniques ($N = 10$), standard navigation ($N = 9$), and the Mazor™ SpineAssist (Mazor Robotics Ltd., Caesarea, Israel) ($N = 18$).[19] Although they found a trend toward improved accuracy in the robotic group (99% Gertzbein and Robbins [GRS] A) compared with the navigated (92% GRS A) and freehand groups (97.5% GRS A), no statistical analysis was performed due to small sample sizes.

Schröder et al performed a literature review of 14 articles comparing the need for intraoperative screw revision or revision surgery for screw malposition in patients undergoing pedicle screw placement with robotic guidance, conventional freehand techniques, or CT/fluoroscopic navigation. They found that intraoperative screw revisions were significantly higher for navigated screws when compared with robot-guided screws ($p < 0.001$, odds ratio [OR] 9.7, 95% confidence interval [CI] 2.9–32.2) and revision surgery for screw malposition was significantly higher for freehand compared with robot-guided screws ($p < 0.001$, OR 8.1, 95% CI 2–33.3).[20]

Most modern robotic spine surgical devices utilize a preoperative CT scan or an intraoperative conebeam CT data set when planning screw trajectories. Little objective evidence exists regarding the superiority of using either a preoperative or intraoperative CT scan for planning. It is interesting to note, however, that Macke et al, after retrospectively evaluating pediatric patients who underwent robot-assisted placement of 662 pedicle screws, found that screw accuracy was significantly higher when the planning CT was taken in the prone position compared with the supine position.[11]

8.2.2 Radiation Exposure

Spinal robots could also theoretically decrease radiation exposure to the patient and surgical team during certain procedures involving spinal instrumentation. Indeed, some series have shown decreased radiation exposure to the surgeon and lower fluoroscopy times per screw when placing pedicle screws with robotic-assistance compared with fluoroscopic guidance,[14,15,16,19,21] though other studies have failed to confirm this.[9,10,12] Solomiichuk et al retrospectively reviewed 70 patients (406 screws) with metastatic spinal disease requiring thoracolumbar instrumentation with the SpineAssist robot ($N = 35$, 192 screws) or conventional, fluoroscopic guidance ($N = 35$, 214 screws) and found that while overall radiation time requirements were comparable between these groups ($p = 0.61$), radiation intensity was higher in the robotic group ($p < 0.01$), a finding they attributed to the need for high-quality fluoroscopy required for the robotic system registration process.[18]

8.2.3 Operative Times and Blood Loss

Although several series have compared operative times with conventional freehand or fluoroscopy-guided pedicle screw placement to robot-assisted pedicle screws, little consensus exists. A single cadaver series found a significantly decreased operative time for pedicle screw placement compared with conventional fluoroscopy,[21] while several other series saw no significant difference between robot-assisted and conventional techniques,[8,15,16] and still others found a significantly increased operative time with robot-assisted screws.[9,12,13] One might expect that procedural modifications involving a new device would lead to longer operative times, at least initially. Over time, as the surgeon and operative staff become more accustomed to the new device and workflow, operative times would be expected to improve.

A single series compared blood loss in a mixed group of open and percutaneous robot-assisted pedicle screw procedures to that seen with open conventional fluoroscopy screw placement and found that blood loss was less in the robotic group.[8]

8.2.4 Other Potential Applications

Bony decompression of the neural elements in patients with pain and neurological deficits is arguably the most important task performed during the vast majority of spinal procedures. Achieving an optimal result can be hindered by spatial disorientation particularly in revision cases and during the learning curve of minimally invasive procedures performed with minimal access retractor systems. Planning the site and extent of decompression preoperatively and using passive or semiactive robots with a drill or osteotome as the end effector could help to optimize the amount of the removal of bone, ligament, and disc desired by the surgeon. Rod-bending is another routine task which could theoretically benefit from robotic assistance as rod-bending involves the conformation of an object to fixed parameters such as screw head location. Given that the stereotactic technology for using optical cameras to facilitate the rod-bending process is already available (Bendini, Nuvasive Inc.), it is not difficult to imagine a robotic device performing a similar process and bending/inserting the rod semiautonomously with the goal of achieving optimal sagittal spinal alignment.

Robotic devices also have a tremendous potential benefit in minimally invasive spine procedures. Certain procedural steps that are difficult for humans to perform through small tubes (e.g., dural closure) could theoretically be performed with greater aptitude by a robotic arm. There is also a significant opportunity to pair robotics with endoscopic spinal surgery to improve efficiency and reproducibility to assist surgeons with a relatively steep learning curve.

Finally, although the field of spinal robotics is still relatively rudimentary, further advancements in robotic technology could enhance our current surgical capabilities and allow for new approaches and treatment possibilities that are currently impractical (▶ Table 8.1). Telesurgery, for instance, or the practice of surgery remote from the patient's location, has been shown to be feasible in other surgical specialties with the use of robotics[22,23] and remote surgery or remote assistance/guidance of other surgeons through robotics could theoretically be a possibility in spine surgery.

8.2.5 Current and Potential Applications

▶ Table 8.1 lists the applications of the robot-assisted surgery.

Table 8.1 Current and potential applications of robotic technology

Screw and implant placement
Bilateral screw placement
Single-stage surgery
Telesurgery/remote surgery
Decompression
Rod-bending
Dural closure

8.2.6 Monetary Costs

Modern robot-assisted pedicle screw placement may confer a modest improvement in screw placement accuracy and other desirable parameters, but the devices themselves also impart a considerable economic cost burden, and this cost may limit the availability and use of such devices to high-volume centers. Little objective data exists regarding the cost-effectiveness of such devices, but data from the use of CT navigation in spine surgery suggests that, in high-volume centers and those performing difficult cases, the relatively high initial cost investment is indeed economically justified by a reduction in the need for costly revision surgeries.[24,25] In addition, reduction in the time required for pedicle screw placement relative to conventional methods further compounds cost savings,[24] as do reductions in the indirect costs likely associated with undue radiation exposure to the patient, surgeon, and staff.

Furthermore, though the robotic spinal systems currently available are fairly limited in scope and application, the utility of these devices will likely grow with time, and with an expanding applicability to a range of difficult spinal procedures, the fiscal efficiency of spinal robotics will concomitantly increase.[26]

8.3 Early Evolution of Spinal Robotics

The use of robotic assistance in spine surgery began in earnest in 2004 with the approval by the U.S. Food and Drug Administration of the Mazor™ SpineAssist system (Mazor Robotics, Caesarea, Israel). As is the case for the majority of spinal robotics systems to follow, the SpineAssist was largely designed to assist with the planning and implementation of a specific trajectory, whether it be for screws, needles, or other instruments. The device itself was mounted to the patient's bony anatomy—either through a clamp attached to a spinous process, a bridge attached through three pins to the patient's posterior superior iliac spine (PSIS) or a device mounted to the surgical bed. Planning took place through a reformatted CT scan of the operative area imported into a planning software suite. The C-arm was then calibrated and various intraoperative fluoroscopy images were taken and merged with the preoperative CT scan. Following this, a robotic arm directed the surgeon's hand to the starting point and angle of the planned trajectory, and a sheath attached to the robotic arm served as a guide for the surgeon's hand during instrument placement.[27]

Several robotic devices intended for use in spine surgery are currently available, and each draws in one way or another on the functionality of SpineAssist; namely, to assist with planning and executing a trajectory with instruments and/or hardware. These include the Mazor™ Renaissance and Mazor™ X (Mazor Robotics, Caesarea, Israel), ExcelsiusGPS (Globus Medical, Inc., Audubon, PA), and ROSA (Medtech Surgical, Inc., New York, NY), among others (▶ Fig. 8.1 and ▶ Fig. 8.2).

The da Vinci Surgical System Robot (Intuitive Surgical, Sunnydale, CA), though popularly known for its use in urological, gynecological, and general surgical procedures, has also been used for transoral odontoidectomy[28] as well as multiple spine procedures in swine (retroperitoneal dissection for anterior lumbar interbody fusion, laminectomy, discectomy, dural closure).[29,30]

8.4 Robot-Assistance and Integrated Navigation

Robotic spine devices and CT/fluoroscopy-based navigation both provide the surgeon with an increased level of awareness and control during surgery, and each has its own unique advantages and disadvantages to consider. Navigation uses a camera and a patient-mounted reference array to give the surgeon information about where an object lies relative to the patient's anatomy. Spinal robotic devices use patient- or table-mounted

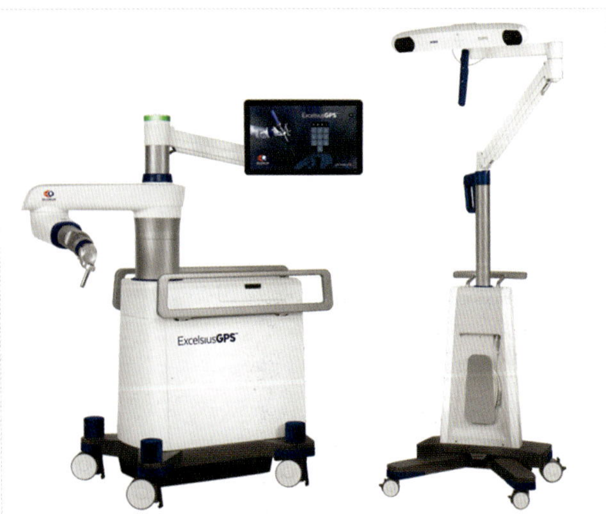

Fig. 8.1 The ExcelsiusGPS surgical system (Globus Medical, Inc., Audubon, PA). This system uses optical tracking and a patient-mounted reference array, obligating the need for the robot to attach directly to the patient or bed. (Image used with permission from Globus Medical.)

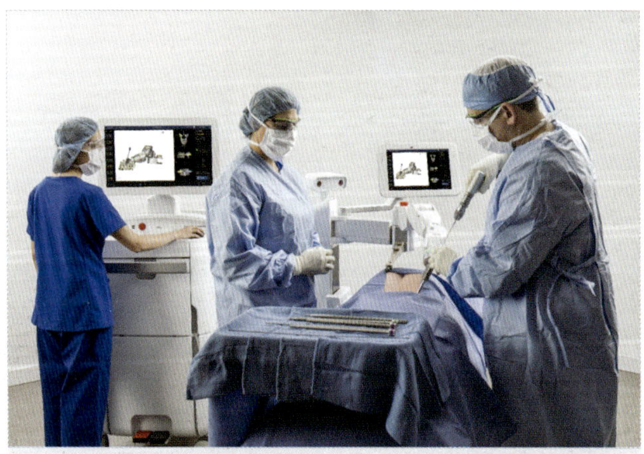

Fig. 8.2 The Mazor™ X surgical system (Mazor Robotics, Caesarea, Israel). This system uses a preoperative or intraoperative computed tomography scan with or without intraoperative calibrated fluoroscopic registration to guide a robotic arm. While currently used primarily for pedicle screw placement, the system is capable of upgrading to include navigation capabilities and bony/disc space work. (Image used with permission from Mazor Robotics, Caesarea, Israel.)

points of fixation to achieve what is essentially the same end, but they provide the surgeon with a robotic arm "guide" to hold instruments in a given orientation. Many currently available robotic systems rely heavily on an optical tracking system similar to that seen in navigation technology, and if necessary, both techniques can often be employed in the same surgical procedure without the need for additional radiation exposure. It is likely that, as time progresses, these "divergent" technologies will become more and more compatible.

One major benefit of modern navigation technology is that it is widely applicable to a variety of uses and procedures. The placement of instrumentation, localization of important landmarks, and removal of bone or other tissues can all be enhanced by the information navigation provides. While most spinal robotic devices assist primarily with pedicle screw placement and will require significant adaptations in order to perform more complex tasks, navigation can be applied to almost any instrument to which a reference array can be affixed, such as a drill, an osteotome, or an interbody graft.

Spinal navigation is not inherently suited to—or marketed as—a preplanned endeavor. Whereas each screw placed with robotic-assistance is planned preoperatively in the office or surgical suite, navigated pedicle screw placement often occurs in "real time."[20] This may be a disadvantage, as hardware constructs created "on the fly" may not take as many variables (e.g., screw cadence and rod-bending) into account. It should be noted that this is not a limitation inherent to the navigation software itself, however, and in-depth surgical plans can in fact be created preoperatively and executed with navigation, if so desired.

The benefit of modern robotic devices is that they provide the surgeon with a relatively stable working channel to guide and hold instruments, relieving the surgeon of the need to maintain an instrument (e.g., a pedicle screw and screwdriver) in a precise location/orientation while also imparting the torque and downward force to drive a screw into the bone. Furthermore, robotic devices also allow the surgeon to look at his own hands and at the operative field rather than at a virtual representation of the instruments and anatomy on an overhead screen.[20]

Both spinal navigation and spinal robot assistance have flaws. Both technologies attempt to impart information about the present state of affairs based on anatomical and radiographic information that was obtained in the past, and thus neither are truly "real-time." Both are susceptible to inaccuracies related to patient movement, movement of the reference frame/array, and human error in general. Navigation and robotics are both tools which should be used for the situation in which their respective limitations and benefits confer the greatest impact on outcome.

8.5 Basic Technique and Workflow

8.5.1 Positioning and Operating Table

Most often the patient will be positioned prone, although some devices have made modifications allowing for the placement of robotic pedicle screws with the patient in the lateral decubitus position. The authors preferentially perform thoracolumbar spinal instrumentation on a Jackson table, although modern robotic devices may be adapted to fit to a variety of operating tables, and some devices do not require fixation to the operating table at all.

8.5.2 Bone-Mounting Platforms

Many of the currently available spinal robotic devices are mounted (either directly or indirectly) to the patient's bony anatomy. This may be through the use of a Schanz screw drilled into the PSIS, or through a number of different spinous process clamps (▶ Fig. 8.3). Often, it is recommended that the bony mount be affixed to an area of the spine in close proximity to operative segments. The Schanz screw method (wherein the mount is secured to the PSIS), for instance, may be used when instrumenting the caudal spine (L3-S2), while more cranial segments may require spinous process clamps. When using spinous process clamps, it is often recommended that the clamp(s) be placed at the center of the segment to be operated.

Other devices (e.g., ExcelsiusGPS, ROSA) utilize an optical tracking system and a reference frame affixed to the patient's bony anatomy and thus, do not require attachment of the robot to the operating table or patient at all.

8.5.3 Planning and Registration

The planning and registration workflow for the large majority of available spinal robotic devices is similar. Planning takes place on a console, wherein CT images (obtained either preoperatively or intraoperatively) are loaded onto a console and virtual representations of hardware (e.g., pedicle screws) or other instruments are projected over the CT images (in axial, sagittal, and coronal views). The orientations of the hardware/instruments are modified by the planning surgeon until the desired orientation, trajectory, and length are achieved and the final plan is set (▶ Fig. 8.4).

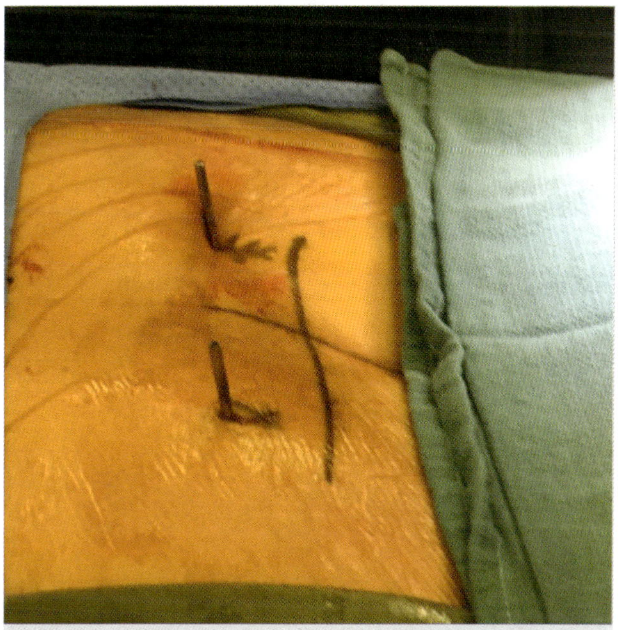

Fig. 8.3 Intraoperative photograph showing Schanz screws placed in a patient's bilateral posterior superior iliac spines. The robot will be affixed to the screws for mounting purposes prior to screw placement.

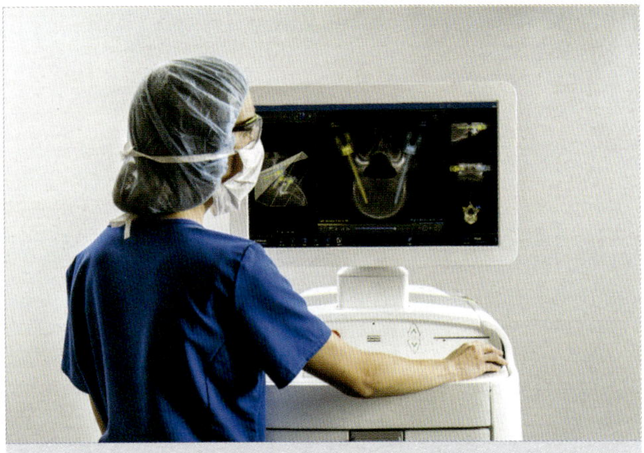

Fig. 8.4 Illustration of intraoperative pedicle screw planning on the Mazor™ X surgical system console. (Image used with permission from Mazor Robotics, Caesarea, Israel.)

When a preoperative CT is used for planning purposes, it must be supplemented by intraoperative anteroposterior and oblique fluoroscopy images taken with a calibrated C-arm, which are together used to create an accurate registration of the orientation and location of the patient's spine relative to the robot in three-dimensional (3D) space (▶ Fig. 8.5). Alternatively, an intraoperative CT-scan may be taken and transferred to the planning console for registration purposes without the need for additional fluoroscopy. One fundamental difference in the registration process of most commercially available robotic spinal systems in comparison with spinal navigation systems is that robotic registration is typically "segmental." This means that each vertebra is registered independent of the position of its neighboring vertebral body. This feature may enhance the accuracy of robotically executed screw insertion in comparison to traditional navigation where error can be introduced when intersegmental motion occurs during the procedure. Because the segmental registration process involves matching a specific level intraoperatively with features seen on the preoperative CT, many surgeons alter the workflow of their pedicle screw insertion technique. Traditional freehand technique is often facilitated by performing medial facetectomies or true Smith-Peterson osteotomies to precisely identify the entry point to the pedicle with the option of palpating the medial wall from within the canal. To maximize the accuracy of registration, many surgeons will reverse this workflow and register with most of the bony anatomy intact, drill and tap, complete their facet work, and place screws as the final step in the process of screw insertion.

Prior to beginning the instrumentation procedure, some robotic devices take additional photographs of the operative field to characterize the 3D space within which the arm is free to move without contacting the patient, surgeon, or other items in the field (▶ Fig. 8.6).

8.5.4 Executing a Trajectory

Moving the arm to a given trajectory is achieved by selecting the desired trajectory on the console. The order of execution can proceed in a variety of sequences, moving from each level, side to side, or moving along all the planned trajectories unilaterally before crossing over to the contralateral side. In percutaneous

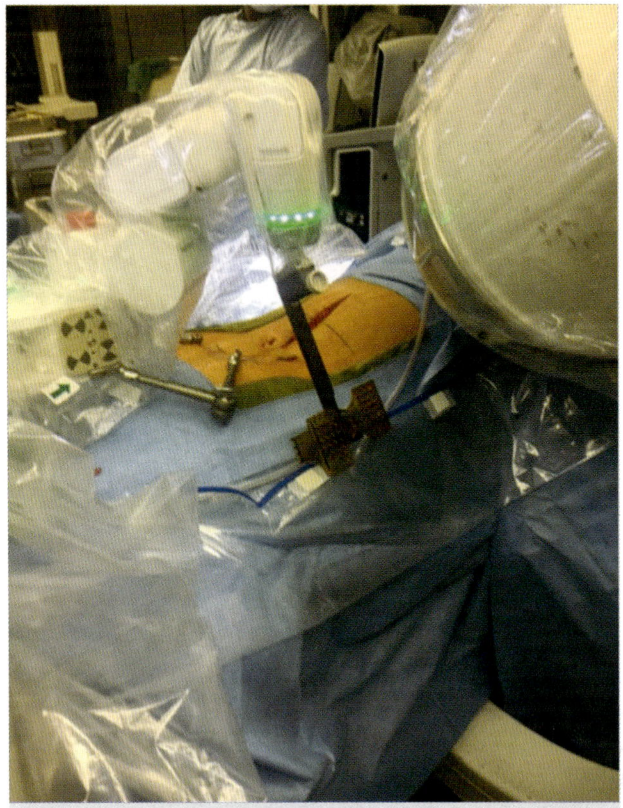

Fig. 8.5 Intraoperative photograph showing an oblique fluoroscopy image being taken for registration purposes.

cases, an incision may be made through the end effector using a specialized scalpel, followed by a series of soft tissue cannulas designed to dilate the fascia and muscle. Drills, taps, and screw drivers may then be placed using the same effector arm, or alternatively, a Kirschner-wire may be placed in the drilled trajectory, to allow subsequent tapping and screw placement with supplemental lateral fluroscopy. The drill guides used often have a serrated—or "reamer"—tip, so that a more secure docking station in the relevant bone can be achieved. This may prevent the guide skiving off irregular bony surfaces, altering the intended trajectory.

8.6 Learning Curve

When new techniques or devices are introduced to the operating room, a there is a period of practitioner and staff learning before maximum confidence and proficiency is achieved. Over time, practitioners and staff become more familiar with workflow and device function and better able to anticipate and react to device-specific idiosyncrasies and limitations. Although placing pedicle screws with robot assistance is no different, the principles underlying the workflow and robot-assisted procedure itself will be familiar to most spine surgeons; particularly those who have experience with CT- or fluoroscopy-guided navigation.

Hu and Lieberman reviewed the first 150 robot-assisted pedicle screw procedures by a single spine surgeon to characterize the learning curve associated with robot-assisted pedicle screw placement.[31] They found that the accuracy of pedicle screws placed with robotic assistance increased considerably

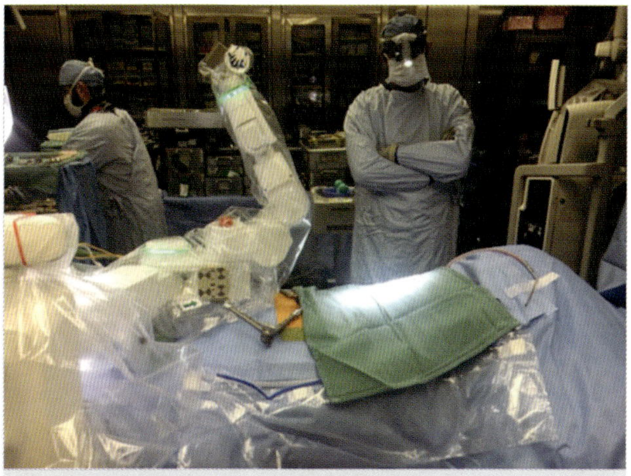

Fig. 8.6 Intraoperative photograph showing the robot taking photographs of the operative field to characterize the three-dimensional space in which it can operate.

(82–93%) after the first 30 cases and remained relatively stable (> 90%) thereafter. Similarly, the number of screws requiring intraoperative conversion from a robot-assisted to a freehand technique decreased (17–7%) after the first 30 cases and remained relatively stable (≤ 8%) over the rest of the study period.

Urakov et al retrospectively evaluated 30 cases with 306 robot-assisted thoracolumbar lumbar pedicle screws placed with resident participation.[32] While no significant difference was seen with regard to time required to place a pedicle screw between junior and senior residents, a trend was seen toward lesser time required per screw with senior residents. Mean time required per screw also increased with relative linearity as the number of robot-assisted cases performed by a given resident increased, although this finding did not reach statistical significance.

Schatlo et al reviewed 258 surgeries in which 1,265 robot-assisted thoracolumbar pedicle screws were placed by 13 surgeons.[33] They found that the number of misplaced pedicle screws rose from a mean of 2.4% in the first 5 surgeries to a peak of 7.1% between 15 and 20 surgeries, thereafter declining steadily. They contribute this finding to a combination of decreased supervision and increased surgeon confidence after the initial few proctored surgeries in surgeons who are left unproctored without having fully mastered the technique.

The learning curve for robot-assisted pedicle screws is also likely to be influenced by an understanding of the inherent limitations of the technique and the associated pitfalls, many of which have been previously described and are discussed below.

8.7 Pearls and Pitfalls

The single most often cited pitfall associated with robot-assisted pedicle screw placement deals with screw inaccuracy associated with imperfect docking of the drill guide or other instruments at the bony site of entry. Often the pedicle screw entry site will be irregular (particularly in patients with advanced spondylosis), and in some cases this can lead to the drill guide or other instruments "skiving" downhill, away from the intended entry point by several millimeters.[8,9,14,18,32] Inexperienced surgeons or those failing to anticipate this pitfall may not detect this small amount of instrument slippage, leading to malpositioned screws. Many authors have suggested that robot-assisted screws in the lumbar spine tend to be malpositioned laterally due to skiving off of the large lumbar facet joints,[8,9,32] whereas robot-assisted screws in the thoracic spine tend to be misplaced medially due to the downward slope of the transverse process.[32,33]

Multiple technical modifications have been suggested to avoid such aberrant movement during docking. First, it is recommended that a relatively flat pedicle screw entry point be chosen at the time of planning. Many times this may be difficult due to patient anatomy, rod-planning purposes, or other considerations. Another suggestion is to level the surface of bony entry manually prior to drilling. This may be done with a drill or rongeur in open cases, but may require a reamer or other device in percutaneous cases. Second, the guide should ideally be engaged with the bony surface under direct visualization to ensure that it does not migrate. Again, in percutaneous cases, this may not be feasible.[18,32] It has also been suggested that additional fluoroscopy should be routinely used during the cannulation process to ensure that the entry points being drilled correlate well with the planned trajectories,[8,18] particularly in the early phase of a surgeon's learning curve with robot-assisted screws. Finally, one should be prepared to convert to conventional or navigated methods at any time in the operation if need be.

Some authors have noted a higher breach rate for robot-assisted pedicle screws placed percutaneously when compared with open robot-assisted screws, a finding that may be accounted for by the inability to flatten bony entry points and directly visualize guide docking, as mentioned above.[31,32] It may be prudent for surgeons unfamiliar with robot-assisted screws to perform their first few cases open for this reason.[33]

Soft-tissue pressure on the robotic arm (e.g., due to inadequate retraction) is another often-cited reason for robot-assisted pedicle screw misplacement.[32] The robotic arms on many modern devices are indeed susceptible to undue mechanical forces placed upon them. A case series by Molliqaj et al noted a higher malposition rate for S1 pedicle screws placed robotically compared with lumbar screws, a finding they attribute to the large lever arm required of the robot to achieve the S1 pedicle trajectory and the degree of soft-tissue retraction needed for placement.[8,17] They suggest using a separate stab incision for sacral screw placement, even when the rest of the procedure is performed open.[17] Stab incisions, in general, should also be sufficiently large to accommodate the guide and should include the fascia.[18,33]

8.8 Future Directions

Although most modern robotic spinal devices engage passively with the operation, the future holds promising possibilities of an expanded role for robots. Given the costs of research and development, however, advances in robotic capabilities will likely progress in a measured and incremental fashion, building successively upon prior platforms and capabilities.[34]

One of the necessary steps toward active robotic participation in spine surgery will be the development of improved

control systems for streamlined transmission of surgeon input to robotic output. Unlike the relatively large cockpit-style console associated with existing systems, such as the da Vinci, virtual and augmented-reality platforms might become an important future element of robotic controller development in spine surgery, easing the transmission of tasks and information from surgeon to robot. Increasingly refined external optics systems or "exoscopes" might capture the surgical field while wearables such as 3D visor displays project preoperative or intraoperative imaging overlay into the surgeon's view. Fiducially tracked and haptic-motor-imbedded gloves could facilitate surgeon–robot interfacing while occupying minimal operating room space and resources. Remote control of a robot by geographically distant cosurgeons would also be logistically feasible with this setup. Pedicles could be sounded, tapped, and instrumented actively and accurately, entirely via telerobotic surgeon control.[35]

Continued miniaturization of articular joints and actuating mechanisms as well as optimization of translational motion scaling will lead to improved robotic capabilities when performing complex tasks through narrow channels.[36] These effector arms would also employ stress and strain force sensors to provide both haptic feedback to the surgeon as well as proprioceptive feedback to the robot.[35] In early stages of implementation, these active systems could be utilized, for instance, to assist with the repair of lateral thecal sac durotomies that are often difficult to suture through minimally invasive access corridors. Drawing on foundational image-guided stereotaxis, active robotic drilling during bony decompression could be safely executed by registering the area of interest while simultaneously defining the boundaries of the thecal sac or spinal canal as a "no-fly zone."[37] A similar application is already emerging in skull base surgery.[38]

Ultimately, sophistication of artificial intelligence software and feedback sensors could facilitate automated assistance for basic procedures such as pedicle screw insertion, uncomplicated bony decompression, and simple dural closure. Integration of multiple technologies into a single robotic unit will also hopefully facilitate a less-crowded operating room. Although cost, learning curve, efficiency, reliability, and safety will always be the main barriers to widespread adaptation of robotics in spine surgery, innovation will continue to drive the field in new directions.

References

[1] Soto E, Lo Y, Friedman K, et al. Total laparoscopic hysterectomy versus da Vinci robotic hysterectomy: is using the robot beneficial? J Gynecol Oncol. 2011; 22(4):253–259

[2] Yaxley JW, Coughlin GD, Chambers SK, et al. Robot-assisted laparoscopic prostatectomy versus open radical retropubic prostatectomy: early outcomes from a randomised controlled phase 3 study. Lancet. 2016; 388 (10049):1057–1066

[3] Wren SM, Curet MJ. Single-port robotic cholecystectomy: results from a first human use clinical study of the new da Vinci single-site surgical platform. Arch Surg. 2011; 146(10):1122–1127

[4] Kang CM, Kim DH, Lee WJ, Chi HS. Conventional laparoscopic and robot-assisted spleen-preserving pancreatectomy: does da Vinci have clinical advantages? Surg Endosc. 2011; 25(6):2004–2009

[5] Tasci AI, Tufek I, Gumus E, et al. Oncologic results, functional outcomes, and complication rates of robotic-assisted radical prostatectomy: multicenter experience in Turkey including 1,499 patients. World J Urol. 2015; 33 (8):1095–1102

[6] Zorn KC, Gofrit ON, Orvieto MA, et al. Da Vinci robot error and failure rates: single institution experience on a single three-arm robot unit of more than 700 consecutive robot-assisted laparoscopic radical prostatectomies. J Endourol. 2007; 21(11):1341–1344

[7] Sarlos D, Kots L, Stevanovic N, Schaer G. Robotic hysterectomy versus conventional laparoscopic hysterectomy: outcome and cost-analyses of a matched case-control study. Eur J Obstet Gynecol Reprod Biol. 2010; 150(1): 92–96

[8] Schatlo B, Molliqaj G, Cuvinciuc V, Kotowski M, Schaller K, Tessitore E. Safety and accuracy of robot-assisted versus fluoroscopy-guided pedicle screw insertion for degenerative diseases of the lumbar spine: a matched cohort comparison. J Neurosurg Spine. 2014; 20(6):636–643

[9] Ringel F, Stüer C, Reinke A, et al. Accuracy of robot-assisted placement of lumbar and sacral pedicle screws: a prospective randomized comparison to conventional freehand screw implantation. Spine. 2012; 37(8):E496–E501

[10] Schizas C, Thein E, Kwiatkowski B, Kulik G. Pedicle screw insertion: robotic assistance versus conventional C-arm fluoroscopy. Acta Orthop Belg. 2012; 78(2):240–245

[11] Macke JJ, Woo R, Varich L. Accuracy of robot-assisted pedicle screw placement for adolescent idiopathic scoliosis in the pediatric population. J Robot Surg. 2016; 10(2):145–150

[12] Lonjon N, Chan-Seng E, Costalat V, Bonnafoux B, Vassal M, Boetto J. Robot-assisted spine surgery: feasibility study through a prospective case-matched analysis. Eur Spine J. 2016; 25(3):947–955

[13] Kim H-J, Jung W-I, Chang B-S, Lee C-K, Kang K-T, Yeom JS. A prospective, randomized, controlled trial of robot-assisted vs freehand pedicle screw fixation in spine surgery. Int J Med Robot. 2016; 13(3):e11779

[14] Keric N, Eum DJ, Afghanyar F, et al. Evaluation of surgical strategy of conventional vs. percutaneous robot-assisted spinal trans-pedicular instrumentation in spondylodiscitis. J Robot Surg. 2017; 11(1):17–25

[15] Kantelhardt SR, Martinez R, Baerwinkel S, Burger R, Giese A, Rohde V. Perioperative course and accuracy of screw positioning in conventional, open robotic-guided and percutaneous robotic-guided, pedicle screw placement. Eur Spine J. 2011; 20(6):860–868

[16] Hyun S-J, Kim K-J, Jahng T-A, Kim H-J. Minimally invasive, robotic vs. open fluoroscopic-guided spinal instrumented fusions: a randomized, controlled trial. Spine. 2016; 42(6):353:358

[17] Molliqaj G, Schatlo B, Alaid A, et al. Accuracy of robot-guided versus freehand fluoroscopy-assisted pedicle screw insertion in thoracolumbar spinal surgery. Neurosurg Focus. 2017; 42(5):E14

[18] Solomiichuk V, Fleischhammer J, Molliqaj G, et al. Robotic versus fluoroscopy-guided pedicle screw insertion for metastatic spinal disease: a matched-cohort comparison. Neurosurg Focus. 2017; 42(5):E13

[19] Roser F, Tatagiba M, Maier G. Spinal robotics: current applications and future perspectives. Neurosurgery. 2013; 72 Suppl 1:12–18

[20] Schröder ML, Staartjes VE. Revisions for screw malposition and clinical outcomes after robot-guided lumbar fusion for spondylolisthesis. Neurosurg Focus. 2017; 42(5):E12

[21] Lieberman IH, Hardenbrook MA, Wang JC, Guyer RD. Assessment of pedicle screw placement accuracy, procedure time, and radiation exposure using a miniature robotic guidance system. J Spinal Disord Tech. 2012; 25(5):241–248

[22] Marescaux J, Rubino F. Transcontinental robot-assisted remote telesurgery, feasibility and potential applications. Teleophthalmology 2006. doi:10.1007/3-540-33714-8_31

[23] Sterbis JR, Hanly EJ, Herman BC, et al. Transcontinental telesurgical nephrectomy using the da Vinci robot in a porcine model. Urology. 2008; 71(5):971–973

[24] Watkins RG, IV, Gupta A, Watkins RG, III. Costeffectiveness of image-guided spine surgery. Open Orthop J. 2010; 4:228:233

[25] Dea N, Fisher CG, Batke J, et al. Economic evaluation comparing intraoperative cone beam CT-based navigation and conventional fluoroscopy for the placement of spinal pedicle screws: a patient-level data cost-effectiveness analysis. Spine J. 2016; 16(1):23–31

[26] Overley SC, Cho SK, Mehta AI, Arnold PM. Navigation and robotics in spinal surgery: where are we now? Neurosurgery. 2017; 80 3S:S86–S99

[27] Barzilay Y, Kaplan L, Libergall M. Robotic assisted spine surgery: a breakthrough or a surgical toy? Int J Med Robot. 2008; 4(3):195–196

[28] Lee JYK, Lega B, Bhowmick D, et al. Da Vinci Robot-assisted transoral odontoidectomy for basilar invagination. ORL J Otorhinolaryngol Relat Spec. 2010; 72 (2):91–95

[29] Ponnusamy K, Chewning S, Mohr C. Robotic approaches to the posterior spine. Spine. 2009; 34(19):2104–2109

[30] Kim MJ, Ha Y, Yang MS, et al. Robot-assisted anterior lumbar interbody fusion (ALIF) using retroperitoneal approach. Acta Neurochir (Wien). 2010; 152 (4):675–679
[31] Hu X, Lieberman IH. What is the learning curve for robotic-assisted pedicle screw placement in spine surgery? Clin Orthop Relat Res. 2014; 472 (6):1839:1844
[32] Urakov TM, Chang KH, Burks SS, Wang MY. Initial academic experience and learning curve with robotic spine instrumentation. Neurosurg Focus. 2017; 42(5):E4
[33] Schatlo B, Martinez R, Alaid A, et al. Unskilled unawareness and the learning curve in robotic spine surgery. Acta Neurochir (Wien). 2015; 157(10):1819–1823, discussion 1823
[34] Joseph JR, Smith BW, Liu X, Park P. Current applications of robotics in spine surgery: a systematic review of the literature. Neurosurg Focus. 2017; 42(5):E2
[35] Madhavan K, Kolcun JPG, Chieng LO, Wang MY. Augmented-reality integrated robotics in neurosurgery: are we there yet? Neurosurg Focus. 2017; 42(5):E3
[36] Ko S, Nakazawa A, Kurose Y, et al. Intelligent control of neurosurgical robot MM-3 using dynamic motion scaling. Neurosurg Focus. 2017; 42(5):E5
[37] Patel V. Future of robotics in spine surgery. Spine. 2018; 43 7S:S28
[38] Couldwell WT, MacDonald JD, Thomas CL, et al. Computer-aided design/computer-aided manufacturing skull base drill. Neurosurg Focus. 2017; 42(5):E6

9 Microscope in MISS

Avelino Parajón, Robert Nicholas Hernandez, Sertac Kirnaz, and Andreas Korge

Summary

Modern microsurgery and minimally invasive spine surgery are no longer conceivable without a surgical microscope. After moderate beginnings starting from the Middle Ages, dramatic technical innovations from the 1950s led in many respects to the surgical microscope becoming an integral part of spinal surgery. Improvements in magnification, illumination, three-dimensional image reproduction, and intraoperative handling have led to increasing acceptance and integration of the microscope into the daily surgical workflow. Modern surgical microscopes already integrate robot-like functions and can be combined with augmented reality. Beyond clinical use, the surgical microscope also serves excellently as a training and teaching tool to train the manual skills of a surgeon outside of intraoperative use.

Keywords: surgical microscope, operating microscope, visualization, magnification, illumination, spinal microsurgery, optics

9.1 Introduction

By definition, microsurgery is performed with the assistance of a surgical microscope. In doing so, the microscope allows surgeons to perform operations through small skin incisions and narrow surgical corridors, with the great advantages and some difficulties due to the narrow surgical corridors. In minimally invasive spine surgery (MISS), the use of the microscope is essential. The use of modern surgical microscopes can save time in surgery, improve the surgical precision and efficiency, facilitate teaching and education, and ergonomically can even help prevent spine surgeons from developing back or neck pain.

9.2 Historical Overview

The first lens believed to have been used as a magnifying glass is the Nimrud lens, found in Nimrud, an ancient Assyrian city, around the 7th century BC.[1] Archimedes in 212 BC is said to have used a burning glass against the Roman fleet which was laying siege to Syracuse. Few studies in optics are found until the 11th century, in which an Arab scholar, Ibn al-Haytham, known in the West as Alhazen, wrote the "Book of Optics" describing the optical principles and anatomy of the eye.[2] In the 13th century, Roger Bacon, an English friar, published the scientific principles of corrective lenses. In 14th century Italy, Friars Giordano da Rivalto and Alessandro della Spina each chronicled or spoke about meeting a man who created the first spectacles. In the 16th century, the most famous spectacle makers in the Netherlands were Zacharias Janssen and Hans Lippershey, who were two of the firsts to invent telescopes by placing two lenses within a sliding tube.[3] In the 17th century in Italy, Galileo Galilei described his "tubum opticum" composed of two lenses, one concave and one convex so that the final image was not inverted. In the same century, Johannes Kepler, a German astronomer, created a telescope composed of two convex lenses so that the final image was inverted but allowed for a much wider field of view than Galileo's telescope.[3,4] Coincident with the development of the telescope, the microscope was also being invented by the same visionaries: Janssen and Lippershey in the Netherlands and Galileo in Italy who described "the occhialino," translated as "the little eye." The term "microscope" was coined by Giovanni Faber who used the term to describe Galileo's compound microscope submitted to the Accademia dei Lincei in 1625. In 1660, Robert Hooke used three lenses to achieve higher magnification, and the first binocular telescope was described by Chérubin d'Orléans in 1671 in his book *La dioptrique oculare*. The main disadvantages of early microscopes were blurry images and spherical aberrations. Additionally, they became more cumbersome with each additional lens. In the late 17th century, the Dutch scientist Antonie van Leeuwenhoek developed smaller and more powerful lenses with fewer aberrations, which led to the creation of a transportable, simple microscope. In the late 18th century, Chester Moore Hall managed to overcome chromatic aberrations by inventing the achromatic lens by placing concave and convex lens together.[5] In 1830, Joseph Jackson Lister, the father of the famous surgeon Joseph Lister, overcame the spherical aberrations by placing a combination of flint glass lenses with crown glass lenses at specific distances. Lister also addressed the problem of vibrations from handheld use by making stands for microscopes, in association with James Smith.[3,6] In 1847, Carl Zeiss produced his first microscope in Jena, Germany. He hired Ernst Karl Abbe, professor of physics at University of Jena, as director of his research center. Abbe made tremendous advancements in the field of microscopy including the invention of the Abbe condenser used for illumination and the development of two critical equations, the Abbe sine condition and the resolution limit of the microscope. Abbe also made great developments in increasing the power of lenses by immersion into oil and later into monobromonaphthalene.[7] Zeiss and Abbe later partnered with Friedrich Otto Schott, who had developed a lithium-based glass. Together they introduced the apochromatic lens, which had improved correction of chromatic and spherical aberrations than the achromatic lens.[7,8] With Abbe's discoveries and equations, the optical qualities of lenses could be calculated and standardized, allowing for the mass production of quality microscopes.

In 1952, Hans Littmann, a physicist working at Zeiss, invented a microscope capable of changing magnification without changing focal length. In 1953, Zeiss made the Zeiss OPMI 1 (Zeiss Operating Microscope 1), a microscope mounted on a stand equipped with a rotating arm and with superior coaxial lighting than other microscopes at the time (▶ Fig. 9.1). Further modifications and improvements were made by users like the Barraquer family, a family of Spanish ophthalmologists who made several contributions to the development of modern microscopes, and Leonard Malis and Gazi Yasargil, who introduced the idea of adjustable multiaxis counterweights with electromagnetic brakes.[5,7,9]

The first clinical use of the microscope dates back to the 17th century when Petrus Borellus described the first use of the microscope in medicine, and Athanasius Kircher used a microscope to examine the blood of individuals affected by the

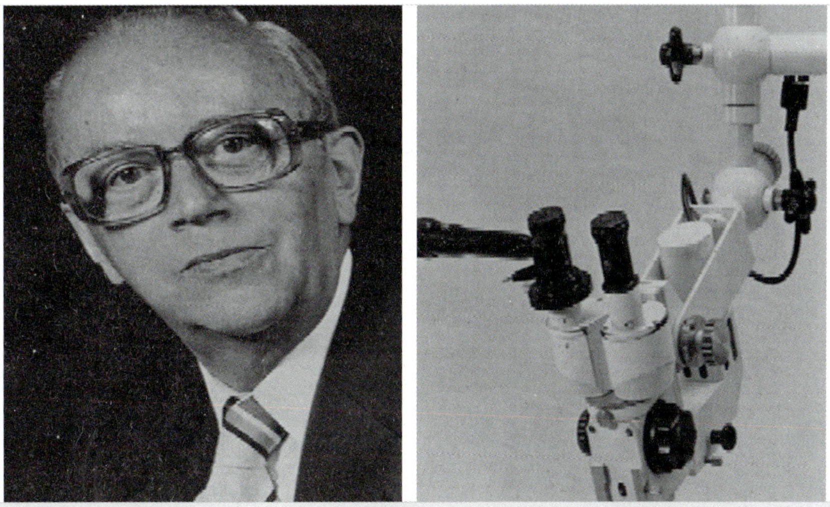

Fig. 9.1 Photographs of Hans Littmann (*left*) and the OPMI 1 Zeiss microscope (*right*). (Reproduced with permission from American Journal of Otolaryngology, 21(6), The History of the Microscope for Use in Ear Surgery, 880-883, Copyright Elsevier, 2000.)

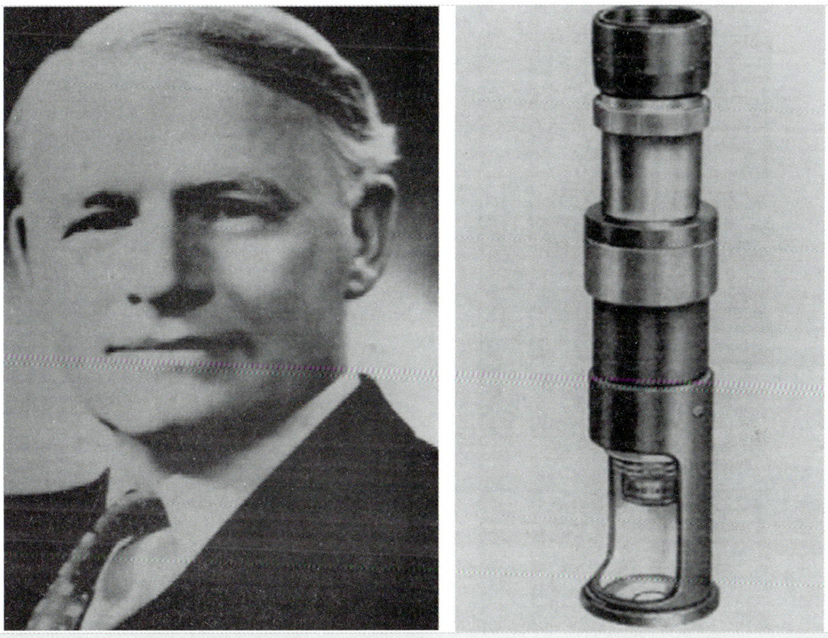

Fig. 9.2 Photographs of Carl-Olof Nylén (*left*) and his first monocular microscope (*right*). (Reproduced with permission from American Journal of Otolaryngology, 21(6), The History of the Microscope for Use in Ear Surgery, 880-883, Copyright Elsevier, 2000.)

plague. The first depicted use of a microscope in clinical practice was Giuseppe Campani's optical viewing system used for the examination of wound in leg.[10] In the 20th century, otolaryngologists were the first to use microscopes in the operating room. A monocular microscope was designed and built by Carl-Olof Nylén in 1921, an otologist from the Stockholm Clinic, and used to treat a patient suffering from chronic otitis media (▶ Fig. 9.2). In 1922, Gunnar Holmgren, Nylén's chief, attached a light source to a microscope and created the first binocular surgical microscope, which overcame the lack of depth perception noticed in the monocular microscope[11,12] (▶ Fig. 9.3). Theodore Kurze became the first neurosurgeon to use the surgical microscope in 1957, and in 1958, R.M.P. Donaghy founded the world's first microsurgery research and training laboratory in Burlington, Vermont, USA.[13] By the mid-1960s the microscope was used in intracranial vascular neurosurgery. In the late 1970s, it was introduced to spine surgery by Caspar, Yasargil, and Williams who published it in different papers.[14,15,16]

9.3 Advantages of Using the Microscope in MISS

The main advantages of using a microscope in spine surgery, and particularly in MISS, can be summarized as follows[17,18] (▶ Table 9.1):

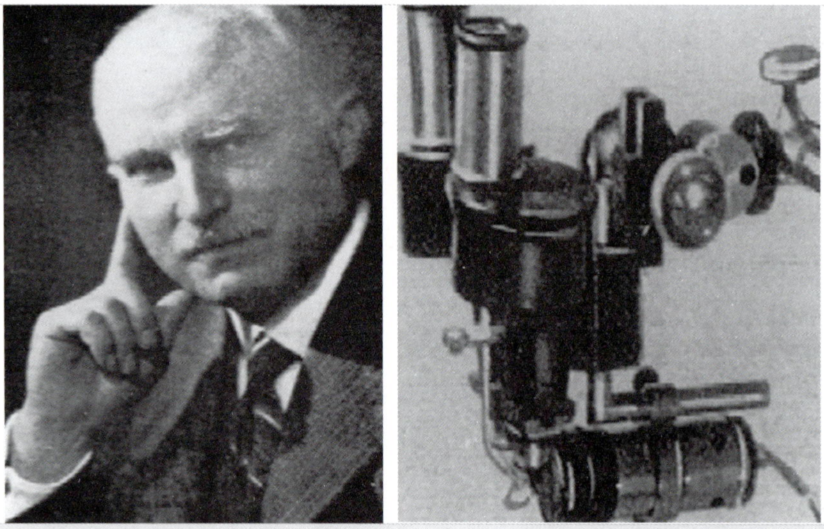

Fig. 9.3 Photographs of Gunnar Holmgren (*left*) and his first binocular microscope (*right*). (Reproduced with permission from American Journal of Otolaryngology, 21(6), The History of the Microscope for Use in Ear Surgery, 880-883, Copyright Elsevier, 2000.)

Table 9.1 Advantages of the operating microscope
1. Increased visualization
2. Improved illumination
3. Improved accuracy of microsurgical procedure
4. Provide ergonomic workflow
5. Digital documentation and education tool

a) **Magnification:** Without any magnification, the resolution (distance at which two objects can be distinguished as separate) of the human eye is 0.2 mm. The operating microscope can decrease this distance to 0.006 mm (▶ Table 9.2). Magnification also results in *improved accuracy and precision*, as both are limited not only by the hands but also by the eyes. Without magnification, a surgeon can make instrument movements 1 to 2 mm at a time. At 20-times magnification, a surgeon may be capable of refining his or her movements to 1 to 20 microns.

b) **Illumination:** This is essential for visualization of deep structures. The microscope illuminates with parallel light in addition to coaxial light, which provides better visualization and less burden on the surgeon's eyes.

c) **Coaxial lighting:** It allows for unobstructed, shadow-free illumination of the operating field.

d) **Three-dimensional image:** The binocular microscope allows the surgeon to view the operative anatomy as a three-dimensional image, including depth perception.

e) **Provides ergonomic workflow:** A microscope allows the surgeon to operate while looking straight ahead without having to bend forward (causing lower back pain) or to look down (causing neck pain). The prevalence rates of neck and back pain in spine surgeons are 59.4 and 62.2%, respectively[19] (▶ Fig. 9.4).

f) **Co-observation by the assistant:** It allows the observer to participate and assist the primary surgeon. Additionally, this allows the surgeon to teach and observe trainees.

g) **Documentation:** Surgeons can take photographs or videos intraoperatively to be used for educational, research, or legal purposes.

h) **Fluorescence imaging techniques:** The magnification and illumination allow the surgeon to perform operations through small skin incisions and access corridors (keyhole surgery), a key concept of MISS.

9.4 Disadvantages of the Microscope

As with every technique or technology used in surgery, there are some disadvantages to its use[17,18,20] (▶ Table 9.3). These disadvantages are not true disadvantages per se, but rather limitations of using the microscope:

a) **Limited visual field:** The visible area is limited and the approach anatomy is usually not visible after having entered the target area. Novice surgeons must learn to be cognizant of structures outside the visual or focal fields to avoid injury to such structures. Due to limited visual and focal fields, detailed planning of the surgical procedure, patient positioning, incision, and angle of approach are needed, and often the microscope must be repositioned so that the working site remains in the visual and focal fields (▶ Fig. 9.5).

b) **Visual axis:** The visual axis must be parallel to the approach axis so that the target area is not obstructed by the surgeon's hand and instruments.

c) **Hand–eye coordination:** Novice surgeons may have difficulty knowing where there hands and instruments are in space when outside the visual field of the microscope. However, the learning curve is easily overcome with repeated use of the microscope.

d) **Price:** Modern microscopes are costly, technologically complex machines and require routine maintenance to maintain optimal performance.

Table 9.2 Magnification and resolution of various magnification systems

Magnification system	Magnification	Resolution (μm)
Human eye	Zero	200
Amsted loupes	1.5 ×	133.33
Low-magnification loupes	2.5 ×	80
Medium power loupes	4 ×	50
Microscope—low magnification	6.4 ×	31
Microscope—medium magnification	10 ×	20
Microscope—high magnification	24 ×	8.33

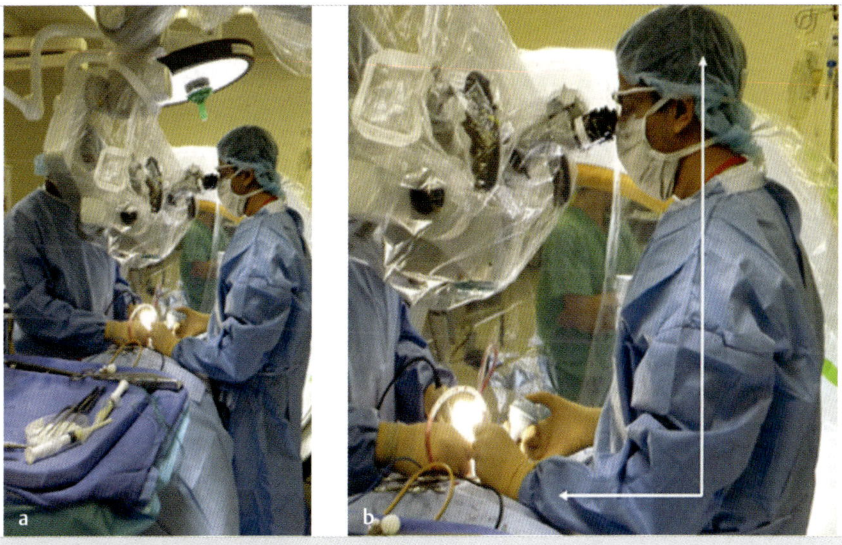

Fig. 9.4 Ergonomic position using the microscope: The surgeon and the assistant are able to maintain a neutral cervical spine **(a)** and upright position **(b)**.

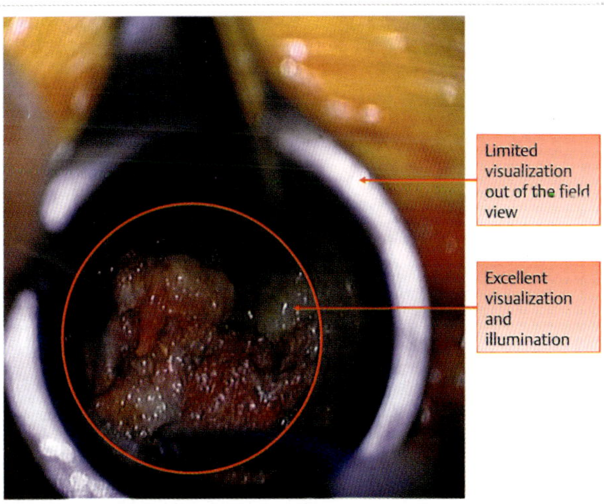

Fig. 9.5 Excellent magnification and illumination in the centered field of view, no visualization outside of the field view.

e) **Light injury to tissue:** Of the listed disadvantages, the one with clinical relevance is the last one. Light sources possess the power to severely damage tissue. In modern microscopes, traditional lighting sources such as incandescent bulbs have been replaced with xenon and halogen lamps. This technologically advanced lighting provides excellent illumination, but this great light energy can damage the illuminated tissue. Secondary damage due to high-intensity lighting has been reported in ophthalmology, plastic surgery, and neurovascular and otologic surgery, and includes blindness, skin burns, and damage to the pedicles and venous occlusion in vascular surgery.[21,22,23] It is therefore important for the surgeon and the operative team to be aware of these potential complications and to know the characteristics of the model used. Light intensity can be measured in two ways:

1. **Radiometric analysis:** It measures the radiant energy produced by a light source, expressed as radiance (radiation emitted, in $W/Sr/m^2$) and irradiance (irradiation of a surface, in W/m^2).
2. **Photometric analysis:** It measures the perceived brightness, expressed in luminance, in lux ($lumen/m^2$).

Tips for lowering the amount of irradiance when using surgical microscopes are[24]:

1. Increasing the working distance: Operate at the greatest working distance which allows safe, effective surgery.
2. Use the lowest microscope intensity setting that provides adequate visualization of the surgical field. In some surgical microscope models, like Pentero (Zeiss), intensity limits can be set automatically.
3. In some microscopes, if spot size changes, the radiance may change. Spot size can be decreased in microscopes by focusing the light into a smaller area or by closing the light

aperture. Focusing the same light energy into a smaller diameter can increase the risk of light injury to the illuminated tissue. Pentero (Zeiss), for example, increases the radiance with decreasing spot size and the intensity should therefore be decreased to limit tissue injury. On the other hand, it is important to use the smallest spot size possible during surgery to decrease thermal injury to the surrounding tissues outside the working field that do not require illumination.

4. There are some patient and instrument factors that may contribute to burns. These include residual betadine or photosensitizing medications. Additionally, metals that remain in the illuminated field may become hot and result in thermal tissue injury. Local injection of anesthetic with vasoconstrictors may decrease the blood supply leading to decreased local heat dissipation. Surgeons may overcome some of these factors by irrigation of the field during surgery.

9.5 Characteristics of Modern Spine/MISS Microscopes

a) Optical system:
   1. Focal length with variable adaptation.
   2. Two binocular tubes, primary and observer (for the surgeon and the assistant).
   3. Camera tube (for documentation).
   4. Adjustable interpupillary distance.

b) Illuminating system: A xenon light source is the standard nowadays (provides homogeneous and coaxial illumination, resembles daylight conditions).[20]

c) Control systems for:
   1. Position.
   2. Focus.
   3. Magnification (zoom).
   4. Working distance.

d) Stands: Electromagnetic coupling of the microscope to the stand (for regular spine surgeries, a standard stand is sufficient).

e) Video technology and documentation.

f) Depth of field: In spine surgery, this can often be great because of the depth of the target and types of instruments used (extended).

9.6 Differences between Microscopes and Loupes

There are several differences between microscopes and loupes. In some types of surgeries where the working field is superficial and there is a primary need for magnification only (versus magnification and illumination), modern loupes are often sufficient, and some studies have shown that there is no difference between the use of surgical loupes and a microscope[25] (▸ Table 9.3). In MISS, in which the depth of the working field can be great and the approach corridors are often narrow, there is a need for both illumination and a high-degree of magnification. In this latter case, microscopes are superior:

a) Magnification: Often loupes 2.5 to 5 ×, microscope 24 ×.

Table 9.3 Disadvantages of the operating microscope

1. Limited field of vision
2. Hand–eye coordination learning curve
3. High cost

b) Focal distance easily adaptable in modern microscopes, without readjusting table height.

c) Improved illumination with the microscope.

d) Improved surgeon ergonomics with the microscope, resulting in less neck and back pain.

9.7 Operating Room Setup and Handling of Microscopes

When using the microscope, standardization of the setup and the operating room workflow is highly recommended. The entire nursing team dealing with the microscope should be carefully trained.

Since the microscope and other technologies used in MISS (e.g., navigation systems or fluoroscopy) are bulky, if these technologies are to be used, the operating room should be large enough to enable the staff to move safely within the room without risking contamination of sterile areas or obstructing access to the patient or critical supplies.

The operating table should be placed in the center of the room. Video equipment, such as a wall-mounted television or the microscope video screen, must be placed in such a way that the scrub nurse has full view of the screen in order to follow the procedure. The best position for the operating microscope is the base of the microscope to be behind the primary surgeon. If fluoroscopy is required, the machine should enter the field opposite the microscope. Since most available surgical microscopes have an asymmetrically constructed optical unit, the primary surgeon's side is always the one with the smaller eye-ocular distance. The height of the table has to be adapted in such a way that the surgeon has his arms at a comfortable 90 degrees flexion at the elbow level. The light in the operating room should be dimmed to increase vision in the surgical field by omitting nonfocal lighting and reducing the diffuse lighting around the oculars. Dimming also increases the contrast of the video monitor. Draping starts with the optical lens, which has a tight-fitting ring around it. The lens must be open for maximum optical quality. Minimal microscope drapes that cover only the handlebars and leave the rest of the equipment unsterile do not fulfill the aseptic requirements of microsurgical spine surgery. The microscope handlebars should be covered tightly with the drape allowing proper handling. Surgeons wearing glasses should choose the shortest ocular length; others should increase it using the long length of the oculars. The usual recommended setup is: medium zoom speed, quick focus speed, maximum light intensity, and full magnification range. Lighting blind should be opened to its maximum at the beginning of the procedures and limited to the retractor size as soon as they are placed. In microscopes that provide lateral movements of the handlebar, the handle for the surgeon's dominant hand should be tilted upward about 45 degrees so that more space for handling of the instruments is obtained; in fact, many surgeons prefer to have both handles at 45 degrees.

Adequate storing of the microscope is essential. All lever arms have to be bent inward to ensure that the space taken up by the device is minimal. The joints and footbrakes must be locked when the microscope is in the idle position for storage. An extra cover, usually provided by the manufacturer, is used for the optical unit to prevent dust accumulation.

9.8 Future

Fluorescence image-guided surgery offers great advantages for tumor resection (e.g., 5 ALA, yellow fluorescence) and for vascular surgery (e.g., indocyanine green [ICG] angiography). Similarly, augmented reality (AR) aims to overlay virtual bony structures and preplanned screw trajectories on patients in the setting of hybrid operating rooms that enable real-time feedback of all instruments in space and also in relation to anatomical structures.[26,27,28,29] It also facilitates the tumor resection by differentiating the surrounding neural tissue and bony landmarks by color, and allowing for the optimal trajectory and laminotomy site to reach the pathology (▶ Fig. 9.6). They are mostly used nowadays in brain surgery, but their use in spine surgery is increasing.

Merging intraoperative microscopic images with navigation systems, combining AR and robotics is another possibility available in the modern microscope. Integration of the operating microscope with navigation systems allows the position of the microscope to be tracked, and the trajectory and field of view can be navigated. Furthermore, the introduction of robotic microscopes avoids the need for the surgeons to take their hands away from the surgical field to reposition the microscope, improving surgical efficiency.[30] Some of the modern models, such as the Kinevo (Zeiss), have introduced this automatization (▶ Fig. 9.7). In addition, this modern surgical microscope allows combining the microscope with the endoscope.

9.9 Training

Microsurgery can be applied in almost every surgical specialty and has become part of surgical training in many institutions. The ability in microsurgery should only be applied in the clinic after a training period in the lab or operating rooms under supervision. Mastering the techniques of microsurgery demands high manual skills, patience, dedication, and continued training. Even a skillful surgeon is not able to perform microsurgery without specialized training. Microsurgical training includes theorical and practical

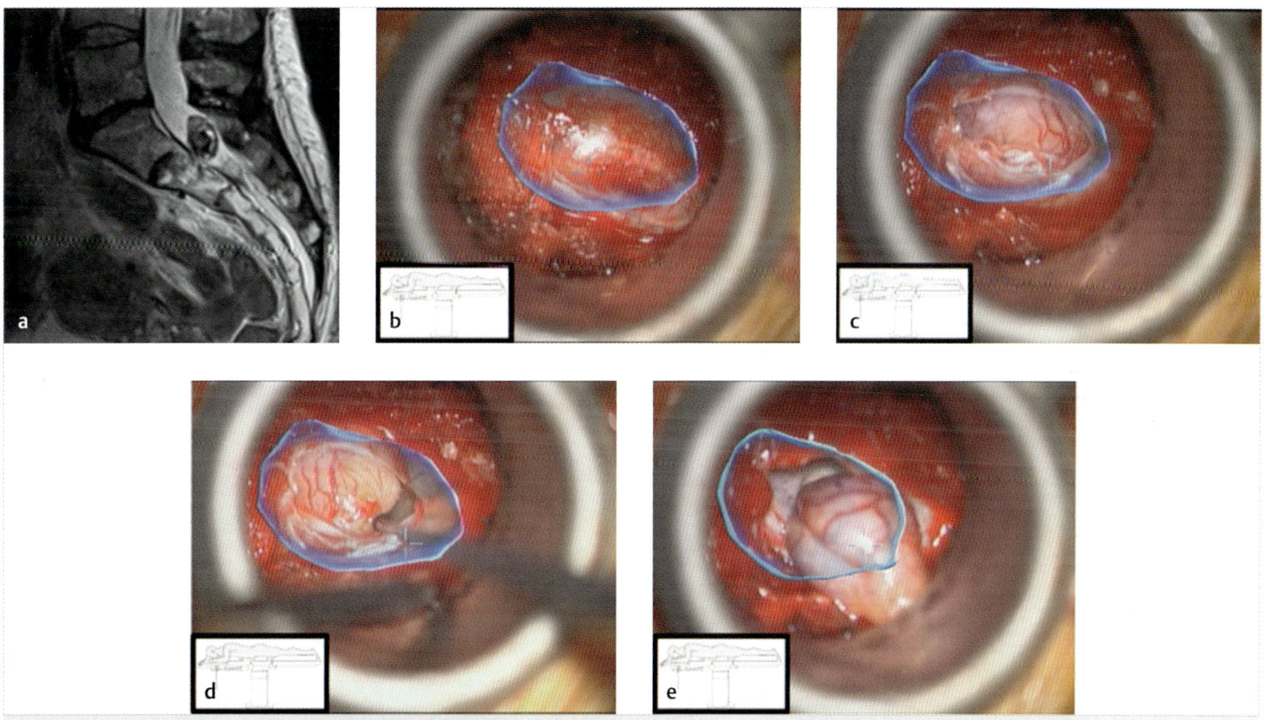

Fig. 9.6 (a–e) Example of an S1–S2 intradural schwannoma resected through a minimally invasive approach using a tubular retractor with augmented reality (AR). Even prior to durotomy, the outline of the tumor is denoted by the *blue* line. Once the durotomy is made, tumor resection is guided by internal debulking, working toward the borders visualized through AR. After excision, the remaining space can be explored using the *blue* AR outline as a perimeter to inspect for confirmation of gross total resection.

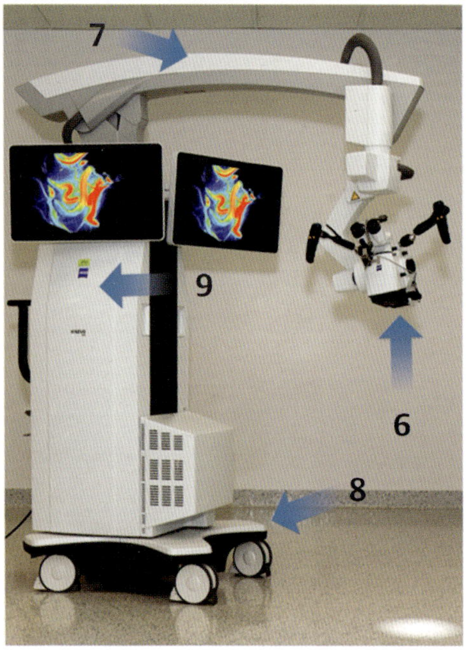

Fig. 9.7 Robotic Visualization System™ – Kinevo®900 from Zeiss. (Reproduced from Microscopes Principles of Operation Operative Microscopes. In: Belykh E, Martirosyan N, Kalani M, Nakaji P, ed. Microsurgical Basics and Bypass Techniques. 1st Edition. New York: Thieme; 2020.)

lectures. It is essential for trainee to learn basic techniques such as positioning, viewing, hand–eye coordination, handling and adjustment of the microscopes, handling micro instruments, and microdissection. The trainee must become accustomed to indirect vision provided by the microscope and be able acquire and refine the coordination of eyes and hands. This training process should be first explored in a cadaver laboratory setting and introduced into the clinical setting only when the surgeon is comfortable with it. However, the training costs are significantly high, and the training is unlike "real" situation cases. In some special circumstances, two surgeons can operate on the same case by using two microscopes simultaneously, such as in tandem microscopic slalom technique, which facilitates the teaching and training of surgeons in MIS[31] (▸ Fig. 9.8). On the other hand, new training techniques have been developed to optimize the learning process such as surgical simulation training system; an example of simulation technique is Realspine® (RSTT Real Surgical Training Technologies GmbH, Leipzig, Germany), which is based on a simulator that offers many surgical scenarios on the spine (▸ Fig. 9.9). Due to its realistic anatomical structures, soft tissues, and intraoperative bleeding system, the simulator is almost as realistic as a real patient. The model can be used with any surgical instrument or technology, since it is life-like. Additionally, other complications can be simulated, for example, an injury to the dura with cerebrospinal fluid flow. By using the simulation system for the training of operations on the lumbar spine, the surgical skills of residents and consultants can be improved in a realistic but risk-free environment for the patient.[32]

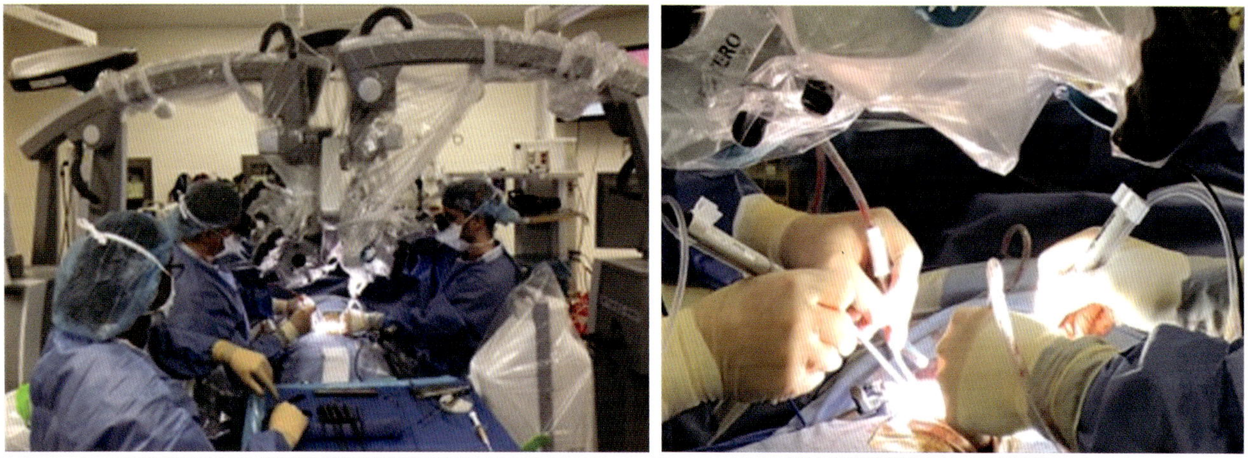

Fig. 9.8 Intraoperative setup with two surgeons working simultaneously with two microscopes, performing the tandem microscopic slalom technique for multilevel lumbar stenosis.

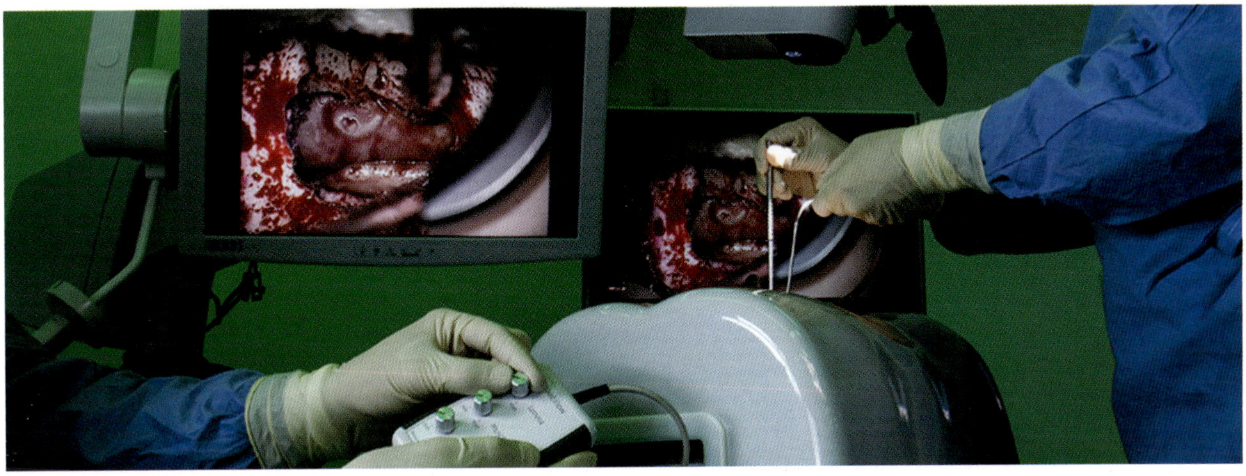

Fig. 9.9 Surgical Simulation Training System, Realspine®, RSTT Real Surgical Training Technologies GmbH, Leipzig, Germany.

References

[1] King HC, Jones HS. The History of the Telescope. New Yok: Courier Dover Publications; 2003

[2] Lindberg DC. Theories of Vision from Al-Kindi to Kepler. Chicago: University of Chicago Press; 1982

[3] Kalderon AE. The evolution of microscope design from its invention to the present days. Am J Surg Pathol. 1983; 7(1):95–102

[4] Drake S. Galileo's first telescopic observations. J Hist Astron. 1976; 7(3):153–168

[5] Uluç K, Kujoth GC, Başkaya MK. Operating microscopes: past, present, and future. Neurosurg Focus. 2009; 27(3):E4

[6] Clarke AR, Eberhardt CN. Microscopy techniques for materials science. Cambridge: Woodhead Publishing Ltd.; 2002

[7] Tamai S. History of microsurgery—from the beginning until the end of the 1970s. Microsurgery. 1993; 14(1):6–13

[8] Volkmann H. Ernst Abbe and his work. Appl Opt. 1966; 5(11):1720–1731

[9] Schultheiss D, Denil J. History of the microscope and development of microsurgery: a revolution for reproductive tract surgery. Andrologia. 2002; 34 (4):234–241

[10] Field JV, James FAJL. Renaissance and Revolution: Humanists, Scholars, Craftsmen and Natural Philosophers in Early Modern Europe. London: Cambridge University Press; 1997

[11] Nylen CO. The microscope in aural surgery, its first use and later development. Acta Otolaryngol Suppl. 1954; 116:226–240

[12] Gelberman RH. Microsurgery and the development of the operating microscope. Contemp Surg. 1978; 13(6):43–46

[13] Kriss TC, Kriss VM. History of the operating microscope: from magnifying glass to microneurosurgery. Neurosurgery. 1998; 42(4):899–907, discussion 907–908

[14] Caspar W. A new microsurgical procedure for lumbar disc herniations causing less tissue damage through a microsurgical approach. Adv Neurosrug. 1977; 4:74–77

[15] Yasargil MG. Microsurgical operation of herniated lumbar disc. Adv Neurosurg. 1977; 7:81

[16] Williams RW. Microlumbar discectomy: a conservative surgical approach to the virgin herniated lumbar disc. Spine. 1978; 3(2):175–182

[17] Mayer HM. Spinal microsurgery, a short introduction. In: Mayer HM, ed. Minimally Invasive Spine Surgery. A Surgical Manual. 2nd ed. Berlin, Heidelberg: Springer; 2006

[18] Hartl R. The four pillars of minimally invasive spine surgery. In: Hartl R, Korge A, eds. MISS, Techniques, Evidence and Controversies. AOSpine, Switzerland and Thieme Verlag Stuttgart and New York; 2012

[19] Auerbach JD, Weidner ZD, Milby AH, Diab M, Lonner BS. Musculoskeletal disorders among spine surgeons: results of a survey of the Scoliosis Research Society membership. Spine. 2011; 36:1715–1721

[20] Rulffes W. Technological advances of surgical microscopes for spine surgery. In: Mayer HM, ed. Minimally Invasive Spine Surgery. A Surgical Manual. 2nd ed. Berlin Heidelberg: Springer; 2006

[21] Boldrey EE, Ho BT, Griffith RD. Retinal burns occurring at cataract extraction. Ophthalmology. 1984; 91(11):1297–1302

[22] Choudhry IK, Kyriakedes J, Foad MB. Iatrogenic burn caused by an operating microscope: case report. J Hand Surg Am. 2013; 38(3):545–547

[23] Kurita M, Okazaki M, Ozaki M, Miyamoto S, Takushima A, Harii K. Thermal effect of illumination on microsurgical transfer of free flaps: experimental study and clinical implications. Scand J Plast Reconstr Surg Hand Surg. 2008; 42(2):58–66

[24] Schutt CA, Redding B, Cao H, Michaelides E. The illumination characteristics of operative microscopes. Am J Otolaryngol. 2015; 36(3):356–360

[25] Serletti JM, Deuber MA, Guidera PM, et al. Comparison of the operating microscope and loupes for free microvascular tissue transfer. Plast Reconstr Surg. 1995; 95(2):270–276

[26] Edstrom E, Burstrom G, Nachabe R, Gerdhem P, Elmi Terander A. A novel augmented-reality-based surgical navigation system for spine surgery in a hybrid operating room: design, workflow, and clinical applications. Oper Neurosurg (Hagerstown). 2020; 18(5):496–502

[27] Edstrom E, Burstrom G, Omar A, et al. Augmented reality surgical navigation in spine surgery to minimize staff radiation exposure. Spine. 2020; 45(1): E45–E53

[28] Elmi-Terander A, Burström G, Nachabe R, et al. Pedicle screw placement using augmented reality surgical navigation with intraoperative 3D imaging: a first in-human prospective cohort study. Spine. 2019; 44(7):517–525

[29] Carl B, Bopp M, Saß B, Nimsky C. Microscope-based augmented reality in degenerative spine surgery: initial experience. World Neurosurg. 2019; 128: e541–e551

[30] Kantelhardt SR, Finke M, Schweikard A, Giese A. Evaluation of a completely robotized neurosurgical operating microscope. Neurosurgery. 2013; 72(51) Suppl 1:19–26

[31] Wipplinger C, Kim E, Lener S, et al. Tandem microscopic slalom technique: the use of 2 microscopes simultaneously performing unilateral laminotomy for bilateral decompression in multilevel lumbar spinal stenosis. Global Spine J. 2020; 10(2) Suppl:88S–93S

[32] Adermann J, Geissler N, Bernal LE, Kotzsch S, Korb W. Development and validation of an artificial wetlab training system for the lumbar discectomy. Eur Spine J. 2014; 23(9):1978–1983

10 Endoscope in MISS: How to Adopt and Change

Albert E. Telfeian

Summary
In this chapter, we review the key features in targeting, technology, and technique necessary to perform endoscopic lumbar spine surgery using a working channel endoscope. Step-by-step descriptions for how to target and treat lumbar pathology through an interlaminar or transforaminal approach are provided in the text and figures.

Keywords: endoscopic lumbar discectomy, transforaminal, interlaminar, working channel endoscope, Kambin's triangle

10.1 Introduction

Endoscopic spine surgery is spine surgery that utilizes an endoscope for visualization. The technique discussed here involves the use of a working channel rigid endoscope. The term "endoscopic spine surgery" indicates a method of visualization rather than a surgical procedure. Lumbar spine surgical procedures, such as discectomy, laminectomy, and fusion, can be performed with visualization by the naked eye, loupes, microscope, or endoscope. When an endoscope is used, the size of the retractor is such that (often a tube is of the size of a number 2 pencil or smaller), it can be placed through a different approach made possible because of the size and accessibility of these very small ports to small spaces. Learning endoscopic spine surgery, therefore, involves much more than becoming familiar with a different method of visualization (think loupes vs. microscope for a lumbar discectomy), it means adapting to an entirely different mode of targeting, technology, and technique.

Minimally invasive spine surgery that utilizes a tubular retractor and a camera with light source attached is known as endoscopic spine surgery, but the tubes used for these procedures are typically 16 mm or greater in diameter and, for the most part, utilize an approach that is similar to non-endoscopic versions of the same procedures. In this chapter, we will discuss endoscopic spine surgery performed through an approximately 7-mm working channel endoscope that can be used for both transforaminal and interlaminar approaches.

Understanding the principles of the targeting, technology, and technique, practicing the technique in a course, and observing a surgeon performing endoscopic spine surgical techniques are good steps in learning to practice these techniques.

10.2 Target

10.2.1 Kambin's Triangle

For transforaminal or interlaminar lumbar endoscopic surgery, the anatomic target is Kambin's triangle. In 1972, Kambin introduced endoscopic intervertebral discectomy by posterolateral approach, defining Kambin's triangle as the site to approach the intervertebral disc.[1] Kambin's triangle is defined as a right triangle over the dorsolateral disc where the hypotenuse is the exiting nerve root, the base (width) is the superior border of the caudal vertebra, and the height is the dura/traversing nerve root. ▶ Fig. 10.1 is photograph of a cadaveric specimen of the L5-S1 neural foramen with the facet removed depicting the anatomical landmarks of Kambin's triangle.[2] The anatomical specimen illustrates the point that the widest area of Kambin's triangle is its base which runs along the superior endplate of the inferior vertebra. The safest target point then to avoid injuring the exiting nerve is to aim for the medial wall of the inferior pedicle to address most foraminal pathology. The distance between the exiting nerve and the inferior pedicle is about 18 mm at the medial wall of the pedicle versus 10 to 11 mm at the lateral wall of the pedicle.[2] Kambin's triangle represents the "safe zone" for avoiding the exiting and traversing nerve roots. For both the transforaminal and interlaminar approaches, Kambin's triangle works as a "landing zone" for the endoscope so that most foraminal pathologies can be visualized from this position. The order for most endoscopic procedures is to first target and access using fluoroscopic guidance and second, once access has been established, begin visualization with the endoscope identifying normal and pathological anatomy.

10.2.2 Foraminal Window

The foramen is bounded by the superior articulating process (SAP) and inferior articulating process of the facet joint superiorly, the pedicles laterally, and the disc and vertebral bodies inferiorly. With loss of disc height or coronal scoliosis, the pedicle-to-pedicle distance and foraminal window narrow in width. With overgrowth of the facet, the foramen can narrow in height. Degenerative disease can cause extreme lateral widening and narrowing of the foramen that makes accessing medial canal pathology from a transforaminal route almost impossible; however, interlaminar

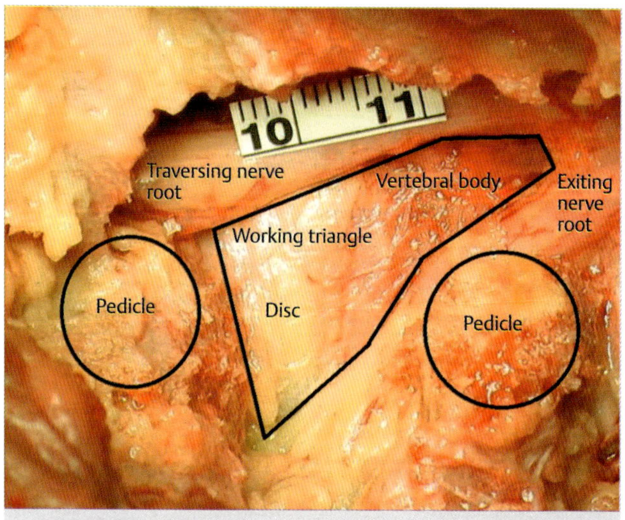

Fig. 10.1 Cadaveric demonstration of the working triangle (Kambin's triangle) in the L5-S1 neural foramen. The working triangle is the triangle between the exiting and the traversing nerve roots above the superior margin of the inferior pedicle.

and contralateral interlaminar approaches then become more feasible for accessing more medial canal pathologies.

10.2.3 Upper Lumbar versus Lower Lumbar

At L5-S1, the iliac crest makes a direct transforaminal approach almost impossible (transiliac crest approaches have been reported). A superior starting point and oblique trajectory become necessary then at L5-S1. This trajectory makes accessing medial superior foraminal pathology difficult.

In the upper lumbar spine as opposed to the lower lumbar spine, the thecal sac widens relative to the bony canal. At L5-S1, the thecal sac ends in an anteroposterior (AP) dimension at the medial wall of the pedicle. At L1–2, the thecal sac ends in an AP dimension at the midpoint of the pedicle. Targeting the medial pedicle wall at L1–2 can potentially lead to dural or neural injury. Special attention to the retroperitoneum also needs to be paid for upper lumbar pathology because the kidneys can be injured if a too lateral approach is taken. In general, for transforaminal approaches, a starting point at 12 to 16 cm off midline is used at L5-S1 and 8 to 10 cm off midline for the upper lumbar segments.

10.2.4 Superior Articulating Process

One of the biggest advances in transforaminal endoscopic spine surgery, arguably, was the addition of circular reamers to remove a portion of the ventral SAP to open the foraminal window for safe targeting and accessing foraminal and canal pathologies. Targeting for maximizing SAP removal using reamers then requires the surgeon to essentially hit and "walk off" the SAP during needle targeting. "Hugging" the SAP during targeting allows for maximal SAP removal, maximal opening for the foraminal window, and maximal access to canal pathology.

10.3 Pathologies Treated

- Herniated discs: Endoscopic spine surgery is an excellent technique for treating lumbar disc herniations. Far-lateral, paracentral, central, and extruded disc herniations are all accessible, but most surgeons start with foraminal disc herniations because they are the most accessible. Far-lateral disc herniations are also very accessible, but these tend to be directly under the exiting nerve root which can add a degree of difficulty to the surgical procedure.
- Stenosis: Foraminal stenosis is treatable with endoscopic drills from both interlaminar and transforaminal approaches. New larger endoscopes with larger working channels for bigger drills and Kerrison punches are now available for treating central stenosis.
- Facet cysts: Facet cysts are treated endoscopically by experienced endoscopic spine surgeons but do not make good "first cases" because they are often adherent to nerves and dura.
- Complex spine problems: Since transforaminal endoscopic spine surgery uses an approach that is different from traditional spine surgery techniques, it can provide an elegant salvage approach for complex spine problems. In the literature there are reports of treating complications from kyphoplasty cement leakage,[3] endplate fractures from artificial disc surgery[4] and lateral fusion surgery,[5] failed lateral recess decompression after fusion,[6] as well as adjacent segment disease.[7]

10.4 Technology

The idea for transforaminal endoscopic spine surgery arose in the 1970s and 1980s from surgeons who thought to apply orthopaedic arthroscopic techniques to spine pathology. Several technological advancements were critical to the reemergence of the technique in the following century: working channel endoscopes with high-definition cameras, continuous irrigation, and specialized instruments for disc and bone removal.

High-definition cameras, rigid fiber optics, continuous irrigation, and radiofrequency cauterization work together to provide incredible visualization to endoscopic spine surgeons. Compared to microscopic surgery where the lens and light source for visualization are about 50 cm away from pathology, putting the lens and light source directly at the target pathology creates a significant opportunity for improved visualization.

Surgical instruments available for endoscopic spine procedures are the similar to those used in open procedures (except smaller): drills, Kerrison punches, graspers, chisels, radiofrequency probes for cautery, and lasers.

Endoscopic spine fusion is an area exploding with commercial interest. Instruments and implants are in current development to (1) navigate the anatomical constraints of Kambin's triangle, (2) decompress disc and foraminal pathologies, and (3) restore foraminal height and provide a substrate for subsequent fusion. The percutaneous nature of this technique makes awake, outpatient spinal fusion a future reality.

Larger working channel endoscopes are available that are 1-cm wide with a 6-mm working channel. These endoscopes are now used to perform awake multilevel cervical and lumbar laminectomies[8,9] through a single 1-cm incision. The large diameter working channel can accommodate drills and Kerrison punches of significantly larger size making larger amounts of bone removal feasible and fast.

10.5 Technique: Step-by-Step

10.5.1 Transforaminal Lumbar

- Position the patient either prone on radiolucent Wilson or Kambin frame or in lateral position with the knees flexed (▶ Fig. 10.2).
- Anesthesia is typically light sedation with Versed and fentanyl. Lidocaine with epinephrine is used for local anesthesia. Patient should be awake enough to respond if he or she feels shooting pain in the legs.
- Targeting is performed with AP and lateral fluoroscopy to determine the skin access point. General rule of thumb is a starting point of 12 cm off midline for L5-S1 pathology, 11 cm off midline for L4–5 pathology, 10 cm off midline for L3–4 pathology, etc. For wider patients the distances are further and for thinner patients the distances are smaller.

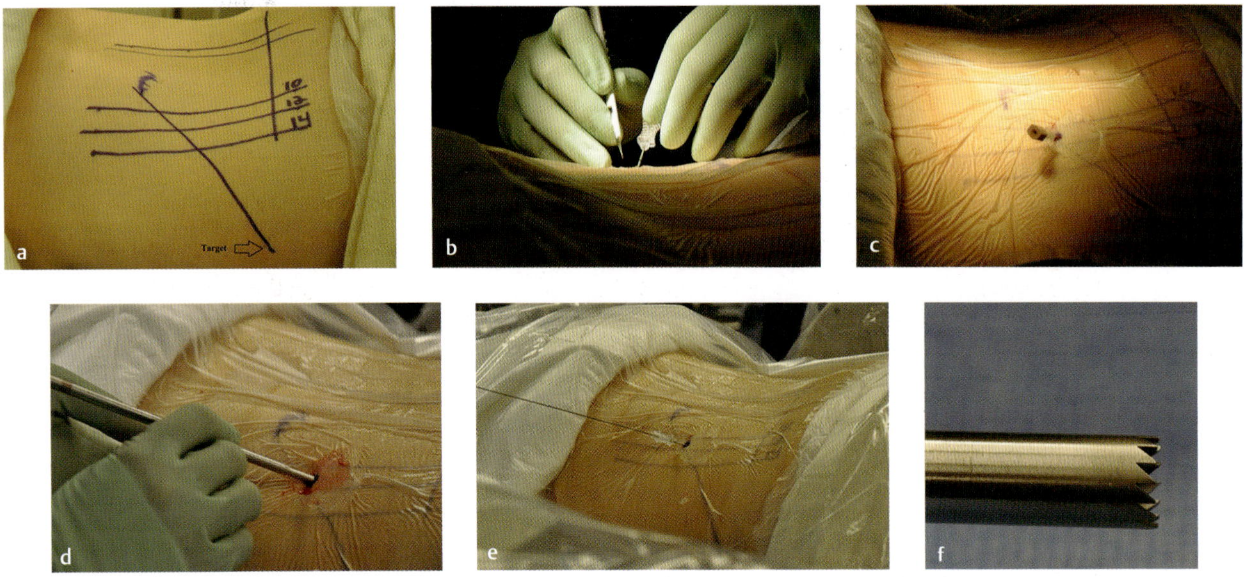

Fig. 10.2 Accessing the foramen—step-by-step. **(a)** Patient is positioned prone (cranial is *left*). Fluoroscopy is used to draw the midline, pedicle line, disc line, and the trajectory to access the disc space. Horizontal lines are drawn 10, 12, and 14 cm from the midline for reference. **(b)** A spinal needle is used to target the disc starting at the point where the target line intersects the appropriate distance off midline (here, about 12 cm). **(c)** A Kirschner wire (K-wire) is placed in the spinal needle. **(d)** A 5-mm incision is made over the spinal needle, and then the spinal needle can be removed, leaving the K-wire in place. **(e)** Sequential dilators are dilated down to the foramen. **(f)** Sequential crown reamers are used over the dilators to remove the ventral portion of the superior articulating process, expanding the foramen.

- A spinal needle (18 gauge, 25 cm) is used to target the top of the superior endplate of the inferior vertebral body touching the endplate on lateral view and at the medial wall of the inferior pedicle on AP view (▶ Fig. 10.3). A transisthmus approach is used to avoid the exiting nerve and maximize the amount of removal of the ventral portion of the SAP with the reamers (▶ Fig. 10.2).
- A Kirschner wire (K-wire) is placed in the needle. A 5-mm stab incision is made over the needle. The needle is removed while pushing in on the K-wire so not to dislodge it. Sequential dilators are placed over the K-wire to dilate the muscle. All but the smallest dilators are removed and reaming begins. Small, medium, and large reamers are used over small, medium, and large dilators. Sequential reaming tends to lead to more effective bony removal and is less painful for the patient (▶ Fig. 10.2).
- A beveled tubular retractor is then placed over the dilators and its position is confirmed on AP and lateral fluoroscopy. The beveled dilator should be laying bevel down on the disc in the epidural space (not in the disc) on lateral view and in the foramen and canal on AP view.
- The working channel endoscope is introduced with irrigation on and the foraminal contents should be visible (▶ Fig. 10.4 and ▶ Fig. 10.5). The ventral portion of the SAP and pedicle are the constant landmarks in this part of the procedure. For far-lateral disc pathologies, the endoscope is held upside down to visualize the exiting nerve.

10.5.2 Interlaminar Lumbar

- Position the patient prone on radiolucent Wilson or Kambin frame.
- Anesthesia is typically light sedation with Versed and fentanyl. Lidocaine with epinephrine is used for local anesthesia. General anesthesia is also used by some practitioners.
- L5-S1 is the easiest level because the interlaminar window is the widest (▶ Fig. 10.6). More superior levels are more challenging. Local anesthetic is infiltrated into the skin and deeper tissue. AP and lateral fluoroscopy are used to the ipsilateral starting point just off the midline and a 5-mm stab incision is made.
- Sequential dilators are used to dilate down to the laminar–facet junction (some surgeons target the inferior lamina, others the superior lamina). At L5-S1, no drilling is necessary. Levels superior to L5-S1 usually require some drilling of the facet–laminar junction to enlarge the interlaminar window.
- The ligamentum flavum is opened with a cutting forcep and the beveled cannula is introduced with its lip lateral to the traversing nerve root.
- The beveled cannula can then be spun 180° and the lip will retract the traversing nerve root medially so that the discectomy can be performed safely.

10.6 Expanding Indications

Endoscopic transforaminal lumbar interbody fusion is probably one of the most exciting areas for expanding the indications for spine endoscopy. The idea would be to access the disc through Kambin's triangle and the technological hurdles to a successful endoscopic fusion surgery would be what I call, "the five Ds":

- Completing a surgery that offers sufficient *decompression* of spine pathology.
- Completing a sufficient *disc preparation* for fusion.
- *Delivering* an interbody device safely through Kambin's triangle without damaging the exiting or traversing nerve roots.

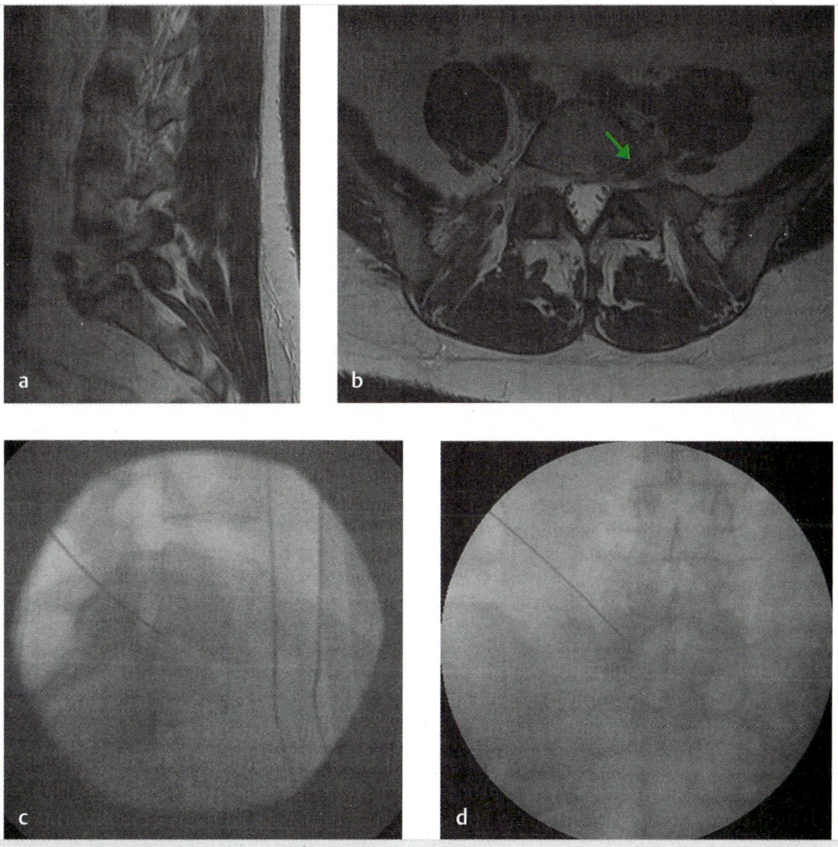

Fig. 10.3 Needle targeting for L5-S1 far-lateral disc herniation. **(a)** Sagittal T2-weighted magnetic resonance imaging (MRI) shows left far lateral disc herniation deforming exiting L5 nerve. **(b)** Axial T2-weighted MRI with *arrow* indicating the far-lateral L5-S1 disc herniation on the left. **(c)** Lateral fluoroscopic and **(d)** anteroposterior (AP) fluoroscopic images demonstrating the needle target position: just entering the disc on the lateral and at the medial wall of the pedicle on the AP image. The actual target is the more inferior aspect of the disc on the lateral view (further away from the exiting nerve) but the superior articulating process deflects the needle.

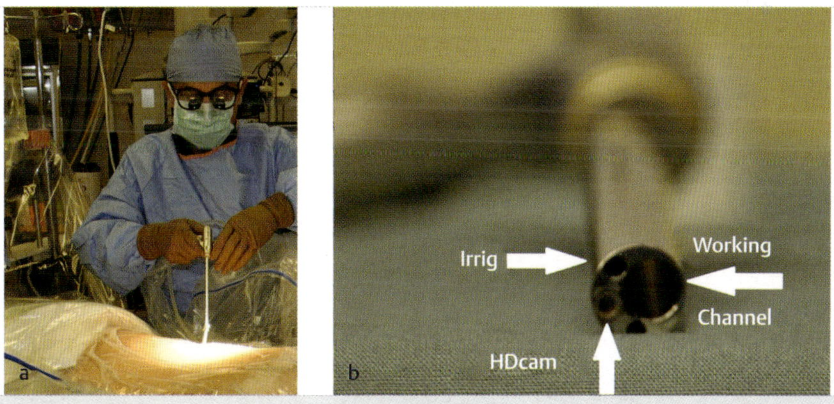

Fig. 10.4 The endoscope. **(a)** Surgeon is shown with the endoscope entering the 7-mm tubular retractor. **(b)** The tip of the working channel endoscope is shown demonstrating the high-definition camera, 3.7-mm working channel for entrance and exit of instruments, and ports for irrigation inflow and outflow.

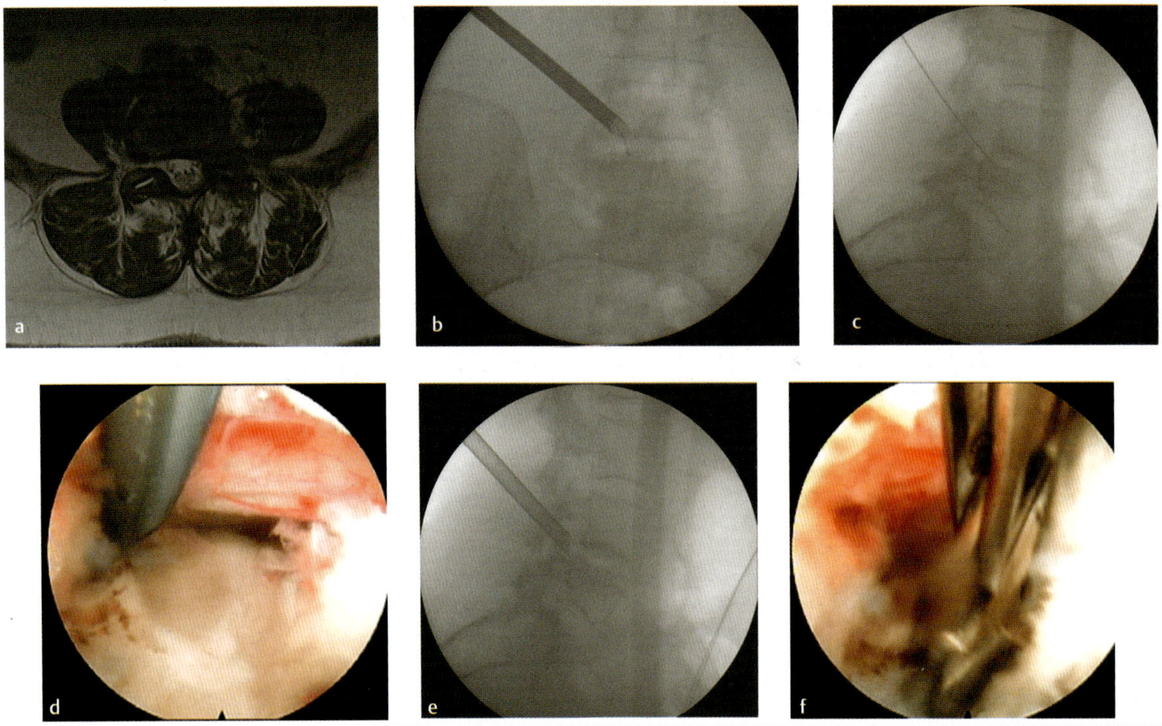

Fig. 10.5 Transforaminal endoscopic surgery. (a) Axial T2-weighted magnetic resonance imaging shows left L4–5 foraminal occlusion by disc and facet pathology. (b) Lateral fluoroscopic image demonstrates the appropriate needle targeting angle for a transisthmus approach targeting the superior endplate of the inferior vertebral body. (c) Lateral fluoroscopic image shows the position of the beveled tubular retractor in the foramen, but not in the disc. (d) Anteroposterior fluoroscopic image shows the ball probe in the canal. (e) Endoscopic camera view of the traversing L5 nerve root, disc, and the radiofrequency probe under the nerve. (f) Endoscopic camera view of the endoscopic grasper removing herniated disc.

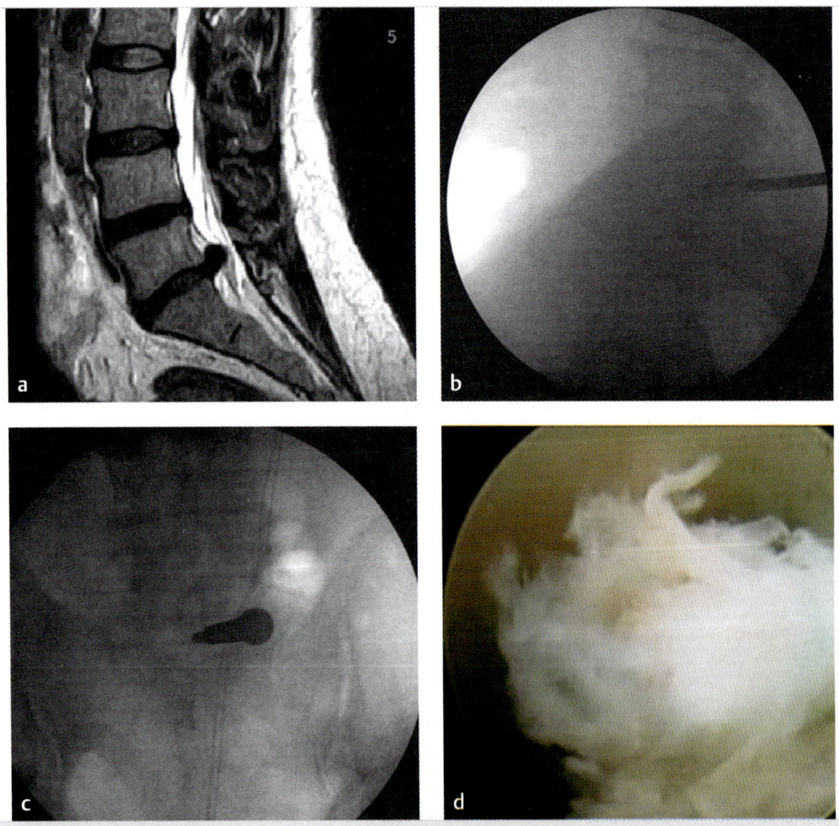

Fig. 10.6 Interlaminar endoscopic surgery. (a) Sagittal T2-weighted magnetic resonance imaging shows a large L5-S1 herniated disc. (b) Anteroposterior fluoroscopic view and lateral fluoroscopic view of the beveled tubular retractor in the interlaminar space and the small dilator in the disc space. (c) Lateral fluoroscopic image shows the endoscopic grasper in the disc space. (d) Endoscopic camera view of the large herniated disc in the tubular retractor.

- Implanting a device that offers enough *disc distraction* that enhances fusion and even offers indirect decompression through restoration of disc height.
- And the fifth D is, *Does it fuse?*

Numerous publications[10,11] have been presented using different techniques and interbody devices, some with the support of biologics to enhance fusion, some with expandable implants, and some with surgery performed without general anesthesia. The future possibility of an ultra-minimally invasive outpatient lumbar spine fusion procedure is lots of spine industry and spine surgeon interest.

10.7 Teaching and Training

10.7.1 Taking a Course

Taking an endoscopic spine surgery course with didactic and hand's on cadaveric instruction is a good introduction to endoscopic spine surgery techniques. Some surgeons take more than one course before feeling comfortable performing their first cases. Many faculty who teach endoscopic spine surgery courses are open to having interested surgeons visit them to witness live cases. Courses are usually offered through major spine societies and through the commercial vendors who supply manufacture endoscopic equipment.

10.7.2 Finding a Mentor

A mentor can be a very useful guiding hand when a surgeon is getting started with endoscopic spine surgery. Many surgeons who teach cadaver laboratories make themselves available to review potential cases and for live case visitations, and some go as far to proctor the new surgeon for his or her first case.

10.7.3 Buying Equipment

Like some of the other minimally invasive spine techniques in this book, endoscopic spine surgery represents a capital equipment purchase for the surgeon or the health care system purchasing the equipment. Nowadays, more companies are manufacturing endoscopic systems. Surgeons can get started with endoscopic spine surgery by buying, trialing, renting, or leasing the equipment.

10.8 Conclusion

The emergence of endoscopic spine surgery techniques is probably very analogous to the earlier emergence of arthroscopy in orthopaedic joint surgery. Advances in tools and visualization made the subfield of orthopaedic surgery possible. Here, we have briefly highlighted some of the key elements to be aware of when considering embarking on learning endoscopic lumbar spine surgical techniques. Understanding the principles of the targeting, technology, and technique, practicing the technique in a cadaver laboratory course, and observing an experienced surgeon in endoscopic spine surgical techniques are good steps in learning to practice these techniques.

References

[1] Kambin P, Sampson S. Posterolateral percutaneous suction-excision of herniated lumbar intervertebral discs. Report of interim results. Clin Orthop Relat Res. 1986(207):37–43

[2] Hardenbrook M, Lombardo S, Wilson MC, Telfeian AE. The anatomic rationale for transforaminal endoscopic interbody fusion: a cadaveric analysis. Neurosurg Focus. 2016; 40(2):E12

[3] Wagner R, Telfeian AE, Iprenburg M. A Transforaminal endoscopic solution to a kyphoplasty complication: case report. World Neurosurg. 2016; 91:195–198

[4] Wagner R, Iprenburg M, Telfeian AE. Transforaminal endoscopic decompression of a postoperative dislocated bone fragment after a two levellumbar total disc arthroplasty: case report. Neurosurg Focus. 2016; 40(2):E8

[5] Wagner R, Telfeian AE, Iprenburg M, Krzok G. Transforaminal endoscopic decompression for a displaced endplate fracture after lateral lumbar interbody fusion: case report. World Neurosurg. 2017; 106:26–29

[6] Telfeian AE, Jasper GP, Francisco GM. Transforaminal endoscopic treatment of lumbar radiculopathy after instrumented lumbar spine fusion. Pain Physician. 2015; 18(2):179–184

[7] Telfeian A. Transforaminal endoscopic surgery for adjacent segment disease after lumbar fusion. World Neurosurg. 2016:Oct 7 pii: S1878-8750(16)30956-1

[8] Wagner R, Telfeian AE. Iprenburg M, Krzok G. A minimally-invasive fully-endoscopic 2-level posterior cervical foraminotomy: technical note. J Spine Surg. 2017; 3(2):260–266

[9] Kim HS, Paudel B, Jang JS, et al. Percutaneous full endoscopic bilateral lumbar decompression of spinal stenosis through uniportal-contralateral approach: techniques and preliminary results. World Neurosurg. 2017; 103:201–209

[10] Lee SH, Erken HY, Bae J. Percutaneous transforaminal endoscopic lumbar interbody fusion: clinical and radiological results of mean 46-month follow-up. BioMed Res Int. 2017; 2017:3731983

[11] Wang MY, Chang PY, Grossman J. Development of an Enhanced Recovery After Surgery (ERAS) approach for lumbar spinal fusion J Neurosurg Spine. 2017; 26(4):411–418

Part IV

MISS Techniques

11	Three Surgical Principles of MISS: Contralateral Decompression, Minimize Instability, and Indirect Decompression	*103*
12	Surgical Techniques and Instrumentation in MISS	*110*
13	Dural Repair in MISS and CSF Leak Management	*114*
14	How to Achieve a Successful Fusion with MIS Techniques	*118*
15	Surgical Tips, Tricks, and Techniques to Minimize Invasiveness; General Advice on How to Handle Fluoroscopy, Blood Loss, and Infection Rates	*126*
16	Perioperative Management; ERAS	*132*
17	Key Elements to Safely Transition from Inpatient to Outpatient Spine Surgery	*136*
18	Posterior Cervical Foraminotomy/Discectomy	*141*
19	Unilateral Tubular Over-the-Top Cervical Laminectomy for Cervical Stenosis	*149*
20	Posterior Cervical Facet Cages DTRAX	*157*
21	MIS Endoscopic Approaches for OC–C1–C2 Pathology	*163*
22	Posterior Muscle Sparing Approaches for Decompression, Laminoplasty, and Laminectomy	*171*
23	Minimally Invasive C1/C2 Fusion	*182*
24	Cervical Three-Dimensional Navigation to Facilitate Minimally Invasive Spine Surgery	*191*
25	Thoracic Vertebroplasty and Kyphoplasty	*197*
26	Thoracic Discectomy: Posterior Transpedicular Tubular Approach	*203*
27	Lateral Retropleural Thoracic Discectomy and Corpectomy	*207*
28	Mini-Open Pedicle Subtraction Osteotomy for Deformity Correction	*214*
29	Posterior Paramedian Endoscopic Thoracic Discectomy	*220*
30	Transpedicular Corpectomy and Fusion for Metastatic Tumor or Infection	*226*
31	Techniques to Decrease the Invasiveness of Thoracic Deformity Correction	*231*
32	Unilateral Lumbar Approach for Over-the-Top Bilateral Decompression	*238*
33	Far-Lateral Lumbar Discectomies	*245*
34	Percutaneous Full-Endoscopic Interlaminar Approach for Lumbar Pathologies: Disc Herniation and Lumbar Spinal Stenosis	*253*

IV

Part IV

MISS Techniques

35	Transforaminal Approach for Endoscopic Decompression	262
36	Endoscopic Interlaminar Lumbar Laminectomy	273
37	LLIF T12/L1-L2	279
38	LLIF L2/3/4/5	286
39	Translumbar Surgery Comparison: Four Surgeons and Regions	293
40	Minimally Invasive Oblique Anterior Lumbar Interbody Fusion	308
41	Maximum Access Surgery Posterior Lumbar Interbody Fusion	314
42	MIS-TLIF with Total Navigation and Expandable Interbody Cages	322
43	MIS-TLIF Comparison: Four Surgeons and Regions	331
44	Percutaneous Pedicle Screw Fixation and MISS SI Joint Fusion	343
45	Intradural Extramedullary Tumors	350
46	Three-Dimensional Navigation in Lumbar Spine to Facilitate Minimally Invasive Spine Surgery	356
47	Strategies to Minimize Invasiveness and Optimize Success: OC Fusion	360
48	Strategies to Minimize Invasiveness and Optimize Success: Cervical Front/Back Surgery for Deformity Correction	367
49	MIS Cervical Pedicle Screws—Percutaneous-Assisted Technique	373
50	Treatment of Degenerative Lumbar Scoliosis with Minimally Invasive Multilevel LLIF in Combination with Lateral ALIF	382
51	Strategies to Minimize Invasiveness and Optimize Success: T10-Pelvis	395
52	Lifestyle Medicine: Optimizing Recovery Following MIS of the Spine	403
53	Three-Dimensional Navigation in MISS	410

IV

11 Three Surgical Principles of MISS: Contralateral Decompression, Minimize Instability, and Indirect Decompression

Ibrahim Hussain, Rodrigo Navarro-Ramirez, Sertac Kirnaz, and Roger Härtl

Summary

There are at least three characteristic surgical principles that are relevant for the vast majority of minimally invasive spine surgeries (MISSs) that recur repeatedly in most MISS procedures. These include:

1. **The idea that it is possible to achieve a bilateral decompression via a unilateral approach:** This is typically done via a tubular or specular retractor or by an endoscope to achieve a bilateral decompression with or without contralateral foraminotomy through a unilateral, minimally invasive approach. This is also frequently called "over the top" decompression. The lumbar tubular decompression procedure has been named "unilateral laminotomy for bilateral decompression" (ULBD). This is a part of several procedures such as MIS transforaminal interbody fusion (TLIF), lumbar stenosis decompression without fusion, contralateral approach for foraminal disc herniation, and synovial cyst resection.
2. **The technique of minimizing iatrogenic instability using "over the top" type decompression approaches:** This reduces the need for instrumentation and fusion surgery. We use this now routinely in patients with lumbar stenosis and stable grade I spondylolisthesis,[1,2] for the contralateral approach for decompression of synovial cysts,[1,3] contralateral approach for decompression of intraforaminal pathology,[3,4,5] and for the treatment of two-level lumbar pathology where one level requires a fusion and the adjacent level with stenosis just a decompression ("one and a half surgery").[6]
3. **The lateral, oblique, or anterior technique of *indirect* decompression of central and foraminal stenosis:** Currently, the challenge is the accurate prediction of successful indirect decompression and to determine which patients should also undergo a direct decompression. This is further covered in Chapters 37 to 40. In addition, these approaches also allow a certain degree of deformity correction depending on the type of implants and techniques used.

Keywords: minimally invasive surgery (MIS), minimally invasive spine surgery (MISS), spine surgery principles, spine concepts

11.1 Introduction

Minimally invasive surgery (MIS) has made enormous strides over the past three decades resulting in advanced patient care while minimizing complications associated with traditional open approaches. Most of the workhorse procedures in neurosurgical and orthopaedic spinal surgeries, including laminectomies, discectomies, and interbody fusions, can now be accomplished via MIS strategies. Within these broad categories lie pertinent principles which help provide guidance when assessing patients in the outpatient setting and are the subject of this chapter. Other surgical technique related topics include, for example, the effective and safe integration of two-dimensional/three-dimensional navigation and robotic surgery into the surgical workflow. Also, the use of special anesthetic enhanced recovery approaches (ERAS) falls into this category and will be covered in subsequent chapters.

11.2 Contralateral Decompression

Unilateral laminotomy for bilateral decompression (ULBD) for lumbar stenosis decompression: ULBD technique has evolved since its earliest description in the late 1990s.[7,8,9] Initially, this was described by McCollough and Spetzger with open surgery but was then modified and combined with tubular surgery by Foley, Fessler, and others.[10,11,12,13,14] A paramedian approach using tubular retractors preserves the posterior tension band, and minimizes muscle cauterization, dissection, and iatrogenic instability. This technique has been shown to significantly improve bilateral symptoms regardless of the side of approach.[15] It can also be used for multi-level decompressions using the "slalom" and "tandem" technique with alternating lateralizing sites of access,[1,16] or at levels above a fusion.[6] Furthermore, a recent meta-analysis demonstrated that patients with lumbar stenosis and degrative spondylolisthesis undergoing ULBD had fewer secondary reoperation rates for fusion, significant decrease in slip progression, and improved clinical outcomes based on pain and disability scoring systems than traditional open laminectomy.[2]

It is important to review the preoperative magnetic resonance imaging (MRI) in order to understand where the spinal stenosis is in relationship to the disc space. This will determine how far caudally the decompression should be carried (▶ Fig. 11.1). In general, we recommend removing a few millimeters of bone of the upper portion of the lamina below. This will ensure that all the ligament has been removed.

When performing the minimally invasive ULBD approach, the contralateral lamina and lateral recess of the level of interest are the primary surgical target. Achieving adequate visualization and technical ergonomics is paramount to achieving this goal. After confirming level localization, a 2.5 to 3 cm incision is made about 1 to 1.5 cm from midline on the side of approach. Typically, 18 or 19 mm tubes are adequate to achieve decompression at L4/L5 and L5/S1 levels. At the higher levels (L1/L2, L2/L3, and L3/L4), a smaller diameter tube inserted close to midline minimizes risk of injury to the pars interarticularis. The initial trocar should be used to carefully identify and palpate the inferior edge of the lamina to be operated on. A characteristic "step-off" should be felt when toggling the trocar cranially-caudally. Sequential dilation with the tubular retractors is then performed (▶ Fig. 11.2), taking note to gently rotate the retractors as they are inserted to allow for adequate muscle

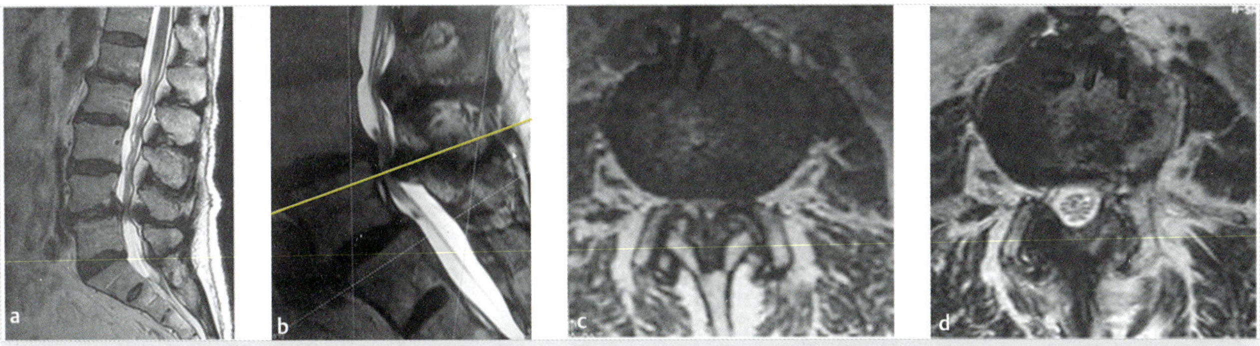

Fig. 11.1 (a–d) Review of preoperative imaging and planning. An image viewer utilizing simultaneous sagittal and axial cuts should be used. The correct level of pathology is identified, and careful attention should be paid to any transitional anatomy. For disc pathology, the size, location, and characteristic of the herniation should be noted. Facet anatomy should be inspected for arthropathy, fluid signal in the joints, and bone spurs which may impair adequate docking of a tubular retractor on the lamina. Spondylolisthesis and ligamentum flavum hypertrophy may cause or exacerbate spinal stenosis. In some situations, the level of stenosis is below the level of the disc space as caudally as the inferior level's pedicle, which should be accounted for in the decompression intraoperatively. Through minimally invasive surgery (MIS) unilateral laminotomy for bilateral decompression (ULBD) approaches, severe bilateral stenosis can be adequately decompressed.

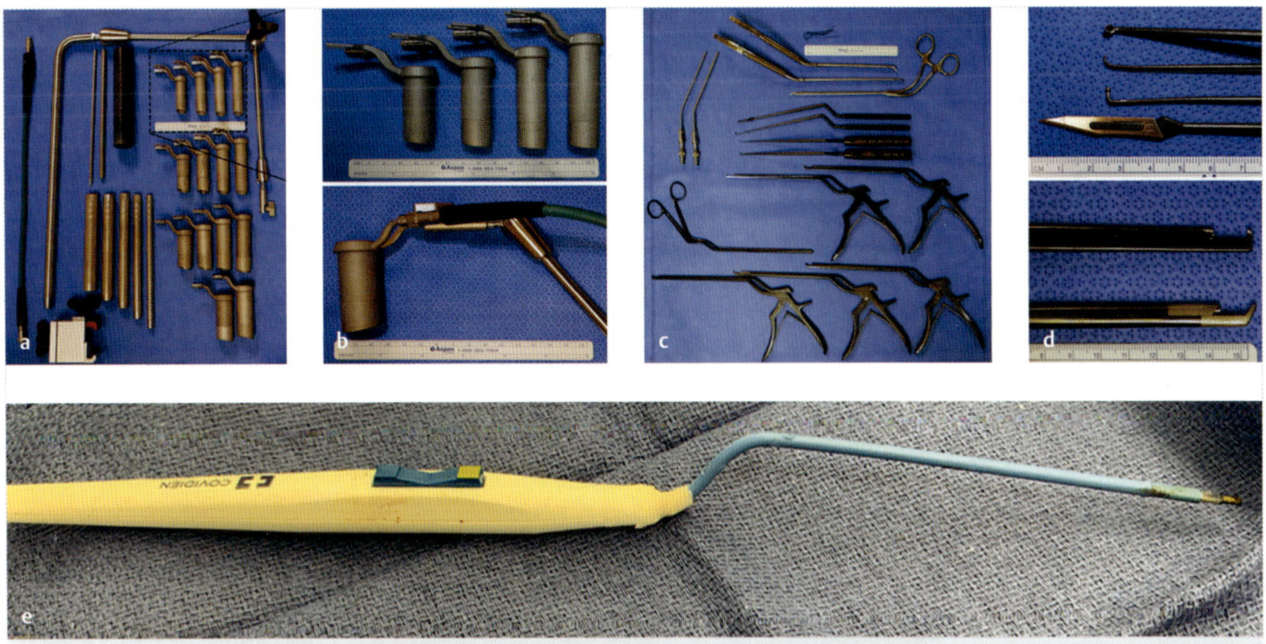

Fig. 11.2 Instruments and equipment for minimally invasive spine surgery (MISS). **(a, b)** Retractor arm and table attachment, trocar, serial dilators, and various size tubular retractors. **(c, d)** 45- and 90-degree bayonetted Kerrison rongeurs, pituitary rongeurs, Frazier suctions, ball-tip probe, nerve hook, 11-blade scalpel on extended handle, and Scanlan tubular dural repair instruments. **(e)** Monopolar cautery device with bayonetted modification and stabilization with strip bandages.

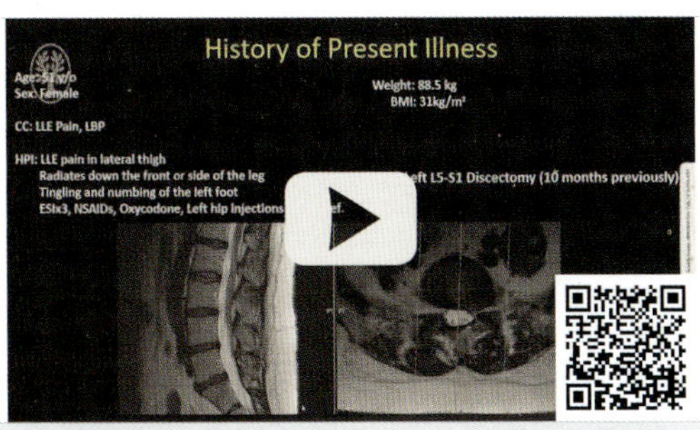

Video 11.1 MIS tubular decompression.

splitting rather than tearing. At this point, the microscope is brought in; exoscope is also an option.

▶ Video 11.1: Our group prefers the use a 3-mm fluted bit on an extended 15-cm curved handle (▶ Fig. 11.3a). The pinky finger of the dominant hand holding the drill is pressed on the body and used to provide stability, while an extended Frazier suction is held in the nondominant hand (▶ Fig. 11.3b). The drill bit is placed inferior to the edge of the lamina and moved cranially, keeping the tip on the ligament as much as possible. This ensures that the ligamentum flavum is always visualized. Caution should be taken when approaching the cranial insertion of the ligamentum flavum since thecal sac will then be directly

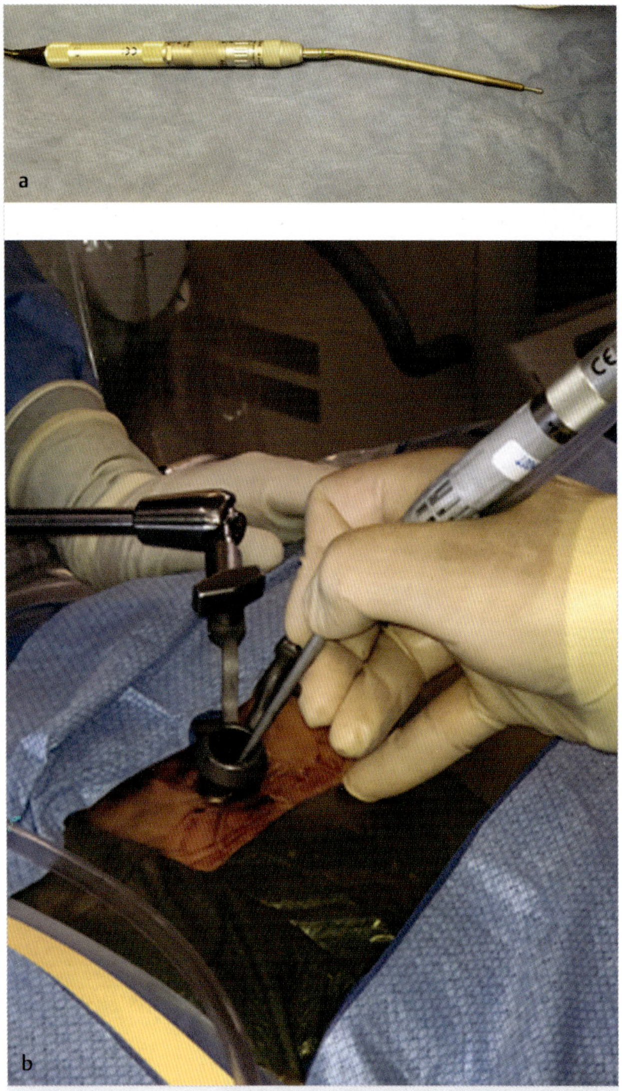

Fig. 11.3 **(a)** 3-mm fluted bit on an extended 15-cm curved handle. **(b)** Stabilization of the hand while drilling by posting the pinky finger on the patient, allowing for suction to be used in the nondominant hand.

underneath the drill bit and is not protected by ligamentum flavum (▶ Fig. 11.4a, b). The cranial insertion of the ligamentum flavum is identified and a ball-tipped dissector can be used to sweep the ligamentum caudally. To bite these superficial tissues away, 3- or 4-mm Kerrison rongeurs can be used (▶ Fig. 11.4c). Along the inner layers of the ligamentum, a ball-tipped dissector or upgoing curette can be used to gently identify a plane in the cranial-caudal direction to identify the underlying epidural fat or thecal sac. To further expose epidural fat or the underlying thecal sac, 2- and 3-mm Kerrison rongeurs are used to slide into this plane and take bites of the ligamentum (▶ Fig. 11.4d). Care should be taken to take bites away from the midline of the thecal sac when possible and to ensure constant upwards pressure when biting to prevent iatrogenic dural injury.

After the ipsilateral decompression is performed, the table is rotated away from the surgeon and the tubular retractor is angled more medially. The operative microscope is adjusted until the contralateral lamina is in a direct line of sight. At this point we switch to a 9-French Frazier suction, which can be used to retract the ligamentum flavum and thecal sac to provide enough working space for drilling without risking dural tears (▶ Fig. 11.4e). After the laminectomy is completed, palpation of the contralateral inferior and superior pedicles confirms adequate decompression caudally and cranially, respectively. The decompression is accomplished once the ligamentum flavum is completely resected (▶ Fig. 11.4f).

Following completion of the contralateral laminotomy, the table is rotated back to neutral position and the tube is angled inferiorly (laterally in terms of the patient) in order to complete the ipsilateral laminotomy. Using 2- and 3-mm Kerrison rongeurs in a backhanded fashion allows the remaining lateral portion of the ipsilateral lamina to be removed. Additional drilling may be required. In some situations, a 90-degree Kerrison rongeur (versus 45 degree) may allow for more deliberate bites (▶ Fig. 11.4f). Extreme caution should be used to prevent iatrogenic injury to the pars interarticularis, which can exacerbate any pre-existing microinstability in that region.

The pars is especially at risk at higher lumbar levels. For this reason, it is advisable to make the skin incision closer to the midline at the L1/L2/L3/L4 levels. It may also be advantageous to use a smaller diameter tube in order to stay away from the pars.

Our experience has shown that decompression of the contralateral lamina can be achieved more thoroughly than the ipsilateral foramen or lateral recess; therefore, in these patients the side of entry should be contralateral to the more symptomatic side. In situations where there are equal bilateral symptoms, it is easier for a right-handed surgeon to approach from the right side and left-handed surgeon to approach from the left side. This is due to the fact that during the procedure the insertion of the ligament is identified at the cranial aspect and the majority of ligamentum flavum resection is carried out in a cranial-caudal direction with Kerrison rongeurs.

"Tubology" Approach Pearls

a) *Foraminal stenosis with radiculopathy due to soft pathology (disc)*
   1. Contralateral "over the top" approach
b) *Central stenosis with neurogenic claudication*
   1. Right-sided approach for right-handed surgeon
   2. Left-sided approach for left-handed surgeon
   3. One to two levels: One incision
   4. Three to four levels: "Slalom" technique
c) *Lateral recess stenosis*
   1. Ipsilateral at L4/L5/S1, consider contralateral at the levels above in order to avoid pars injury
d) *Unilateral disc herniation*
   1. Ipsilateral approach
e) *Synovial cyst*
   1. Contralateral approach

For experienced MIS surgeons, ULBD techniques can be adopted for decompression of cervical stenosis as well. This technique is more challenging due to limited ability to manipulate the cervical thecal sac, and consequently can cause greater iatrogenic

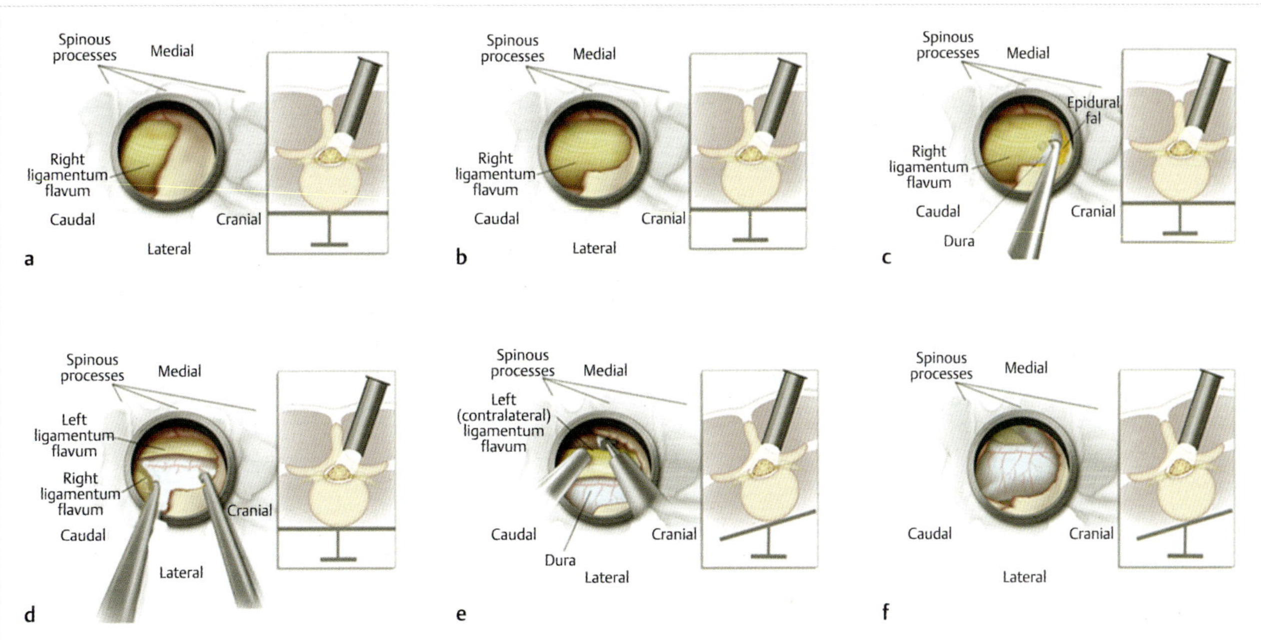

Fig. 11.4 (a–f) Step-by-step schematic of the unilateral laminotomy for bilateral decompression (ULBD) technique.

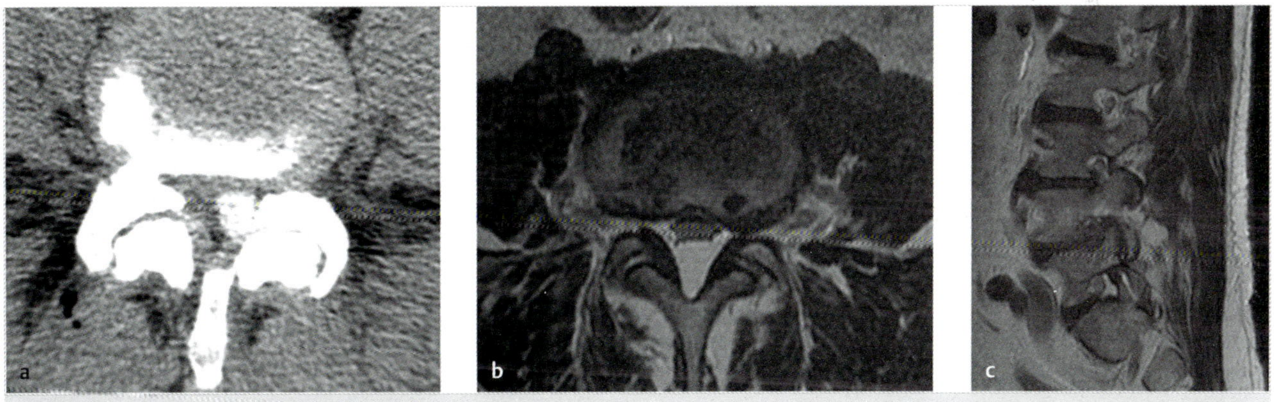

Fig. 11.5 Unilateral laminotomy for bilateral decompression (ULBD) can be utilized to treat contralateral foraminal pathology. **(a)** Axial computed tomography (CT) cut demonstrating a calcified synovial cyst, which is best approached via a contralateral approach in order to dissect the dura off the cyst wall and avoid a cerebrospinal fluid (CSF) leak. **(b, c)** Axial and sagittal T2 magnetic resonance imaging (MRI) demonstrating lumbar stenosis due to epidural lipomatosis and a left foraminal soft disc herniation. Both pathologies can be treated effectively via a right-sided approach for bilateral decompression and resection of the left foraminal disc herniation.

neurologic injury. Patient selection is important; only patients with preserved cervical lordosis and no evidence of spinal instability on dynamic X-rays should be considered candidates. Typically, this procedure can be accomplished through a 15- or 16-mm tubular retractor. The general steps are similar to those in lumbar ULBD, and have been extensively described in recent publications.[17,18]

11.3 Minimizing Instability

The first principle above is closely related to the principle of preservation of spinal stability. The “over the top” type decompression utilized in ULBD procedures preserves important stabilizing structures in the spine, such as the interspinous ligaments and medial facet joints. This reduces the need for instrumentation and fusion surgery. We use this now routinely in patients with lumbar stenosis and stable grade I spondylolisthesis.[1,2] Patients are selected for this procedure primarily based on the absence of mechanical low back pain and stability on dynamic lumbar flexion/extension films. Other procedures where we apply the principle of preserving stability with the “over the top” ULBD decompression technique is the contralateral approach for decompression of synovial cysts,[1,3] contralateral approach for decompression of intraforaminal pathology,[3,4,5] and for the treatment of two-level lumbar pathology where one level requires a fusion and the adjacent level with stenosis just a decompression (“one and a half surgery”)[6] (▶ Fig. 11.5). In this regard, MISS allows us to reduce the number of spinal fusions that need to be performed.

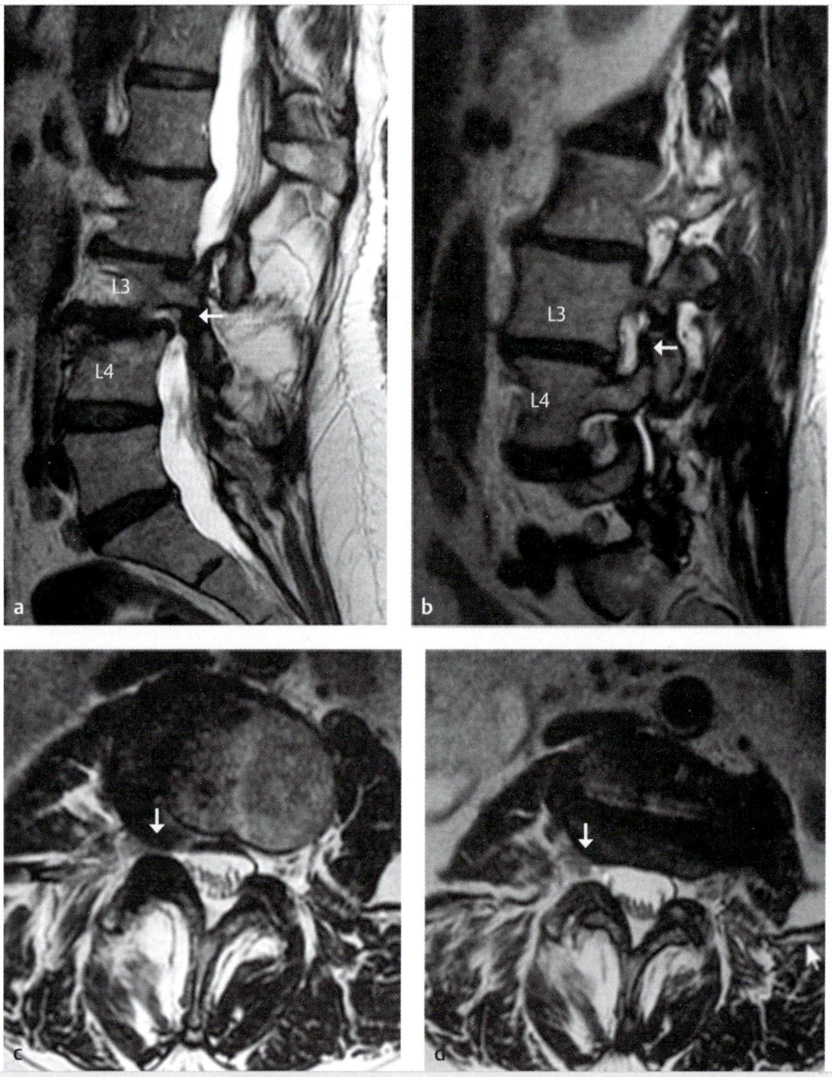

Fig. 11.6 Indirect decompression with interbody grafts can be used for foraminal nerve compression. **(a)** Sagittal and **(c)** axial preoperative cuts demonstrating right L3/L4 foraminal compression of the exiting L3 nerve root. Following L3/L4 lateral lumbar interbody fusion (LLIF), there is significant indirect decompression of the nerve root **(b, d)** due to elevation of disc height.

MISS = Minimally invasive spine surgery, but also "Minimal Instrumentation Spine Surgery"

11.4 Indirect Decompression

Among the primary advantages of indirect decompression is treating the symptomatic pathology while minimizing iatrogenic injury. In this respect, the bilateral neural foramina and the central spinal canal are the targets in these procedures. Placing interbody cages through any approach (transforaminal, translumbar [Lateral lumbar interbody fusion (LLIF)], anterior lumbar interbody fusion [ALIF], anterior psoas [pre/oblique] lateral interbody fusion [APLIF]) results in an elevation of intervertebral height, and thus increase in volume of the associated foramen. With the foraminal volume increased, the exiting nerve roots are decompressed, relieving pain and neurologic symptoms[19] (▶ Fig. 11.6). Important steps during these procedures are thorough discectomy and end plate preparation. The sequential placement of trial implants also allows the surgeon to adequately assess the width and height of the permanent cage to be used and also helps stretch the soft tissues and ligaments that may limit the larger cage placement. It is imperative that the end plate is not violated during these procedures, as this can lead to subsidence and pseudarthrosis. For anterior and laterally placed cages, the addition of plate is at the discretion of the surgeon and based on anatomic factors. Instead of lateral plates, we prefer placing pedicle screws because they are biomechanically more stable. More recently, stand-alone cages with screw implants built into them have been developed which circumvent the need for additional plate systems (for anterior lumbar interbody fusions). The development of expandable interbody cages will likely further facilitate this

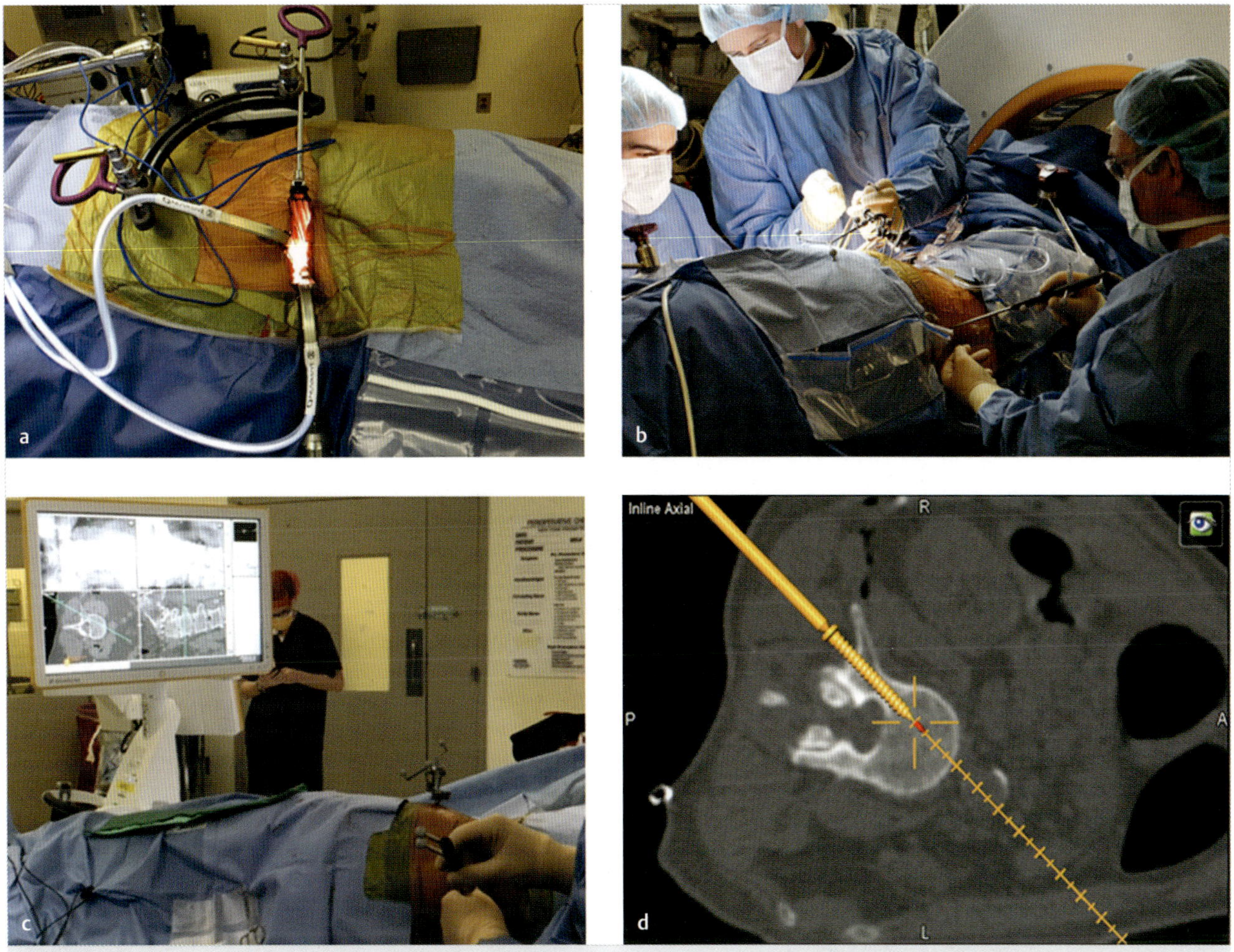

Fig. 11.7 (a, b) Simultaneous single-stage lateral approach anterior lumbar interbody fusion (ALIF) and posterior percutaneous pedicle screw placement with three-dimensional navigation (c, d).

procedure. These indirect procedures are in contrast to direct decompression procedures such as foraminotomies, which place the nerve root at significantly higher risk during bony resection with a drill or Kerrison rongeurs. Furthermore, studies have also suggested that central canal stenosis can be relieved through indirect decompression procedures. Distraction of the posterior longitudinal ligament coupled with unbuckling of lax ligamentum flavum can contribute to reconstituting the thecal sac and pressure on traversing nerve roots in this respect. Work from our group has shown that using lateral translumbar cage placement increases the average volume of the foramen and central canal by 20 to 25%.[19] The most important factor affecting successful indirect decompression is cage width; the wider the cage the less subsidence and the completer and more sustained is the indirect decompression.[20] Cage height is not a significant factor determining indirect decompression. Based on a review of the literature, indirect decompression fails in approximately 10% of patients. These patients have persistent symptoms from foraminal or central stenosis and may require more surgery and direct decompression. Severe lateral recess stenosis is a factor that predicts failure of indirect decompression.[21] Recent advances in workflow, instrumentation technology, and navigation have made it possible to improve the efficiency of lateral translumbar surgery by performing front/lateral/back surgery in single stage and single position. With the patient positioned laterally, the L4/L5/S1 levels can be accessed from the front (ALIF), the levels L4/L5 can be accessed from the side or via APLIF, and screws can be placed with navigation or robotic surgery posteriorly (▶ Fig. 11.7). If necessary, a tubular direct decompression can be added as well. Further discussion of LLIF and APLIF can be found in Chapters 37, 38, and 40.

Indirect decompression interbody approaches:

- ALIF = Anterior lumbar interbody fusion
- LLIF = Lateral lumbar interbody fusion (transpsoas)
- APLIF = Anterior psoas (pre/oblique) lateral interbody fusion

Direct decompression interbody approaches:

- PLIF = Posterior lumbar interbody fusion
- TLIF = Transforaminal interbody fusion

11.5 Conclusion

The three main principles of MISS include the idea of performing a bilateral decompression via a unilateral approach, the observation that by doing this "over the top," using tubular retractors or the endoscope, iatrogenic instability associated with traditional open surgery is minimized, and finally the idea of replacing direct decompression for foraminal and central canal stenosis with indirect decompression via cage placement. These, together with a few others such as percutaneous pedicle screw placement, are the recurrent themes that lay the foundation for MISS. A surgeon familiar with these principles will be able to minimize the necessity of fusion surgery in his or her patients and perform surgery that requires fusion in a less invasive and more efficient and targeted way.

References

[1] Boukebir MA, Berlin CD, Navarro-Ramirez R, et al. Ten-step minimally invasive spine lumbar decompression and dural repair through tubular retractors. Oper Neurosurg (Hagerstown). 2017; 13(2):232–245

[2] Schöller K, Alimi M, Cong GT, Christos P, Härtl R. Lumbar spinal stenosis associated with degenerative lumbar spondylolisthesis: a systematic review and meta-analysis of secondary fusion rates following open vs minimally invasive decompression. Neurosurgery. 2017; 80(3):355–367

[3] James A, Laufer I, Parikh K, Nagineni VV, Saleh TO, Härtl R. Lumbar juxtafacet cyst resection: the facet sparing contralateral minimally invasive surgical approach. J Spinal Disord Tech. 2012; 25(2):E13–E17

[4] Alimi M, Njoku I, Jr, Cong GT, et al. Minimally invasive foraminotomy through tubular retractors via a contralateral approach in patients with unilateral radiculopathy. Neurosurgery. 2014; 10 Suppl 3:436–447, discussion 446–447

[5] Kirnaz S, Wipplinger C, Schmidt FA, Hernandez RN, Hussain I, Hartl R. Minimally invasive laminotomy for contralateral "over-the-top" foraminal decompression using 3-dimensional total navigation: 2-dimensional operative video. Oper Neurosurg (Hagerstown). 2020; 19 3:E296

[6] Wipplinger C, Melcher C, Hernandez RN, et al. "One and a half" minimally invasive transforaminal lumbar interbody fusion: single level transforaminal lumbar interbody fusion with adjacent segment unilateral laminotomy for bilateral decompression for spondylolisthesis with bisegmental stenosis. J Spine Surg. 2018; 4(4):780–786

[7] Costa F, Sassi M, Cardia A, et al. Degenerative lumbar spinal stenosis: analysis of results in a series of 374 patients treated with unilateral laminotomy for bilateral microdecompression. J Neurosurg Spine. 2007; 7(6):579–586

[8] Moisi M, Fisahn C, Tkachenko L, et al. Unilateral laminotomy with bilateral spinal canal decompression for lumbar stenosis: a technical note. Cureus. 2016; 8(5):e623

[9] Spetzger U, Bertalanffy H, Naujokat C, von Keyserlingk DG, Gilsbach JM. Unilateral laminotomy for bilateral decompression of lumbar spinal stenosis. Part I: Anatomical and surgical considerations. Acta Neurochir (Wien). 1997; 139(5):392–396

[10] Perez-Cruet MJ, Foley KT, Isaacs RE, et al. Microendoscopic lumbar discectomy: technical note. Neurosurgery. 2002; 51(5) Suppl:S129–S136

[11] Palmer S, Turner R, Palmer R. Bilateral decompression of lumbar spinal stenosis involving a unilateral approach with microscope and tubular retractor system. J Neurosurg. 2002; 97(2) Suppl:213–217

[12] Guiot BH, Khoo LT, Fessler RG. A minimally invasive technique for decompression of the lumbar spine. Spine. 2002; 27(4):432–438

[13] Spetzger U, Bertalanffy H, Reinges MH, Gilsbach JM. Unilateral laminotomy for bilateral decompression of lumbar spinal stenosis. Part II: Clinical experiences. Acta Neurochir (Wien). 1997; 139(5):397–403

[14] McCulloch JA. Microsurgery for Lumbar Spinal Canal Stenosis. Essentials of Spinal Microsurgery. Lippincott-Raven; 1998:475–480

[15] Alimi M, Hofstetter CP, Torres-Campa JM, et al. Unilateral tubular approach for bilateral laminotomy: effect on ipsilateral and contralateral buttock and leg pain. Eur Spine J. 2017; 26(2):389–396

[16] Mayer HM, Heider F. "Slalom": microsurgical cross-over decompression for multilevel degenerative lumbar stenosis. BioMed Res Int. 2016; 2016:9074257

[17] Hernandez RN, Wipplinger C, Navarro-Ramirez R, et al. Ten-step minimally invasive cervical decompression via unilateral tubular laminotomy: technical note and early clinical experience. Oper Neurosurg (Hagerstown). 2020; 18(3):284–294

[18] Kirnaz S, Wipplinger C, Wong T, Schmidt FA, Nangunoori R, Härtl R. Less invasive cervical decompression via unilateral tubular laminotomy using 3-dimensional total navigation: 2-dimensional operative video. Oper Neurosurg (Hagerstown). 2020:opaa059

[19] Navarro-Ramirez R, Berlin C, Lang G, et al. A new volumetric radiologic method to assess indirect decompression after extreme lateral interbody fusion using high-resolution intraoperative computed tomography. World Neurosurg. 2018; 109:59–67

[20] Lang G, Navarro-Ramirez R, Gandevia L, et al. Elimination of subsidence with 26-mm-wide cages in extreme lateral interbody fusion. World Neurosurg. 2017; 104:644–652

[21] Lang G, Perrech M, Navarro-Ramirez R, et al. Potential and limitations of neural decompression in extreme lateral interbody fusion—a systematic review. World Neurosurg. 2017; 101:99–113

12 Surgical Techniques and Instrumentation in MISS

Robert Nicholas Hernandez, Sertac Kirnaz, and Michael S. Virk

Summary
This chapter highlights an essential part of MISS, Surgical Techniques and Instrumentation. Due to the small working corridor of MISS and the proximity to critical anatomical structures, instruments should be able to facilitate the field of view of the surgeon and not obstruct any of the relevant anatomy. To achieve this, MISS often utilizes smaller instruments that are often curved or bayoneted to further increase the available viewing angle; to provide examples, the following instruments/scenarios are discussed: visualization, retractors, power drills, bone scalpel, endoscopic techniques, and CSF leak repair.

Keywords: CSF leak, endoscopy, instruments, laminotomy, minimally invasive spine surgery, tubular retractors, ULBD

12.1 Introduction

The surgical principles of minimally invasive spine surgery (MISS) revolve around minimizing the operative footprint while achieving the same goals as traditional open approaches. Specifically, minimizing tissue disruption and instability, achieving bilateral decompression via a unilateral approach, and achieving indirect neural element decompression have driven the evolution and advancement of MISS techniques and instrumentation. As the field advances to better achieve the goals of MISS, instruments that facilitate safe and efficient procedures through narrow, highly targeted access corridors inherent in MISS approaches are mandatory. The design of MISS instruments, therefore, must abide by the following principles:

- Provide variable extension in order to reach the target.
- Offer bayoneted or curved design that does not obscure the surgeon's line-of-sight.
- Present more precision and specialized tissue interfaces with variable angles or degrees of manipulation.
- Offer enhanced ergonomics.

With these characteristics in mind, this chapter will discuss the instrumentation required for the performance of MISS techniques.

12.2 Bayoneted or Curved Instrumentation

Bayoneted or curved designs allow the surgeon to comfortably hold instruments without obstructing the surgeon's view as he or she operates down the operative corridor. It is a fundamental design principle of MISS. Bayoneted instruments also offer extension to allow the surgeon's hands to work above the operative field while at the same time reaching the target, which can be located several centimeters deep. This is particularly necessary in obese patients, in whom minimally invasive procedures have proven to be advantageous over open techniques,[1] as the depth of tubular retractor can reach 10 cm or greater. Lateral approaches also require extended length instruments. The basic set of extended, bayoneted, or curved instruments includes (▶ Fig. 12.1 and ▶ Fig. 12.2):

- Suction tips and suction retractors.
- Bipolar and monopolar electrocautery (the extended monopolar base can be bent slightly to create a bent or curved-like instrument).
- High-speed power drills.
- 45° and 90° Kerrison rongeurs.
- Microinstruments such as ball-tip probes, nerve hooks, curettes, microdissectors, etc.

12.3 Retractors

12.3.1 Tubular Retractors

The advent of tubular retractors propelled MISS and allowed for marked proliferation. Since the introduction by Foley and Smith in 1997,[2] tubular retractors have been applied for the treatment of disease at all levels of the spinal column. Tubular retractor systems consist of a table clamp, a rigid arm, a series of dilating tubes of sequentially enlarging diameter, and the tubular retractors (▶ Fig. 12.3). The tubular retractors come in various depths and diameters, often ranging from 15 to 24 mm in diameter and 40 to 100 mm in depth. Typically, we use a 15-mm retractor for lumbar

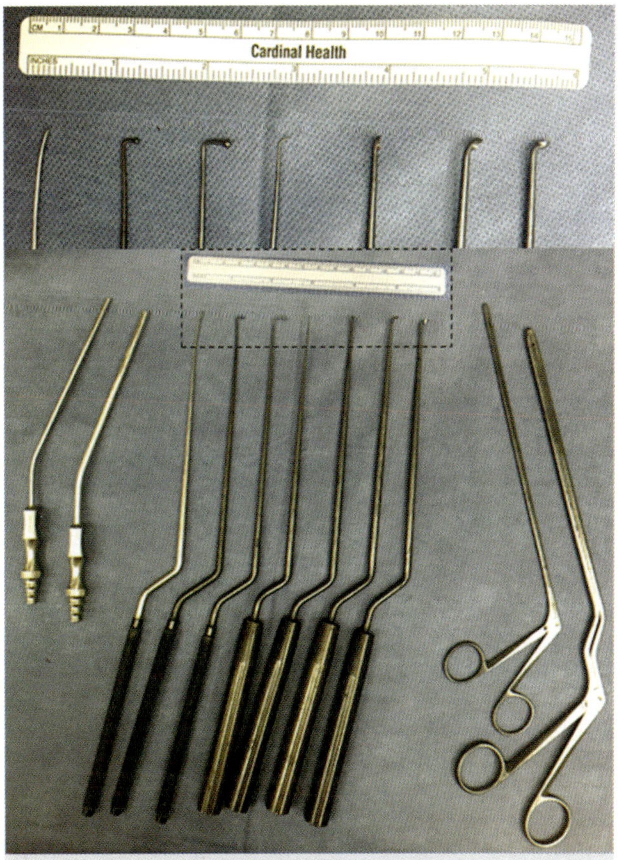

Fig. 12.1 Bayoneted microinstruments.

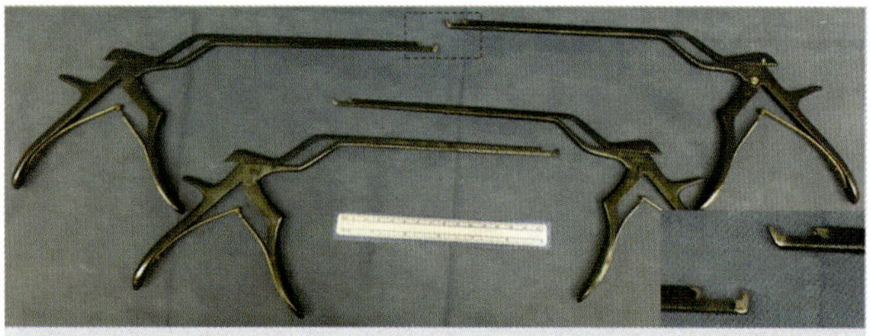

Fig. 12.2 Bayoneted Kerrison rongeurs.

microdiscectomy and cervical foraminotomy, an 18-mm retractor for laminectomies at all levels, and a 21-mm retractor for transforaminal lumbar interbody fusion. After sequential dilation of the soft tissue and musculature, the depth to the target is identified and the appropriate tubular retractor is passed over the dilators and secured in position by the rigid table arm. In this manner, the retractor is fixed in place but can be "wanded" or redirected in any direction to achieve additional visualization and exposure outside the fixed diameter of the tubular retractor. This "wanding" technique is critical to achieving the goals of MISS when using tubular retractors. It permits visualization of multiple regions beyond the initial docking site through a single corridor. See also Chapter 5 in this book.[3]

12.4 Drills

12.4.1 Power Drills

High-speed power drills used in MISS include curved and extended drill shafts and bits that attach to the same power sources used in open surgeries. This allows the drill to reach the target while affording the surgeon line-of-sight and ergonomic use. In our practice, we use a 15-cm curved drill shaft. In addition, self-irrigating drills are also available.

Two drill bits lend themselves well to use in MISS. The 3-mm fluted matchstick drill bit is a side-cutting burr that has a blunt tip. This drill bit is particularly useful for minimally invasive laminectomy; the blunt tip can safely rest atop the ligamentum flavum while the lamina is drilled away in a side-cutting fashion (▶ Fig. 12.4). In this manner, the ligamentum flavum can be entirely exposed and acts as a protective layer from injury to the underlying dura.[4]

The diamond burr is another drill bit useful in MISS. This drill bit can be used in a side-cutting manner, similar to the matchstick; also it can drill with gentle downward pressure. With the appropriate amount of pressure, the diamond burr will drill away bone but not ligamentum flavum, rather pushing the soft tissue away. Thus, similar to the matchstick bit, the ligamentum flavum can be exposed and kept intact to protect the underlying dura. One advantage of the diamond burr is that due to the heat it gives off, bony bleeding is minimized through thermal coagulation. However, continuous irrigation is required to avoid thermal injury to adjacent neural structures.

While extended drill shafts are necessary for tubular MISS, the long distance between the surgeon's hand and the tip of the drill can result in poor drill control. To improve control, the drill should be held with the hand resting on the patient to stabilize the hand and the shaft of the drill resting on the edge of the

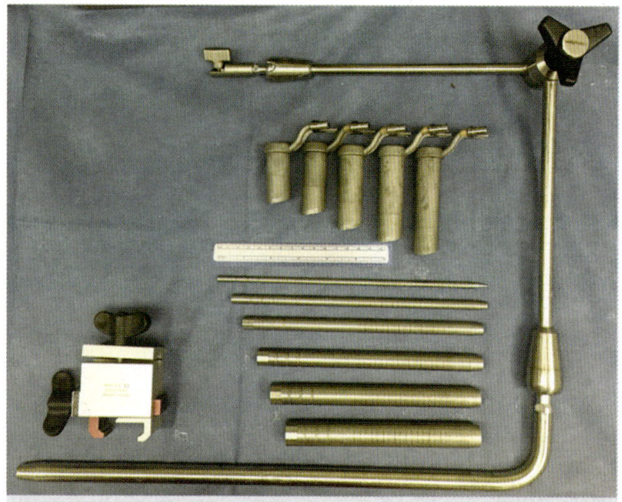

Fig. 12.3 Tubular retractor system.

tubular retractor to stabilize the tip of the drill. Only very small movements of the hand are required.

12.4.2 Bone Scalpel

The ultrasonic bone scalpel has been used in a variety of open spine surgeries and has demonstrated decreased blood loss compared with traditional high-speed drills[5,6] with similar rates of incidental durotomy.[7] Bone scalpels on thin, curved, extended shafts are available for MISS (▶ Fig. 12.5). While still too bulky for 16- to 18-mm tubular retractors, they are compatible with expandable and mini-open retractors. The potential advantages of decreased blood loss, decreased heat generation when operating near neural structures, and decreased mechanical injury to neural tissue[8,9] are attractive.

12.5 Visualization

Though the access ports in MISS are small and the working depth can be great, surgeons must have a method to obtain high-quality visualization and magnification of the surgical anatomy. Foley and Smith's original description of microdiscectomy via tubular retractors utilized an endoscope to provide direct visualization of the operative anatomy from just a few centimeters away.[2] The endoscope continues to be coupled with tubular retractors to provide direct visualization, magnification, and illumination as well as to use angled scopes to look around fixed retractors or anatomical elements. The operative microscope was applied to tubular microdiscectomy in the early 2000s and thereafter gained widespread use.[10] Advantages of the operative microscope over the endoscope include that the coaxial microscope provides depth perception and therefore a three-dimensional view of the operative field, compared with the two-dimensional views obtained with an endoscope, and the microscope can be moved in addition to "wanding" of the tubular retractor, thus granting wider visualization of the anatomy than "wanding" alone. In addition, an assistant can work opposite the operating surgeon with direct visualization of the anatomy via the observer microscope attachment. Regardless of

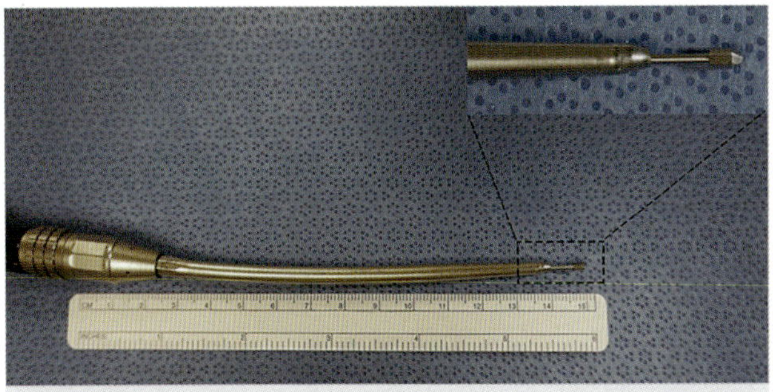

Fig. 12.4 Curved matchstick drill bit.

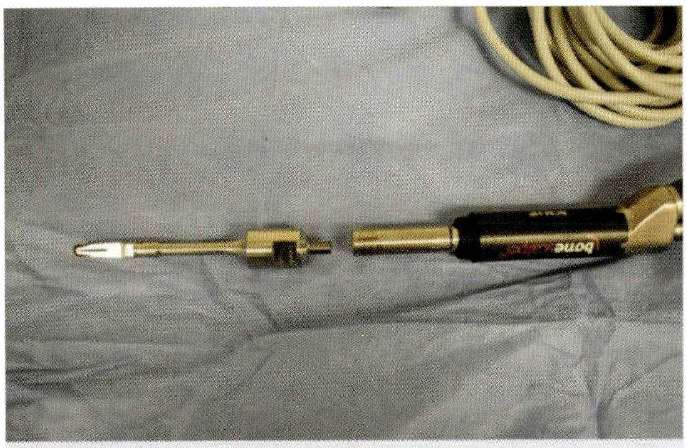

Fig. 12.5 Bone scalpel.

preference for endoscope versus microscope, the use of one is mandatory when performing MISS via tubular retractors.

12.6 Endoscopic Spine Surgery

Spine surgery performed through a working channel within an endoscope has recently begun to enjoy a renewed surge of interest within the field of MISS. Through a stab incision in the skin, a dilator and sheath are passed to the anatomical region of interest, and through the sheath an endoscope with a working channel is inserted. The outer diameter of endoscopes can range from 6 to 10 mm depending on the application. The surgeon then has a magnified, illuminated view of the surgical site from just a few millimeters away. Instruments are passed through the back of the endoscope via working channels while continuous irrigation, a light source, and a camera operate through separate channels to provide illumination and clear visualization of the operative field (▶ Fig. 12.6).

See also Chapters 9, 28, 33, 34, and 35 in this book.[11,12,13,14,15]

12.7 Cerebral Spinal Fluid Leak Repair

The most common complication associated with MISS is incidental durotomy, with reported rates ranging from 2.7 to 7.2%. Primary repair with traditional instruments can often be challenging due to the limited exposure and narrow working channel afforded by tubular retractors and minimal access corridors.

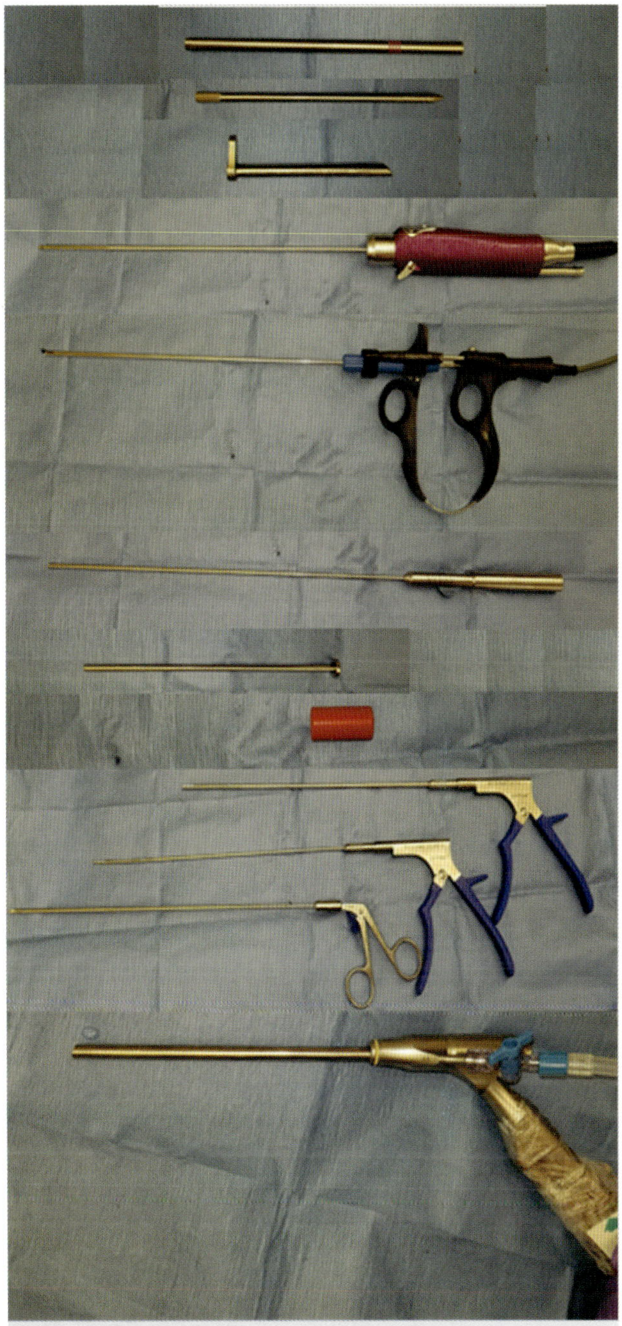

Fig. 12.6 Endoscopic spine instruments.

Several instrument kits exist for the specific purpose of dural closure in MISS. The Scanlan® dural closure kit (Scanlan International, Inc., St. Paul, MN, USA) is particularly useful for this indication as the instruments are bayoneted and extended. A "knot pushing" instrument to allow knot tying down the depth of the tubular retractor is available. We use a 4–0 Nurulon TF-5 "fishhook" suture (Ethicon, Inc., Somerville, NJ, USA).[4] Alternatively, Chou et al have described using a micropituitary rongeur as a needle driver with a 5–0 Prolene suture (Ethicon, Inc., Somerville, NJ, USA) and a laparoscopic knot pusher to aid in suture tying.[16] This chapter is dedicated to dural repair and cerebral spinal fluid leak management (▶ Fig. 12.7).

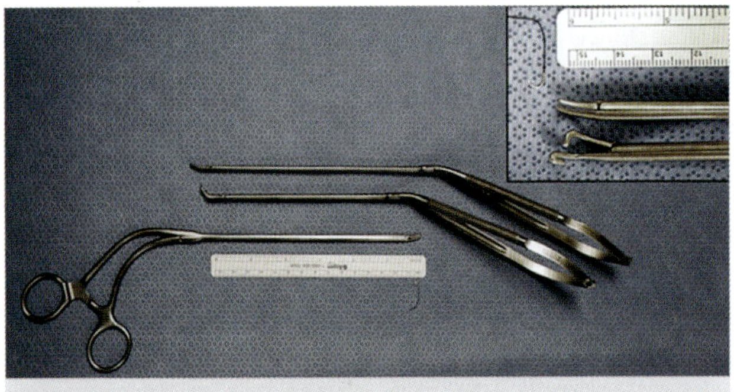

Fig. 12.7 Dural repair instruments. (Used with permission of Oxford University Press from Boukebir et al. Ten-Step Minimally Invasive Spine Lumbar Decompression and Dural Repair Through Tubular Retractors. *Oper Neurosurg*. 2017;13:232–245.)

12.8 Conclusion

MISS aims to achieve similar surgical outcomes as realized by traditional open surgeries while minimizing the operative footprint via small approach corridors and minimal collateral tissue disruption. In accomplishing these goals, compared with open approaches, patients experience less postoperative pain and narcotic use, less intraoperative blood loss, shorter hospitalization and recovery, and decreased infection rates.[17,18,19,20,21,22,23,24,25,26] Instrumentation used in MISS, due to the narrow access ports, must often be finer than traditional open instruments and bayoneted or curved so as to not obscure the surgeon's view. They must also offer longer extension in order to reach the operative target, while at the same time offering enhanced ergonomics so that they can be held and easily manipulated for long periods of time. This chapter has reviewed the basic instruments that are mandatory for the safe and effective performance of MISS procedures. Technological advances in design and function of MISS instruments facilitate the application of these techniques to even more complex and technically demanding indications.

References

[1] Xie Q, Zhang J, Lu F, Wu H, Chen Z, Jian F. Minimally invasive versus open transforaminal lumbar Interbody fusion in obese patients: a meta-analysis. BMC Musculoskelet Disord. 2018; 19(1):15

[2] Foley KT, Smith MM. Microendoscopic discectomy. Tech Neurosurg. 1997; 3:301–307

[3] Wipplinger C, Lener S, Kirnaz S, Abdelsalam A, Härtl R, Thomé C. Tubular and Specular Retractors in Minimally Invasive Spine Surgery. In: Hartl R, Navarro-Ramirez R. Ten Step Techniques for Minimally Invasive Spine Surgery. New York, NY: Thieme. 2021

[4] Boukebir MA, Berlin CD, Navarro-Ramirez R, et al. Ten-step minimally invasive spine lumbar decompression and dural repair through tubular retractors. Oper Neurosurg (Hagerstown). 2017; 13(2):232–245

[5] Onen MR, Yuvruk E, Akay S, Naderi S. The reliability of the ultrasonic bone scalpel in cervical spondylotic myelopathy: a comparative study of 46 patients. World Neurosurg. 2015; 84(6):1962–1967

[6] Bartley CE, Bastrom TP, Newton PO. Blood loss reduction during surgical correction of adolescent idiopathic scoliosis utilizing an ultrasonic bone scalpel. Spine Deform. 2014; 2(4):285–290

[7] Bydon M, Xu R, Papademetriou K, et al. Safety of spinal decompression using an ultrasonic bone curette compared with a high-speed drill: outcomes in 337 patients. J Neurosurg Spine. 2013; 18(6):627–633

[8] Nakagawa H, Kim SD, Mizuno J, Ohara Y, Ito K. Technical advantages of an ultrasonic bone curette in spinal surgery. J Neurosurg Spine. 2005; 2(4):431–435

[9] Hazer DB, Yaşar B, Rosberg HE, Akbaş A. Technical aspects on the use of ultrasonic bone shaver in spine surgery: experience in 307 patients. BioMed Res Int. 2016; 2016:8428530

[10] Palmer S. Use of a tubular retractor system in microscopic lumbar discectomy: 1 year prospective results in 135 patients. Neurosurg Focus. 2002; 13 (2):E5

[11] Telfeian A. Technology: endoscope in MISS; how to adopt and change. In: Hartl R, Navarro-Ramirez R. Ten Step Techniques for Minimally Invasive Spine Surgery. New York, NY: Thieme. In press

[12] Nangunoori R, Jho DH, Jho DH, Jho H. 10 steps: endoscopic posterior thoracic discectomy/decompression. In: Hartl R, Navarro-Ramirez R. Ten Step Techniques for Minimally Invasive Spine Surgery. New York, NY: Thieme. In press

[13] Quillo-Olvera J, Kim J. 10 steps: interlaminar approach endoscopic decompression; discectomy/laminectomy. In: Hartl R, Navarro-Ramirez R. Ten Step Techniques for Minimally Invasive Spine Surgery. New York, NY: Thieme. In press

[14] Wagner R. 10 steps: transforaminal approach endoscopic decompression. In: Hartl R, Navarro-Ramirez R. Ten Step Techniques for Minimally Invasive Spine Surgery. New York, NY: Thieme. In press

[15] Hofstetter C. 10 steps: endoscopic decompression lumbar stenosis. In: Hartl R, Navarro-Ramirez R. Ten Step Techniques for Minimally Invasive Spine Surgery. New York, NY: Thieme. In press

[16] Chou D, Wang VY, Khan AS. Primary dural repair during minimally invasive microdiscectomy using standard operating room instruments. Neurosurgery. 2009; 64(5) Suppl 2:356–358, discussion 358–359

[17] Ghobrial GM, Theofanis T, Darden BV, Arnold P, Fehlings MG, Harrop JS. Unintended durotomy in lumbar degenerative spinal surgery: a 10-year systematic review of the literature. Neurosurg Focus. 2015; 39(4):E8

[18] Goldstein CL, Macwan K, Sundararajan K, Rampersaud YR. Perioperative outcomes and adverse events of minimally invasive versus open posterior lumbar fusion: meta-analysis and systematic review. J Neurosurg Spine. 2016; 24 (3):416–427

[19] Ross DA. Complications of minimally invasive, tubular access surgery for cervical, thoracic, and lumbar surgery. Minim Invasive Surg. 2014; 2014:451637

[20] Phan K, Mobbs RJ. Minimally invasive versus open laminectomy for lumbar stenosis: a systematic review and meta-analysis. Spine. 2016; 41(2):E91–E100

[21] Wong AP, Shih P, Smith TR, et al. Comparison of symptomatic cerebral spinal fluid leak between patients undergoing minimally invasive versus open lumbar foraminotomy, discectomy, or laminectomy. World Neurosurg. 2014; 81 (3–4):634–640

[22] Dasenbrock HH, Juraschek SP, Schultz LR, et al. The efficacy of minimally invasive discectomy compared with open discectomy: a meta-analysis of prospective randomized controlled trials. J Neurosurg Spine. 2012; 16(5):452–462

[23] He J, Xiao S, Wu Z, Yuan Z. Microendoscopic discectomy versus open discectomy for lumbar disc herniation: a meta-analysis. Eur Spine J. 2016; 25 (5):1373–1381

[24] Schöller K, Alimi M, Cong GT, Christos P, Härtl R. Lumbar spinal stenosis associated with degenerative lumbar spondylolisthesis: a systematic review and meta-analysis of secondary fusion rates following open vs minimally invasive decompression. Neurosurgery. 2017; 80(3):355–367

[25] Wong AP, Smith ZA, Stadler JA, III, et al. Minimally invasive transforaminal lumbar interbody fusion (MI-TLIF): surgical technique, long-term 4-year prospective outcomes, and complications compared with an open TLIF cohort. Neurosurg Clin N Am. 2014; 25(2):279–304

[26] Wu RH, Fraser JF, Härtl R. Minimal access versus open transforaminal lumbar interbody fusion: meta-analysis of fusion rates. Spine. 2010; 35(26):2273–2281

13 Dural Repair in MISS and CSF Leak Management

Ramin A. Morshed, Young M. Lee, and Dean Chou

Summary
Durotomies are intraoperative complications that can significantly impact a patient's postoperative recovery and are difficult to repair during minimally invasive spine surgery (MISS). In this chapter, we review management approaches for intraoperative durotomies during MISS as well as repair techniques.

Keywords: dural tear, durotomy, cerebrospinal fluid leak, minimally invasive spine surgery, repair

13.1 Introduction

Dural tears are intraoperative complications that can significantly impact a patient's postoperative recovery and clinical course after spine surgery. Symptoms of a cerebrospinal fluid (CSF) leak include positional headaches, dizziness, and visual impairment, but consequences may be as severe as the formation of a subdural hematoma or hygroma due to intracranial hypotension. CSF leakage from an incision may cause wound breakdown or a surgical site infection, necessitating reoperation. Furthermore, herniation of nerve roots through a pseudomeningocele may cause neurological deficits. Nandyala et al reported longer hospitalization and greater incidence of perioperative complications including high rates of neurological injury in patients with incidental durotomies during spine surgery.[1]

Although reportedly less frequent than in open procedures, dural tears occur in up to 1.6 to 6.6% of minimally invasive spine surgeries (MISS).[2,3,4,5] However, primary dural closure in these cases can be challenging given the narrow surgical working area during MISS. Thus, novel techniques for dural closure are needed. Here, we review several intraoperative techniques for management of CSF leaks in MISS as well as postoperative management considerations.

> Repair of an intraoperative CSF leak is possible in MISS despite limitations placed on surgeons by the tube-retractor system. Conversion to open surgery is usually not necessary. Small openings with only CSF leakage can be repaired with dural sealants. If there are nerve roots extruded, this requires careful reinsertion and primary closure.

13.2 Techniques for Repair (▶ Video 13.1)

The following steps for repair are summarized in ▶ Table 13.1. When a CSF leak is identified intraoperatively, the extent of injury must be adequately assessed immediately before proceeding with the remainder of the operation. In order to allow for better visualization, the surgical corridor may be expanded using larger diameter tubes, the intraoperative microscope may need to be brought in if not already used, and adequate lighting of the area may be achieved through the use of a fiberoptic light source. If intrathecal elements (e.g., nerve rootlets) are noted to have herniated through the dural defect, care must be taken to push these gently back intradurally. Positioning techniques such as placing the patient in Trendelenburg position may allow for relaxation of the thecal sac to allow for more facile dural edge approximation. In some instances, additional bone may need to be removed in order to completely expose the entirety of the defect.

The technique used for repair depends on the size of the defect and whether primary repair is possible based on location. Often, for small dural tears with slow rates of CSF leakage, adhesive sealant closure with agents such as fibrin glue or polyethylene glycol-based hydrogel products may be attempted with postapplication observation to ensure that the leak is not ongoing. Of note, rare reports demonstrate expansion of hydrogels after applications resulting in spinal cord or cauda equina compression.[6,7] With larger tears associated with more brisk flow of CSF, application of adhesive sealant may not be sufficient and primary closure must be attempted.

For slightly larger dural tears, various techniques have been reported in the literature. Shibayama et al described a patch technique using bioabsorbable polyglactin 910 and fibrin glue. Small squares of 3 to 10 mm in size were soaked in fibrinogen solution and placed over the defect, sometimes in multiple layers. Thrombin was then applied reacting with the fibrinogen to seal the defect. This technique was used in seven patients with adequate closure of the dural defect with no evidence of a CSF leak postoperatively on MRI and no need for reoperation.[8] Other groups have used self-closing U-clips for closure of small defects, and Ferroli et al reported no evidence of persistent CSF leakage in seven patients with intraoperative durotomy using this device.[9,10] These devices will approximate the dural edges together to achieve closure, but it is critical to choose the correct size to ensure the edges are tightly approximated.

However, primary closure with sutures may be required for CSF leaks due to dural injury. In MISS, the use of a Castroviejo needle driver is limited because opening and closing of this microinstrument may be impaired with the additional limitation of inadequate needle rotation to throw sutures at the correct angle. Instead, a micropituitary rongeur can be used as a needle driver, a technique adapted from arthroscopic surgery.[11] We typically use a 5–0 prolene suture to perform a figure-of-eight

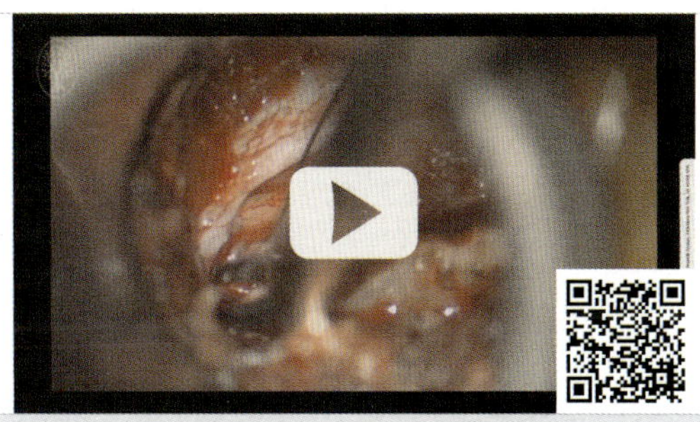

Video 13.1 CSF-leak MIS dural repair.

Table 13.1 Surgical steps for management of CSF leak in MISS

1. Identification of leak	• Determine the extent and location of leak to see if primary closure is possible • Identify the size of dural opening
2. Obtain adequate exposure	• Expand surgical corridor with larger diameter tubes • Remove excess ligament or bone to better isolate area of leak and expose edges of the dura to allow closure
3. Protect critical structures	• Consider placement of paddies to cover and reduce any herniating nerve roots through the dural defect • Place patient in Trendelenburg position to allow for relaxation of thecal sac to aide in reducing any herniating nerve roots
4. Small dural defect	• Consider applying adhesive sealant • Perform Valsalva maneuver check to ensure no further leakage after repair
5. Large dural defect (nerve root sticking out)	• Drain CSF and reinsert nerve roots • Patch technique • Apply self-closing U-clips • Primary closure with suture with appropriate surgical instrumentation; consider adjuvant adhesive sealant and paraspinal muscle • Perform Valsalva maneuver check to ensure no further leakage after repair
6. Postoperative management	• Recommend bedrest for 2 to 5 days depending on size of leak • Patient positioning: Upright positioning is recommended for cervical durotomies; flat positioning is recommended for lumbar durotomies • Consideration of a lumbar drain at the time of surgery if there is high suspicion that primary closure will fail. May consider percutaneous lumbar drain placement at a later time if patient continues to have ongoing symptoms of a CSF leak or develops bogginess around the incision. The drain must be placed at a lumbar level that was not involved in the operation. We would recommend drainage of 10 to 15 mL of CSF per hour with a lower rate if patients develop low-pressure headaches • Obtain a head CT if patient develops severe, worsening headaches or a focal neurological deficit

Abbreviations: CSF, cerebrospinal fluid; CT, computed tomography; MISS, minimally invasive spine surgery.

Table 13.2 Summary of reports detailing dural closure techniques in MISS

Study	Technique	Study size
Shibayama et al[8]	Patch technique using bioabsorbable polyglactin 910 and fibrin glue	7
Song et al[10]	U-clips for closure	2
Ferroli et al[9]	U-clips for closure	1
Chou et al[11]	Standard surgical instruments for primary closure	1
Ruban et al[13]	Small/partial thickness: • Repaired with fibrin glue Large/full thickness: • If primary repair not possible, then gelfoam + fibrin glue • If primary repair possible, then suture used with fibrin glue overlay; paraspinal muscle/collagen matrix used if dural closure not watertight	53
Tan et al[12]	Specialized MIS instruments (Scanlan) for primary closure; use of adjuvant fibrin glue overlying suture line; paraspinal muscle/collagen matrix used if dural closure not watertight	23
Haque et al[14]	Specialized MIS instruments (Scanlan) for primary closure	2
Boukebir et al[15]	Specialized MIS instruments (Scanlan) for primary closure; currently our group uses CV-6 Gore-Tex suture because the needle is smaller than the suture, therefore reducing the risk of leakage around the suture	31

Abbreviations: MIS, minimally invasive surgery; MISS, minimally invasive spine surgery.

suture over the tear. Other sutures that could be used include neurolon or Gore-Tex (Ethicon).[12] The suture can then be tied completely outside the wound and pushed down using a laparoscopic knot pusher. Tan et al reported primary dural closure on intended durotomies with specialized MIS Scanlan instruments (Scanlan International, St. Paul, Minnesota) with adjuvant fibrin glue with no patients having a pseudomeningocele and no patient requiring revision surgery. For more information about the specific instruments and management of CSF leaks via MIS Scanlan instruments, please refer to Chapter 11, Fig. 11.6. In this report, a Scanlan dural repair kit was used which included a special curved needle holder, Jacobson needle holder, Chitwood knot pusher, and modified suture scissors.[12] To bolster an irregular, nonlinear defect, a small piece of paraspinal muscle may be harvested and used to plug the dural defect in between a figure-of-eight stitch. Some groups advocate for adjuvant adhesive sealant application over the suture line, regardless of whether it is watertight after repair.[13] Finally, if the dural tear is very large and primary closure through the tube is not possible despite the abovementioned techniques, conversion to an open procedure with more exposure may be needed. A summary of reports addressing dural closure in MIS cases can be found in ▶ Table 13.2 with ▶ Fig. 13.1 providing an illustration of these techniques.

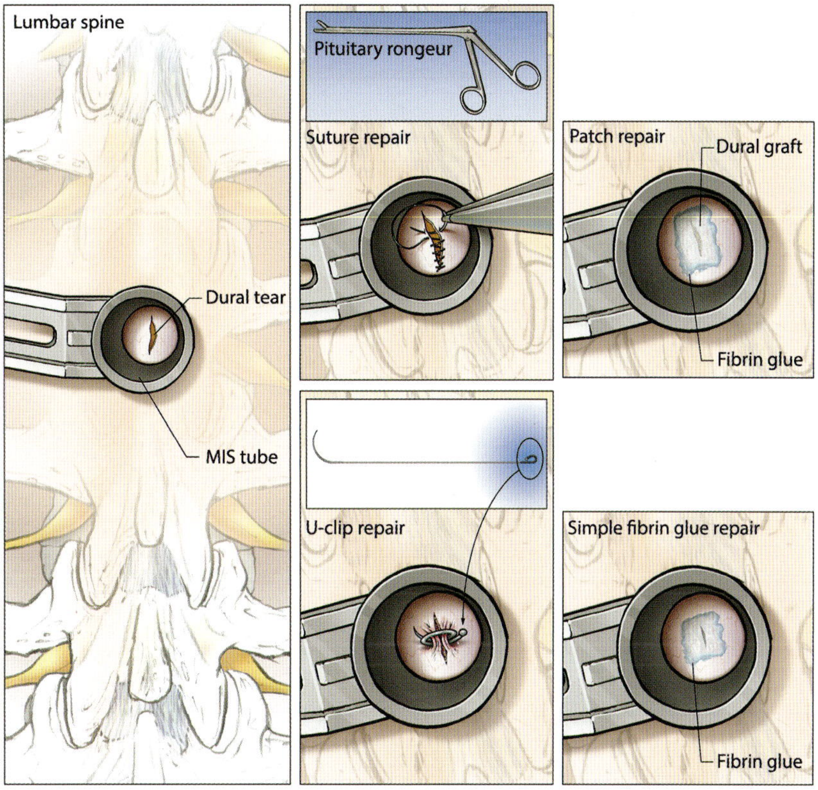

Fig. 13.1 Illustration of four techniques for durotomy closure in minimally invasive spine surgery (MISS). *Top middle panel*: Primary closure using suture and a micropituitary rongeur; *top right panel*: patch repair using bioabsorbable material and fibrin glue; *bottom middle panel*: U-clip application; or *bottom right panel*: simple fibrin glue application.

No matter which technique is employed, it is important to confirm with the microscope that all knots are tight and that there is no evidence of a spinal fluid leak with a Valsalva maneuver. Of utmost importance is tight closure of the fascial, subcutaneous, and cutaneous soft tissue layers. If the wound is closed properly and tightly, even if a pseudomeningocele forms, it will hopefully not result in CSF leakage from the incision requiring revision.

If there is a concern for ongoing CSF leakage or if evidence of a CSF leak is identified postoperatively, several management decisions should be considered. A patient should be kept on bed rest for 2 to 5 days to avoid excess drainage through the defect when standing. Various bed positions may be employed depending on suspected leak location. For a suspected lumbar leak, the patient should be kept flat, whereas for cervical durotomies, an upright position decreases intrathecal pressure in this region. A lumbar subarachnoid drain may also be placed to minimize the formation of a CSF fistula. However, we do not recommend placement of a lumbar subarachnoid drain unless there is very high suspicion that a primary closure will fail or in the event that a primary repair has already failed once.

13.3 Conclusion

Repair of an intraoperative CSF leak is possible in MISS despite limitations placed on surgeons by the tube-retractor system. Conversion to open surgery is usually not necessary. Dural repair should be undertaken after identification to prevent postoperative complications including pseudomeningocele formation, wound breakdown, and symptoms of low intracranial pressure due a CSF leak. A variety of techniques have been employed to allow for both small and large defect closure, and primary closure with suturing can be achieved with both standard surgical instruments as well as specialized MISS dural closure instruments.

References

[1] Nandyala SV, Elboghdady IM, Marquez-Lara A, Noureldin MNB, Sankaranarayanan S, Singh K. Cost analysis of incidental durotomy in spine surgery. Spine. 2014; 39(17):E1042–E1051

[2] Parikh K, Tomasino A, Knopman J, Boockvar J, Härtl R. Operative results and learning curve: microscope-assisted tubular microsurgery for 1- and 2-level discectomies and laminectomies. Neurosurg Focus. 2008; 25(2):E14

[3] Wu X, Zhuang S, Mao Z, Chen H. Microendoscopic discectomy for lumbar disc herniation: surgical technique and outcome in 873 consecutive cases. Spine. 2006; 31(23):2689–2694

[4] Phan K, Huo YR, Hogan JA, et al. Minimally invasive surgery in adult degenerative scoliosis: a systematic review and meta-analysis of decompression, anterior/lateral and posterior lumbar approaches. J Spine Surg. 2016; 2 (2):89–104

[5] Wong AP, Shih P, Smith TR, et al. Comparison of symptomatic cerebral spinal fluid leak between patients undergoing minimally invasive versus open lumbar foraminotomy, discectomy, or laminectomy. World Neurosurg. 2014; 81 (3–4):634–640

[6] Thavarajah D, De Lacy P, Hussain R, Redfern RM. Postoperative cervical cord compression induced by hydrogel (DuraSeal): a possible complication. Spine. 2010; 35(1):E25–E26
[7] Mulder M, Crosier J, Dunn R. Cauda equina compression by hydrogel dural sealant after a laminotomy and discectomy: case report. Spine. 2009; 34(4): E144–E148
[8] Shibayama M, Mizutani J, Takahashi I, Nagao S, Ohta H, Otsuka T. Patch technique for repair of a dural tear in microendoscopic spinal surgery. J Bone Joint Surg Br. 2008; 90(8):1066–1067
[9] Ferroli P, Franzini A, Messina G, Tringali G, Broggi G. Use of self-closing U-clips for dural repair in mini-invasive surgery for herniated disc. Acta Neurochir (Wien). 2008; 150(10):1103–1105
[10] Song D, Park P. Primary closure of inadvertent durotomies utilizing the U-Clip in minimally invasive spinal surgery. Spine. 2011; 36(26):E1753–E1757
[11] Chou D, Wang VY, Khan AS. Primary dural repair during minimally invasive microdiscectomy using standard operating room instruments. Neurosurgery. 2009; 64(5) Suppl 2:356–358, discussion 358–359
[12] Tan LA, Takagi I, Straus D, O'Toole JE. Management of intended durotomy in minimally invasive intradural spine surgery: clinical article. J Neurosurg Spine. 2014; 21(2):279–285
[13] Ruban D, O'Toole JE. Management of incidental durotomy in minimally invasive spine surgery. Neurosurg Focus. 2011; 31(4):E15
[14] Haque RM, Hashmi SZ, Ahmed Y, Uddin O, Ogden AT, Fessler R. Primary dural repair in minimally invasive spine surgery. Case Rep Med. 2013; 2013:876351
[15] Boukebir MA, Berlin CD, Navarro-Ramirez R, et al. Ten-step minimally invasive spine lumbar decompression and dural repair through tubular retractors. Oper Neurosurg (Hagerstown). 2017; 13(2):232–245

14 How to Achieve a Successful Fusion with MIS Techniques

Nickul S. Jain and Jeffrey C. Wang

Summary

Arthrodesis procedures make up a significant portion of spinal procedures and can be used to treat pathologies secondary to degenerative disease, trauma, and deformity. With the marked increase in minimally invasive procedures including fusion techniques, ensuring successful fusion is critical to prevent the problems associated with symptomatic pseudoarthrosis. While outcomes between minimally invasive and traditional techniques are generally considered to be similar, minimally invasive techniques are limited by decreased visualization and exposure that may reduce both local autograft harvest as well as surface area for arthrodesis. In order to mitigate this potentially higher risk of psueodarthrosis, biologic bone graft extenders have become increasingly popular to help achieve successful fusion in minimally invasive techniques, particularly in minimally invasive transforaminal lumbar interbody fusion.

Keywords: biologics, bone graft extenders, bone morphogenic protein, BMP, MIS TLIF

14.1 Introduction

Spine fusion or arthrodesis is a critical aspect of many spine surgical procedures. As minimally invasive techniques have increased in popularity and have been shown to provide better immediate postoperative outcomes, their use will not positively affect patient clinical outcomes unless the surgeon can achieve a successful and stable arthrodesis. Failure of fusion can result in severe clinical symptoms and pseudoarthrosis rates in spine surgery have been reported up to 30% of lumbar spine fusions.[1] Despite the advent of improved rigid internal fixation, fusion promoting materials such as bone morphogenic protein (BMP), and improved surgical techniques, pseudoarthrosis still remains a significant cause of negative patient outcomes and results in higher medical costs, morbidity, and rates of revision surgery. Achieving a successful fusion requires a balance of biological, technical, and biomechanical factors including an optimization of host factors, low-strain mechanical environment, vascularization of the fusion bed, osteoinduction, osteoconduction, osteogenesis, and appropriate surgical technique for graft bed preparation.

14.2 Host Factors

It is imperative for the surgeon to recognize that successful fusion, regardless of surgical technique, is dependent on multiple factors. Patient factors such as age, bone density, metabolic disorders, hormonal imbalance, nicotine and smoking use, and comorbidities are equally as important as technical surgeon-controlled factors in achieving a successful union. Regardless of open versus minimally invasive surgery (MIS), these factors must be examined and optimized preoperatively by the operating surgeon in order to achieve a successful arthrodesis. Osteoporosis, for example, should be suspected especially in elderly women and treated accordingly before surgery.

> Interbody fusion is the "sine qua non" when arthrodesis is pursued via MISS techniques. The use of powerful biologics to improve fusion rates will not obviate the need for careful and thorough discectomy, endplate preparation, and adequate carpentry of the implant.

14.2.1 Biomechanics

Ideal biomechanics are essential to successful arthrodesis in spine surgery. A low-strain environment combined with solid internal fixation and instrumentation that allows load sharing between host and graft tissues are critical principles.[2] Pedicle screw constructs have now been established as the gold standard for rigid internal fixation in the thoracolumbar spine and have shown significantly higher successful arthrodesis rates when compared with noninstrumented fusions.[3,4,5] MIS fixation techniques include navigated and percutaneous pedicle screw placement to avoid the traditional open soft-tissue dissection and are outside of the scope of this chapter but are critical for achieving rigid fixation in minimally invasive lumbar fusion.

14.2.2 Biologics

In achieving a successful fusion, the surgeon must not only optimize biomechanical considerations of low-strain and rigid fixation, but also must create an environment conducive to osteogenesis across a motion segment. Various biologics can be added to the fusion bed to aide in this process. The principles of osteogenesis require osteoconduction, osteoinduction, and osteogenesis. Osteoconductivity refers to the ability of graft material to act as a scaffold or matrix to support osteoblasts and osteoprogenitor (OPG) cells. Osteoinduction refers to the ability of a graft to signal and induce osteoblastic differentiation of OPG stem cells. Osteogenic potential of a graft refers to the ability of a graft to directly provide bone-forming cells to the fusion bed. All biologics have at least one if not more of these properties with the ideal graft combining all of these aspects.

The traditional gold standard for spine fusion has long been iliac crest bone autograft (ICBG) as it combines cancellous bone, structural cortical bone, and autogenous bone marrow cells. However, due to finite supply and patient morbidity, its utility in spine fusion procedures has steadily decreased given up to a reported 30% complication rate including pain, infection, hematoma, and neurovascular injury.[6,7,8,9,10,11,12] Minimally invasive procedures in particular aim to limit patient morbidity and soft-tissue dissection, and have made ICBG nearly prohibitory for use.

Local autograft, while more limited in quantity in minimally invasive procedures when compared with traditional open surgery, is still an integral part of obtaining a successful fusion and should be maximized in quantity during any fusion procedure. The surgeon should make all attempts during decompressive

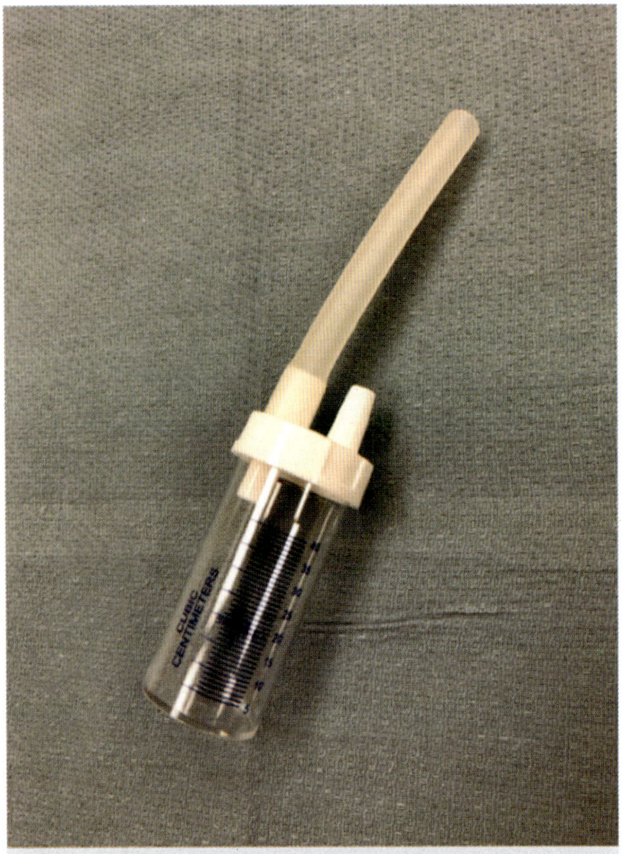

Fig. 14.1 Lukens trap used for collection of bone shavings during minimally invasive lumbar fusion procedures.

surgery to preserve, collect, and reuse as much local autograft as possible given its potential for osteoinduction, osteoconduction, and osteogenesis. Particularly in minimally invasive transforaminal lumbar interbody fusion (MIS TLIF), ample amount of local autograft can be obtained through careful surgical technique. Specific techniques to the preservation of autograft include minimizing burr use, using a Lukens trap (▶ Fig. 14.1) to collect bone shavings, preserving bone chips from decompression performed with a Kerrison rongeur, and cutting both the inferior and superior articular processes with an osteotome, and removing them whole to be used as a significant source of structural local autograft.[13] Local bone shavings have been shown to have preserved histological properties with no significant damage at a cellular level to potential osteogenic cells; however, they likely have inferior osteogenic potential when compared with local autograft bone chips obtained from Kerrison rongeurs.[14,15] Kasliwal et al used isolated local autograft collected with a Lukens trap during MIS TLIF in a retrospective series with a 67% fusion rate in 40 patients with a 1-year follow-up assessed with thin-cut computed tomography (CT) scan.[16]

Bone allografts function as bone extenders to help aide in fusion in cases without adequate autograft. Their benefits have been well described in the literature and include elimination of donor site morbidity and ample supply, but they are not without risks including disease transmission and antigenicity that can induce host reactions.[17] Various alternatives to autograft exist: demineralized bone matrix (DBM), ceramics, composite grafts, BMPs, and mesenchymal stem cells (MSCs). Careful graft selection is critical for a successful outcome in fusion and an understanding of the variety of graft materials is an important consideration for the surgeon during minimally invasive procedures.

14.2.3 Allograft

Cadaver allograft is available in both a structural and nonstructural varieties. It is processed after harvest to reduce antigenicity as well as disease transmission; however, this eliminates their osteogenic potential. Advantages include abundance of supply and avoidance of autograft donor site morbidity. Disadvantages include disease transmission risk, however this has been reduced to less than 1 in 1.5 million. They are an osteoconductive scaffold and weakly osteoinductive, and when used in isolation in a recent meta-analysis obtained a collective fusion rate of 52% in posterolateral lumbar fusion.[18]

DBM is obtained by acid extraction demineralization of allograft bone. This process results in a matrix of isolated Type 1 collagen and noncollagenous proteins and growth factors that may have osteoconductive properties and potentially weak osteoinductive properties while sacrificing structural support. DBMs are available commercially in many forms including moldable putty, injectable gel, and flexible strips. There is a wide variety of osteoinductive qualities between graft vendors and even lot numbers that has previously been well described.[19,20] This variability leads to limitations in their osteoinductive capabilities. Their isolated use for fusion is also not recommended as they require combination with mechanically resistant materials to avoid migration or excess motion.[21] However, they do have a strong track record of success as a bone graft extender when combined with autograft.[22]

14.2.4 Ceramics

Ceramics such as calcium carbonate and beta-tricalcium phosphate provide osteoconductive scaffold for new bone formation but lack osteoinductive and structural support qualities. Hydroxyapatite coating of ceramic grafts may promote bony ingrowth and slow resorption rates.[23] Advantages of ceramics include synthetic nature resulting in unlimited supply and lack of antigenicity or disease transmission risk. Disadvantages include brittle structure and requirement of supplemental fixation to protect against excess forces. In addition, they require large surface areas of decorticated bone for success.[24] Their routine isolated use for lumbar arthrodesis has been attempted with some success; however, acceptable fusion rates with ceramics in the lumbar spine have been described when used in combination with bone marrow aspirate and local bone graft.[25] A recent meta-analysis of ceramics demonstrated an 85% fusion rate in posterolateral lumbar fusion when combined with an osteoinductive source of autologous cells.[18] Further study is needed into their use as an isolated bone graft substitute.

14.2.5 Bone Marrow Aspirate

Bone marrow aspirate allows for collection and concentration of growth factors and MSCs which have osteogenic potential due to their ability to differentiate into OPG cell lines. Their

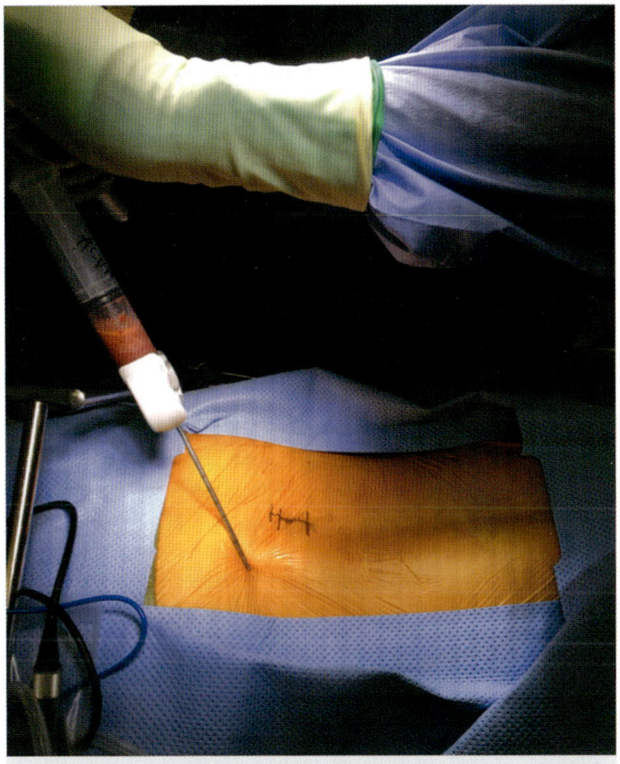

Fig. 14.2 Bone marrow aspiration from the posterior superior iliac spine.

osteogenic properties were first described by Burwell in 1964.[26] It is readily available and can be harvested percutaneously from the posterior superior iliac spine (PSIS; ▶ Fig. 14.2) among other sites of the body. Selective cell retention technology can be used to increase the number of OPG cells by three to four times.[27] Bone marrow aspiration (BMA) does require a osteoconductive carrier or scaffold to obtain optimal fusion mass.

In combination with local autograft, BMA has been shown to be a viable alternative to ICBG autograft with similar fusion rates in open posterolateral spine fusions.[28,29] Equivalent clinical outcomes and fusion rates with BMA combined with a collagen carrier compared with ICBG and BMP-2 in single-level revision posterolateral lumbar fusion has also previously been demonstrated.[30] A combination analysis of 2 studies totaling 40 patients undergoing posterolateral fusion resulted in 85% fusion rate when a concentrated BMA protocol with osteoconductive ceramic or allograft was used.[18]

Some disadvantages of BMA include: variations in the osteoblast colony-forming units per individual, inability to extract more than 2 mL per location due to dilution in blood, and unclear evidence for clinical advantages of centrifugation and concentration.[31,32,33]

14.2.6 Bone Morphogenic Protein

BMP is an osteoinductive growth factor first described by Urist in 1965.[34] It has been commercially available in its recombinant form since 2002 and provides significant osteoinductive capabilities to promote spinal arthrodesis in multiple human studies.[35,36,37,38,39,40,41,42,43] It has been well described for both primary and revision lumbar fusion surgery for its benefits in environments with limited local autograft.[30,44]

While it has significant osteogenic potential, it lacks structural and osteoconductive ability and requires combination with a carrier matrix to prevent dissolution from the operative site. It is commercially available in multiple forms; however, the most commonly utilized is rhBMP-2, which has been approved by Food and Drug Administration (FDA) for use in anterior lumbar interbody fusion procedures. Use of rhBMP-2 in the posterior lumbar spine is physician-directed and not FDA approved. However, there is evidence suggesting that rhBMP-2 produces better clinical and radiographic results than allograft alone, and has equivalent or better fusion rates and clinical results when compared with ICBG, with fusion rates as high as 94 to 100% being reported in the posterolateral lumbar spine.[18,36,45,46] Despite the clinical evidence supporting its use to promote fusion, there have been several reported complications.

BMP Complications

Several complications have been reported regarding rhBMP use.

Temporary ipsilateral postoperative inflammatory radiculitis has been seen in up to 11% of patients undergoing MIS-TLIF with rhBMP-2 use.[47] All resolved in 6 weeks with nonoperative treatment. It has been theorized to occur due to the chemotactic and proinflammatory characteristics of BMP that make it such an effective osteoinductive factor.[48] While a known complication of TLIF without BMP, there is a suggestion that there is a higher rate of radiculitis in patients undergoing TLIF with BMP use.[49]

Aggressive, early vertebral body osteolysis has also been described with use of BMP in the interbody space in lumbar surgery. It has been seen in up to 44 to 69% of operated levels undergoing TLIF procedures with rhBMP-2 and resulted in both significant back pain (often treated conservatively) as well as graft migration and pseudarthrois.[50,51] It has been theorized that this osteolysis and resorption is a part of the normal osteoclastic remodeling process that is amplified by BMP; however, it has been associated with both spontaneous resolution as well as cage migration, subsidence, and nonunion.[48,52] Overstuffing of the joint, BMP dosing, L5-S1 level with high inclination, and endplate violation have all been proposed as possible causes of the excess osteolysis seen in these patients.[51]

Excess and heterotopic bone formation resulting in neural compression has also been described in relation to BMP-2 use in the lumbar spine. It has been attributed to BMP leaking from the intervertebral space into the epidural space and resulting in either canal or foraminal compression.[53] Cage placement within 2 mm of the posterior vertebral cortex was associated with excess extradiscal bone formation with BMP-treated patients undergoing posterior lumbar interbody fusion (PLIF).[40] A systemic review has identified the rate of extradiscal heterotopic bone formation associated with BMP use of approximately 8%. Whether or not these patients required reoperation due to heterotopic bone formation is not as clear.[51]

De novo cancer as a result of BMP use has also been described in the literature by the Yale Open Data Access project with nearly a double risk of development of cancer in patients receiving rhBMP-2.[54] Contradictory studies have demonstrated no significant increase in cancer rates.[55,56] A conclusive link between BMP and de novo cancer rates has yet to be established.

Additional complications such as postoperative wound seromas, extradural cyst formations, and anterior cervical swelling and dysphagia have additionally been described.[51]

BMP Dosing

Many efforts have been made to counteract some of the negative aspects of BMP including reduced and low dosing BMP. Most studies describing the use of BMP in the interbody space describe typical BMP use of 4.0 to 12.0 mg/level.[40,47] However, many authors have purported that decreasing BMP dosing can still achieve successful fusion in order to mitigate the potential side effects of vertebral osteolysis and ectopic bone formation in low levels.[51] Optimal dosing for BMP use is yet to be defined.

14.3 Interbody Fusion

In the past three decades, circumferential fusion utilizing the interbody space in the lumbar spine has had increasing popularity in degenerative conditions. Purported benefits include increased surface area for bony fusion. The interbody space can be accessed from the anterior, lateral, and posterior approaches. Specifically, MIS for the posterior lumbar spine via a transforaminal approach (MIS TLIF) has gained popularity due to its potential for improved short-term patient outcomes when compared with open TLIF.[57,58,59,60] Advantages include decreased estimated blood loss, shorter length of stay, and avoidance of the morbidity seen with both anterior and minimally invasive lateral transpsoas procedures for interbody fusion.

The axis of rotation in flexion and extension within the lumbar spine is at the anterior aspect of the disc space. Limiting motion as close to this axis as possible limits the length of the lever arm of forces against the fusion location.[2,61] Increased distance from this lever arm creates increased distractive forces and can predispose to pseudoarthrosis. Interbody fusion provides increased bony surface areas and compression loading across grafts to aide in fusion.[62] Wolff's law states that bone develops in response to mechanical stress and interbody fusion helps allow for fusion across a region of the spine that is loaded in compression as opposed to tension (as seen in the posterior elements). In addition, there are the purported benefits of restoration of segmental lordosis that may prevent adjacent segment degeneration.[63]

Interbody fusion combined with posterior instrumentation (pedicle screws) has been shown to have increased stability which allows for a more favorable low-strain environment for fusion.[64] While the theoretical benefits of interbody fusion are well described, definitive studies showing that posterior interbody fusion decreases pseudoarthroiss rates have not yet been established. Technical factors are critical to the success of interbody fusion and include appropriate discectomy, vertebral body endplate preparation, and thorough removal of cartilaginous structures.

14.3.1 Minimally Invasive Transforaminal Lumbar Interbody Fusion

MIS TLIF combines many of the aforementioned techniques and theories in order to obtain a successful lumbar arthrodesis while preserving the midline ligamentous tension band and potentially still restoring sagittal alignment. Moreover, TLIF avoids the high rates of iatrogenic nerve injury seen in PLIF, allows for circumferential arthrodesis entirely from a posterior approach, and avoids the morbidity associated with anterior and lateral approaches to the interbody space. Ideal bone grafting in this situation is debated among surgeons and highly dependent on surgeon preferences; however, general principles of creating a vascularized fusion bed with a bone graft with ostoeconductive, osteoindiuctive, and osteogenic potential remain critical.

Choosing graft material in MIS TLIF is a complex question with limited data. Kasliwal et al examined using solely local autograft shavings combined with interbody cage in a small series of MIS TLIF patients and saw a 67.5% fusion rate, however, there was noted to be good clinical outcomes in 92% of patients.[16]

A recent meta-analysis of MIS TLIF patients including 1,533 patients over 40 series demonstrated high fusion rates (> 90%) overall regardless of graft choice.[65] Subgroup analysis showed the addition of rhBMP to autologous local bone graft increased the fusion rate from 91.8 to 95.3%. The highest fusion rates were seen when BMP was combined with local autologous bone as well as bone graft extenders (99.1%). The highest fusion rate without the use of rhBMP was seen with autologous local bone and bone extender (93.1%). This suggests that high arthrodesis rates can be achieved without routine BMP use; however, the addition of BMP can further enhance overall fusion rates in MIS procedures. However, its use is not without complications as described previously.

14.3.2 Simultaneous Posterolateral Fusion in MIS TLIF

Posterolateral fusion using the transverse processes, pars interarticularis, and facet joint was first described by Watkins in 1953.[66] It has widely become standard for posterior lumbar fusion procedures as it allows movement of the fusion mass anteriorly, closer to the axis of rotation of the lumbar spine, decreasing micromotion and tensile forces on graft material.[2]

MIS TLIF has been well described and can be performed with simultaneous posterolateral fusion by furthering dissection around facet joints and exposing and decorticating the transverse processes. While one critique of MIS TLIF includes difficult access to the intertransverse window for posterolateral fusion, we find that retractor systems can be easily used to achieve concomitant posterolateral fusion during MIS TLIF with a careful docking technique centered on the facet (▶ Fig. 14.3).

More recently, some authors have questioned the need for posterolateral fusion during MIS TLIF. A meta-analysis by Bevevino et al described an overall CT-confirmed fusion rate of 94.7% in patients undergoing MIS TLIF without posterolateral fusion.[67] Avoiding posterolateral fusion has purported advantages of decreased operative time, blood loss, and muscle dissection. One alternative includes fusion of the facet joints alone which can be done on the contralateral side as TLIF during MIS TLIF.

14.4 Authors' Preferred Technique for MIS TLIF

Preoperative patient optimization is performed of all medical comorbidities and patient screening for host factors for pseudoarthrosis risk is performed. Once in the operating room, patients

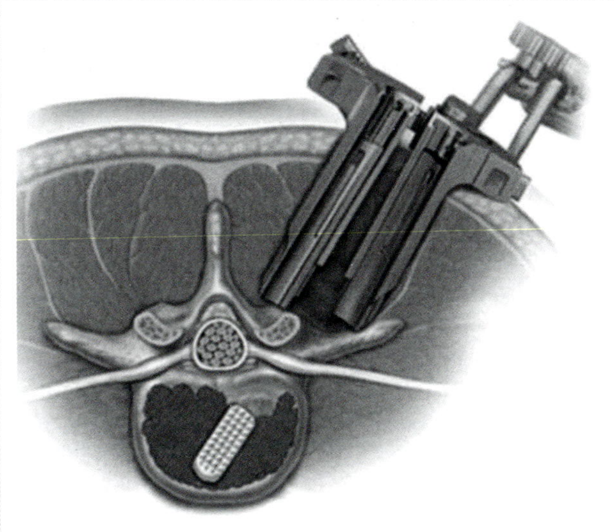

Fig. 14.3 Minimally invasive surgery retractor system docking over the facet allowing for both transforaminal lumbar interbody fusion procedure and posterolateral intertransverse fusion. (Reproduced from Pipeline Expandable Access System (DePuy). In: Sandhu F, Voyadzis J, Fessler R, ed. Decision Making for Minimally Invasive Spine Surgery. 1st Edition. New York: Thieme; 2011.)

are positioned in a standard fashion, prone on a four-post Jackson frame taking care to extend the hips and maximize lumbar lordosis. Bilateral MIS retractor system table attachments are placed on the bed prior to patient positioning. Bone marrow aspirate is then harvested from the PSIS using a three-hole Jamshidi needle that is advanced 2 cm every 6 mL of aspirate to avoid hemodilution of the bone marrow aspirate (▶ Fig. 14.2).[32] It is then passed off for concentration and then placed onto a collagen carrier. Bilateral retractor systems are then placed via sequential dilation in a standard fashion after localization over the facet joint of the level to be fused in a standard Wiltse-type approach, typically 3.5 to 4.5 cm off midline on each side of the spine. After muscle dissection and exposure of the lamina, pars interarticularis, facet joints, and transverse processes of each level to be fused, pedicle screws are then placed on the side contralateral to the planned TLIF. At this point, if significant segmental lordosis is desired, bilateral Smith-Peterson osteotomies can be performed using a combination of osteotomes and Kerrison rongeurs with all bone saved for use as local autograft. If not, the facet joint, pars interarticularis, and transverse processes are then decorticated using a high-speed drill with irrigation to prevent thermal necrosis. A combination of locally harvested autograft, bone marrow aspirate with a collagen carrier, and DBM is used to pack the posterolateral gutter and decorticated facet. A temporary rod is placed to allow for maintenance of disc height during the TLIF procedure.

On the side of the TLIF, the inferior articular process is harvested in its entirety using a Chevron cut with an osteotome (▶ Fig. 14.4) and morcellized for autograft. The superior articular process is removed to the base of the pedicle using a combination of drill and Kerrison rongeours. A Lukens trap is used to collect bone dust and shavings during drill use. Once the interbody space is exposed via Kambin's triangle, thorough discectomy is performed with a combination of shavers, dilators, and both straight and angled curettes to adequately remove disc and prepare the vertebral endplates, taking care not to violate the

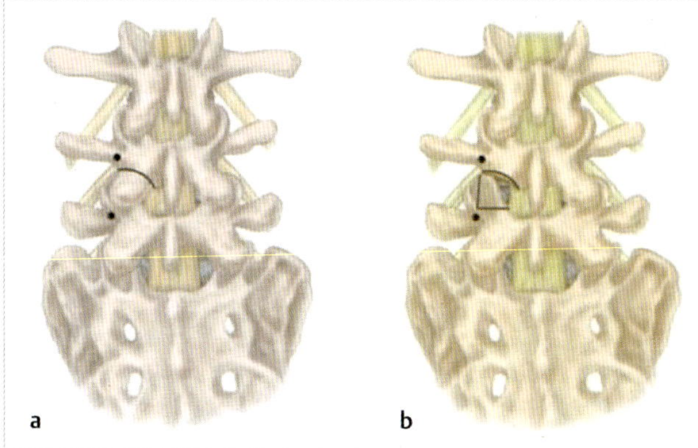

Fig. 14.4 (a, b) Technique of inferior articular process resection as one en bloc piece for reuse as autograft. (Reproduced from Instrumentation. In: Kim D, Fessler R, Regan J, ed. Endoscopic Spine Surgery and Instrumentation. 1st Edition. New York: Thieme; 2004.)

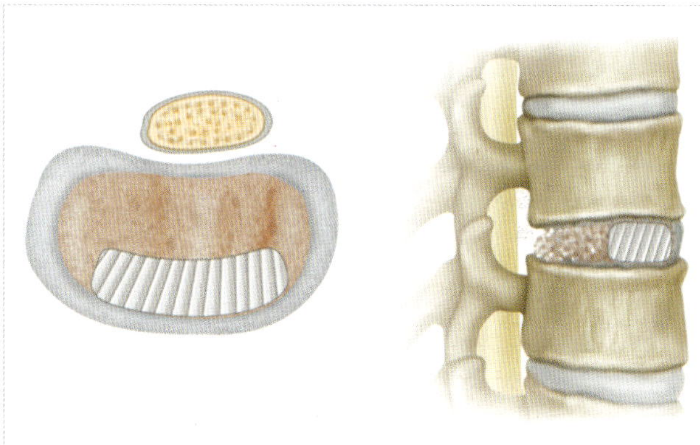

Fig. 14.5 Technique of anterior cage placement to allow for segmental lordosis restoration and room for bone graft placement. (Reproduced from Tips, Pearls, and Lessons Learned. In: Vaccaro A, Albert T, ed. Spine Surgery: Tricks of the Trade. 3rd Edition. New York: Thieme; 2016.)

endplates. Navigated instruments for disc preparation are commercially available for use if desired. Discectomy is a critical portion of the procedure as successful fusion mandates adequate disc removal and endplate preparation. Typical disc preparation takes minimum 15 to 30 minutes of dedicated operative time.

Once discectomy is complete, interbody graft trialing is performed. The appropriate cage is selected and packed with local autograft and harvested BMA with collagen carrier. BMA with collagen carriers is packed into the anterior disc space prior to cage placement. The cage is then placed as anterior as possible and centrally within the disc space, more than 2 mm from the margin of the posterior vertebral cortex (▶ Fig. 14.5). In cases with high pseudoarthrosis risk and no history of malignancy, off-label physician-directed use of low-dose BMP (1.5–2.5 mg) is chosen. It is split in half and one half placed into the interbody cage and other half anterior to it within the disc space. BMP is not used behind the cage in order to limit potential side effects of heterotopic/ectopic bone formation or in the posterolateral gutter on the side of the TLIF to avoid radiculitis.[68] At this point, a small amount of bone graft is placed into the posterolateral gutter, taking care not to overstuff over the open exiting

nerve root in the foramen. A standard closure is then performed after thorough irrigation. Choice of biologics and interbody cage graft material are debatable and based on surgeon preference. We do not routinely use BMP unless there is an increased risk of pseudoarthrosis.

14.4.1 Bracing

Postoperative bracing after lumbar fusion with minimally invasive techniques is not well reported in the literature. However, there have been high-quality studies looking at the effect of bracing on clinical and radiographic outcomes following traditional lumbar fusion. Dailey et al completed a review of bracing in the setting of lumbar spine pathology and concluded that bracing following instrumented lumbar fusion was not recommended as outcomes were unchanged by brace use, primarily based on the Level I evidence by Yee et al.[69,70] These findings were echoed by Zhu et al.[71] As such, routine bracing after thoracolumbar fusions for degenerative pathology, performed either minimally invasively or traditionally, is not recommended as it does not seem to affect arthrodesis rates.

14.4.2 Bone Stimulators

Electrical and electromagnetic energy have a proven therapeutic benefit on bone healing and arthrodesis. Both invasive and noninvasive electrical stimulation have been described and studied in the literature to assist in achieving a solid arthrodesis. Invasive stimulation is via direct current stimulation (DCS) with electrodes placed into the fusion mass intraoperatively. Noninvasive stimulation is performed through pulsed electromagnetic field stimulation (PEMFS) or capacitive coupled electrical stimulation (CCES).

Overall, there is a paucity of literature to support or refute routine use of bone stimulation via either invasive or noninvasive methodology for either traditional open or MIS surgery. The *Journal of Neurosurgery Spine* has published guidelines for the performance of fusion procedures for degenerative disease of the lumbar spine and potentially recommended DCS as an option for patients younger than 60 years of age but recommended against it in patients older than 60 years undergoing lumbar fusion; however, the quality of evidence was low for these recommendations. There was also insufficient evidence to either support or reject routine use of noninvasive PEMFS or CCES stimulation in primary or revision surgery for pseudoarthrosis. Further study with a randomized clinical trial was recommended by the guideline committee.[72] While bone stimulation can be considered a potential adjunct, the invasiveness of DCS and the high cost of noninvasive methods, such as PEMFS, may offset the potential benefits on arthrodesis rates.

14.4.3 Percutaneous Fixation for Traumatic Injuries

Minimally invasive percutaneous fixation for traumatic injuries or oncologic disease has been well described for the thoracolumbar spine with a relatively low rate of complications and benefit for faster patient mobilization and potentially overall outcomes in patients who do not require open neurologic decompression or fracture reduction.[73] Many authors advocate for the routine removal of instrumentation after percutaneous fixation for traumatic injuries after bony union has occurred of the fracture and avoidance of formal fusion typically in the setting of burst fractures as clinical results have been similar to open fusion.[74] However, some authors have described adding bone graft to potentially allow for fusion across motion segments in percutaneous fixation via nasal speculums.[75] Achieving union of thoracolumbar fractures not requiring open reduction or neurologic decompression with percutaneous pedicle screw fixation appears to be successful without formal bone grafting; however, it can be performed if desired by the surgeon. Data and techniques on concurrent fusion at the time of percutaneous pedicle screw fixation is lacking in the literature.

14.4.4 Medication Augmentation

The process of inducing fusion across motion segments in the spine is a biological process, and medication adjuncts may provide the surgeon significant benefit in the goals of achieving fusion as well as instrumentation fixation within bone. Bisphosphonates such as alendronate and anabolic medications such as teriparatide (synthetic parathyroid hormone) have been studied in the setting of spine fusion. Bisphosphonates such as alendronate have been studied both in preclinical animal models and clinical trials. Animal studies revealed lower bone mass in animals treated with alendronate.[80] Clinically, there are conflicting reports with some authors reporting increased fusion rates with alendronate and others suggesting a possible decrease in fusion rates.[81,82] Based on this conflicting data and preclinical animal studies, we do not recommend routine use of the bisphosphonates to aide in fusion during MIS surgery.

Multiple clinical studies have been performed comparing bisphosphonates and teriparatide in the setting of postmenopausal osteoporosis and spine fusion with promising results of teriparatide in reducing rates of hardware loosening, increasing insertional screw torque, and potentially reducing time to fusion.[76,77,78] The importance of pretreatment with these medications (some authors recommending at least 3 months in osteoporotic patients and others more than 6 months) emphasizes the necessity for ideal preoperative optimization of patients to achieve successful fusion.[79,83] In addition, there appears to be some high-quality data suggesting that treatment with teriparatide in the postoperative period in the setting of osteoporosis can improve fusion rates and time to union.

14.5 Discussion

Bone graft selection is a critical portion of spine fusion surgery. Osteobiologics, including rhBMP-2, are powerful methods to achieve successful arthrodesis and can be used in a surgeon's armamentarium during minimally invasive procedures. Successful fusion is dependent on patient factors and surgeon-controlled technical factors, and surgeons should have a good understanding of the various bone graft options in order to improve patient outcomes via successful arthrodesis during minimally invasive techniques. Future novel osteobiologic agents such as BMP-2-binding peptide amphiphiles may further improve arthrodesis and allow for continued advancement of fusion in MIS procedures.

References

[1] Cleveland M, Bosworth DM, Thompson FR. Pseudarthrosis in the lumbosacral spine. J Bone Joint Surg Am. 1948; 30A(2):302–312

[2] Reid JJ, Johnson JS, Wang JC. Challenges to bone formation in spinal fusion. J Biomech. 2011; 44(2):213–220

[3] Zdeblick TA. A prospective, randomized study of lumbar fusion. Preliminary results. Spine. 1993; 18(8):983–991

[4] Thomsen K, Christensen FB, Eiskjaer SP, Hansen ES, Fruensgaard S, Bunger CE. The effect of pedicle screw instrumentation on functional outcome and fusion rates in posterolateral lumbar spinal fusion: a prospective, randomized clinical study. Spine. 1997; 22(24):2813–2822

[5] Dickman CA, Fissler RG, MacMillan M, Haid RW. Transpedicular screw-rod fixation of the lumbar spine: operative technique and outcome in 104 cases. J Neurosurg. 1992; 77:860–870

[6] Arrington ED, Smith WJ, Chambers HG, Bucknell AL, Davino NA. Complications of iliac crest bone graft harvesting. Clin Orthop Relat Res. 1996 (329):300–309

[7] Banwart JC, Asher MA, Hassanein RS. Iliac crest bone graft harvest donor site morbidity. A statistical evaluation. Spine. 1995; 20(9):1055–1060

[8] Fernyhough JC, Schimandle JJ, Weigel MC, Edwards CC, Levine AM. Chronic donor site pain complicating bone graft harvesting from the posterior iliac crest for spinal fusion. Spine. 1992; 17(12):1474–1480

[9] Kurz LT, Garfin SR, Booth RE, Jr. Harvesting autogenous iliac bone grafts. A review of complications and techniques. Spine. 1989; 14(12):1324–1331

[10] Shin AY, Moran ME, Wenger DR. Superior gluteal artery injury secondary to posterior iliac crest bone graft harvesting. A surgical technique to control hemorrhage. Spine. 1996; 21(11):1371–1374

[11] Summers BN, Eisenstein SM. Donor site pain from the ilium. A complication of lumbar spine fusion. J Bone Joint Surg Br. 1989; 71(4):677–680

[12] Sasso RC, LeHuec JC, Shaffrey C, Spine Interbody Research Group. Iliac crest bone graft donor site pain after anterior lumbar interbody fusion: a prospective patient satisfaction outcome assessment. J Spinal Disord Tech. 2005; 18 Suppl:S77–S81

[13] Steffen T, Downer P, Steiner B, Hehli M, Aebi M. Minimally invasive bone harvesting tools. Eur Spine J. 2000; 9 Suppl 1:S114–S118

[14] Patel VV, Estes SM, Naar EM, Lindley EM, Burger E. Histologic evaluation of high speed burr shavings collected during spinal decompression surgery. Orthopedics. 2009; 32(1):23

[15] Eder C, Chavanne A, Meissner J, et al. Autografts for spinal fusion: osteogenic potential of laminectomy bone chips and bone shavings collected via high speed drill. Eur Spine J. 2011; 20(11):1791–1795

[16] Kasliwal MK, Deutsch H. Clinical and radiographic outcomes using local bone shavings as autograft in minimally invasive transforaminal lumbar interbody fusion. World Neurosurg. 2012; 78(1–2):185–190

[17] Lord CF, Gebhardt MC, Tomford WW, Mankin HJ. Infection in bone allografts. Incidence, nature, and treatment. J Bone Joint Surg Am. 1988; 70(3):369–376

[18] Hsu WK, Nickoli MS, Wang JC, et al. Improving the clinical evidence of bone graft substitute technology in lumbar spine surgery. Global Spine J. 2012; 2 (4):239–248

[19] Wang JC, Alanay A, Mark D, et al. A comparison of commercially available demineralized bone matrix for spinal fusion. Eur Spine J. 2007; 16(8):1233–1240

[20] Bae HW, Zhao L, Kanim LE, Wong P, Delamarter RB, Dawson EG. Intervariability and intravariability of bone morphogenetic proteins in commercially available demineralized bone matrix products. Spine. 2006; 31(12):1299–1306, discussion 1307–1308

[21] Gazdag AR, Lane JM, Glaser D, Forster RA. Alternatives to autogenous bone graft: efficacy and indications. J Am Acad Orthop Surg. 1995; 3(1):1–8

[22] Cammisa FP, Jr, Lowery G, Garfin SR, et al. Two-year fusion rate equivalency between Grafton DBM gel and autograft in posterolateral spine fusion: a prospective controlled trial employing a side-by-side comparison in the same patient. Spine. 2004; 29(6):660–666

[23] Wenisch S, Stahl JP, Horas U, et al. In vivo mechanisms of hydroxyapatite ceramic degradation by osteoclasts: fine structural microscopy. J Biomed Mater Res A. 2003; 67(3):713–718

[24] Gitelman A, Basho R, Rebholz BK, McAllister BD, Wang JC. Bone Graft Substitutes/Biologics. In: Anderson DG, Vaccaro AR. Decision Making in Spinal Care. 2nd ed. New York, NY: Thieme; 2013

[25] Yamada T, Yoshii T, Sotome S, et al. Hybrid grafting using bone marrow aspirate combined with porous β-tricalcium phosphate and trephine bone for lumbar posterolateral spinal fusion: a prospective, comparative study versus local bone grafting. Spine. 2012; 37(3):E174–E179

[26] Burwell RG. Studies in the transplantation of bone. Vii. The fresh composite homograft-autograft of cancellous bone: an analysis of factors leading to osteogenesis in marrow transplants and in marrow-containing bone grafts. J Bone Joint Surg Br. 1964; 46:110–140

[27] Muschler GF, Nitto H, Matsukura Y, et al. Spine fusion using cell matrix composites enriched in bone marrow-derived cells. Clin Orthop Relat Res. 2003 (407):102–118

[28] Niu CC, Tsai TT, Fu TS, Lai PL, Chen LH, Chen WJ. A comparison of posterolateral lumbar fusion comparing autograft, autogenous laminectomy bone with bone marrow aspirate, and calcium sulphate with bone marrow aspirate: a prospective randomized study. Spine. 2009; 34(25):2715–2719

[29] Neen D, Noyes D, Shaw M, Gwilym S, Fairlie N, Birch N. Healos and bone marrow aspirate used for lumbar spine fusion: a case controlled study comparing healos with autograft. Spine. 2006; 31(18):E636–E640

[30] Taghavi CE, Lee KB, Keorochana G, Tzeng ST, Yoo JH, Wang JC. Bone morphogenetic protein-2 and bone marrow aspirate with allograft as alternatives to autograft in instrumented revision posterolateral lumbar spinal fusion: a minimum two-year follow-up study. Spine. 2010; 35(11):1144–1150

[31] Muschler GF, Nitto H, Boehm CA, Easley KA. Age- and gender-related changes in the cellularity of human bone marrow and the prevalence of osteoblastic progenitors. J Orthop Res. 2001; 19(1):117–125

[32] Muschler GF, Boehm C, Easley K. Aspiration to obtain osteoblast progenitor cells from human bone marrow: the influence of aspiration volume. J Bone Joint Surg Am. 1997; 79(11):1699–1709

[33] Odri GA, Hami A, Pomero V, et al. Development of a per-operative procedure for concentrated bone marrow adjunction in postero-lateral lumbar fusion: radiological, biological and clinical assessment. Eur Spine J. 2012; 21 (12):2665–2672

[34] Urist MR. Bone: formation by autoinduction. Science. 1965; 150(3698):893–899

[35] Glassman SD, Carreon L, Djurasovic M, et al. Posterolateral lumbar spine fusion with INFUSE bone graft. Spine J. 2007; 7(1):44–49

[36] Dimar JR, Glassman SD, Burkus KJ, Carreon LY. Clinical outcomes and fusion success at 2 years of single-level instrumented posterolateral fusions with recombinant human bone morphogenetic protein-2/compression resistant matrix versus iliac crest bone graft. Spine. 2006; 31(22):2534–2539, discussion 2540

[37] Luhmann SJ, Bridwell KH, Cheng I, Imamura T, Lenke LG, Schootman M. Use of bone morphogenetic protein-2 for adult spinal deformity. Spine. 2005; 30 Suppl 17:S110–S117

[38] Schwender JD, Holly LT, Rouben DP, Foley KT. Minimally invasive transforaminal lumbar interbody fusion (TLIF): technical feasibility and initial results. J Spinal Disord Tech. 2005; 18 Suppl:S1–S6

[39] Mummaneni PV, Pan J, Haid RW, Rodts GE. Contribution of recombinant human bone morphogenetic protein-2 to the rapid creation of interbody fusion when used in transforaminal lumbar interbody fusion: a preliminary report. Invited submission from the Joint Section Meeting on Disorders of the Spine and Peripheral Nerves, March 2004. J Neurosurg Spine. 2004; 1(1):19–23

[40] Haid RW, Jr, Branch CL, Jr, Alexander JT, Burkus JK. Posterior lumbar interbody fusion using recombinant human bone morphogenetic protein type 2 with cylindrical interbody cages. Spine J. 2004; 4(5):527–538, discussion 538–539

[41] Baskin DS, Ryan P, Sonntag V, Westmark R, Widmayer MA. A prospective, randomized, controlled cervical fusion study using recombinant human bone morphogenetic protein-2 with the CORNERSTONE-SR allograft ring and the ATLANTIS anterior cervical plate. Spine. 2003; 28(12):1219–1224, discussion 1225

[42] Boakye M, Mummaneni PV, Garrett M, Rodts G, Haid R. Anterior cervical discectomy and fusion involving a polyetheretherketone spacer and bone morphogenetic protein. J Neurosurg Spine. 2005; 2(5):521–525

[43] Meisel HJ, Schnöring M, Hohaus C, et al. Posterior lumbar interbody fusion using rhBMP-2. Eur Spine J. 2008; 17(12):1735–1744

[44] Hsu WK, Wang JC. The use of bone morphogenetic protein in spine fusion. Spine J. 2008; 8(3):419–425

[45] Hurlbert RJ, Alexander D, Bailey S, et al. rhBMP-2 for posterolateral instrumented lumbar fusion: a multicenter prospective randomized controlled trial. Spine. 2013; 38(25):2139–2148

[46] Boden SD, Kang J, Sandhu H, et al. Use of recombinant human bone morphogenic protein-2 to achieve posterolateral lumbar spine fusion in humans, a prospective randomized clinical pilot trial. Spine. 2002; 27(23):2662–2673

[47] Mindea SA, Shih P, Song JK. Recombinant human bone morphogenetic protein-2-induced radiculitis in elective minimally invasive transforaminal lumbar interbody fusions: a series review. Spine. 2009; 34(14):1480–1484, discussion 1485

[48] Mannion RJ, Nowitzke AM, Wood MJ. Promoting fusion in minimally invasive lumbar interbody stabilization with low-dose bone morphogenic protein-2—but what is the cost? Spine J. 2011; 11(6):527–533

[49] Rihn JA, Gates C, Glassman SD, Phillips FM, Schwender JD, Albert TJ. The use of bone morphogenetic protein in lumbar spine surgery. J Bone Joint Surg Am. 2008; 90(9):2014–2025

[50] McClellan JW, Mulconrey DS, Forbes RJ, Fullmer N. Vertebral bone resorption after transforaminal lumbar interbody fusion with bone morphogenetic protein (rhBMP-2). J Spinal Disord Tech. 2006; 19(7):483–486

[51] Mroz TE, Wang JC, Hashimoto R, Norvell DC. Complications related to osteobiologics use in spine surgery: a systematic review. Spine. 2010; 35(9) Suppl: S86–S104

[52] Lewandrowski KU, Nanson C, Calderon R. Vertebral osteolysis after posterior interbody lumbar fusion with recombinant human bone morphogenetic protein 2: a report of five cases. Spine J. 2007; 7(5):609–614

[53] Benglis D, Wang MY, Levi AD. A comprehensive review of the safety profile of bone morphogenetic protein in spine surgery. Neurosurgery. 2008; 62(5) Suppl 2:ONS423–ONS431, discussion ONS431

[54] Simmonds MC, Brown JV, Heirs MK, et al. Safety and effectiveness of recombinant human bone morphogenetic protein-2 for spinal fusion. Ann Intern Med. 2013; 158:877–889

[55] Kelly MP, Savage JW, Bentzen SM, Hsu WK, Ellison SA, Anderson PA. Cancer risk from bone morphogenetic protein exposure in spinal arthrodesis. J Bone Joint Surg Am. 2014; 96(17):1417–1422

[56] Cahill KS, McCormick PC, Levi AD. A comprehensive assessment of the risk of bone morphogenetic protein use in spinal fusion surgery and postoperative cancer diagnosis. J Neurosurg Spine. 2015; 23(1):86–93

[57] Wang J, Zhou Y, Zhang ZF, Li CQ, Zheng WJ, Liu J. Comparison of one-level minimally invasive and open transforaminal lumbar interbody fusion in degenerative and isthmic spondylolisthesis grades 1 and 2. Eur Spine J. 2010; 19(10):1780–1784

[58] Lee JC, Jang HD, Shin BJ. Learning curve and clinical outcomes of minimally invasive transforaminal lumbar interbody fusion: our experience in 86 consecutive cases. Spine. 2012; 37(18):1548–1557

[59] Gu G, Zhang H, Fan G, et al. Comparison of minimally invasive versus open transforaminal lumbar interbody fusion in two-level degenerative lumbar disease. Int Orthop. 2014; 38(4):817–824

[60] Tian NF, Wu YS, Zhang XL, Xu HZ, Chi YL, Mao FM. Minimally invasive versus open transforaminal lumbar interbody fusion: a meta-analysis based on the current evidence. Eur Spine J. 2013; 22(8):1741–1749

[61] Rolander SD. Motion of the lumbar spine with special reference to the stabilizing effect of posterior fusion. An experimental study on autopsy specimens. Acta Orthop Scand. 1966 Suppl 90:90–, 1–144

[62] Boden SD. Overview of the biology of lumbar spine fusion and principles for selecting a bone graft substitute. Spine. 2002; 27(16) Suppl 1:S26–S31

[63] Heo Y, Park JH, Seong HY, et al. Symptomatic adjacent segment degeneration at the L3–4 level after fusion surgery at the L4–5 level: evaluation of the risk factors and 10-year incidence. Eur Spine J. 2015; 24(11):2474–2480

[64] Ames CP, Acosta FL, Jr, Chi J, et al. Biomechanical comparison of posterior lumbar interbody fusion and transforaminal lumbar interbody fusion performed at 1 and 2 levels. Spine. 2005; 30(19):E562–E566

[65] Parajón A, Alimi M, Navarro-Ramirez R, et al. Minimally invasive transforaminal lumbar interbody fusion: meta-analysis of the fusion rates. what is the optimal graft material? Neurosurgery. 2017; 81(6):958–971

[66] Watkins MB. Posterolateral fusion of the lumbar and lumbosacral spine. J Bone Joint Surg Am. 1953; 35-A(4):1014–1018

[67] Bevevino AJ, Kang DG, Lehman RA, Jr, Van Blarcum GS, Wagner SC, Gwinn DE. Systematic review and meta-analysis of minimally invasive transforaminal lumbar interbody fusion rates performed without posterolateral fusion. J Clin Neurosci. 2014; 21(10):1686–1690

[68] Glassman SD, Howard JM, Sweet A, Carreon LY. Complications and concerns with osteobiologics for spine fusion in clinical practice. Spine. 2010; 35 (17):1621:1628

[69] Dailey AT, Ghogawala Z, Choudhri TF, et al. Guideline update for the performance of fusion procedures for degenerative disease of the lumbar spine. Part 14: brace therapy as an adjunct to or substitute for lumbar fusion. J Neurosurg Spine. 2014; 21(1):91–101

[70] Yee AJ, Yoo JU, Marsolais EB, et al. Use of a postoperative lumbar corset after lumbar spinal arthrodesis for degenerative conditions of the spine. A prospective randomized trial. J Bone Joint Surg Am. 2008; 90(10):2062–2068

[71] Zhu MP, Tetreault LA, Sorefan-Mangou F, Garwood P, Wilson JR. Efficacy, safety, and economics of bracing after spine surgery: a systematic review of the literature. Spine J. 2018; 18(9):1513–1525

[72] Kaiser MG, Eck JC, Groff MW, et al. Guideline update for the performance of fusion procedures for degenerative disease of the lumbar spine. Part 17: bone growth stimulators as an adjunct for lumbar fusion. J Neurosurg Spine. 2014; 21(1):133–139

[73] Gasbarrini A, Cappuccio M, Colangeli S, Posadas MD, Ghermandi R, Amendola L. Complications in minimally invasive percutaneous fixation of thoracic and lumbar spine fractures and tumors. Eur Spine J. 2013; 22 Suppl 6:S965–S971– Epub 2013 Sep 21

[74] Dai LY, Jiang LS, Jiang SD. Posterior short-segment fixation with or without fusion for thoracolumbar burst fractures. a five to seven-year prospective randomized study. J Bone Joint Surg Am. 2009; 91(5):1033–1041

[75] Grossbach AJ, Dahdaleh NS, Abel TJ, Woods GD, Dlouhy BJ, Hitchon PW. Flexion-distraction injuries of the thoracolumbar spine: open fusion versus percutaneous pedicle screw fixation. Neurosurg Focus. 2013; 35(2):E2

[76] Ohtori S, Inoue G, Orita S, et al. Teriparatide accelerates lumbar posterolateral fusion in women with postmenopausal osteoporosis: prospective study. Spine. 2012; 37(23):E1464–E1468

[77] Ohtori S, Inoue G, Orita S, et al. Comparison of teriparatide and bisphosphonate treatment to reduce pedicle screw loosening after lumbar spinal fusion surgery in postmenopausal women with osteoporosis from a bone quality perspective. Spine. 2013; 38(8):E487–E492

[78] Inoue G, Ueno M, Nakazawa T, et al. Teriparatide increases the insertional torque of pedicle screws during fusion surgery in patients with postmenopausal osteoporosis. J Neurosurg Spine. 2014; 21(3):425–431

[79] Chaudhary N, Lee JS, Wu JY, Tharin S. Evidence for use of teriparatide in spinal fusion surgery in osteoporotic patients. World Neurosurg. 2017; 100:551–556

[80] Lehman RA, Jr, Kuklo TR, Freedman BA, Cowart JR, Mense MG, Riew KD. The effect of alendronate sodium on spinal fusion: a rabbit model. Spine J. 2004; 4(1):36–43

[81] Nagahama K, Kanayama M, Togawa D, Hashimoto T, Minami A. Does alendronate disturb the healing process of posterior lumbar interbody fusion? A prospective randomized trial. J Neurosurg Spine. 2011; 14(4):500–507

[82] Kim SM, Rhee W, Ha S, Lim JH, Jang IT. Influence of alendronate and endplate degeneration to single level posterior lumbar spinal interbody fusion. Korean J Spine. 2014; 11(4):221–226

[83] Ohtori S, Orita S, Yamauchi K, et al. More than 6 months of teriparatide treatment was more effective for bone union than shorter treatment following lumbar posterolateral fusion surgery. Asian Spine J. 2015; 9(4):573–580

15 Surgical Tips, Tricks, and Techniques to Minimize Invasiveness; General Advice on How to Handle Fluoroscopy, Blood Loss, and Infection Rates

Eric H. Elowitz

Summary

Surgical tips, tricks, and techniques to minimize invasiveness are reviewed with special emphasis on how to handle fluoroscopy, blood loss, and infection rates. Minimally invasive spine surgery (MISS) offers many potential advantages for patients. However, for the surgeon, there are unique considerations to best achieve the successful performance of these lesser invasive surgeries. Thorough preoperative planning, patient selection criteria, and review of radiological studies are critical. Additionally, there is typically a reliance on intraoperative imaging, including fluoroscopy or computerized-image guidance, requiring the surgeon to have an additional level of technologic sophistication. Avoidance of blood loss and a knowledge of vascular anatomy are also essential. Although the infection rate has been shown to be lower with minimally invasive surgeries than more conventional spine procedures, attention to proper sterile technique in the operating room has particular challenges in minimally invasive procedures.

Keywords: minimally invasive spine surgery, fluoroscopy, radiation exposure, infection, incision planning, surgical navigation

The topics discussed in this chapter are relevant for a variety of procedures and pathologies encountered in MISS. A seasoned expert in MISS provides valuable pearls that are relevant for surgeons at any stage of the procedure; especially preoperative planning and careful patient and procedure selections are stressed. Overall, a surgeon's attention to detail is critical for successful MISS.

15.1 Introduction

Over the past several decades, minimally invasive techniques for spine surgery have gained acceptance and increased popularity.[1] Advancements in technology, as well as unique approaches to the spine, have fueled the growth in this area. More and more surgeons are adopting these techniques in their practice for the benefit of their patients. As has been widely quoted, minimally invasive spine surgery (MISS) techniques involve smaller incisions,[2] less muscle dissection and trauma,[3,4] shorter hospital stays,[5] and decreased infection rates.[6,7] However, as with all new surgical areas, MISS does offer unique challenges. The learning curve can often be lengthy and may temporarily increase complication rates.[8] New technologies must be evaluated with long-term outcomes. Over time, MISS techniques need to be validated and be shown to be equivalent, or superior, to more conventional approaches.

In many ways, MISS techniques require a mindset in practitioners of innovation and technique advancement. The safe performance of these procedures offers unique challenges. Although the incisions may be smaller, often multiple incisions are required. Change of patient position under anesthesia also has potential risks. The intraoperative setup and positioning time is frequently lengthier than conventional, open spine surgery. Additionally, the need for fluoroscopy, and other image guidance, requires a technological sophistication on the part of the surgeon as well as a reliance on radiology technologists and the proper operation of this equipment. Successful performance of MISS requires a great attention to detail. Surgeons must have a willingness to use and adapt new technologies and techniques for the benefits of their patients and the advancement of spinal care.

15.2 Patient Evaluation and Selection

The key elements to successful spine surgery start well before the day of surgery. Patient history, physical examination, and evaluation of radiological imaging must be carefully considered. Nonsurgical treatment is often recommended initially for patients with pain and degenerative spinal conditions; however, based on the imaging and clinical status of the patient, surgery may be offered. It is important to listen to patients in order to ascertain their concerns and goals of treatment when surgery is being considered. Frequently, a frank discussion between the patient and surgeon is necessary to help guide a shared-decision process.

The overall condition and age of the patient are important presurgical considerations. For example, older patients who have spinal stenosis and a minimal spondylolisthesis may be appropriate candidates for a simple tubular decompression, while younger, more active, patients may be more appropriate for a spinal fusion. Additionally, evaluation for any prior spine surgery is necessary.

A thorough evaluation of radiological imaging is also a requirement. The pathology demonstrated needs to be correlated with a patient's complaints and physical findings. Frequently, multilevel spinal pathology is present and clinical judgment is required to best determine which levels may be responsible for the patient's symptoms. In some cases, the decision may be made to treat just the perceived symptomatic level while in other patients, a more global approach to the spinal problem would be optimal.

Magnetic resonance imaging (MRI) is the mainstay for spine evaluation. Additionally, there are many instances where computed tomography (CT) can be of benefit; in situations where there is concern for bony anatomy, or if there has been prior surgery, CT scanning may be helpful. For patients who have had prior spinal instrumentation, CT may be used to evaluate the degree of fusion as well as hardware positioning. X-ray imaging

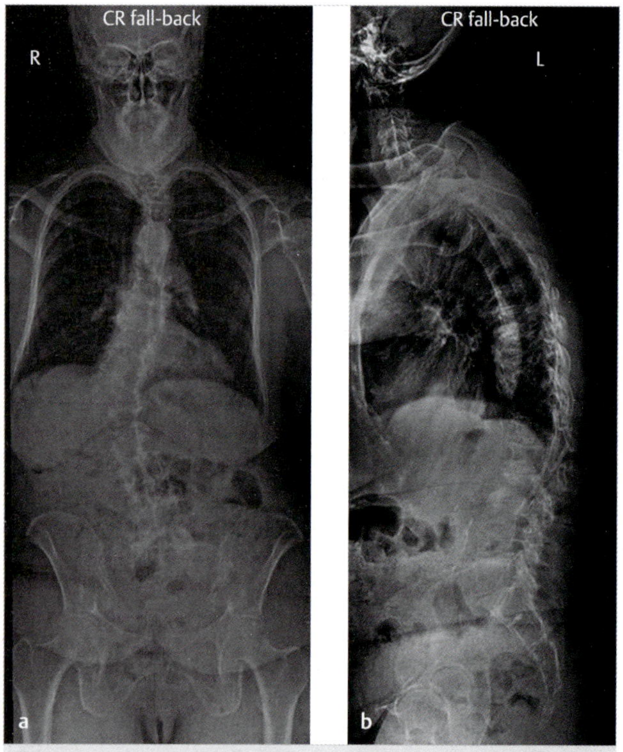

Fig. 15.1 Full-spine scoliosis films are ordered to evaluate global coronal and sagittal balance: (a) anteroposterior (AP) image; (b) lateral image.

also plays a role, particularly when dynamic views are ordered; flexion-extension X-rays can be of benefit to evaluate a mobile spondylolisthesis. Full-body scoliosis films are ordered to evaluate global coronal and sagittal balance (▶ Fig. 15.1). Recently, there has been a greater appreciation of the role of proper spinal alignment for successful surgical outcomes.[9]

When considering surgery for a patient, the goals of surgery should be clearly considered. Commonly this includes a decompression when there is impingement of neural structures. Fusion, in cases of instability or extensive planned bone removal, may be a goal. Proper correction of spinal alignment, or restoration of disc height, may also be goals to be considered. For the spinal surgeon who favors MISS, it is necessary to consider whether the goals of the surgery can be accomplished through these lesser invasive surgeries; even for the experienced MISS surgeon, not all pathologies can best be fully addressed using these techniques and more conventional open approaches may need to be considered. It is critical to configure the MISS techniques to the goals of surgery rather than vice versa; a surgeon should not readjust the surgical goals just for the sake of making a surgery smaller.

In preoperative evaluation and selection, there are many situations where special considerations are necessary. As an example, in patients who are being considered for a lateral lumbar interbody fusion (LLIF), it is critical to ask whether they have had prior abdominal or retroperitoneal surgery; for patients who have had major abdominal surgeries, a different approach may be best advised to reduce the risk of bowel injury. Additionally, patients who have had previous surgeries should be physically examined in order to assess their prior wounds for proper healing as well as planning of any subsequent incisions.

15.3 Preoperative Planning

It has been said, "A surgery can fail even before the patient arrives in the operating room." For the successful performance and outcome of any surgery, thoughtful preoperative planning is required. MISS has unique considerations and often requires additional preoperative planning. The surgeon must visualize, in advance, the surgery itself as well as the needs of the operation. MISS often requires significant equipment and technology, and this needs to be considered and ordered well before the surgical date.

Some MISS surgeons may use a mental, or even a physical, checklist to prepare for a surgery. Some of the important considerations are:

- Approach.
- Patient positioning.
- Equipment.
- Personnel.
- Equipment placement.
- Intraoperative imaging.
- Intraoperative neurophysiology monitoring.
- Bone for fusion.
- Navigation.
- Postoperative care.

15.4 Incision Planning and Tubular Considerations

Conventional lumbar spine surgery generally involves a single midline incision with significant muscle dissection and retraction. However, MISS employs smaller, but often multiple, incisions to approach the spine. As the incisions are smaller and the corridors to the spine more limited, in many ways, the incision location is even more critical than in open surgery. Intraoperative MISS incision planning requires the use of image guidance, either fluoroscopy or computerized navigation.

Tubular retractors are frequently employed during MISS. The benefit of these retractors is that incisions are not only smaller but also they use dilation rather than cutting of muscle.[3] The length of the skin incision is dependent on the size of the tube being used. Although smaller incisions are clearly preferable, it is important to keep the incision adequate enough to avoid excess pressure on the skin edges, which can lead to necrosis and poor wound healing. In my experience, a 16- or 18-mm tube is appropriate for microdiscectomies while a 22-mm tube is used for decompressive laminectomies. Spinal endoscopy often requires little more than a stab incision.

The side of approach is another important preoperative planning decision. Although the incision is often ipsilateral to the side of the pathology, such as a paracentral herniated disc, there are situations where a contralateral approach may be considered. Some authors have advocated the use of a contralateral tubular approach for the resection of lumbar synovial cysts.[10] In LLIF procedures, the incision and side of approach may be contralateral to the patient's symptoms if there is a

scoliosis or partial disc collapse; in some cases, the relationship of the disc space to the iliac crest may dictate the side of approach. Also, anterior cervical discectomy incisions are frequently contralateral to the patient's radiculopathy. In all surgeries where the planned incision is contralateral to the patient's symptoms, a discussion with the patient prior to surgery is helpful to avoid the misperception of a "wrong"-sided approach.

In tubular MISS, the incision's lateral distance from the spine also needs to be planned. An endoscopic discectomy may require an incision almost at the midline in order to gain more lateral visualization through the endoscope. For a tubular microdiscectomy, the incision is generally 1 cm lateral to midline; however, for an extraforaminal approach, where tube docking is performed on the pars interarticularis, a 2 cm distance is preferred.[11]

15.5 Incision Planning for Lumbar Fusions

Lumbar spinal fusions performed using MISS techniques offers benefits to the patient over conventional, open surgery.[1,12] There are several different possible approaches and the surgical plan should be customized depending on the needs of each patient. One of the first MISS techniques described, the MISS transforaminal lumbar interbody fusion (TLIF),[2] is routinely performed via a slightly lateral incision, approximately 3 cm off midline. Contralateral pedicle screws are placed through a separate incision.

The percutaneous placement of pedicle screws is a common MISS procedure. However, the nature of the skin incisions can vary. For a one- or two-level fusion, a lateral incision, frequently 3 cm off the midline, is performed. At the lower lumbar levels (L4/L5 and L5/S1), a single lateral incision is usually performed on each side as the lumbar lordosis brings the percutaneous entry points very close. However, in the middle and upper lumbar levels (such as L2/L3 and L3/L4), smaller separate incisions may be employed and the rod passed under the skin and fascia. In cases of multilevel fusion with percutaneous screw placement, some authors advocate for a single midline skin incision and multiple lateral fascial incisions.[13] This is particularly the case in multilevel percutaneous screw placement for deformity correction.

In LLIF surgery, skin incision placement is also critical. The skin incision is marked out with the use of lateral and anteroposterior (AP) fluoroscopy to gain a direct trajectory to the disc via the tubular retractor path. This will prevent being off-plane to the disc, which could compromise interbody graft placement. It is this surgeon's bias that for a single LLIF a transverse incision is performed, while in a multiple level LLIF, a longitudinal skin incision is performed with separate transverse fascial incisions.

15.6 Fluoroscopy/Radiation Exposure

As MISS is highly dependent on small incision and frequently tubular approaches, image guidance is a necessity. Most surgeons rely on intraoperative fluoroscopy for tube placement as well as pedicle screw trajectory. The use of fluoroscopy does pose a risk of continued and frequent radiation exposure to the spine surgeon and operative team. There have been many reports describing the potential health risks to the operating room personnel related to radiation exposure.[14,15]

It is critical that all of the operating room personnel wear protective radiation shields and, in particular, thyroid collars. One drawback to heavy lead gowns is the length of time that many of these procedures require by placing physical strain on the staff. Lighter weight materials that are protective are now available.[16] Radiation protective glasses should also be considered, particularly in procedures employing multiple fluoroscopy images, such as percutaneous pedicle screw placement. Radiation exposure to the eyes has been linked to early cataract development.[17] Some surgeons use radio-opaque gloves to minimize radiation exposure to their hands, although the thickness of these gloves can diminish tactile feedback.

Other strategies can be used to minimize radiation exposure to both the patient and operative team.[18] Live fluoroscopy should be used only selectively and, in fact, is rarely needed in MISS procedures. The use of magnification on the fluoroscope significantly increases the radiation dose and should be limited. Thoughtful use of fluoroscopy in order to minimize the number of images obtained is also important. Collimation of the field is another effective way of limiting radiation and may improve image quality as well (▶ Fig. 15.2). Newer technologies, such as LessRay (NuVasive, San Diego, CA), are being developed to reduce radiation exposure.

15.7 Navigation and Robotics

Computerized stereotactic navigation is being used increasingly in spine surgery with several systems and technologies available.[19] Some systems rely upon preoperative CT imaging and fuse those to intraoperative fluoroscopy. The use of intraoperative CT scans and three-dimensional imaging is also an effective way of minimizing radiation exposure to the operative team, although there is some concern that this can increase the exposure to the patient. The Airo intraoperative CT scan (Brainlab AG, Munich, Germany) (▶ Fig. 15.3) and the O-arm (Medtronic, Minneapolis, MN) are used to obtain intraoperative imaging, with the data then being transferred to the stereotactic navigation system (▶ Fig. 15.4). A reference array for frameless stereotaxy is used. This array is attached either to a spinous process or, in the case of many MISS, to iliac crest pins as the midline spinous process may not be exposed. Robotics is also being explored to facilitate the accurate placement of percutaneous instrumentation.[20] Another advantage of intraoperative CT imaging is that screw placement can be evaluated while the patient is still in the operating room and instrumentation can be repositioned, if needed.

15.8 Blood Loss Minimization

Another potential advantage of MISS over more traditional spine surgery techniques is limited blood loss. Still, special considerations need to be applied. As with any surgery, meticulous hemostasis throughout the procedure is required. MISS often requires multiple skin incisions, so an awareness of potential

AOSPINE

	Radiation to Pt	Relative to CXR
MRI	0	0
Chest X-ray	20 mrems	1 x
Hip X-ray	100	5 x
Spine X-ray	130	6.5 x
Bone X-ray	4000	200 x
Spine CT	5000	250 x
Cerebral embolization	34,000	1700 x
Cardiac cath	150,000	7500 x
C-arm (spine)	3,000/min	

Fig. 15.2 Table presented by Dr. Roger Härtl that summarizes the radiation dose of each of the imaging modalities. Abbreviations: CXR, chest X-ray.

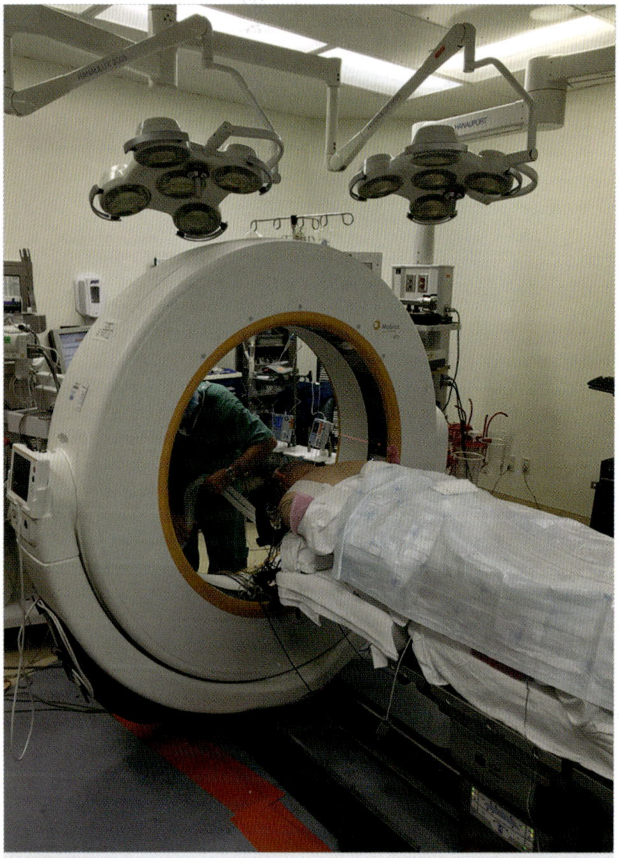

Fig. 15.3 The Airo intraoperative computed tomography (CT) scan (Brainlab AG, Munich, Germany) is used to obtain imaging before and after placement of instrumentation.

bleeding in another open wound while working is important; it is possible that the surgeon might overlook bleeding in another location as he or she is focused on the primary site.

Evaluation of preoperative imaging for vascular anatomy is also necessary. This is particularly the case with lateral lumbar surgery, as there is a potential risk of injury to the iliac vessels. Patients with a significant rotatory scoliosis may offer a particular challenge; extra attention should be paid to assure a true lateral approach based on the AP fluoroscopic imaging for each level addressed. Also, in the patients undergoing LLIF surgery, it is necessary to evaluate the preoperative imaging for vasculature anatomy as injury could lead to potentially catastrophic hemorrhage.

When tubular retractors are used during MISS, blood vessels in the muscle may be tamponaded. However, once the tube is removed, there is possibility of bleeding. Care must be taken to remove the tube slowly while the microscope is still employed and any bleeding points cauterized. There is a potential risk of continued bleeding and postoperative hemorrhage even in relatively limited surgeries. Retroperitoneal hemorrhage has been reported after endoscopic spine procedures.[21] ▶ Fig. 15.5 illustrates a large postoperative epidural hematoma causing new symptoms 3 days following a tubular resection of synovial cyst. Hemorrhages have also been described after LLIF surgery, making inspection of the psoas muscle necessary, as the lateral retractor is being withdrawn, for safe surgical technique.

15.9 Infection Rates

Multiple studies have indicated that a clear benefit of MISS over traditional techniques is a decrease in infection rate.[6,7] It has been postulated that as the muscle is not dissected from the bone, there better vascularization is maintained. Additionally, there is far less "dead space" where blood products can accumulate. Still, infections can occur and adherence to proper surgical principles of sterility is necessary. Preoperative antibiotic administration and antibiotic irrigation are used to minimize the infection risk.

MISS techniques do pose particular concerns relating to maintenance of operative sterility. Often there is a significant

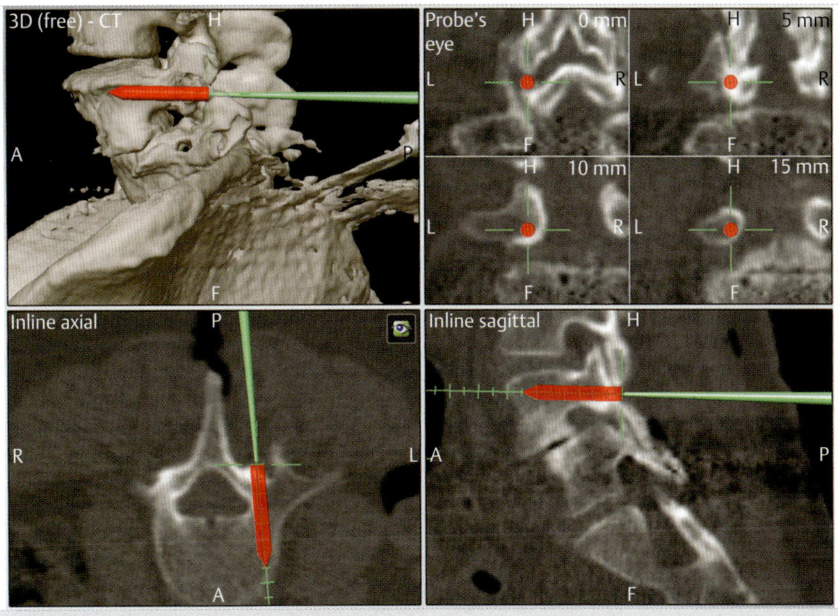

Fig. 15.4 Stereotactic navigation screen used for planning and placement of laterally guided cortical pedicle screws using the Brainlab frameless system (Brainlab AG, Munich, Germany).

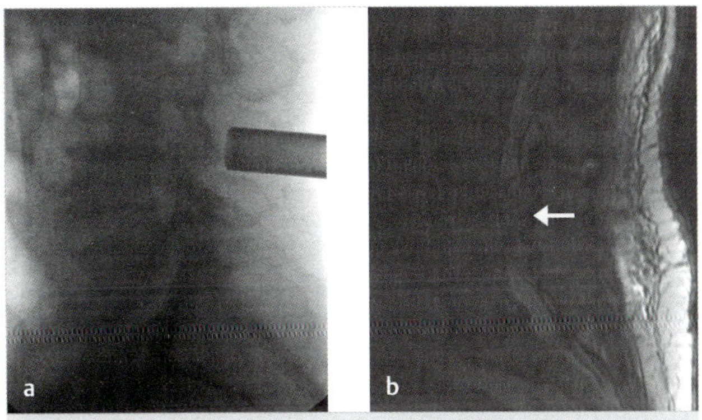

Fig. 15.5 **(a)** Intraoperative fluoroscopic image of tubular retractor placed during resection of L3/L4 synovial cyst; **(b)** Sagittal T2-weighted magnetic resonance imaging (MRI) image obtained 3 days after resection of L3/L4 synovial cyst with new, large epidural hematoma causing thecal sac compression.

extra equipment in the operating room. Table-mounted retractors may require perforating the sterile draping and these cut areas need to be carefully covered. Additional personnel staffing leads to more foot traffic, potentially increasing contamination risks. Also, MISS frequently requires many open equipment trays and extra instrumentation, leading to more concern.

Proper draping of fluoroscopy and CT units in the operating room has to be incorporated into the workflow. Fluoroscopy drapes are used; but in cases where AP views are obtained, as in percutaneous pedicle screw placement, a lateral drape is necessary to prevent the contaminated C-arm from returning to the operative field in the lateral position.

15.10 Conclusion

Successful outcomes in MISS depend on a number of factors. Frequently, MISS procedures require significant preoperative planning. As with any surgery, patient evaluation and selection are critical. Discussion with the patient regarding the goals of treatment is important and may influence the type of surgery offered. Proper radiologic imaging studies need to be reviewed and may include full-spine X-rays to evaluate global alignment. When surgery is scheduled, surgeons must consider the needs of the procedure ahead of time to ensure that the proper equipment and instrumentation are available. As MISS employs smaller incisions, and often tubular retractors, incision planning must be thought over; in some cases, the incisions may be contralateral to the pathology. MISS lumbar fusions offer great benefits to patients but have their own, unique considerations including choice of approach and bone graft materials. Image guidance is also a necessity for MISS and requires additional attention from the surgeon. Fluoroscopy is frequently used but does pose a risk to the surgeon and operating room team due to radiation exposure. Although there are several methods to limit radiation during fluoroscopy, computerized stereotactic navigation offers the possibility of eliminating the need for fluoroscopy use during many procedures. Intraoperative CT imaging also has the benefit of evaluating instrumentation placement while still in the operating room. Blood loss minimization is another advantage of MISS procedures; steps to reduce the risk of postoperative hemorrhage also plays an important role in successful outcomes. Attention to sterile technique and proper draping of equipment can help to reduce an already low infection rate. Overall, a surgeon's attention to detail is critical for successful MISS with positive patient outcomes.

References

[1] Härtl RH, Korge A, eds. Minimally Invasive Spine Surgery Techniques, Evidence and Controversies. New York, NY: Thieme; 2012

[2] Schwender JD, Holly LT, Rouben DP, Foley KT. Minimally invasive transforaminal lumbar interbody fusion (TLIF): technical feasibility and initial results. J Spinal Disord Tech. 2005; 18 Suppl:S1–S6

[3] Tomasino A, Parikh K, Steinberger J, Knopman J, Boockvar J, Härtl R. Tubular microsurgery for lumbar discectomies and laminectomies in obese patients: operative results and outcome. Spine. 2009; 34(18):E664–E672

[4] Khoo LT, Fessler RG. Microendoscopic decompressive laminotomy for the treatment of lumbar stenosis. Neurosurgery. 2002; 51(5) Suppl:S146–S154

[5] Parker SL, Mendenhall SK, Shau DN, et al. Minimally invasive versus open transforaminal lumbar interbody fusion for degenerative spondylolisthesis: comparative effectiveness and cost-utility analysis. World Neurosurg. 2014; 82(1–2):230–238

[6] McGirt MJ, Parker SL, Lerner J, Engelhart L, Knight T, Wang MY. Comparative analysis of perioperative surgical site infection after minimally invasive versus open posterior/transforaminal lumbar interbody fusion: analysis of hospital billing and discharge data from 5170 patients. J Neurosurg Spine. 2011; 14(6):771–778

[7] O'Toole JE, Eichholz KM, Fessler RG. Surgical site infection rates after minimally invasive spinal surgery. J Neurosurg Spine. 2009; 11(4):471–476

[8] Sclafani JA, Kim CW. Complications associated with the initial learning curve of minimally invasive spine surgery: a systematic review. Clin Orthop Relat Res. 2014; 472(6):1711–1717

[9] Schwab F, Patel A, Ungar B, Farcy JP, Lafage V. Adult spinal deformity-postoperative standing imbalance: how much can you tolerate? An overview of key parameters in assessing alignment and planning corrective surgery. Spine. 2010; 35(25):2224–2231

[10] James A, Laufer I, Parikh K, Nagineni VV, Saleh TO, Härtl R. Lumbar juxtafacet cyst resection: the facet sparing contralateral minimally invasive surgical approach. J Spinal Disord Tech. 2012; 25(2):E13–E17

[11] Virk MS, Elowitz E. A minimally invasive approach to the lumbar neural foramen and extraforaminal compartment: modified surgical technique. J Spine. 2014; 4(1):1000:203–1000–208

[12] Park P, Foley KT. Minimally invasive transforaminal lumbar interbody fusion with reduction of spondylolisthesis: technique and outcomes after a minimum of 2 years' follow-up. Neurosurg Focus. 2008; 25(2):E16

[13] Wang MY. Improvement of sagittal balance and lumbar lordosis following less invasive adult spinal deformity surgery with expandable cages and percutaneous instrumentation. J Neurosurg Spine. 2013; 18(1):4–12

[14] Ahn Y, Kim CH, Lee JH, Lee SH, Kim JS. Radiation exposure to the surgeon during percutaneous endoscopic lumbar discectomy: a prospective study. Spine. 2013; 38(7):617–625

[15] Lee K, Lee KM, Park MS, Lee B, Kwon DG, Chung CY. Measurements of surgeons' exposure to ionizing radiation dose during intraoperative use of C-arm fluoroscopy. Spine. 2012; 37(14):1240–1244

[16] McCaffrey JP, Shen H, Downton B, Mainegra-Hing E. Radiation attenuation by lead and nonlead materials used in radiation shielding garments. Med Phys. 2007; 34(2):530–537

[17] Chodick G, Bekiroglu N, Hauptmann M, et al. Risk of cataract after exposure to low doses of ionizing radiation: a 20-year prospective cohort study among US radiologic technologists. Am J Epidemiol. 2008; 168(6):620–631

[18] Srinivasan D, Than KD, Wang AC, et al. Radiation safety and spine surgery: systematic review of exposure limits and methods to minimize radiation exposure. World Neurosurg. 2014; 82(6):1337–1343

[19] Shin BJ, James AR, Njoku IU, Härtl R. Pedicle screw navigation: a systematic review and meta-analysis of perforation risk for computer-navigated versus freehand insertion. J Neurosurg Spine. 2012; 17(2):113–122

[20] Roser F, Tatagiba M, Maier G. Spinal robotics: current applications and future perspectives. Neurosurgery. 2013; 72 Suppl 1:12–18

[21] Ahn Y, Kim JU, Lee BH, et al. Postoperative retroperitoneal hematoma following transforaminal percutaneous endoscopic lumbar discectomy. J Neurosurg Spine. 2009; 10(6):595–602

16 Perioperative Management; ERAS

G. Damian Brusko, Karthik Madhavan, and Michael Y. Wang

Summary

Recent implementation of Enhanced Recovery After Surgery (ERAS) pathways in spine surgery have resulted in improved outcomes for patients. These perioperative protocols incorporate several basic and evidence-based principles of enhanced recovery that aim to reduce postoperative narcotics consumption, decrease complications, and shorten length of stay. When ERAS pathways are combined with minimally-invasive spine surgery (MISS) approaches, an even greater benefit may be demonstrated. This chapter discusses the key components of ERAS and how to successfully implement them within an MISS practice.

Keywords: Enhanced Recovery After Surgery (ERAS), implementation, minimally invasive, outcomes, perioperative, spine surgery

16.1 Introduction

Enhanced Recovery After Surgery (ERAS) pathways aim to improve outcomes, accelerate recovery times, and reduce health care costs through multidisciplinary management of the perioperative course. The gradual adoption of ERAS protocols in numerous specialties has gained considerable momentum since its inception in the late 1990s for colorectal surgery. However, neurosurgery has been slower to integrate ERAS principles into practice, despite the growing body of evidence in support of its efficacy in other specialties. Spinal neurosurgery, in particular, would greatly benefit from measures geared toward reducing postoperative pain and narcotic use, as well as mobilizing patients earlier after surgery to enhance recovery. Recent advancements in neurosurgical techniques, particularly minimally invasive spine surgery (MISS), now enable incorporation of these fast-track surgical pathways into routine practice. This chapter discusses the core principles of ERAS, examine key features of ERAS within spine surgery, and finally, outline steps for successful pathway implementation.

16.2 Basic Principles of Enhanced Recovery

Henrik Kehlet first described a multimodal pathway for colorectal surgery patients in 1997 that centered around reducing the physiologic response to stress following surgery.[1] He postulated that the body's inflammatory cascade is responsible for pathogenesis of the morbidities associated with major surgery, and concluded that modulation of these mediators could improve recovery. His investigations spawned the development of a multimodal approach for minimizing postoperative recovery time starting from the preoperative period with proper nutrition prior to surgery, progressing to interventions to reduce pain and generalized patient discomfort due to nausea and vomiting, and concluding with exercise regimens to mobilize patients in the early postoperative period.

The most important of the physiologic derangements following surgery is the development of insulin resistance. Catecholamine release and impaired immune function combine to induce a state of insulin resistance that negatively impacts glucose metabolism. Both increased hepatic glucose production and decreased insulin-dependent peripheral uptake lead to hyperglycemia.[2] The increased levels of circulating glucose are transported into immune cells, neurons, and endothelial cells because glucose transport in these cells is concentration dependent. Accumulation of glucose within the cells is responsible for oxygen radical production, altered gene expression, and inflammation.[3] Managing the development of key pathogenic factors, particularly insulin resistance, is paramount to speed up recovery time and improve outcomes. Preoperative optimization of the patient's health, use of minimally invasive surgical techniques, nonnarcotic pain management, and early mobilization all contribute to reducing the surgical stress response. The core physiologic principles of ERAS are summarized in ▶ Fig. 16.1.

16.3 Incorporating ERAS into Minimally Invasive Spine Surgery

More recently, spine surgery has begun to explore the implementation of ERAS principles. An increased demand for major spinal surgery and global variations in length of stay, recovery, and complication rates make spine surgery a solid candidate to benefit from a fast-track recovery protocol.[4] Spine surgery is associated with especially high pain levels postoperatively, with lumbar fusions and complex reconstructions rated as three of the top six most painful surgical procedures.[5] In addition, rising health care costs over the past decade for spine surgeries may potentially be due to the greater number of procedures and increased length of stay.[4,6] Each of these factors demonstrates the utility of an ERAS protocol for spine surgery.

The following sections examine a perioperative approach that spine surgeons may consider for implementation of ERAS. Additional focus is placed on a few specific aspects that can easily be incorporated into a spine surgeon's daily practice. It should be noted that, at present, no official ERAS guidelines for spine surgery have been published, but there is a growing body of literature suggesting the effectiveness of many of the interventions described below. A sample ERAS protocol adapted from our institution is applicable to many standard spine procedures ranging from one-level decompression to multilevel fusion, as it focuses primarily on the pre- and postoperative components (▶ Fig. 16.2).

16.3.1 Preoperative Preparation

The patient's journey through ERAS begins at the time of surgical consult in the clinic. ERAS protocols can be applied to all

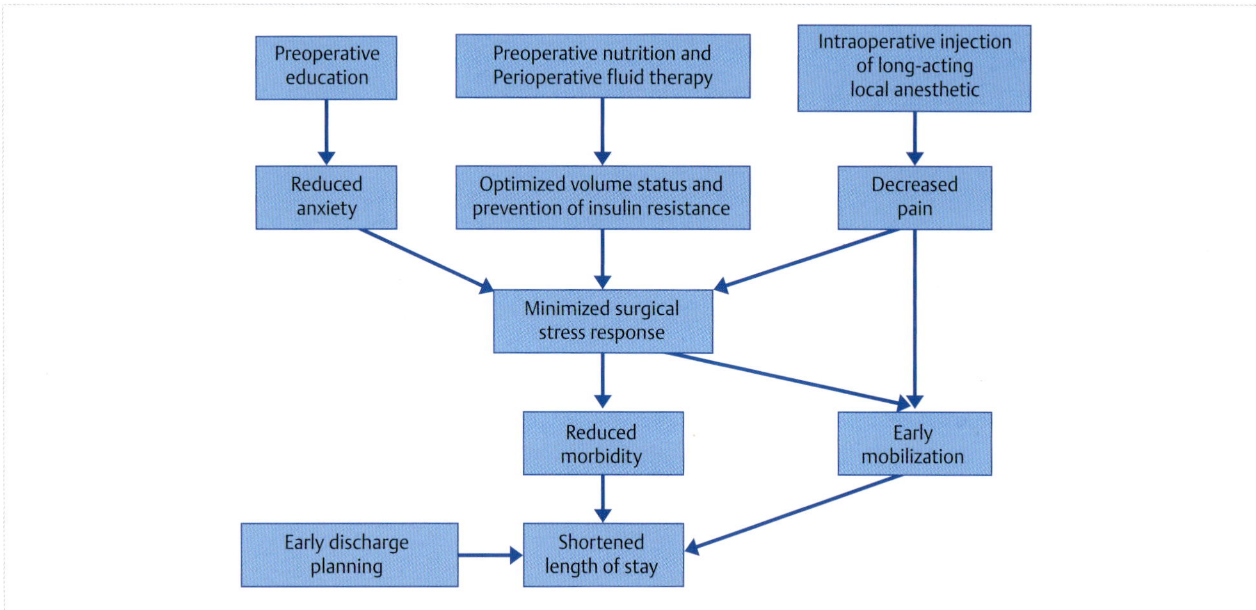

Fig. 16.1 Physiological principles of Enhanced Recovery After Surgery®.

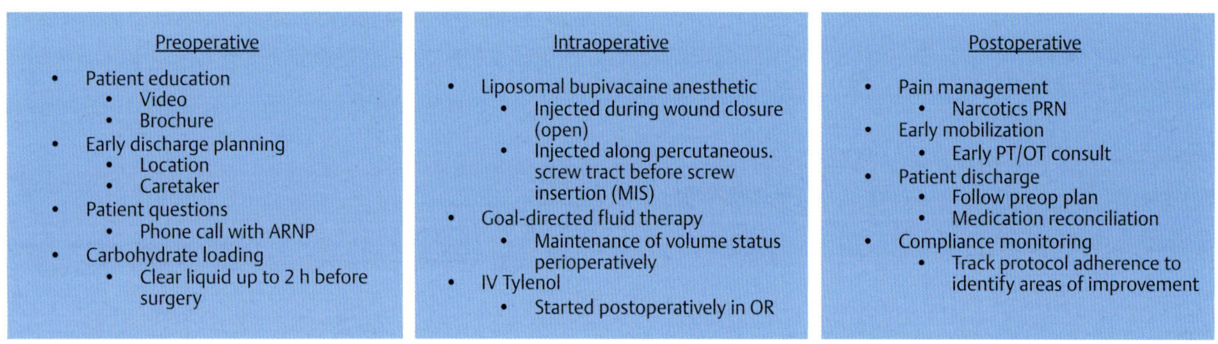

Fig. 16.2 Sample Enhanced Recovery After Surgery® protocol for elective spine surgery.

patients undergoing any elective spine surgery, regardless of age or comorbidities. However, during the early implementation phase at our institution, we chose to include all patients undergoing only posterior lumbar fusion procedures (▶ Table 16.1). Once a patient enters the ERAS pathway, expectations regarding the surgery and recovery process must be detailed. The surgeon should describe all aspects of the process, from preoperative preparations to the recovery process and early discharge. Surgeons must assess the patient's current health status and develop a plan for optimization of health before surgery. Patients should be educated on smoking and alcohol cessation for 30 days prior to surgery and advised to walk for 30 minutes each day. In addition to lifestyle modifications aimed at improving physical health status, patients must be prepared mentally for each aspect of surgery. This includes reducing fear and anxiety about surgical and anesthetic procedures and preparing patients for a decreased hospital stay. Patients should understand that recovery only happens with their participation in the protocol. Both physical and mental preparations prior to surgery, in combination with preadmission discharge planning, are the essential first steps in an efficacious ERAS pathway.

Table 16.1 Sample ERAS inclusion and exclusion criteria for posterior lumbar instrumented fusion

Inclusion criteria	Exclusion criteria
Elective surgery	ER-hospital admissions
1–3 levels	4 or more levels
Open and MIS procedures	Staged (multiday) procedures
Revision procedures	Front/back procedures

Abbreviations: ER, emergency department; ERAS, Enhanced Recovery After Surgery; MIS, minimally invasive surgery.

Another essential component of ERAS is perioperative, goal-directed fluid management, which prevents hypotension and maintains adequate oxygen delivery to tissues. Hydration with a clear carbohydrate drink up to 2 hours before surgery is recommended to reduce gluconeogenesis, prevent insulin resistance, and limit anxiety. This practice is also supported by the current American Society of Anesthesiologists guidelines on

preoperative fasting.[7] During surgery, the body's natural reaction to blood loss is to conserve sodium and consequently water via activation of the renin–angiotensin–aldosterone system. However, the body is more efficient at conservation of sodium compared to elimination. Therefore, intravenous (IV) infusion of lactated Ringer's solution, blood loss, and urine output during surgery should all be maintained in a balanced 1:1 ratio, optimizing volume status and preventing common surgical complications.[8] Maintenance of volume status is the key; an association with weight gain of 5 lb or more has been shown to lengthen hospital stay and increase complications, thus directly opposing the core principles of ERAS.[9]

16.3.2 Intraoperative Technique

Specific surgical techniques are directed based on the diagnosis and surgeon preference, but within ERAS, should utilize minimally invasive approaches, many of which are described in this book. There are, however, important intraoperative aspects that are unique to ERAS, including awake anesthesia, percutaneous screws, and use of a long-acting local anesthetic that have previously been described for endoscopic minimally invasive spine transforaminal lateral interbody fusion (MIS TLIF).[10] Awake anesthesia reduces both postoperative stress and memory loss. Injection of a long-acting sodium blocker, specifically liposomal bupivacaine, along the pedicle screw tracts before screw insertion is recommended. The use of liposomal bupivacaine has been shown to reduce postoperative narcotic consumption and length of stay in patients undergoing TLIF.[10,11] Future development of similar ultra-minimally invasive surgical procedures will likely increase the feasibility of incorporating ERAS into spine surgery.

16.3.3 Postoperative Management

The key aspects of postoperative management within ERAS include nonnarcotic pain control, prevention of ileus and nausea, and early mobilization. Patients are given oral acetaminophen prior to surgery and IV acetaminophen for pain control immediately following surgery. This strays from the traditional paradigm of patient-controlled analgesia with opioids and instead only supplies narcotics on an "as needed" basis. Our institution has recently implemented a similar analgesic protocol for an awake MIS TLIF described above. Early results have demonstrated significant reductions in average total daily narcotic usage on postoperative days 0 and 1, and overall narcotic usage as compared with conventional MIS TLIF, with additional reductions in length of stay, operative time, and blood loss. The 72-hour duration of liposomal bupivacaine combined with IV acetaminophen in the early postoperative period should provide adequate pain relief for patients, obviating the need for opioids and enabling the next essential phase in the enhanced recovery process—early mobilization.

Fear of movement following surgery, both pre- and postoperatively, is associated with increased pain and disability and overall poorer quality of life scores, thus highlighting the importance of early mobilization.[12,13] The combination of prehabilitation and early rehabilitation programs, with optimized multimodal elements of intense mobilization the day of surgery, analgesic control, and enteral nutrition, resulted in reduced morbidity, length of stay, pain, and increased patient satisfaction.[14,15] Such interventions aim to assuage patients' fears about poor postoperative mobility and ready them for an earlier discharge from the hospital.

> The editors find that one of the most important and frequently neglected components of ERAS is the preoperative education of patients in order to create realistic expectations as per length of stay, pain, etc. Intramuscular injection of liposomal bupivacaine is frequently quoted but not widely popular because of high costs and little evidence for effectiveness. Many surgeons who perform ambulatory surgery use a combination of bupivacaine or lidocaine with epinephrine intramuscular injection very successfully.

16.4 Implementation of ERAS in Spine Surgery

This chapter outlines many measures which may be taken to incorporate elements of ERAS into the practice of MISS. ERAS requires coordination from the patient, surgeon, and providers in other facets of care to fully realize the multimodal approach. Therefore, each of the published ERAS guidelines includes a section outlining the framework for an audit system, which functions to track compliance and various outcomes over time, creating an iterative, results-based pathway. Compliance has recently been identified as a major factor in promoting optimal recovery.[16] In addition, significant reduction of acute care costs resulting from shorter operating times, reduced intensive care unit complications, and decreased length of stay for an ERAS-centered MIS TLIF compared with conventional MIS TLIF has been shown.[17] Reduced costs may, therefore, provide a necessary incentive for health care networks to adopt ERAS pathways, removing another potential barrier to implementation. Future improvements in the form of clinical trials, cost analyses, and new specialty guidelines will likely further strengthen the ERAS framework.

16.5 Conclusion

MISS is a growing area of innovation and interest among neurosurgeons. Novel techniques and devices continue to emerge, contributing to better outcomes and increased patient satisfaction. The addition of an ERAS protocol complements MIS spinal procedures, furthering the improvement of outcome measures such as length of stay, narcotic usage, and clinical improvement. Fundamentally, ERAS consists of multidisciplinary interventions aimed at reducing the surgical stress response, improving outcomes, and reducing hospitalization time, culminating in increased patient satisfaction and curbed health care costs. Future development of spine-specific guidelines will provide the foundation necessary for global implementation of ERAS within the discipline.

References

[1] Kehlet H. Multimodal approach to control postoperative pathophysiology and rehabilitation. Br J Anaesth. 1997; 78(5):606–617

[2] Thorell A, Nygren J, Hirshman MF, et al. Surgery-induced insulin resistance in human patients: relation to glucose transport and utilization. Am J Physiol. 1999; 276(4):E754–E761

[3] Carli F. Physiologic considerations of Enhanced Recovery After Surgery (ERAS) programs: implications of the stress response. Can J Anaesth. 2015; 62 (2):110–119

[4] Wainwright TW, Immins T, Middleton RG. Enhanced Recovery After Surgery (ERAS) and its applicability for major spine surgery. Best Pract Res Clin Anaesthesiol. 2016; 30(1):91–102

[5] Gerbershagen HJ, Aduckathil S, van Wijck AJM, Peelen LM, Kalkman CJ, Meissner W. Pain intensity on the first day after surgery: a prospective cohort study comparing 179 surgical procedures. Anesthesiology. 2013; 118 (4):934–944

[6] Deyo RA, Mirza SK, Martin BI, Kreuter W, Goodman DC, Jarvik JG. Trends, major medical complications, and charges associated with surgery for lumbar spinal stenosis in older adults. JAMA. 2010; 303(13):1259–1265

[7] Practice Guidelines for Preoperative Fasting and the Use of Pharmacologic Agents to Reduce the Risk of Pulmonary Aspiration: Application to Healthy Patients Undergoing Elective Procedures: An Updated Report by the American Society of Anesthesiologists Task Force on Preoperative Fasting and the Use of Pharmacologic Agents to Reduce the Risk of Pulmonary Aspiration. Anesthesiology. 2017; 126(3):376–393

[8] Bellamy MC. Wet, dry or something else? Br J Anaesth. 2006; 97(6):755–757

[9] Lowell JA, Schifferdecker C, Driscoll DF, Benotti PN, Bistrian BR. Postoperative fluid overload: not a benign problem. Crit Care Med. 1990; 18(7):728–733

[10] Wang MY, Grossman J. Endoscopic minimally invasive transforaminal interbody fusion without general anesthesia: initial clinical experience with 1-year follow-up. Neurosurg Focus. 2016; 40(2):E13

[11] Kim J, Burke SM, Kryzanski JT, et al. The role of liposomal bupivacaine in Reduction of Postoperative Pain after Transforaminal Lumbar Interbody Fusion: A Clinical Study. World Neurosurg. 2016; 91:460–467

[12] den Boer JJ, Oostendorp RA, Beems T, Munneke M, Evers AW. Continued disability and pain after lumbar disc surgery: the role of cognitive-behavioral factors. Pain. 2006; 123(1–2):45–52

[13] Abbott AD, Tyni-Lenné R, Hedlund R. The influence of psychological factors on pre-operative levels of pain intensity, disability and health-related quality of life in lumbar spinal fusion surgery patients. Physiotherapy. 2010; 96 (3):213–221

[14] Nielsen PR, Andreasen J, Asmussen M, Tønnesen H. Costs and quality of life for prehabilitation and early rehabilitation after surgery of the lumbar spine. BMC Health Serv Res. 2008; 8:209

[15] Epstein NE. A review article on the benefits of early mobilization following spinal surgery and other medical/surgical procedures. Surg Neurol Int. 2014; 5 Suppl 3:S66–S73

[16] Aarts M-A, Rotstein OD, Pearsall EA, et al. iERAS group. Postoperative ERAS interventions have the greatest impact on optimal recovery: experience with implementation of ERAS across multiple hospitals. Ann Surg. 2018; 267 (6):992–997

[17] Wang MY, Chang HK, Grossman J. Reduced acute care costs with the ERAS® minimally invasive transforaminal lumbar interbody fusion compared with conventional minimally invasive transforaminal lumbar interbody fusion. Neurosurgery. 2018; 83(4):827–834

17 Key Elements to Safely Transition from Inpatient to Outpatient Spine Surgery

Richard Wohns

Summary

This chapter is a guide to build and transition from the inpatient to the outpatient setting. This is a common practice in some well-developed countries. However, we are certain that using this chapter, the readers not only in the US but around the world would be able to potentially replicate the model suggested by the author.

Keywords: ambulatory surgery, ambulatory center, outpatient surgery, outpatient spine surgery, ambulatory spine surgery, spine center

17.1 Proper Procedure Choices

The cost-effectiveness of select outpatient spine procedures is well documented.[1,2,3,4] However, the keys to success lie in patient and case selection. Ambulatory surgery and outpatient surgery can be used as synonyms. However, in this chapter, we will refer to outpatient procedures to those that are done inside a special "outpatient facility" by following specific anesthesia protocols (▶ Table 17.1). On the other hand, "ambulatory" are those procedures performed inside a hospital and where patients may or may not require to stay overnight. In the following paragraphs, we will provide a guide for specific spine procedures that can safely and effectively be transitioned to the outpatient setting.

17.2 Lumbar Spine

17.2.1 Laminoforaminotomy with or without Microdiscectomy

Zahrawi was the first to report performing an outpatient lumbar microdiscectomy in 1985. He reported on 103 consecutive patients on whom which he performed this procedure via a 1-inch incision and patients were discharged a few hours after the procedure. He reported 88% excellent and good results and concluded that this procedure can be safely performed as an outpatient procedure.[1] This was further corroborated by Asch et al.[2] However, via bivariate and multivariate analyses, they found workers' compensation status and older age had a negative effect on outcome. A larger cohort of patients (713) who underwent outpatient microdiscectomy reported that the complication rate following outpatient microdiscectomy is low, consisting mostly of recurrent herniation (6.4%).[3] Pugely et al found higher unadjusted and adjusted overall complication rates in patients who underwent microdiscectomy in the inpatient setting versus those who underwent surgery in the outpatient setting.[4] In fact, inpatient hospital stay was an independent risk factor. Other risk factors included older age, presence of diabetes mellitus, preoperative wound infection, blood transfusion, and operative time.[4]

Because of reported regional ischemia associated with even short duration microdiscectomies in young patient, minimally invasive technical refinements have been advocated toward the transition to outpatient spine surgery, specifically via tube surgery. However, a prospective randomized trial that compared outcomes of tubular microdiscectomies with conventional microdiscectomies found no difference in disability.[5] Although patients undergoing tube surgery reported higher visual analog scale (VAS) back and leg pain, this difference was not clinically significant. There was no difference in reoperation rates between the two groups.

Bekelis et al assessed the cost of inpatient compared to outpatient microdiscectomy and reported mean total charges of inpatient microdiscectomy to be $29,906, compared to $13,107 for outpatient microdiscectomies.[6]

As demonstrated, microdiscectomy is likely more cost-effective when performed in the outpatient setting compared to the inpatient setting. Actually, performing these procedures in the inpatient setting may be an independent risk factor for postoperative complications. Patient variables that may portend a higher complication rate include older age, history of diabetes mellitus, preoperative wound infection, anemia, and workers'

Table 17.1 Outpatient anesthesia protocol example

1. Specific protocols should be established for pre-, intra-, and postsurgery
2. An overall anesthesia and analgesia plan should be established preoperatively
3. Patient should be allowed to eat solids for up to 6 hours prior to surgery
4. Preoperative analgesia is mandatory to reduce nausea postoperatively
5. Analgesia and anesthesia protocols will be different, depending on the surgery/insult expected (MIS TLIF vs. MIS tubular decompression)
6. Patients should be educated to manage mild or strong analgesics after surgery
7. The panel of anesthesiologist should approve the protocols
8. Patients with any of the following are **EXCLUDED** from "outpatient" management:
   - NYHA 3–4
   - Angina
   - ASA grade 4
   - Excessive anxiety during medical procedures
   - Inability to take care of themselves or not having someone at home to take care of them for at least the first 24 hours post procedure

Abbreviations: ASA, American Society of Anesthesiologists; MIS TLIF, minimally invasive transforaminal lumbar interbody fusion; NYHA, New York Heart Association.

compensation status. We recommend that patients with these risk factors be operated on in the inpatient setting.

Outpatient and ambulatory surgeries are becoming increasingly prevalent, as are corresponding surgery centers. The success of this type of surgery as well as the recent interest in the wake of spinal fusion surgery is based on advances made in the perioperative management of pain, as outlined in Michael Wang's Chapter 16 on ERAS.

17.2.2 Laminectomy (One or Two Level) and Interspinous Process Devices (IPD)

Multiple studies have reported that multilevel laminectomies can be safely performed in the outpatient setting. Yen and Albargi reported on 41 and 82 patients who underwent single or multilevel laminectomies before and after full implementation of their outpatient spine surgery protocol respectively.[7] In the postprotocol cohort, patients were assigned to outpatient surgery based on two factors: (1) American Society of Anesthesiologists (ASA) of 3 or less and (2) availability of someone to help perform homemaking activities. None of the patients designated to have outpatient surgery required overnight stay. Also, there were no 30-day readmissions in this cohort.

To further hone in on patient selection, one study assessed a database of 2,358 patients who underwent laminectomy for lumbar spinal stenosis between 2011 and 2012.[8] They reported independent risk factors for prolonged hospital stay after multivariate analysis were increased age, increased body mass index (BMI), ASA class of 3–4, and preoperative hematocrit of less than 36.0.

From a technical standpoint, the merit of minimally invasive unilateral laminectomy for bilateral decompression toward minimizing soft tissue trauma, and hence improving postoperative outcomes, has been a point of contention. Phan and Mobbs performed a systematic review and meta-analysis comparing this approach with the traditional open laminectomy. They reported a higher satisfaction rate, lower VAS back pain score, less blood loss, and shorter hospital stay in the minimally invasive approach compared to the traditional approach.[9] Furthermore, Schöller et al reported that minimally invasive decompression in patients with degenerative spondylolisthesis, compared to traditional open laminectomy, is associated with lower reoperation and fusion rates, less slip progression, and greater patient satisfaction.[10]

For low-demand elderly patients with good general health and minimal comorbidities who are candidates for decompressive surgery, an IPD may be a viable option. A little over a decade ago, IPDs were introduced as a minimally invasive method for treating lumbar spinal stenosis (LSS) in patients who were poor surgical candidates and whose symptoms abated with forward flexion.[11,12] The biomechanical rationale behind these devices is fairly intuitive. IPDs were subsequently introduced into the market showing promise with pain and functional outcomes between minimally invasive surgery (MIS) decompression and X-STOP (early generation IPD) being equivalent.[13] However, over time, X-STOP was found to be associated with unacceptably high revision rates of up to 30%.[14,15] Most recently, a systematic review and meta-analysis of randomized controlled trials comparing IPD alone to decompressive surgery for LSS concluded that IPD alone was less cost-effective than traditional decompression alone.[16]

Newer generation technologies have been more encouraging; most notably the Coflex Interlaminar Stabilizing System (ILS). A recent meta-analysis showed decompression and Coflex was more effective than decompression and instrumented fusion in terms of Oswestry Disability Index (ODI), length of stay, and blood loss for patients with stenosis due to degenerative spondylolisthesis.[17] However, the role of IPDs is still being defined in the spectrum of surgical treatment options for LSS with or without instability and should be cautiously utilized in the outpatient setting.

In conclusion, we believe most one- and two-level laminectomies and IPD implants can be safely transitioned to the outpatient setting. Utilizing minimally invasive techniques may enhance this transition. We recommend to be cautious when performing these outpatient procedures on patients > 60 years of age, with a BMI > 35, ASA class 3–4, and with preoperative anemia. Perhaps, these procedures should be performed in the inpatient setting.

17.2.3 MIS TLIF with Percutaneous Pedicle Screw Fixation

Given the recent paradigm shift toward reducing hospital stay after spinal surgery, the importance of determining whether same-day discharge following lumbar fusion can be performed safely, reliably, and effectively cannot be overemphasized and has not been aggressively explored until recently. MIS techniques, especially for fusions that otherwise require significant soft tissue stripping and are associated with increased morbidity, show promise toward this end. Most pronouncedly, minimally invasive transforaminal lumbar interbody fusion (MIS TLIF) has repeatedly demonstrated equivalent efficacy in pain and functional outcomes compared to open TLIFs. However, MIS TLIF is associated with decreased blood loss, short-term back pain, postoperative length of stay, and infection rates[18]—all factors previously considered as barriers to performing fusions in the outpatient setting. This was further corroborated by Eckman et al who reported on 1,114 consecutive MIS TLIF patients who were offered to be discharged home the same day of the procedure, resulting in a 73% same-day discharge rate.[19] The mean age of patients discharged on the same day was 52 years, compared to 64 years for those who stayed in the hospital. The hospital stay cohort was statistically significantly older and had a higher preoperative back pain score. In addition, they reported a higher medical complication and readmission rate in patients > 65 years old who were among the inpatient cohort. They concluded that experienced surgeons can consider MIS TLIF in an outpatient setting for younger patients with good general health. Recently, a prospective registry study comparing MIS to open TLIF reported reduced blood loss and shorter length of stay for one-level fusion favoring MIS TLIF after propensity matching.[20] Another study demonstrated cost savings in favor of MIS fusion ranging from 2.5 to 49.3%, especially when performed in the outpatient setting[21] (▶ Table 17.2).

We believe one-level, nonrevision MIS TLIF with percutaneous screw fixation can be safely, reliably, and effectively

Table 17.2 Outpatient concept

Outpatient candidates	Outpatient ideal	Outpatient possible	Outpatient NOT an option
	• <65 years (healthy) • Lover BMI (~<30) • ASA 1, 2	• >65 years (healthy) • BMI (~>35–<40) • ASA 3	• >65 years + any comorbidities (CV disease, sleep apnea, opioid dependence, substance abuse) • BMI (~>40) • ASA 4
Procedure examples:	Ideal	Possible	NOT an option
	• Microdiscectomy (tubular or endoscopic)	• ACDF	• Tumors
	• Tubular decompression	• Single-level MIS TLIF	• Multilevel fusions
	• Single-level MIS TLIF	• Lateral single-level fusions	• Complex osteotomies (VCR, PSO)

Abbreviations: ACDF, anterior cervical discectomy and fusion; BMI, body mass index; CV, cardiovascular; MIS TLIF, minimally invasive transforaminal lumbar interbody fusion.

performed in the outpatient setting for patients younger than 65 years old and with minimal comorbidities.

17.2.4 Lateral Lumbar Interbody Fusion (LLIF)

LLIF was popularized as a minimally invasive alternative to perform lumbar spine fusion via the lateral approach, effectively avoiding morbidity associated with anterior and posterior approaches. LLIF has most robustly been adopted for degenerative lumbar spinal pathologies and spinal deformity. This adoption has not been without consequence, as LLIF is intrinsically associated with up to a 60% incidence of postoperative anterior thigh pain, numbness, and weakness due to lumbar plexus neuropraxia, most often following L4–L5 LLIF.[22,23] However, these symptoms are often short lived and rarely permanent.[24,25]

LLIF is frequently performed in the hospital setting, and there is a paucity of data assessing its feasibility in the outpatient setting. The study by Chin et al is the only study to date comparing outcomes following inpatient versus outpatient LLIF.[26] They compared, in a retrospective cohort study, 40 patients (Group I) who underwent this procedure in the hospital setting to 30 patients (Group II) who underwent the procedure in the outpatient setting. Inclusion criteria included: (1) BMI ≤ 42.2; (2) chronically ill patients had to be stable and cleared for surgery by their primary medicine doctor (PMD); (3) patients with a cardiac history must be cleared for surgery by their cardiologist via an echocardiogram and/or stress test; and (4) ASA 1–3. Exclusion criteria included: (1) History of malignancy, spinal infections, and congenital disease; (2) history of major acute trauma, major deformities (severe scoliosis and ankylosis spondylitis); and (3) previous lumbar spine surgery.

At final follow-up in 2 years, both groups displayed improved VAS back pain; however, ODI scores did not change within each group. Between-group analysis showed a significant improvement in ODI score in group 2 (outpatient) compared to group 1. Fusion rate was 100% in both groups. Operative time and blood loss were less in group 2 compared to group 1.

Although this is a level IV study, it at least demonstrates noninferiority of LLIF in the outpatient setting compared to the inpatient setting and sets the framework for further safety and feasibility studies.

Ultimately, when considering LLIFs in the outpatient setting, patient selection is paramount. BMI should be < 42, the operation should be limited to one level, L5–S1 LLIF should be avoided, L4–L5 LLIF should be carefully selected (radiographic anatomy should be rigorously scrutinized), and previously mentioned exclusion criteria should be considered.[27,28,29]

17.3 Cervical Spine

17.3.1 Anterior Cervical Decompression and Fusion with either Cage or Allograft/Plate (One to Four Levels)

Anterior cervical discectomy and fusion (ACDF) accounts for 68% of spine surgeries performed in the outpatient setting, which is the largest proportion.[30] Stieber et al compared ACDF with plate fixation for one- or two-level cervical radiculopathy recalcitrant to conservative treatment performed in a freestanding ambulatory surgery center (ASC) compared to the inpatient setting.[31] They reported no major complications. Readmission was required for 7% of patients in the inpatient group for minor complications, whereas none in the outpatient group required readmission.

Although catastrophic complications requiring emergent medical intervention following ACDF rarely occurs, results from a recent Delphi Panel suggests that there is an acceptable range of time from 3 to 6 hours for post-op observation following this procedure.[32] Tally et al reported average hospital stays of 4.7 hours for single-level ACDF and 5.4 hours for two-level ACDF in the ASC, with no major complication or readmission. Villavicencio et al published a highly cited study in 2006 examining outpatient with one or more levels of instrumented ACDF.[33] Median discharge time was 8 hours, far below the 23-hour limit for outpatient procedures in many states. Four patients stayed under observation for longer than 23 hours after undergoing three-level ACDF. Jossefer et al reported on a series of 390 outpatient ACDF patients with no major complications and an average of 3 hours post-operative observation period.[34] In a more recent series of 1,000 outpatient ACDFs, Adamson et al described 629 one-level procedures and 365 two-level procedures performed in a single ASC.[35] All patients spent 4 hours in the ASC's postanesthesia care unit and most were discharged

home; 0.8% were transferred to a hospital for either postoperative pain control, profound chest weakness, or surgical re-exploration. One patient reported a postoperative hematoma. None of the patients died due to surgical complications. In another large series by McGirt et al comparing a propensity matched cohort of 1,442 patients who underwent ACDFs, 650 inpatients and 792 outpatients reported major morbidity rate of 3.1% versus 1.4% ($p = 0.03$), and return to operating room rate of 1.4% versus 0.34% ($p = 0.04$), respectively.[36]

One- or two-level stand-alone (with screw integration) ACDF, or ACDF with plate fixation can be safely, effectively, and reliably performed in the outpatient setting. Outcomes following outpatient ACDF is at least equivalent; however, it is sometimes reported as superior due to scant reports of lower complication and readmission rates compared to those performed in the inpatient setting. Patient factors that may preclude outpatient ACDF include ASA 4, significant cardiovascular disease, sleep apnea requiring continuous positive airway pressure (CPAP), opioid dependence, and substance abuse. Three-level ACDFs are sometimes performed in the outpatient setting but may be associated with a higher complication and admission rate. Four-level and revision ACDFs can be performed in the outpatient setting by experienced outpatient spine surgeons.

17.3.2 Disc Arthroplasty (One or Two Levels)

Cervical disc arthroplasty (CDR) is also gaining notoriety as a motion preserving alternative to ACDF that can safely be performed in the outpatient setting as extrapolated from the ACDF literature. A 2010 study described 27 patients who underwent cervical disc replacement at an ASC where all patients reported improved symptoms postoperatively.[37] Average operative time was 40 minutes and patients spent a minimum of 3 hours recovering. None of the patients had major complications, and there were no reports of worsening or persistent pain. Outpatient cervical disc arthroplasties cost 62% less than inpatient cervical disc arthroplasties and outcomes were similar among all groups.

Again, patient selection for outpatient CDR is of paramount importance. General health variables for excluding patients from having CDR in the outpatient setting are similar to those reported for outpatient ACDF. However, patients indicated for CDR should often demonstrate no segmental instability (< 3 mm translation, or < 11 mm angular motion) or kyphosis, preserved disc height, and minimal spondylosis and facet joint degeneration. CDR should be avoided in osteoporotic patients as well. Currently, one implant is approved for one- and two-level CDRs in the US, both in the inpatient and outpatient settings, although three- and four-level CDRs are sometimes performed in Europe with reported good outcomes.[38]

Although dysphagia is common and usually transient following anterior cervical spinal surgery, the incidence and severity of dysphagia may be lower after arthroplasty, likely secondary to lower profile implants utilized.[39] The risk of high-grade heterotopic ossification (HO) following CDR can be as high as 60%, although patients with HO typically do not fare worse clinically compared to those without.[40] Nonsteroidal anti-inflammatory drugs (NSAIDs) may be given toward decreasing the risk of heterotopic ossification.[41]

References

[1] Zahrawi F. Microlumbar discectomy. Is it safe as an outpatient procedure? Spine. 1994; 19(9):1070–1074

[2] Asch HL, Lewis PJ, Moreland DB, et al. Prospective multiple outcomes study of outpatient lumbar microdiscectomy: should 75 to 80% success rates be the norm? J Neurosurg. 2002; 96(1) Suppl:34–44

[3] Best NM, Sasso RC. Success and safety in outpatient microlumbar discectomy. J Spinal Disord Tech. 2006; 19(5):334–337

[4] Pugely AJ, Martin CT, Gao Y, Mendoza-Lattes SA. Outpatient surgery reduces short-term complications in lumbar discectomy: an analysis of 4310 patients from the ACS-NSQIP database. Spine. 2013; 38(3):264–271

[5] Arts MP, Brand R, van den Akker ME, et al. Tubular discectomy vs conventional microdiscectomy for the treatment of lumbar disc herniation: 2-year results of a double-blind randomized controlled trial. Neurosurgery. 2011; 69 (1):135–144, discussion 144

[6] Bekelis K, Missios S, Kakoulides G, Rahmani R, Simmons N. Selection of patients for ambulatory lumbar discectomy: results from four US states. Spine J. 2014; 14(9):1944–1950

[7] Yen D, Albargi A. Results and limitations of outpatient and overnight stay laminectomies for lumbar spinal stenosis. Can J Surg. 2017; 60(5):329–334

[8] Basques BA, Varthi AG, Golinvaux NS, Bohl DD, Grauer JN. Patient characteristics associated with increased postoperative length of stay and readmission after elective laminectomy for lumbar spinal stenosis. Spine. 2014; 39 (10):833–840

[9] Phan K, Mobbs RJ. Minimally invasive versus open laminectomy for lumbar stenosis: a systematic review and meta-analysis. Spine. 2016; 41(2):E91–E100

[10] Schöller K, Alimi M, Cong G-T, Christos P, Härtl R. Lumbar spinal stenosis associated with degenerative lumbar spondylolisthesis: a systematic review and meta-analysis of secondary fusion rates following open vs minimally invasive decompression. Neurosurgery. 2017; 80(3):355–367

[11] Chiu JC. Interspinous process decompression (IPD) system (X-STOP) for the treatment of lumbar spinal stenosis. Surg Technol Int. 2006; 15:265–275

[12] Lauryssen C. Appropriate selection of patients with lumbar spinal stenosis for interspinous process decompression with the X STOP device. Neurosurg Focus. 2007; 22(1):E5

[13] Lønne G, Johnsen LG, Rossvoll I, et al. Minimally invasive decompression versus x-stop in lumbar spinal stenosis: a randomized controlled multicenter study. Spine. 2015; 40(2):77–85

[14] Verhoof OJ, Bron JL, Wapstra FH, van Royen BJ. High failure rate of the interspinous distraction device (X-Stop) for the treatment of lumbar spinal stenosis caused by degenerative spondylolisthesis. Eur Spine J. 2008; 17(2):188–192

[15] Tuschel A, Chavanne A, Eder C, Meissl M, Becker P, Ogon M. Implant survival analysis and failure modes of the X-Stop interspinous distraction device. Spine. 2013; 38(21):1826–1831

[16] Zhao X-W, Ma JX, Ma XL, et al. Interspinous process devices (IPD) alone versus decompression surgery for lumbar spinal stenosis (LSS): a systematic review and meta-analysis of randomized controlled trials. Int J Surg. 2017; 39:57–64

[17] Li A-M, Li X, Yang Z. Decompression and coflex interlaminar stabilisation compared with conventional surgical procedures for lumbar spinal stenosis: a systematic review and meta-analysis. Int J Surg. 2017; 40:60–67

[18] Vazan M, Gempt J, Meyer B, Buchmann N, Ryang Y-M. Minimally invasive transforaminal lumbar interbody fusion versus open transforaminal lumbar interbody fusion: a technical description and review of the literature. Acta Neurochir (Wien). 2017; 159(6):1137–1146

[19] Eckman WW, Hester L, McMillen M. Same-day discharge after minimally invasive transforaminal lumbar interbody fusion: a series of 808 cases. Clin Orthop Relat Res. 2014; 472(6):1806–1812

[20] McGirt MJ, Parker SL, Mummaneni P, et al. Is the use of minimally invasive fusion technologies associated with improved outcomes after elective interbody lumbar fusion? Analysis of a nationwide prospective patient-reported outcomes registry. Spine J. 2017; 17(7):922–932

[21] Goldstein CL, Phillips FM, Rampersaud YR. Comparative effectiveness and economic evaluations of open versus minimally invasive posterior or transforaminal lumbar interbody fusion: a systematic review. Spine. 2016; 41 Suppl 8:S74–S89

[22] Patel VC, Park DK, Herkowitz HN. Lateral transpsoas fusion: indications and outcomes. ScientificWorldJournal. 2012; 2012:893608

[23] Guérin P, Obeid I, Bourghli A, et al. The lumbosacral plexus: anatomic considerations for minimally invasive retroperitoneal transpsoas approach. Surg Radiol Anat. 2012; 34(2):151–157

[24] Barbagallo GMV, Albanese V, Raich AL, Dettori JR, Sherry N, Balsano M. Lumbar lateral interbody fusion (LLIF): comparative effectiveness and safety versus PLIF/TLIF and predictive factors affecting LLIF outcome. Evid Based Spine Care J. 2014; 5(1):28–37

[25] Moller DJ, Slimack NP, Acosta FL, Jr, Koski TR, Fessler RG, Liu JC. Minimally invasive lateral lumbar interbody fusion and transpsoas approach-related morbidity. Neurosurg Focus. 2011; 31(4):E4

[26] Chin KR, Pencle FJ, Coombs AV, et al. Lateral lumbar interbody fusion in ambulatory surgery centers: patient selection and outcome measures compared with an inhospital cohort. Spine. 2016; 41(8):686–692

[27] Ozgur BM, Aryan HE, Pimenta L, Taylor WR. Extreme lateral interbody fusion (XLIF): a novel surgical technique for anterior lumbar interbody fusion. Spine J. 2006; 6(4):435–443

[28] Chin KR, Coombs AV, Seale JA. Feasibility and patient-reported outcomes after outpatient single-level instrumented posterior lumbar interbody fusion in a surgery center: preliminary results in 16 patients. Spine. 2015; 40(1): E36–E42

[29] Hofer RE, Kai T, Decker PA, Warner DO. Obesity as a risk factor for unanticipated admissions after ambulatory surgery. Mayo Clin Proc. 2008; 83 (8):908–916

[30] Baird EO, Egorova NN, McAnany SJ, Qureshi SA, Hecht AC, Cho SK. National trends in outpatient surgical treatment of degenerative cervical spine disease. Global Spine J. 2014; 4(3):143–150

[31] Stieber JR, Brown K, Donald GD, Cohen JD. Anterior cervical decompression and fusion with plate fixation as an outpatient procedure. Spine J. 2005; 5 (5):503–507

[32] Mohandas A, Summa C, Worthington WB, et al. Best practices for outpatient anterior cervical surgery: results from a Delphi Panel. Spine. 2017; 42(11): E648–E659

[33] Villavicencio AT, Pushchak E, Burneikiene S, Thramann JJ. The safety of instrumented outpatient anterior cervical discectomy and fusion. Spine J. 2007; 7 (2):148–153

[34] Jossefer S, Shin P, Wohns RNW. Outpatient anterior cervical discectomy and fusion: indications and clinical experience in a consecutive series of 390 patients. Neurosurg Quart 2010 20(2): 107–110

[35] Adamson T, Godil SS, Mehrlich M, Mendenhall S, Asher AL, McGirt MJ. Anterior cervical discectomy and fusion in the outpatient ambulatory surgery setting compared with the inpatient hospital setting: analysis of 1000 consecutive cases. J Neurosurg Spine. 2016; 24(6):878–884

[36] McGirt MJ, Godil SS, Asher AL, Parker SL, Devin CJ. Quality analysis of anterior cervical discectomy and fusion in the outpatient versus inpatient setting: analysis of 7288 patients from the NSQIP database. Neurosurg Focus. 2015; 39(6):E9

[37] Wohns R. Safety and cost-effectiveness of outpatient cervical disc arthroplasty. Surg Neurol Int. 2010; 1:77

[38] Huppert J, Beaurain J, Steib JP, et al. Comparison between single- and multilevel patients: clinical and radiological outcomes 2 years after cervical disc replacement. Eur Spine J. 2011; 20(9):1417–1426

[39] McAfee PC, Cappuccino A, Cunningham BW, et al. Lower incidence of dysphagia with cervical arthroplasty compared with ACDF in a prospective randomized clinical trial. J Spinal Disord Tech. 2010; 23(1):1–8

[40] Sundseth J, Jacobsen EA, Kolstad F, et al. Heterotopic ossification and clinical outcome in nonconstrained cervical arthroplasty 2 years after surgery: the Norwegian Cervical Arthroplasty Trial (NORCAT). Eur Spine J. 2016; 25 (7):2271–2278

[41] Mehren C, Suchomel P, Grochulla F, et al. Heterotopic ossification in total cervical artificial disc replacement. Spine. 2006; 31(24):2802–2806

18 Posterior Cervical Foraminotomy/Discectomy

Luca Papavero

Summary

Posterior cervical foraminotomy (PCFo) is a clinically effective, cost effective, motion preserving, and time-proven surgical treatment for intraforaminal disc herniation and narrow root canal. In the past, the main disadvantage of the technique was the burdening postoperative neck pain due to the extensive subperiosteal dissection of the neck muscles from the midline. Nowadays, the blunt transmuscular approach has been borrowed from endoscopy and blended with the microsurgical/microendoscopic technique through a tubular retractor. This development, described here, has significantly reduced the surgical traumatization while keeping all the advantages of PCFo unchanged.

Keywords: cervical spine, posterior cervical foraminotomy, tubular retractor, minimally invasive spine surgery

18.1 Introduction

Cervical radiculopathy that does not improve with conservative treatment can be addressed surgically with implant-free anterior or posterior cervical foraminotomy (PCFo), or with implant-dependent fusion (anterior cervical discectomy and fusion [ACDF]) or total disc replacement. It is evident that there is no single technique that can best treat all types of this pathology. Good clinical practice recommends that the procedure best suited to the patient's needs should be chosen.

In the daily practice, the average cost of an ACDF is 89% more than a PCFo. Provided a comparable patient outcome for either procedure, from a health care economics standpoint, a minimally invasive PCFo (mi-PCFo) should be considered in the treatment of cervical radiculopathy.[1]

Both the ventral and dorsal approaches offer certain advantages and disadvantages.

PCFo is a motion-preserving procedure that has been found to relieve symptoms due to foraminal soft disc fragment, bony spur, or synovial cyst in roughly 90% of patients.[2,3,4] It avoids the complications associated with anterior approaches such as dysphagia, hoarseness, and adjacent segment disease. Furthermore, fusion-threatening smoking, short-neck, location of pathology below C7 or above C3 are less burdening risk factors in the posterior than in the anterior route. However, one of the drawbacks of conventionally performed PCFo is significant subperiosteal muscle dissection and retraction to expose the lamino-facet junction, which may result in postoperative neck pain, muscle spasm, and malalignment of the spine.[5] Recently, minimally invasive approaches for PCFo have been introduced to reduce the problems related to extensive soft-tissue dissection.[5,6] mi-PCFo is intended as a microsurgical procedure from skin to skin via a small paramedian incision, comprehensive of a blunt muscle-splitting approach with placement of a tubular or a miniaturized speculum retractor and decompression of the foraminal root (▶ Video 18.1).

18.2 Patient Selection: Indications, Contraindications

Indications:

- Intraforaminal soft disc herniations, provided that ≥ 2/3 of their mass is lateral to the dural sac (▶ Fig. 18.1a–d).
- Bony narrowing of the root canal (▶ Fig. 18.1e, f).

Relative indications:

- Paramedian disc herniations with a prevalent intraforaminal component which is clinically relevant.
- Intraforaminal synovial cysts and tumors.
- Increased risk factors for anterior surgery: professional singer, smoking, extensive scarring post thyroid surgery, location of pathology caudal to C7 and cranial to C3 in short neck.

Contraindications:

- Kyphotic malalignment or instability of the index level.
- Anomalous course of vertebral artery at the target level.
- Ossification of the posterior longitudinal ligament.

Relative contraindications:

- Recurrent disc and bilateral pathology.

For the well-selected patient, this operation can be extremely satisfying especially since the alternative involves anterior surgery and permanent implants. After the keyhole drilling has been performed, the editors find it helpful to identify next the medial border of the pedicles above and below, as they will define the foramen and the exiting nerve root in between. Be aware that sometimes there may be two nerve roots, a sensory and a motor branch in separate dural sleeves. This is an excellent description by one of the masters in the field.

18.3 Preoperative Planning

Preoperative planning includes:

- Preoperative imaging of the C-spine should answer the following questions:
  - Biplanar X-ray with additional flexion/extension: spontaneous fusion of the target level? Labeling of the target level feasible in the operating room (OR; shoulder blade artifact C7-T1)?

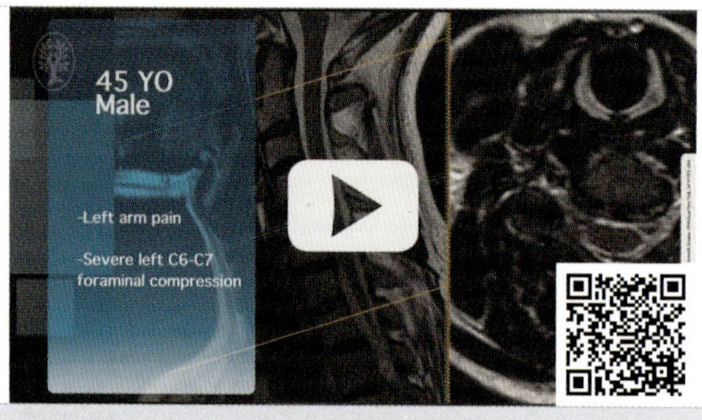

Video 18.1 Posterior cervical foraminotomy.

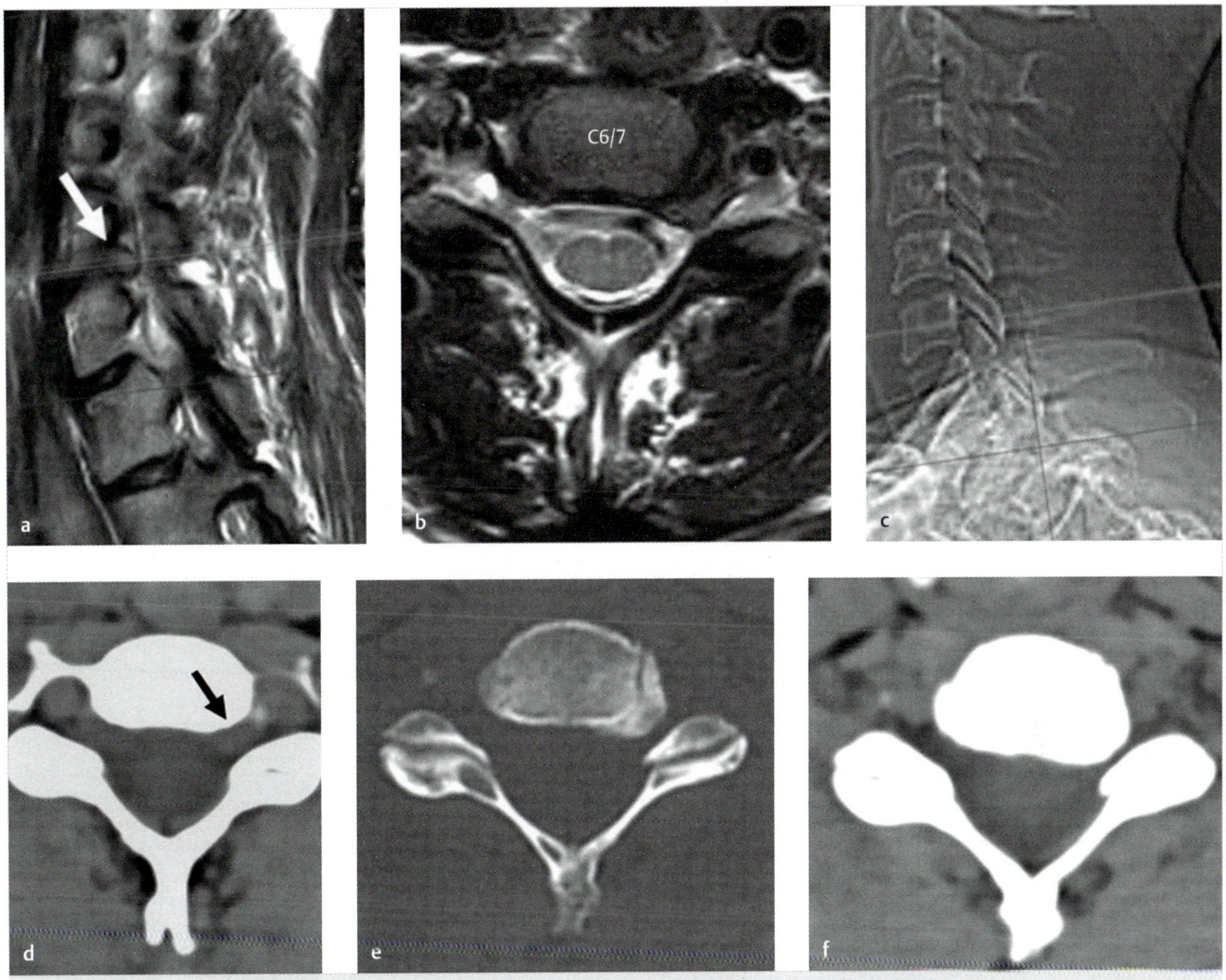

Fig. 18.1 **(a)** Paramedian left-sided sagittal T2-weighted magnetic resonance imaging showing an intraforaminal disc herniation C6/C7 (*white arrow*) confirmed by **(b)** the axial slice; **(c)** computed tomography-scout view with *white* reference line corresponding to the intraforaminal disc herniation; **(d)** *black arrow*; **(e, f)** an example of left-sided narrow root canal.

- Computed tomography (CT) scan: calcified disc herniation? Additional bony narrowing of the root canal?
- Magnetic resonance imaging (MRI): relationship between the space-occupying lesion and the neural structures? Location of the vertebral artery at the target level?

18.4 Patient Positioning and Labeling of the Disc Space

After having performed the dorsolateral foraminotomy over years with the patient in sitting or in prone position, since two decades we favor the so-called Concorde positioning. It consists a reverse Trendelenburg which offers the advantage of a decreased epidural venous congestion but avoids the need of cardiac catheter to prevent air embolism (▶ Fig. 18.2). Nowadays, the sitting position is an option for very obese patients or those affected by ventilatory disturbances.

Labeling of the disc space: whenever possible in lateral fluoroscopy with a spinal needle inserted contralateral to the intended surgical site about one finger breadth paramedian. Labeling of caudal levels in short-neck patients may be accomplished with anteroposterior (AP)-fluoroscopy: in this case attention should be paid to the angle between C-arm and skin!

The OR-setup shown in ▶ Fig. 18.3 has proved to be effective but can be modified according to local requirements.

18.5 Surgical Technique

18.5.1 mi-PCFo Steps

1. Micro from skin to skin: 25-mm skin incision roughly 15-mm paramedian centered on the puncture point of the labeling spinal needle.
2. Incision of the dorsal fascia and holding sutures. See Tips & Tricks (T&T) no. 2.
3. Blunt splitting of the fascial planes and muscle layers. See T&T no. 3. Splitting is performed with the help of two slim retractors (6-mm width) and of the tip of a scissor rigorously according to the fiber direction of the different muscle layers. This step is bloodless.

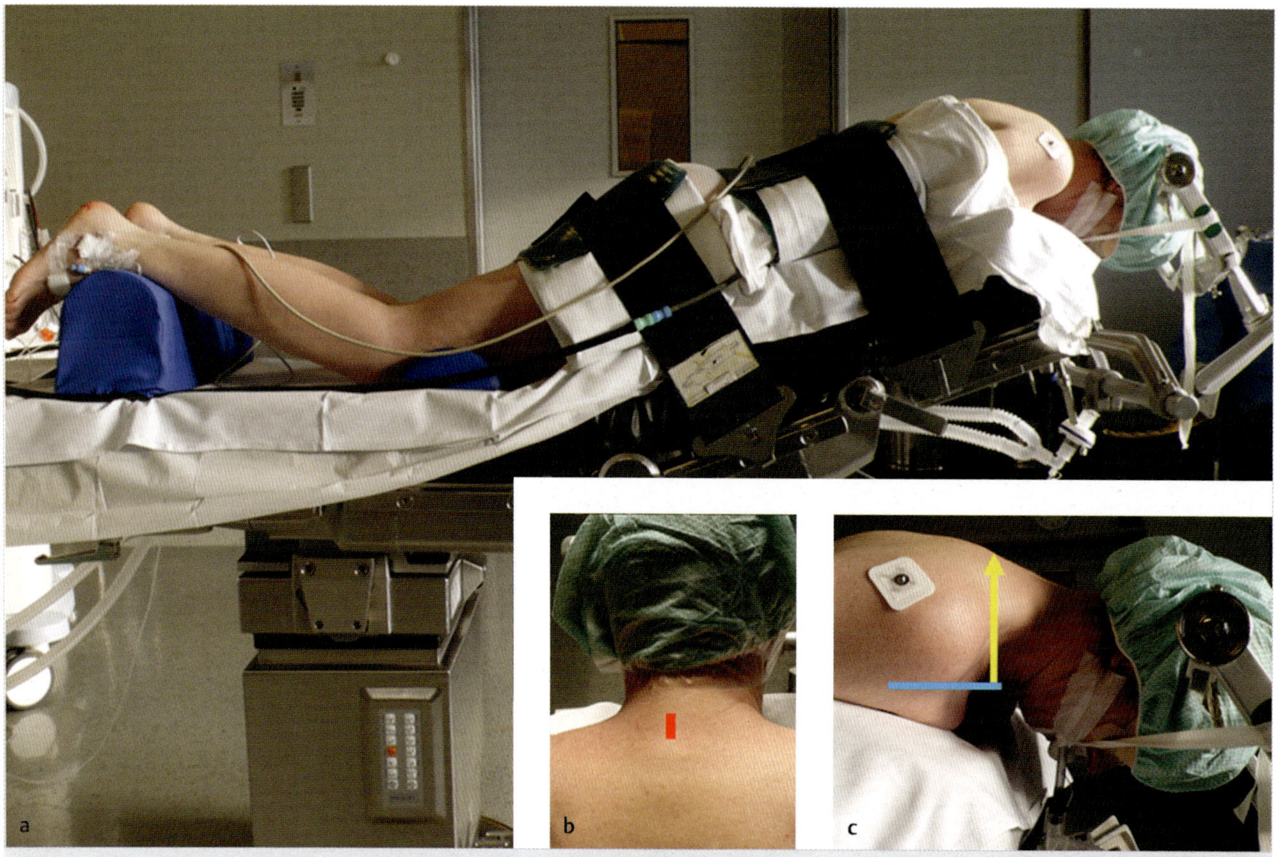

Fig. 18.2 **(a)** Concorde positioning with the head fixed with Mayfield-clamp; **(b)** skin incision (*red line*) for the C6/C7 disc herniation shown in ▸ Fig. 18.1; **(c)** the OR-situs (*yellow arrow*) is about 15 cm above the right-sided atrium (*blue line*). A moderate flexion of the head (chin on chest) opens the interlaminar space. A strap placed from arm to arm and behind the buttocks keeps the patient in place.

4. Inserting the expandable tubular or speculum retractor (▸ Fig. 18.4). The tubular retractor (⌀15 mm) is inserted and then opened with diverging half-shells on the target area (⌀24 mm). The speculum retractor is smaller (width 5 mm) and can be opened up to 35 mm. Both retractors are fixed with a table-mounted holding arm (▸ Fig. 18.5).
5. Fluoroscopy: Confirming the right target level.
6. Bone resection 1: Drilling the keyhole (▸ Fig. 18.6). Use a 3-mm bit coated with diamond dust.
7. Lateral flavectomy and coagulation of the epidural veins. The goal is to expose the lateral border of the dural sac. See T&T no 4.
8. Bone resection 2: Decompression of the root enables less traumatizing manipulation of the root during the removal of disc fragments.
9. Exploring the epidural space looking for the disc fragment/s. See T&T no 5. Discectomy is usually not necessary.
10. Wrapping the root with Gelfoam soaked with steroid and closure by layers.

18.6 Postoperative Care

Patient mobilization is allowed few hours following surgery. Oral analgesia is administered on demand. No collar is worn. Isometric neck muscle exercises are started the morning after surgery. No routine postsurgical imaging is required. Patients are discharged earliest. In my practice they stay for two days after surgery because of reimbursement regulations, but they could be discharged sooner. Return to work is usually scheduled at 2 weeks after discharge for white and at 4 weeks for blue collars. The follow-up examination 8 weeks after surgery concludes a regular treatment.

18.7 Complications and Avoidance

In the following some hazards at the beginning of the learning curve are addressed:

- Postsurgical segmental instability following excessive drilling of the facet joint (▸ Fig. 18.7).
- Injury of the branch of the accessory spinal nerve crossing the fascia of the trapezoid muscle (▸ Fig. 18.8).
- Bipolar coagulation of small radiculomedullary vessel into the intrarachidian plexus (▸ Fig. 18.9).

18.8 Tips and Tricks

1. Labeling of a caudal disc space in short-neck patients with the C-arm: Use the AP instead of the lateral view and pay attention to the degree of tilt of the C-arm! If three-dimensional navigation should be available, labeling of the target disc could be performed in a very elegant way.

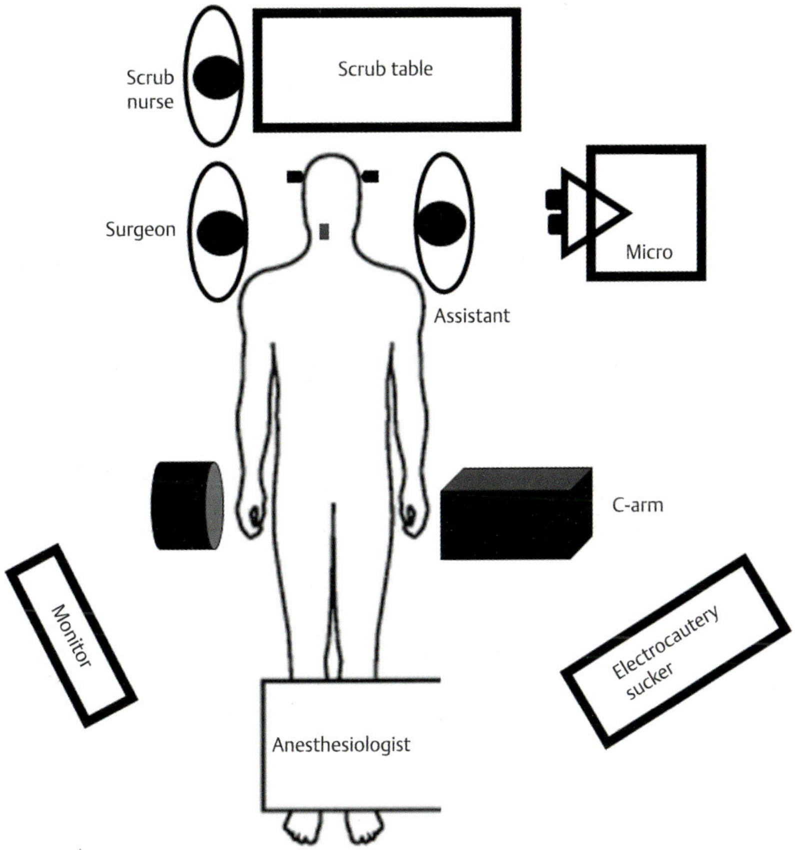

Fig. 18.3 The optimal operating room setup depends on the specific location. That shown here requires from 12 to 15 m^2. After draping the patient, the table-mounted retractor unit is fixed at the opposite side of the skin incision.

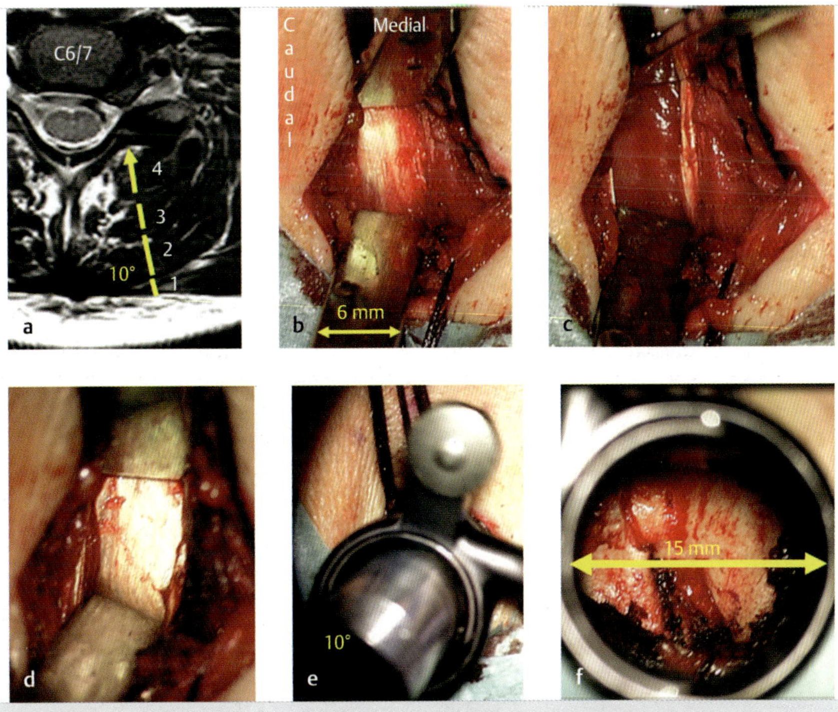

Fig. 18.4 **(a)** The blunt muscle-splitting approach (1: trapezius muscle, 2: splenius muscle, 3: semispinalis muscle, 4: multifidus muscle) requires 10° convergence to the midline. It starts with **(b)** opening the superficial fascia of the trapezoid muscle; **(c)** splitting the muscle fibers according to their direction; **(d)** the superficial fascia of the m. splenius appears; **(e)** the expandable tubular retractor is inserted under optical control and fluoroscopy is limited to the confirmation of the target level; **(f)** the diameter of the tubular retractor is 15 mm but the expandable half-shells allow for 24 mm in the depth.

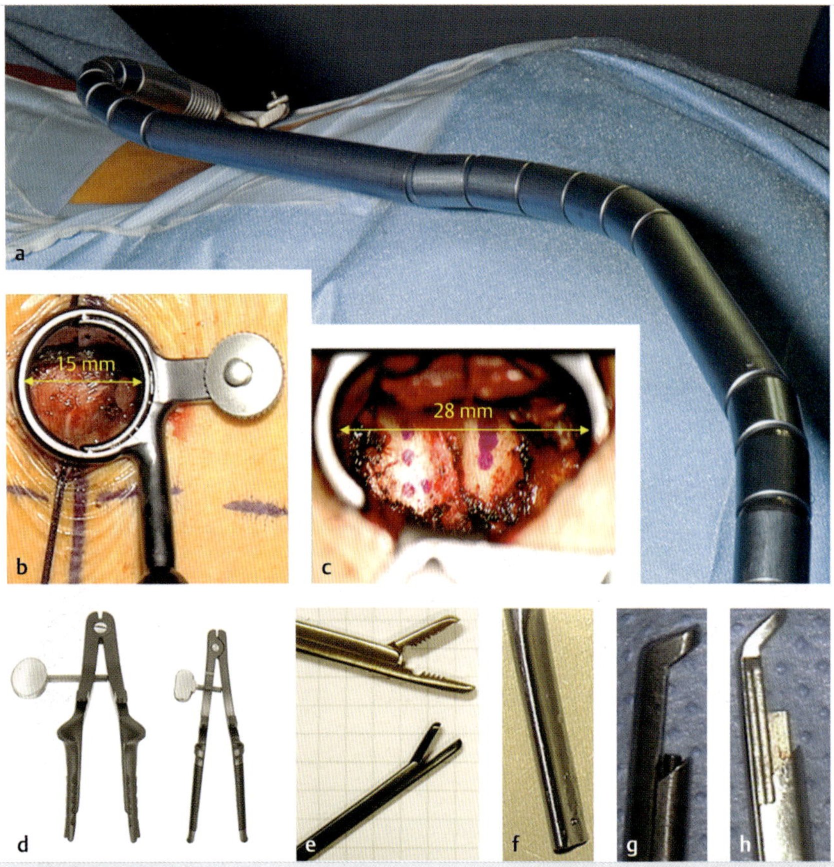

Fig. 18.5 **(a)** The self-holding arm may fix, **(b)** an expandable tubular retractor, or **(c)** a miniaturized speculum retractor. Both retractors are inserted via a blunt muscle-splitting approach. **(d)** Caspar-speculum retractor on the left and minimally invasive surgery (MIS)-adapted on the right; **(e)** miniaturized black forceps compared with conventional forceps; **(f)** flat sucker for retracting the root; **(g)** conventional thin-foot plate punch, and **(h)** MIS-miniaturized punch (manufacturer of the MIS-instruments: Medicon eG, Tuttlingen, Germany; www.medicon.de).

2. Be very careful incising the superficial cervical fascia: a branch of the spinal accessory nerve may cross to the superior border of the trapezoid muscle (▶ Fig. 18.8).
3. During blunt splitting of the muscle layer keep a 10° convergent direction to the midline. A too convergent direction may lead you the spinous process what is of no harm. A too divergent direction may lead you to pass laterally the facet joint favoring an injury of the vertebral artery.
4. To prevent excessive drilling of the facet, stop bone resection a couple of millimeters lateral to the lateral border of the dural sac. Proceed with epidural exploration to find the axilla of the root. Then continue with bone resection corresponding to the course of the root.
5. How to know that the decompression has been carried out laterally enough, especially in bony foraminal stenosis without soft disc? Measure the distance from the lateral border of the dural sac to the lateral border of the bony foraminal narrowing by preoperative MRI or CT-scan. Cut a cottonoid accordingly. Put the cottonoid on the unroofed root and proceed as necessary. Probe the remaining root canal with a hook.
6. When you explore the epidural space underneath the root with a hook looking for the extruded disc fragment do not rotate the hook like a hockey stick: there is the risk to tear epidural veins. Explore the area with back and forward movements of the hook and changing direction.
7. Be aware of the fact that, although very rarely, dorsal and ventral root sleeves are arranged in a distinct superficial-deep manner. Under such circumstances the deep soft bulging may be taken for the contained soft disc herniation. To prevent damage to concealed neural structures, structure incise always the assumed or real disc herniation parallel to the root direction. In so doing even if you accidentally open the ventral root, transection of the rootlets will be avoided.[7]
8. Take your time performing epidural hemostasis with Gelfoam, cottonoids, and rinsing with saline. Coagulate as little as possible near to the root: in some cases small medullary vessels may run atypically along the root.
9. Split the muscles blunt whenever possible! Neck muscle share with the extrinsic eye muscles the highest density of spindle receptors.[9] Furthermore, the postsurgical neck pain is less if muscles are not sharply incised (▶ Fig. 18.10).

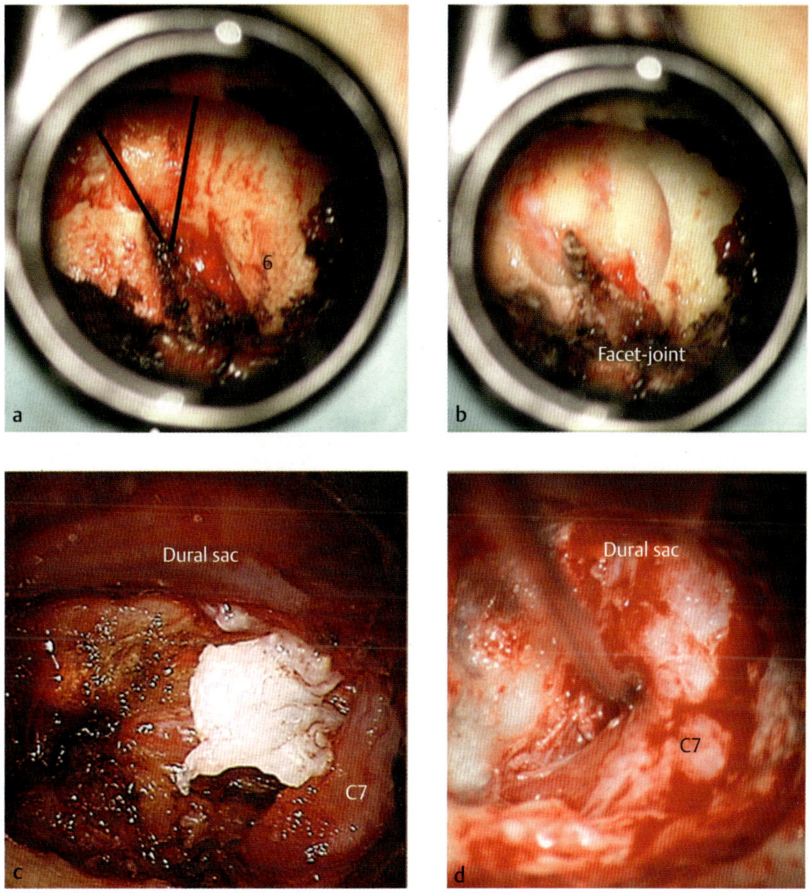

Fig. 18.6 Right-sided posterior foraminotomy C6/C7: **(a)** The interlaminar yellow ligament is shaped as a triangle; **(b)** the keyhole has been drilled and will be completed with a punch; **(c)** usually the intraforaminal disc fragment is located underneath the axilla of the target root; **(d)** the epidural space ventral to the root should be explored between the adjacent pedicles with hooks of different lengths.

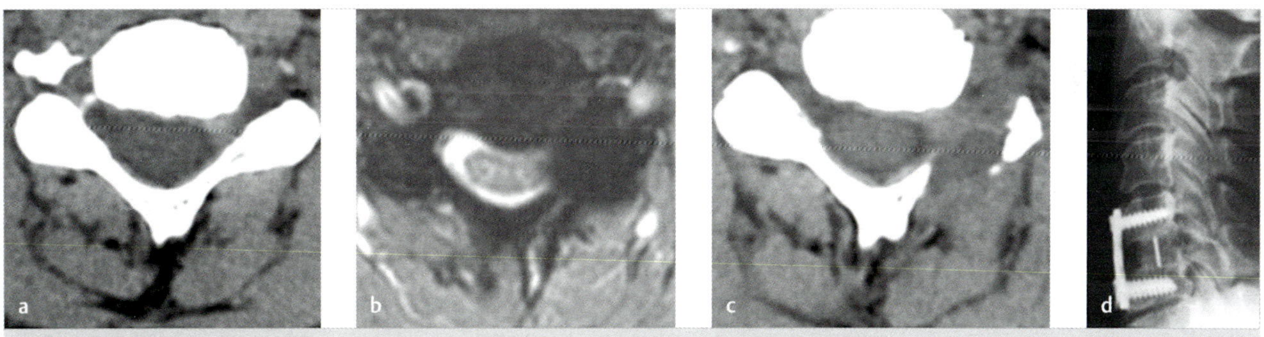

Fig. 18.7 Teaching case: **(a)** A 46-year-old woman complained about C6 pain and biceps muscle 3/5 palsy. The computed tomography (CT) scan showed an intraforaminal disc herniation C5/C6. As the pain was resistant to CT-guided infiltrations, minimally invasive posterior cervical foraminotomy was performed; **(b)** after surgery the weakness improved. A mild hypoesthesia C6 persisted. A new severe load-depending neck pain over 3 weeks occurred which improved with a Philadelphia collar. The magnetic resonance imaging showed metallic dust in the surgical target area; **(c)** The CT excluded a hematoma or intraspinal bone fragments but confirmed the extensive drilling of the facet joint causing mechanical neck pain; **(d)** After anterior cervical-dependent fusion C5C/C6, the patient recovered completely except for the mild hypoesthesia C6. Take home message: do not resect more than 50% of the facet joint![8]

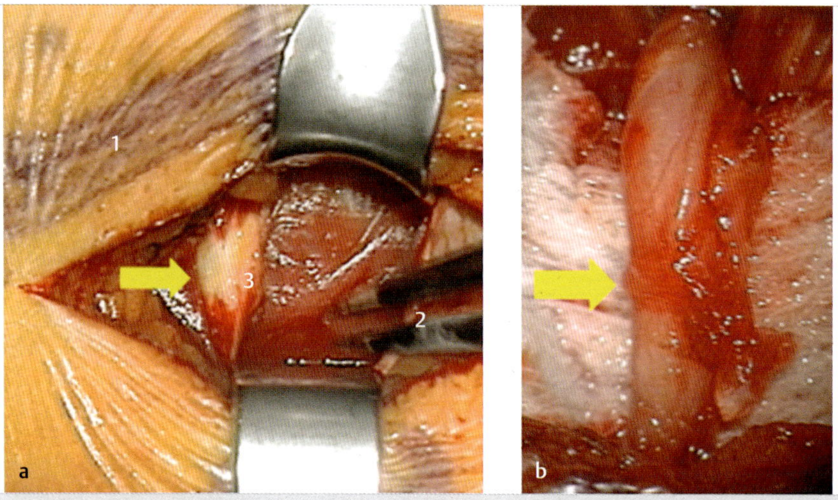

Fig. 18.8 **(a)** Left-sided transmuscular approach: midline labeling (1), superficial fascia (2), and belly (3) of the trapezoid muscle. The *yellow arrow* points to a neural structure crossing the fascia; **(b)** further dissection shows the branch of the accessory spinal nerve heading to the cranial part of the trapezoid muscle.

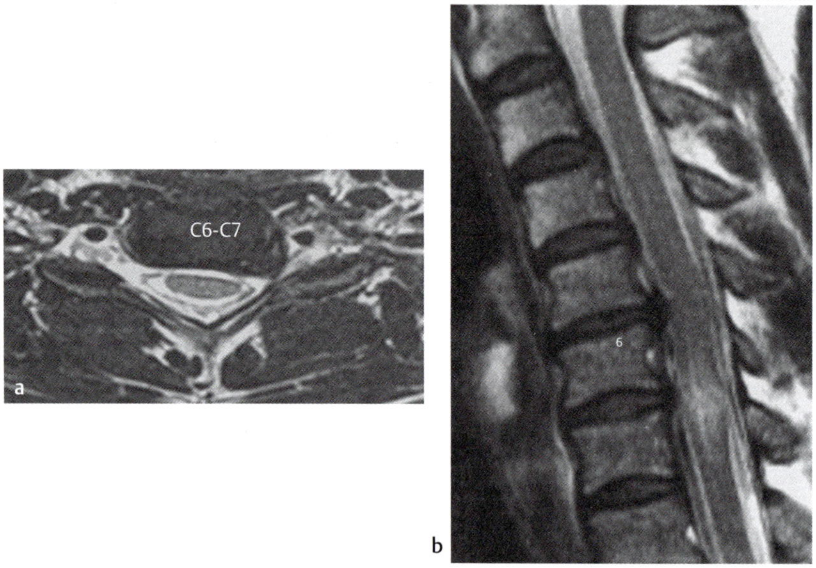

Fig. 18.9 **(a)** A 52-year-old patient complained about a left-sided C7 pain and triceps muscle weakness. The magnetic resonance imaging (MRI) confirmed an intraforaminal disc herniation at C6/C7. The surgery was without excessive retraction of the nerve root but with repeated bipolar coagulation in the axillary area. The first postoperative day the patient complained about gait disturbance and paresthesia of the upper and lower extremities, whereas the triceps muscle weakness improved; **(b)** the postsurgical MRI showed an intramedullary hyperintensity at the level C6/C7, probably an ischemic lesion. Following steroids and rheological treatment, a partial recovery occurred within 1 week.

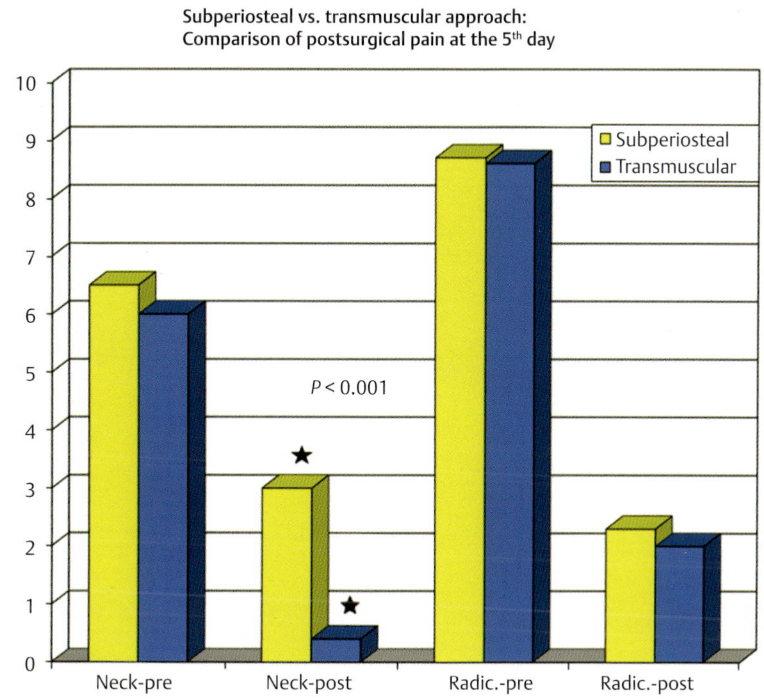

Fig. 18.10 Unpublished results of a prospective cohort study comparing 40 patients treated with posterior foraminotomy via a conventional subperiosteal approach versus 52 patients treated via a transmuscular approach. The postsurgical decrease of the radicular pain was remarkable and comparable in both groups. The early postoperative neck pain was significant less in the second group.

References

[1] Mansfield HE, Canar WJ, Gerard CS, O'Toole JE. Single-level anterior cervical discectomy and fusion versus minimally invasive posterior cervical foraminotomy for patients with cervical radiculopathy: a cost analysis. Neurosurg Focus. 2014; 37(5):E9

[2] Henderson CM, Hennessy RG, Shuey HM, Jr, Shackelford EG. Posterior-lateral foraminotomy as an exclusive operative technique for cervical radiculopathy: a review of 846 consecutively operated cases. Neurosurgery. 1983; 13 (5):504–512

[3] Murphey F, Simmons JC. Ruptured cervical disc. Experience with 250 cases Am Surg. 1966; 32(2):83–88

[4] Zeidman SM, Ducker TB. Posterior cervical laminoforaminotomy for radiculopathy: review of 172 cases. Neurosurgery. 1993; 33(3):356–362

[5] Adamson TE. Microendoscopic posterior cervical laminoforaminotomy for unilateral radiculopathy: results of a new technique in 100 cases. J Neurosurg. 2001; 95 Suppl 1:51–57

[6] Fessler RG, Khoo LT. Minimally invasive cervical microendoscopic foraminotomy: an initial clinical experience. Neurosurgery. 2002; 51 Suppl 5:S37–S45

[7] Zrinzo L, Ashkan K, Johnston F. Unusual cervical nerve root arrangement exposed during surgery: case report and review of the literature. Br J Neurosurg. 2004; 18(6):624–626

[8] Skovrlj B, Gologorsky Y, Haque R, Fessler RG, Qureshi SA. Complications, outcomes, and need for fusion after minimally invasive posterior cervical foraminotomy and microdiscectomy. Spine J. 2014; 14(10):2405–2411

[9] Kulkarni V, Chandy MJ, Babu KS. Quantitative study of muscle spindles in suboccipital muscles of human foetuses. Neurol India. 2001; 49(4):355–359

19 Unilateral Tubular Over-the-Top Cervical Laminectomy for Cervical Stenosis

Robert Nicholas Hernandez, Sergio Soriano-Solis, and José-Antonio Soriano-Sánchez

Summary

Unilateral Tubular Over-the-Top Cervical Laminectomy for Cervical Stenosis addresses the technical aspects of performing a minimally invasive cervical laminectomy for central cervical stenosis via tubular retractor. This chapter discusses indications and contraindications, preoperative planning, the surgical technique formatted into an easy-to-understand technique, and postoperative care. In addition, tips and tricks to facilitate safe and efficient performance of the technique as well as complication avoidance are discussed.

Keywords: cervical laminectomy, minimally invasive laminectomy, minimally invasive spine surgery, technique, tubular retractor

19.1 Introduction

The association between cervical spondylosis and spinal cord compression with myelopathy was first described in 1952 by Brain,[1] now termed as cervical spondylotic myelopathy (CSM). CSM refers to impaired function of the spinal cord caused by degenerative changes of the anatomy within the cervical spine. The original treatment was open laminectomy, but associated complications included the development of cervical kyphosis, gross instability, infection, postlaminectomy membrane formation, and neurological deterioration.[2] This led to the development of other surgical options including anterior and posterior approaches.[3] Although improvements have been made, postoperative axial neck pain is still a common patient complaint with open techniques.[4] With the advancements of minimally invasive spine surgery (MISS) in the past two decades,[5] minimally invasive techniques and approaches to spine have been developed and continue to evolve. The concept of achieving bilateral spinal decompression via a unilateral approach was first applied to open lumbar surgery in 1997.[6] Minimally invasive unilateral laminotomy for bilateral decompression (ULBD) using tubular retractors was introduced for the treatment of lumbar spinal stenosis in 2002.[7,8,9] Since then, the concept of ULBD has become a key surgical principle of MISS, with its application recently extending to all levels of the spinal column including the treatment of CSM.[10,11,12,13,14,15] Potential advantages of a minimally invasive laminectomy compared with open laminectomy include less blood loss, less muscle disruption, and bony removal which may in return result in decreased rates of postlaminectomy kyphosis or secondary fusion, less postoperative pain, infection, and shorter recovery and hospital stay. However, concerns and risks exist, most importantly the risk of intraoperative injury to the dura, spinal cord, and nerves.

This chapter provides a detailed description of the step-by-step microsurgical technique for the performance of the minimally invasive cervical laminectomy via a unilateral approach for bilateral decompression.

19.2 Indications

The main indication for this technique is single- or multilevel CSM with or without accompanying radiculopathy. This procedure is particularly useful for patients with a posterior compression vector (e.g., ligamentum flavum [LF] hypertrophy and/or buckling). As with most MISS decompression procedures, this technique can be particularly beneficial for obese and/or elderly patients in whom open surgery may carry greater than acceptable surgical risk.[16,17]

19.3 Contraindications

The contraindications for MIS cervical laminectomy include those for open laminectomy:

- Fixed cervical kyphosis.
- Gross cervical instability.
- Severe medical comorbidities with unacceptable risk for surgery.

Relative contraindications for MIS cervical laminectomy include:

- Flexible cervical kyphosis.
- Prior posterior cervical surgery at the index level with scar tissue/fibrosis.
- Predominantly anterior spinal cord compression. Patients with adequate cervical lordosis may undergo MIS cervical laminectomy with good outcome if the surgeon is confident that the spinal cord will adequately fall posterior, away from the anterior compression.

19.4 Preoperative Planning

19.4.1 Target (Patient Selection)

Radiographic evaluation should include magnetic resonance imaging and flexion/extension radiographs (▶ Fig. 19.1), and a computed tomography (CT) scan should be obtained for any patient with suspected ossification of the posterior longitudinal ligament. Assessment of the cervical spinal alignment and lordosis, identification of the level of stenosis, and detection of accompanying foraminal stenosis with nerve root involvement are necessary. Radiographic findings should be correlated to the clinical findings on history and physical examination.

19.4.2 Technology

The instruments required to perform this procedure include:

- Tubular retractor system with multiple dilators of increasing diameter, a rigid holding arm, and a table clamp. We use a 15- to 18-mm tubular retractor to perform the laminectomy.
- Bayoneted 45- and 90-degree 2-, 3-, and 4-mm kerrison rongeurs.
- Bayoneted 2- and 3-mm kerrison rongeurs.

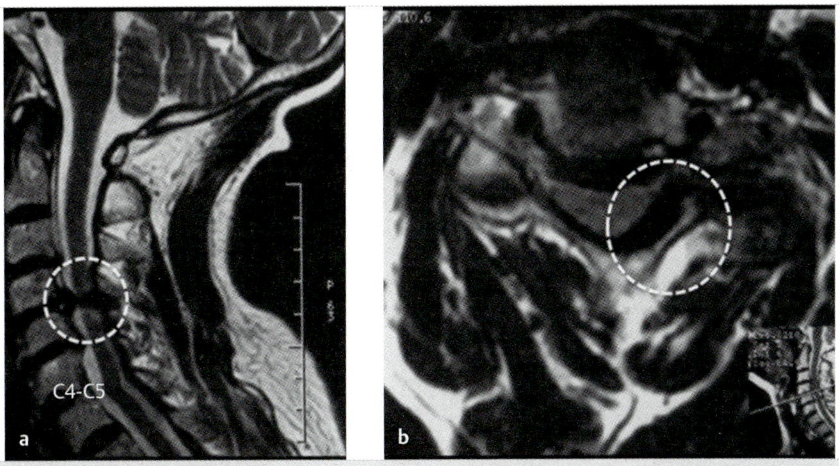

Fig. 19.1 Preoperative sagittal **(a)** and axial **(b)** T2-weighted magnetic resonance imaging demonstrating severe spinal stenosis at C4–C5 with significant posterior compression from ligamentum flavum hypertrophy and buckling.

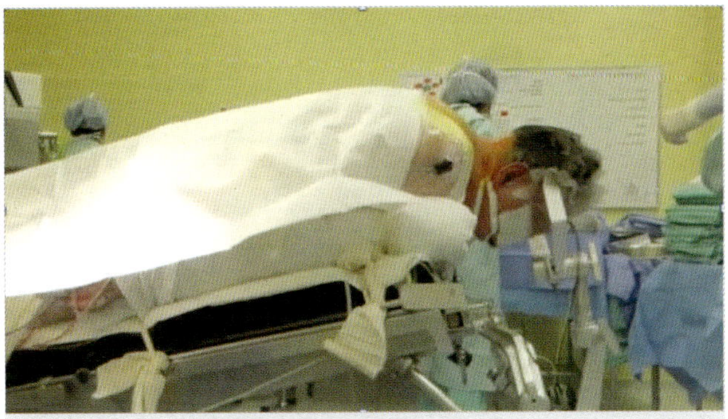

Fig. 19.2 Photograph demonstrating the patient positioning.

- Bayoneted ball-tip probe or blunt nerve hook.
- Angled surgical drill with a 15-cm curved drill shaft: we prefer a 3-mm fluted side-cutting matchstick drill bit with blunt tip.
- Operative microscope.
- Size 12 and 9 metal suction tips.
- Extended monopolar electrocautery.
- Extended bayoneted bipolar electrocautery.
- Fluoroscopy or computer-assisted navigation.
- Hemostatic agents: Thrombin Gelfoam, Surgiflo, Cottonoids, etc.

19.5 Surgical Steps

19.5.1 Patient Positioning

Step 1: Patient Positioning

The patient is positioned in the prone position on a radiolucent table with the head immobilized in a 3-pin skull clamp attached to the operating table. The neck is neutral or slightly flexed to unshingle the cervical laminae (▶ Fig. 19.2). Intraoperative neuromonitoring (IOM) can be utilized and may be especially helpful and reassuring in the beginning of the learning curve.

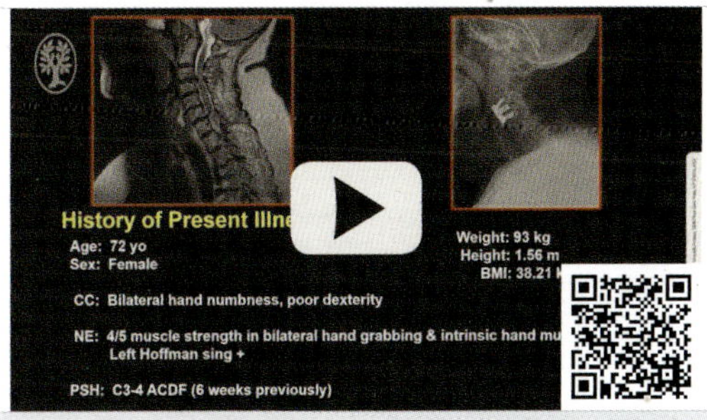

Video 19.1 MIS tubular cervical laminectomy.

Countertraction of the shoulders with tape is applied to facilitate fluoroscopy.

19.5.2 Incision

Step 2: Incision

Lateral fluoroscopy or navigation is used to identify the incision site. A metal instrument or spinal needle should be aimed at the disc space of interest. Keep the instrument perpendicular to the floor so that the working angle will also be perpendicular to the floor. Once the target facet joint and disc space has been identified, local anesthetic with epinephrine is injected into the skin 2-cm off midline. A linear 2.5-cm incision is then made (▶ Fig. 19.3a).

19.5.3 Technique (▶ Video 19.1)

Step 3: Approach

Monopolar electrocautery or sharp dissection is continued until the fascia is identified. The fascia is incised sharply in a linear manner so as to facilitate closure at the conclusion of the procedure. Care should be taken to avoid incising the underlying musculature to avoid bleeding. Using a Metzenbaum scissor or blunt clamp, a corridor through the cervical musculature to the cervical lamina is created (▶ Fig. 19.3b). This blunt dissection

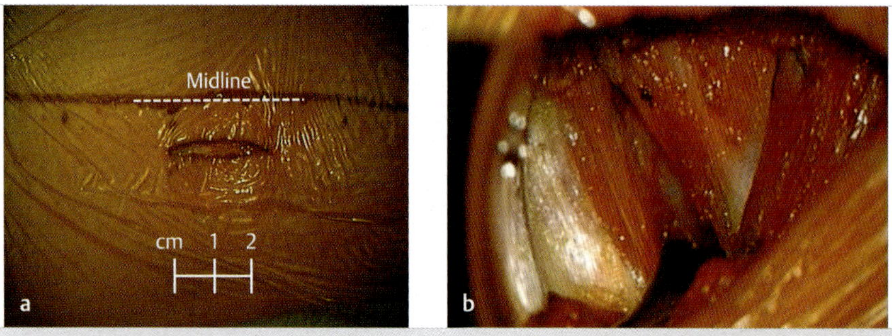

Fig. 19.3 (a) Photograph demonstrating the incision. (b) Intraoperative photograph after the muscular dissection has been completed demonstrating the access corridor to the cervical spine.

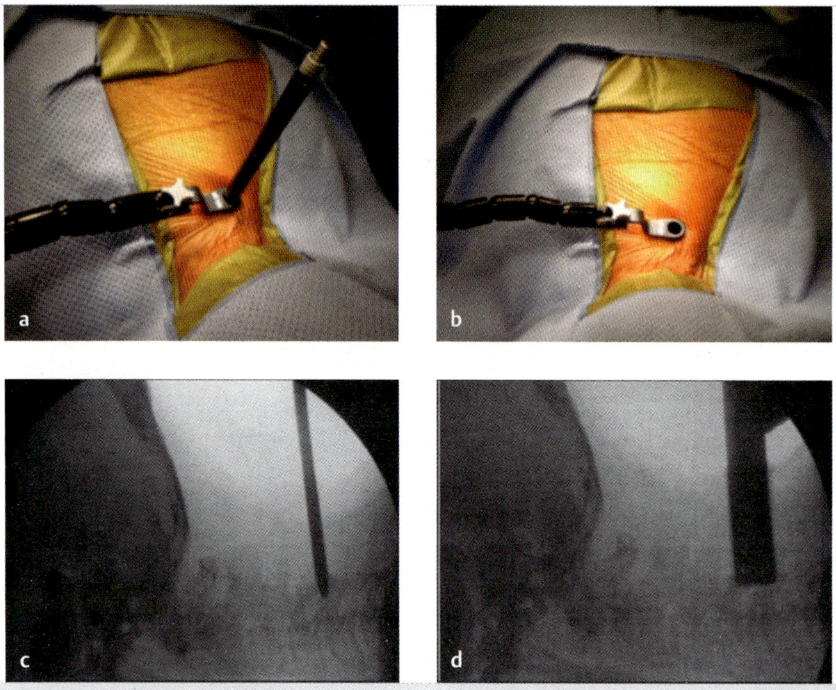

Fig. 19.4 Intraoperative photographs showing serial dilation and tubular retractor placement (a, b) and confirmation of the correct level with lateral X-ray (c, d).

helps limit the amount of muscular bleeding, which can be significant in the cervical spine. Bipolar electrocautery is used to control bleeding.

Step 4: Serial Dilation and Tubular Retractor Placement

Under direct visualization through the created muscular corridor, the first tubular dilator is placed directly onto the cervical lamina. Dilators of increasing size are then passed over one another to dilate the corridor through the soft tissue (▶ Fig. 19.4a). The surgeon should keep gentle downward pressure on the first dilator to keep it on the lamina. Care should be taken to avoid slipping of the dilator into the interlaminar space. Once the last dilator is passed, the surgeon can measure the depth and pass the appropriate sized tubular retractor onto the lamina and secure it in place with the table attachment (▶ Fig. 19.4b). Lateral fluoroscopic images are obtained to confirm the correct level has been targeted (▶ Fig. 19.4c, d).

Step 5: Exposure of Bony Anatomy

The extended monopolar tip is used to remove any remaining soft tissue overlying the cervical bony anatomy (▶ Fig. 19.5a). Start by identifying the spinous process and continuing the dissection laterally along the lamina. The exposure should include the target lamina, base of the spinous process, medial 50% of the lateral mass, and the superior one-third of the lamina caudal to the target lamina as it is shown in ▶ Video 19.1. The triangle formed by the target and caudal lamina and laminofacet junction should be identified (▶ Fig. 19.5b).

Step 6: Ipsilateral Laminectomy

The general principle for the decompression is the following: the spinal cord compression is typically caused by buckling and/or hypertrophy of the LF between the target and caudal lamina. The goal, therefore, is to identify the cranial insertion of the LF and follow the LF caudally until the insertion into the caudal lamina where is it completely removed. Drilling begins

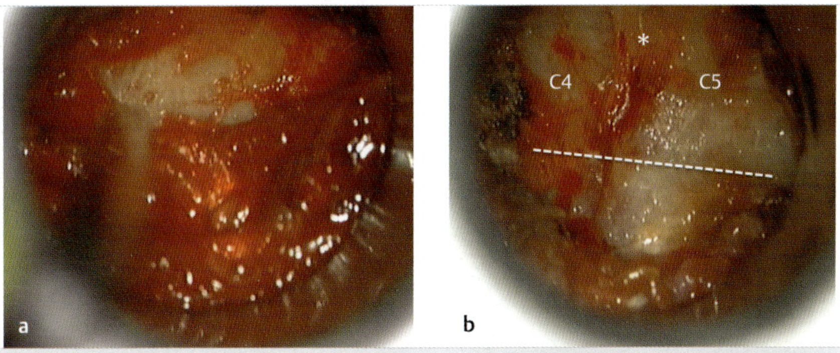

Fig. 19.5 Intraoperative photographs demonstrating removal of the soft tissue overlying the bony anatomy **(a)** and the anatomical landmarks **(b)**. The *asterisk* represents the interlaminar space and LF. The *dashed line* represents the laminofacet junction.

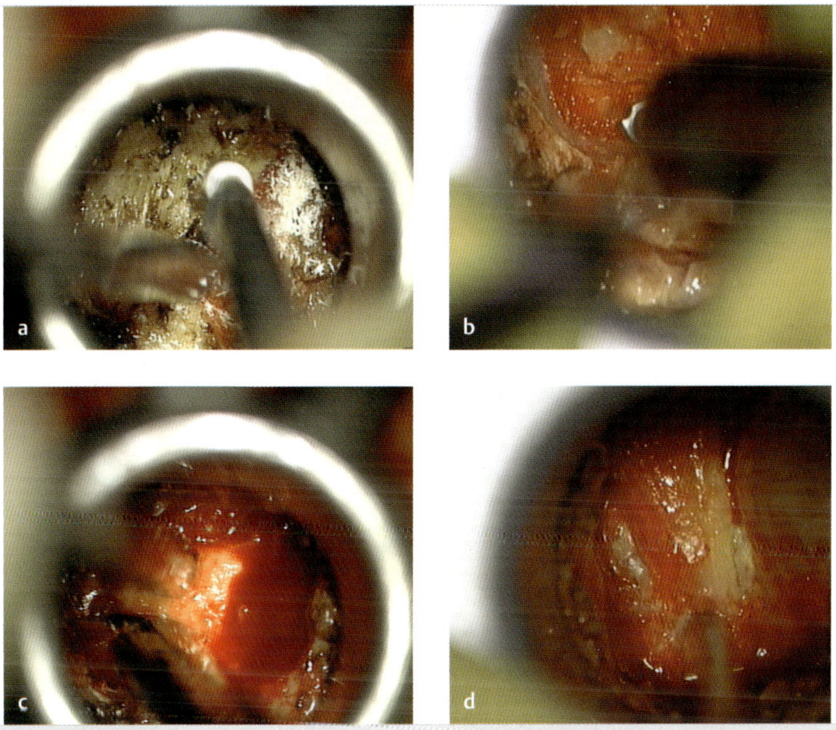

Fig. 19.6 Intraoperative photographs of the ipsilateral laminectomy. Drilling begins within the interlaminar space atop the LF **(a)**. Drilling extends cephalad and caudad until the attachments of the LF are identified **(b, c)**. A Kerrison rongeur is used to complete the cephalad laminectomy to avoid drill injury to the dura **(c)**. Up to 50% of the medial ipsilateral facet can be drilled away to expose LF **(d)**.

atop the LF in the exposed interlaminar space (▶ Fig. 19.6a). By keeping the tip of the drill atop LF and using the side of the drill to remove bone, the dura is protected by the LF (▶ Fig. 19.6b). Safe drilling technique becomes especially crucial at this point. The cranial-caudal drilling should continue until the cranial attachments of the LF are identified, often indicated by epidural fat. We typically extend this a few millimeters cranially, which can be safely performed with a Kerrison rongeur, to expose the dura just cranial to the attachment of LF (▶ Fig. 19.6c). Drilling should continue laterally taking care to not drill more than 50% of the ipsilateral facet (▶ Fig. 19.6d).

Step 7: Contralateral Laminectomy

The tubular retractor should be tilted to aim medially and the operating table should be rotated away from the surgeon to grant the surgeon an appropriate trajectory for the performance of the contralateral decompression (▶ Fig. 19.7a). Drilling should begin at the base of the spinous process and proceed in an ipsilateral-to-contralateral direction. Using the LF and the suction as a protective barrier, the ventral surface of the contralateral lamina is drilled away (▶ Fig. 19.7b). Alternatively, a trough in the ventral lamina can be created, leaving a thin rim of bone atop the LF. This will protect the dura and spinal cord from accidental injury from the drill bit. This rim can then be removed with a straight curette using an upward-oriented force vector, away from the cervical spinal cord.

Step 8: Ligamentum Flavum Resection

A ball-tip probe or blunt nerve hook is used to strip the LF away from its bony attachments (▶ Fig. 19.8a). Epidural fat marks the

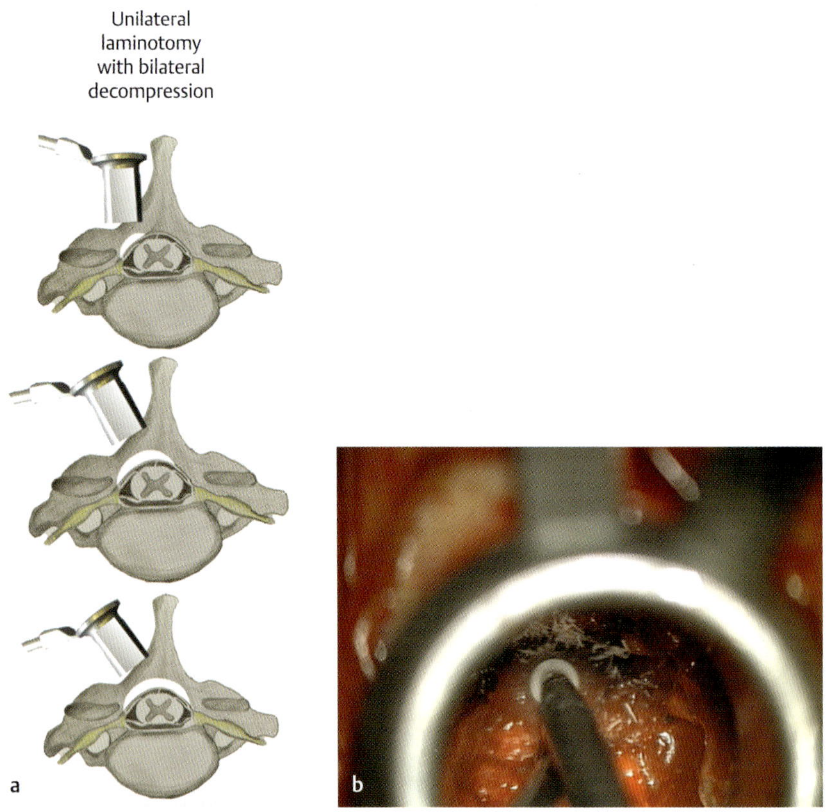

Fig. 19.7 (a) Diagram depicting “wanding” the tubular retractor medially to perform the over-the-top contralateral decompression. (b) Intraoperative photograph demonstrating drilling of the contralateral lamina.

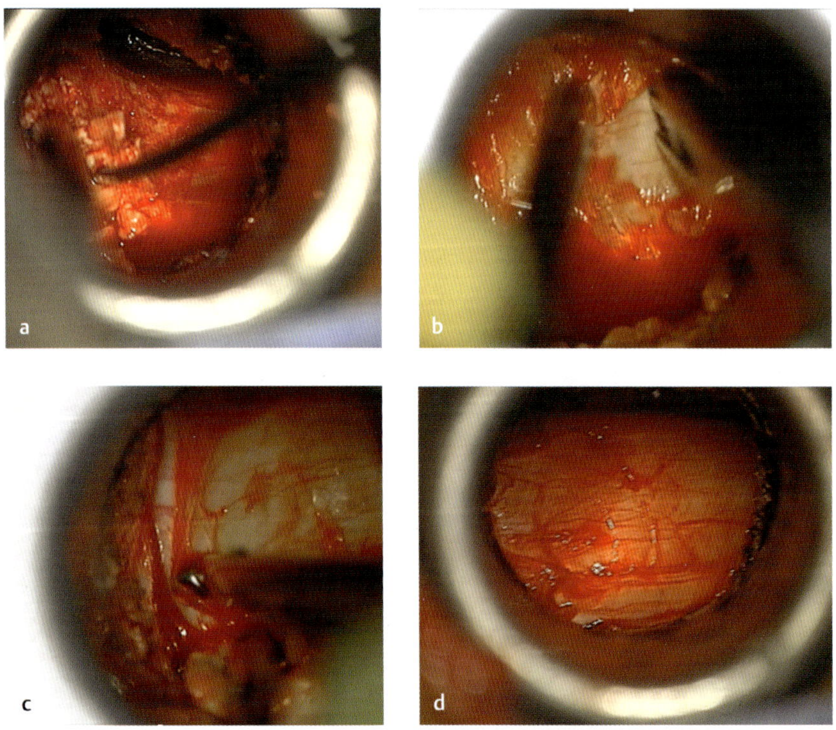

Fig. 19.8 Intraoperative photographs demonstrating resection of the LF. (a) A ball-tip probe is used to strip the LF from its bony attachments, creating a plane between dura and LF. (b) Kerrison rongeurs are used to resect the LF. (c) Taking time to create a plan between LF and dura reduces the risk of durotomy. (d) The final decompression demonstrating complete resection of the LF.

midline between the two leaves of the LF. Once the LF has been mobilized away from its attachments, Kerrison rongeurs are used to resect the LF (▶ Fig. 19.8b). Care must be taken to avoid downward pressure and avoid dural injury while performing this resection. The contralateral decompression is the step, during the procedure, at greatest risk for obtaining a cerebrospinal fluid (CSF) leak. Taking time to create a plane between LF and dura with the probe will help decrease the risk of CSF leak (▶ Fig. 19.8c). For a successful decompression, always identify the insertions of the LF in every direction (cranial, caudal, and lateral) and avoid drilling beyond those landmarks.

Step 9: Inspect Decompression

Once the LF has been resected, the surgeon should inspect the decompression by tilting the tubular retractor in all directions (▶ Fig. 19.8d). The contralateral decompression should extend to the medial border of the contralateral pedicle. This can be confirmed with direct palpation, fluoroscopy, or computer-assisted navigation.

19.5.4 Closure

Step 10: Hemostasis and Closure

Strict hemostasis should be achieved using bipolar electrocautery and hemostatic agents. The tubular retractor should slowly be removed and any soft-tissue bleeding should be addressed. The fascial layer is reapproximated. The deep dermal layer is then reapproximated with buried knots and the skin surface is closed with a subcuticular running stitch (▶ Fig. 19.9). If hemostasis is inadequate or the patient is at elevated risk for a postoperative hematoma, a subfascial drain should be placed, however this is rarely necessary.

19.6 Postoperative Care

- Patients are observed in the hospital overnight and discharged within 23 hours of surgery.

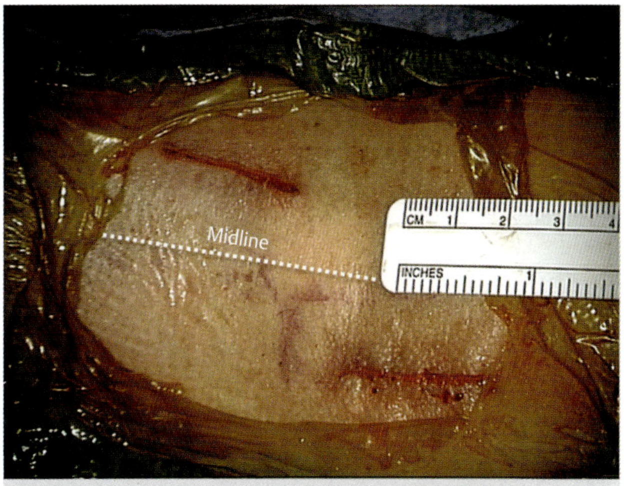

Fig. 19.9 Intraoperative photograph depicting the skin incisions at closure.

- A postoperative CT with sagittal and coronal reconstructions for use as a baseline study for future follow-up is recommended.
- After the stitches are removed at 2 weeks postoperatively, isometric exercises are recommended. In addition, analgesic, anti-inflammatory physical therapy is prescribed, including ultrasound, transcutaneous electrical nerve stimulation, and anti-inflammatory subtle massage.
- Patients are instructed to follow-up at 2 weeks, 6 weeks, and 1 year postoperatively.

19.7 Complication Avoidance

While there are few reports in the literature on minimally invasive cervical laminectomy, the complication rates that are reported are low ranging from 0 to 6.5%.[10,11,12,13,14,15] The following section summarizes methods to avoid potential complications.

19.7.1 Patient Selection

The most important factor associated with complications in the vast majority of spine surgeries is patient selection. Appropriate patient selection for minimally invasive over-the-top cervical laminectomy should take into account the indications and contraindications discussed above. Patients should have adequate cervical lordosis, be expected to have adequate decompression of the spinal cord with a posterior release, and most importantly, have clinical symptoms/findings that match the radiographic findings.

19.7.2 Intraoperative Neuromonitoring

Although in our experience neurological complications with the procedure are rare, IOM allows for the real-time detection of neurologic injury. Theoretically, overly aggressive shoulder taping could result in a brachial plexopathy which could be detected with IOM and treated with release of shoulder countertraction.[18] If during the procedure IOM detects signal decrease, the surgeon may explore intraoperatively to identify the cause, such as kinking of the cervical cord on adjacent levels or epidural hematoma.

19.7.3 No Kirschner Wires

We strongly advise against the use of Kirschner wires during the approach. The risk of injury to the cervical dura, spinal cord, and/or spinal nerve roots is not insignificant.[19] We rather encourage surgeons to use blunt dissection to create a plane through the cervical musculature which allows the surgeon to dock on the cervical lamina under direct visualization and helps limit the amount of muscle bleeding.

19.7.4 Avoid Downward Pressure

It is imperative for the surgeon to be aware of and avoid downward pressure on the cervical spinal cord throughout the procedure. The lack of attention to this technical detail can result in devastating consequences. Hand ergonomics are crucial for

surgeon comfort and for the avoidance of mechanical trauma to the neurologic structures, as well as for proper drilling of the bone. The hand should rest on the patient with the shaft of the drill resting on the edge of the tubular retractor. This stabilizes the hand and drill and allows for safe and controlled drilling.

19.7.5 Hemostasis

Careful attention to hemostasis is required to avoid the complication of postoperative hematoma and the devastating neurologic injury that can result. Prior to removal of the tubular retractor, ensure venous epidural bleeding is controlled with the use of hemostatic agents, gentle pressure, and time. Bony bleeding can be controlled with thrombin gelatin foam or bone wax. The tubular retractor should be removed slowly under direct visualization, and any soft-tissue bleeding noted upon retractor removal should be addressed immediately. If adequate hemostasis is unable to be achieved or if there is a higher-than-normal risk for postoperative hematoma (e.g., aspirin use, pre-existing coagulopathy, etc.), a subfascial drain should be left in place and can be removed the following day if the output is low.

19.7.6 Cerebrospinal Fluid Leak

As in lumbar decompression via tubular retractor, accidental durotomy with CSF leak is a potential complication of minimally invasive cervical laminectomy.[11] We find that the contralateral LF resection is the step during the procedure at greatest risk for obtaining a CSF leak. Taking time to create a plane between LF and dura with the probe will help decrease the risk of CSF leak. If CSF leak does occur, there are a number of methods for management. If the durotomy is accessible, a primary repair can be attempted with a minimally invasive dural closure set.[20] If primary repair is not feasible, gelatin foam or dural substitute can be placed atop the durotomy followed by fibrin sealant. If immediate cessation of CSF egress is not achieved intraoperatively, one should consider immediate placement of a lumbar drain with 3 to 5 days of external CSF diversion.

19.8 Tips and Tricks

19.8.1 Tilting

Moving the tubular retractor, or tilting, medially is necessary in order to change one's working trajectory and facilitate the over-the-top contralateral laminectomy (▶ Fig. 19.7a). In addition, the tubular retractor should be tilted cranial and caudad in order to identify the attachments of the LF after drilling and after the decompression is completed in order to inspect the adequacy of decompression.

19.8.2 Tilting the Bed

While performing the ipsilateral laminectomy, the table should be in a neutral position. Once the surgeon is ready to perform the contralateral laminectomy, the bed should be rotated away from the surgeon to improve the surgical view and working trajectory. In combination with tilting the tubular retractor, this provides the surgeon with an appropriate working trajectory.

19.8.3 "Slalom" Technique

If more than one level is to be addressed, a "slalom" technique can be utilized wherein the laminectomies are approached from alternating sides (▶ Fig. 19.10).[21] This technique has multiple advantages. First, approaching the subsequent laminectomy from the opposite side eliminates the risk of passing the dilator into the newly created laminectomy defect, therefore decreasing the risk of iatrogenic cervical spine injury. Second, performing laminectomies from opposite sides theoretically results in less destabilization, a key principle of MISS. Finally, if there are two experienced MISS surgeons and microscopes available, the "slalom" technique allows two surgeons to work simultaneously, thus decreasing operative time.

19.8.4 Start Big and Using a Diamond Drill Bit

We typically use a 17- or 18-mm tubular retractor to perform the decompression, which is sufficient to achieve the goal of surgery. Initially, surgeons may find it easier to begin with a larger 20-mm diameter tubular retractor and can downsize once they have become comfortable with the procedure.

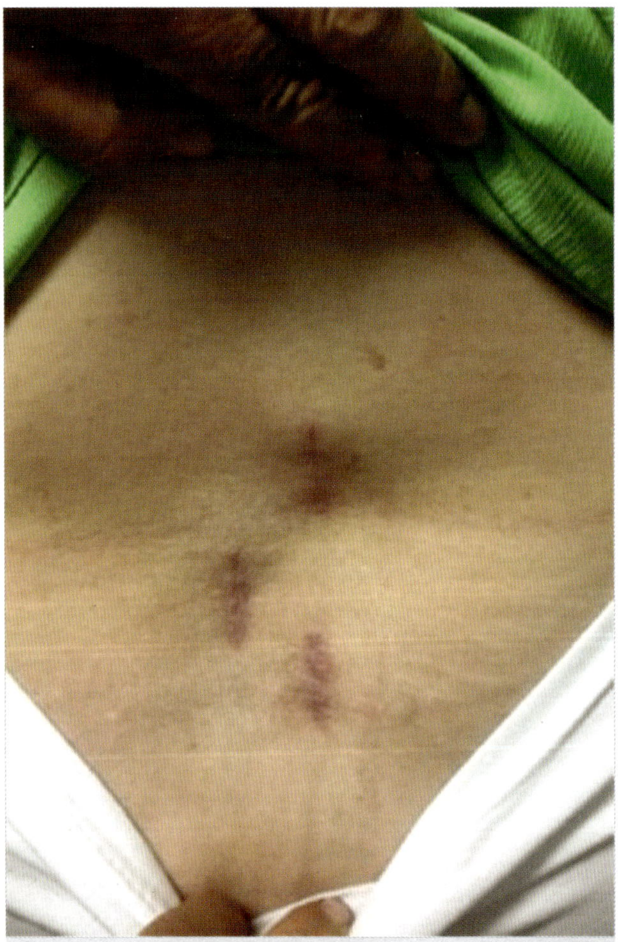

Fig. 19.10 Postoperative image showing healed scars from alternating incisions in the lumbar spine. Same distribution is observed in the cervical spine approach (▶ Fig. 19.9).

19.9 Conclusion

CSM is a common disorder of the cervical spine, associated with the normal aging process and resultant degenerative changes. Cervical stenosis occurs as a result of anterior compression from disc bulges and osteophyte formation and/or posterior compression from facet and LF hypertrophy. Surgical approaches for the treatment of CSM include anterior approach, such as anterior cervical discectomy and fusion, and posterior approach, such as traditional open laminectomy or laminoplasty. Open posterior surgery requires dissection of the cervical musculature away from the posterior bony elements and, with laminectomy, requires removal of the posterior tension band. This can result in the development of postoperative kyphotic deformity necessitating secondary fusion. The minimally invasive cervical laminectomy preserves the posterior muscle attachments and the posterior tension band, and requires less bony removal than open techniques. The hypothesized effect of this minimally disruptive approach is a decreased rate of postlaminectomy kyphosis compared with open laminectomy. This, in turn, may result in a lower rate of secondary fusion following minimally invasive cervical laminectomy.

The presented step-by-step technique provides a reference guide for surgeons wishing to undertake this approach for the treatment of CSM. The learning curve associated with surgery through tubular retractors can be challenging to overcome and requires patience and adequate education. Abiding by the four Ts presented earlier in this book will facilitate the successful performance of MISS techniques. Importantly, patient selection (target) remains a critical factor for the clinical success of MISS and a significant amount of time must be spent with the patient during history and physical examination, as well as careful review of the imaging studies with correlation to clinical findings. With these concepts in mind, unilateral tubular over-the-top cervical laminectomy can be a safe and effective technique for the minimally invasive spine surgeon to add to his or her armamentarium.

References

[1] Brain WR, Northfield D, Wilkinson M. The neurological manifestations of cervical spondylosis. Brain. 1952; 75(2):187–225

[2] Geck MJ, Eismont FJ. Surgical options for the treatment of cervical spondylotic myelopathy. Orthop Clin North Am. 2002; 33(2):329–348

[3] Bakhsheshian J, Mehta VA, Liu JC. Current diagnosis and management of cervical spondylotic myelopathy. Global Spine J. 2017; 7(6):572–586

[4] Riew KD, Raich AL, Dettori JR, Heller JG. Neck pain following cervical laminoplasty: does preservation of the C2 muscle attachments and/or C7 matter? Evid Based Spine Care J. 2013; 4(1):42–53

[5] Oppenheimer JH, DeCastro I, McDonnell DE. Minimally invasive spine technology and minimally invasive spine surgery: a historical review. Neurosurg Focus. 2009; 27(3):E9

[6] Spetzger U, Bertalanffy H, Reinges MHT, Gilsbach JM. Unilateral laminotomy for bilateral decompression of lumbar spinal stenosis. Part II: clinical experiences. Acta Neurochir (Wien). 1997; 139(5):397–403

[7] Guiot BH, Khoo LT, Fessler RG. A minimally invasive technique for decompression of the lumbar spine. Spine. 2002; 27(4):432–438

[8] Khoo LT, Fessler RG. Microendoscopic decompressive laminotomy for the treatment of lumbar stenosis. Neurosurgery. 2002; 51 Suppl 5:S146–S154

[9] Palmer S, Turner R, Palmer R. Bilateral decompressive surgery in lumbar spinal stenosis associated with spondylolisthesis: unilateral approach and use of a microscope and tubular retractor system. Neurosurg Focus. 2002; 13(1):E4

[10] Dahdaleh NS, Wong AP, Smith ZA, Wong RH, Lam SK, Fessler RG. Microendoscopic decompression for cervical spondylotic myelopathy. Neurosurg Focus. 2013; 35(1):E8

[11] Abbas SF, Spurgas MP, Szewczyk BS, Yim B, Ata A, German JW. A comparison of minimally invasive posterior cervical decompression and open anterior cervical decompression and instrumented fusion in the surgical management of degenerative cervical myelopathy. Neurosurg Focus. 2016; 40(6):E7

[12] Hur JW, Kim JS, Shin MH, Ryu KS. Minimally invasive posterior cervical decompression using tubular retractor: the technical note and early clinical outcome. Surg Neurol Int. 2014; 5:34

[13] Chung HJ, Hur JW, Ryu KS, Kim JS, Seong JH. Clinical outcomes of minimally invasive posterior cervical decompression using a tubular retractor for the treatment of cervical spondylotic myelopathy: single-center experience with a minimum 12-month follow-up. Nerve. 2016; 2:48–53

[14] Minamide A, Yoshida M, Simpson AK, et al. Microendoscopic laminotomy versus conventional laminoplasty for cervical spondylotic myelopathy: 5-year follow-up study. J Neurosurg Spine. 2017; 27(4):403–409

[15] Vergara P. Minimally invasive microscopic posterior cervical decompression: simple, safe, and effective. J Neurol Surg A Cent Eur Neurosurg. 2017; 78 (5):440–445

[16] Wang T, Han C, Jiang H, Tian P. The effect of obesity on clinical outcomes after minimally invasive spine surgery of the spine: a systematic review and meta-analysis. World Neurosurg. 2017; 106:790–805

[17] Avila MJ, Walter CM, Baaj AA. Outcomes and complications of minimally invasive surgery of the lumbar spine in the elderly. Cureus. 2016; 8(3):e519

[18] Than KD, Mummaneni PV, Smith ZA, et al. Brachial plexopathy after cervical spine surgery. Global Spine J. 2017; 7 Suppl 1:17S–20S

[19] Furuhata R, Nishida M, Morihita M, Yanagimoto S, Tezuka M, Okada E. Migration of a Kirschner wire into the spinal canal: a case report and review of the literature. J Spinal Cord Med. 20 20; 43:272–275– [Epub ahead of print]

[20] Boukebir MA, Berlin CD, Navarro-Ramirez R, et al. Ten-step minimally invasive spine lumbar decompression and dural repair through tubular retractors. Oper Neurosurg (Hagerstown). 2017; 13(2):232–245

[21] Mayer HM, Heider F. "Slalom": microsurgical cross-over decompression for multilevel degenerative lumbar stenosis. BioMed Res Int. 2016; 2016:9074257

20 Posterior Cervical Facet Cages DTRAX

Melissa Meyer, John B. Ferraro, and Rahul V. Shah

Summary

DTRAX posterior cervical facet cages provide a minimally invasive, tissue sparing approach to performing posterior cervical fusion (PCF) surgery without significantly disrupting cervical paraspinal musculature or significantly affecting the posterior tension band. Traditional open PCF surgery with lateral mass fixation has been wrought with postoperative complications, particularly in older patients with multiple comorbidities. One study analyzing 3,401 patients who underwent traditional open PCF surgery with lateral mass screw (LMS) fixation exhibited a 30-day readmission rate of 6.20%.[1] Of these, 4.97% of the patients required a return to the operating room.[1] Postoperative infection was the most common complication in 17.06% patients.[1] DTRAX provides an alternative posterior approach for a select patient population. This innovative, tissue sparing, minimally invasive posterior cervical approach allows for faster recovery time, shorter hospital stay, and negligible blood loss.[2] Furthermore, a 2013 study by McCormack evaluating 60 patients who underwent DTRAX surgery illustrated zero vertebral artery injuries, nerve root injuries, spinal cord injuries, or reoperations.[3] In addition, research has demonstrated that minimally invasive PCF with facet cages yields stability similar to traditional open PCF surgery with LMSs.[4]

Keywords: DTRAX, facet, cages, posterior, cervical, fusion, minimally invasive, tissue, sparing

20.1 Introduction

DTRAX posterior cervical facet cages provide a minimally invasive, tissue sparing approach to performing posterior cervical fusion (PCF) surgery without significantly disrupting cervical paraspinal musculature or significantly affecting the posterior tension band. Traditional open PCF surgery with lateral mass fixation has been wrought with postoperative complications, particularly in older patients with multiple comorbidities.[1] One study analyzing 3,401 patients that underwent traditional open PCF surgery with lateral mass screw (LMS) fixation exhibited a 30-day readmission rate of 6.20%.[1] Of these, 4.97% of the patients required a return to the operating room.[1] Postoperative infection was the most common complication in 17.06% patients.[1] DTRAX provides an alternative posterior approach for a select patient population. This innovative, tissue sparing, minimally invasive posterior cervical approach allows for faster recovery time, shorter hospital stay, and negligible blood loss.[2] Furthermore, a 2013 study by McCormack evaluating 60 patients who underwent DTRAX surgery illustrated zero vertebral artery injuries, nerve root injuries, spinal cord injuries, or reoperations.[3] In addition, research has demonstrated that minimally invasive PCF with facet cages yields similar stability to traditional open PCF surgery with LMSs.[4]

20.2 Indications

- Indicated for C3–C7 levels.
- Foraminal stenosis with radiculopathy that has improved temporarily with injections.
- Facet-mediated pain not responsive to nonoperative measures.
- Pseudoarthrosis.
- Adjunct to multilevel anterior decompression and fusion.
- Adjacent level compromise following prior anterior cervical discectomy and fusion (ACDF).

20.3 Contraindications

- Facet joint tumors or trauma destroying facet joint.
- Active infection.
- Spondylolisthesis greater than grade 1 signifying flexion/extension instability.

20.4 Preoperative Planning

- Utilize neuromonitoring to monitor somatosensory evoked potential, maximum expiratory pressure as indicated.
- Anteroposterior (AP)/lateral cervical radiographs with flexion and extension views to rule out underlying instability.
- Computed tomography (CT) scan to identify extent of facet hypertrophy, facet autofusion, and posterior facet osteophyte complexes.
- CT scan/magnetic resonance imaging will help to determine severity of the foraminal stenosis. These findings will allow the surgeon to determine if it may be more appropriate to perform the DTRAX portion of a staged anterior and posterior fusion first.

20.5 Patient Positioning

- A Skytron/Maquet table typically works best and allows for best flouro access.
- Two blanket rolls or gel rolls are placed under the patient's chest and pelvis.
- Cervical visualization harness is placed on the table prior to positioning the patient. The harness will help to optimize fluoroscopic visualization of the lower cervical levels in larger patients and patients with broad shoulders.
- A tuck sheet is placed at the middle of the table so that the patient's arms may be adequately secured by the patient's side.
- Wrist restraints are placed at the foot of the table. These will be used to gently traction the patient's arms and further pull the shoulders out of the field of view (▸ Fig. 20.1).
- The patient is placed in the prone position with a foam face pillow.
- The patient's head is gently taped to the bed to minimize intraoperative rotation.
- The wrist restraints are secured and tractioned. The arms are tucked at the patient's side. The shoulder harness is tractioned and secured at the foot of the bed.

- The knees should be bent with legs flexed. Note that this maneuver will loosen the wrist restraint traction. You must again increase the traction on the wrist restraints once the legs have been flexed. Intraoperatively you may now use the bed control to further extend the knees and traction shoulders out of the field of view.
- The patient is placed in slight reverse Trendelenburg to accentuate the point of cervical flexion and allow for better access.

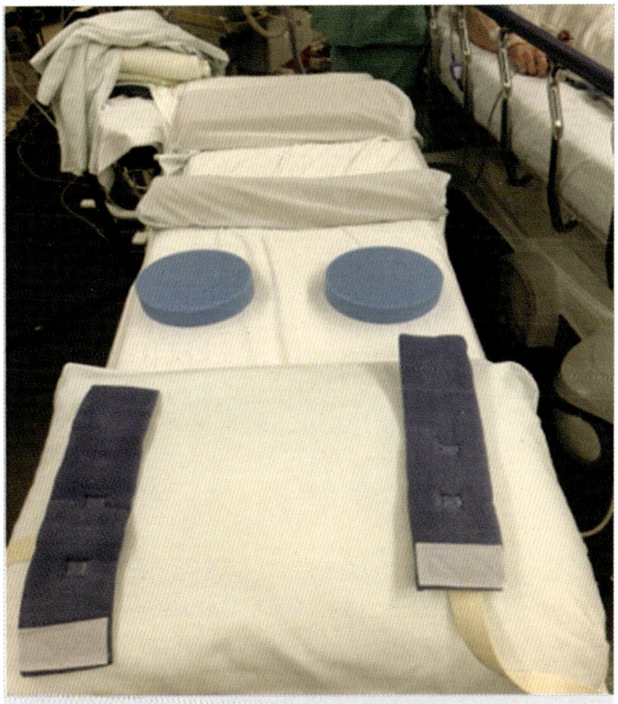

Fig. 20.1 Intraoperative table setup for patient position demonstrating chest and pelvis rolls, foam pads for the knees, and wrist restraints attached distally to allow for traction.

- At this point, the two C-arms are brought into position. One is placed at the head of the table for AP view and the other comes in laterally (▶ Fig. 20.2).
- Once the C-arms are in position, take initial lateral C-arm shots to assess for adequate visualization of the appropriate levels.

20.6 Surgical Technique

- Obtain clear imaging.
- Identify and optimize the lateral view first (▶ Fig. 20.3a):
  - Utilize the table tilt in order to superimpose the facet joints.
  - If necessary, wag the C-arm in order to better visualize the facet clear space.
- Identify and optimize the AP view (▶ Fig. 20.3b):
  - If the lateral view is precise, then the AP view should be crisp and well aligned at 90 degrees.
  - If there is a need to tilt the C-arm on the AP view, then this implies either a cervical scoliotic deformity or a suboptimal lateral view.
- Identify and optimize the on-fos view (▶ Fig. 20.3c):
  - This view is obtained by orienting the C-arm for the AP view in line with the angle and orientation of the facet joints. This is approximately 64 ± 6 degrees off the axial plane[5] (▶ Fig. 20.2c).
  - The on-fos view is considered to be the most reliable radiographic view utilized in this case.
  - It is easy to get thrown off with straight AP and lateral views. Always confirm the location of the instrumentation by assessing the on-fos view.
- Once clear imaging has been obtained, mark out the landmarks for the medial and lateral aspect of the facet using fluoro and a marking stick.
- Next the patient is prepped and draped in routine fashion. Be sure to prep and drape out the patient's lumbosacral region as well if electing to obtain autograft from the patient's iliac crest. Local anesthetic is injected (▶ Video 20.1).

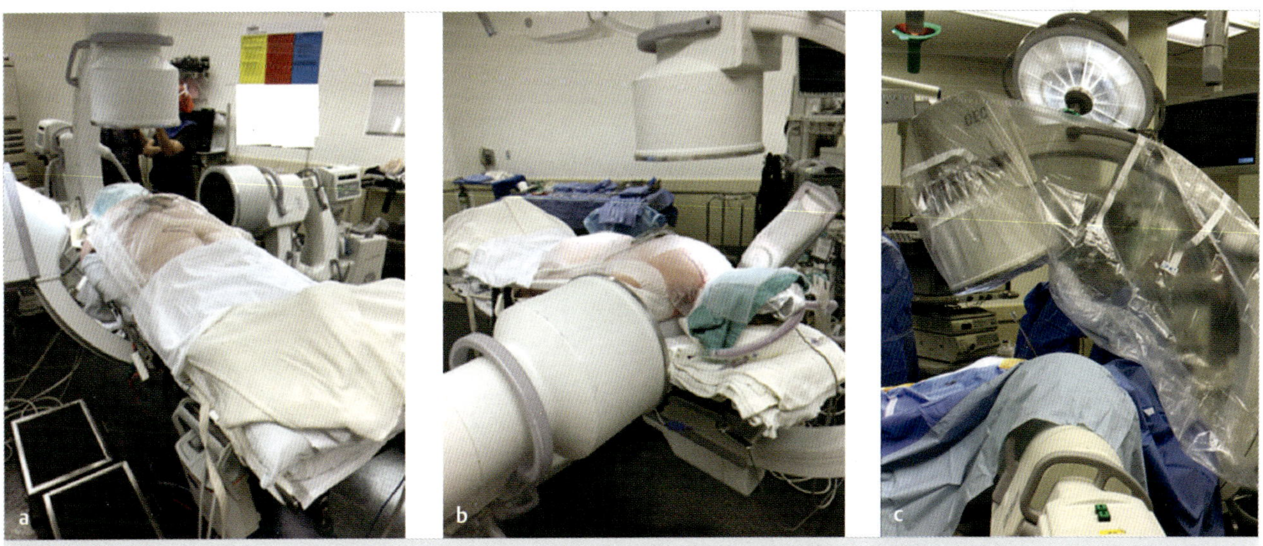

Fig. 20.2 Fluoroscopy C-arm positioning (a, b) in orthogonal orientation. (c) C-arm position to obtain the on-fos view.

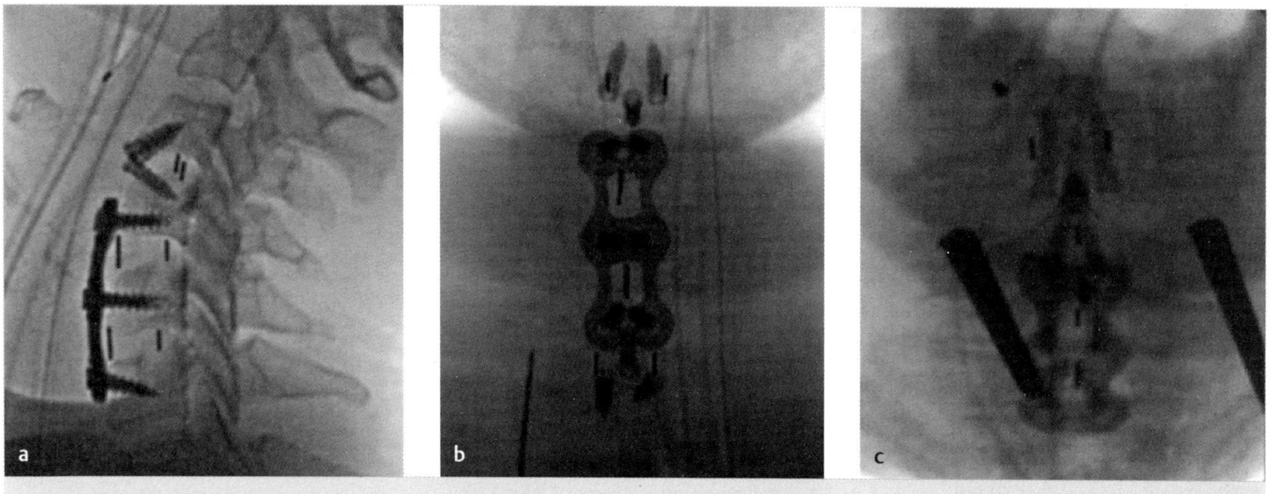

Fig. 20.3 Intraoperative fluoroscopy with desired **(a)** lateral, **(b)** anteroposterior, and **(c)** on-fos views. A spinal needle aligned with the midpoint of the facet may also be seen in **(b)**.

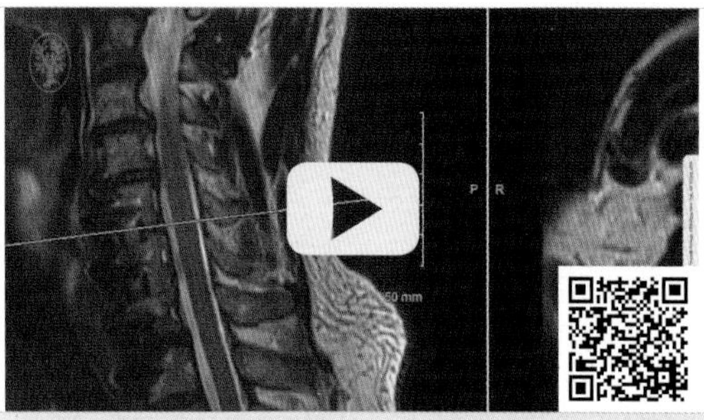

Video 20.1 This video demonstrates steps for the DTRAX procedure, beginning with room setup. Patient positioning and C-arm set up is shown. The step-by-step procedure for DTRAX placement is then reviewed.

- Step 1: Autograft harvest (if necessary)
  - If you have elected to obtain autograft from the patient's iliac crest, it is best to get this done first. Utilize a bone-harvesting device to obtain the autograft material. On the back table mix the autograft with allograft, if necessary. This graft material will then be used to fill the implants.
- Step 2: Targeting and incision
  - It is important to target the appropriate levels before making the incision. This is best achieved by utilizing a spinal needle and fluoroscopy. It is best practice to make the incision about two levels or two fingerbreadths inferior to the target level. A spinal needle is advanced toward the midpoint of the facet on the AP view (▶ Fig. 20.3b) and toward the inferior tip of the facet on the lateral view. Once this has been achieved, the first incision is made along the same trajectory as the spinal needle (▶ Fig. 20.4a–c).
- Step 3: Accessing the facet
  - Introduce the access chisel in line with the muscle fibers in order to make a vertical path through the thoracodorsal fascia.
  - Utilize AP and lateral fluoroscopy while approaching the facet joint. Rotate the access chisel so that it is collinear with the facet joint (▶ Fig. 20.5a).
  - It is important that the access chisel enter into the facet joint in a medial to lateral trajectory. The goal is to position the chisel more toward the lateral aspect of the facet joint. Once in the joint, confirm that there is medial facet clear space with on-fos imaging (▶ Fig. 20.5b).
  - In addition, confirm that the tip of the chisel is at the anterior margin of the superior articular facet with lateral imaging (▶ Fig. 20.5c).
- Step 4: Decortication of the facet joint capsule
  - Once the access chisel is in position, the chisel handle is removed to allow the decortication trephine to slide down over the chisel and onto the facet (▶ Fig. 20.6).
  - Decorticate the joint capsule using the trephine.
  - While decorticating, work on the inferior and superior facet joints deliberately with no medial or lateral decortication as this will displace the orientation of the access chisel.
  - Once decortication is complete the trephine is removed.
- Step 5: Guide tube placement
  - Introduce the guide tube/working cannula over access chisel such that medial clear space is maintained and the anterior margin of superior articular facet is respected.
  - The guide tube is then advanced into the facet joint utilizing the fork mallet.
  - Evaluate the depth of the guide tube within the facet by assessing the small notches at the base of the guide tube prongs.
- Step 6: Decortication of the facet joint surface
  - The access chisel is then removed and the guide tube is left in place within the facet joint.
  - If the guide tube is still proud relative to the facet joint, use the flat-tipped rasp to advance the guide tube further into the joint. If the guide tube does appear to have adequate depth within the facet joint, you may skip the flat-tipped rasp and go directly to the next step (▶ Fig. 20.7a).
  - Ream out the inside of the facet joint using the pineapple-tipped decortication bur (▶ Fig. 20.7b).
- Step 7: Implant/cage preparation and delivery
  - The burr is removed.

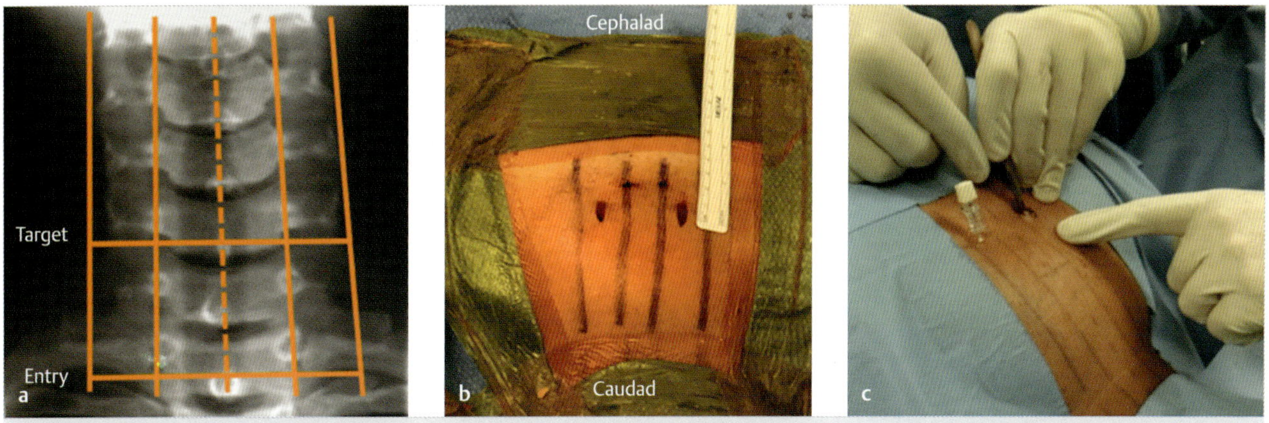

Fig. 20.4 X-ray and clinical images depicting **(a)** medial and lateral aspects of the facets with entry level, two levels below target level; **(b)** intraoperative image of medial and lateral facet markings and skin incisions with ruler to demonstrate incision size; and **(c)** spinal needle used to asses trajectory prior to incision and subsequent incision in line with that trajectory.

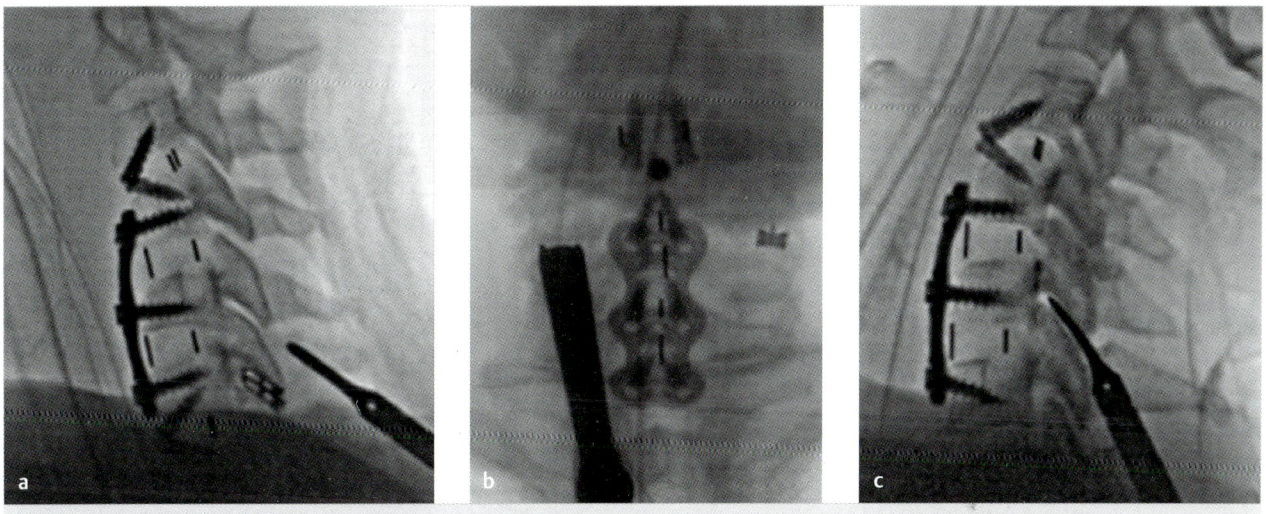

Fig. 20.5 Intraoperative fluoroscopy demonstrating **(a)** the chisel rotated collinear with the facet joint on the lateral view, **(b)** medial facet clear space seen on the on-fos view, **(c)** the tip of the chisel at the anterior margin of the facet on lateral view.

- The cage should be filled with graft material prior to delivery.
- Deliver the appropriately sized implant. Remember to identify the orientation of the facet screw prior to insertion. There is a small arrow on the implant delivery device indicating the direction of the facet screw. Direct it superiorly or inferiorly, as the patient's anatomy dictates.
- Assess the depth of the implant prior to unlocking it from the delivery system device. Once appropriate depth has been achieved, unlock the implant.

- Step 8: Locking screw placement
  - Introduce the bone screw through locking mechanism. Reorient hand such that the screw trajectory is divergent from the cage trajectory. The bone screw acts to lock the implant into the inferior articular facet (▶ Fig. 20.8).
- Step 9: Bone graft insertion
  - After the locking screw has been placed, the screw delivery system is removed and the guide tube is left in place within the facet joint.

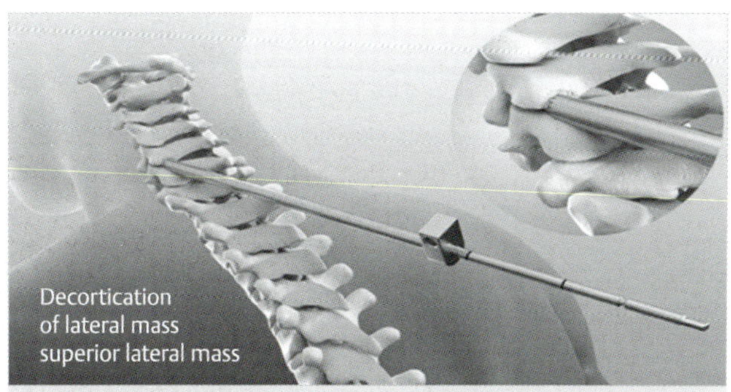

Fig. 20.6 The trephine is advanced over the access chisel in order to decorticate the lateral mass. (Used with permission from Providence Medical Technology.)

  - Deliver some of the bone graft material through the guide tube. Utilize the tamp to deliver the graft down the guide tube and into the joint (▶ Fig. 20.9).
  - The guide tube and tamp are removed.

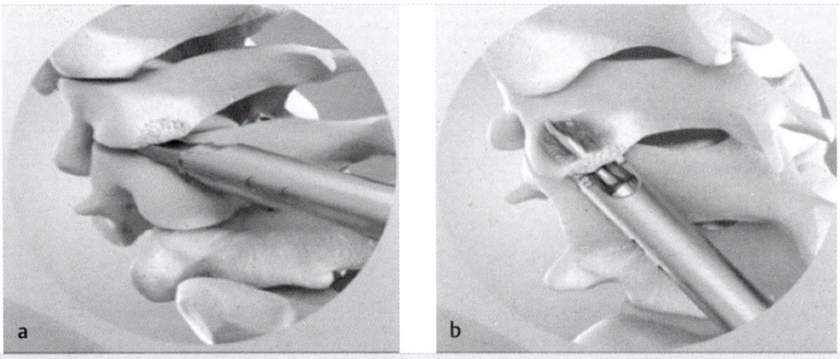

Fig. 20.7 Decortication of the facet joint is achieved utilizing the (a) flat-tipped rasp and (b) decortication burr. (Used with permission from Providence Medical Technology.)

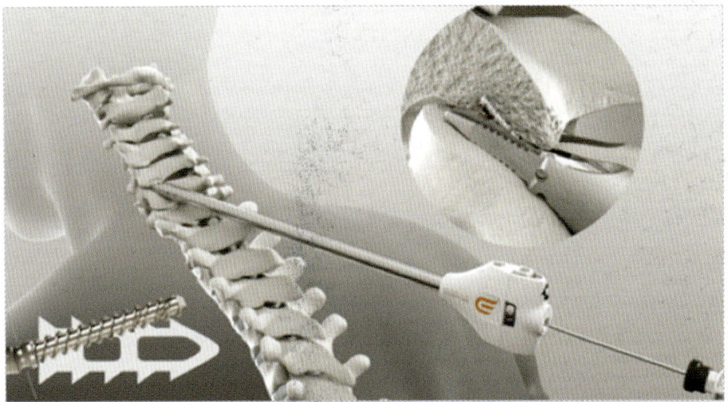

Fig. 20.8 Superiorly directed locking screw can be seen diverging from the cage trajectory. (Used with permission from Providence Medical Technology.)

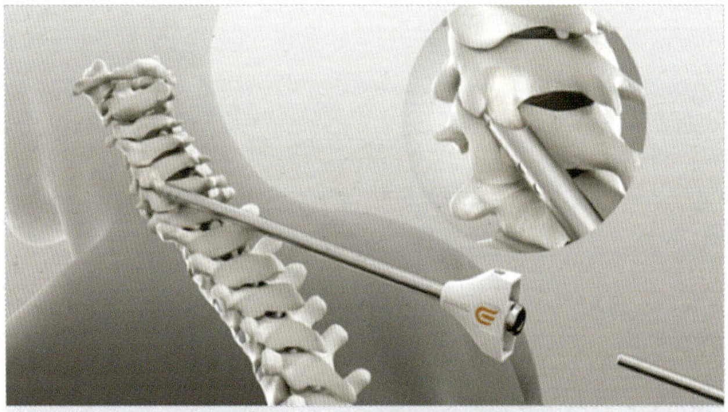

Fig. 20.9 Bone graft is delivered through the guide tube and advanced using the tamp. (Used with permission from Providence Medical Technology.)

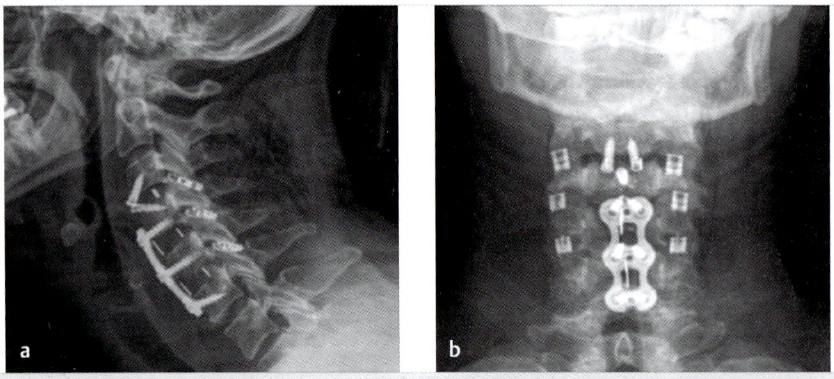

Fig. 20.10 (a) Lateral and (b) anteroposterior postoperative radiographs demonstrating a patient status post-C3–C6 anterior cervical discectomy and fusion and subsequent DTRAX placement.

- Step 10: Irrigation, closure, and final radiographs
  - Irrigate and close skin incisions in layered fashion. Obtain final radiographs (▶ Fig. 20.10).

20.7 Postoperative Care

- Multilevel DTRAX surgery, when done alone without concurrent ACDF, can oftentimes be done outpatient.
- Can immediately collar or brace for 2 to 4 weeks depending on preference.
- Begin isometric neck strengthening exercises in 2 to 4 weeks.
- Begin formalized therapy if/when warranted.
- Avoid any anti-inflammatory medications for 3 months postoperatively.
- Patient follow-up at 2, 4, and 8 to 10 weeks; 14 to 16 weeks; 6 months; and 1 year postoperative.

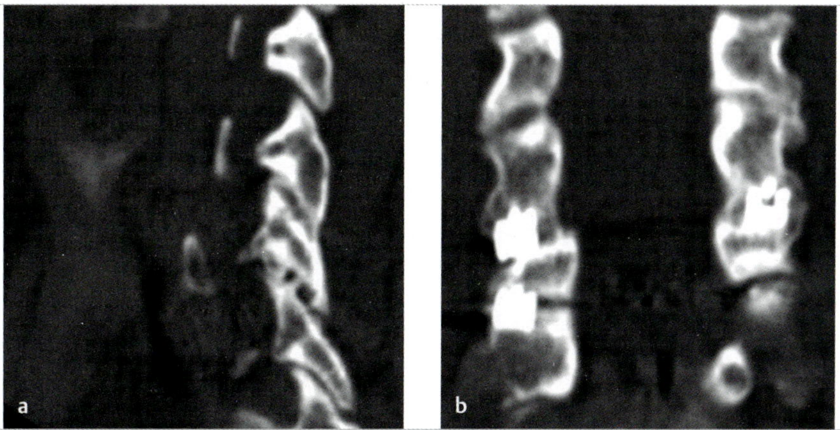

Fig. 20.11 Sagittal **(a)** and coronal **(b)** cuts of a postoperative computed tomography scan demonstrating fusion around the DTRAX construct.

- Monitor facet joint arthrodesis with routine cervical radiographs. May also obtain postop CT scan to further assess arthrodesis if warranted (▶ Fig. 20.11).

20.8 Complications and Avoidance

- Medial positioning of implants can result in nerve root injury:
  - Remember to check the on-fos imaging throughout the case in order to ensure medial to lateral position of the implant, and to confirm the presence of facet medial clear space.
  - Utilize a medial to lateral trajectory while advancing the instrumentation into the facet joint.
- Patient with significant flexion/extension instability.

20.9 Tips and Tricks

- When positioning the patient's head, not having any significant cervical deformity, ensure that ears and shoulders are level with one another.
- Using the shoulder harness in larger patients helps to pull the shoulders down and out of the way for optimal radiographic visualization.
- Tape the head gently to the table to help stabilize it and avoid intraoperative rotation.
- On-fos view:
  - Useful in assessing medial clear space within the facet joint.
  - In patients with dental implants, it helps to use the on-fos view to visualize above and below the implant and confirm placement of the instrumentation.
- Start on one side and if unable to gain access into the facet joint, attempting to access the contralateral side first may help.
- Establishing clear fluoroscopy on AP, lateral, and on-fos views is imperative:
  - May need to wag the C-arm and table tilt in order to achieve optimal, clear imaging of the facet joints.
  - When performing a multilevel posterior fusion, it may be difficult to superimpose all of the adjacent facet joints and visualize the facet clear space at consecutive levels.
  - If you run into this problem, it is best practice to optimize visualization at the most inferior level first, then adjust while working caudal to cranial utilizing the bed controls as necessary.

References

[1] Choy W, Lam SK, Smith ZA, Dahdaleh NS. Predictors of 30-day hospital readmission after posterior cervical fusion in 3401 patients. Spine. 2018; 43 (5):356–363

[2] Siemionow KB, Glowka P, Blok RJ, et al. Perioperative complications in patients treated with posterior cervical fusion and bilateral cages. J Craniovertebr Junction Spine. 2017; 8(4):342–349

[3] McCormack BM, Bundoc RC, Ver MR, Ignacio JMF, Berven SH, Eyster EF. Percutaneous posterior cervical fusion with the DTRAX facet system for single-level radiculopathy: results in 60 patients. J Neurosurg Spine. 2013; 18 (3):245–254

[4] Voronov LI, Siemionow KB, Havey RM, Carandang G, Patwardhan AG. Biomechanical evaluation of DTRAX(®) posterior cervical cage stabilization with and without lateral mass fixation. Med Devices (Auckl). 2016; 9:285–290

[5] Rong X, Liu Z, Wang B, Chen H, Liu H. The facet orientation of the subaxial cervical spine and the implications for cervical movements and clinical conditions. Spine. 2017; 42(6):E320–E325

21 MIS Endoscopic Approaches for OC–C1–C2 Pathology

Rafael Uribe, Sertac Kirnaz, and Theodore H. Schwartz

Summary

Craniocervical junction is closely related to critical neurovascular structures including the carotid and vertebral arteries, brainstem, and upper spinal cord, as well as critical prevertebral structures including the oropharynx, esophagus, and trachea. Anterior craniocervical pathology is complicated by virtue of the many important anatomic structures that reside in that region. This chapter will illustrate possible anterior MIS approaches to the OC–C1–C2 region. These approaches are: the endoscopic endonasal approach, the transoral approach, and the endoscopic transcervical approach. Each of these have their own indications, advantages, and limitations, but all MISS approaches share the common goal of minimizing local tissue disruption and maximizing effectiveness in a confined working window.

Keywords: anterior cervical spine, craniocervical junction, endoscopic endonasal approach, endoscopic transcervical approach, transoral approach

21.1 Introduction

The craniocervical junction (CCJ) is a highly complex anatomic region. It is closely related to critical neurovascular structures including the carotid and vertebral arteries, brainstem, and upper spinal cord, as well as critical prevertebral structures including the oropharynx, esophagus, and trachea. The CCJ is seat to a myriad of pathologies including primary and metastatic tumors, degenerative and autoimmune spinal diseases, traumatic lesions, infections, and congenital malformations.[1,2,3,4,5] Surgical approaches to this region vary depending on the pathology being addressed but generally fall into two broad categories depending on the anatomic route that is used: anterior and posterior approaches. This chapter will focus on minimally invasive treatment approaches to the ventral CCJ: the endoscopic endonasal approach (EEA), the transoral approach, and the endoscopic transcervical approach.

> Anterior approaches to the craniovertebral junction have undergone significant evolution with the introduction of less invasive open microsurgical techniques using the operating microscope and especially more recently using minimally invasive endoscopic technology.

21.2 Indications

21.2.1 Endoscopic Endonasal Approach

The EEA to the skull base and CCJ is the result of the technological evolution that allowed ear, nose, and throat (ENT) surgeons and neurosurgeons to access the ventral skull base through natural orifices. As suggested in the introduction to the chapter, ventral approaches to the CCJ can address primary extradural (e.g., metastatic tumors, inflammatory conditions,[2] degenerative spine disease, basilar impression),[6,7,8] infections, osteomyelitis, epidural abscess[9,10], or congenital malformations (e.g., retroflexed odontoid),[11] extra- and intradural diseases (e.g., chordomas,[12] chondrosarcomas[13]) or intradural tumors (e.g., brainstem gliomas,[4] epidermoid/dermoid tumors,[14] meningiomas[15]), and vascular lesions.[16,17] The upper limit of this approach is the highest of all approaches, reaching up to the frontal sinus, while the inferior limit is generally the base of the odontoid.

21.2.2 Transoral Approach

The indications for the transoral approach are similar to those mentioned for the EEA.[18,19,20,21] However, a potential advantage of the transoral approach compared with the EEA is the possibility of reaching more lesions. This approach allows limited superior access not only above the odontoid but also the base of C2 and often C3. When further exposure is necessary, the sphenoid and inferior clivus can be accessed cranially through an open-door maxillotomy. However, that approach is invasive and can be replaced by EEAs for rostrally located lesions. C3 and C4 can be exposed via a median transmandibular and transglottic approach.[22,23] The transoral approach is not ideal for patients who have mouth opening limitations (e.g., temporomandibular joint pathologies) or restrictions of cervical spine flexion (e.g., deformity).

21.2.3 Endoscopic Transcervical Approach

The indications for the endoscopic transcervical approach are basilar invagination and atlantoaxial dislocations with high cervical myelopathy.[24,25,26,27] In contrast with the transoral approach, the entire cervical spine can be accessed with this approach with the advantage of a sterile surgical corridor. Obese patients and patients with thoracic abnormalities (such as barrel chest, severe kyphosis) are not suitable for this technique.

21.3 Techniques

21.3.1 Endoscopic Endonasal Approach

The EEA approach to the CCJ proceeds in the same way that is used for other approaches along the sagittal plane of the skull base. Patients are placed in supine position with the head fixed in a Mayfield three-pin head holder.[28] The head is usually rotated approximately 15 degrees in three planes: lateral rotation, lateral tilt, and neck extension. For a conventional approach to the sellar region, the patient's chin will point to the patient's right foot. However, for clivus and craniocervical approaches, the head has to be flexed more than usual in order to provide comfortable visualization. It is our practice for the surgeon to stand on the right side of the patient (i.e., for right-handed surgeons). An endoscope holder is placed on the contralateral side of the bed, opposite from the surgeon. Fiberoptic

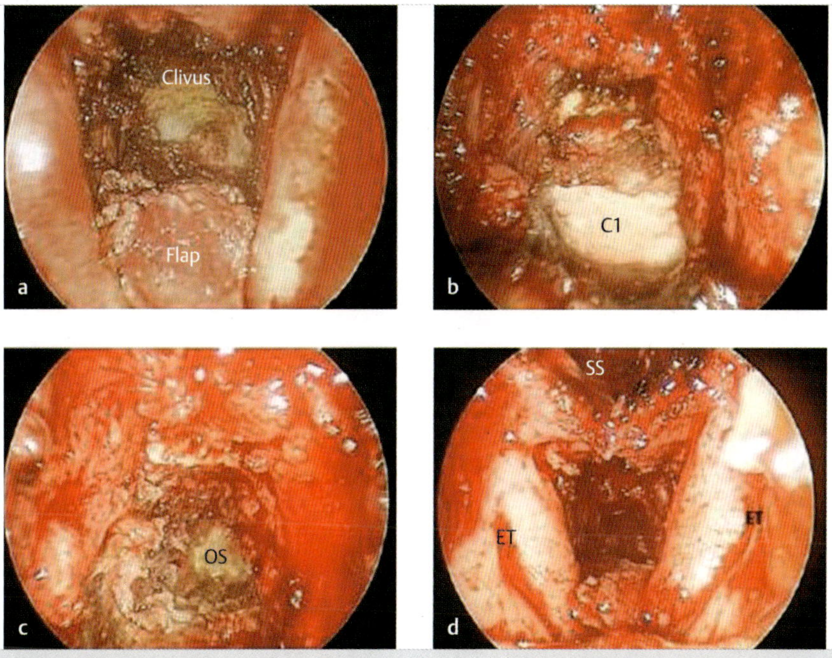

Fig. 21.1 Intraoperative views of an endoscopic endonasal approach for odontiodectomy. **(a)** Intraoperative endoscopic views of the craniovertebral junction demonstrating the clivus and the inferiorly reflected nasopharyngeal mucosal flap. **(b)** Further dissection inferior to the clivus reveals the anterior arch of C1. **(c)** After removal of the anterior arch of C1, an os odontoideum (OS) can be visualized. **(d)** A nonmagnified view demonstrates the sphenoid sinus (SS), the lateral limits of the exposure determined by the Eustachian tubes (ET), and the epidural space after removal of C1 and the odontoid process. (Reproduced from Härtl R and Korge A. Minimally Invasive Spine Surgery: Techniques, Evidence, and Controversies. Thieme, 2012.)

orotracheal intubation is preferred if there is evidence of craniocervical instability. The tube is secured to the left side of the mouth to provide an unobstructed view of the surgical field. Neuromonitoring will be used depending on the type of pathology being addressed; we do not use neuromonitoring for routine extradural cases. Doppler ultrasound and frameless stereotactic navigation are commonly used and become especially relevant to appropriately identify the trajectory of the carotid arteries which may be unusually displaced. Close attention must be paid to the final location of the navigation system reference array. We routinely place it contralateral to the side where the surgeon is standing and make sure it does not obstruct the surgical field. The abdomen is always prepped in the event when a fat graft needs to be harvested for closure. The leg is also prepped for a fascia lata graft in cases where a large intradural opening is expected and there is a chance for a high-flow cerebrospinal fluid (CSF) leak. After registration and surgical site prepping is completed, the nasal phase of the procedure is begun by the ENT surgeon who will harvest a nasoseptal flap if needed at the end of the case for reconstruction. For cases that involve resection of the dens, a vertical incision is made in the basopharyngel fascia in the midline between the Eustachian tubes. Intraoperative computed tomography scanning is a useful adjunct in order to ensure complete resection of the odontoid process.[6] The underlying longus colli and longus capitis muscles are mobilized laterally in order to expose the anterior arch of C1 and the body of C2. Anatomical landmarks are identified including the C1/2 interspace, anterior ring of the atlas, inferior edge of the clivus, and the odontoid process (▶ Fig. 21.1 and ▶ Fig. 21.2). The apical and alar ligaments are sharply divided. A diamond drill may be used with care to avoid any injury to the dura. When the bone has been thinned, pituitary and Kerrison rongeurs can be used to remove the remaining bony elements. If a rheumatoid pannus is present, it must be removed with special care to avoid any injury to the dura. For larger approaches that involve intradural exploration, the pharyngeal mucosa can be incised in an inverted U shape to improve lateral visualization. At the end of the procedure, if there is no CSF leak such as with an odontoid resection, nonabsorbable stitches are placed to reapproximate the mucosa and a bioresorbable nasal dressing is left in place (Nasopore® Stryker Corporation, Kalamazoo, MI). If there is a small leak, fat can be placed over the defect and covered with fibrin glue before closing the mucosa. If a large CSF leak occurs as a result of removing intradural pathology, a button or gasket seal closure is performed and covered with a nasoseptal flap (▶ Fig. 21.3).[29,30] Temporary lumbar drainage is also often used to decrease pulsatile pressure on the closure.

21.3.2 Transoral Approach

For transoral approaches, the patient is intubated awake with fiberoptic scope assistance via a nasotracheal[20] or orotracheal route.[22] The patient is positioned supine on the operating table, the head is fixed in a three-point Mayfield head holder. The neck is slightly extended, the head is tilted to the contralateral side of the surgeon, and rotated to the ipsilateral side. The chin will point to the patient's right foot, as described above for the EEA. The reference array is attached to the Mayfield head clamp. In order to prevent postoperative swelling, the retractor

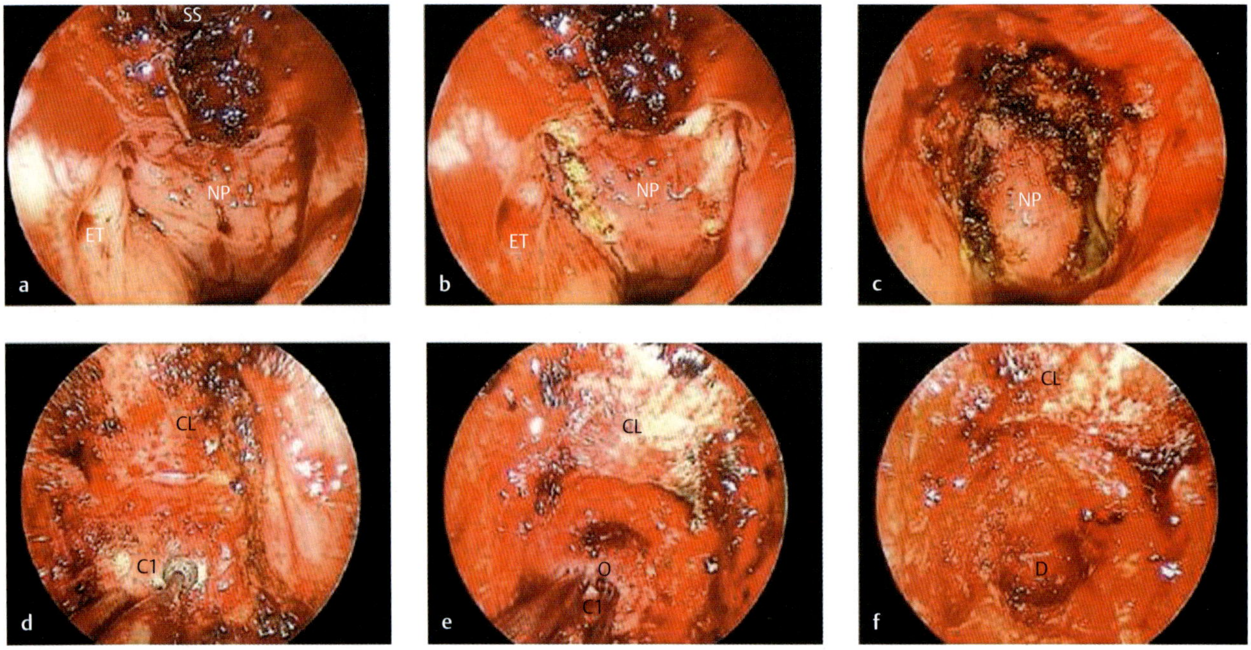

Fig. 21.2 Intraoperative endoscopic views of the endoscopic endonasal approach to the craniovertebral junction. **(a)** Endoscopic view after exposure of the sphenoid sinus (SS) with identification of the Eustachian tube (ET) and the nasopharyngeal (NP) mucosa. **(b, c)** The NP mucosa is incised in a U-shaped flap with the lateral limits demarcated by the opening of the ET. **(d)** After inferior reflection of the mucosal flap, the clivus (CL) and anterior arch of C1 are identified. **(e)** After removing the anterior arch of C1 and the surrounding ligamentous attachments at the top, the odontoid process (O) is identified. **(f)** Further drilling of the arch of C1 reveals the body of the dens (D) at the bottom of the exposure. (Reproduced from Härtl R and Korge A. Minimally Invasive Spine Surgery: Techniques, Evidence, and Controversies. Thieme, 2012.)

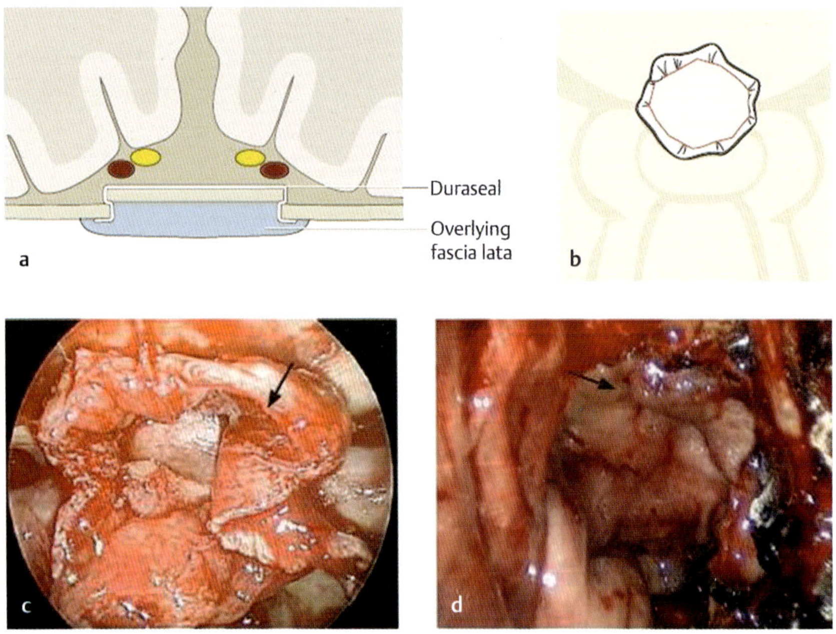

Fig. 21.3 **(a)** A coronal view of suprasellar contents and closure of the skull base defect with a gasket seal alone. The countersunk rigid buttress is cut to a size slightly larger than the skull base defect and countersunk with overlying fascia lata for a watertight seal. A final layer of DuraSeal is applied to hold the construct in position to ensure a watertight closure. **(b)** Illustration of a gasket-seal closure similar to **(c)**. **(c)** Intraoperative view of a gasket-seal reconstruction of the skull base. Note the large margin of overhanging fascia lata (*black arrow*) and the countersunk bone. **(d)** Intraoperative view shows a rotated nasoseptal flap (*black arrow*) secured in a place over a gasket-seal closure. The edges of the nasoseptal flap are secured in place with dural sealant material to hold the flap in position over the gasket-seal closure. (Reproduced from Härtl R and Korge A. Minimally Invasive Spine Surgery: Techniques, Evidence, and Controversies. Thieme, 2012.)

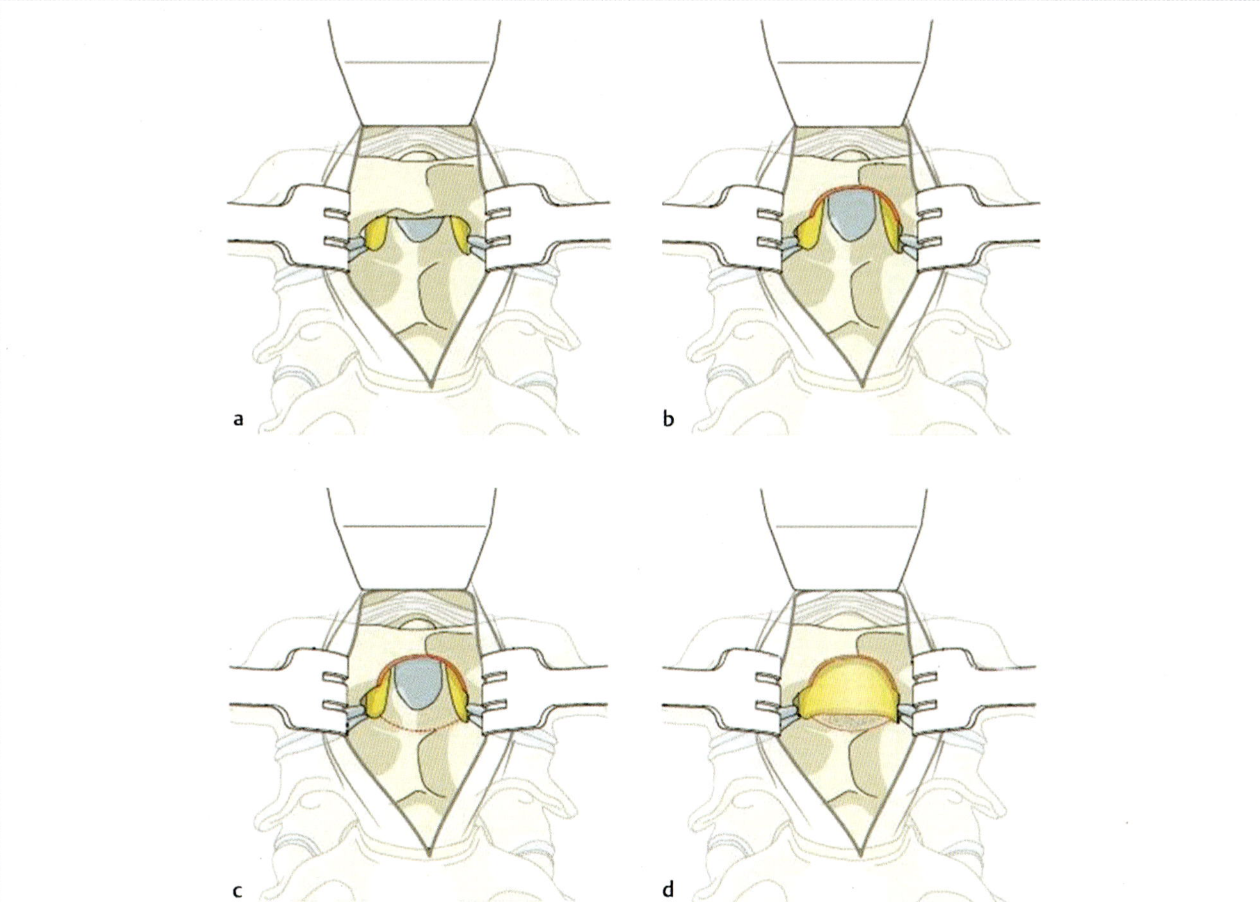

Fig. 21.4 Transoral approach to the craniovertebral junction. (a) A vertical incision is made in the median raphe of the oropharynx, exposing the anterior arch of C1 and the body of C2. (b) The inferior portion of the C1 arch is drilled off to expose the base of the odontoid. (c) The dens is drilled down, starting at its base. (d) The dens is carefully removed to complete the decompression, with care being taken to avoid any injury to the dura. (Reproduced from Härtl R and Korge A. Minimally Invasive Spine Surgery: Techniques, Evidence, and Controversies. Thieme, 2012.)

system (Dingman oral retractor) should be place carefully; any undue pressure to the soft tissues must be avoided. In addition, the tongue is retracted downward to avoid pressing it against the teeth. A curved retractor blade can be used to elevate the soft palate and avoid a palatal incision. The tubercle of C1 is identified using stereotactic neuronavigation. A vertical incision is made in the median raphe of the oropharynx and retracted with a pharyngeal retractor system. The underlying longus colli and longus capitis muscles are mobilized laterally in order to expose the anterior arch of C1 and the body of C2. Anatomical landmarks are identified similar to the endonasal endoscopic approach (▶ Fig. 21.4). The vertebral arteries and bony landmarks can be located using stereotactic neuronavigation if the normal anatomy is deformed. If the dura has been opened, it can be attempted to close the dural edges with sutures and cover with Surgicel and fibrin glue. In addition, a dural substitute and/or fascia lata graft can be placed over the defect when a large CSF leak is identified. Fibrin glue is used to fix them in place and ensure a watertight closure. Mucosal layers are closed with 3-0 vicryl interrupted sutures. In cases that require significant bone drilling where expected craniocervical instability is expected, a separate posterior stabilization procedure will be necessary following the initial anterior decompression.

21.3.3 Endoscopic Transcervical Approach

The patient is intubated using either an endotracheal[26] tube or a nasotracheal fiberoptic scope[24] and is positioned supine on a radiolucent operating table. This approach is often performed with somatosensory- and motor-evoked potential monitoring. A shoulder roll is placed under the patient in order to extend the patient's neck. The patient's head is positioned in a halo ring and fixed in neutral position with a Mayfield halo adapter. The stereotactic neuronavigation reference array is attached to the halo ring. Prophylactic antibiotics are administered intraoperatively. The patient's neck is cleaned, prepared, and draped in standard fashion for an anterior cervical approach. The approach can be performed from either side of the spine depending on the surgeon's laterality. All screens are placed on the contralateral side. A transverse incision is made starting at the midline and extending laterally for 3.5 cm at approximately the C4/5 level. Dissection is carried out in a standard fashion for a Cloward approach. The spine is exposed cranially until the C1 tubercle is palpated with the aid of Kittner dissectors and a 22-mm tubular retractor (30° bevel) is placed. The most cranial tip of the retractor is anchored to the C1 tubercle and the caudal

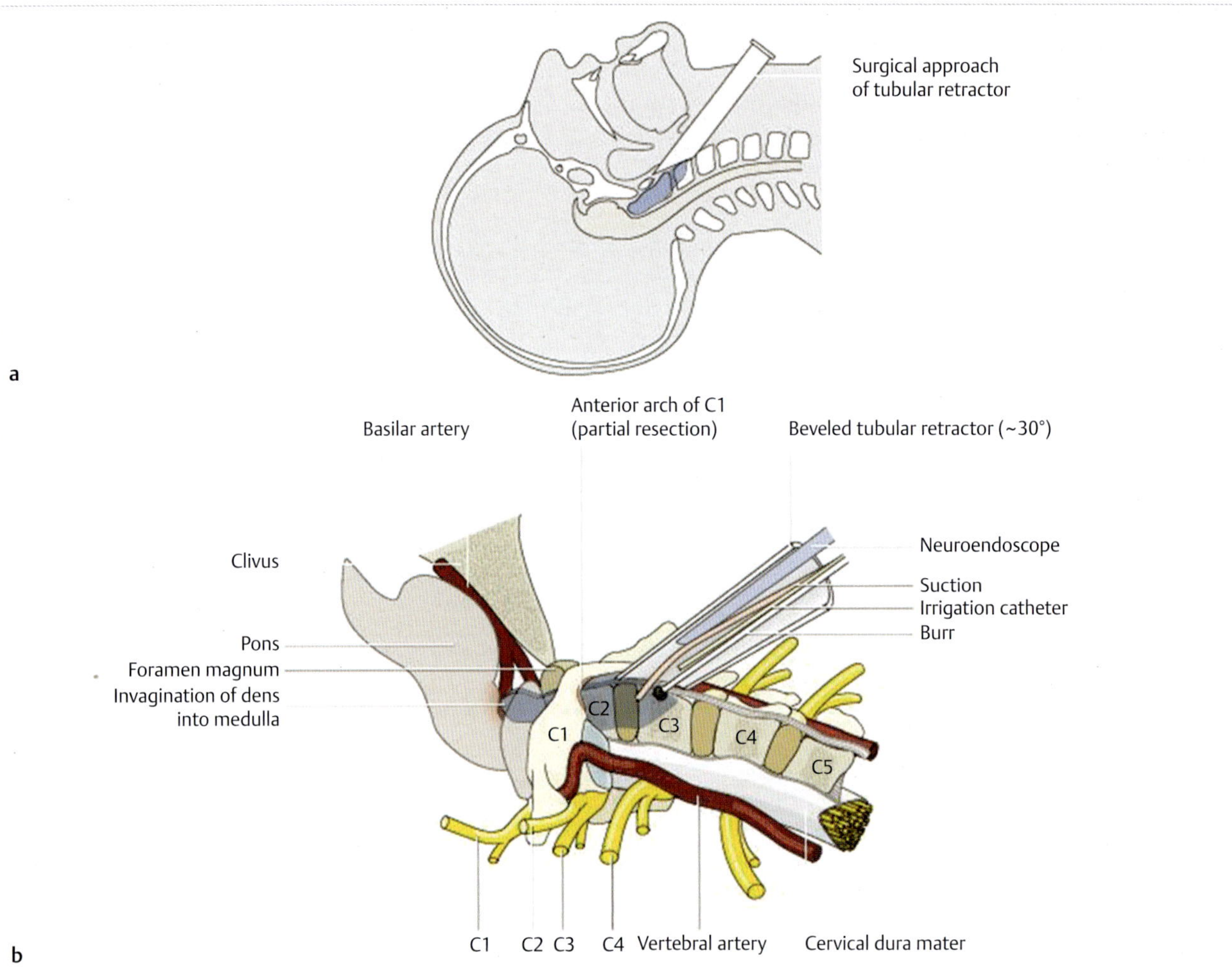

Fig. 21.5 Endoscopic transcervical odontoidectomy. **(a)** Trajectory of the tubular retractor on the sagittal plane. **(b)** Relation of the tubular retractor to neighboring anatomical structures. (Reproduced from Härtl R and Korge A. Minimally Invasive Spine Surgery: Techniques, Evidence, and Controversies. Thieme, 2012.)

aspect is positioned over the C3 vertebral body. Stereotactic neuronavigation can be utilized to ensure that the tubular retractor is positioned accurately. A 30-degree endoscope is introduced to the field; it can be held either by an assistant or attached to an endoscope holder. The longus colli muscles are swept off laterally and then, the lateral aspects of the odontoid are identified (▶ Fig. 21.5). At this point, it is important to pay attention to the location of the vertebral arteries to avoid inadvertent injury. After determining the junction of the odontoid process and C2 vertebral body, initial drilling starts at the base of C2. During the resection of osseous elements, the apical and transverse ligaments are preserved for the purpose of utilizing them as a protective barrier over the dura. The resection proceeds toward the ventral aspect of C2, posterior of the C1 arch until the tip of the odontoid is reached. Remaining part of the resection is performed in a "top–down" fashion along the length of the odontoid. This approach prevents free-floating of the odontoid which could cause challenges and complications. Once the removal of all bony elements is complete, the ligaments (posterior longitudinal ligament, transverse ligament, and nuchal ligament) are resected to expose underlying dura. The platysma and skin closure are completed following removal of the retractor. The patient can then be repositioned to the prone position for the posterior instrumentation and fusion.

21.4 Complication Avoidance and Management

The anatomic corridors used for the EEA and transoral approach are naturally contaminated, so prophylactic antibiotic use is of the utmost importance. A third-generation cephalosporin (typically ceftriaxone) is used for most cases. We only use double antibiotics (ceftriaxone and vancomycin) in cases with a high risk of CSF leak that will require the use of a lumbar drain. In cases with a high risk of vascular injury (e.g., clival chordomas that invade the carotid arteries), a Foley catheter is kept in the room in case of intraoperative hemorrhage. If hemorrhage occurs, the catheter is introduced through the nose and the balloon inflated to pack off the bleeding while more definitive treatment measures are instituted (i.e., endovascular sacrifice of the carotid).

In cases where a CSF leak is expected or considered to be high risk, there must be adequate planning regarding the appropriate closure technique. A conversation with the ENT specialist must happen ahead of the case to determine the need to harvest a nasoseptal flap and decide the optimal place to store it during the case (i.e., nasopharynx or maxillary sinus depending on the surgical target). The need for fat or fascia lata grafts must always be contemplated and prepped for.

In cases where bone resection is extensive (e.g., odontoidectomy), attention to the potential for new craniocervical instability is important. Patients should be immobilized with a hard cervical collar and spine precautions exercised until definitive spine fusion is completed. In our practice, stabilization is frequently performed in advance to the endoscopic decompression.

21.5 Postoperative Care

The postoperative care of patients who undergo surgery of the CCJ is usually straightforward and does not require special assistance. Patients who undergo endonasal surgery can be fed and extubated right away but usually require saline flushes to avoid nasal crusting. Early follow-up after discharge is usually performed by the ENT surgeon. Patients who underwent a dural opening procedure should avoid strenuous physical activity after surgery including weight-lifting to decrease the risk of CSF leak. Patients who undergo transoral approaches require evaluation by a speech and language pathologist during admission to assess the capacity to swallow and avoid aspiration episodes. In contrast to the endonasal patients, these patients are often extubated and also fed a few days after surgery.[2,31] Odontoidectomy patients will require cervical immobilization until spinal fusion is completed. It is our practice to complete the fusion first, either the same day or within a short time frame, to avoid progressive cranial settling and C1/C2 subluxation.[32]

21.6 Case Examples

21.6.1 Case 1

This patient presented with compression of the upper spinal cord secondary to os odontoideum and atlantoaxial instability (▶ Fig. 21.6).

21.6.2 Case 2

This patient presented with compression of the upper cervical spinal cord and brainstem secondary to basilar invagination and cranial settling (▶ Fig. 21.7).

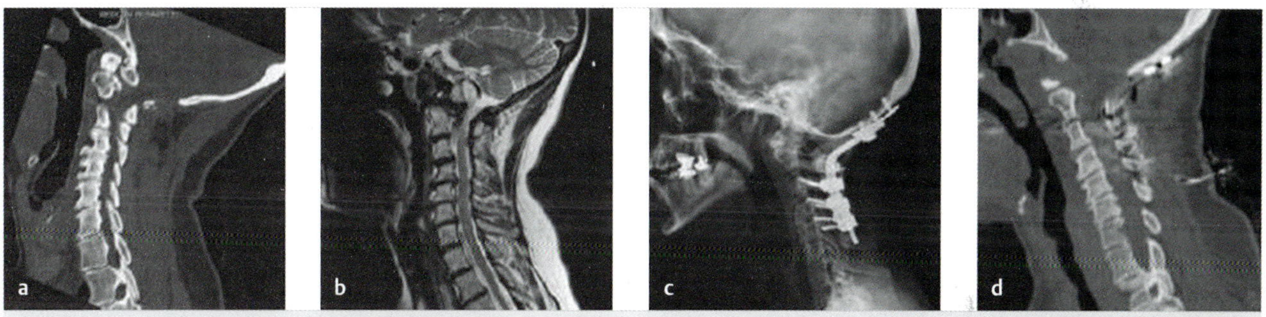

Fig. 21.6 Preoperative sagittal computed tomography (CT) scan **(a)** and magnetic resonance imaging **(b)** demonstrating severe cord compression. Postoperative lateral X-ray demonstrating the occipitocervical fusion **(c)** which was followed by endonasal endoscopic removal of the odontoideum and anterior arch of C1 depicted on the CT scan **(d)**. (Reproduced from Härtl R and Korge A. Minimally Invasive Spine Surgery: Techniques, Evidence, and Controversies. Thieme, 2012.)

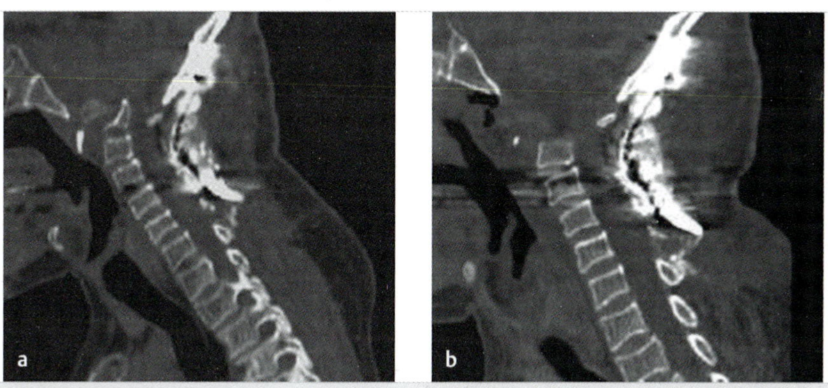

Fig. 21.7 Pre- and postoperative sagittal computed tomography (CT) scans. **(a)** Preoperative sagittal CT scan demonstrating the previous occipitocervical fusion with basilar invagination and severe brainstem and upper cervical cord compression. **(b)** Postoperative CT scan demonstrating decompression of the craniovertebral junction with removal of the anterior arch of C1 and odontoid process up to the body of C2 using an endonasal endoscopic approach. (Reproduced from Härtl R and Korge A. Minimally Invasive Spine Surgery: Techniques, Evidence, and Controversies. Thieme, 2012.)

21.6.3 Case 3

This patient presented with myelopathy due to severe basilar invagination (▶ Fig. 21.8).

21.6.4 Case 4

This patient presented with progressive myelopathy due to compression at multiple levels of the cervical spine (▶ Fig. 21.9).

21.7 Conclusion

Anterior craniocervical pathology is complicated by virtue of the many important anatomic structures that reside in that region. Ventral, minimally invasive approaches afford the possibility of addressing these conditions with less tissue disruption and faster recovery times. These techniques should be part of the surgical armamentarium of all neurosurgeons who deal with pathology at this level.

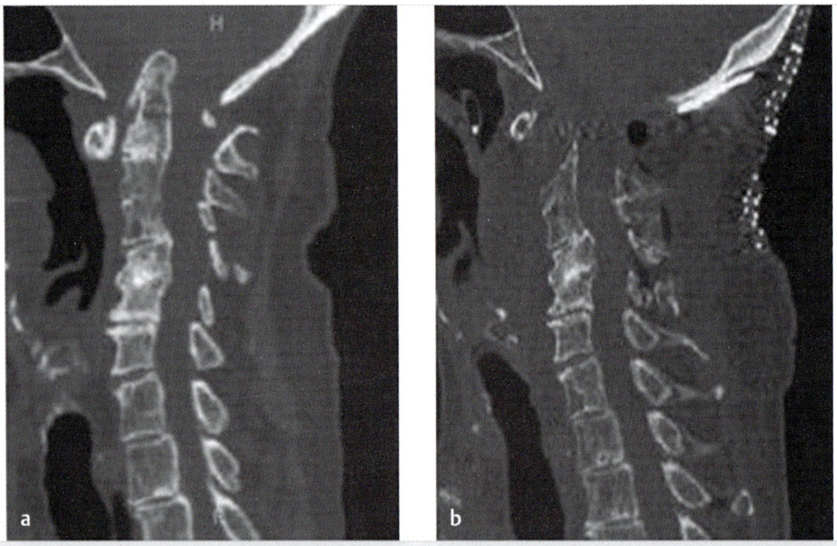

Fig. 21.8 **(a)** Preoperative computed tomography (CT) scan demonstrating severe basilar invagination with brainstem compression. **(b)** Postoperative CT scan after endoscopic transcervical odontoidectomy, demonstrating resection of C2, and decompression of basilar invagination. (Reproduced from Härtl R and Korge A. Minimally Invasive Spine Surgery: Techniques, Evidence, and Controversies. Thieme, 2012.)

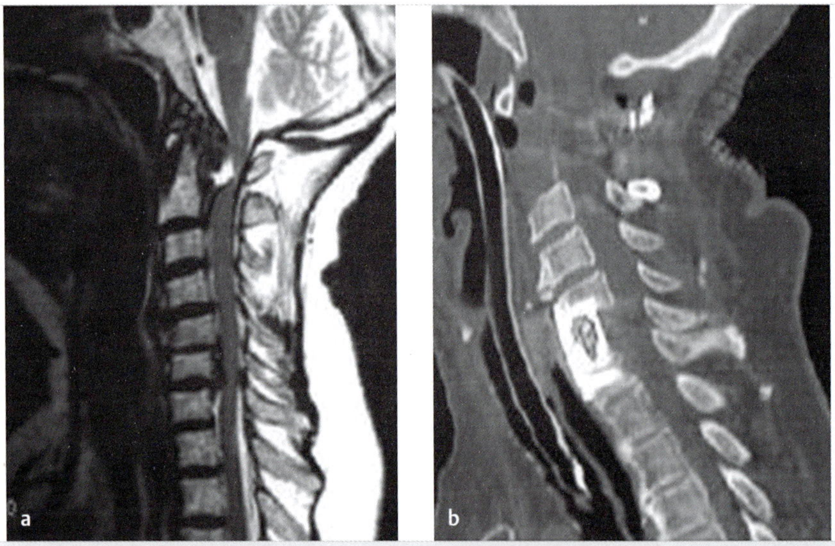

Fig. 21.9 **(a)** Preoperative magnetic resonance imaging showing C2 pannus and C6 stenosis. **(b)** Postoperative computed tomography scan showing resection of C2 and pannus via endoscopic transcervical odontoidectomy and C6 corpectomy with C5–C6 anterior reconstruction, all performed through the same incision. (Reproduced from Härtl R and Korge A. Minimally Invasive Spine Surgery: Techniques, Evidence, and Controversies. Thieme, 2012.)

References

[1] Riley K, Singh H, Meyer SA, Jenkins AL , III. Minimally invasive surgical approach for odontoid lesions: a technical description in a case of high cervical osteomyelitis and abscess. World Neurosurg. 2016; 91:332–339

[2] Goldschlager T, Härtl R, Greenfield JP, Anand VK, Schwartz TH. The endoscopic endonasal approach to the odontoid and its impact on early extubation and feeding. J Neurosurg. 2015; 122(3):511–518

[3] Morales-Valero SF, Serchi E, Zoli M, Mazzatenta D, Van Gompel JJ. Endoscopic endonasal approach for craniovertebral junction pathology: a review of the literature. Neurosurg Focus. 2015; 38(4):E15

[4] Rajappa P, Margetis K, Sigounas D, Anand V, Schwartz TH, Greenfield JP. Endoscopic endonasal transclival approach to a ventral pontine pediatric ependymoma. J Neurosurg Pediatr. 2013; 12(5):465–468

[5] Visocchi M, Signorelli F, Liao C, et al. Endoscopic endonasal approach for craniovertebral junction pathologic conditions: myth and truth in clinical series and personal experience. World Neurosurg. 2017; 101:122–129

[6] Singh H, Rote S, Jada A, et al. Endoscopic endonasal odontoid resection with real-time intraoperative image-guided computed tomography: report of 4 cases. J Neurosurg. 2018; 128(5):1486–1491

[7] Leng LZ, Anand VK, Hartl R, Schwartz TH. Endonasal endoscopic resection of an os odontoideum to decompress the cervicomedullary junction: a minimal access surgical technique. Spine. 2009; 34(4):E139–E143

[8] Laufer I, Greenfield JP, Anand VK, Härtl R, Schwartz TH. Endonasal endoscopic resection of the odontoid process in a nonachondroplastic dwarf with juvenile rheumatoid arthritis: feasibility of the approach and utility of the intraoperative Iso-C three-dimensional navigation. Case report. J Neurosurg Spine. 2008; 8(4):376–380

[9] Shawky Abdelgawaad A, Kellner G, Elnady B, Ezzati A. Odontoid-sparing transnasal approach for drainage of craniocervical epidural abscess; a novel technique and review of the literature. Spine J. 2018; 18(3):540–546

[10] Burns TC, Mindea SA, Pendharkar AV, Lapustea NB, Irime I, Nayak JV. Endoscopic transnasal approach for urgent decompression of the craniocervical junction in acute skull base osteomyelitis. J Neurol Surg Rep. 2015; 76(1):e37–e42

[11] Liu JK, Patel J, Goldstein IM, Eloy JA. Endoscopic endonasal transclival transodontoid approach for ventral decompression of the craniovertebral junction: operative technique and nuances. Neurosurg Focus. 2015; 38(4):E17

[12] Holzmann D, Reisch R, Krayenbühl N, Hug E, Bernays RL. The transnasal transclival approach for clivus chordoma. Minim Invasive Neurosurg. 2010; 53(5-6):211–217

[13] Moussazadeh N, Kulwin C, Anand VK, et al. Endoscopic endonasal resection of skull base chondrosarcomas: technique and early results. J Neurosurg. 2015; 122(4):735–742

[14] Forbes JA, Banu M, Lehner K, et al. Endoscopic endonasal resection of epidermoid cysts involving the ventral cranial base. J Neurosurg. 2018:1–10

[15] Wang WH, Abhinav K, Wang E, Snyderman C, Gardner PA, Fernandez-Miranda JC. Endoscopic endonasal transclival transcondylar approach for foramen magnum meningiomas: surgical anatomy and technical note. Oper Neurosurg (Hagerstown). 2016; 12(2):153–162

[16] Dallan I, Battaglia P, de Notaris M, Caniglia M, Turri-Zanoni M. Endoscopic endonasal transclival approach to a pontine cavernous malformation: case report. Int J Pediatr Otorhinolaryngol. 2015; 79(9):1584–1588

[17] Enseñat J, Alobid I, de Notaris M, et al. Endoscopic endonasal clipping of a ruptured vertebral-posterior inferior cerebellar artery aneurysm: technical case report. Neurosurgery. 2011; 69(1) Suppl Operative:E121–E127, discussion E127–E128

[18] Crockard HA, Pozo JL, Ransford AO, Stevens JM, Kendall BE, Essigman WK. Transoral decompression and posterior fusion for rheumatoid atlanto-axial subluxation. J Bone Joint Surg Br. 1986; 68(3):350–356

[19] Menezes AH, VanGilder JC. Transoral-transpharyngeal approach to the anterior craniocervical junction. Ten-year experience with 72 patients. J Neurosurg. 1988; 69(6):895–903

[20] Visocchi M, Doglietto F, Della Pepa GM, et al. Endoscope-assisted microsurgical transoral approach to the anterior craniovertebral junction compressive pathologies. Eur Spine J. 2011; 20(9):1518–1525

[21] Husain M, Rastogi M, Ojha BK, Chandra A, Jha DK. Endoscopic transoral surgery for craniovertebral junction anomalies. Technical note. J Neurosurg Spine. 2006; 5(4):367–373

[22] Qiuhang Z, Feng K, Bo Y, et al. Transoral endoscopic odontoidectomy to decompress the cervicomedullary junction. Spine. 2013; 38(14):E901–E906

[23] Visocchi M, Signorelli F, Liao C, et al. Transoral versus transnasal approach for craniovertebral junction pathologies: never say never. World Neurosurg. 2018; 110:592–603

[24] Dasenbrock HH, Clarke MJ, Bydon A, et al. Endoscopic image-guided transcervical odontoidectomy: outcomes of 15 patients with basilar invagination. Neurosurgery. 2012; 70(2):351–359, discussion 359–360

[25] McGirt MJ, Attenello FJ, Sciubba DM, Gokaslan ZL, Wolinsky JP. Endoscopic transcervical odontoidectomy for pediatric basilar invagination and cranial settling. Report of 4 cases. J Neurosurg Pediatr. 2008; 1(4):337–342

[26] Wolinsky JP, Sciubba DM, Suk I, Gokaslan ZL. Endoscopic image-guided odontoidectomy for decompression of basilar invagination via a standard anterior cervical approach. Technical note. J Neurosurg Spine. 2007; 6(2):184–191

[27] Yadav YR, Ratre S, Parhihar V, Dubey A, Dubey NM. Endoscopic technique for single-stage anterior decompression and anterior fusion by transcervical approach in atlantoaxial dislocation. Neurol India. 2017; 65(2):341–347

[28] Fraser JF, Nyquist GG, Moore N, Anand VK, Schwartz TH. Endoscopic endonasal minimal access approach to the clivus: case series and technical nuances. Neurosurgery. 2010; 67(3) Suppl Operative:ons150–ons158, discussion ons158

[29] Leng LZ, Brown S, Anand VK, Schwartz TH. "Gasket-seal" watertight closure in minimal-access endoscopic cranial base surgery. Neurosurgery. 2008; 62 (5) Suppl 2:E342–E343, discussion E343

[30] Garcia-Navarro V, Anand VK, Schwartz TH. Gasket seal closure for extended endonasal endoscopic skull base surgery: efficacy in a large case series. World Neurosurg. 2013; 80(5):563–568

[31] Komotar RJ , Sr, Raper DMS, Anand VK, Schwartz TH. Endonasal versus transoral odontoid resection: systematic meta-analysis of outcomes. Innovative Neurosurgery. 2013; 1:37–47

[32] Hussain I, Schwartz TH, Greenfield JP. Endoscopic endonasal approach to the upper cervical spine for decompression of the cervicomedullary junction following occipitocervical fusion. Clin Spine Surg. 2018; 31(7):285–292

22 Posterior Muscle Sparing Approaches for Decompression, Laminoplasty, and Laminectomy

Lionel N. Metz, Martin H. Pham, Kevin M. Hwang, and K. Daniel Riew

Summary
Laminoplasty is a powerful operation for treating cervical stenosis while maintaining cervical motion. By implementing the muscle-sparing techniques described and depicted in this chapter, one can offer effective treatment of myelopathy while avoiding instability and postoperative pain. This chapter describes the combination of laminectomy, open door laminoplasty, and foraminotomy to relieve stenosis while sparing motion. The essential aspects of this procedure are meticulous dissection to minimize muscle necrosis and facet destabilization, safe decompression, avoidance of interlaminar impingement to maintain intersegmental motion, and restoration of anatomy with multilayered wound closure. The addition of foraminotomies to the procedure allows for the extended application of laminoplasty to patients with co-existing, symptomatic foraminal stenosis in addition to central stenosis.

Keywords: laminoplasty, cervical myelopathy, cervical laminectomy, posterior cervical decompression, neck pain

22.1 Introduction

By definition, laminoplasty of multiple levels is not a minimally invasive operation, in the usual sense of the term. It requires a relatively large incision and encompasses multiple levels. However, one can use muscle-sparing techniques to minimize the invasiveness of the procedure. Muscle sparing is a critical aspect of the successful deployment of motion sparing decompression in the cervical spine. Posterior-based motion-preserving surgery in the cervical spine includes foraminotomy, laminectomy, and laminoplasty when performed without fusion. These procedures are commonly used in conjunction with one another to achieve spinal cord and nerve root decompression, while preserving both cervical motion and segmental stability in the subaxial cervical spine.

Preservation of the intrinsic and extrinsic cervical musculature to the greatest possible degree is critical to maintaining motion, proprioception, and stability in the cervical spine. Disruption of the posterior musculature and nonanatomic reconstruction of the muscular attachments have been implicated in axial and periscapular pain postoperatively and impaired postoperative outcome scores. In our practice, meticulous dissection, preservation of muscular attachments when possible, and anatomic multilayered closure are cornerstones for successful surgical approaches. Our techniques and methods will be discussed in detail below.

During a surgical approach, the intrinsic muscles are most at risk during subperiosteal exposure of the dorsal elements. Insult to these muscles includes disruption of the muscle origin, disruption of the muscular insertion, denervation, thermal injury to muscle fibers, and nonanatomic reattachment of healing of muscles. We will describe methods to mitigate approach-related morbidity during laminoplasty of the subaxial spine with foraminotomy and laminectomy performed as indicated on a patient-specific basis. With appropriate combination of these techniques, adequate decompression of the spinal canal and neuroforamen can be achieved while preserving both segmental stability and cervical motion.

Cervical laminoplasty is well-established treatment for cervical myelopathy and myeloradiculopathy resulting from congenital stenosis, spondylotic stenosis, and ossification of the posterior longitudinal ligament (OPLL). Laminoplasty was originally performed in 12 myelopathic patients by Tsuji in 1982 where he cut the lamina bilaterally at the stenotic levels and allowed the resultant "lamina-flap" to "float" on top of the dura thus expanding the spinal canal.[1] Subsequently, various laminoplasty methods have been described since his technique which have provided more reliable results, including French-door laminoplasty, dome-shaped laminoplasty, and open-door laminoplasty. Methods to stabilize the laminar hinges have also evolved to include miniplate fixation, suture–anchor stabilization, and ceramic plate stabilization among others.[2,3,4]

Hirabayashi et al first described the open-door laminoplasty in 1983, and since then it has become the most widely used laminoplasty.[5] The technique involves cutting the lamina unilaterally while hinging the other side to expand the spinal canal thus creating more space for the spinal cord. Laminoplasty achieves direct decompression of dorsal impingement and indirect decompression of ventral compression and therefore is most powerful when performed over several segments in the subaxial cervical spine with lordotic alignment. Lordotic alignment augments the ability of the spinal cord to drift dorsally to away from compressive ventral pathology. Laminoplasty can still achieve adequate decompression for patients with neutral alignment (< 10 degree kyphosis). Suda et al found that when local cervical kyphosis was greater than 13 degree patient had inferior clinical outcome with laminoplasty.[6] The use of the "K-line" and "modified K-line" can also help to predict if adequate spinal cord decompression can be achieved with laminoplasty.[7,8,9] Recently, it has been shown that increased C2–C7 sagittal vertical alignment and higher T1 slope are correlated with loss of cervical lordosis after laminoplasty.[10]

22.2 Patient Selection: Indications, Contraindications

22.2.1 Indications

Cervical laminoplasty with posterior foraminotomy can provide effective decompression for multilevel cervical stenosis resulting from cervical spondylosis, congenital spinal stenosis, or OPLL. It is important to note that the effect of laminoplasty on axial neck pain is less predictable particularly when axial neck pain is attributed to cervical spondylosis and facet arthropathy. Patients with severe axial neck pain are not ideal candidates for

laminoplasty. Nonetheless, a more recent study demonstrated that patients may have substantial improvements in total Neck Disability Index (NDI) score, as well as the NDI pain score after laminoplasty.[11] Thus, laminoplasty may still be a good option in patients who desire motion preservation but have mild to moderate neck pain, as long as they have appropriate expectations regarding the goals of surgery.

Compared with laminectomy alone, laminoplasty decreases the risk of postoperative kyphosis by allowing paraspinal muscles to heal to bone and restoring soft-tissue tension.[12] Laminoplasty offers several advantages over laminectomy and fusion for patients with cervical stenosis without predominant axial neck pain. Motion preservation is the most significant advantage. Laminoplasty mitigates the risk of cervical pseudoarthrosis in patients with risk factors for nonunion. In addition, it prevents soft-tissue scarring on to the dura by preserving the protective bony elements which prevents soft tissue and scar bucking into spinal and provides bony landmarks during dissection in revision surgery. Furthermore, exposure for laminoplasty is less morbid and instrumentation is less extensive compared with laminectomy and fusion, which is associated with a faster recovery.[13]

22.2.2 Contraindications

Cervical kyphosis in the region of planned posterior decompression is a contraindication to laminoplasty as the cord may remain draped over the kyphotic segment without lordotic alignment to allow cord drift back. However, in setting of mild kyphosis and circumferential stenosis, laminoplasty can still be a good treatment option as dorsal compression can be relieved directly. These patients must understand that if laminoplasty results in suboptimal clinical improvement from persistent ventral pathology anterior decompression and fusion to address ventral pathology or posterior fusion for realignment may subsequently be indicated.

An important concept to understand is that for myelopathic patients with kyphotic alignment and anterior compression who have adequate cerebrospinal fluid dorsally, draping of the cord over the ventral pathology must be alleviated to achieve clinical success. This phenomenon is best illustrated by the concept of the "K-line," introduced by Fujiyosh et al. He described a straight line drawn between by connecting the midpoint of the spinal canal at C2 and C7 on standing neutral lateral cervical X-rays, to predict the position of the spinal cord after laminoplasty and correlated this measurement to clinical success in patients with OPLL.[7] They found that when anterior compression crossed the "K-line" neurological recovery was worse.

Taniyama et al similarly described the modified "K-line" differing in that it was based on a sagittal magnetic resonance imaging (MRI) which allow for better assessment of ventral pathologies that were not visible on X-rays. He demonstrated that patients with < 4 mm between the modified K-line and the anterior compressive pathology had much higher risk for persistent anterior spinal cord compression after laminoplasty.[8,9] In select cases, laminoplasty can be combined with an instrumented posterior fusion to address multilevel stenosis with kyphotic deformity. This has the advantages of increasing surface area for fusion and preserving the protective bony elements, though this concept has not been studied extensively.

In patients with cervical myeloradiculopathy, posterior foraminotomies can be used along with laminoplasty to relieve the nerve root compression, particularly when symptomatic root compression is unilateral. The axial imaging, MRI, and computed tomography (CT) should be studied carefully to determine if foraminotomy is likely to provide adequate root decompression on a case-by-case basis. Although bilateral foraminotomies have been performed with open-door laminoplasty, foraminotomy on the hinge side is technically demanding and may lead to a higher rate of hinge fracture.

Severe axial neck pain is a contraindication to laminoplasty. Although, interscapular and upper trapezial pain are often results of radiculopathy due to foraminal stenosis, that usually improve after posterior foraminotomies at the appropriate levels. Hosono et al reported postoperative axial neck pain prevalence to be 60% following laminoplasty as compared with 19% following anterior fusion operations.[14] Contrastingly, Yoshida et al found that French-door laminoplasty had no effect on either the development or resolution of neck or shoulder pain.[15] For patients with preoperative neck pain, it is imperative to discuss appropriate postoperative expectations prior to surgery. Laminoplasty may also be performed in patients with degenerative spondylolisthesis if there is no gross instability present. Shigematsu et al fount that spondylolisthesis in elderly patients was not associated with worse outcome after laminoplasty; this finding is reflected in our experience as well.[16]

22.3 Preoperative Planning

A thorough patient evaluation should be performed prior to surgery. A complete history and relevant physical examination should be performed. All indicated diagnostic imaging modalities should be reviewed.

The relevant history included the onset and progression of symptoms of myelopathy in the upper and lower extremities. With prompting patients may endorse weakness or numbness, reduced fine motor skills often noted with handwriting or buttoning a shirt, changes to gait or balance, falls, or changes to bowel or bladder function. Discrete radicular symptoms may be superimposed. The distribution of neck pain and arm pain or numbness should be noted.

Physical exam begins with observation of the patient's seated and standing balance, the width, breadth, and cadence of their gait with and without assistive devices. Range of motion in the neck should be noted in addition to positions or motions that exacerbate neck or arm pain. Muscle strength should be graded from 0 to 5, and sensation should be tested with light touch and pin prick along the standard dermatome test areas. Finally, reflexes should be documented in the upper and lower extremities and pathologic reflexes should be documented if present including Hoffman's, inverted brachioradialis, ankle clonus, and Babinski.

It is critical to understand the range of motion as well as the resting cervical alignment. Thus, plain radiographs should include anteroposterior (AP) and lateral radiographs, flexion and extension lateral radiographs, and oblique radiographs (to visualize the neural foramen) of the cervical spine. In addition to cervical alignment and range of motion, radiographs are used to assess spondylosis, instability, and spondylolisthesis,

developmental stenosis, foraminal stenosis, autofusions, and other pathologies of the cervical spine. MRI is used to evaluate the cranial and caudal and extent of stenosis and the severity of central and foraminal stenosis. The etiology of stenosis at each segment should be noted including disc bulging, uncovertebral and facet arthrosis, hypertrophy and infolding of the ligamentum flavum, underlying developmental stenosis, deformity, or OPLL. CT of the cervical spine is indicated when OPLL is suspected and to further characterize osseous foraminal stenosis from uncovertebral or facet arthrosis. A topical three-dimensional (3D) reconstruction of the CT scan can be used to understand the bony surface anatomy and shape of the spinal canal. If MRI is contraindicated, CT myelography can help to evaluate the severity of canal stenosis.

> We favor using bivector traction involving two ropes attached to the Gardner–Wells tongs at different vectors, one which will extend the head and neck and one which will keep the neck in gentle flexion. The procedure begins with 15 pounds applied to the Gardner–Wells tongs on the flexion rope to optimize surgical exposure and then extended using the extension rope to as necessary to assess range of motion prior to closure.

22.4 Patient Positioning

Our preferred patient positioning is on a Jackson table with four bolsters and a leg sling in the prone position. Proximally, pads are placed at the level of the sternum, distally, pads are placed at the anterior superior iliac spine, and the lower extremities are supported on pillows on top of a sling. Arms are padded and tucked at the sides. Hyperextension of the neck must be avoided during the intubation for patients with cervical stenosis to minimize risk of spinal cord injury. Mean arterial pressure should be maintained above 70 mmHg or perhaps higher if patient has baseline hypertension to ensure cord perfusion. A bite block is used and the endotracheal tube is secured prior to placement of Gardner–Wells tongs. Transcranial motor-evoked potentials and somatosensory-evoked potentials are utilized and preflip baseline values may be established if indicated.

Bivector traction involves two ropes attached to the Gardner–Wells tongs at different vectors, one which will extend the head and neck and one which will keep the neck in gentle flexion. The flexion rope is aligned with the external auditory meatus and cranial vertex which will place the cervical spine in slight flexion; the extension rope is routed over an elevated crossbar at the head of the Jackson frame, and will gently extend the neck when it is bearing the weight. The procedure begins with 15 pounds weight applied to the Gardner–Wells tongs on the flexion rope to optimize surgical exposure (▶ Fig. 22.1) and then extended using the extension rope to as necessary to assess range of motion prior to closure.

Once the patient is secured to the frame with the abdomen hanging free, the bed should be put in slight to reverse Trendelenburg to reduce venous pressure at the wound, as well as facial and laryngeal edema. A forced-air warming blanket is most effective when placed beneath the patient and Jackson frame as the rising warm air will prevent ventral thermal losses and prevents the blanket from interfering with the drapes. The posterior neck is prepped and draped from the occiput proximally to the upper thoracic spine with sufficient skin exposure on either side to allow lateral passage of drains at the distal edges of the wound.

> Preservation of the cervical musculature to the greatest possible degree is critical to maintaining motion, proprioception, and stability in the cervical spine. Disruption of the posterior musculature and nonanatomic reconstruction of the muscular attachments have been implicated in axial and periscapular pain postoperatively and impaired postoperative outcome scores. In our practice, meticulous dissection, preservation of muscular attachments when possible, and anatomic multilayered closure are cornerstones for successful surgical approaches.

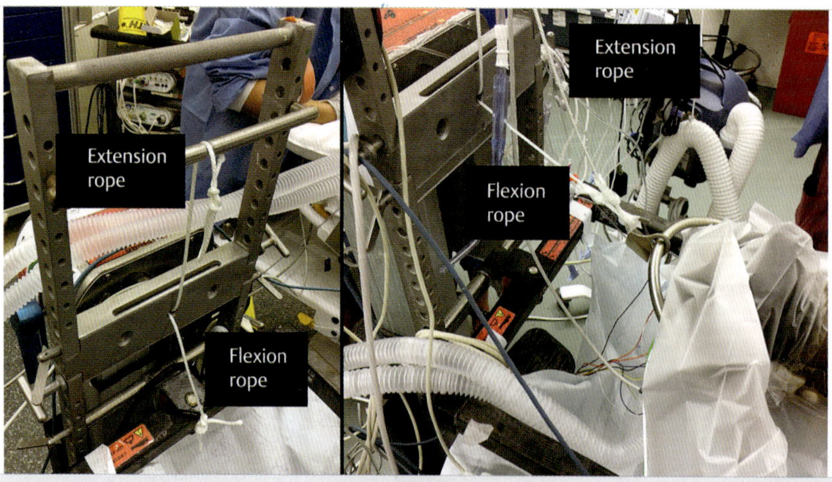

Fig. 22.1 A photograph demonstrating the bivector cervical traction setup with Gardner–Wells tongs.

22.5 Surgical Technique

22.5.1 Surgical Exposure

Uncompromised visualization of the surgical field requires excellent magnification and illumination. While cervical decompression can be performed using surgical loupes with a headlamp, we favor use of an operating microscope for the entire procedure from skin incision to wound closure. The microscope provides unparalleled visualization and illumination of the surgical field and optimizes depth perception and anatomic identification which allows decompression in the safest possible manner while also enhancing surgical ergonomics. This section describes the exposure of the subaxial cervical spine from C3 to C7, and this approach should be adjusted as needed depending on the location of pathology.

Prior to incision, surgical levels are identified using the lateral fluoroscopy. The skin is incised from C3 to C7 in the midline centered over the spinous processes (▶ Fig. 22.2). All subcutaneous dissection are done with electrocautery. Repalpation of the spinous processes ensures that dissection remains in the exact midline where an avascular plane can be exploited. The aponeurosis of the extrinsic cervical muscles (trapezius, rhomboids, and levator scapulae) form a relatively avascular plane along the central raphe. Blood loss can be minimized by careful dissection in the midline. Metzenbaum scissors can be used to spread in line with muscle fibers to identify and develop the avascular midline raphe. Meticulous dissection and attention to the tissue planes maximize potential for wound healing and reduce the pain associated with muscle injury.

Muscle injury occurs with detachment of the origin, detachment of the insertion, denervation, or direct injury to the muscle fibers. With cervical laminoplasty using open-door technique, disruption of the intrinsic muscle insertion is inevitable; however, injury to the origin can be limited by minimizing the extent of lateral dissection and denervation and muscle fiber injury can be avoided with careful technique.

After the superficial paraspinal muscles are separated in the midline down to the level of the spinous processes, the monofid and bifid spine processes can be palpated. The spinous process can be marked with a clamp and the level of dissection verified with lateral fluoroscopy. The monofid spinous processes of C7 and at times C6, the midline of the dorsal process is exposed with electrocautery down to the level of the lamina, followed by sharp dissection using a Cobb elevator assisted by electrocautery to release tendinous attachments. The anatomy of the bifid spinous process can be utilized to enter the subperiosteal plane of dissection. Cautery is used along the midline sulcus of the bifid spinous processes dorsally, leaving muscle attachments at the dorsal tips and lateral edges of these processes (▶ Fig. 22.3).

Next, a small bone cutter is used to cut each bifid process at the level of the sulcus (▶ Fig. 22.3). When performing the osteotomy, the bone cutter should be held horizontally to the wound and advanced across the bifid process from a midline-to-lateral direction so as not to risk cutting ventrally into the lamina or entering the spinal canal. Because only the bifid tips of the spinous processes are cut, the bases are left for manipulation during laminoplasty procedures. Alternatively, a half-inch osteotome can be used to perform the osteotomy of the spinous processes as described originally by Shiraishi et al.[17] We favor a small sharp bone cutter to avoid percussion over an often myelopathic spinal cord. Cutting the bifid spinous processes facilitates visualization across the surgical field and aids in subperiosteal dissection and in reapproximation of the paraspinal muscles at the time of wound closure. To facilitate closure, the bony fragments are tagged with sutures or marked at the time of osteotomy. These sutures can reapproximate the bony fragments at each corresponding level at the time of wound closure.

If a CT scan is available, a 3D surface reconstruction of the posterior elements, especially the spinous processes, may serve as a useful confirmatory adjunct to fluoroscopic localization. The spinous process osteotomies substantially facilitate subperiosteal dissection in an atraumatic fashion. A small Cobb elevator is then used to elevate the paraspinal muscles from the

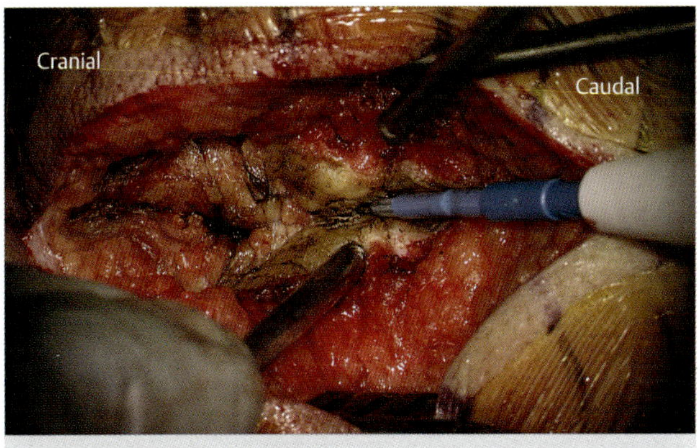

Fig. 22.2 Incision viewed through the magnification of the operative microscope. Cranial is to the image's *left* side. Routine palpation and blunt finger dissection is performed to ensure that exposure occurs down the avascular midline plane. Demonstrated is dissection along the avascular midline plane during exposure to minimize blood loss when performed in this manner.

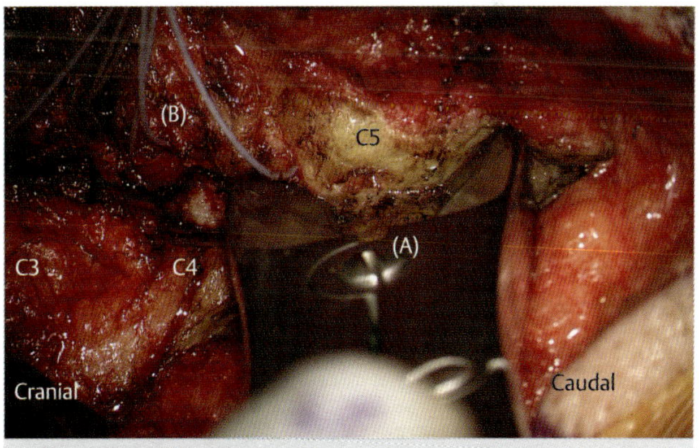

Fig. 22.3 Magnified view of the exposure down to the spinous process minimizing blood loss. Electrocautery is used to dissect down to the bifid spinous processes dorsally, leaving muscle attachments at the dorsal tips and lateral edges intact. A small bone cutter (marked A) is used to cut the tip of each bifid process at each level. Once the tip of the bifid process is cut, it is tagged with a nonabsorbable braided tagging suture (marked B). This is repeated at each caudal level. Shown here is one entire side with tagged bifid bone fragments. This is repeated again on the contralateral side until both sides of the wound have tagged bone fragments.

lamina while tethering fibers are released with electrocautery. As the medial facet capsule is encountered over the lateral mass, great care should be taken to dissect superficial to the facet joint capsule. The goal of lateral dissection should be to leave the facet capsule mentally disturbed; elevate only the muscle origin lateral enough to perform the decompression and plating, and avoid electrocautery laterally where muscle innervation is found.

After dissection is carried to the lateral mass, gentle placement of blunt tipped, self-retaining retractors, such as a McCulloch retractor, helps to avoid unnecessary bleeding and muscle and soft-tissue trauma. Retractor blades should be oriented in a parasagittal fashion to maintain well-distributed retraction. Meticulous hemostasis will maximize the safety and efficiency of the operation. Various agents may be used for hemostasis; however, those which inhibit bone healing such as bone wax should not be used on bony surfaces that are intended to heal, such as the hinge region of the laminoplasty.

22.5.2 Decompression

Posterior foraminotomy is frequently performed with laminoplasty to address foraminal stenosis and may expand the efficacy of laminoplasty in patients with myeloradiculopathy. We prefer to perform foraminotomies prior to performing the laminoplasty. Although we no longer perform routine prophylactic bilateral foraminotomies at C4–C5 to prevent C5 nerve palsy, we do perform foraminotomies at symptomatic levels with foraminal stenosis amenable to decompression with foraminotomy.

It is critical to have a 3D understanding of the anatomic boundaries to neural foramen to perform a safe and effective foraminotomy. The ventral boundary of the neuroforamen is the lateral intervertebral disc and uncovertebral joint and the dorsal boundary is the superior articular process (SAP) of the caudal vertebra (e.g., the SAP of C6 at the C5–C6 foramen). Cranially and caudally, the neuroforamen is bound by the adjacent pedicles. Posterior foraminotomy unroofs the neuroforamen by the removal of the SAP from its medial aspect up to the lateral margins of the pedicles allowing the nerve root to drift dorsally away from ventral compression. Adequate decompression entails resection of the SAP out to the lateral margins of the pedicles. Underresection of the SAP may lead to residual foraminal stenosis; however, overaggressive resection may lead to facet joint instability. A key landmark both for foraminotomy and subsequent laminoplasty is the interlaminar "V," which is the point at which the distal aspect of the cranial lamina intersects the leading edge of the caudal lamina (▶ Fig. 22.4).

First the distal-medial portion of the overlying inferior articular process (IAP) is resected until the cranial edge of the SAP is visualized. This can be accomplished quickly by using a high-speed burr (▶ Fig. 22.5). At least 50% of the mediolateral width of the facet should be retained to ensure stability. Cervical flexion helps to uncover the underlying SAP as the IAP translates cranially. Next, the exposed medial aspect of the SAP is removed with a burr by cutting an L-shaped trough (▶ Fig. 22.6), with the vertical limb of the "L" cut along the lateral border of the pedicle, and the horizontal limb cut just cranial to the caudal pedicle. A "sickle-shaped" decompression may result from failure to visualize the cranial border of the C6 superior articular facet and thus underresection which may lead to persistent nerve root compression (▶ Fig. 22.7). To avoid this scenario, the cranial border of the C6 facet should be exposed before the decompression begins. Adequate visualization of the SAP can be achieved by flexion of the neck and adequate resection of the IAP. Generous irrigation can prevent thermal injury to the nerve root.

A high-speed burr is used for the majority of the foraminotomy as it minimizes introduction of space-occupying instruments, such as a Kerrison rongeur, into an already stenotic foramen. Once the root is decompressed by unroofing the foramen, a 1-mm Kerrison punch or a small curette (Codman 1B or 2B curette) can be used to remove any overhanging bone (▶ Fig. 22.8). After the foraminotomy, the lateral walls of the cranial and caudal pedicles should be readily palpable with a nerve hook or a small curette. There should be no overhanging

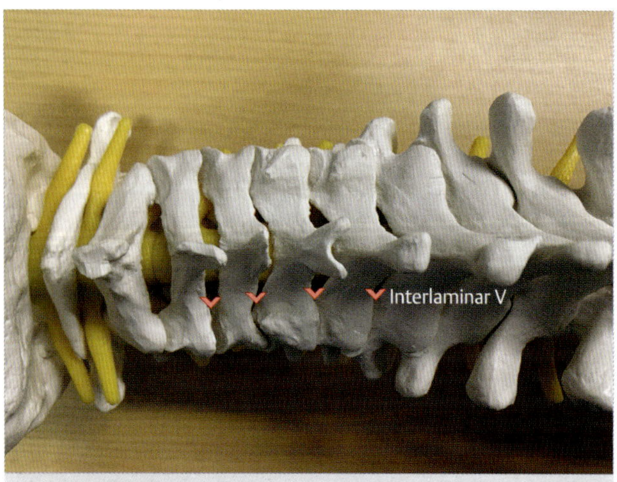

Fig. 22.4 The interlaminar "V," a key landmark for both foraminotomy and laminoplasty, is delineated by the distal aspect of the cranial lamina intersecting the leading edge of the caudal lamina.

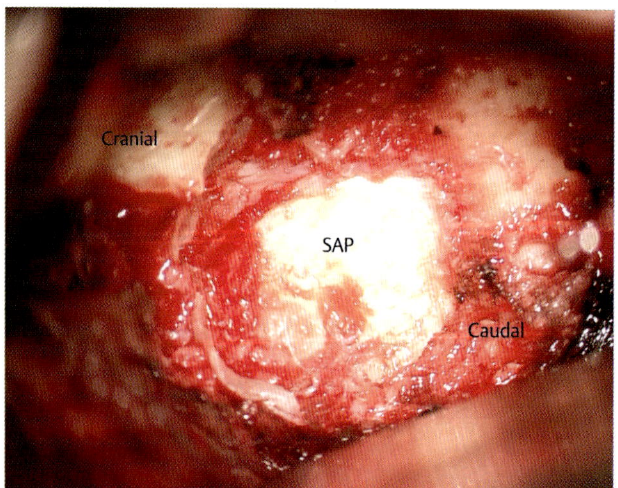

Fig. 22.5 An intraoperative photograph demonstrating the removal of the medial half of the C5 inferior articular process, and visualization of the underlying medial half of the C6 superior articular process (SAP).

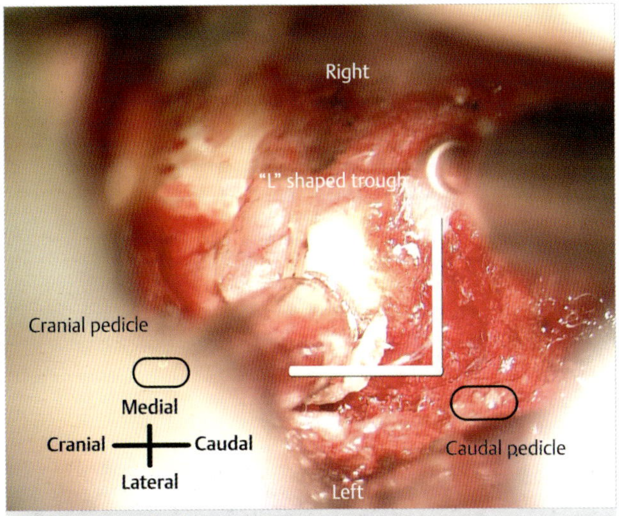

Fig. 22.6 An intraoperative photograph showing the "L"-shaped trough, with the vertical cut along the lateral border of the pedicle, and the horizontal cut just cranial to the caudal pedicle.

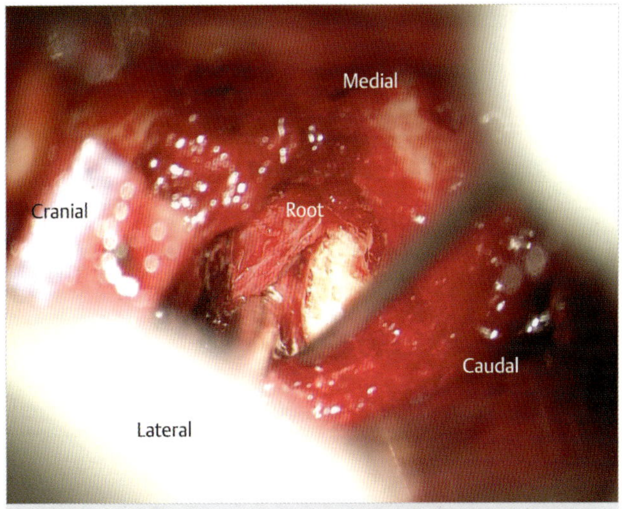

Fig. 22.8 An intraoperative photograph demonstrating adequate removal of superior articular process with decompression of the exiting nerve root.

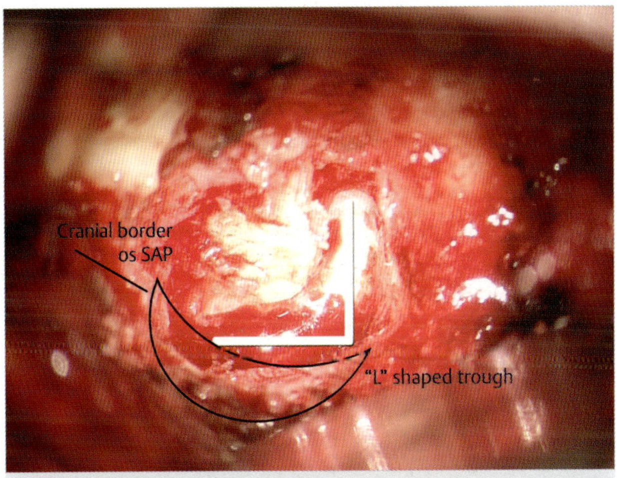

Fig. 22.7 Failure to visualize the cranial border of the superior articular process (SAP) can result in a "sickle-shaped" decompression, which leads to persistent nerve root compression by the cranial–medial portion of the residual SAP.

bone medially or at the cranial aspects of the caudal pedicle. After completing the foraminotomy, meticulous hemostasis is obtained with local hemostatic agents such as powdered thrombin or Gelfoam (Pfizer).

22.5.3 Laminectomy and Laminoplasty

The following text describes the treatment of myelopathy due to multilevel spondylotic stenosis from C2–C3 to C6–C7 with a C3 laminectomy and C4, C5, and C6 open-door laminoplasty. The steps outlined below may be in conjunction with a partial C2 dome laminectomy (a dome-like excision of the distal and ventral lamina up to the origin of the ligamentum flavum) and/or partial C7 laminectomy, depending on the proximal and distal extents of the stenosis. The levels addressed during the decompression depend on the pathology unique to each patient.

First, to address stenosis of C2–C3, the distal portion of C2 is resected with a matchstick burr using a side-to-side sweeping motion. This resection proceeds from distal to proximal until the ligamentum insertion is reached and it can be easily released with a curette. Next, a C3 laminectomy is performed by cutting troughs along the lamina–lateral mass junction using the burr. Extra precaution should be taken when cutting the trough at the proximal third of the lamina as there is no ligamentum to protect the underlying dura. The ligamentum flavum is then detached from the cranial portion of the dorsal C4 lamina with a burr or curette without transmitting excessive force to the spinal cord.

The C4–C6 laminoplasties begin with a full thickness cut through the lamina on the open side of the open-door laminoplasty using the burr. The opening side of the laminoplasty is generally the side with more severe cord compression or the side that requires one or more foraminotomies. The cut-line of the open side is first defined with electrocautery, which is the line that delineates the lamina–facet junction by connecting the interlaminar Vs at the corresponding level. The first pass using the burr should be to depth that removes the dorsal cortical bone along with much of the underlying cancellous bone. The second pass removes the remaining cancellous bone and thins the ventral cortical lamina to a shell. Both passes can be safely and quickly completed with some practice. Bone wax placed on a cottonoid patty can be used to effectively stop bone bleeding from the trough. The final pass with the burr completes the cut at each lamina, as evidenced by movement across the cut at each level with gentle pressure on the spinous process. If there is uncertainty regarding the completion of the cut through the ventral cortex, a small curette can be used to verify the presence of remaining bony bridges.

When the lamina cuts are completed on the open side (▸ Fig. 22.9), the high-speed burr is used to detach the ligamentum flavum from the cranial portion of the dorsal C7 lamina and perform a partial C7 laminectomy if necessary. The cranial portion of C7 can be thinned with a burr and resected if necessary depending on the extent of stenosis. The ligamentum

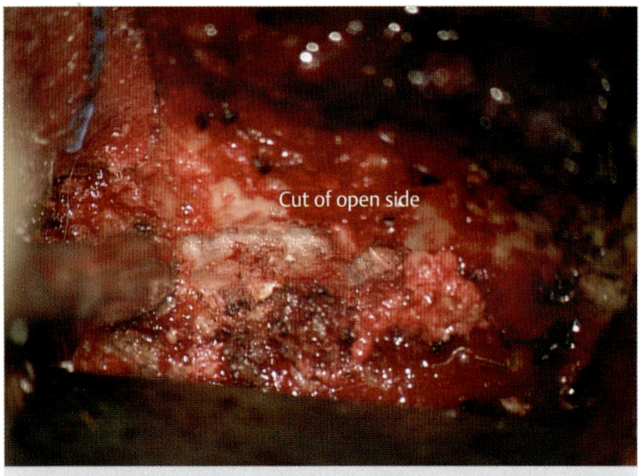

Fig. 22.9 An intraoperative photograph showing the cut on the open side after second pass with the high-speed burr leaving only a thin shell of ventral cortical bone; bone wax is applied with a small cottonoid patty for hemostasis before a final pass with the high-speed burr to complete the cut. The trough on the hinge side is completed by first creating two notches at the adjacent interlaminar "V"s, and then connecting these notches with high-speed burr to remove the dorsal cortical bone while leaving an adequate amount of cancellous bone and the ventral cortical bone intact.

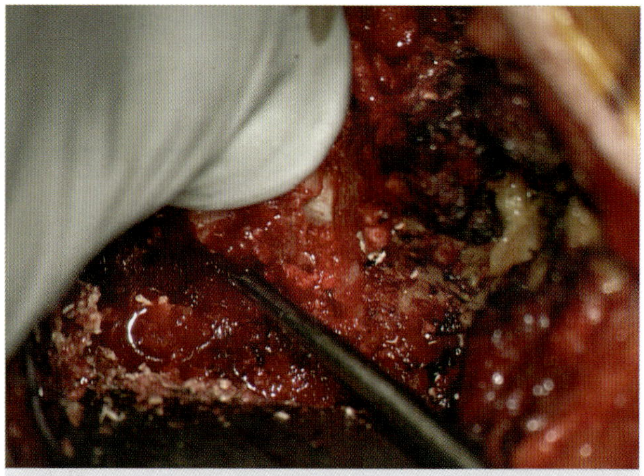

Fig. 22.10 Hinging of the lamina should be completed with the thumb pushing on the stump of the spinous process toward the hinge side, while the other hand gently lifting the lamina up with a small curette on the open side.

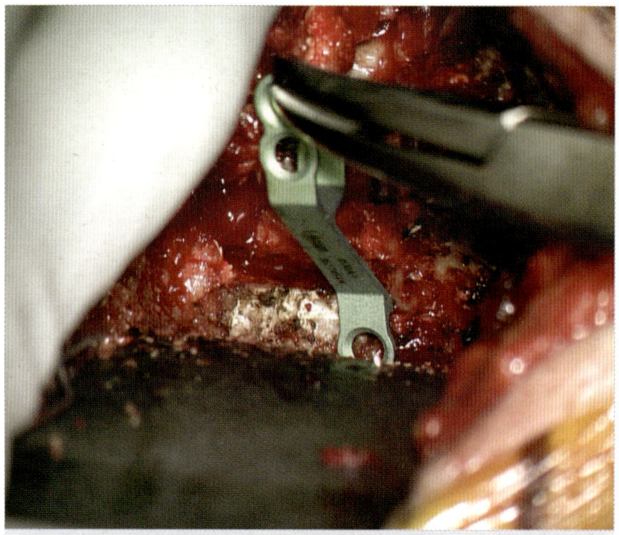

Fig. 22.11 The laminoplasty plate is introduced onto the lamina on the tip of a long-handled, fine-tipped hemostat as shown in photograph.

flavum is thinned with the burr and released between C6 and C7 with a curette or Kerrison rongeur. Next, attention is directed to the hinge side of the laminoplasty. First, the burr is used to notch the cranial and caudal edges of each lamina through its full thickness along the planned hinge line. These regions of the lamina are tricortical and therefore provide the greatest resistance to hinging. Second, a trough is then made by removing the dorsal cortex and a small amount of the underlying cancellous bone between the two previously made laminar notches. If done appropriately, hinging of the lamina should be easily achievable with gentle pressure.

Hinging of the lamina requires great care and finesse. If done too forcefully, the lamina can easily fracture off on the hinge side. In addition, sudden recoil of the lamina during hinging may cause iatrogenic spinal cord injury with the potential for devastating neurological sequelae. Therefore, this part of the procedure should be done with both hands, with the thumb of one hand pushing on the stump of the spinous process toward the hinge side, while the other hand gently lifting the lamina up with a small curette under the lamina (▶ Fig. 22.10). Several factors may complicate this step of the procedure: (1) residual ligamentum flavum attachments to bony elements, (2) adhesions to the underlying dura, or (3) an inadequately thinned ventral lamina on the hinge side preventing opening of the lamina. Because bone is viscoelastic, the lamina should be hinged slowly and gradually. We routinely mobilized the hinges from distal to proximal, first hinging C6 and then C5 and C4 sequentially and gradually, repeating this process three or more times, to obtain adequate laminar opening.

Each lamina is stabilized on the opening side with a laminoplasty plate. The plate is introduced onto the lamina on the tip of a long-handled, fine-tipped hemostat (▶ Fig. 22.11) and stabilized with the surgeon's thumb by the surgeon and with a curette held by the assistant at the lateral mass. A 7-mm-deep hole is then drilled and screw inserted at the upper one-third of the lateral mass in a slightly cranial and lateral trajectory. This will help to obtain a 7-mm trajectory with minimal change of violating the joint above or below. A second screw is then inserted through the plate into the lateral mass in parallel to the first screw. Shorter, 5-mm screws are placed through the laminar side of the plate to stabilize it to the lamina (▶ Fig. 22.12). In the event if the laminar hinge breaks, the hinge can be repaired to the lateral mass with a hinge plate which will allow the hinge to heal. These steps are repeated at each segment. After plate fixation, the spinous processes excised flush to the lamina and the cranial-caudal width of the lamina is narrowed with the burr to allow improved motion and aid in wound closure (▶ Fig. 22.13).

Range of motion must be verified after plate fixation is completed to ensure that there is no block to extension. While the Gardner–Wells tongs are stabilized through the drape by the surgeon, the anesthesia team switches the weight to the

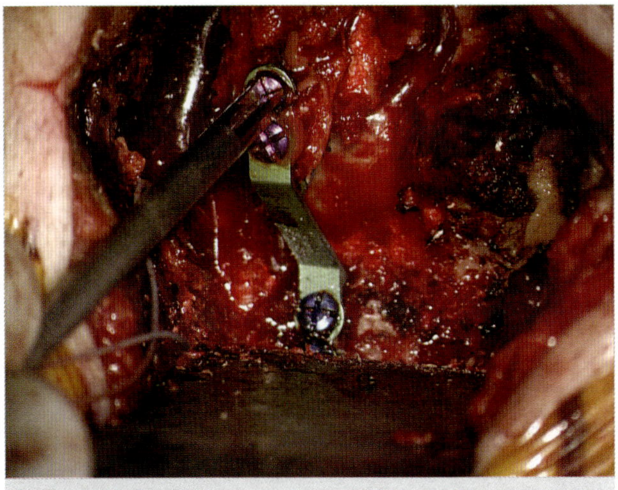

Fig. 22.12 Two 7-mm-deep holes are drilled through the plate into the lateral mass, and two 7-mm-long screws are inserted to secure the laminoplasty plates onto the lateral mass. The plates are secured to the lamina by two 5-mm-long screws at each level.

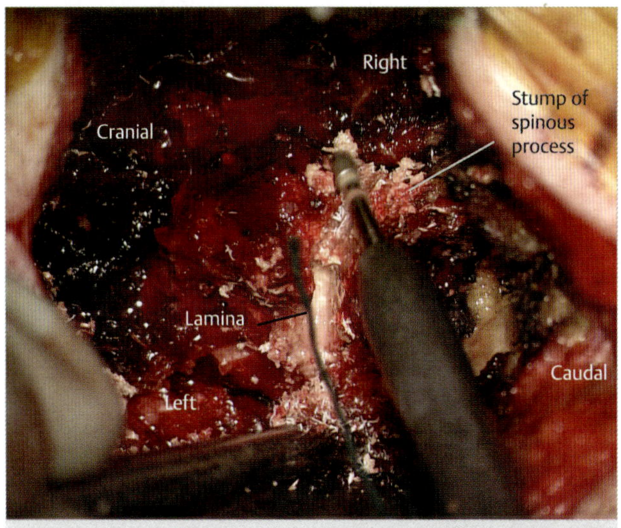

Fig. 22.13 The spinous processes are removed with the burr to prevent bony block and facilitate wound closure.

extension rope and full extension can be noted with direct visualization of the surgical field. If needed, additional lamina is removed or the ligamentum flavum is thinned until full extension is unimpeded. The Gardner–Wells tongs are reattached to the flexion rope for wound closure. The dura is examined to rule out compression and dural pulsations are noted to indicate adequate decompression. The wound is thoroughly irrigated to ensure that no bone debris remains to stimulate unintended autofusion.[18]

Prior to closure, meticulous hemostasis is achieved. We carefully inject methylprednisolone acetate (40 mg in 1 cm^3 solution) under the caudal intact lamina with an 18-gauge angiocatheter. The same dose of methylprednisolone is injected into the subcutaneous tissue from with the wound to aid in pain relief for the first 1 to 2 weeks after the procedure. A deep drain is then placed and 1 g of vancomycin powder is sprinkled into the wound prior to closure. Surgiflo and Surgicel are placed along the retracted cuff of muscles as the retractors are removed as this is a predictable place for bleeding. We place a thrombin-soaked Gelfoam over the laminoplasty levels to aid hemostasis but not directly over the dura as expansion of the material near dura can cause cord compression. Meticulous hemostasis, muscle-sparing dissection, and use of steroids help to minimize pain and wound drainage allowing patients to be discharged the following day.

22.5.4 Closure

Meticulous closure is facilitated by deliberate exposure. Careful delineation of anatomic planes at the time of exposure renders clarity to the approximation of those planes at the time of closure (▶ Fig. 22.14). First, the previously cut bone fragments are reapproximated by bringing the tagging sutures together. This preliminary closure is reinforced with a large braided slow-absorbing suture at each level through the tendinous portion of the semispinalis capitis tendons. Next, the remaining paraspinal muscles are reapproximated in 8 to 10 layers with No. 1 Vicryl

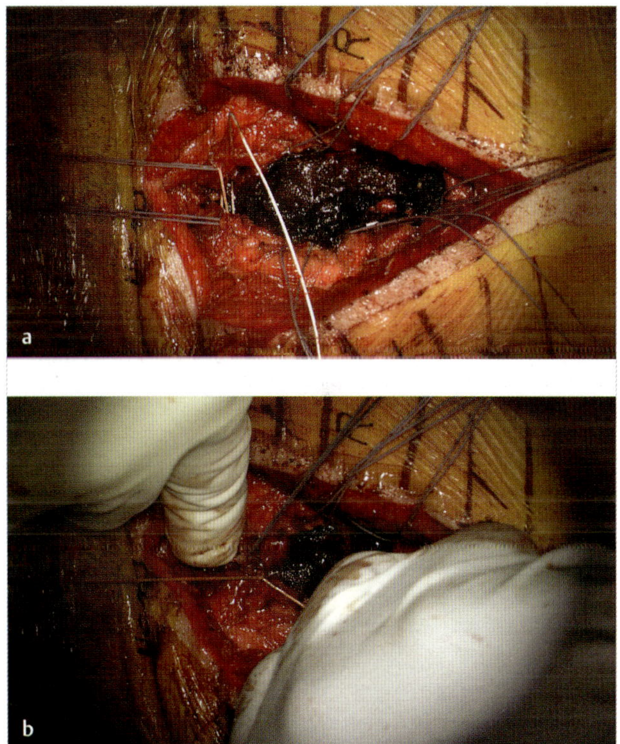

Fig. 22.14 (a) Postoperative wound bed showing meticulous hemostasis with Surgiflo, Gelfoam, and Surgicel. The previously cut bone fragments are seen with *blue* nonabsorbable braided tagging sutures and are reinforced with another suture shown as the nondyed vicryl suture. (b) Both sutures are tied together at the same time, with the tagging suture allowing appropriate reapproximation of the anatomic plane and cut bifid spinous process and the vicryl suture allowing for reinforcement and closure of the paraspinal muscular and fascial level. Wound showing the multilayer closure in progress with many sutures. In addition to being introduced into the wound bed prior to the initiation of closure, vancomycin continues to be used throughout the closure in the fascial and superficial layers as well.

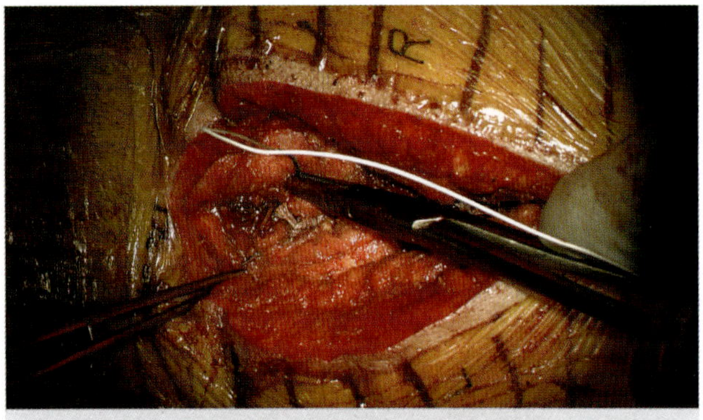

Fig. 22.15 Shown here is the introduction of the suture needle into the tissues without any intervening space, dead space from the needle swage to its point. The body of the needle is not seen and shows an appropriately small shallow bite for a continued multiple multilayer tissue closure.

(Ethilon, Cornelia, Georgia, USA), minimizing the dead space in the wound. Only small bits of tissue are used in muscle reapproximation, and sutures are not overtightened to avoid vascular compromise and muscle necrosis.

The fascial layer is closed with large, braided, slow-absorbing suture such as No. 1 Vicryl in a watertight manner. After closure of the fascia, the wound is again irrigated with saline and a small portion of vancomycin may be again dispersed in the wound bed at the discretion of the surgeon. We recommend placement of a superficial drain in situations where the subcutaneous fat layer exceeds 2 cm in depth. The subcutaneous tissues are reapproximated in layers with small-caliber braided absorbable sutures, leaving no dead space (▶ Fig. 22.15). The skin is closed with a subcuticular 3–0 monofilament followed by a dry dressing of the surgeon's choice.

We routinely use over 120 to 150 individual sutures to close an incision from C3 to C7 and this practice has essentially eliminated infections or other wound complications. With the muscle-sparing dissection and anatomic, layered closure described above, we find that posterior cervical procedures can have the same low risk of infection as anterior cervical procedures. We have also found that this technique limits postoperative pain and allows for early motion when combined with the muscle-sparing dissection technique described above. Patients are routinely discharged on postoperative day 1 or 2 with minimal pain.

22.5.5 Postoperative Care

As a general practice, patients are provided with a soft collar which they wear only for comfort and should wean as tolerated. Hard collars are unnecessary and may contribute to muscle atrophy. There are no specific precautions aside from performing activities as tolerated. Prior to discharge home, wound drainage should not exceed 20 cm^3 per 8 hour shift, pain should be controlled with oral medications, and patient should be able to perform routine self-care at home with the aid of family. Patients require an overnight admission for pain control and to ensure that drain output is low. They may begin mobilizing with nursing and physical therapy a few hours after surgery. An AP and lateral cervical spine X-ray is taken the evening of surgery. Most patients are discharged on postoperative day 1 and instructed to return to the clinic 6 weeks after their surgery.

22.5.6 Complications and Avoidance

Complications associated with muscle-sparing approaches in posterior cervical spine surgery are uncommon but can have a major effect on quality of life and surgical outcomes.

Postoperative C5 palsy has been reported in the literature with an incidence of 2 to 10%.[19,20] In a study of 1,858 patients who underwent laminoplasty, Imagama et al found that 67% of patients with postoperative C5 palsy completely recovered without further surgical intervention at a mean follow-up of 4.1 months.[21] Many mechanisms have been proposed to explain this postoperative condition, including traction of the C5 ventral nerve roots due to the dorsal postdecompression "floating" of the spinal cord, spinal cord ischemia, and reperfusion injury. No conclusive evidence points to one mechanism over another. In a prospective study of 141 patients undergoing open-door laminoplasty with prophylactic bilateral foraminotomies, Ohashi et al reported a postoperative C5 palsy incidence of 1.7% as compared with 7.0% in a retrospectively reviewed nonforaminotomy control group ($p = 0.043$).[22] Our institution performed a retrospective review of risk factors of C5 palsy in the setting of prophylactic bilateral foraminotomies and found preoperative symptom duration and T2 cord signal change on MRI as statistically significant risk factors.[23] At our institution, it is no longer our routine practice to perform prophylactic bilateral foraminotomies as we found it made no difference in the risk of C5 palsy. However, we perform foraminotomies at all the symptomatic levels in which preoperative imaging clearly demonstrating foraminal stenosis. Cadaveric studies have shown that shoulder depression increases C5 nerve root tension.[24] Careful patient positioning neuromonitoring may assist in ameliorating this risk especially if the surgeon is notified by the neuromonitoring team that there are signal abnormalities in the C5 innervated muscle groups being monitored.

Axial neck pain is another commonly reported finding in patients after posterior cervical spine surgery and usually encompasses the periscapular and trapezial regions. In a comparative study between anterior and posterior cervical spine procedures, Hosono et al showed a substantially higher incidence of neck pain with posterior approaches and reported that 26% of patients who underwent laminoplasty continued to experience neck pain for an average of 5.5 months with their postoperative protocol of 2 to 3 months of a rigid cervical collar.[14] At our institution, patients are not placed into rigid cervical collars after motion-preserving surgery and instead are given soft collars as needed for early postoperative comfort and counseled to utilize their range of motion as tolerated. In addition, preservation of the cervical extensors and semispinalis attachments at the C2 and C7 spinous processes have been associated with decreased postoperative neck pain.[25] Our practice is to perform partial C3 laminectomy instead of C3 laminoplasty, allowing for less cranial dissection and preservation of the semispinalis attachment at the C2 spinous process. In situations where exposure is required, we perform an osteotomy of the C2 spinous process to preserve this attachment and facilitate bone-to-bone healing.

Postoperative kyphosis after laminoplasty has been reported in as many as 10% of patients and this loss of lordosis has been associated with worsened clinical outcomes.[26] The literature suggests that preservation of the semispinalis cervicis, especially at the C2 attachment, is strongly correlated with the preservation of lordotic alignment.[27] It is our practice to preserve the insertional anatomy onto the C2 spinous process to preserve the dynamic stabilizers of the cervical spine. When these structures require detachment, they are either taken by bony osteotomy of the C2 spinous process or marked with suture and individually repaired on closure.

Surgical site infections following cervical spine surgery overall have been reported to range from 1 to 7%,[28,29,30] but posterior cervical spine surgery as compared with anterior surgery has been reported to be as high as 18%.[31] We introduced a protocol in a prior publication that significantly reduced the postoperative infection rate in posterior cervical surgery with the addition of a preliminary preparation of alcohol foam, a suprafascial drain in obese patients, and vancomycin powder placed locally in the wound.[32] It is possible that the addition of a suprafascial drain in obese patients helps to reduce dead space and seroma formation which impedes wound healing and provides a bed for infection. The reduction and elimination of dead space during wound closure in all patients can be facilitated through the multilayered closure described above and may be a contributing reason for the extremely low infection rate observed in the senior author's experience.

22.6 Tips and Tricks

The following surgical pearls and pitfalls were gained through extensive and repetitive experience of the senior authors. They are presented in bullet format for brevity and to facilitate rapid review.

22.6.1 Patient Positioning

- Airway and intubation:
  - For high-risk patients, consider fiberoptic intubation and neuromonitoring.
  - Maintain in-line traction and avoid chin-lift and jaw-thrust maneuvers.
- Bed preparation:
  - To optimize reverse Trendelenberg positioning, place the head portion of the bed on a high rung and the foot portion of the bed on the lowest rung. This will allow more flexibility in subsequent bed controls with the patient in the prone position.
  - Place the warming blanket on the patient's ventral surface (underneath the patient) where the greatest amount of heat loss occurs. This has the added benefit of not interfering with the drapes when the blanket is inflated.
- Prone positioning (bivector traction):
  - Have both a neutral/flexion rope and an extension rope setup. It may be helpful to flag the extension rope on the anesthesia side with a piece of tape to assist in communication during surgery of "which rope" to manipulate or exchange weights. Predraping review with anesthesia of the traction setup may also help to facilitate intraoperative communication.
  - The optimum position of the patient's head in reference to the top of the table is not so close as to interfere with intraoperative microscope positioning, but not so far away that the extension vector rope cannot be utilized appropriately.
  - Slight reverse Trendelenberg positioning decreases blood loss and intraocular pressure to reduce the risk of blindness, and allows for a comfortable and intuitive operating posture for the surgeon.
  - Use of the bivector traction will depend upon the type and stage of surgery. Flexion assists in exposure for foraminotomy while extension allows for assessment for postlaminoplasty range of motion and bony impingement.

22.6.2 Exposure

- Palpate regularly with a finger or bovie tip to ensure that dissection is performed precisely in the midline. It is helpful to start the dissection caudally where the most caudal midline spinous process rises most superficially and then proceed cranially once this is found. Intermittent blunt finger dissection also allows the opportunity for muscles to split down their natural potential planes atraumatically.
- At C2, avoid detaching the semispinalis cervicis from its spinous process.

Preserve all facet capsules during bony dissection by staying superficial to their capsular fibers.

22.6.3 Foraminotomy

- Approximately 50% of the medial IAP must be removed to expose the underlying SAP.
- To avoid a "sickle-shaped decompression" that may lead to persistent nerve root compression, the cranial border of the SAP should be visualized and identified as the cranial border of the decompression.
- Subsequently, adequate decompression of the nerve requires removal of the SAP in an L-shaped trough that extends to the lateral border of the pedicle.

22.6.4 Laminectomy and Laminoplasty

- Resect the ligamentum flavum as this can prevent opening of the lamina during the laminoplasty.
- The patient's most symptomatic side should determine which side to open for the laminoplasty for more decompression, with the hinge placed on the patient's less symptomatic side.
- Placement of the open and hinge troughs should be made just medial to the pedicle wall.
- Drill the open side first. This will provide the surgeon an idea of lamina thickness when subsequently drilling the hinge side.
- When drilling the hinge side, intermittently test the "springiness" of the spinous process so that just enough bone is removed in the trough to allow for careful opening of the lamina. This can help avoid a broken hinge.

- Unless contraindicated on preoperative imaging, we use 7-mm screws in the lateral masses and 5-mm screws on the lamina. Owing to the small size of screws, less manipulation of drilled screw tracts is ideal. Intraoperative fluoroscopy should confirm that the lateral mass screws have not violated the facet joints.
- In lieu of a formal laminoplasty, partial laminectomies or undercutting of the cranial and caudal segments can allow for additional decompression with shorter operative times, less muscle disruption, and less postoperative pain.

22.6.5 Closure

- Deep and superficial hemovac drains are placed. Thorough hemostasis will decrease hematoma and seroma formation and reduce total time for drains. Drains are left in place until less than 30 cm^3 of output in 12 hours for each drain, in most cases these criteria are met on postop day 1.
- A meticulous multilayered closure will reduce postoperative pain and optimize outcomes. This is accomplished through small shallow bites of the tissue that will reduce the potential for muscle necrosis and minimize dead space in the wound.

22.6.6 Postoperative Care

- Patients are encouraged to return to regular activities as tolerated and instructed to avoid painful positions.
- Soft collars may facilitate pain control and protect soft tissues in the early postoperative period.

References

[1] Tsuji H. Laminoplasty for patients with compressive myelopathy due to so-called spinal canal stenosis in cervical and thoracic regions. Spine. 1982; 7 (1):28–34

[2] O'Brien MF, Peterson D, Casey AT, Crockard HA. A novel technique for laminoplasty augmentation of spinal canal area using titanium miniplate stabilization. A computerized morphometric analysis. Spine. 1996; 21(4):474–483, discussion 484

[3] Hase H, Watanabe T, Hirasawa Y, et al. Bilateral open laminoplasty using ceramic laminas for cervical myelopathy. Spine. 1991; 16(11):1269–1276

[4] Tsuzuki N, Abe R, Saiki K, Iizuka T. Tension-band laminoplasty of the cervical spine. Int Orthop. 1996; 20(5):275–284

[5] Hirabayashi K, Watanabe K, Wakano K, Suzuki N, Satomi K, Ishii Y. Expansive open-door laminoplasty for cervical spinal stenotic myelopathy. Spine. 1983; 8(7):693–699

[6] Suda K, Abumi K, Ito M, Shono Y, Kaneda K, Fujiya M. Local kyphosis reduces surgical outcomes of expansive open-door laminoplasty for cervical spondylotic myelopathy. Spine. 2003; 28(12):1258–1262

[7] Fujiyoshi T, Yamazaki M, Kawabe J, et al. A new concept for making decisions regarding the surgical approach for cervical ossification of the posterior longitudinal ligament: the K-line. Spine. 2008; 33(26):E990–E993

[8] Taniyama T, Hirai T, Yamada T, et al. Modified K-line in magnetic resonance imaging predicts insufficient decompression of cervical laminoplasty. Spine. 2013; 38(6):496–501

[9] Taniyama T, Hirai T, Yoshii T, et al. Modified K-line in magnetic resonance imaging predicts clinical outcome in patients with nonlordotic alignment after laminoplasty for cervical spondylotic myelopathy. Spine. 2014; 39(21): E1261–E1268

[10] Zhang JT, Li JQ, Niu RJ, Liu Z, Tong T, Shen Y. Predictors of cervical lordosis loss after laminoplasty in patients with cervical spondylotic myelopathy. Eur Spine J. 2017; 26(4):1205–1210

[11] Mesfin A, Park M-S, Piyaskulkaew C, et al. Neck pain following laminoplasty. Global Spine J. 2015; 5(1):17–22

[12] Nowinski GP, Visarius H, Nolte LP, Herkowitz HN. A biomechanical comparison of cervical laminaplasty and cervical laminectomy with progressive facetectomy. Spine. 1993; 18(14):1995–2004

[13] Lau D, Winkler EA, Than KD, Chou D, Mummaneni PV. Laminoplasty versus laminectomy with posterior spinal fusion for multilevel cervical spondylotic myelopathy: influence of cervical alignment on outcomes. J Neurosurg Spine. 2017; 27(5):508–517

[14] Hosono N, Yonenobu K, Ono K. Neck and shoulder pain after laminoplasty. A noticeable complication. Spine. 1996; 21(17):1969–1973

[15] Yoshida M, Tamaki T, Kawakami M, et al. Does reconstruction of posterior ligamentous complex with extensor musculature decrease axial symptoms after cervical laminoplasty? Spine. 2002; 27(13):1414–1418

[16] Shigematsu H, Ueda Y, Takeshima T, et al. Degenerative spondylolisthesis does not influence surgical results of laminoplasty in elderly cervical spondylotic myelopathy patients. Eur Spine J. 2010; 19(5):720–725

[17] Shiraishi T, Fukuda K, Yato Y, Nakamura M, Ikegami T. Results of skip laminectomy-minimum 2-year follow-up study compared with open-door laminoplasty. Spine. 2003; 28(24):2667–2672

[18] Hyun S-J, Riew KD, Rhim S-C. Range of motion loss after cervical laminoplasty: a prospective study with minimum 5-year follow-up data. Spine J. 2013; 13(4):384–390

[19] Chiba K, Ogawa Y, Ishii K, et al. Long-term results of expansive open-door laminoplasty for cervical myelopathy: average 14-year follow-up study. Spine. 2006; 31(26):2998–3005

[20] Yonenobu K, Hosono N, Iwasaki M, Asano M, Ono K. Neurologic complications of surgery for cervical compression myelopathy. Spine. 1991; 16(11):1277–1282

[21] Imagama S, Matsuyama Y, Yukawa Y, et al. Nagoya Spine Group. C5 palsy after cervical laminoplasty: a multicentre study. J Bone Joint Surg Br. 2010; 92 (3):393–400

[22] Ohashi M, Yamazaki A, Watanabe K, Katsumi K, Shoji H. Two-year clinical and radiological outcomes of open-door cervical laminoplasty with prophylactic bilateral C4-C5 foraminotomy in a prospective study. Spine. 2014; 39(9):721–727

[23] Liu G, Reyes MR, Riew KD. Why does C5 palsy occur after prophylactic bilateral C4-5 foraminotomy in open-door cervical laminoplasty? A risk factor analysis. Global Spine J. 2017; 7(7):696–702

[24] Alonso F, Voin V, Iwanaga J, et al. Potential mechanism for some postoperative C5 palsies: an anatomical study. Spine. 2018; 43(3):161–166

[25] Takeuchi K, Yokoyama T, Aburakawa S, et al. Axial symptoms after cervical laminoplasty with C3 laminectomy compared with conventional C3-C7 laminoplasty: a modified laminoplasty preserving the semispinalis cervicis inserted into axis. Spine. 2005; 30(22):2544–2549

[26] Suk K-S, Kim K-T, Lee J-H, Lee S-H, Lim Y-J, Kim J-S. Sagittal alignment of the cervical spine after the laminoplasty. Spine. 2007; 32(23):E656–E660

[27] Iizuka H, Shimizu T, Tateno K, et al. Extensor musculature of the cervical spine after laminoplasty: morphologic evaluation by coronal view of the magnetic resonance image. Spine. 2001; 26(20):2220–2226

[28] Olsen MA, Nepple JJ, Riew KD, et al. Risk factors for surgical site infection following orthopaedic spinal operations. J Bone Joint Surg Am. 2008; 90(1):62–69

[29] Watanabe M, Sakai D, Matsuyama D, Yamamoto Y, Sato M, Mochida J. Risk factors for surgical site infection following spine surgery: efficacy of intraoperative saline irrigation. J Neurosurg Spine. 2010; 12(5):540–546

[30] Sebastian A, Huddleston P, III, Kakar S, Habermann E, Wagie A, Nassr A. Risk factors for surgical site infection after posterior cervical spine surgery: an analysis of 5,441 patients from the ACS NSQIP 2005–2012. Spine J. 2016; 16 (4):504–509

[31] Mehta AI, Babu R, Sharma R, et al. Thickness of subcutaneous fat as a risk factor for infection in cervical spine fusion surgery. J Bone Joint Surg Am. 2013; 95(4):323–328

[32] Pahys JM, Pahys JR, Cho SK, et al. Methods to decrease postoperative infections following posterior cervical spine surgery. J Bone Joint Surg Am. 2013; 95(6):549–554

23 Minimally Invasive C1/C2 Fusion

Marcus Richter

Summary

Minimally invasive atlantoaxial fixation and fusion with posterior transarticular screws C1/C2 represents a modification of established and traditional techniques and screw trajectories. Reduced approach morbidity is achieved by percutaneous-assisted screw placement with significantly reduced incision length and reduced muscle trauma of the approach. Using an atlas-claw, rigidly fixed at the transarticular screws C1/C2, further reduces operative time, and complications, as no sublaminar wiring and no structural bone graft are needed.[1] The use of spinal navigation for the placement of the transarticular screws C1/C2 allows for further reduction of the approach size and reduces the rate of screw misplacement.[2]

Keywords: cervical spine, atlantoaxial fixation, transarticular screw fixation, posterior instrumentation, claw fixation, spinal navigation, minimally invasive spine surgery

23.1 Introduction

Many different techniques for atlantoaxial fixation and fusion via anterior, bilateral, and posterior approaches have been described. Several posterior wiring techniques and modifications were published. These techniques differ in number of sublaminar wires, wire position, graft position, and bone graft shape. As a disadvantage, all of these wiring techniques are associated with potential risks due to the use of wires. Furthermore, the primary stability of wiring techniques is poor and therefore, long-lasting postoperative immobilization is necessary and the rate of nonunion as well as loss of reduction is high.[3] Other techniques tried to avoid these risks by using clamp or claw constructs.[4] These techniques do not have the risks associated to wiring but biomechanical stability is still not sufficient. In 1987, Magerl and Seemann[5] introduced a new technique using posterior transarticular screws through the C1/C2 articulation. In several studies, this technique showed biomechanical stability superior to that of different wire fixations.[3] Although biomechanical stability is high for axial rotation and lateral bending, there is still a deficit for flexion/extension. Therefore, in case of intended atlantoaxial fusion, the transarticular screws should be combined with a posterior interlaminar stabilization to provide a three-point fixation. The standard for additional posterior interlaminar stabilization is the Gallie procedure with a cortical bone graft and sublaminar wiring. The clinical results with this combined three-point fixation were excellent with increased fusion rates.[6] The disadvantage of this technique is the need for a cortical bone graft and the risks associated to sublaminar wiring. To avoid these disadvantages of the Gallie technique, C1 arch clamps fixed to the transarticular screws (atlas-claw) were introduced. This new technology reduces the morbidity and risk of the procedure significantly. Operation time, blood loss, and donor site morbidity were reduced and biomechanical stability improved.[3] Anatomic and radiological studies of the atlantoaxial region have suggested that in up to 20% of the cases a safe placement of transarticular screws is not possible, mostly because of a high-riding transverse foramen.[7] Alternative techniques such as a combination of lateral mass screws C1 with pedicle screws C2[8] or translaminar screws C2[9] have been described. The biomechanical stability of these techniques is nearly comparable to that of transarticular screws C1/C2 in combination with an atlas-claw[3,10] but the lateral mass screw C1 can irritate the dorsal root ganglion of C2 and the blood loss can be significant due to the epidural venous plexus near the facet joint C1/C2. Nevertheless in situations where a transarticular screw C1/C2 cannot be placed safely, these alternative techniques are very helpful. In the author's practice, transarticular screws C1/C2 with atlas-claw is the standard operation for instrumented C1/C2 fusion. The second-line option is the combination of lateral mass screws C1 with pedicle-screws C2, if pedicle screws C2 are not possible for anatomic reasons translaminar screws are used. Owing to reduced operative time, incision length, and blood loss, the authors' prefer the transarticular C1/C2 + atlas-claw option.

23.2 Indications

In general, this technique can be used for all patients requiring C1/C2 stabilization, either only for the level C1/C2 or in combination with fixation to the occiput or the subaxial spine. Indications are instabilities, degenerative changes, and tumor involvement. The following indications have to be taken into consideration:

- Rheumatoid arthritis instability C1/C2 (anteroposterior or/and lateral instability).
- Rheumatoid arthritis instability C0/C2 with basilar impression (fixation to the occiput in combination with transarticular screws C1/C2).
- Unstable odontoid nonunion.
- Odontoid fracture (type Anderson II or III) in special cases: that is, poor bone quality, extensive comminution, associated intra-articular fracture C1/C2, associated Jefferson fracture, high thoracic marked kyphosis (anterior approach not possible), unsuitable fracture line for anterior odontoid screw fixation.
- Unstable Jefferson fracture.
- Unstable rotatory dislocation C1/C2 or recurrent rotatory dislocation C1/C2 after conservative therapy with closed reduction and immobilization.
- Atlanto-occipital dislocation.
- Tumor involvement C1/C2 (metastasis or primary bone tumor) with pathological fracture or imminent pathological fracture as well as compression of the spinal cord.

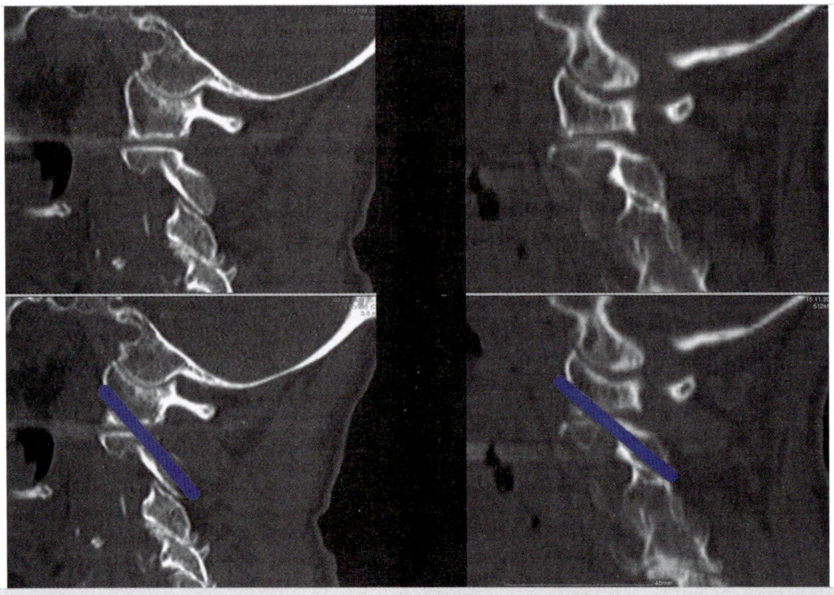

Fig. 23.1 Preoperative computed tomography (CT) with reconstruction in the screw axis: on the left side the anatomy is suitable for a transarticular screw C1/C2, on the right side vertebral artery anomaly called "high-riding transverse foramen" is shown, therefore a transarticular screw C1/C2 would injure the vertebral artery.

- Congenital atlantoaxial instabilities.
- Osteoarthritis of the C1/C2 facet joints.

23.3 Contraindications

- Infection of the surgical site.
- Poor health prohibiting general anesthesia.
- Anatomical variations of the vertebral artery in C2 which make the placement of a transarticular screws C1/C2 impossible ("high riding transverse foramen"). To detect variations of the vertebral artery, a preoperative computed tomography (CT) or CT angiography with multiplanar reconstructions is always recommended.

23.4 Preoperative Planning

Clinical assessment including neurological status should be done.

The following imaging studies are needed:

- X-ray in ap- and lateral projection and transoral ap-view.
- Extension/flexion in lateral projection X-rays.
- Lateral bending X-rays in ap projection (if lateral instability is suspected).
- CT/CT angio occiput–C3 with multiplanar reconstruction.
- Magnetic resonance imaging (MRI) if spinal cord compression is suspected or in tumor cases.

Preoperative screw planning is done based on the CT scan and multiplanar reconstructions in the axis of the transarticular screws C1/C2 with determination of the vertebral artery course and planning of angulation and length of the screws (▶ Fig. 23.1). If transarticular screws C1/C2 are not possible due to anatomical variants on one or both sides, the planning in the multiplanar CT reconstructions is recommended for C2 pedicle screws. If none of these options is possible, translaminar screws at C2 are always a good option.

23.5 Patient Positioning

General endotracheal anesthesia with muscle relaxation is mandatory. Once the patient is in supine position, disinfection of the pin sites is done and the Mayfield clamp is fixed to the occiput in the standard technique and location. Positioning of the head without using a Mayfield head holder may also be possible but is not recommended as the possibilities of reduction and fixation in reduced position are limited with the head over an unsteady surface. Then the patient is flipped to the prone position over a gel-filled mattress; support of the thorax and pelvis is done using foam pillows. The arms are fixed with adhesive tapes. In our center, we also used pulley systems and 2.5-kg traction on each side. Prior to surgery, shaving of the surgical area is performed using a clipper.Reduction is achieved under lateral X-ray visualization. After the positioning is finished, appropriate surgical site localization should be checked with a straight metal instrument to confirm if the planned screw trajectory is possible under X-ray control, otherwise repositioning should be done until adequate positioning has been achieved (▶ Fig. 23.2a, b). Intraoperatively, ap X-ray control will be needed at least once. Thus, it should be tested if ap-view is possible before the patient is draped and the position of the image intensifier should be marked on the floor. Doing this will improve the workflow during the operation once the patient is draped. The Mayfield clamp position in relation to the intensifier needs to be rechecked before draping the patient to confirm that it can be moved from anteroposterior to lateral position freely (▶ Fig. 23.3).

Perioperative antibiotic prophylaxis is given once 20 to 30 minute prior the skin incision.

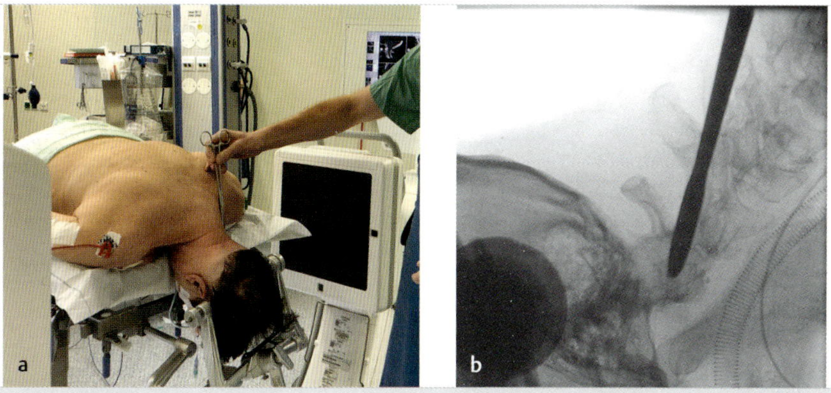

Fig. 23.2 (a) Patient in prone position on a gel-filled mattress, support of the thorax and pelvis is done with foam pillows. The arms are fixed by adhesive tapes and continuously pulled with a pulley system and 2.5 kg each side. Check with a straight metal instrument if the planned screw trajectory is possible under X-ray control. **(b)** X-ray control shows that the optimal screw trajectory for the transarticular screws C1/C2 is possible.

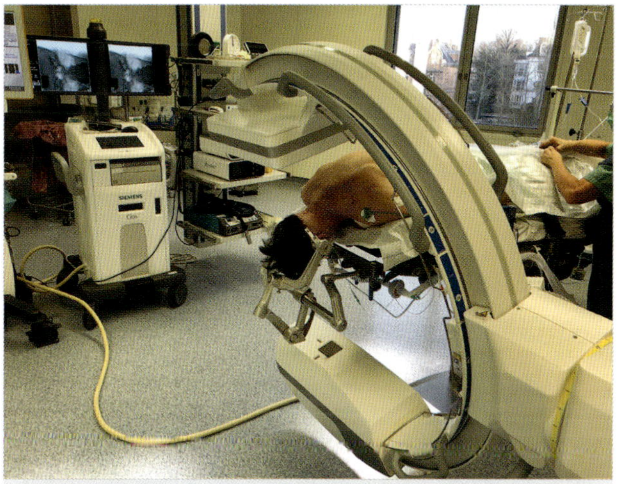

Fig. 23.3 Preoperative test if ap-view is possible and the position of the image intensifier for the ap-view should be marked on the floor, so that this position can be found easily during operation if the patient is draped.

The described method for C1/C2 fixation is microsurgical due to the reduced approach morbidity: short incision, percutaneous-assisted screw placement, and three-point fixation with an atlas-claw. For minimal invasive instrumentation, a cannular system for percutaneous-assisted screw placement is needed in order to limit the incision length.

23.6 Surgical Steps

23.6.1 Incision

1. After prepping and draping with the image intensifier in the lateral view, a midline incision is made from the posterior arch C1 to the spinous process C2. The length of the incision is dependent on the patient's weight, on average the incision length is 3 to 4 cm.
2. After subcutaneous preparation, incision of the fascia in the midline is done and subperiosteal exposure of the posterior arch of C1 and the spinous process as well as the posterior arch of C2. It is important to stay exactly in the midline to reduce blood loss and muscle trauma.
3. The preparation can be done using an electrocautery knife. To reduce further blood loss and tissue trauma, the use of a harmonic scalpel is beneficial.

23.6.2 Technique

1. The described method for C1/C2 fixation is microsurgical due to the reduced approach morbidity: short incision, percutaneous-assisted screw placement, and three-point fixation with an atlas-claw. Owing to the small size of the approach, a headlamp is beneficial for good illumination of the situs. Before describing the various surgical steps, the trajectory and insertion point of the transarticular screws must be explained (▶ Fig. 23.4). The entry point for the transarticular C1/C2 screw lies in a straight sagittal line in the center of the isthmus (connection between the cranial and caudal joint facet) at the inferior border of the caudal facet of C2, 2 mm cranial and lateral to the medial border. The medial border of the isthmic part of C2 can be determined with a dissector in the spinal canal lateral to the dura or with ap X-ray view.
2. The trajectory is aimed toward the cranial part of the anterior tubercle of C1. The exact screw direction should be planned preoperatively using the CT with multiplanar reconstructions.
3. For minimal invasive instrumentation, a cannular system for percutaneous-assisted screw placement is needed because otherwise due to the recommended screw angulation the incision would not be 4 cm but 20 cm for open screw placement. There are several cannulated systems on the market either with cannulated screws which are placed over Kirschner wires (K-wires) or noncannulated screws which are placed after preparing the screw hole with a drill.
4. After preparation and draping of the surgical field, the insertion point for the trocar system is determined. This is done by holding the trocar lateral to the neck and looking for the correct screw direction in the lateral X-ray view. Then a stab

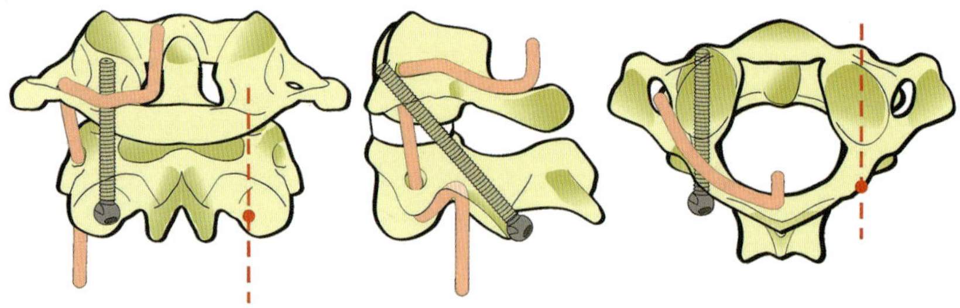

Fig. 23.4 Transarticular C1/C2 screw positioning according to Magerl, the entry points as well as the screw trajectory is shown.

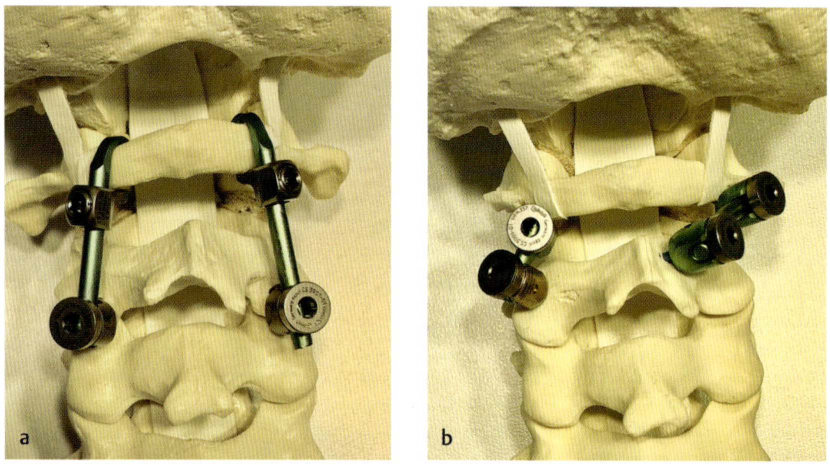

Fig. 23.5 (a) Completed instrumentation with transarticular C1/C2 screws and atlas claws for three-point fixation. **(b)** Alternative instrumentation if transarticular screws are not possible: *left side*: lateral mass screws C1 + pedicle screw C2; *right side*: lateral mass screws C1 + translaminar screw C2.

incision is made approximately 1 cm lateral to the spinous process on each side and the trocar system is introduced percutaneously to the screw insertion point.

5. If a closed reduction is not possible or not sufficient in most cases, open reduction can be done by manipulating the C2 arch with a clamp. In most types of instabilities with anterior dislocation of C1 over C2, C2 can be pushed anteriorly to complete the reduction. In case of posterior dislocation of C1 over C2, the C2 can be pulled back with the clamp. After adequate reduction is done, the trocar system is placed at the insertion point of the screw and the position is checked by X-ray in the lateral view. The insertion point can clearly be identified through the midline incision, flouro is not necessary.
6. Then the K-wire or drill is placed on the first side with X-ray control in the lateral view. The K-wire tip should not penetrate the anterior cortical border. After placement of the first K-wire, the procedure is repeated on the other side. Following bilateral placement of the K-wires or drills, the correct position is checked by biplanar X-ray. After correct position has been shown, self-drilling screws are inserted over the K-wires through the cannula system with the screwdriver and then the K-wires are removed. When using noncannulated screws, the drill is removed on one side first and the first screw is placed through the trocar system. Then the other screw is placed after drill removal. When using noncannulated screws, you have to be careful to have no movement between C1 and C2 after removing the drill, especially in high-grade instabilities. After placement of both screws X-rays in ap and lateral must be done to document the correct screw position.
7. For three-point fixation in minimally invasive technique, atlas-claws which are fixed to the posterior arch of C1 are rigidly connected to the transarticular screws C1/C2 (▸ Fig. 23.5a). For fusion, the posterior arches of C1 and C2 are decorticated and bone substitute is placed in onlay technique. Cancellous bone from the posterior iliac crest can also be used, but then the morbidity is increased.

If the used implant system does not have the possibility of fixing an atlas-claw, a Gallie procedure should be done with sublaminar wires at C1 and a cortical bone graft harvested from the posterior iliac crest. If no posterior three-point fixation is performed the risk of nonunion as well as implant failure is increased and a three-point fixation is strongly recommended.

Transarticular screws C1/C2 can be placed with adequate accuracy in the above described minimally invasive technique. Nevertheless, there are potential risks of iatrogenic damage to the vertebral artery or the spinal cord due to screw misplacement. Furthermore, the lateral mass of C1 should be fixed properly to ensure adequate biomechanical stability. In patients

with a vertebral artery anomaly, where transarticular screws cannot be placed safely on one or both sides alternative stabilization methods should be used that are described now.

If a pedicle screw C2 is possible, this screw can be combined with a lateral mass screw C1.[8] In some cases, with severe anomaly of the vertebral artery or significant bony destructions, a pedicle screw C2 may also not be possible. In these cases, a translaminar screw C2 should be used and combined with a lateral mass screw C1. The translaminar screw C2 crosses the posterior lamina to the opposite side and is possible in all cases (▶ Fig. 23.5b).[9]

23.6.3 Spinal Navigation

In 1993, computer navigation systems (CAS) were first presented for the installation of pedicle screws in the lumbar spine based on reports of misplacement rates between 5 and 40% using conventional techniques. In vitro studies showed that misplacement rates of lumbar pedicle screws could be significantly reduced when using spinal navigation. In vivo studies confirmed these results. As in vitro as well as in vivo studies have shown that cervical pedicle screws and transarticular screws C1/C2 can be safely applied using a spinal navigation system,[6,11,12] this technique should also be described although spinal navigation is not mandatory for placement of transarticular screws C1/C2.

The CAS system is positioned on the right side of the patient in front of the head once the posterior aspect of the spine has been approached. The monitor with the touch screen is positioned, so that the surgeon has a good view and can easily reach the draped touch screen. To ensure a good line of sight, the camera is positioned over on the left side of the head for transarticular C1/C2 screws. The surgeon stands at the left side of the patient for transarticular C1/C2 screws.

After the posterior approach is done, the reference clamp is fixed to the spinous process of C2. There is another option when the Brainlab software is used and then, the dynamic reference base can be fixed at the Mayfield headholder. Nevertheless, I prefer the spinous process of C2 to achieve better accuracy. In cases where the spinous process C2 is fractured, I use the spinous process C1 or C3, depending on the pathology.

Next, registration of the vertebra is performed using the surface matching algorithm, where a predicted accuracy < 1.0 mm is acceptable. If the predicted accuracy is > 1.0 mm, a repeated registration procedure should be done until accuracy < 1.0 mm is achieved. After registration of the vertebra, verification has to be done to ensure that the virtual reality of the spinal navigation system corresponds with the surgical reality. This is easily done by tipping with the pointer at points on the posterior surface of the vertebra which are easy to find and clearly identifiable and then control if the position of the pointer shown by the spinal navigation system corresponds to the pointer position in the situs. If verification is accurate, the navigated instrumentation can begin. If verification is inaccurate, the whole registration procedure must be repeated.

The spinal navigation system can be used to find the ideal position for the stab incision for percutaneous-assisted screw placement. The pointer with offset-setting of 8 to 10 cm is used to identify the optimal position for the stab incision (▶ Fig. 23.6a, b). After the stab incision is done, the calibrated trocar system is introduced, the screw is planned, and the K-wire is placed (▶ Fig. 23.7a).

When using K-wires, the spinal navigation system can only visualize the trajectory of the K-wire and not the K-wire itself due to its bending. Therefore, the image intensifier in the lateral view should be used to control the position of the K-wire. Because only one surgical object can be navigated, the instruments can only be navigated in C2, when using the spinal navigation system, the image intensifier is also necessary to control the K-wire/drill position in C1 (▶ Fig. 23.7b). After implanting the K-wires bilateral or if planned only unilateral, the correct position of the K-wires should be controlled by biplanar X-ray (▶ Fig. 23.7c, d). After the correct K-wire

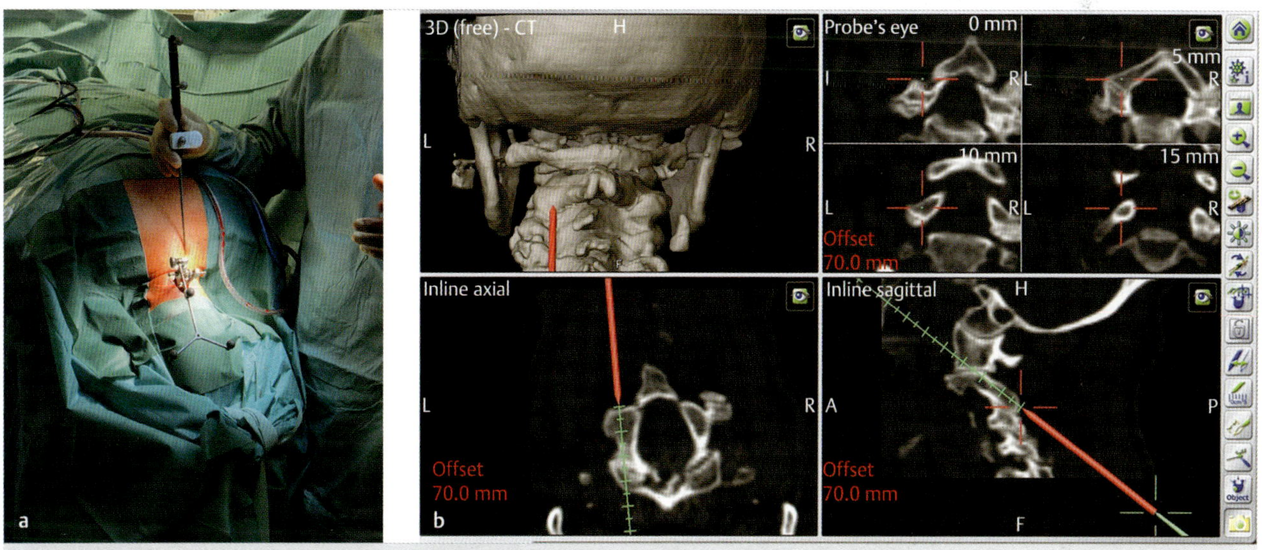

Fig. 23.6 (a) Intraoperative setup for computer-assisted screw placement. After the posterior approach is done, the reference clamp is fixed to the spinous process of C2, the navigation system is placed at the head of the patient. The correct position for the stab incision for the percutaneous screw placement is determined using the pointer with offset setting. **(b)** Intraoperative screenshot of the navigation system while the correct position for the stab incision for the percutaneous screw placement is determined using the pointer with offset setting.

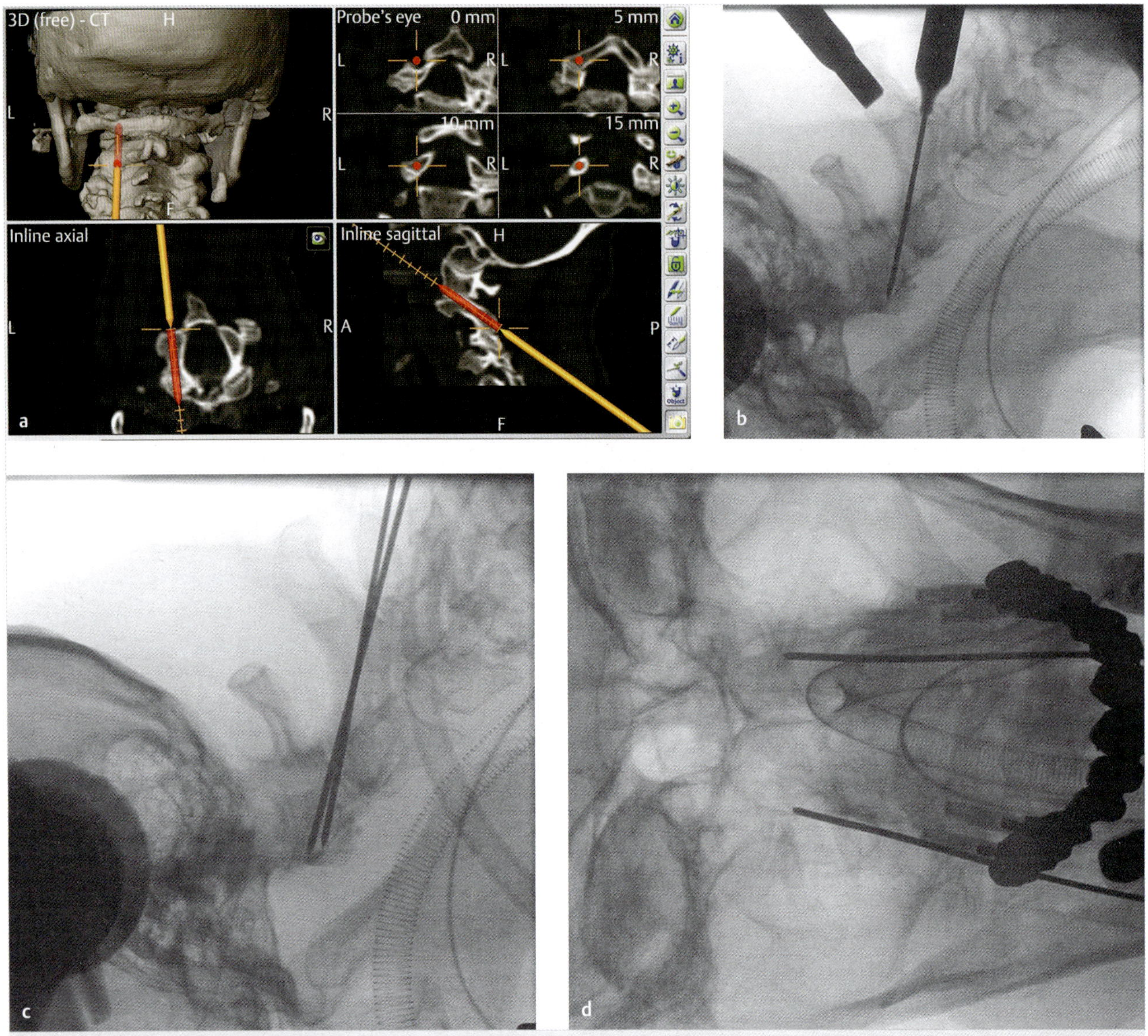

Fig. 23.7 **(a)** Intraoperative screenshot of the screw planning after percutaneous-assisted placement of the K-wire using the precalibrated and verified trocar system. **(b)** Intraoperative lateral X-ray control after percutaneous-assisted placement of the K-wire using the precalibrated and verified trocar system. **(c, d)** Intraoperative biplanar X-ray control of the bilaterally placed K-wires.

position is shown, the planned screws are implanted and the K-wire removed. For three-point fixation in minimally invasive technique atlas-claws which are fixed to the posterior arch of C1 are rigidly connected to the transarticular screws C1/C2 (▸ Fig. 23.8a, b). For fusion, the posterior arches of C1 and C2 are decorticated and bone substitute is placed in onlay technique (▸ Fig. 23.8c, d).

23.6.4 Closure

Wound closure is done over a subfascial drain. Skin closure should be done with interrupted sutures. The cannulas are removed after wound closure of the midline incision and the stab incisions are closed with subcutaneous suture and skin suture.

After turning the patient, the Mayfield clamp is removed and sterile draping of the pin sites should be done.

23.7 Postoperative Care

Owing to the excellent biomechanical stability of the transarticular screws C1/C2 in combination with a three-point fixation, no postoperative collar is needed. If a three-point fixation is not performed, a postoperative immobilization with a cervical collar should follow for 6 weeks. The drain can be removed 2 days postoperative, skin sutures are removed 14 days postoperatively. X-ray controls are recommended before discharge and after 3 and 12 months.

23.8 Complication Avoidance

The main complications of the posterior C1/C2 instrumentation with transarticular screws are related to misplacement of one or both screws or placement of screws in a patient with unsuitable

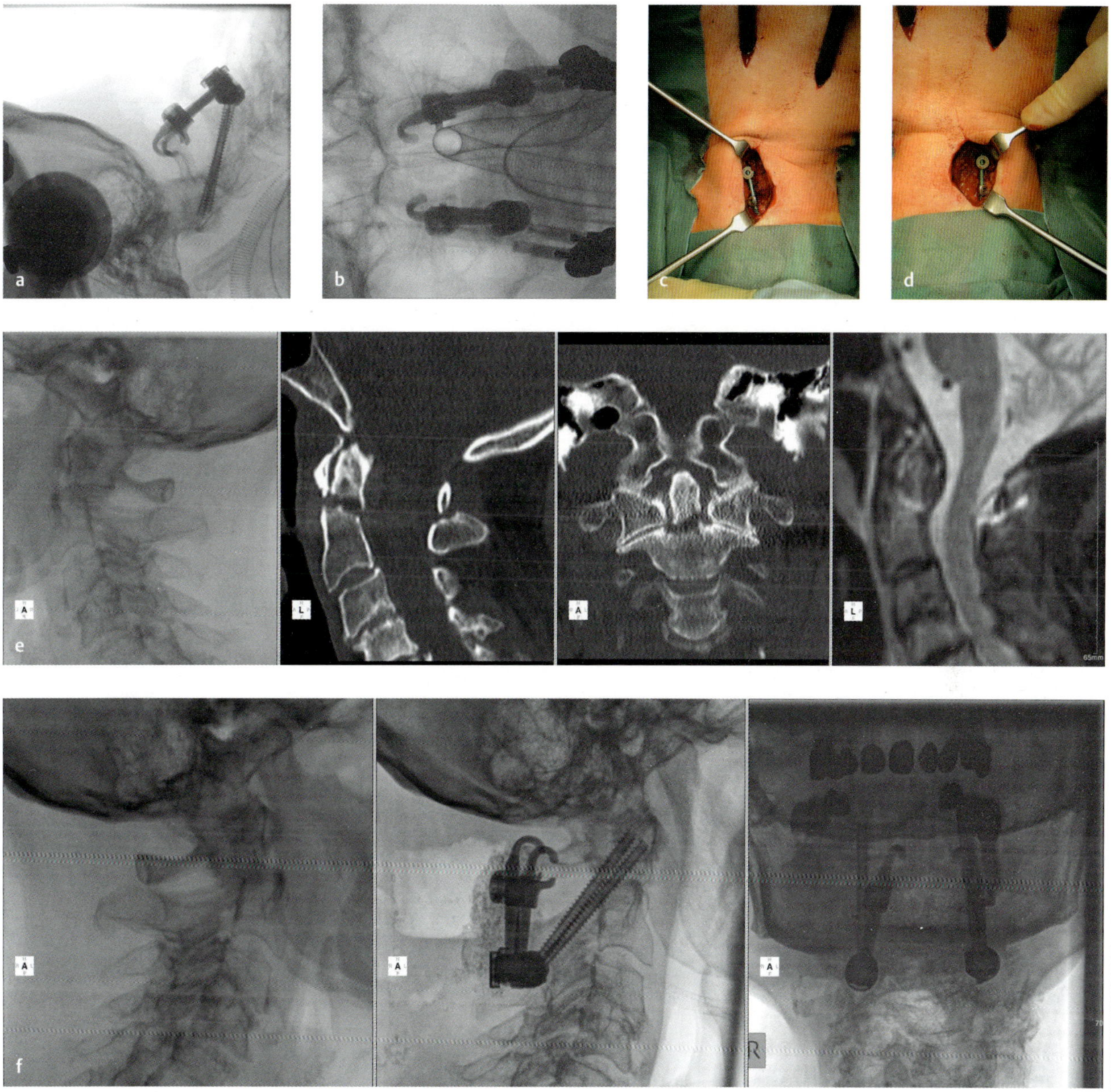

Fig. 23.8 **(a, b)** Intraoperative biplanar X-ray control of the completed instrumentation. **(c, d)** Intraoperative view after completed instrumentation, due to the minimal invasive approach only one side can be shown, note the radiolucent cannulas for percutaneous-assisted placement of the transarticular screws C1/2. **(e, f)** The presented case: 78-year-old woman with unstable odontoid fracture (Anderson 2) **(e)** preoperative lateral X-ray, computed tomography and magnetic resonance imaging showing an unstable odontoid fracture **(f)** preoperative X-ray lateral view and postop biplanar X-ray control.

anatomy for transarticular screws C1/C2. The most frequent reason for unsuitable anatomy is an abnormal course of the vertebral artery in C2 called "high-riding transverse foramen."

Vertebral artery injury, reported in approximately 2 to 4% of patients, may lead to arteriovenous fistula, occlusion, narrowing or dissection of the vertebral artery, which may remain asymptomatic or lead to transient ischemic attacks, stroke, or death.[2,13,14] The best strategy to reduce the risk of vertebral artery injury is thorough preoperative planning with preoperative CT (▶ Fig. 23.1) and exclusion of the patients with vertebral artery variations which are unsuitable for transarticular screws C1/C2 on one or both sides.[7]

The placement of a transarticular screw in a patient with a "high-riding transverse foramen" can lead to an injury of the vertebral artery. To identify these anatomical variations, a preoperative CT of the craniocervical junction with multiplanar reconstructions in the proposed screw axis is mandatory. The course of the vertebral artery can normally be identified in the normal CT as the vertebral groove is seen on the CT (▶ Fig. 23.1). If there are any doubts concerning the course of the vertebral artery, an angio-CT or angio-MRI should be done. In patients with a vertebral artery anomaly, where transarticular screws cannot be placed safely on one or both sides alternative stabilization methods should be used. If a pedicle screw C2 is possible

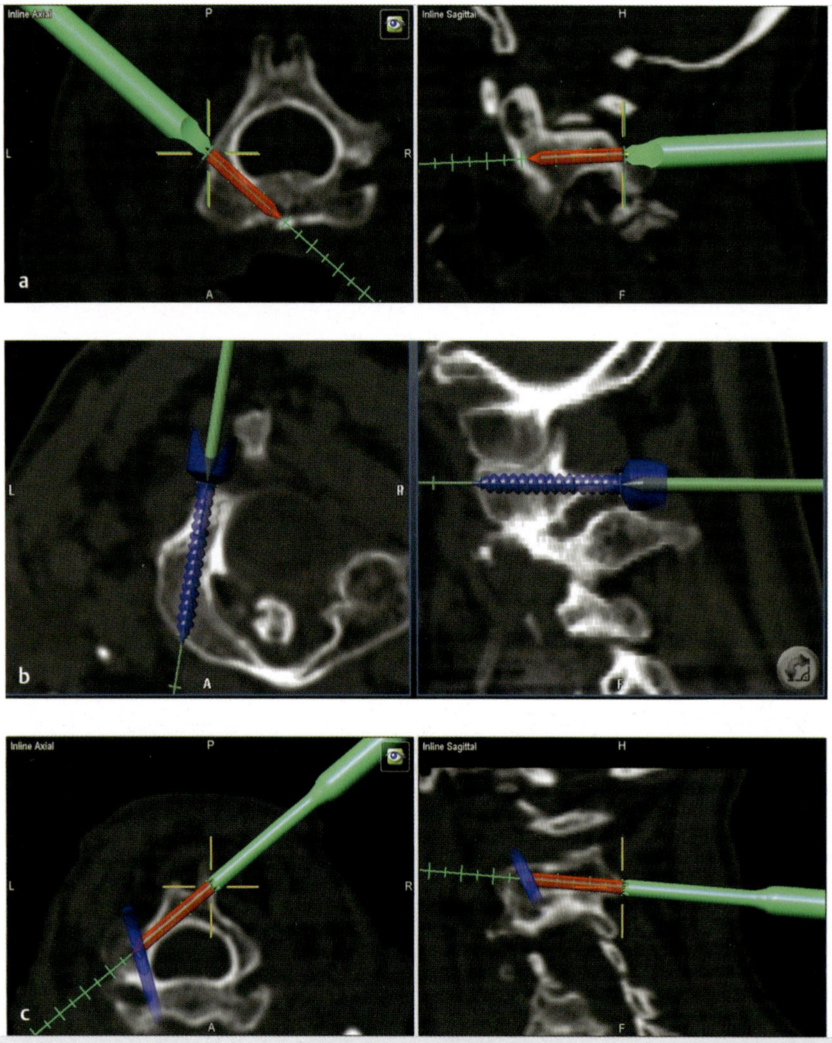

Fig. 23.9 (a) Intraoperative screenshot of a pedicle screw C2. **(b)** Intraoperative screenshot of a lateral mass screw C1. **(c)** Intraoperative screenshot of a translaminar screw C2.

(▸ Fig. 23.9a), this screw can be combined with a lateral mass screw C1[8] (▸ Fig. 23.5b *left* side and ▸ Fig. 23.9b). In some patients with severe anomaly of the vertebral artery, a pedicle screw C2 is also not possible. In these patients, a translaminar screw C2 should be used. This screw crosses the posterior lamina to the opposite side and is possible in all cases (▸ Fig. 23.5b *right* side and ▸ Fig. 23.9c).[9]

The misplacement of a transarticular screw C1/C2 in a patient with suitable anatomy determined by preoperative CT can also lead to an injury of the vertebral artery, especially if the screw angle related to the endplate of C2 is too small. In case of an injury of the vertebral artery on one side, the screw on this side should be inserted to stop the bleeding. A repair of the vertebral artery in this location is not possible. If the vertebral artery was injured on the side of the first screw, a screw should be chosen for the other side which makes an injury of the vertebral artery impossible. The safest screw in this situation is a translaminar crossing screw, as described above.

The misplacement of a transarticular screw can also cause an impaired biomechanical stability if the lateral mass of C1 is not fixed properly with the screw. This normally happens if the screw angle is too small, more rarely the reason is a too laterally or too medially placed screw.

To prevent a misplacement of the screws the correct positioning of the patient is important. In older patients with a high-thoracic kyphosis, the positioning can be especially difficult. It is helpful to check the positioning of the patient in the lateral view of the image intensifier with a straight instrument held lateral to the patient if the optimal screw angulation is possible (▸ Fig. 23.2). If it is not possible, the positioning of the patient should be changed until the needed screw angulation can be achieved. Normally a higher foam pillar under the chest of the patient helps to allow more inclination of the cervical spine.

If the positioning of the patient is correct, other possible reasons for screw misplacement are wrong entry point or wrong screw trajectory. To prevent screw misplacement, thorough knowledge of the three-dimensional anatomy of C1/C2 is mandatory.

To identify a wrong entry point or screw trajectory, X-ray control ap and lateral should be done as early as possible after

placement of both K-wires or drills (▶ Fig. 23.7c, d). If a wrong placement is shown, the drill or K-wire position can be changed before a screw is implanted.

Another approach-related complication is injury to the vertebral artery during dissection of the posterior arch of C1. To be safe, dissection should not be carried out more than 16 mm lateral to the midline on both sides.

Other possible complications are typical complications of spine stabilization such as wound healing problems or infections. Due to the minimally invasive approach these complications are less frequent as compared with traditional approaches. In case of wound healing disturbances, early revision with debridement and perhaps vacuum suction helps to avoid deep infections. In case of deep infection of the implant site, early revision is also beneficial. Implant removal is not necessary but placement of local antibiotics, such as septopal chains, is recommended.

23.9 Tips and Tricks

- Thorough preoperative planning using CT with multiplanar reconstruction to ensure that transarticular screws C1/C2 are possible: Exclude high-riding transverse foramen or other anomalies of the vertebral artery. If transarticular screws C1/C2 are not possible without increased risk for vertebral artery injury, use lateral mass screws C1 in combination with pedicle screws C2 or translaminar screws C2.
- Correct positioning of the patient: Ensure that placement of the cannulas for the percutaneous-assisted placement of the transarticular screws C1/C2 is possible, otherwise correct the positioning if possible, if not possible use lateral mass screws C1 in combination with pedicle screws C2 or translaminar screws C2.
- If possible use spinal navigation for placement of the K-wires.
- Always check the correct position of the K-wires or drills with biplanar X-ray before implanting the screws.
- If you are in doubt that the vertebral artery could be injured on one side, place the screw on this side and use alternative screws without the risk of vertebral artery injury on the opposite side.
- In case of possible vertebral artery injury intraoperatively, postoperative angiography is mandatory to rule out a fistula or pseudoaneurysm which could be treated by endovascular techniques.
- The correct length of the transarticular screws C1/C2 should be planned preoperatively in the CT with multiplanar reconstructions in the planned screw trajectory or intraoperatively with spinal navigation. If the screws are too long, injury to the hypoglossal nerve or the carotid artery is possible.

23.10 Conclusion

- Posterior transarticular screws C1/C2 in combination with posterior three-point fixation allow a stable C1/C2 fixation with the highest biomechanical stability compared to all other techniques.
- The use of atlas-claws fixed to the transarticular screws C1/C2 for three-point fixation reduces the risk and morbidity as sublaminar wires C1 and cortical bone grafts are not needed.
- Percutaneous-assisted screw placement in combination with a small midline incision reduces the approach-related morbidity and makes the correct screw placement easier.
- Computer navigation is not needed for screw placement, but reduces the risk of screw misplacement.

References

[1] Richter M. Posterior instrumentation of the cervical spine for instability using the neon occipito-cervical system. Part 1: atlanto-axial instrumentation. Orthop Traumatol. 2003; 1:70–89

[2] Weidner A, Wähler M, Chiu ST, Ullrich CG. Modification of C1-C2 transarticular screw fixation by image-guided surgery. Spine. 2000; 25(20):2668–2673, discussion 2674

[3] Richter M, Schmidt R, Claes L, Puhl W, Wilke HJ. Posterior atlantoaxial fixation: biomechanical in vitro comparison of six different techniques. Spine. 2002; 27(16):1724–1732

[4] Mitsui H. A new operation for atlanto-axial arthrodesis. J Bone Joint Surg Br. 1984; 66(3):422–425

[5] Magerl F, Seemann P. Stable posterior fusion of the atlas and axis by transarticular screw fixation. In: Kehr P, Weidner A, eds. Cervical Spine Vol. 1. Strassbourg, Wien, New York: Springer Verlag; 1987:322–327

[6] Grob D, Jeanneret B, Aebi M, Markwalder TM. Atlanto-axial fusion with transarticular screw fixation. J Bone Joint Surg Br. 1991; 73(6):972–976

[7] Paramore CG, Dickman CA, Sonntag VK. The anatomical suitability of the C1–2 complex for transarticular screw fixation. J Neurosurg. 1996; 85(2):221–224

[8] Goel A, Laheri V. Plate and screw fixation for atlanto-axial subluxation. Acta Neurochir (Wien). 1994; 129(1–2):47–53

[9] Wright NM. Posterior C2 fixation using bilateral, crossing C2 laminar screws: case series and technical note. J Spinal Disord Tech. 2004; 17(2):158–162

[10] Melcher RP, Puttlitz CM, Kleinstueck FS, Lotz JC, Harms J, Bradford DS. Biomechanical testing of posterior atlantoaxial fixation techniques. Spine. 2002; 27(22):2435–2440

[11] Richter M, Mattes T, Cakir B. Computer-assisted posterior instrumentation of the cervical and cervico-thoracic spine. Eur Spine J. 2004, 13(1):50–59

[12] Amiot LP, Labelle H, DeGuise JA, Sati M, Brodeur P, Rivard CH. Computer-assisted pedicle screw fixation. A feasibility study. Spine. 1995; 20(10):1208–1212

[13] Wright NM, Lauryssen C, American Association of Neurological Surgeons/Congress of Neurological Surgeons. Vertebral artery injury in C1–2 transarticular screw fixation: results of a survey of the AANS/CNS section on disorders of the spine and peripheral nerves. J Neurosurg. 1998; 88(4):634–640

[14] Prabhu VC, France JC, Voelker JL, Zoarski GH. Vertebral artery pseudoaneurysm complicating posterior C1–2 transarticular screw fixation: case report. Surg Neurol. 2001; 55(1):29–33, discussion 33–34

24 Cervical Three-Dimensional Navigation to Facilitate Minimally Invasive Spine Surgery

Maziyar A. Kalani, Iain H. Kalfas, and Michael P. Steinmetz

Summary

As three-dimensional spinal navigation becomes more pervasive, its role in cervical spine surgery continues to evolve. Although the indications for performing surgery in the cervical spine remain dependent on the patient-specific pathology and complaints, surgical navigation acts as a powerful adjunct in helping address challenging anatomy and pathology. This technology may be applied to anterior and posterior approaches, from the craniocervical down to the cervicothoracic junction; it may be applied to degenerative and bony pathology and to intradural cysts and tumors. Although computed tomography (CT) imaging is the standard data set used for spinal navigation, magnetic resonance imaging (MRI) and ultrasonography may play a greater role in its future. In this chapter, we discuss the role of navigation in facilitating cervical spine surgery, including our experience, pearls, and pitfall avoidance.

Keywords: cervical spine surgery, intraoperative computed tomography, surgical navigation, minimally invasive spine surgery, transarticular screw, craniocervical junction, atlantoaxial instability, cervical spine deformity

24.1 Introduction

The presence of the spinal cord, nerve roots, carotid and vertebral arteries as well as small bony fixation points in the cervical spine provide an opportunity for exploring the use of spinal navigation to facilitate the safety and effectiveness of instrumentation. A very well-known risk in instrumenting the upper cervical spine is that of vertebral artery injury during transarticular screw placement; a major vascular complication rate is reported to be as high as 4.1%, resulting in a movement away from this biomechanically favorable screw toward the potentially safer C1 lateral mass and C2 pars/pedicle instrumentation.[1] In addition to critical neural and vascular structures, the other remaining challenges to cervical spine surgery include appropriate localization, particularly in the lower cervical spine, and maintenance of alignment in order to prevent iatrogenic deformity during instrumentation. Although these issues may be addressed with larger incisions, the use of image guidance and navigation may mitigate the need for further invasion of soft tissue. Herein, we discuss the role of navigation in facilitating cervical spine surgery, highlighting the relative indications and contraindications, complication avoidance as well as tips and tricks to aid spine surgeons.

Similar to cranial navigation, spinal navigation relies on frameless stereotaxy. Indeed the first case of frameless stereotactic spinal navigation was performed at the Cleveland Clinic in 1994.[2,3] The first reported feasibility study for the use of three-dimensional fluoroscopic-based stereotactic navigation in the cervical spine was reported by Holly and Foley, where screws were placed at C1–C2 (transarticular), C3–C6 (lateral mass), and C7 (pedicle) with 97.6% accuracy with only one of 42 screws demonstrating a cortical breech (C7 pedicle screw).[4] Since then, numerous cadaveric and clinical feasibility studies have reported lower rates of misplaced instrumentation in the cervical spine for translaminar, transarticular, lateral mass, and transpedicular screws with overall lower blood loss.[5,6,7,8,9] The rate of poor screw placement was 12.5 to 17.9% higher without the use of three-dimensional navigation.[10,11,12] A similar study demonstrated the safety and feasibility of using three-dimensional computer-assisted navigation in the instrumentation of pediatric cervical spines.[1314,15]

Anterior cervical corpectomy may be performed with shorter operative time and reduced morbidity when assisted by three-dimensional navigation.[14,15] Moreover, computer-assisted navigation has facilitated both anterior and posterior approaches for minimally invasive foraminotomies.[16,17,18] Often, patients' body habitus may make localization of lower cervical foraminotomies challenging. The use of image guidance not only eases correct level surgery, but also helps delineate the boundaries of decompression, allowing for a safe and efficacious operation to be performed at the intended level.

Traumatic injuries to the cervical spine may distort normal anatomy significantly. Anatomic consideration and reduced room for error in hardware placement make traumatic cervical spine injuries an area where navigation is highly used. Three-dimensional navigation has been used to treat hangman's fractures,[19,20] Jefferson-variant fractures,[21] atlantoaxial instability,[22,23] as well as uncomplicated injuries to the subaxial spine.[22,23]

Adult degenerative cervical deformity is an interesting area of potential application of three-dimensional navigation. There is little description of its use in the literature so far; although it may not help facilitate minimally invasive surgery due to challenges such as spinal cord and vascular considerations, it has ample uses in open cervical deformity correction such as placement of instrumentation or osteotomy planning.

Three-dimensional navigation is of particular utility in the craniocervical junction. Frameless stereotaxis has successfully facilitated the decompression of anterior transcervical, transoral, and transnasal odontoidectomy,[24,2526,27] as well as resection of malignancies of the craniocervical junction.[28]

Beyond utilizing three-dimensional navigation for bony decompression and arthrodesis, image guidance may be utilized for fenestration of intradural arachnoid cysts,[29,30,31] and intra- and extramedullary tumors.[32,33,34,35]

24.2 Indications

The decision whether to use three-dimensional navigation for cervical spine surgery dovetails with the indications for surgical intervention. Indications typically include decompression of the spinal cord and/or nerve roots, correction of deformity, stabilization of instability causing mechanical pain, and, in the case of malignancy and infection, for diagnostic purposes. There is no absolute indication for the use of this technology; relative indications include revision surgery or irradiation where the anatomy is

distorted, presence of trauma, and as an adjunct for en bloc resection or complex osteotomies in deformity correction.

24.3 Contraindications

Relative contraindications include a lack of static structure to affix the reference array, inability to fixate the head using a three-point holder, patient habitus resulting in poor image acquisition, and lack of appropriate surgical table which may result in poor resolution images.

24.4 Preoperative Planning

In order to prepare for operative intervention, standard preoperative imaging is obtained to aid in the surgical plan. Magnetic resonance imaging (MRI) and computed tomography (CT) scans are helpful in determining the pathology as well as normal anatomy with respect to the pathology. Standing upright radiographs may be useful in better understanding alignment and stability; dynamic noninvasive imaging with MRI and CT may be considered to give further insight into the specific patient's complaints. Other preoperative ancillaries may include choice of specific instrumentation, use of autograft versus allograft, incorporation of intraoperative neurophysiologic monitoring, patient positioning, and necessity of an approach surgeon (for transnasal or high-risk anterior cervical approaches).

Surgical table selection is particularly important for cervical three-dimensional navigation assisted surgery. Careful selection of the appropriate bed will allow for ease of workflow while acquiring the necessary intraoperative imaging; certain table designs and radiolucent head holder dimensions may hinder the ability to acquire intraoperative cone-beam CT for three-dimensional navigation (▶ Fig. 24.1). Both the standard surgical table with the pedestal at the caudal end as well as a carbon frame table allow for appropriate positioning of the intraoperative O-arm CT (Medtronic, Dublin, Ireland) to acquire imaging and provide for appropriate maintenance of alignment and deformity correction. Alternatively, the Airo CT scanner system (Brainlab, Munich, Germany) has an integrated surgical bed to which a radiolucent three-point cranial fixation may be attached.

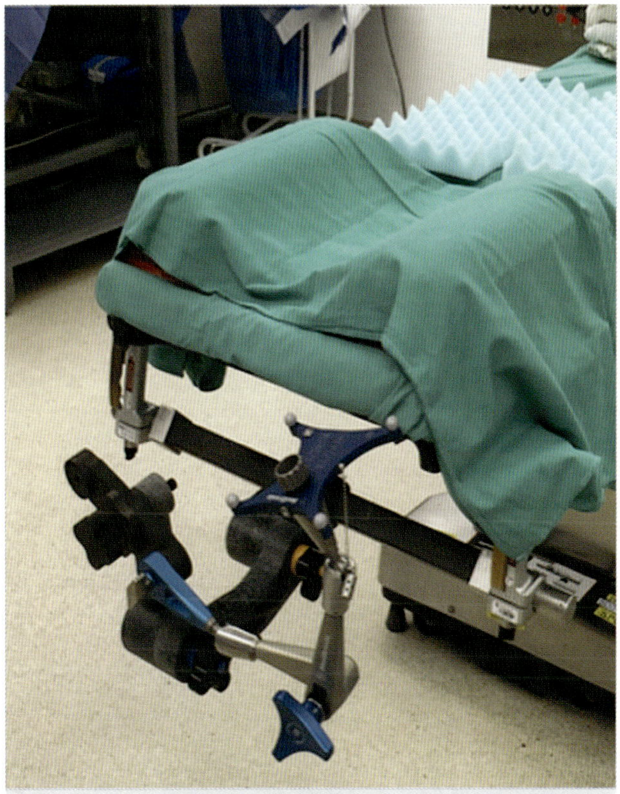

Fig. 24.1 Standard surgical bed with bolsters is shown with a radiolucent three-pin head holder. Rigid fixation of the reference array to the radiolucent head holder is demonstrated.

In the cervical spine, three-dimensional navigation can be helpful for the planning and placement of transarticular C1–C2 screws, C1 lateral mass screws, C2 translaminar screws, C2 pars/pedicle screws, lateral mass screws, and C7 pedicle screws. In addition, it can also be used for occipital screw placement and for localization of pathology, for example, for cervical foraminotomies. Navigation is especially useful for localization of the correct level in the lower cervical spine due to the shoulder blade artifact seen with fluoroscopy during conventional surgical techniques.

24.5 Patient Positioning

Appropriate patient positioning is dependent on the surgical approach that is determined by the surgeon. The most common approach used in conjunction with three-dimensional navigation is the posterior cervical approach (▶ Fig. 24.2). Anterior approaches may be performed with standard supine positioning. Regardless of the approach, patient factors such as body habitus and the presence of an adequate rigid structure to attach the reference array are important. Obese patients pose a challenge for performing three-dimensional navigation assisted cervical spine surgery due to the difficulty in obtaining optimal beam penetration, which may confound image quality and the accuracy of instrumentation positioning.

The use of a radiolucent three-pin head holder not only allows for rigid cranial fixation and preservation of spinal alignment but also limits metallic interference during imaging. All pressure points are padded including the chest, anterior superior iliac spine, and knees; the feet are elevated as to not put pressure on the toes. The patient's head should be above the level of the heart and the ankles positioned at the level of the hips, with the knees flexed to minimized bleeding and increase venous return. Mechanical venous thrombosis prophylaxis is also recommended.

24.6 Surgical Steps

24.6.1 Step 1: Incision

After patient positioning, the navigation reference array can be attached to the three-point head holder and left exposed following surgical draping. Alternatively, the array can be attached

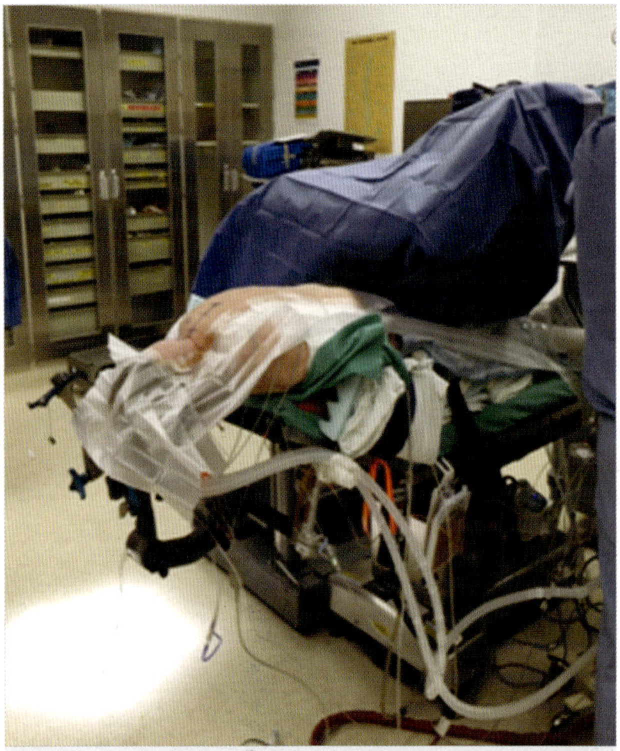

Fig. 24.2 A patient undergoing C2–C3 stabilization for hangman's fracture with anterolisthesis of C2 on C3 is shown with the cervical spine in the neutral position. The head is immobilized with a radiolucent head holder with an affixed reference array.

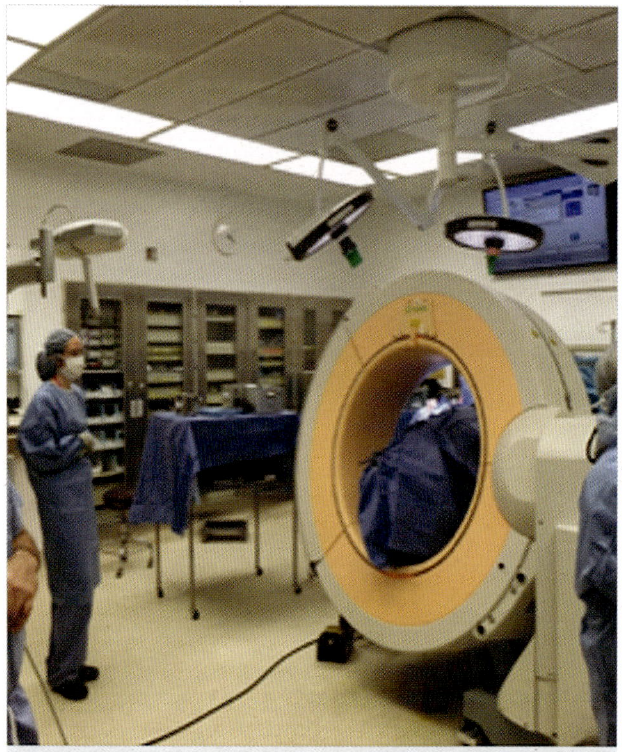

Fig. 24.3 Operating room setup demonstrating the intraoperative O-arm in position for image acquisition. Note the navigation camera to the top left and the exposed reference array.

to a spinous process in the surgical field following exposure. If the array is screwed into the spinous process, it is important to apply a counter-rotational torque to the base of the array in order to prevent fracturing of the spinous process and disruption of point of fixation rigidity. Ideally, the reference array should be placed close to the working area within the exposure. Accuracy may decrease with increasing distance between the array and the operative area of navigational interest.[36,37,38] Since localization is less of an issue with high-definition CT imaging, shoulder traction or other means to lower the shoulders is not necessary.

The operative incision may be planned using preincision imaging or may be made using anatomical landmarks.

24.6.2 Step 2: Navigation Setup

Following a standard midline incision, a subperiosteal dissection is used to expose the bony spine. The surgical field is draped and the intraoperative CT scanner positioned for image acquisition (▶ Fig. 24.3). The wound retractors may be left in position or removed prior to imaging. Movements during image acquisition may cause distortion during acquisition and make registration more challenging. We recommend asking the anesthesiologist to hold the patient's respirations (apnea) during the acquisition process.

Navigational and instrumentation accuracy are both dependent on high-quality image acquisition and reproducible registration of instrumentation to the acquired three-dimensional imaging. Registration is the critical step of spinal navigation in that it establishes the precise spatial relationship of the image data with the physical space of the patient's corresponding surgical anatomy. Registration of the image data set to the spinal anatomy occurs automatically with intraoperative CT navigation. With preoperative CT-based navigation, the surgeon performing surgical exposure must carry out registration. Pre-selected registration points in the image data are individually matched to their corresponding points in the surgical field. In either registration methods, placing a navigation tool onto any discreet landmark in the surgical field and confirming that the same point is highlighted on the navigation workstation screen validates the accuracy of the registration process.

24.6.3 Step 3: Screw Trajectory Confirmation

After satisfactory image acquisition and registration, navigation for the selection of appropriate screw trajectories is performed. Confirming the navigation acquisition with normal, visible anatomy reduces inaccuracies; spinous processes, lateral masses, and facet joints may be used along with the reference array itself.

24.6.4 Step 4: Screw Insertion

In the cervical spine, these screw trajectories navigation can be carried out for the placement of transarticular C1–C2 screws, C1 lateral mass screws, C2 translaminar screws, C2 pars/pedicle screws, lateral mass screws, and C7 pedicle screws; navigation

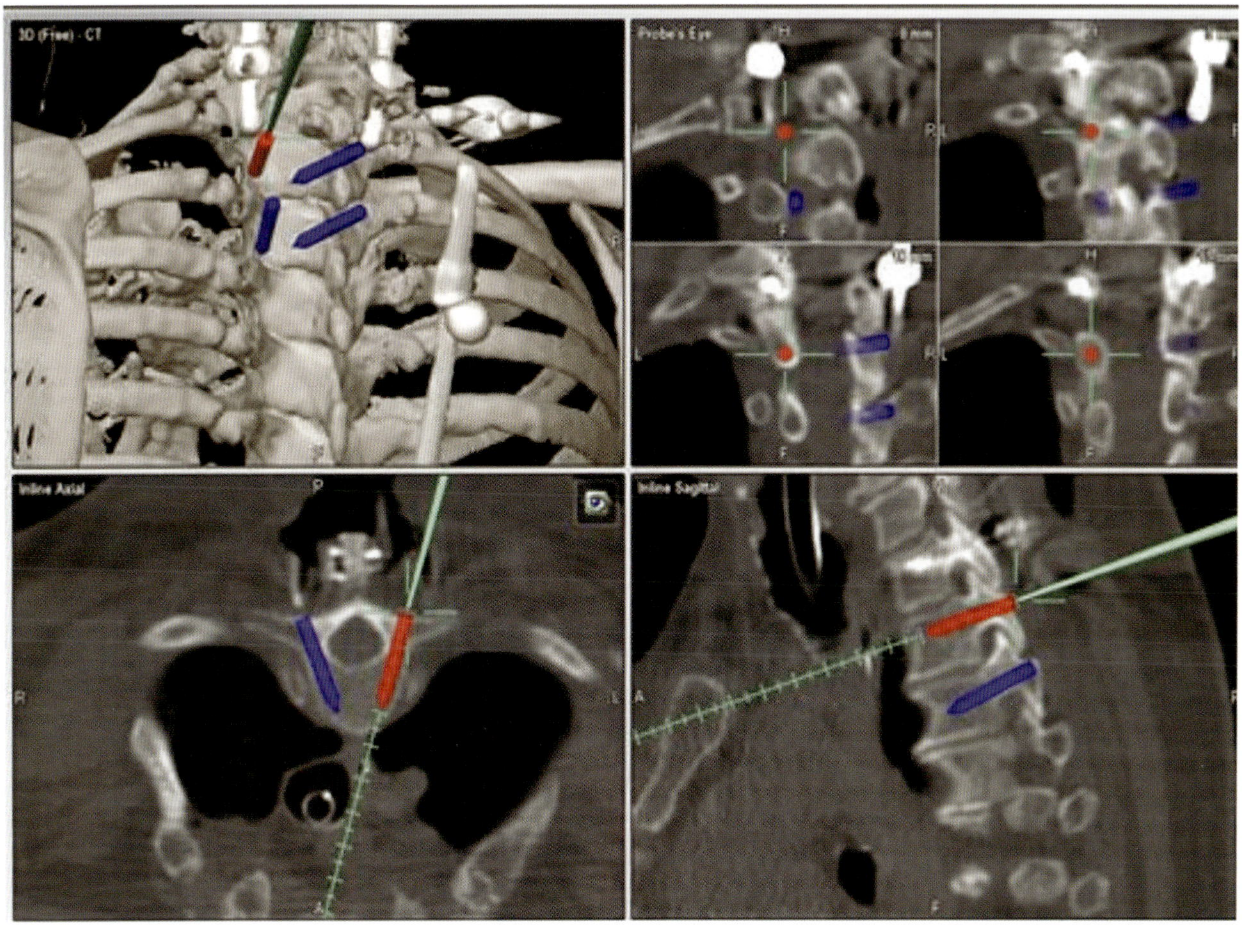

Fig. 24.1 Navigation screenshot. Demonstrating the utility of this technology specially in areas where lateral fluoroscopy is complicated (T1-T5).

is especially useful in this case due to the shoulder blade artifact seen on conventional surgical techniques (▶ Fig. 24.4). For ease of workflow and to reduce perioperative radiation exposure, flat-plate or intraoperative fluoroscopy is used to evaluate instrumentation; a repeat intraoperative scan is not unreasonable if there are concerns. Navigation can also be used to monitor the extent of decompression particularly through a transoral or endonasal approach (▶ Video 24.1).

24.6.5 Step 5: Closure

Prior to initiating closure, we utilize vancomycin powder when instrumentation is placed. Furthermore, to allow for evacuation of any compressive hematoma and to facilitate a tension-free closure, subfascial drains are placed. Closure is performed in a standard manner beginning with closure of the deep and superficial fascial layers, followed by closure of the dermal and subdermal layers. Dermal adhesive glue is used to close the skin and the subfascial drain is secured with an anchoring stitch and Roman sandal relaxation ties.

24.7 Postoperative Care

Standard postoperative care includes pain control with intravenous and oral opioids with or without antispasmodics.

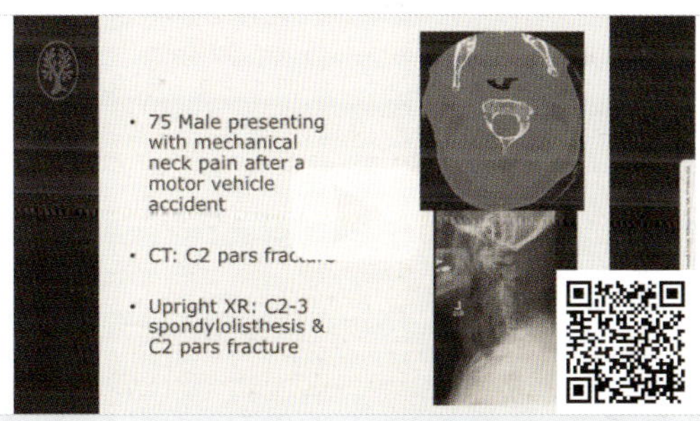

Video 24.1 Cervical 3D navigation to facilitate MISS.

Subfascial drains are typically removed when output reaches 50 cc or less per 8-hour shift. Weight-bearing upright radiographs are obtained prior to discharge in order to assess cervical alignment and hardware if it is placed.

24.8 Complication Avoidance

The most common complication of spinal navigation is the failure to achieve or maintain accurate registration of the surgical field. This typically results from movement of the reference array following image acquisition or, in the setting of preoperative CT-based navigation, following manual registration.

Therefore, it is important that the reference array be firmly attached prior to navigation. It is also important to routinely and regularly validate the registration accuracy throughout the navigation process. This helps to avoid any errors that may occur following an unrecognized displacement of the array. It also serves as means of secondary confirmation of the selected trajectories.

With intraoperative CT navigation, it is important to be aware of standard radiation safety techniques for all operating room personnel given the higher radiation dosing used for CT imaging compared to traditional fluoroscopy or radiography.[39] Each O-arm image acquisition spin is the equivalent of up to 65 chest X-rays. A standard O-arm spin is approximately 65 chest X-rays; in that regard, they were able to reduce it to nearly 10% of a standard default run and therefore 6 to 7 X-rays in their pediatric protocol. Thus, adequate exposure prior to image acquisition is important to prevent the need for repetitive spins. This may be facilitated by a preincision flat plate or fluoroscopic image to help delineate the incision. However, radiation exposure to the operating room attendant is mitigated, so long as 10 feet distance is maintained between the attendant and the scanner.[39] It is also important to note that the radiation exposure to the surgeon may be significant and cumulative on an annual basis, while that to the patient is generally not due to the focal nature of the use of image guidance in the operation.

24.9 Tips and Tricks

Developing and maintaining a consistent workflow for patient positioning, image acquisition, and instrument registration are essential for reproducible efficiency and effectiveness when applying three-dimensional navigation to the surgeon's armamentarium. Teamwork is vital to make sure every step is done correctly every time. It is critical to maintain a high level of vigilance for avoiding dislodgment of the reference array. Since the potential for array dislodgment increases with time, we recommend performing navigation immediately following image acquisition when intraoperative CT navigation is used. It is also important to be persistent and routinely validate registration and navigational tool accuracy throughout the navigation process, which may be done against visible, fixed landmarks within the exposed field or using the reference array.

Three-dimensional navigation is a safe and effective technology for facilitating improved accuracy during cervical spine surgery. Navigation has successfully been applied to challenging cervical anatomy, trauma, malignancies, and complex deformity correction. Developing a consistent intraoperative, team-based workflow, rigid reference array fixation, and persistent audit for accuracy are pearls for success in using navigation to facilitate cervical spine surgery.

References

[1] Madawi AA, Casey AT, Solanki GA, Tuite G, Veres R, Crockard HA. Radiological and anatomical evaluation of the atlantoaxial transarticular screw fixation technique. J Neurosurg. 1997; 86(6):961–968

[2] Murphy MA, McKenzie RL, Kormos DW, Kalfas IH. Frameless stereotaxis for the insertion of lumbar pedicle screws. J Clin Neurosci. 1994; 1(4):257–260

[3] Kalfas IH, Kormos DW, Murphy MA, et al. Application of frameless stereotaxy to pedicle screw fixation of the spine. J Neurosurg. 1995; 83(4):641–647

[4] Holly LT, Foley KT. Percutaneous placement of posterior cervical screws using three-dimensional fluoroscopy. Spine. 2006; 31(5):536–540, discussion 541

[5] Hitti FL, Hudgins ED, Chen HI, Malhotra NR, Zager EL, Schuster JM. Intraoperative navigation is associated with reduced blood loss during C1-C2 posterior cervical fixation. World Neurosurg. 2017; 107:574–578

[6] Barsa P, Fröhlich R, Šercl M, Buchvald P, Suchomel P. The intraoperative portable CT scanner-based spinal navigation: a viable option for instrumentation in the region of cervico-thoracic junction. Eur Spine J. 2016; 25(6):1643–1650

[7] Rajasekaran S, Avadhani A, Shetty AP. Axial translaminar screw placement using three-dimensional fluoroscopy-based navigation. Singapore Med J. 2011; 52(1):15–18

[8] Ishikawa Y, Kanemura T, Yoshida G, et al. Intraoperative, full-rotation, three-dimensional image (O-arm)-based navigation system for cervical pedicle screw insertion. J Neurosurg Spine. 2011; 15(5):472–478

[9] Ishikawa Y, Kanemura T, Yoshida G, Ito Z, Muramoto A, Ohno S. Clinical accuracy of three-dimensional fluoroscopy-based computer-assisted cervical pedicle screw placement: a retrospective comparative study of conventional versus computer-assisted cervical pedicle screw placement. J Neurosurg Spine. 2010; 13(5):606–611

[10] Suchomel P, Hradil J, Frölich R, Barsa P, Lukás R. [Navigation techniques in surgery of cranio-cervical junction and upper cervical spine]. Acta Chir Orthop Traumatol Cech. 2009; 76(2):137–148

[11] Grob D, Jeanneret B, Aebi M, Markwalder TM. Atlanto-axial fusion with transarticular screw fixation. J Bone Joint Surg Br. 1991; 73(6):972–976

[12] Tian W, Liu Y, Zheng S, Lv Y. Accuracy of lower cervical pedicle screw placement with assistance of distinct navigation systems: a human cadaveric study. Eur Spine J. 2013; 22(1):148–155

[13] Rajasekaran S, Kanna PRM, Shetty AP. Safety of cervical pedicle screw insertion in children: a clinicoradiological evaluation of computer-assisted insertion of 51 cervical pedicle screws including 28 subaxial pedicle screws in 16 children. Spine. 2012; 37(4):E216–E223

[14] Yao N, Wang C, Wang W, Wang L. Full-endoscopic technique for anterior cervical discectomy and interbody fusion: 5-year follow-up results of 67 cases. Eur Spine J. 2011; 20(6):899–904

[15] Ruetten S, Komp M, Merk H, Godolias G. Full-endoscopic anterior decompression versus conventional anterior decompression and fusion in cervical disc herniations. Int Orthop. 2009; 33(6):1677–1682

[16] Del Curto D, Kim J-S, Lee S-H. Minimally invasive posterior cervical microforaminotomy in the lower cervical spine and C-T junction assisted by O-arm-based navigation. Comput Aided Surg. 2013; 18(3–4):76–83

[17] Fessler RG, Khoo LT. Minimally invasive cervical microendoscopic foraminotomy: an initial clinical experience. Neurosurgery. 2002; 51(5) Suppl:S37–S45

[18] Kim J-S, Eun SS, Prada N, Choi G, Lee S-H. Modified transcorporeal anterior cervical microforaminotomy assisted by O-arm-based navigation: a technical case report. Eur Spine J. 2011; 20(2) Suppl 2:S147–S152

[19] Lang Z, Tian W, Liu Y, Liu B, Yuan Q, Sun Y. Minimally invasive pedicle screw fixation using intraoperative 3-dimensional fluoroscopy-based navigation (CAMISS technique) for hangman fracture. Spine. 2016; 41(1):39–45

[20] Buchholz AL, Morgan SL, Robinson LC, Frankel BM. Minimally invasive percutaneous screw fixation of traumatic spondylolisthesis of the axis. J Neurosurg Spine. 2015; 22(5):459–465

[21] Malcolm JG, Tan LA, Johnson AK. Image-guided internal fixation of an oblique sagittal split fracture of C1 lateral mass with motion preservation: a technical report. Cureus. 2017; 9(7):e1496

[22] Stein G, Schiffer G, Bredow J, Meyer C. [3D fluoroscopy-navigated Magerl fusion of the 1st and 2nd cervical vertebra]. Z Orthop Unfall. 2016; 154 (6):636–637

[23] Czabanka M, Haemmerli J, Hecht N, et al. Spinal navigation for posterior instrumentation of C1-2 instability using a mobile intraoperative CT scanner. J Neurosurg Spine. 2017; 27(3):268–275

[24] Leng LZ, Anand VK, Hartl R, Schwartz TH. Endonasal endoscopic resection of an os odontoideum to decompress the cervicomedullary junction: a minimal access surgical technique. Spine. 2009; 34(4):E139–E143

[25] Kaibara T, Hurlbert RJ, Sutherland GR. Intraoperative magnetic resonance imaging-augmented transoral resection of axial disease. Neurosurg Focus. 2001; 10(2):E4

[26] Dasenbrock HH, Clarke MJ, Bydon A, et al. Endoscopic image-guided transcervical odontoidectomy: outcomes of 15 patients with basilar invagination. Neurosurgery. 2012; 70(2):351–359, discussion 359–360
[27] Wolinsky J-P, Sciubba DM, Suk I, Gokaslan ZL. Endoscopic image-guided odontoidectomy for decompression of basilar invagination via a standard anterior cervical approach. Technical note. J Neurosurg Spine. 2007; 6 (2):184–191
[28] Hsu W, Kosztowski TA, Zaidi HA, Gokaslan ZL, Wolinsky J-P. Image-guided, endoscopic, transcervical resection of cervical chordoma. J Neurosurg Spine. 2010; 12(4):431–435
[29] Takahashi S, Saruhashi Y, Odate S, Matsusue Y, Morikawa S. Percutaneous aspiration of spinal terminal ventricle cysts using real-time magnetic resonance imaging and navigation. Spine. 2009; 34(6):629–634
[30] Takahashi S, Morikawa S, Saruhashi Y, Matsusue Y, Kawakami M. Percutaneous transthoracic fenestration of an intramedullary neurenteric cyst in the thoracic spine with intraoperative magnetic resonance image navigation and thoracoscopy. J Neurosurg Spine. 2008; 9(5):488–492
[31] Takahashi S, Morikawa S, Egawa M, Saruhashi Y, Matsusue Y. Magnetic resonance imaging-guided percutaneous fenestration of a cervical intradural cyst. Case report. J Neurosurg. 2003; 99(3) Suppl:313–315
[32] Stefini R, Peron S, Mandelli J, Bianchini E, Roccucci P. Intraoperative spinal navigation for the removal of intradural tumors: technical notes. Oper Neurosurg (Hagerstown, Md). 2018; 15(1):54–59
[33] Vasudeva VS, Abd-El-Barr M, Pompeu YA, Karhade A, Groff MW, Lu Y. Use of intraoperative ultrasound during spinal surgery. Global Spine J. 2017; 7 (7):648–656
[34] Hussain I, Navarro-Ramirez R, Lang G, Härtl R. 3D navigation-guided resection of giant ventral cervical intradural schwannoma with 360-degree stabilization. Clin Spine Surg. 2018; 31(5):E257–E265
[35] Mannion RJ, Nowitzke AM, Efendy J, Wood MJ. Safety and efficacy of intradural extramedullary spinal tumor removal using a minimally invasive approach. Neurosurgery. 2011; 68(1) Suppl Operative:208–216, discussion 216
[36] Holly LT, Bloch O, Johnson JP. Evaluation of registration techniques for spinal image guidance. J Neurosurg Spine. 2006; 4(4):323–328
[37] Scheufler K-M, Franke J, Eckardt A, Dohmen H. Accuracy of image-guided pedicle screw placement using intraoperative computed tomography-based navigation with automated referencing, part I: cervicothoracic spine. Neurosurgery. 2011; 69(4):782–795, discussion 795
[38] Quiñones-Hinojosa A, Robert Kolen E, Jun P, Rosenberg WS, Weinstein PR. Accuracy over space and time of computer-assisted fluoroscopic navigation in the lumbar spine in vivo. J Spinal Disord Tech. 2006; 19(2):109–113
[39] Su AW, Luo TD, McIntosh AL, et al. Switching to a pediatric dose O-arm protocol in spine surgery significantly reduced patient radiation exposure. J Pediatr Orthop. 2016; 36(6):621–626

25 Thoracic Vertebroplasty and Kyphoplasty

Justin Schwarz, Srikanth Boddu, Ibrahim Hussain, Alejandro Santillan, and Athos Patsalides

Summary

Thoracic vertebroplasty and kyphoplasty are vertebral augmentation procedures (VAPs) that are safe and effective minimally invasive treatments of symptomatic mechanically stable thoracic vertebral compression fractures (VCFs). VCFs are a highly prevalent disease that cause significant morbidity, especially in the elderly and cancer populations. VAPs have shown significant utility in treating symptomatic VCFs with a relatively recent paradigm shift toward early surgical intervention. In this chapter, appropriate patient evaluation and patient selection are discussed, as well as the indications and contraindications of VAP. Detailed step-by-step VAP instructions are provided, specifically highlighting the key to maximizing a favorable clinical outcome while avoiding potential complications.

Keywords: vertebral compression fractures (VCFs), vertebral augmentation procedure (VAP), osteoporosis, kyphosis, vertebroplasty, kyphoplasty, polymethylmethacrylate (PMMA)

25.1 Introduction

Vertebral compression fractures (VCFs) are a highly prevalent disease affecting approximately 700,000 people in the United States each year.[1,2] These fractures have a profoundly negative impact on patient function and quality of life with approximately 30 to 40% of VCF patients developing disabling pain, resulting in 150,000 annual hospitalizations.[3,4] Vertebroplasty and kyphoplasty are vertebral augmentation procedures (VAPs) that are effective percutaneous minimally invasive techniques for treating VCF and ameliorating symptoms. In both procedures, cement is injected into the fractured bone where it hardens and congeals the fracture fragments, providing immediate stability and pain relief.[5,6,7] Kyphoplasty includes an additional step prior to cement injection where a balloon is gently inflated within the fractured vertebral body to create a cavity for the cement and restore vertebral body height.[8]

25.2 Indications

Thoracic VCF with symptoms that are not adequately controlled on oral pain medications are considered for kyphoplasty or vertebroplasty. The typical presentation of a symptomatic thoracic compression fracture is an acute onset of mechanical back pain that roughly correlates with the vertebral level of the osteoporotic or pathologic VCF. This mechanical back pain is often accompanied by muscle spasm pain and pain that radiates along the respective spinal level's intercostal distribution.

The majority of patients who suffer from osteoporotic or pathologic VCF are elderly and have multiple medical comorbidities, such as arthritis or metastatic cancer, which may make the assessment of pain difficult. In such cases, it may be difficult to determine if a newly diagnosed compression fracture is truly symptomatic. A thorough clinical history is necessary to determine the time frame and potential mechanism of injury, which can help ascertain if a VCF is the etiology of a patient's pain. Determining the chronicity of symptoms and correlating the clinical history with physical examination and radiographic findings are important. A dedicated thoracic spine computed tomography (CT) or magnetic resonance imaging (MRI) is preferred for diagnosis. Plain films are inadequate for proper diagnosis, but have limited utility as an initial screening tool. The time frame of injury can be determined by comparing current imaging with past radiologic studies, including previous X-rays, CT, or MRI. If no comparison imaging is available, an MRI is obtained to determine acuity. Short tau inversion recovery (STIR) hyperintensity within the vertebral body of interest suggests a relatively recent fracture, and identifies a vertebral body that is amenable to intervention. Subacute and acute compression fractures respond well to VAP, whereas chronic fractures are unlikely to have a favorable response. MRI aids in the assessment of the stability of the fracture, as well as the chronicity. A1, A2, and A3 fractures in the AO classification scheme respond well to VAP. A4 fractures can also be good candidates for VAP as long as there is no symptomatic retropulsion or significant alignment abnormalities that would suggest disruption of the posterior tension band. In regard to the thoracolumbar injury classification and severity score (TLICS) classification, vertebroplasty can be attempted in patients with a TLICS 4 injury to achieve symptom improvement, but results can be highly variable. If vertebroplasty is to be attempted in such a case, care needs to be taken during the procedure to ensure that there is no leakage of cement into the spinal canal.

25.3 Contraindications

Vertebroplasty and kyphoplasty are typically reserved for patients with osteoporotic or pathologic VCF that are mechanically stable. Patients with unstable thoracic fractures do not respond to VAP and continue to have significant pain despite VAP. These patients, with unstable as opposed to stable fractures, typically require open surgical intervention for stabilization. Retropulsion with symptomatic cord compression is an absolute contraindication to VAP, as these patients require open surgical intervention for decompression and stabilization. Asymptomatic patients with retropulsion are still candidates for vertebroplasty. In this patient population, cement injection is performed cautiously to avoid any worsening of the retropulsion and prevent any neurologic deterioration. Other absolute contraindications to VAP include active osteomyelitis at the fracture area or an allergy to cement, polymethylmethacrylate (PMMA).

Typically, fractures involving T5 through T12 are amenable to VAP because the vertebral anatomy is easily visualized using frontal and lateral fluoroscopy for these spinal levels. In certain situations, T3 and T4 can be visualized well enough to attempt VAP, but this is dependent upon the patient's body habitus and anatomy. In these situations, the operator often will not know if the T3 or T4 level can be successfully visualized to perform VAP until the patient is positioned.

25.4 Preoperative Planning

25.4.1 Anesthesia Planning

VAP is performed with the assistance of an anesthesiologist. Ideally, the procedure is performed under monitored anesthesia care (MAC), but endotracheal intubation with general anesthesia is used in select patients. MAC is used for relatively healthy and cooperative patients undergoing a one- or two-level kyphoplasty or vertebroplasty. General anesthesia is used if three or more levels are being treated, the patient is unable to cooperate, or systemic medical issues necessitate endotracheal intubation with general anesthesia.

25.4.2 Procedure Location

Thoracic VAP is most efficiently performed using biplane fluoroscopy, but can also be performed using single-plane fluoroscopy in either an interventional procedure room or the operating room using "C-arm" fluoroscopy or two C-arms simultaneously (AP and lateral views). Biplane fluoroscopy typically reduces the procedural time significantly by obviating the need for equipment repositioning, especially when switching between anterior-posterior and lateral fluoroscopic projections.

25.4.3 Unipedicular versus Bipedicular Approach

An effective result can be obtained utilizing either a uni- or bipedicular approach. In the majority of cases, a bipedicular approach is preferred to allow for maximal and uniform distribution of cement. A unipedicular approach is used in certain situations, such as when one of the pedicles is destroyed by tumor invasion or is significantly fractured, the vertebral body is sufficiently small to allow for adequate cement filling through one cannula, or when the patient's anatomy allows for an appropriate transpedicular trajectory into the medial and anterior vertebral body. The unipedicular approach has the advantage of reducing procedure time because only one cannula needs to be navigated into the affected vertebral body. For this reason, the unipedicular technique may be used in patients needing treatment of multiple levels, or those with significant medical comorbidities where minimizing procedural time is imperative.

25.5 Patient Positioning

Patients are placed in the prone position on the procedure table prior to the administration of moderate sedation or following endotracheal intubation and administration of general anesthesia. Two large bolsters are placed transversely for adequate support during the procedure. One large bolster is placed at the level of the iliac crest and the second is placed at the level of the chest, typically just superior to the nipple line. The exact position of these bolsters varies slightly depending upon body habitus. A pillow is placed under the patient's head, with the head rotated toward the anesthesia team for easy access during the procedure. The arms are positioned above the head, with the elbows bent at approximately 90 degrees with the forearms overlapping above the patient's head. An additional bolster, or multiple pillows, is placed under the distal shins, just proximal to the patient's ankles to minimize pressure on the patient's feet. Pressure points, including the forearms, elbows, knees, and abdomen, are carefully inspected and padded. It is important to prevent any excessive rotation of the patient's spine that could make visualization with fluoroscopy more difficult. The patient is then secured in position with a safety belt across the buttocks and fabric tape across the waist, shoulders, and elbows to minimize movement during the procedure (▶ Fig. 25.1a). The procedure and its important steps are narrated and illustrated in ▶ Video 25.1.

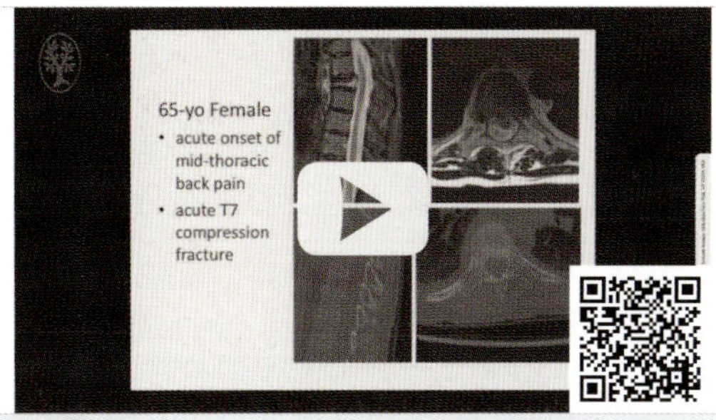

Video 25.1 Thoracic vertebroplasty and kyphoplasty.

> Thoracic vertebroplasty and kyphoplasty are VAPs that are effective and safe percutaneous, minimally invasive treatment options for symptomatic mechanically stable thoracic VCFs.

25.6 Surgical Steps

25.6.1 Preparation

The patient's back is prepped widely using chlorhexidine or betadine and sterilely draped (▶ Fig. 25.1b). The patient is dosed with weight-based antibiotics as per the institutional protocol.

25.6.2 Localization

The appropriate level is localized using frontal and lateral fluoroscopy by counting rostrally from the sacrum or caudally from the occiput. Preoperative imaging is analyzed closely, making note of any transitional anatomy to ensure accurate localization. Pre-existing deformities on preoperative imaging, such as large osteophytes, significant antero- or retrolisthesis, compression deformities, or previous VAP or spinal instrumentation, can help confirm accurate localization (▶ Fig. 25.2a, b).

25.6.3 Image Optimization

Once the appropriate level or levels are identified, the fluoroscopic image is optimized in the frontal and lateral projections to ensure that the end plates, pedicles, and ribs are well aligned and visualized by adjusting the cranial-caudal and oblique

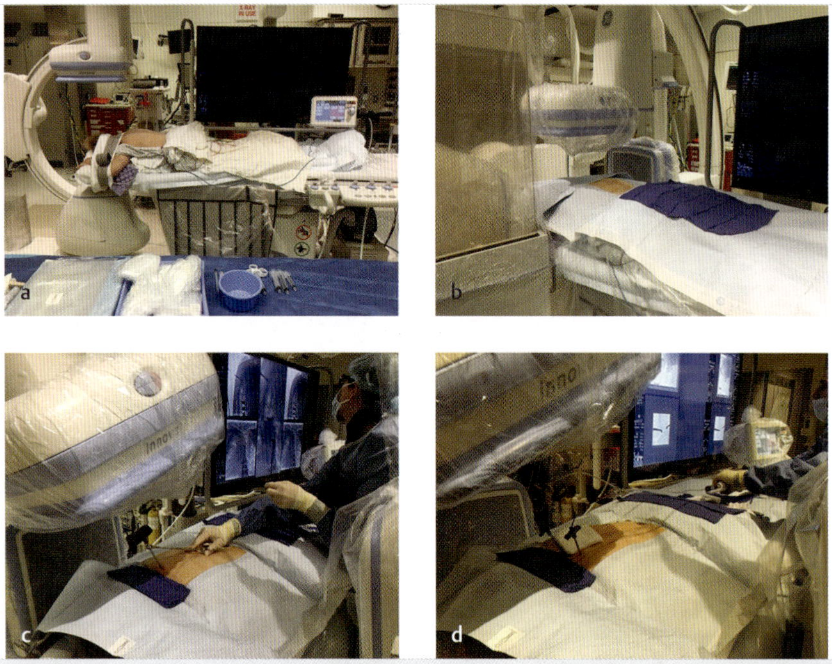

Fig. 25.1 (a) The patient is positioned prone, with care taken to ensure that all pressure points are well padded. (b) Biplane fluoroscopy is used with anesthesia positioned on the other side of the large monitor. (c) 10-gauge cannula is guided down the thoracic pedicle with an oblique, "down the barrel" view under intermittent fluoroscopy. (d) Balloons are slowly inflated with radiopaque material under continuous fluoroscopy to ensure adequate expansion within the vertebral body.

angles in each plane independently. If possible, the fluoroscopic image is collimated so that only the spinal level of interest is included to minimize radiation exposure to the patient and surgeon (▶ Fig. 25.2c–h).

25.6.4 Skin Entry Point Identification

A large clamp is used to identify the optimal skin entry point using fluoroscopy in the frontal and lateral planes. The oblique frontal plane is used to look "down the barrel" of the pedicle (▶ Fig. 25.1c). The optimum skin entry point in the medial-lateral plane correlates with the lateral aspect of the pedicle on oblique frontal fluoroscopy. The rostral-caudal skin access point should allow for ultimate positioning of the cannula within the anterior and medial aspect of the vertebral body, while still being entirely contained within the pedicle. This point is marked with a surgical marking pen and local anesthetic (1% lidocaine) is injected subcutaneously.

25.6.5 Trajectory Planning

A 22-gauge spinal needle is used to establish an appropriate cannula trajectory. The spinal needle is advanced under intermittent fluoroscopy until bone is reached, with the final position of the needle tip at the lateral aspect of the pedicle on the oblique frontal projection (▶ Fig. 25.2c). The lateral projection confirms a trajectory that will allow for a final cannula position within the anterior and medial vertebral body. Next, bupivacaine and dexamethasone are injected through the spinal needle. The spinal needle is removed, and an 11-blade scalpel is used to make a skin incision at the desired point of entry.

25.6.6 Cannula Insertion and Navigation

A 10-gauge cannula is inserted through the skin incision under intermittent fluoroscopy in a trajectory that mimics that of the spinal needle (▶ Fig. 25.2d, e). A large clamp is used to manipulate the cannula to minimize radiation exposure to the surgeon during the procedure (▶ Fig. 25.1c). Once the appropriate starting location is reached, a mallet is used to advance the cannula into the bone, taking care to prevent slippage. Once the cannula has good purchase into the bone, intermittent frontal and lateral fluoroscopy is used while navigating the cannula with the mallet through the pedicle in a slightly medial direction. Typically, the frontal projection is brought back to "true" AP from the slightly oblique position to ensure appropriate medialization of the cannula. Slight adjustments often need to be made to the trajectory to ensure that the cannula remains within the pedicle with an ultimate trajectory leading to the medial aspect of the anterior vertebral body (▶ Fig. 25.2e). If large adjustments need to be made, the inner cannula can be removed and replaced with a special slanted tip which allows for more substantial cannula redirection. It is important that intermittent fluoroscopy is utilized while navigating through the pedicle to ensure that the medial, inferior, and superior walls of the pedicle are not breached. Typically, a more lateral starting point and more aggressive medialization are needed for a unipedicular

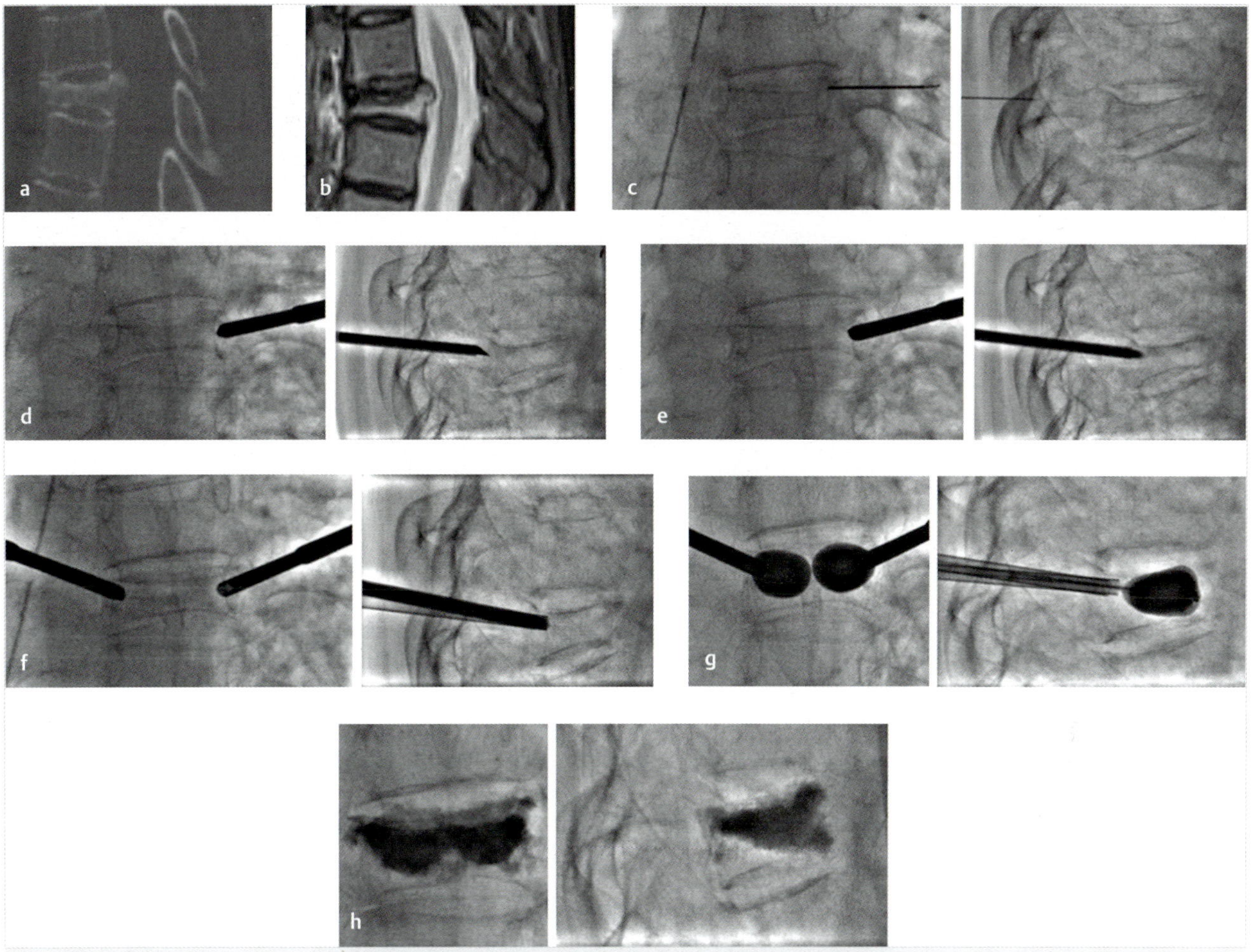

Fig. 25.2 Bipedicular thoracic kyphoplasty. **(a)** Sagittal computed tomography (CT) thoracic spine showing a T7 compression fracture with retropulsion. **(b)** Magnetic resonance imaging (MRI) thoracic spine sagittal short tau inversion recovery (STIR) sequence showing hyperintensity within the T7 vertebral body, signifying an acute fracture. **(c)** Localization of bone entry point on the right side using a 22-gauge spinal needle in the frontal and lateral projections. **(d)** Navigated trocar in a transpedicular trajectory just past the spinal canal, with verification that the medial wall of the pedicle has not been breached. **(e)** Final positioning of the right-sided trocar within the T7 vertebral body. **(f)** Final positioning of bilateral transpedicular trocars, just prior to bone biopsy and drilling. **(g)** Balloon inflation within the T7 vertebral body, following bone core biopsy and drilling. **(h)** T7 vertebral body following cement injection, with the anterior two-thirds of the vertebral body filled with cement from the superior to inferior end plate.

approach to obtain the best radiologic and clinical outcome (▶ Fig. 25.3a). Once the cannula has traversed the pedicle and the tip of the cannula is safely past the spinal canal, the cannula can be more aggressively medialized to ensure a desirable end position (▶ Fig. 25.2f).

25.6.7 Biopsy and Drilling

The inner cannula is removed and a 12-gauge biopsy needle is advanced past the end of the cannula and into the central aspect of the vertebral body (▶ Fig. 25.3a). The biopsy needle is removed under gentle aspiration to obtain a core bone biopsy that is sent to pathology. A 12-gauge drill is advanced past the end of the cannula and into the central and anterior aspect of the vertebral body under intermittent fluoroscopy, ensuring not to breach the anterior wall of the vertebral body. The entire process described above is then repeated on the contralateral side for a bipedicular approach.

25.6.8 Balloon Inflation (Kyphoplasty)

A balloon is introduced through the cannula (bilateral for bipedicular approach) and into the vertebral body, again ensuring that the anterior aspect of the vertebral body is not breached. The balloons are slowly inflated with radiopaque material under continuous fluoroscopy to ensure adequate expansion within the vertebral body to make space for the cement and restore vertebral body height without violation of the end plates (▶ Fig. 25.1d, ▶ Fig. 25.2g, and ▶ Fig. 25.3b). Following adequate expansion of the balloons, the balloons are deflated and removed.

25.6.9 Cement Injection

Cement is injected slowly through the cannulas under intermittent fluoroscopy until the vertebral body is adequately filled with cement. This typically consists of complete filling of the anterior

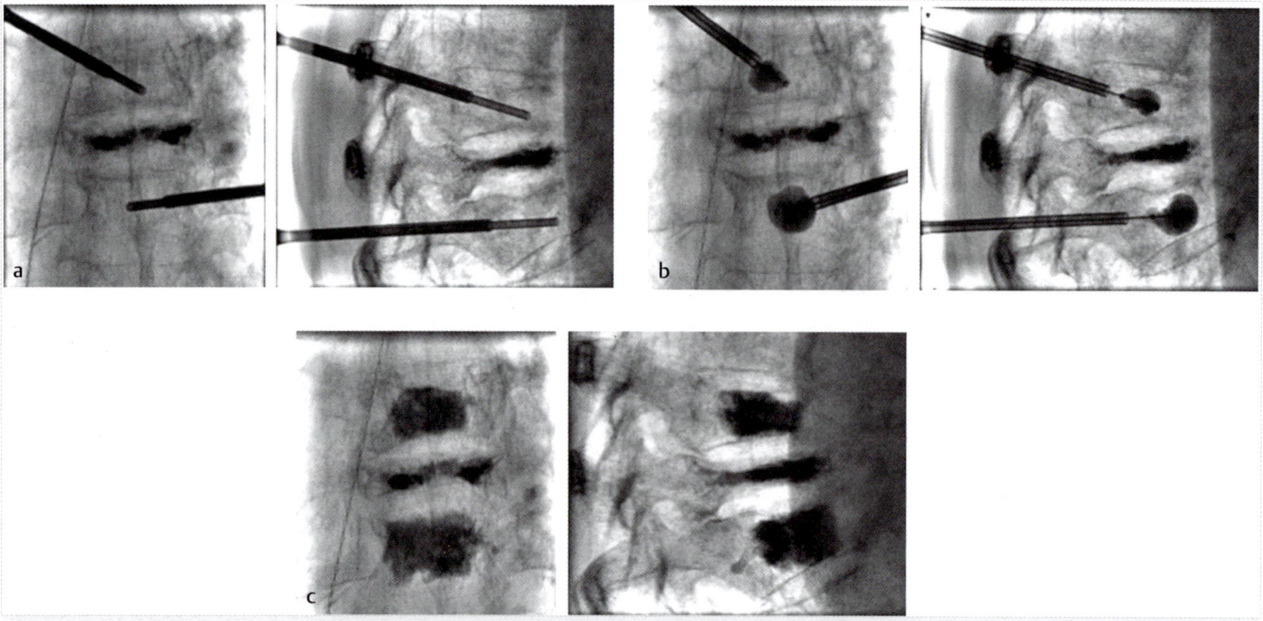

Fig. 25.3 Unipedicular thoracic kyphoplasty. Previous T8 kyphoplasty with acute T7 and T9 compression fractures. **(a)** Left-sided T7 unipedicular approach and right-sided unipedicular approach to T9. There are 12-gauge biopsy needles extending into the T7 and T9 medial and anterior vertebral bodies. The trocars are more aggressively medialized than in the bipedicular approach, as evidenced by the frontal projections. **(b)** Balloon inflation within the T7 and T9 vertebral bodies, with care taken to prevent fracture of the superior and inferior end plates. **(c)** Final radiographic result with anterior two-thirds of the T7 and T9 vertebral body filled from the superior to inferior end plates.

two-thirds of the vertebral body from superior to inferior end plate, including the medial aspect of the vertebral body (▶ Fig. 25.2h and ▶ Fig. 25.3c). Care is also taken that the cement does not track posteriorly into the spinal canal, superiorly or inferiorly into the disc space, or anteriorly beyond the extent of the vertebral body. The oblique lateral projection can be used to visualize in between the cannulas in a bipedicular approach to ensure that the cement is not tracking posteriorly toward the spinal canal. Although there are electric injectors available, the authors prefer manual hand injection because there is better tactile feedback.

25.6.10 Closure

Once adequate vertebral body filling of the body has been accomplished, the inner cannulas are replaced and the trocars are completely removed. Replacing the inner cannulas prior to removal prevents the cement from tracking posteriorly out of the vertebral body. Once the trocars are removed, gentle pressure is applied to the incisions and the patient's back is cleaned using sterile water or saline. A small amount of bacitracin is applied to the incisions and a gentle pressure dressing is applied, typically consisting of gauze and a coverlet (▶ Fig. 25.4).

25.7 Postoperative Care

Postoperative patients are monitored in the recovery room with frequent neurologic, vital sign, and pain assessments. For the first 2 hours, patients are placed on strict bed rest and are kept flat to allow the cement adequate time to cure and appropriately harden. Patients are then slowly encouraged to sit up and ambulate. Prior to the VAP, patients are fitted with a thoracolumbosacral orthosis (TLSO) brace and are instructed to wear it when out of bed and ambulating for 2 weeks postoperatively. Patients with severe osteoporosis and at high risk for future insufficiency fractures are referred to their primary care physicians or an endocrinologist to address the patients' underlying etiology. Patients undergoing VAP are typically discharged home on the same day of the procedure. Patients who are admitted for pain control prior to the VAP are usually observed overnight and are discharged the following day, pending a physical therapy evaluation and adequate pain control. Dressings are removed 48 hours after the procedure, and patients are instructed to avoid any lifting over 5 pounds and excessive bending and twisting for 2 weeks. Patients are evaluated at an outpatient clinic visit 2 weeks postoperatively or sooner if their symptoms fail to improve or worsen.

25.8 Complication Avoidance

The most severe potential complication of VAP is neurologic injury, and careful consideration is taken when selecting patients and performing the procedure to minimize this risk. Frequent fluoroscopy and trajectory manipulation are vital to ensure that the VAP cannula does not violate the medial, inferior, and superior borders of the pedicle. This ensures that the cannula does not breach into the spinal canal or neuroforamina, where there is potential to cause neurologic injury. Frequent fluoroscopy is also important during biopsy, drilling, and balloon inflation to ensure that the boundaries of the vertebral body are not violated, which could potentially lead to vascular, thoracic, or abdominal injury.

Symptomatic cement embolism and cement extravasation into the spinal canal, although rare, are other potential complications that necessitate procedural precaution. Cement is injected slowly

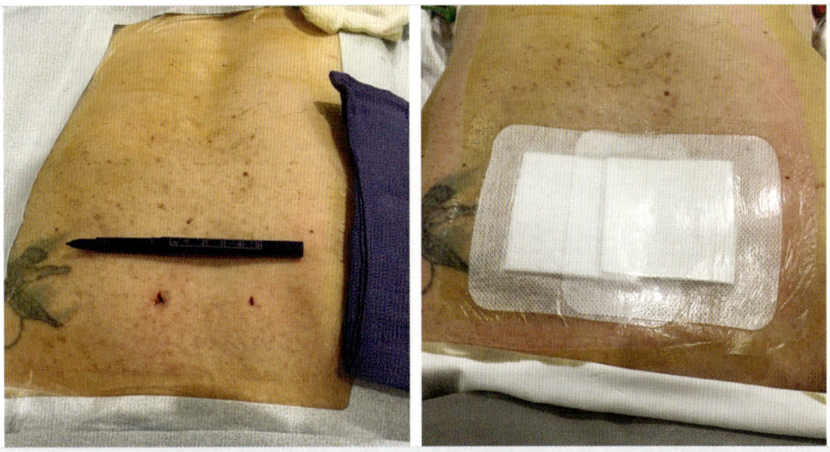

Fig. 25.4 Small incisions on a patient's thoracic back following kyphoplasty. Bacitracin ointment is applied to the incisions and covered with gauze and a standard coverlet dressing.

into the vertebral body under frequent intermittent fluoroscopy to ensure that the cement is not traveling outside of the boundaries of the vertebral bodies, such as posteriorly into the spinal canal or into veins. If any of these circumstances are encountered, further cement injection is contraindicated.

To minimize the risk of perioperative bleeding, patients are instructed to hold any anticoagulant prior to the procedure. These medications can usually be restarted on postoperative day one. It is safe to perform the procedure on prophylactic aspirin dosing, but any additional antiplatelet therapy is held for 1 week prior to the procedure as long as it is reasonably safe from a medical perspective.

25.9 Tips and Tricks

Minimizing radiation exposure is important for the patient and surgeon. Collimating the fluoroscopic image and use of appropriate leaded shields, glasses, and garments are essential to minimizing radiation exposure. Biplane fluoroscopy minimizes the time and effort needed to successfully navigate the trocar, while ensuring procedural safety. It is also helpful to check the cement consistency to ensure that it is the appropriate viscosity prior to injection.

25.10 Conclusion

Thoracic vertebroplasty and kyphoplasty are VAPs that are effective and safe percutaneous, minimally invasive treatment options for symptomatic mechanically stable thoracic VCF.

References

[1] Ensrud KE, Schousboe JT. Clinical practice. Vertebral fractures. N Engl J Med. 2011; 364(17):1634–1642

[2] Cooper C. Epidemiology and public health impact of osteoporosis. Baillieres Clin Rheumatol. 1993; 7(3):459–477

[3] Lindsay R, Silverman SL, Cooper C, et al. Risk of new vertebral fracture in the year following a fracture. JAMA. 2001; 285(3):320–323

[4] Fink HA, Milavetz DL, Palermo L, et al. Fracture Intervention Trial Research Group. What proportion of incident radiographic vertebral deformities is clinically diagnosed and vice versa? J Bone Miner Res. 2005; 20(7):1216–1222

[5] Voormolen MHJ, Mali WPTM, Lohle PNM, et al. Percutaneous vertebroplasty compared with optimal pain medication treatment: short-term clinical outcome of patients with subacute or chronic painful osteoporotic vertebral compression fractures. The VERTOS study. AJNR Am J Neuroradiol. 2007; 28(3):555–560

[6] Wardlaw D, Cummings SR, Van Meirhaeghe J, et al. Efficacy and safety of balloon kyphoplasty compared with non-surgical care for vertebral compression fracture (FREE): a randomised controlled trial. Lancet. 2009; 373(9668):1016–1024

[7] Klazen CAH, Lohle PNM, de Vries J, et al. Vertebroplasty versus conservative treatment in acute osteoporotic vertebral compression fractures (Vertos II): an open-label randomised trial. Lancet. 2010; 376(9746):1085–1092

[8] Van Meirhaeghe J, Bastian L, Boonen S, Ranstam J, Tillman JB, Wardlaw D, FREE investigators. A randomized trial of balloon kyphoplasty and nonsurgical management for treating acute vertebral compression fractures: vertebral body kyphosis correction and surgical parameters. Spine. 2013; 38(12):971–983

26 Thoracic Discectomy: Posterior Transpedicular Tubular Approach

Christopher D. Witiw, Brian T. David, and Richard G. Fessler

Summary
The posterior transpedicular tubular approach is one among the several options available for treatment of a symptomatic thoracic disc herniation. It serves as an effective minimally invasive corridor of access through a trajectory that is very familiar to spinal surgeons. It may be performed using a microscope or an endoscope for visualization. This chapter describes the procedure in a detailed step-by-step manner.

Keywords: thoracic, disc herniation, posterior, minimally invasive, transpedicular

26.1 Introduction

The surgical management of thoracic disc herniations presents a substantial clinical challenge. Owing to the lesser incidence of thoracic disc herniations compared with those of the cervical or lumbar spine, surgeons typically have less familiarity with this pathology. Moreover, surgery is technically challenging because of the anatomical constraints imposed by the narrow thoracic spinal canal, the need to avoid spinal cord manipulation, and the frequently calcified nature of the disc herniations.

Multiple corridors of access have been described. These include anterior thoracotomy or thoracoscopy-based approaches, lateral retropleural approaches, or any of a contingent of posterior-lateral approaches. Of these posterior-lateral approaches, two in particular are highly amenable to minimally invasive tubular retractor-based access. One is the microendoscopic thoracic discectomy starting lateral to the facet joint,[1] which will be described in Chapter 29. This chapter will focus on the posterior transpedicular approach to the thoracic disc.

The transpedicular approach was initially described by Patterson and Arbit in 1978.[2] This involves accessing the posterior-lateral aspect of the spinal dura via hemilaminotomies and a medial facetectomy (▶ Fig. 26.1a) followed by a partial resection of the pedicle, thereby providing the surgeon exposure to the disc space and allowing decompression of the disc fragment without undue spinal cord manipulation (▶ Fig. 26.1b). Traditionally, the exposure was provided via a midline incision and lateral retraction of the paraspinal muscles. However, with the advancement of minimally invasive techniques, the exposure has been adapted to incorporate tubular muscle dilation and visualization with either a microscope or endoscope.[3,4] This chapter will serve to provide an overview of the indications, surgical considerations, and techniques for those planning to perform a minimally invasive, tubular retractor based transpedicular approach to a herniated thoracic disc.

26.2 Indications

The primary indication for a posterior transpedicular thoracic discectomy is a symptomatic midline or paramedian thoracic disc herniation.

26.3 Contraindications

Most thoracic disc herniations are accessible with a unilateral posterior tubular approach. However, certain broad-based herniations resulting in bilateral compression of the spinal cord may necessitate a bilateral transpedicular approach with instrumented fusion. Additionally, in rare cases of an intradural thoracic disc herniation an anterior or lateral extracavitary approach might be considered to ensure the appropriate trajectory to retrieve the disc fragment.

26.4 Preoperative Planning

A detailed clinical history and physical examination are critical prior to any plan for surgical intervention. Patients with a symptomatic thoracic disc herniation will present with complaints consistent with a radiculopathy localizable to a thoracic level, a myelopathy involving the lower extremities, or a combination of both. In cases without strong clinical–radiographic correlation, an alternative source of the neurological dysfunction should be ruled out prior to proceeding to surgical intervention at the thoracic level.

As part of a comprehensive presurgical workup, all patients should have magnetic resonance (MR) and computed tomography (CT) imaging of the thoracic spine. The MR imaging serves to assess the degree and direction of spinal cord deformation from the disc herniation, while the CT images serve to identify any evidence of calcification within the herniated fragment.

These images should include either the sacrum or the second cervical vertebrae to ensure accurate localization of the level of the pathology. All patients must also have a preoperative chest radiograph to account for the possibility of an additional rib, as

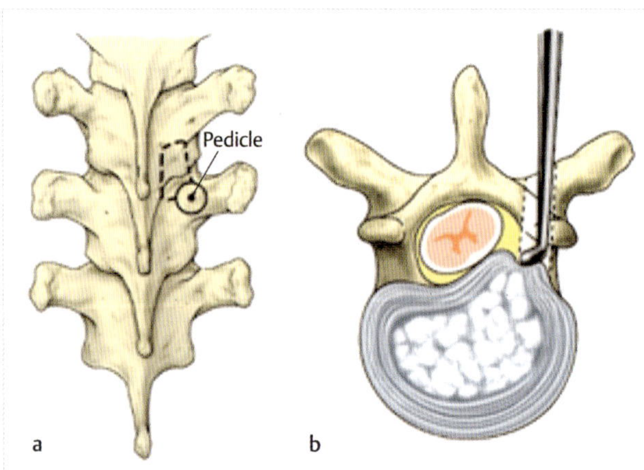

Fig. 26.1 (a) Posterior view of the thoracic spinal column. Dashed lines represent the posterior bone decompression performed via hemilaminotomy and medial facetectomy. **(b)** Partial resection of the pedicle permits access to the herniated disc. (Adapted from Bilsky et al. Neurosurg Focus. 2000 Oct 15;9(4):e3.)

well as lumbosacral radiographs to assess for the presence of a lumbosacral transitional vertebra. Taking these steps prior to surgery will serve to mitigate the risk of operating at an incorrect thoracic level.

26.5 Patient Positioning

The patient should be positioned prone on a Jackson table. This permits unencumbered access for C-arm fluoroscopy both in the anteroposterior (AP) and lateral orientations. The choice of frame may be based on the surgeon's preference. The patient can be positioned on either an open Jackson frame with chest and hip bolsters or on a traditional Wilson frame. An open Jackson frame ensures maximal decompression of the abdomen, which may reduce epidural venous plexus bleeding during the surgery and also ensures full AP radiographic visualization of all thoracic levels. A Wilson frame matches the natural kyphotic contour of the thoracic spine and may provide a more anatomic configuration of the thoracic levels. However, one should be aware of the position of any radiopaque components of the Wilson frame as these may obstruct AP fluoroscopic images intraoperatively.

Once the patient is positioned, the accurate localization of the level of pathology is of paramount importance; this is particularly true in the thoracic spine, where the risk of wrong-level surgery is particularly high. Fluoroscopic localization with multiple cues from AP and lateral images should be utilized. An upward count from the sacrum is preferred because intraoperatively it is easier to count in a cranial direction from the sacrum or from the lowest rib because the pectoral girdle can obstruct fluoroscopy of the lower cervical and upper thoracic spine.

There are multiple options available to the spine surgeon faced with the management of a symptomatic thoracic disc herniation. The posterior transpedicular tubular approach described in this chapter provides an effective minimally invasive access corridor to the pathology. This procedure can be performed using either microscopic or endoscopic visualization. In the editor's experience, the use of intraoperative CT guidance can be helpful for localization and for final intraoperative confirmation of successful decompression.

26.6 Surgical Steps

26.6.1 Incision

The skin incision should be made 2.5 cm off the midline. In very obese patients, it is helpful to mark the true midline on the skin using AP fluoroscopy. The area should be infiltrated with local anesthetic with epinephrine to help with initial hemostasis and postoperative pain.

26.6.2 Technique

1. Once the incision is made, the dissection should be carried down to the posterior thoracolumbar fascia. This should be opened longitudinally using monopolar electrocautery.
2. Then the first dilating tube can be gently passed through the erector spinae muscles, being sure to stay away from the midline to avoid the risk of traversing the interlaminar space and entering the spinal canal. If there is any concern during this step, a lateral fluoroscopic image should be taken to confirm the depth of the tip of the dilator.
3. The initial boney docking site should be the facet joint. From here, the dilator can be gently walked medially to identify the spinous process–lamina junction (▶ Video 26.1).
4. Sequential dilation should be performed, and the final working channel should be placed after reconfirming localization with lateral fluoroscopy.
5. At this point the monopolar electrocautery should be used to resect any remaining muscle overlying the bone of the ipsilateral lamina and the facet joint.
6. The decompression should begin by identifying the caudal aspect of the lamina of the level above the disc space of interest (▶ Fig. 26.2a). Then using a combination of Kerrison rongeurs and high-speed drill, an ipsilateral hemilaminotomy should be performed at the cranial and caudal lamina followed by a resection of the medial half of the facet joint (label **F** in ▶ Fig. 26.2b).
7. Next the high-speed drill may be used to carefully remove the medial and cranial aspect of the pedicle. Up to two-thirds of the medial and cranial aspect of the pedicle may be safely removed without concern for segmental destabilization. This should provide sufficient medial visualization for the intervertebral disc without requiring any manipulation of the spinal cord (▶ Fig. 26.2c).
8. Bipolar electrocautery may be used to coagulate the epidural veins.
9. Next the lateral/paramedian annulus of the disc should be incised and any soft disc should be removed to create additional space. Up to 10% of the cranial and caudal vertebral bodies adjacent to the disc may be removed using the high-speed drill to create a cavity around the disc.
10. At this point, the herniated fragment can be carefully mobilized away from the dura and into the space created in the vertebral bodies using a downward angled curette. Once the fragment is free from the dura and in the vertebral body cavity, it may be removed using a pituitary rongeur. This may be repeated until all herniated disc material is removed (▶ Fig. 26.2d). Sufficient spinal cord decompression may be assured by sliding an angled instrument carefully along the ventral aspect of the dura.

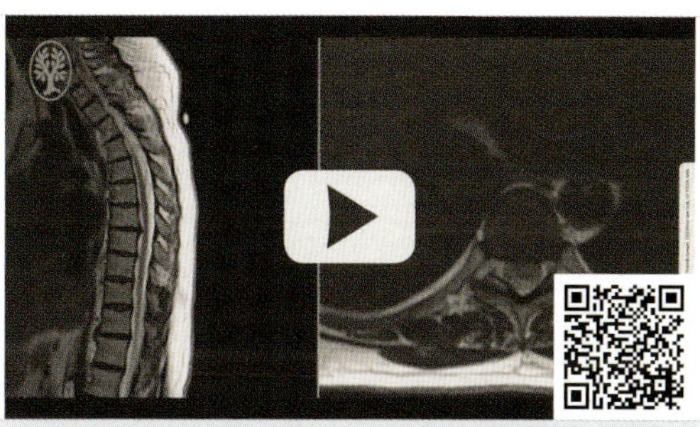

Video 26.1 Decompression of a symptomatic T7/8 disc herniation via a right-sided posterior transpedicular tubular approach.

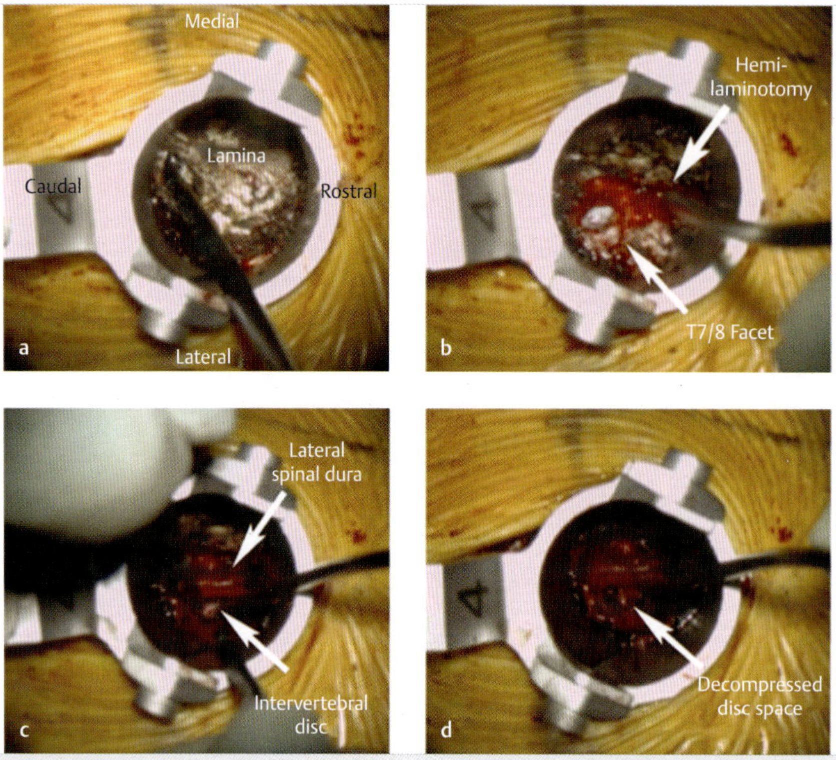

Fig. 26.2 **(a)** View through tubular working channel of rostral laminal and medial zygoapophyseal joint; **(b)** hemilaminotomy of rostral and caudal levels with initial view of lateral spinal cord dura under ligamentum flavum; **(c)** view of the intervertebral disc and partial resection of the cranial and medial aspects of the pedicle; **(d)** view of the disc space following discectomy.

26.6.3 Closure

The tubular working channel should be removed slowly as one unit. Bipolar electrocautery should be used to control any evident bleeding points. The posterior thoracolumbar fascia should be closed with a 0 absorbable suture and the subcutaneous planes with a 2–0 absorbable suture. The skin should be reapproximated with a 4–0 absorbable suture and then a dry sterile dressing or surgical adhesive glue may be applied to the skin surface.

26.7 Postoperative Care

Patients may ambulate following surgery and may be discharged home as soon as they are doing so safely, and able to void their bladder normally. Prior to discharge, patients should have a routine noncontrast CT of the thoracic spine to assess the degree of decompression. In instances of insufficient decompression, reoperation may be considered. In cases where significant preoperative neurological dysfunction was present, initial mobilization should be done under careful supervision to ensure safety. Consultation with physical and occupational therapy services may facilitate appropriate postoperative rehabilitation.

If an incidental dural breach and cerebrospinal fluid (CSF) leak occurred intraoperatively, these patients should be kept on bed rest for 24 hours. After this, the patient may be slowly mobilized. In the case where a lumbar drain is placed for CSF diversion, these patients should remain on bed rest for 3 to 5 days.

26.8 Complication Avoidance

Any surgical intervention in close proximity to the spinal cord presents an inherent risk of spinal cord injury. However, in myelopathic patients this is even higher since the spinal cord has already sustained an injury. To mitigate the risk of iatrogenic injury, all patients should have neurophysiological monitoring at the time of positioning and throughout the surgical intervention. This should include somatosensory evoked potentials and motor evoked potentials. To ensure an unconfounded assessment of the evoked potentials, the general anesthetic should not include any neuromuscular paralysis (beyond what is needed for the initial induction stages). Clear and open communication between the surgeon and the neuromonitoring technologist should occur throughout the surgery.

The anatomic location of a herniated thoracic disc may result in anterior spinal artery compression and ensuing spinal cord hypoperfusion. This places the patient at risk for an anterior spinal cord syndrome. The anesthesia team should be hypervigilant to avoid any episodes of hypotension (systolic blood pressure less than 90 mmHg), particularly during the induction stages. Furthermore, they should also endeavor to keep the mean arterial pressure greater than 80 mmHg through the operation.

26.9 Tips and Tricks

During localization, it is best to avoid the use of a K-wire as there is a potential risk of passing the K-wire through the

intralaminar space and inadvertently injuring the spinal cord. The authors prefer to open a linear incision in the dorsal layer of the thoracolumbar fascia and gently pass the first dilator tube down to the docking site on the zygoapophyseal joint.

During resection of the cranial and medial aspects of the pedicle, it is safest to use the high-speed drill to core out the cancellous portion of the pedicle first while leaving a thin cortical rim intact to protect the adjacent nerve root and lateral aspect of the spinal cord dura. Once a cavity has been created then a downward angled curette can be used to carefully tamp the remaining thin cortical rim of bone away from the neural elements and into the cavity. This reduces the risk of a dural injury from the high-speed drill.

An incidental linear durotomy located along the posterior or posterior-lateral aspect of the spinal dura may be directly repaired using a 5–0 Gore-Tex suture with instruments appropriate for suturing through a tubular retractor. Conversely, direct repair of incidental ventral durotomies or large dural defects from adherent calcified disc herniations should not be attempted. Onlay dural substitutes in combination with dural sealants may be considered, based on surgeon's preference. For large ventral defects, a lumbar drain for CSF diversion may be placed while the patient is still under anesthesia from the surgery. In general, the lack of dead space due to the minimally invasive approach via muscle dilation is the best measure to address these defects, making symptomatic CSF leaks relatively uncommon.

26.10 Conclusion

There are multiple options available to the spine surgeon faced with the management of a symptomatic thoracic disc herniation. The posterior transpedicular tubular approach described in this chapter provides an effective minimally invasive access corridor to the pathology. The posterior trajectory is a familiar to spine surgeons and avoids the potential complications associated with entering the thoracic cavity and does not necessitate an instrumented fusion. Moreover, this procedure can be performed using either microscopic or endoscopic visualization. Regardless of what approach a surgeon selects to address this challenging pathology, a systematic approach is needed to ensure accurate localization within the thoracic spine and avoid iatrogenic neurological injury to the already vulnerable thoracic spinal cord.

References

[1] Perez-Cruet MJ, Kim BS, Sandhu F, Samartzis D, Fessler RG. Thoracic microendoscopic discectomy. J Neurosurg Spine. 2004; 1(1):58–63

[2] Patterson RH , Jr, Arbit E. A surgical approach through the pedicle to protruded thoracic discs. J Neurosurg. 1978; 48(5):768–772

[3] Jho HD. Endoscopic microscopic transpedicular thoracic discectomy. Technical note. Neurosurg Focus. 1998; 4(2):e7

[4] Chi JH, Dhall SS, Kanter AS, Mummaneni PV. The mini-open transpedicular thoracic discectomy: surgical technique and assessment. Neurosurg Focus. 2008; 25(2):E5

27 Lateral Retropleural Thoracic Discectomy and Corpectomy

David S. Xu, Jakub Godzik, S. Harrison Farber, Shashank V. Gandhi, Ernest J. Wright, Courtney Hemphill, Sebastian Uribe, and Juan S. Uribe

Summary

Lateral retropleural thoracic discectomy and corpectomy is a minimally invasive surgical strategy to treat thoracic disc herniations. Open anterolateral transthoracic approaches have traditionally been the gold standard surgical strategy to perform thoracic discectomies, but perioperative morbidity and postoperative chest wall pain syndromes are significant associated risks. In efforts to reduce the morbidity associated with open thoracotomy, the mini-open lateral retropleural approach has been developed to achieve maximal exposure of the herniated disc without obstruction by the thecal sac. In this chapter, we outline patient selection, preoperative planning, and intraoperative workflow to safely and efficiently execute a mini-open lateral retropleural thoracic discectomy.

Keywords: corpectomy, discectomy, minimal invasive surgery, mini-open lateral, retropleural, spine, thoracic

27.1 Introduction

Thoracic disc herniations are uncommon and comprise less than 1% of all symptomatic disc herniations.[1,2] Based on historical studies, less than 25% of patients with herniated thoracic discs are symptomatic.[3] When symptoms do present, the clinical manifestations are protean and depend on the anatomic configuration of the herniated disc. Large central herniations may cause spinal cord compression, leading to motor deficits and myelopathy, while paracentral herniation may impinge on thoracic nerve roots leading to radiculopathy or dysesthetic pain along the chest wall, abdomen, or viscera.[4,5]

Early surgical management of thoracic disc herniations relied on laminectomy alone and resulted in high rates of major morbidity ranging from 18 to 75% in different series.[1,6] These poor results are most likely due to iatrogenic injuries incurred during manipulation of the thecal sac to visualize the disc space. Consequently, in the 1960s, anterior approaches via thoracotomy quickly became the gold standard by permitting wide exposure of herniated discs, unimpeded by neural structures, allowing the removal of even heavily calcified and transdural lesions.[7] However, an open thoracotomy carries a risk of morbidity, with over 30% of patients developing significant thoracic pain more than 4 years postoperatively.[8] Thoracoscopic discectomy emerged to reduce the morbidity of open transthoracic exposures but has had limited acceptance due to the specialization and high cost of equipment, the steep learning curve, and limitations of the technique in managing intraoperative complications such as hemorrhage or cerebrospinal fluid (CSF) leaks.[9,10]

Recently, a lateral mini-open retropleural approach to the thoracic spine was developed as an intermediate option between open thoracotomy and minimally invasive thoracoscopy.[11,12] Through specialized retractors, the lateral mini-open approach enables direct visualization of the thoracic disc with less exposure-associated morbidity, while enabling the use of standard instruments in a familiar operative corridor. In this chapter, the authors provide a detailed description of the operative planning, execution, and postoperative care of patients undergoing a mini-open lateral thoracic retropleural discectomy.

27.2 Indications

Thoracic discectomy is indicated in patients with declining motor function or progressive myelopathy attributable to spinal cord or conus compression by a herniated thoracic disc. Furthermore, intractable pain or discomfort caused by thecal sac or nerve root compression that is unresponsive to conservative measures is also an indication for discectomy.

27.3 Contraindications

Significant scoliosis is a contraindication for a lateral approach because the coronal deformity may prevent a perpendicular approach to the disc space. Previous thoracic surgery is a relative contraindication due to the presence of scar tissue between the parietal pleura and the endothoracic fascia, forcing an intrapleural approach. Knowledge of and familiarity with lateral approach surgeries are paramount and are the primary determinant of what types of disc herniations are amenable to surgical resection. Small, paracentral disc herniations are less technically demanding and can be undertaken by surgeons early in the learning curve. Removal of large central disc herniations or those that are heavily calcified should be undertaken only by surgeons well accomplished with the approach and equipment.

27.4 Preoperative Planning

A preoperative magnetic resonance imaging (MRI) or computed tomography (CT) myelography of the thoracic spine is required to define the neural elements and level to be treated. In addition, noncontrast CT imaging of the thoracic spine should be done to determine the degree of disc calcification as well as to facilitate accurate level localization. In patients with variant anatomy or large body habitus that the surgeon anticipates might cause difficulty with intraoperative localization, a radiopaque fiducial can be placed in the pedicle or rib head adjacent to the treated level before surgery. In all patients, neuromonitoring with somatosensory and motor evoked potentials is mandatory.

27.5 Patient Positioning

After induction of general anesthesia and intubation, the patient is positioned in the lateral decubitus position with the side of the approach facing upward (▶ Fig. 27.1a). The patient's

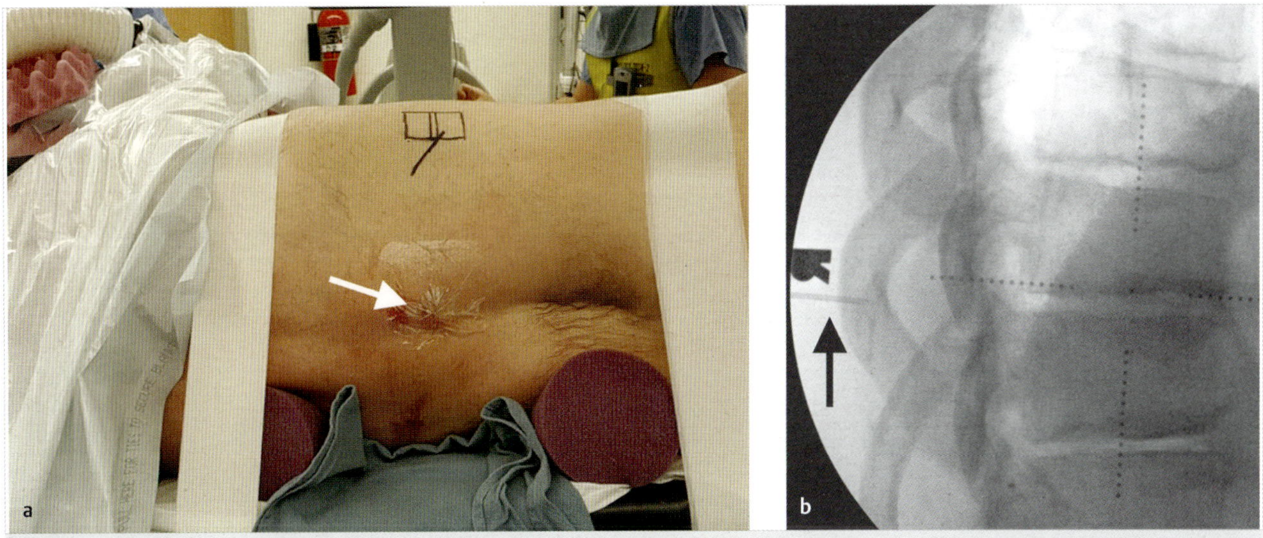

Fig. 27.1 Patient positioning and fiducial placement. **(a)** The patient is positioned for a right-sided approach with the left flank facing downward and the head on the left-hand side of the image. A purple foam roll is placed under the axilla to decompress the brachial plexus and above the downfacing iliac crest to facilitate torso bending during table breakage. A 14-gauge needle (*arrow*) is inserted into the spinous process directly overlaying the disc space to act as a fiducial. **(b)** Lateral radiograph shows the fiducial (*arrow*) in line with the disc space to be treated. (Used with permission from Barrow Neurological Institute, Phoenix, Arizona.)

height on the bed should be adjusted to ensure that the thoracic level to be treated rests above the table break. An axillary roll is placed to decompress the brachial plexus, and an optional roll can be placed just above the underlying iliac crest to promote torso bending. The table is then subtly broken to increase the intercostal distance. At this point, the fluoroscope is brought in to verify the level of localization, and the bed should be repositioned to achieve perfect anteroposterior (AP) and lateral radiographs of the level to be treated, without requiring changes to the tilt or arc of the fluoroscope. A 16 gauge needle can be inserted into the spinous process overlying the level to be treated, which acts as an in-situ fiducial (▶ Fig. 27.1a, b).

Incision planning proceeds by drawing the lateral projection of the disc space and adjacent vertebra on the patient's flank (▶ Fig. 27.2a, b). A 5-cm incision begins at the posterior margin of the disc space and runs parallel to the underlying rib or intercostal space. This incision ensures that the retractor will be centered on the interface between the disc space and thecal sac (▶ Fig. 27.2c).

27.6 Step-by-Step Surgical Technique with Example

27.6.1 Incision and Exposure

Step 1: The planned incision is made, and the underlying intercostal space is exposed. If the intercostal space is not large enough to accommodate a working corridor, a 5- to 7-cm segment of the bordering rib is resected. Upon removal of the rib, the parietal pleura is visualized and deflected anteriorly along with the underlying lung by digital or blunt retraction (▶ Fig. 27.3a).

Step 2: A retropleural corridor is then created by carefully dissecting the medial and deep planes of the parietal pleura from the adjacent endothoracic fascia in an extracavitary fashion (▶ Fig. 27.3b).

Step 3: Once the dissection approaches the rib head attached to the vertebral body inferior to the disc space, sequential blunt dilators are inserted to allow placement of a split blade retractor (MaXcess, NuVasive Inc.) that is then docked and opened.

Step 4: The rib head is then resected to expose the underlying pedicle (▶ Fig. 27.4a, b), and the retractor is opened to the final working diameter. The size of the final exposed operative field consists of a superior-inferior border delimited by the inferior margin of the pedicles of the vertebral bodies adjacent to the disc space to be treated, the posterior border marked by the transverse processes of the spine, and the anterior border marked at the midpoint of the disc space (▶ Fig. 27.4c).

Lateral retropleural thoracic discectomy is a safe and efficacious procedure with reduced surgical consequences compared to traditional open thoracotomies. The use of an appropriate lateral access retractor as well as a well-defined, structured workflow are key to the success of the procedure. Keeping the retropleural plane can be technically challenging. In the authors' experience, localization of the pathology can be greatly facilitated by using intraoperative CT navigation.

27.6.2 Technique

Step 5: Resection of the herniated disc proceeds under the operating microscope. First, the lateral surface of the thecal sac is exposed by drilling through the pedicle of the inferior vertebral body (▶ Fig. 27.5a). During drilling, AP fluoroscopy aids in providing feedback on drill bit positioning to avoid breaching the deep cortical margin of the pedicle

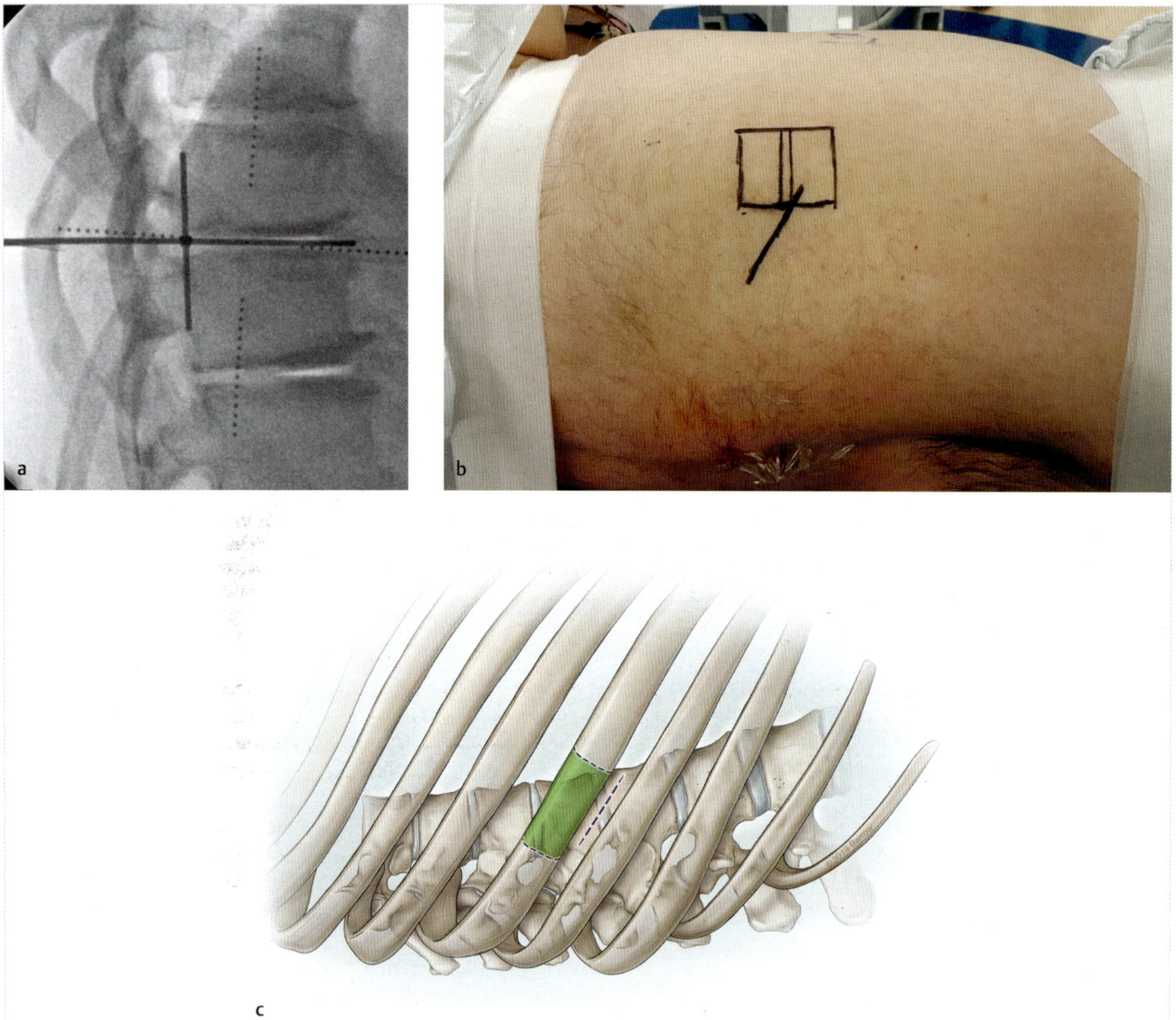

Fig. 27.2 Incision planning. **(a)** Lateral radiograph shows a reference cross on the patient's skin in line with the posterior margin of the vertebral body and the disc space to aid in planning the incision. **(b)** Photograph of the planned incision shows the outline of the disc space to be treated as well as the adjacent vertebra. The incision itself is a slanted line that intersects the posterior margin of the disc space and runs along the groove of the underlying rib or intercostal space. **(c)** The illustration shows the superimposed image of the planned incision and the underlying thoracic structures. The incision is centered posterior to the disc space to allow easier dissection of the retropleural plane and anterior retraction of the pleura and lung. (Used with permission from Barrow Neurological Institute, Phoenix, Arizona.)

(▶ Fig. 27.5b). After the pedicle is removed, the underlying ligamentum flavum is divided with a small curet to expose the lateral surface of the thecal sac. A Kerrison rongeur is then used to resect the ligament cranially and caudally, spanning the area of the disc herniation (▶ Fig. 27.5c).

Step 6: A partial corpectomy is created to enlarge the working space for the discectomy. The size of the corpectomy should span 1 to 2 cm superiorly and inferiorly to the disc space, anteriorly to one-third of the distance of the disc space, and to the depth of the medial border of the contralateral pedicle to ensure that the cavity will span the width of the spinal canal. To begin the corpectomy, we find it helpful to use an ultrasonic cutter (BoneScalpel, Misonix, Inc., Farmingdale, NY) to make linear cuts demarcating the margins of the bone to be removed (▶ Fig. 27.6a).

Step 7: A large coarse or extra coarse diamond drill bit is then used to drill down to the deep margin of the corpectomy, which is referenced at the level of the contralateral pedicle, with verification by AP fluoroscopy (▶ Fig. 27.6b). The disc space and end plates are not amenable to drilling and instead are removed with a rongeur as the bone above and below is removed by drilling. Posteriorly, the bone should be removed until the ventral posterior longitudinal ligament (PLL) is exposed. When the corpectomy is completed (▶ Fig. 27.6c), the remaining disc and end plate are suspended in front of the cavity by the PLL above and below the disc space.

Step 8: The PLL above and below the herniated disc is divided. This step can be one of the most dangerous portions of the procedure because manipulation of the PLL may transmit movement to the herniated disc and into the spinal cord. To

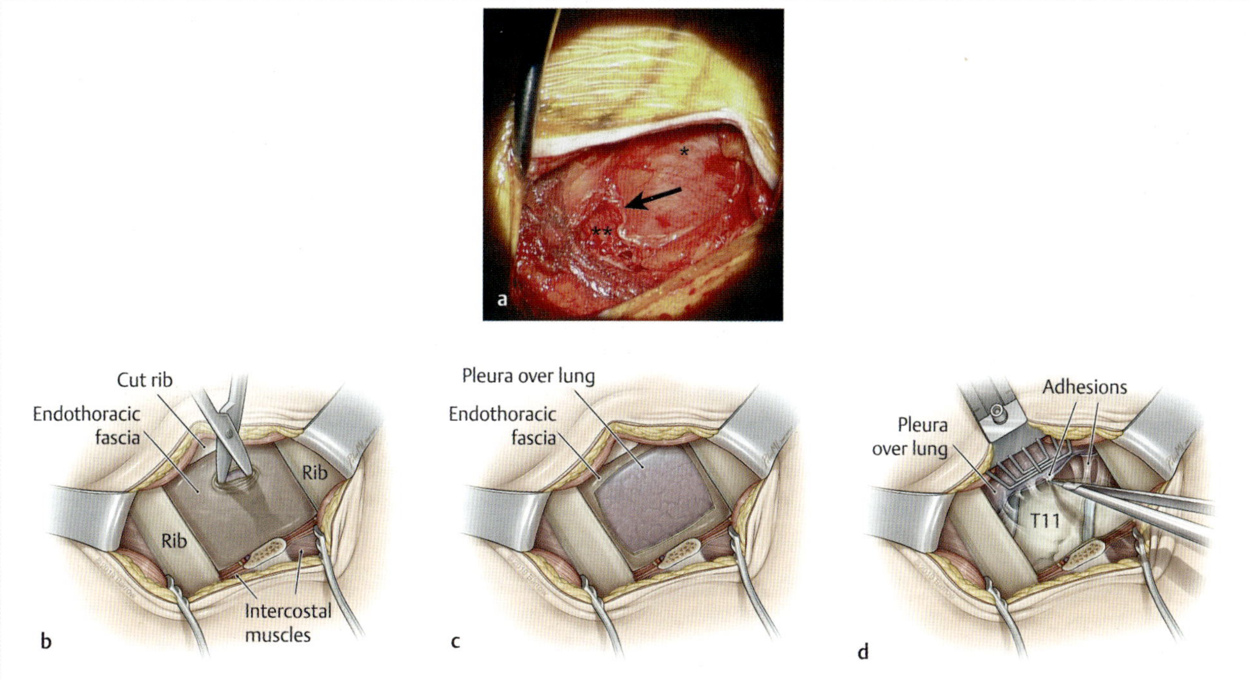

Fig. 27.3 Retropleural approach. (a) Intraoperative photograph after the underlying rib is removed shows the exposed pleural surface (*), the endothoracic fascia (**), and the plane of dissection between those two layers (*arrow*). (b) Illustration shows the dissection plan. The pleura is very delicate and has multiple small adhesions to the endothoracic fascia. We recommend using a blunt instrument or finger dissection to develop the plane widely, with sharp dissection reserved for dense fibrous connections. (c) Illustration showing the intercostal space and dissection of the endothoracic fascia, exposing the pleura. (d) Illustration of the intercostal space after the fascia is dissected and the lung is retracted, exposing the thoracic spine vertebra. (Used with permission from Barrow Neurological Institute, Phoenix, Arizona.)

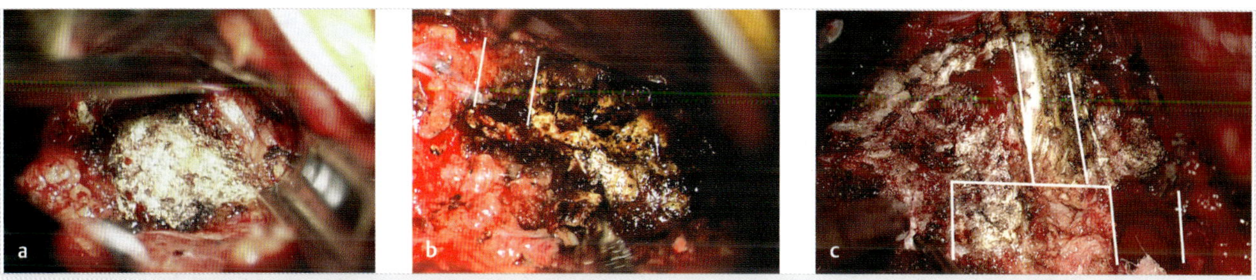

Fig. 27.4 Final exposure. (a) Intraoperative photograph after the initial deployment of the retractor shows the rib head overlying the pedicle of the vertebra inferior to the disc space to be treated. (b) Using either an osteotome or high-speed drill, the rib head is removed, exposing the underlying pedicle of the vertebral body below the disc space (*solid lines*). (c) Intraoperative photograph shows the final exposure with some preliminary drilling of the inferior pedicle. The outlines of the vertebral bodies and disc space (*solid lines*) are highlighted, showing that the bone is exposed from inferior borders of both pedicles as well as half the anterior distance of the vertebral body. (Used with permission from Barrow Neurological Institute, Phoenix, Arizona.)

excise the PLL, the surgeon uses a sharp straight curet to puncture multiple holes in the PLL (▶ Fig. 27.7a). A Kerrison rongeur can then be used to "hook" through those holes, dividing the PLL in a piecemeal fashion (▶ Fig. 27.7b).

Step 9: Finally, after the PLL is transected, the herniated disc is pushed ventrally into the corpectomy cavity (▶ Fig. 27.7c). Care must be taken during manipulation of the disc, as a sudden application or removal of force can cause "rebounding" of the disc into the thecal sac. As the PLL is pushed ventrally, adhesions along the ventral thecal sac are carefully divided (▶ Fig. 27.7d), and the contralateral PLL is detached with Kerrison rongeurs or other sharp instruments (▶ Fig. 27.7e), allowing separation of the disc. If the disc is solidly calcified into the dura or if there is evidence of transdural herniation, we do not recommend any further dissection. Instead, the herniated disc fragment should be left "floating" in the corpectomy cavity after it has been circumferentially disconnected from the PLL and vertebral bodies (▶ Video 27.1).

27.6.3 Closure

Step 10: After discectomy, hemostasis of the bone margins should be achieved with wax or other hemostatic agents. The retractor is withdrawn with careful inspection of the pleura and primary closure of small tears with absorbable suture. A drain is placed in the surgical bed and tunneled

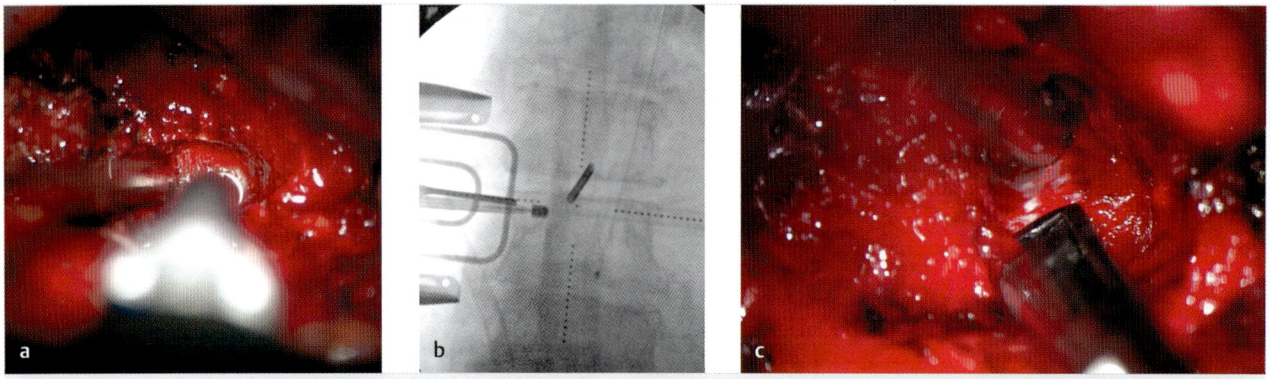

Fig. 27.5 Exposing the lateral thecal sac. **(a)** Intraoperative photograph depicts drilling of the inferior pedicle. **(b)** Anteroposterior fluoroscopy during pedicle resection expedites pedicle drilling by showing when the medial cortical wall of the pedicle is reached. **(c)** After exposing the dura as depicted in this photograph, a Kerrison rongeur can be used to complete the pedicle resection and extend the dural exposure cranially and caudally. (Used with permission from Barrow Neurological Institute, Phoenix, Arizona.)

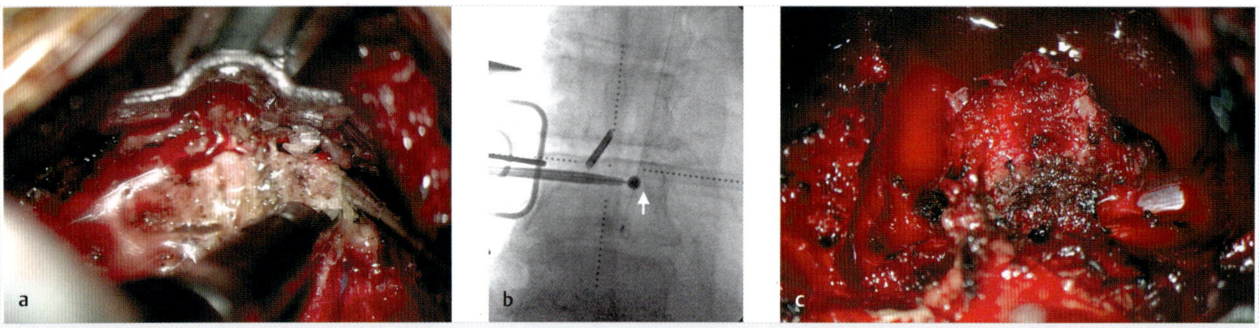

Fig. 27.6 Corpectomy. **(a)** An ultrasonic scalpel is used to cut the initial borders of the corpectomy. **(b)** During cutting and drilling of the corpectomy, an anteroposterior radiograph can be obtained to check on the depth of the corpectomy, which does not need to extend beyond the medial border of the contralateral pedicle (*arrow*), delineating the span of the spinal canal. **(c)** After completion of the corpectomy, residual disc and end plate attached to the herniation are suspended by the exposed posterior longitudinal ligament above and below the disc space. (Used with permission from Barrow Neurological Institute, Phoenix, Arizona.)

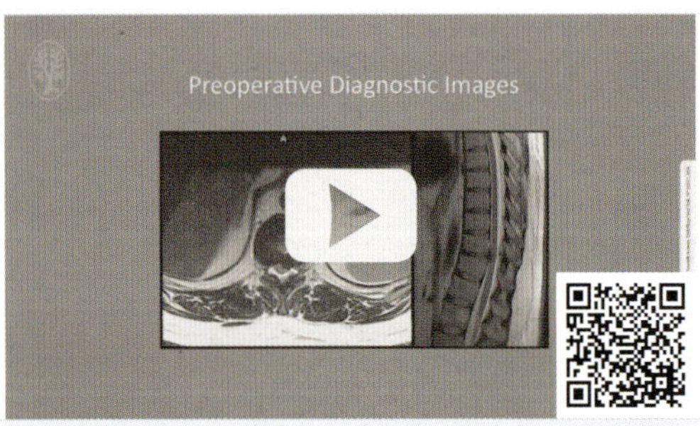

Video 27.1 Minimally invasive lateral retropleural thoracic discectomy.

subcutaneously away from the incision site. If there is a significant pleural violation, a chest tube should be used instead. For postoperative pain control, a local intercostal nerve block can be administered using 0.5% bupivacaine along the two ribs bordering the working corridor. The superficial intercostal muscles and fascia are then closed, followed by the skin. The drain or chest tube is then water sealed, and multiple Valsalva maneuvers are performed to evacuate air and fully expand the lung.

27.7 Postoperative Care

After extubation, a chest radiograph should be obtained to verify full expansion of the lung. Patients are admitted to the intensive care unit for the first night and are mobilized as soon as possible. The surgical drain or chest tube is removed when there is less than 50 mL of output in a 12-hour period. In our experience, most patients can be discharged home within 48 hours. Lastly, we routinely obtain postoperative MRI and CT imaging to assess the degree of decompression as well as critique the bone work performed (▶ Fig. 27.8a–d).

27.8 Complications and Avoidance

27.8.1 Durotomy

Dural tears can occur at any point during surgery, and due to the risk of a pleural CSF fistula, all durotomies should be repaired as aggressively as possible. Typically, tears that occur along the lateral thecal sac can be repaired primarily, sometimes requiring the use of long cardiothoracic suturing instruments. However, ventral dural tears are difficult to suture. If

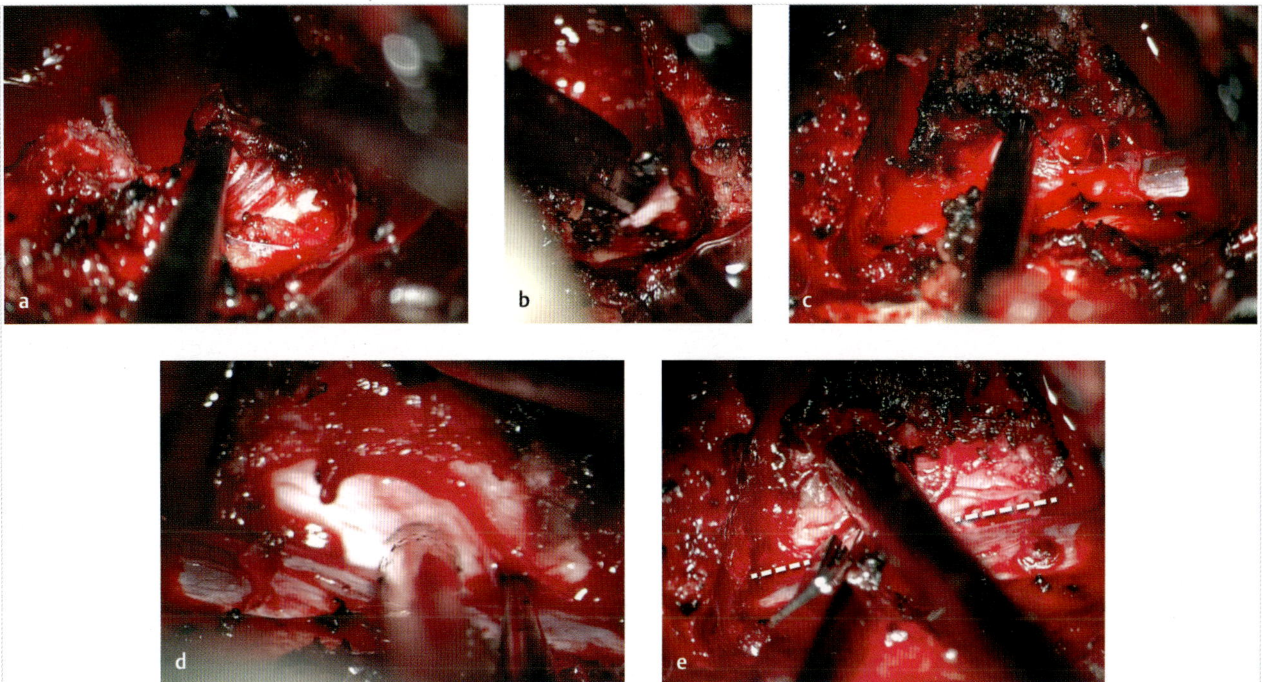

Fig. 27.7 Resection of the posterior longitudinal ligament (PLL) and discectomy. **(a)** A straight or upcurving curet is used to puncture multiple holes in the PLL. **(b)** A Kerrison rongeur is then used to hook through the puncture site and resect the PLL in a piecemeal fashion. **(c)** After the release of the PLL, the disc fragment along with the attached end plate or residual bone is pushed ventrally into the corpectomy cavity. **(d)** During mobilization of the disc, ventral adhesions can be resected with a curet or another sharp instrument. If there is fusion of the disc to the dura, no further dissection is attempted. **(e)** After the disc fragment is mobilized, the contralateral PLL attachment (*dashed line*) can be cut sharply with a knife, as pictured, or resected with a Kerrison rongeur. (Used with permission from Barrow Neurological Institute, Phoenix, Arizona.)

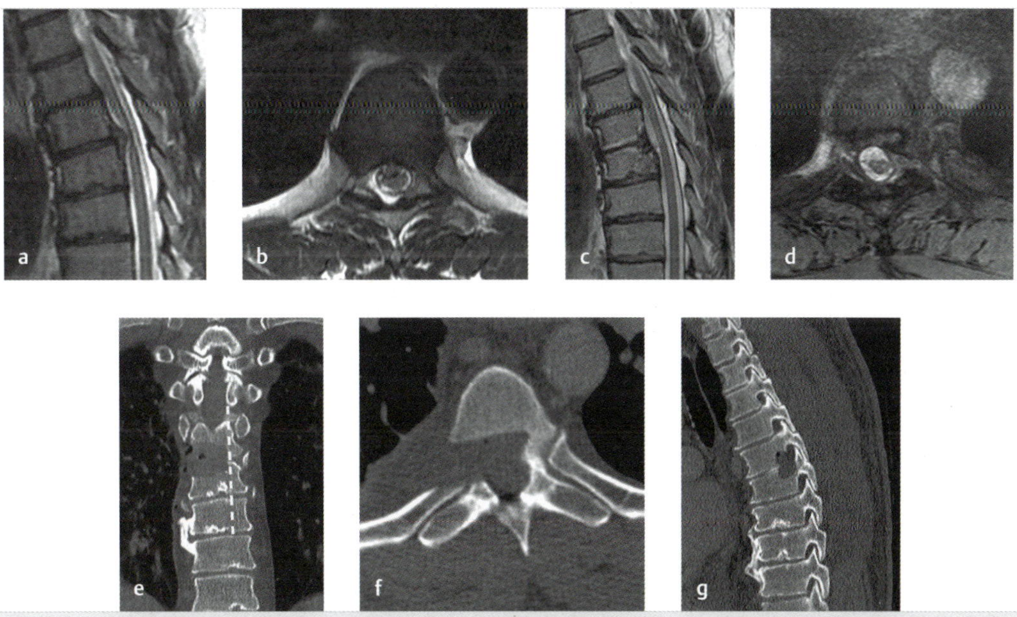

Fig. 27.8 Case example. Preoperative **(a)** sagittal and **(b)** axial T2-weighted magnetic resonance imaging (MRI) of a patient with progressive paraparesis reveals a T6–T7 herniated disc causing spinal cord compression. Postoperative **(c)** sagittal and **(d)** axial T2-weighted MRI obtained after a right-sided lateral retropleural discectomy shows full resection of the herniated disc and expansion of the thecal sac. Postoperative CT imaging reveals the extent of the bone work. **(e)** Coronal image shows the corpectomy depth extends to the medial border of the contralateral pedicle (*dotted line*), which serves as the distal margin of the spinal canal, as seen in **(f)** axial imaging. **(g)** Sagittal image shows the pedicle of the inferior vertebral body has been drilled away exposing the lateral surface of the thecal sac. The length of the corpectomy spans from the inferior border of the superior and inferior pedicle, and the width approximates one-third of the anteroposterior length of the disc space. (Used with permission from Barrow Neurological Institute, Phoenix, Arizona.)

primary repair is not able to be achieved, a small piece of dural onlay matrix (Integra Duragen, Integra LifeSciences, Plainsboro, NJ) is inserted through the hole into the subdural space to act as a gasket, and an additional piece of the matrix is placed epidurally and secured with fibrin glue.

27.8.2 Spinal Cord Injury

Due to ongoing compression from the herniated disc, the spinal cord has an extremely low tolerance of manipulation or pressure. The risk is amplified due to the narrow and long working corridor that encumbers delicate surgical manipulations. To minimize the risk of iatrogenic spinal cord injury, the surgeon must slowly, deliberately, and with the utmost care insert and withdraw any instrument on tissues in the operative site.

27.8.3 Retropleural Effusion

Because the operative bed is in the retropleural space, postoperative fluid and oozing is not exposed to the pleural cavity and can accumulate. Consequently, we recommend placement of either a surgical drain or chest tube in all patients. Even after drain removal, accumulation of postoperative fluid in the retropleural space is common and should not be evacuated unless patients are symptomatic or there is a concern for either CSF leak or infection.

27.9 Tips and Tricks

27.9.1 Retropleural Dissection

The parietal pleura is very thin and susceptible to tears during dissection from the endothoracic fascia. Typically, we find that the initial small blunt dilator used in the MaXcess (NuVasive, Inc., San Diego, CA) set is useful to gently push and mobilize the plane of dissection between the pleura and fascia. Furthermore, dissection should sweep superiorly and inferiorly as much as possible, undercutting adjacent ribs to reduce the tension on the interface of the pleura and fascia.

27.9.2 Need for Fusion

When the senior author (Juan S. Uribe) began performing lateral retropleural discectomies, all patients underwent concurrent posterior fixation with pedicle screws and interbody arthrodesis across the operative disc space. However, within the past 5 years, the staged procedure has taken precedence over performing the concurrent instrumented fusion on any discectomy patient. Theoretically, only the middle column of the spine is disrupted with the mini-open lateral approach, with preservation of the anterior longitudinal lligament and the posterior facet complexes. If fusion is necessary, the operative workflow changes in two ways. First, more anterior exposure should be obtained, and a full discectomy with end plate preparation is performed before the corpectomy. Second, after the discectomy is completed, a lateral interbody cage can be inserted into the disc space followed by a second stage surgery with placement of pedicle screws and rods.

27.9.3 Postoperative Costal Pain

Compression neuropathy can be caused by compression of the costal neurovascular bundle into the rib. After placement and expansion of the retractor, the adjacent costal nerves should be inspected to ensure there is no significant compression against an adjacent rib. If significant compression is found, additional rib resection should be performed.

27.10 Conclusion

Lateral retropleural thoracic discectomy is a safe and efficacious procedure with reduced surgical consequences compared to traditional open thoracotomies. In a large multicenter study examining 60 patients undergoing mini-open lateral discectomies across five institutions, only one patient (5%) experienced an adverse neurologic outcome following surgery.[12] Keys to the success of the procedure include the use of an appropriate lateral access retractor as well as a well-defined, structured workflow that includes (1) exposure of the lateral thecal sac, (2) creation of a workspace through a partial corpectomy, (3) resection of the PLL above and below the herniated disc, and (4) dissection of the disc into the corpectomy cavity. Above all, proper patient selection compatible with the surgeon's comfort level with the technique is vital for safety and proper surgical execution.

References

[1] McCormick WE, Will SF, Benzel EC. Surgery for thoracic disc disease. Complication avoidance: overview and management. Neurosurg Focus. 2000; 9(4): e13

[2] Dietze DD, Jr, Fessler RG. Thoracic disc herniations. Neurosurg Clin N Am. 1993; 4(1):75–90

[3] Brown CW, Deffer PA, Jr, Akmakjian J, Donaldson DH, Brugman JL. The natural history of thoracic disc herniation. Spine. 1992; 17(6) Suppl:S97–S102

[4] Shirzadi A, Drazin D, Jeswani S, Lovely L, Liu J. Atypical presentation of thoracic disc herniation: case series and review of the literature. Case Rep Orthop. 2013; 2013:621476

[5] Lara FJP, Berges AF, Quesada JQ, Ramiro JAM, Toledo RB, Muñoz HO. Thoracic disc herniation, a not infrequent cause of chronic abdominal pain. Int Surg. 2012; 97(1):27–33

[6] Fessler RG, Sturgill M. Review: complications of surgery for thoracic disc disease. Surg Neurol. 1998; 49(6):609–618

[7] Perot PL, Jr, Munro DD. Transthoracic removal of midline thoracic disc protrusions causing spinal cord compression. J Neurosurg. 1969; 31(4):452–458

[8] Karmakar MK, Ho AM. Postthoracotomy pain syndrome. Thorac Surg Clin. 2004; 14(3):345–352

[9] Burke TG, Caputy AJ. Treatment of thoracic disc herniation: evolution toward the minimally invasive thoracoscopic technique. Neurosurg Focus. 2000; 9 (4):e9

[10] Han PP, Kenny K, Dickman CA. Thoracoscopic approaches to the thoracic spine: experience with 241 surgical procedures. Neurosurgery. 2002; 51(5) Suppl:S88–S95

[11] Khoo LT, Smith ZA, Asgarzadie F, et al. Minimally invasive extracavitary approach for thoracic discectomy and interbody fusion: 1-year clinical and radiographic outcomes in 13 patients compared with a cohort of traditional anterior transthoracic approaches. J Neurosurg Spine. 2011; 14(2):250–260

[12] Uribe JS, Smith WD, Pimenta L, et al. Minimally invasive lateral approach for symptomatic thoracic disc herniation: initial multicenter clinical experience. J Neurosurg Spine. 2012; 16(3):264–279

28 Mini-Open Pedicle Subtraction Osteotomy for Deformity Correction

Cory Hartman, Jakub Godzik, Esteban Quiceno, and Juan S. Uribe

Summary

Adult spinal deformity is becoming a commonly diagnosed pathology because of the increasing elderly population. There are many different surgical approaches to correct these dimensional deformities; most of these approaches are associated with high morbidity and high rates of complications. This chapter reviews the indications and surgical technique for a mini-open pedicle subtraction osteotomy (PSO), a component of a hybrid minimally invasive approach to spinal deformity management. PSO is a valid option that can reduce blood loss, prolonged hospitalizations, and prolonged surgical times associated with traditional open surgical approaches for correcting fixed kyphotic deformity.

Keywords: adult spinal deformity, kyphosis, minimally invasive spine surgery, osteotomy, pedicle subtraction osteotomy

28.1 Introduction

Adult spinal deformity (ASD) is a common pathology; it has been reported in up to 60% of the older population.[1] The surgical treatment associated with correction of sagittal imbalance in ASD is associated with improved quality of life and patient outcome scores. A wide range of osteotomies are employed to achieve an adequate improvement in sagittal balance and spinopelvic parameters; however, these surgical techniques are associated with a complication rate of 39%.[2,3]

There are six different types of osteotomies classified by Schwab (▶ Fig. 28.1). (1) Grade 1 is a partial facet resection, such as the Smith-Peterson osteotomy; with this procedure, about 5 to 10 degrees of correction can be gained at each level.[2] (2) Grade 2 osteotomy is a complete facet resection; the typical example is the Ponte osteotomy, which was described in 1987

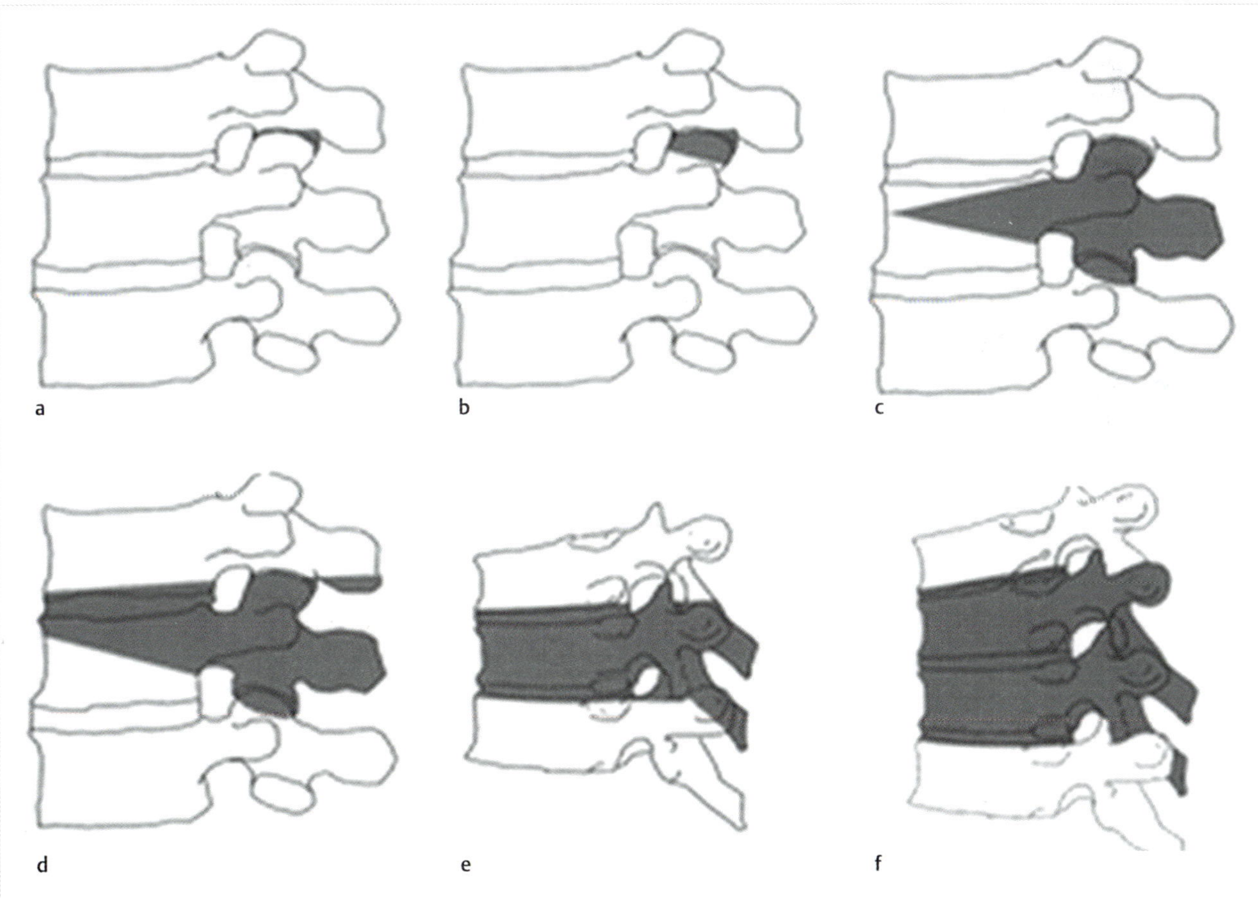

Fig. 28.1 Schematic of the comprehensive anatomic spinal osteotomy classification proposed by Schwab et al. **(a)** Partial facet. **(b)** Complete facet. **(c)** Pedicle and partial vertebrectomy. **(d)** Pedicle, partial vertebrectomy, and disc. **(e)** Complete vertebrectomy and adjacent discs. **(f)** Multilevel complete vertebrectomy and discs. (Adapted from AOSpine Master Series, Vol 4: Adult Spinal Deformities.[5])

Table 28.1 Advantages and disadvantages of MIS PSO

	MIS PSO
Advantages	• Reduced blood loss • Less collateral tissue damage • Potentially faster recovery than open procedures • Faster surgical workflow
Disadvantages	• Development of special skills • Increased radiation (X-rays) • Special hardware, tools, instruments • Questionable capacity to perform posterolateral bone preparation (arthrodesis)

Abbreviation: MIS PSO, minimally invasive surgery pedicle subtraction osteotomy.

and consists of wide resection of the thoracic facet joints and laminae and the complete removal of the ligamentum flavum.[4] (3) Grade 3 osteotomy is the pedicle subtraction osteotomy (PSO), which extends the resection of the posterior vertebral elements into the vertebral body. (4) Grade 4 osteotomy includes a disc resection. (5) Grade 5 osteotomy includes the complete body and disc resection, and (6) grade 6 includes multiple vertebral body and disc resections.[2]

The PSO was first described in a series of 11 patients with ankylosing spondylitis. The procedure involves a three-column osteotomy with a transpedicular wedge resection extending from the posterior elements through the vertebral body, but the anterior cortex is left intact.[6] Currently, the PSO is widely used to correct kyphotic deformities and, in some cases, flat back syndrome. Recent evidence suggests that PSO is more effective in achieving good clinical outcomes in patients with kyphotic deformities than in patients with flat back syndrome who have had previous lumbar surgeries. Patients with flat back syndrome may also develop more surgical complications.

With advances in technology, new minimally invasive surgery (MIS) techniques have been developed to improve clinical outcomes and reduce surgical time, blood loss, and morbidity. MIS techniques, such as interbody fusion associated with posterolateral stabilization, have been used as a treatment for ASD, but these techniques are of limited use when the surgeon faces fixed kyphotic deformities.[7] The mini-open PSO technique is an element of the hybrid MIS-open approach to management of ASD. The mini-open PSO allows for a PSO to be performed through a smaller opening, reducing blood loss. The remaining construct is created via MIS techniques, such as percutaneous pedicle screws and anterolateral arthrodesis.

We describe a minimally invasive form of PSO that allows for a smaller incision, less blood loss, and less surgical time (▶ Table 28.1).

28.2 Indications

a) Correction of > 25 degrees of lordosis desired (degenerative scoliosis with loss of lumbar lordosis).
b) Spine stiffness (unable to achieve correction as shown on extension radiographs).
c) Fixed deformity.
d) Coronal malalignment in a fused spine.
e) > 10 cm of sagittal imbalance.[6]

The PSO is commonly performed below the conus in the lumbar spine. In the past, it was performed only between L3 and L5 to recreate physiological lordosis and to avoid spinal cord manipulation during the closure of the wedge osteotomy. However, with the improvement of surgical technique and new technological aids, a PSO can be performed in the cervical and thoracic spine. The PSO should be performed at the level of the kyphotic deformity.[6] The osteotomy should be performed at the level of the apex of the kyphosis or fixed deformity to maximize lordosis. In cases of lumbar kyphosis or hypolordosis, the PSO should be performed in the lower lumbar spine. This location provides more physiologic lumbar lordosis because 60% of the lordosis is between L4 and S1.

28.3 Contraindications

a) Medical contraindications.
b) Poor bone quality (all patients must have a recent bone density scan).

In cases that require more than 40 degrees of correction, additional methods including interbody cages or additional osteotomies, such as Smith-Peterson, may be used with a PSO to achieve spinopelvic balance.

PSO is an essential surgical tool for the surgeon for correcting ASD. Even when done using less invasive techniques such as outlined in this chapter, it can still be associated with a significant rate of complications. New MIS techniques such as ultrasonic bone scalpel and navigation have allowed for modifications of the PSO. These modifications lead to less blood loss and shorter surgical times, which are important factors to consider, especially for older patients.

28.4 Preoperative Planning

Proper physical evaluation and clinical history are crucial in the management of patients with ASD. Image evaluation is essential for preoperative planning. Standing spinal radiographs showing posteroanterior and lateral views are mandatory for achieving the proper correction.[8] Sagittal balance should be measured using these radiographs because it is closely related to quality-of-life scores, and one of the goals of the surgery is to correct the malalignment.[9]

The goals of ASD correction include a sagittal vertical axis of 40 to 50 mm, pelvic incidence minus lumbar lordosis within 10 degrees, and a pelvic tilt of less than 20 degrees; however, older patients require less rigorous alignment objectives.[9] These preoperative measurements are critical because the surgeon uses them to determine what surgical strategies are needed based on the required restoration of lumbar lordosis. A PSO restores 30 to 40 degrees of lumbar lordosis.[6]

Long flexion and hyperextension radiographs allow one to assess the flexibility of the kyphotic segment of the spine.

Supine radiographs can be helpful in determining the flexibility of the deformity in the sagittal and coronal planes. The amount of correction necessary can be reevaluated if the spine corrects significantly in the supine position.[8] This step can be performed in the operating room during patient positioning.

Magnetic resonance imaging (MRI) provides information on soft-tissue anatomy; it indicates the presence of arachnoiditis, periradicular fibrosis, or pseudomeningocele in patients with a previous history of lumbar surgery—conditions that are associated with a less favorable outcome. The presence of lumbar spinal stenosis, either central or foraminal, can be identified and adequately decompressed during surgery.

Computed tomography (CT) provides a complementary view of the bony anatomy; it is useful for planning the placement of spinal instrumentation and shows disc osteophytes, fixed deformities, and calcifications. We do not advocate the routine use of CT myelography but reserve it for situations in which MRI does not provide adequate visualization or cannot be performed.

28.5 Patient Positioning

The patient is positioned in the standard prone position, with the bony prominences well-padded and the abdomen free during surgery. A bed that flexes can be useful during the closing of the deformity. Anterior and lateral fluoroscopy is performed to ensure adequate positioning and to determine the extent of the reduction of the deformity. Previous stages of surgery may have involved lateral or supine positioning for an anterolateral interbody fusion.

28.6 Surgical Steps

The mini-open PSO is a hybrid technique combining percutaneous and open technique with a primary goal of mitigating blood loss.

28.6.1 Incision

After the appropriate surgical level is localized using anteroposterior or lateral fluoroscopy, an incision is made in the midline just long enough to expose the transverse process of the adjacent levels of the PSO vertebra to facilitate a standard PSO technique and placement of pedicle screws above and below the osteotomy.

28.6.2 Technique

1. Bilateral subperiosteal dissection is performed exposing the posterior elements and the transverse process of the desired level, the superior joint of the lower level, and the inferior joint of the superior vertebral level.
2. Open pedicle screw placement is performed at the levels cranial and caudal to the PSO. The pedicle screws may be placed by a freehand technique, by imaging guidance, or by robot.
3. Screw placement is verified on intraoperative fluoroscopy. We recommend these screws be placed deeper in the pedicle than the other pedicle screws in the overall construct to facilitate stability of the final construct.
4. The remaining pedicle screws may be placed via MIS techniques (▶ Fig. 28.2a). Additionally, deeper screw placement is required for satellite rod placement (discussed below).
5. After removing the spinous process of the index vertebra and the level above, the surgeon proceeds with laminectomy and complete facetectomy of all joints of the index level using a rongeur and Kerrison punch.
6. The decompression laminectomy is performed to expose the pedicles above and below the proposed pedicle resection. At the level of the PSO, the transverse processes are detached from the vertebral body using a Kerrison rongeur, and the ligamentum flavum is also removed. At this point, the vertebral body is isolated, and the nerve roots are completely visualized (▶ Fig. 28.2b).
7. Next, the lateral surface of the vertebral body is exposed with Cobb or Penfield dissectors. If lateral segmental vessels are seen, bipolar cautery is used to control the bleeding. The plane between the lateral aspect of the vertebral body and the adjacent soft tissue is maintained with retractors. The nerve roots are visualized and are protected during the resection of the pedicles, which can be done with a rongeur.
8. A temporary deep-seated, satellite rod is placed across the PSO from the superior to the inferior pedicle screws to prevent translation and neural injury. Eventually, the satellite rods serve as the final rods in the construct, and the primary rods lie above them. It is essential for the surgeon to deeply seat the pedicle screws at the levels above and below the PSO to avoid interference with the primary rods. The wedge osteotomy can be performed using a variety of tools. At our institution, we favor using an ultrasonic oscillating bone scalpel to reduce blood loss and surgical time as well as to maximize the amount of bone available for autografting. Fluoroscopic guidance is used to maintain orientation when creating the wedge. Wedge angulation is dependent on the surgical goals, ranging in the literature from 25 to 40 degrees.[6] When resecting the vertebral body, one must take care to begin by creating a thin posterior cortical wall anteriorly to facilitate closure of the osteotomy. Using an oscillating bone scalpel instead of a high-speed drill allows one to obtain a large amount of autograft from the vertebral body resection. Once the majority of the osteotomy is performed with the ultrasonic oscillating bone scalpel, curettes may be used to complete the resection (▶ Fig. 28.2c, d).
9. A curved Freer elevator can be used to remove any dural adhesions to the posterior wall to prevent injury to the anterior portion of the dura. Once the resection of the lateral wall is complete, an angled curet or downward pusher can be used to fracture the thinned posterior wall into the osteotomy site. The anterior vertebral cortex must be preserved to avoid vascular and visceral injuries (▶ Fig. 28.2e). Before closing the osteotomy, the surgeon must remove bone fragments that could compress the nerve roots.
10. Closure of the wedge osteotomy can be accomplished by sequential compression maneuvers across the satellite rods bilaterally, bending of the table, and lifting of the patient's feet. With advances in technology and pedicle screw reduction systems, one may use towers on the tulip heads to reduce both sides simultaneously. This technique allows for compression without the use of a compressor tool, which can slip off the rod if compression is not done appropriately.

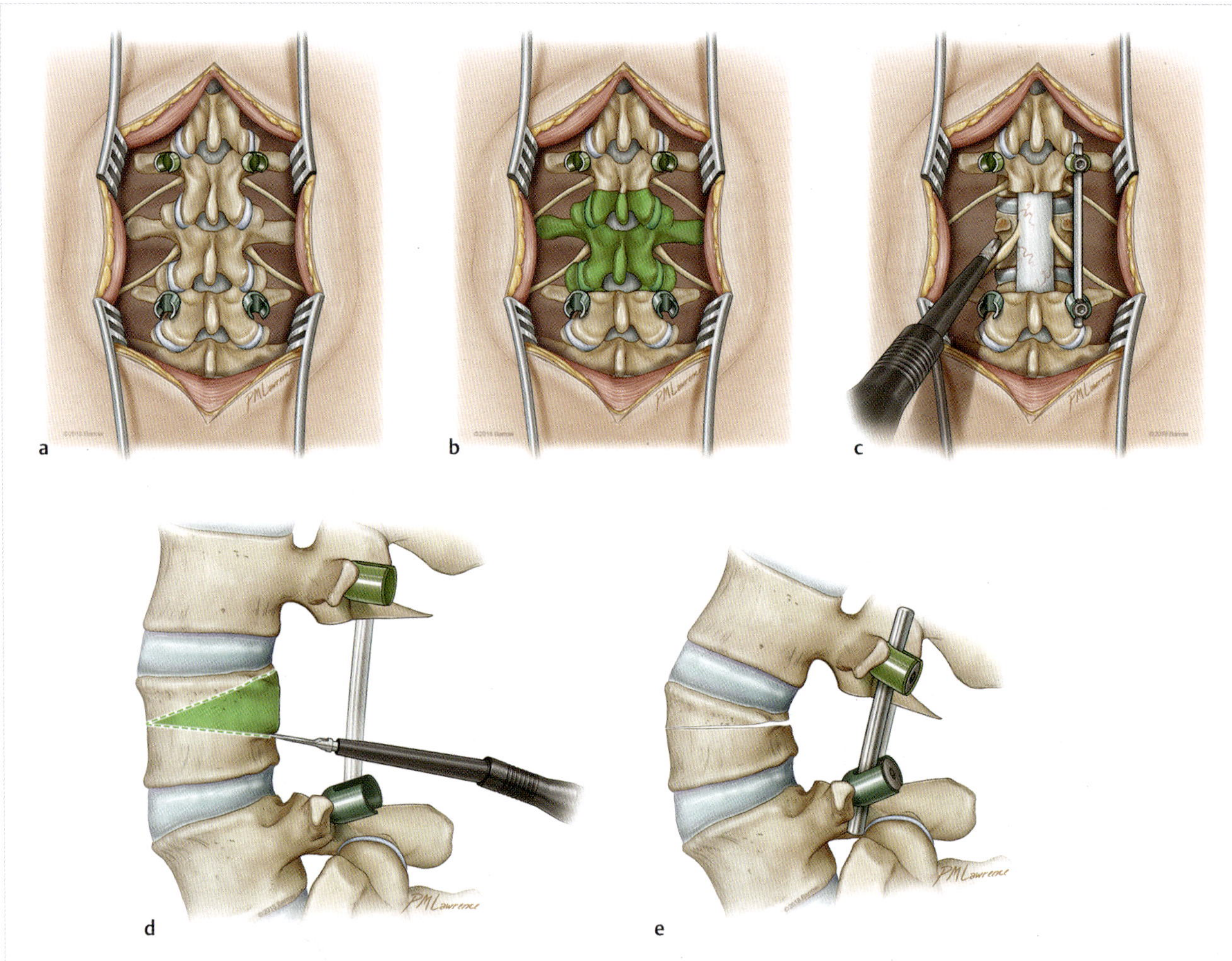

Fig. 28.2 Illustrations depicting the basic steps of a wedge osteotomy. **(a)** Posteroanterior view of the exposure of the vertebrae and placement of the pedicle screws. **(b)** Area of bone and ligaments to be removed (*green*). **(c)** Posteroanterior view with bone removed from the vertebra, revealing spinal cord and nerve roots below. **(d)** Sagittal view of bone wedge removed from the vertebral body (spinal cord not shown). **(e)** Sagittal view of lumbar spine with normal curvature and pedicle screws and rods in place. (Used with permission from Barrow Neurological Institute, Phoenix, Arizona.)

We recommend this maneuver be done under strict visual inspection and neuromonitoring to prevent injury to neural structures.

In the final construct, the deep-seated satellite rods connect the upper and lower pedicles over the PSO level. The primary rods that connect the other fixation points across the spine (placed percutaneously) do not attach to the pedicle screws immediately above and below the PSO. This arrangement avoids the severe bending of the long rods, which may predispose the rod to fatigue and fracture, and provides increased rod density across a biomechanically vulnerable portion of the surgical construct. The long rods are contoured with a navigated spinal rod bending system that expedites manual rod manipulation via computer-assisted bending instructions, which are then placed via MIS and secured (▶ Fig. 28.3).

28.6.3 Closure

The incisions are closed in the usual fashion, with a watertight closure of the fascia and deep dermal layers. Drains are routinely left in place.

28.7 Postoperative Care

We recommend postoperative imaging and overnight hospitalization in the intensive care unit. If there were any neuromonitoring changes during surgery, the mean systolic blood pressure should be kept above 85 mm Hg. Patients are monitored postoperatively at 6 weeks, 3 months, 6 months, 1 year, and 2 years with repeated standing spinal radiographs to evaluate the construct and progression of fusion.

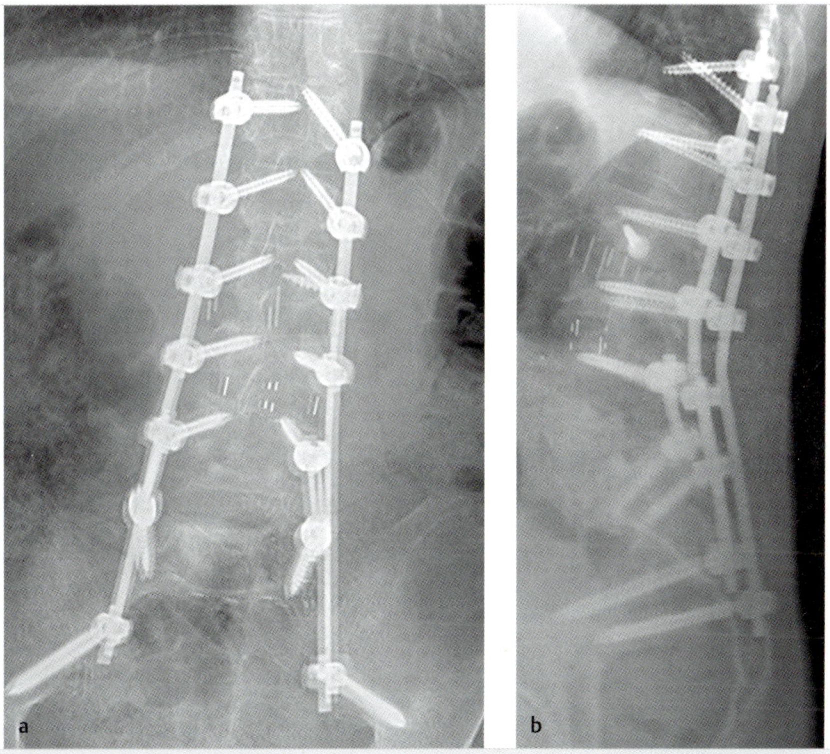

Fig. 28.3 Standing radiographs of a patient who underwent a mini-open pedicle subtraction osteotomy of an L3–L4 deformity. **(a)** Posteroanterior view. **(b)** Sagittal view. (Used with permission from Barrow Neurological Institute, Phoenix, Arizona.)

28.8 Complication Avoidance

Open PSO procedures have a complication rate of 38%.[10] The rate of neurological complication with open PSO is 11%, and intraoperative blood loss is variable, but approximately 19% of patients have excessive bleeding (> 5,000 mL). Previously described minimally invasive PSO techniques[11] have demonstrated decreased blood loss. Wang and Bordon[12] have described an average blood loss of 843 mL per patient.

The most crucial surgical step to avoid neurologic deficit is the careful closure of the wedge osteotomy. It is essential to have adequate neuromonitoring. Extreme buckling of the dura should be avoided. Pseudarthrosis is a major concern in traditional open PSO. With the use of satellite rods and MIS techniques for the majority of the construct, we hope the rates of pseudarthrosis will decrease for the mini-open hybrid technique. Other expected complications during or after surgery include conversion to open surgery because of ineffective reduction of the deformity, unintentional durotomy resulting in a cerebrospinal fluid (CSF) leak, and proximal junctional kyphosis. The only series of mini-open PSO reported in the literature describes the outcomes of 16 patients and 6 complications, including CSF leak, wound infection, iliac screw dislodgement, and graft extrusion.[12]

28.9 Tips and Tricks

ASD surgery has a high complication rate, and patient selection is crucial for successful outcomes. The use of standing and bending spinal radiographs is critical for determining the appropriate surgery for each patient.

In our experience, the use of a small incision and less exposure of subcutaneous tissue lead to decreased blood loss and a lower rate of infections. The size of the incision must be weighed against the difficulties associated with the placement of the pedicle screws and performing safe surgery.

An oscillating scalpel is useful when performing the wedge osteotomy. We have found that it reduces blood loss, allows for more precise bone cut, and maximizes autograft yield.

Strict neuromonitoring is required, particularly during the closing of the wedge osteotomy, which is when most of the neurological complications take place because of neural compression. Extreme dural buckling should be avoided, and the intrathecal contents can be shortened up to one-third of the vertebral body.

Lastly, we routinely bend the long rod with a computer-assisted bending system that expedites manual rod manipulation and helps in passing the rod in an MIS fashion. This technique allows one to easily contour the rod to transverse posteriorly to the satellite rods.

28.10 Conclusion

PSO is an essential surgical tool for the surgeon for correcting ASD. Unfortunately, it is associated with a high rate of complications. New MIS techniques have allowed for modifications of the PSO. These modifications lead to less blood loss and shorter surgical times, which are important factors to consider, especially for older patients affected by ASD.

Acknowledgment

The authors thank the staff of Neuroscience Publications at Barrow Neurological Institute for assistance with manuscript preparation.

References

[1] Schwab F, Ungar B, Blondel B, et al. Scoliosis Research Society-Schwab adult spinal deformity classification: a validation study. Spine. 2012; 37(12):1077–1082

[2] Diebo B, Liu S, Lafage V, Schwab F. Osteotomies in the treatment of spinal deformities: indications, classification, and surgical planning. Eur J Orthop Surg Traumatol. 2014; 24 Suppl 1:S11–S20

[3] Charosky S, Guigui P, Blamoutier A, Roussouly P, Chopin D, Study Group on Scoliosis. Complications and risk factors of primary adult scoliosis surgery: a multicenter study of 306 patients. Spine. 2012; 37(8):693–700

[4] Ponte A, Orlando G, Siccardi GL. The true Ponte osteotomy: by the one who developed it. Spine Deform. 2018; 6(1):2–11

[5] Sciubba DM. AOSpine Masters Series, Volume 4: Adult Spinal Deformities. Luiz Roberto Vialle, Kenneth MC Cheung, Lawrence G. Lenke. New York, NY: Thieme; 2015. In: Elsevier; 2016

[6] Gupta S, Gupta MC. The nuances of pedicle subtraction osteotomies. Neurosurg Clin N Am. 2018; 29(3):355–363

[7] Wang MY. Miniopen pedicle subtraction osteotomy: surgical technique and initial results. Neurosurg Clin N Am. 2014; 25(2):347–351

[8] Gupta MC, Kebaish K, Blondel B, Klineberg E. Spinal osteotomies for rigid deformities. Neurosurg Clin N Am. 2013; 24(2):203–211

[9] Diebo BG, Varghese JJ, Lafage R, Schwab FJ, Lafage V. Sagittal alignment of the spine: what do you need to know? Clin Neurol Neurosurg. 2015; 139:295–301

[10] Auerbach JD, Lenke LG, Bridwell KH, et al. Major complications and comparison between 3-column osteotomy techniques in 105 consecutive spinal deformity procedures. Spine. 2012; 37(14):1198–1210

[11] Fanous AA, Liounakos JI, Wang MY. Minimally invasive pedicle subtraction osteotomy. Neurosurg Clin N Am. 2018; 29(3):461–466

[12] Wang MY, Bordon G. Mini-open pedicle subtraction osteotomy as a treatment for severe adult spinal deformities: case series with initial clinical and radiographic outcomes. J Neurosurg Spine. 2016; 24(5):769–776

29 Posterior Paramedian Endoscopic Thoracic Discectomy

Raj Nangunoori, Diana H. Jho, David H. Jho, and Hae-Dong Jho

Summary

In this chapter, the reader will find a thorough guide on the background, rationale, surgical technique, postoperative care, and tricks on how to perform thoracic discectomies via an endoscopic transthoracic technique. The surgical treatment of thoracic disc herniations is challenging. The authors not only achieve a good description of the procedure but also walk the reader step-by-step on how to perform this technique safely.

Keywords: thoracic disc herniation, thoracic endoscopic discectomy, thoracic disc endoscopic surgery, thoracoscopic surgery

29.1 Introduction

Posterior paramedian endoscopic discectomy is a minimally invasive surgical technique for thoracic disc herniation. Surgical treatment for thoracic disc herniation has been considered more technically challenging with potentially higher risks than cervical or lumbar disc herniation, in part due to decreased buffer space for the neural elements and increased sensitivity with more tenuous vascular supply of the spinal cord in this region. The senior author's (H.-D. Jho) experience with posterior paramedian approach to thoracic disc herniation has evolved from a modified transpedicular approach to the current posterior paramedian approach in his practice over time. The posterior paramedian endoscopic approach is probably most analogous to the surgical approach for lumbar disc herniation, but there are some key technical differences that are critical for procedural safety. A paramount consideration is that the disc herniation is often ventral to the spinal cord in a relatively narrow spinal canal, and the disc may be associated with osteophytes and calcifications, reducing the capacity or safety of thecal retraction. The use of an endoscope with fixed pneumatic holder can provide a direct ventral view of the anterior aspect of the dura. The details of the surgical technique are described.

29.2 Evolution of the Paramedian Approach

Surgical treatments for symptomatic thoracic disc herniations have historically been complicated by anatomic and physiologic factors of the thoracic spine region, which include potentially tenuous and anatomically variable vascular supply, anatomic challenges in safely accessing the ventral aspect of the spinal canal while limiting morbidity and without compromising biomechanical stability, and the limited capacity and tolerance of the thoracic spinal cord to retraction, which may additionally be worsened by the presence of significant disc calcifications or osteophytes. The earliest clinical description of thoracic disc herniation was in 1938 by Key, although the first attempt at surgical decompression was not until 1922.[1,2] Early thoracic disc surgery was performed with basic midline laminectomy techniques. Spinal cord damage occurred with high frequency in midline laminectomy techniques, which emphasized the need to develop different approaches to treat thoracic disc herniations.[3,4] To avoid iatrogenic injury to the spinal cord, various approaches were developed with the common goal of treating the compressive component of disc herniation, with minimal manipulation of the spinal cord. These surgical approaches included: (1) Posterior approaches such as transpedicular or transfacet techniques, (2) posterolateral approaches such as costotransversectomy or lateral rachotomy or lateral extracavitary approach, (3) lateral transthoracic approaches such as transpleural or extrapleural techniques, and (4) anterior approaches such as transsternal or thoracoscopic techniques.[5,6,7,8,9,10] Most of the posterolateral, lateral transthoracic, and anterior approaches typically involve more invasiveness and increased tissue dissection compared to posterior approaches or thoracoscopic techniques, such that some surgeons further developed thoracoscopic techniques to potentially reduce morbidities and to reduce postoperative healing periods.[11] However, the steep learning curve and specialized equipment, including the differences in surgical instruments for thoracoscopic surgery versus conventional spine surgery, can make the incorporation of thoracoscopic approaches into routine practice challenging.

In regards to posterior approaches, Patterson and Arbit first described the transpedicular approach in a series of three patients in 1978.[12] Stillerman et al introduced a transfacet pedicle-sparing approach in 1995, in which the medial portion of the facet complex was removed for exposure.[13] However, since the dura covering the thoracic spinal cord abuts the pedicle of the vertebral body just below the target level disc herniation, the surgical exposure may be inadequate without removal of the superior-medial portion of the pedicle despite a partial facetectomy. In order to acknowledge and honor the original report of the transpedicular approach, we had initially published our technique as a variant of the transpedicular approach, as a hybrid technique with partial drilling of the pedicle and medial facets for exposure. Medial facetectomy combined with drilling of the superior-medial portion of the lower pedicle provides surgical access of approximately 3 to 5 mm lateral to the spinal cord. Once the drilling is complete, the exposed lateral dura corresponds to the subarachnoid space of approximately 2 to 3 mm width lateral to the spinal cord, allowing for some potential gentle retraction of the dura medially, which can provide more working space. The bony exposure combined with the lateral subarachnoid space provides a total working window width of 5 to 8 mm lateral to the spinal cord, and this posterior paramedian endoscopic thoracic discectomy was developed by the senior author (H.-D. Jho) as a minimally invasive alternative using endoscopy to mitigate the risks of spinal cord manipulation.[14] The term "paramedian approach" is used to describe this approach, which utilizes natural anatomic corridors while minimizing risk for iatrogenic instability.

The main advantage of this approach is that it utilizes normal tissue planes and minimizes the risk of causing instability. The use of an endoscope can provide a direct ventral view of the anterior aspect of the dura. However, these advantages come at a significant cost, as this is a technically very demanding approach that requires adequate training. Calcified and midline thoracic discs would not be good targets.

29.3 Patient Selection

Symptomatic thoracic disc herniations are relatively rare compared to cervical and lumbar disc herniations, with incidence rates in the literature widely ranging from 0.1 to 0.0001%.[13,15] Clinical presentation for thoracic disc herniation may be variable, and up to 37% of patients with radiographic evidence of a disc herniation may be incidental and clinically asymptomatic.[16,17,18,19] Surgical indications for thoracic disc herniations can include myelopathy, radiculopathy, and focal paraspinal back pain, depending on the overall clinical scenario. Patients with myelopathy may classically present with sensory disturbances (e.g., hypesthesia, paresthesia, dysesthesia), motor disturbances such as progressive paraparesis or paraplegia, spastic gait disturbances, rarely Brown-Séquard syndrome, and/or bowel and bladder dysfunction.[20,21,22,23] The goal of surgery for myelopathy is decreasing or preventing further progression of spinal cord dysfunction, although some neurologic improvement may be seen on a variable spectrum. The patients should be counseled in advance that the symptoms of myelopathy may not improve completely. Another surgical indication may be thoracic radiculopathy, which may manifest as a radicular band of pain, intercostal neuralgia, or point tenderness. Thoracic disc herniation symptoms may occasionally overlap with referred pain from cardiac, intra-abdominal, or even pelvic pathologies.[24,25,26,27] Thoracic disc disease may very rarely mimic neurogenic claudication, which is much more typical in the context of lumbar spinal stenosis.[28] It is especially important in unusual cases to use a thorough history and physical examination to correlate radiographic findings with clinical symptoms. When diagnostic measures are sufficiently exhausted and thoracic disc herniation is the only significant pathology seen on imaging, surgical intervention might be carefully considered in those cases. When midline thoracic back pain is the only symptom, surgery can be performed only if the location of pain matches with the level of pathology, and pain is truly intractable. But these patients should know that axial thoracic back pain might not be completely resolved despite successful surgical decompression at the region of the herniated disc.

The endoscopic technique described is designed to be versatile and has been utilized by the senior author (H.-D. Jho) with customized adjustments made to the degree of ventral bone drilling depending on the medial to lateral location of the disc and calcified versus soft disc material. In general, a soft disc or lateral location of the disc makes thoracic disc surgery more favorable, similar to other approaches for thoracic disc herniations. If the general principles described are utilized, this approach may be used regardless of the location or degree of calcification due to the versatility of the approach and direct visualization provided by the endoscope.

29.4 Preoperative Planning and Patient Positioning

One of the problems that may be encountered preoperatively is the lack of sagittal scout imaging views that include the entire spine. Sometimes the level of disc herniation is variably counted from the top down or from the sacrum up on radiology reports or labeling or levels. Sometimes there may be anatomic variations such as 4 or 6 lumbar vertebrae, transitional lumbosacral vertebra, 11 or 13 thoracic vertebrae with associated ribs, Klippel-Feil deformity or other segmentation variations in the spine, and other anatomic anomalies that could potentially complicate the accurate localization of levels. These variations highlight the necessity for at least a complete sagittal scout image to accurately localize the level of pathology.

Surgical instruments for performing this procedure include: an endoscope tower which contains a monitor, light source, and video recording system, motorized lens cleansing device, 4-mm rod-lens endoscopes (0-, 30-, and 70-degree lenses), a gas-powered endoscope holder, and a slender high-speed drill (▶ Fig. 29.1a, b). For surgery, the patient is initially placed in lateral position with the pathology side facing up while under general endotracheal anesthesia, with initial lateral positioning for localization before turning the patient and/or rotating the table ventrally approximately 30 degrees for the operative position, such that the coronal plane of the patient forms a 60-degree angle with the horizontal plane (which will be termed the "60-degree position"). The 60-degree position is most similar to but not as much ventrally rotated as the three-quarter prone or park bench position. An axillary roll is placed under the dependent side, and the patient is padded and gently secured to the table with tape. Two or three 18-gauge spinal needles are placed in serial fashion (counting upwards from the sacrum) against the laminar bone at the spinolaminar junction just lateral to midline, and the surgical level is confirmed using fluoroscopy or alternatively overlapping X-rays. Usually the first needle is placed at the upper lumbar region, and a second needle is placed rostral to the first needle in the thoracic spine and adjusted to the target site. For upper thoracic levels, a third needle may be required. Once the correct level of surgery is localized with the spinal needles, the target site needle is used for injection of 0.5 mL of methylene blue into the soft tissue at the target level. Another 18-gauge spinal needle is inserted 5 cm lateral to the midline on the target side and the tip is placed at the laminar bone at the spinolaminar junction. The midline needles are removed, but the single laterally inserted needle is kept and draped into the field. The laterally inserted needle and methylene blue serve as landmarks to confirm the surgical level intraoperatively (▶ Fig. 29.2a, b).

Then the patient is tilted to a ventrally inclined lateral decubitus position which is 60 degrees from the horizontal plane, somewhat similar to the three-quarter lateral or park bench position (▶ Fig. 29.3). Neuromonitoring such as somatosensory evoked potentials is used only if the degree of spinal cord compression is excessively severe. An endoscope holder is mounted to the operating table so that the surgeon can use two hands for

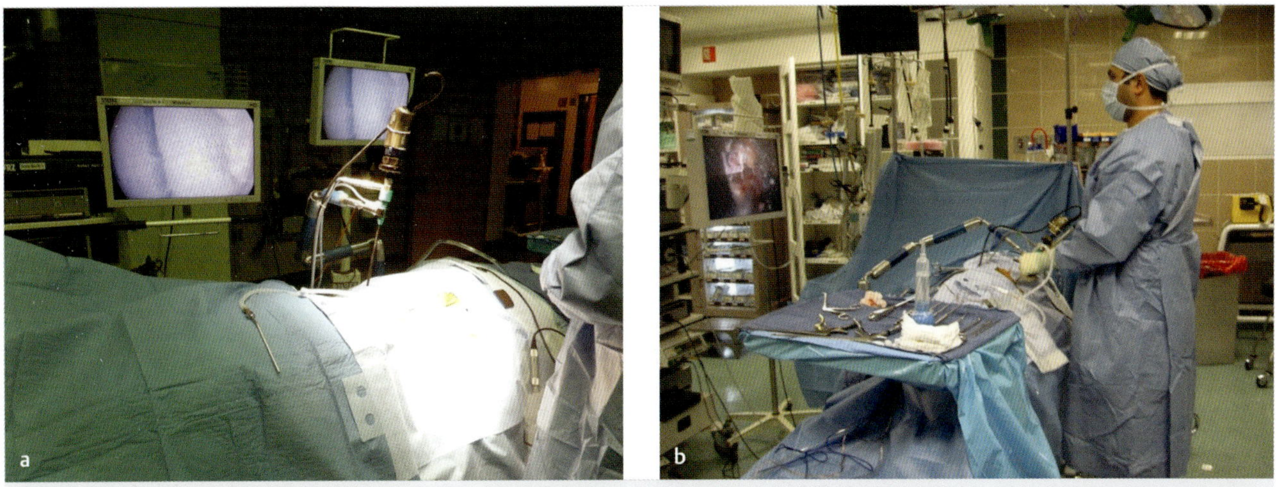

Fig. 29.1 The photos demonstrate an operating room setup, **(a)** with draping and preparation for endoscopic thoracic discectomy for a left-sided approach with the surgeon standing on the left side of the patient, and **(b)** intraoperative setup for a left-sided approach on a different patient with the surgeon standing to the left side of the patient.

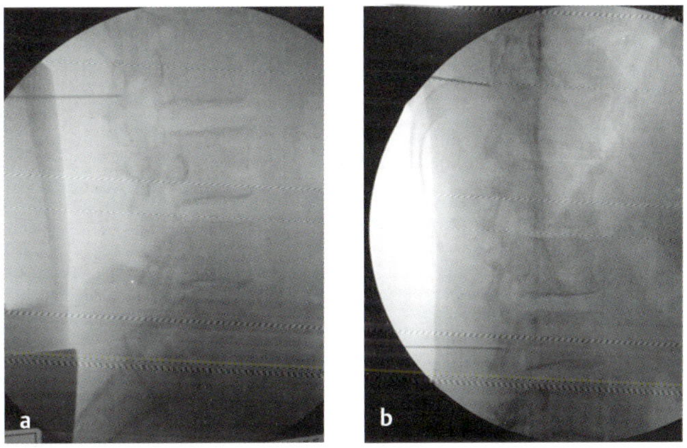

Fig. 29.2 Intraoperative radiographic marking is demonstrated. **(a)** A localizing needle at the upper lumbar region is shown. **(b)** A needle placed rostrally to localize the T10–T11 level is demonstrated. A patient is in lateral position with two serial midline needles and a lateral needle 5 cm from the midline at the target level.

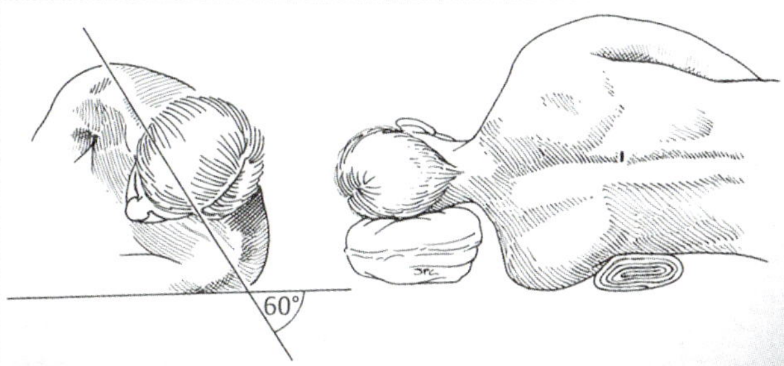

Fig. 29.3 Schematic drawings demonstrate patient positioning. Initially, the patient is placed in direct lateral position for radiographic localization. After target marking is complete, the position is tilted with ventral inclined lateral decubitus position at 60 degrees from the horizontal plane. In our experience, this "60-degree position" has been optimal for the paramedian endoscopic approach.

surgery, and the endoscope tower, endoscope cleansing device, and drill system are connected.

29.5 Surgical Technique

a) A 2-cm transverse incision is made from the lateral edge of the spinous process. The fascia is opened perpendicular to the skin incision, with vertically oriented opening made in the fascia with Metzenbaum scissors, and the ipsilateral paraspinal muscles are dissected away from the lamina. A 1.5-cm tubular threaded trocar (▸ Fig. 29.4) is introduced, providing exposure to the lateral edge of the lamina and medial facet joint.
b) The correct target level for surgery is confirmed as the tip of the laterally placed spinal needle and the methylene blue in the soft tissue of the region should be encountered. The

lamina, the medial 2 to 3 mm portion of the ipsilateral facet complex, and the rostromedial 2 to 3 mm portion of the lower pedicle inferior to the herniated disc are drilled using a 2-mm diamond drill bit under direct visualization using a 0-degree endoscope. We use a slender and slightly curved tubular drill to maneuver in the narrow surgical corridor. When bony removal is completed, 2 to 3 mm of the lateral portion of the dura mater covering the spinal cord at the spinal canal is exposed (▸ Fig. 29.5a–c). The exposed lateral dura corresponds to the subarachnoid space, which in the thoracic spine is typically 3 to 5 mm in this region.

c) The width of the subarachnoid space and configuration of the spinal cord in relation to cerebrospinal fluid (CSF) compartments around the spinal cord within the thecal sac are well reviewed before surgery on the T2-weighted axial views of the patient's magnetic resonance imaging (MRI). The ipsilateral nerve root is identified either immediately above the disc or just rostral to the lower pedicle and extends laterally through the neural foramen but may have a slightly ascending or descending course depending on the thoracic level. Ideally, when bony drilling is complete, the exposed spinal cord dura mater should correspond to the subarachnoid space while the remaining lamina protects the spinal cord (▸ Fig. 29.5c).

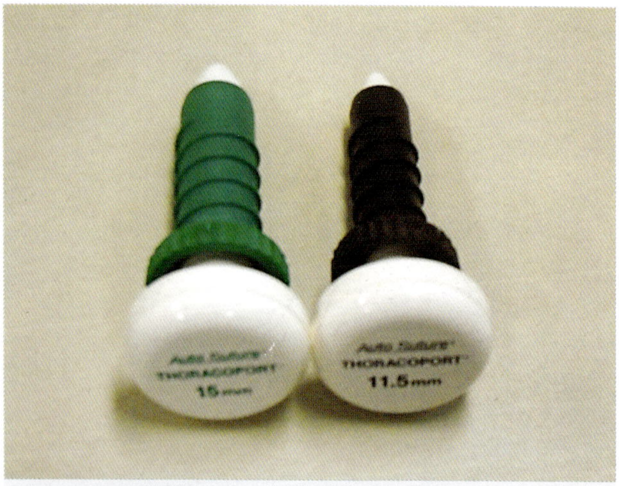

Fig. 29.4 Threaded trocars, measuring 15 or 11.5 mm in working space diameter, are utilized for this procedure.

d) Then the drilled portion of the pedicle is further drilled into the vertebral body just caudal to the disc, approximately 5 mm in depth. A similar way, the vertebral body rostral to the disc is also drilled approximately 5 mm in depth. Connecting the drilled cavity across the disc by drilling, a 5-mm-depth cavity is created lateral to the spinal cord dura mater approximately 5 mm rostral and caudal to the disc space.

e) Using various curettes, the herniated or calcified discs (with or without associated spondylotic bone spurs) are removed or separated away from the ventral aspect of the spinal cord (▸ Fig. 29.6). A 0-degree endoscope is used to initially visualize the ventral aspect of the spinal cord dura mater toward the lateral border. For paracentral or lateral disc herniations, the procedure could be performed entirely with a 0-degree endoscope. However, the 30- and 70-degree endoscopes can be used for improved medial visualization for more central or midline disc herniations ventral to the spinal cord. The cavity created for buffer space laterally and ventrally, combined with exposure of the lateral dura limited mostly to the subarachnoid space while preserving some bony protection of lamina, helps prevent inadvertent spinal cord injury.

f) If the 30- and 70-degree endoscopes are brought into the field, they can be used to directly visualize the midline ventral dura mater during decompression. Curved surgical instruments are used to accommodate around the shape of the spinal cord dura mater. Using various down-angled curettes, the herniated or calcified disc with osteophytes is pushed away from the spinal cord and removed. The down-angled curette and a pituitary rongeur are then used to push this remaining portion into the lateral cavity that was previously created. Direct visualization with the angled endoscopes can provide an added measure of safety to ensure that there is not excessive pressure placed on the ventral cord during decompression.

g) When sufficiently decompressed, the ventral dura will relax and bulge into the created cavity. Hemostasis may be achieved in various standard ways, including bipolar

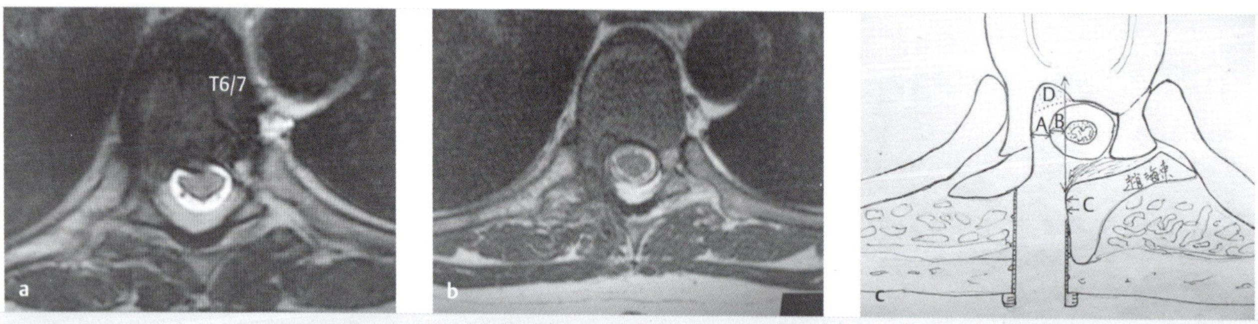

Fig. 29.5 Preoperative T2-weighted magnetic resonance imaging (MRI) axial views show a right-paracental and central disc herniation at the T6–T7 level **(a)**, which has been resected with postoperative imaging shown **(b)**. Schematic drawing demonstrates the surgical exposure for the posterior paramedian endoscopic thoracic discectomy **(c)**. The superior-medial portion of the ipsilateral pedicle at the lower vertebral body is drilled to create a space approximately 3 to 5 mm lateral to the spinal cord (label A), which may be combined with 2 to 3 mm of medial dural retraction (label B) to create a working space of approximately 5 to 8 mm in width to the target site (label D). The remaining lamina may also help limit excessive dural retraction (label C) during disc and osteophyte removal. When the superior-medial portion of the ipsilateral pedicle is drilled, the depth is typically around 5 mm into the vertebral body but may be customized to the pathology as needed.

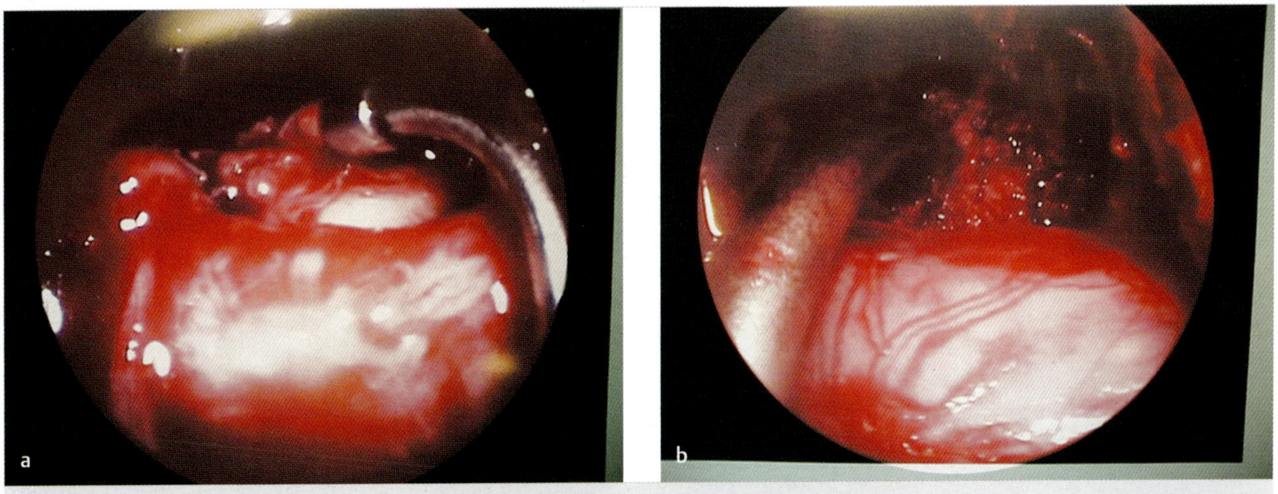

Fig. 29.6 Intraoperative photos under view of a 70-degree endoscope demonstrate the herniated disc ventral to the spinal cord (a) and the decompressed cavity after removal of the herniated disc (b).

coagulation for epidural venous bleeding and selective bone wax for cancellous bone bleeding. A small piece of noncompressed absorbable gelatin is placed at the decompression cavity.

h) The trocar is gradually removed with intermittent hemostasis of the surrounding muscle with electrocautery as needed. Local anesthetic can be used to infiltrate the surrounding muscle to reduce some postoperative pain. The fascia and subcutaneous layers are closed with absorbable sutures. The skin is approximated with adhesive surgical glue, and a small bandage is applied.

29.6 Postoperative Care

After typical surgery, patients can be discharged home later that same day or admitted to the hospital overnight. Patients with preoperative myelopathy are typically admitted to the hospital overnight for observation and postoperative evaluation prior to discharge the following day. A few days of oral pain medications are prescribed, and routine postoperative MRI is done in 6 weeks.

29.7 Complications and Avoidance

In general, complications related to thoracic disc surgery may vary, partly related to the approach used. Potential complications for any thoracic spine surgery include spinal cord injury, durotomy, hematoma, infection, spinal instability, wrong-level surgery, and failure of preoperative symptom resolution. In the experience of the senior author (H.-D. Jho), the posterior paramedian endoscopic technique can potentially minimize these risks due to the ability to directly visualize the ventral dura mater during decompression, and the small region of required dissection minimizes postoperative pains and risk of spinal instability.

29.8 Tips and Tricks

a) Endoscopic surgery requires additional training and practice, as endoscopic visualization is different from the stereoscopic visualization with a standard operating microscope. A surgeon who has relatively limited endoscopic experience will rely more on alternative visual cues to aid with depth perception. The visual screen representation is akin to video games in which a three-dimensional world is depicted in a two-dimensional rendering. There is also an analogous separation of space between the hand performance site and visual perception site remotely on the monitor, which has noticeable technical differences from microscopic surgery. The endoscope has some advantages of mobility close to the surgical site and seeing around corners, with excellent visualization of the ventral dura mater.

b) Surgical tools required to perform this procedure include rod-lens endoscope (0, 30, and 70 degrees), endoscope holder, lens-cleansing device, a slender tubular drill, and various configurations of curettes.

c) The laminotomy and drilling of the medial facet to expose the dura mater must be appropriately sized to optimally protect the spinal cord. However, if a precise exposure is not initially obtained or if the bony opening is larger than described, then the surgeon may take extra caution to avoid unnecessary retraction on the spinal cord.

References

[1] Key CA. On paraplegia depending on disease of the ligaments of the spine. Guys Hosp Rep. 1838; 3:17–34

[2] Mixter W, Barr J. Rupture of the intervertebral discs with involvement of the spinal canal. N Engl J Med. 1934; 211:210–215

[3] Fessler RG, Sturgill M. Review: complications of surgery for thoracic disc disease. Surg Neurol. 1998; 49(6):609–618

[4] Simpson JM, Silveri CP, Simeone FA, Balderston RA, An HS. Thoracic disc herniation. Re-evaluation of the posterior approach using a modified costotransversectomy. Spine. 1993; 18(13):1872–1877

[5] Hulme A. The surgical approach to thoracic intervertebral disc protrusions. J Neurol Neurosurg Psychiatry. 1960; 23:133–137
[6] Campbell WC, Edmonson AS, Crenshaw AH. Campbell's Operative Orthopaedics. 6th ed. St. Louis: CV Mosby; 1980
[7] Fessler RG, Dietze DD , Jr, Millan MM, Peace D. Lateral parascapular extrapleural approach to the upper thoracic spine. J Neurosurg. 1991; 75(3):349–355
[8] McCormick PC. Retropleural approach to the thoracic and thoracolumbar spine. Neurosurgery. 1995; 37(5):908–914
[9] McCormick WE, Will SF, Benzel EC. Surgery for thoracic disc disease. Complication avoidance: overview and management. Neurosurg Focus. 2000; 9(4): e13
[10] Perot PL , Jr, Munro DD. Transthoracic removal of midline thoracic disc protrusions causing spinal cord compression. J Neurosurg. 1969; 31(4):452–458
[11] Burke TG, Caputy AJ. Treatment of thoracic disc herniation: evolution toward the minimally invasive thoracoscopic technique. Neurosurg Focus. 2000; 9 (4):e9
[12] Patterson RH , Jr, Arbit E. A surgical approach through the pedicle to protruded thoracic discs. J Neurosurg. 1978; 48(5):768–772
[13] Stillerman CB, Chen TC, Couldwell WT, et al. Trans-facet pedicle-sparing approach. In: Benzel EC, Stillerman CB, eds. The Thoracic Spine. St Louis, MO: Quality Medical; 1999:338–345
[14] Jho HD. Endoscopic transpedicular thoracic discectomy. J Neurosurg. 1999; 91(2) Suppl:151–156
[15] Brown CW, Deffer PA , Jr, Akmakjian J, Donaldson DH, Brugman JL. The natural history of thoracic disc herniation. Spine. 1992; 17(6) Suppl:S97–S102
[16] Carson J, Gumpert J, Jefferson A. Diagnosis and treatment of thoracic intervertebral disc protrusions. J Neurol Neurosurg Psychiatry. 1971; 34(1):68–77
[17] Love JG, Schorn VG. Thoracic-disc protrusions. JAMA. 1965; 191:627–631
[18] Russell T. Thoracic intervertebral disc protrusion: experience of 67 cases and review of the literature. Br J Neurosurg. 1989; 3(2):153–160
[19] Wood KB, Blair JM, Aepple DM, et al. The natural history of asymptomatic thoracic disc herniations. Spine. 1997; 22(5):525–529, discussion 529–530
[20] Abbott KH, Retter RH. Protrusions of thoracic intervertebral discs. Neurology. 1956; 6(1):1–10
[21] Arseni C, Nash F. Thoracic intervertebral disc protrusion: a clinical study. J Neurosurg. 1960; 17:418–430
[22] Logue V. Thoracic intervertebral disc prolapse with spinal cord compression. J Neurol Neurosurg Psychiatry. 1952; 15(4):227–241
[23] Love JG, Kiefer EJ. Root pain and paraplegia due to protrusions of thoracic intervertebral discs. J Neurosurg. 1950; 7(1):62–69, illust
[24] Eleraky MA, Apostolides PJ, Dickman CA, Sonntag VK. Herniated thoracic discs mimic cardiac disease: three case reports. Acta Neurochir (Wien). 1998; 140(7):643–646
[25] Georges C, Toledano C, Zagdanski AM, et al. Thoracic disc herniation mimicking renal crisis. Eur J Intern Med. 2004; 15(1):59–61
[26] Whitcomb DC, Martin SP, Schoen RE, Jho HD. Chronic abdominal pain caused by thoracic disc herniation. Am J Gastroenterol. 1995; 90(5):835–837
[27] Xiong Y, Lachmann E, Marini S, Nagler W. Thoracic disc herniation presenting as abdominal and pelvic pain: a case report. Arch Phys Med Rehabil. 2001; 82 (8):1142–1144
[28] Morgenlander JC, Massey EW. Neurogenic claudication with positionally dependent weakness from a thoracic disc herniation. Neurology. 1989; 39 (8):1133–1134

30 Transpedicular Corpectomy and Fusion for Metastatic Tumor or Infection

Young M. Lee, Ramin A. Morshed, and Dean Chou

Summary
Tumors and infections of the spine are often indications for the use of transpedicular corpectomy and fusion. The use of open transpedicular corpectomies for these indications is a well-developed technique. In this chapter, we review the technique of minimally invasive transpedicular corpectomy along with patient selection, preoperative planning, postoperative care, and complication avoidance.

Keywords: transpedicular corpectomy, minimally invasive surgery, trap door osteotomy, rib head osteotomy, tumor

30.1 Introduction

The use of transpedicular corpectomy allows for an anterior surgery to be performed, but from a posterior approach. Common indications for the use of transpedicular corpectomy include stabilization, neurologic function preservation, pain relief, and resection of tumor or removal of infectious nidus. The use of open transpedicular corpectomies is a well-developed technique,[1,2,3,4] but one important variation includes the minimally invasive technique.

30.2 Patient Selection: Indications and Contraindications

Typical indications for transpedicular corpectomy typically include a lesion (tumor or infection nidus) that is anterior to the spinal canal. However, trauma and the need for stabilization/pain relief can be another indication for transpedicular corpectomy. The use of the minimally invasive transpedicular corpectomy has a particular advantage which is true for patients at high risk of morbidity/mortality from a larger operation, such as the obese or the elderly. A relative contraindication to the minimally invasive transpedicular approach is in the case of complex revision cases, during which extensive scarring and destruction of normal anatomy may make surgery difficult.

30.3 Preoperative Planning

Preoperative planning should include review of magnetic resonance imaging (MRI) and computed tomography (CT) scans to evaluate the location of infection and/or tumor. Routine presurgical laboratory tests, including chemistry, complete blood cell count, and coagulation panel with type and screening for blood products should be performed. Neuromonitoring should be available and the procedure is typically performed under somatosensory evoked potential (SSEP), motor evoked potential (MEP), and electromyography (EMG) monitoring. Anesthesiology teams should be made aware that neuromonitoring will be performed so that paralytic agents can be avoided during the critical portions of the case when neuromonitoring is required. The fluoroscopic C-arm should be made available as it is critical in the localization of the correct level and the placement of percutaneous pedicle screws.

30.4 Patient Positioning

After induction with general anesthesia, a urinary catheter is inserted, neuromonitoring equipment is set up, and then the patient is positioned prone. This is typically done on a Jackson table to minimize abdominal compression and associated venous hypertension. For thoracic levels, a Wilson frame may be more suited to the natural kyphosis at these levels. The head can be position in a padded head frame or horseshoe but care must be taken to avoid excess orbital pressure. Some authors advocate for Mayfield fixation to avoid this.[5] Anesthesiologist must also have access to manage airway issues, so a neutral neck position is ideal. The arms are positioned forward at right angles with elbows in-line with the shoulders. Padded chest and hip rests in addition to knee and ankle padding prevent pressure sores from developing during long operative times. Fluoroscopy is set up in the room, and the desired level is localized using a C-arm and marked externally.

This is a hybrid minimally invasive surgery (MIS) approach that, if done technically well, can significantly reduce blood loss, tissue disruption, and infection rates from metastatic tumor resection. Three-dimensional navigation can be extremely helpful—also for the corpectomy portion—to identify the healthy end plates above and below and confirm good bilateral and anterior decompression, as well as for screw placement. Preoperative embolization may be helpful. If significant blood loss is encountered it may be safer to place bone cement instead of a structural cage.

30.5 Surgical Technique with Illustration/Example

30.5.1 Step 1: Incision

After preoperative fluoroscopy is utilized to localize the correct level, a midline skin incision is performed with preservation of the fascia (▶ Fig. 30.1 and ▶ Video 30.1).

30.5.2 Step 2: Pedicle Screw Insertion

Percutaneous pedicle screws are placed two levels above and below the planned corpectomy site using Jamshidi needles,

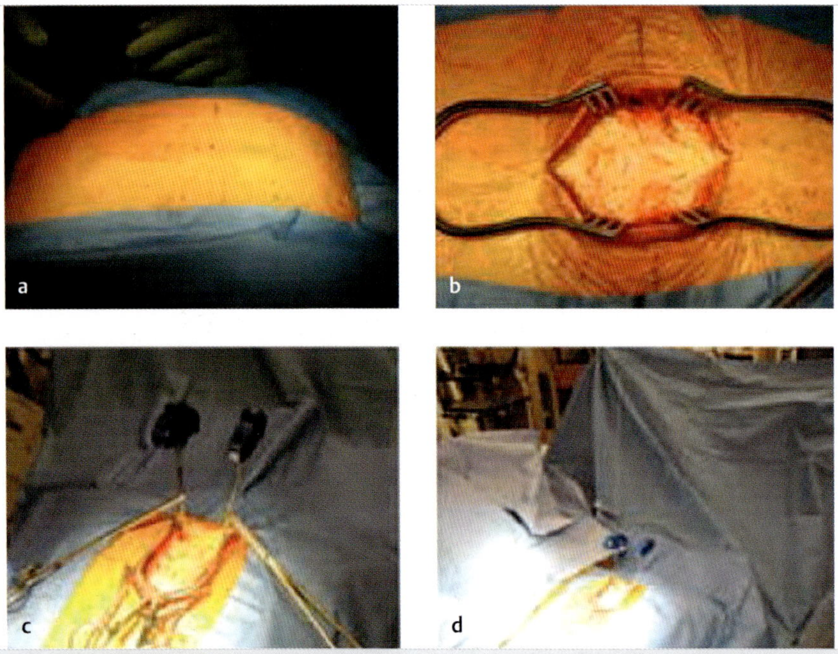

Fig. 30.1 (a) The skin incision is planned based on the radiographs. **(b)** The skin incision is made while preserving the fascia and retraction is performed **(c)** and **(d)** K-wires are inserted under fluoroscopic guidance.

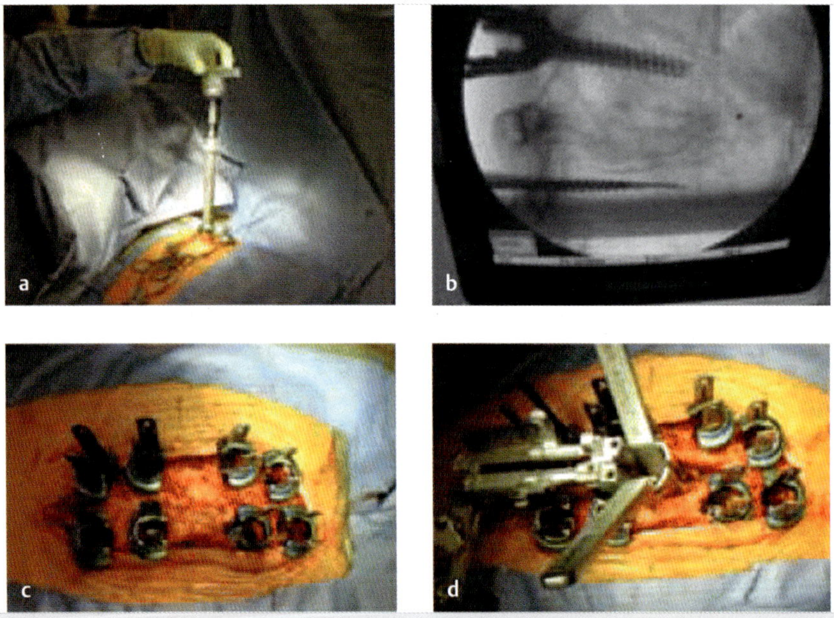

Fig. 30.2 (a) After the pedicle is tapped and the K-wire is inserted, cannulated screws are inserted. **(b)** The cannulated screws are inserted two levels above and below the planned corpectomy site. **(c)** A midline fascial opening is performed and **(d)** a retractor is placed.

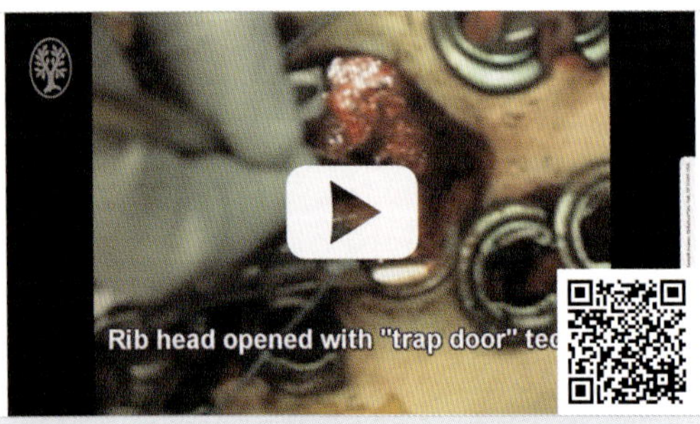

Video 30.1 Mini-open transpedicular corpectomy.

Kirschner wires, and cannulated screw system under fluoroscopic guidance (▶ Fig. 30.2).

30.5.3 Step 3: MIS Ipsilateral Transpedicular Corpectomy

A midline fascial opening is performed over the corpectomy level and partial exposure of the lamina above and below is performed. At this point, an expandable tubular retractor or a standard cerebellar retractor can be placed (▶ Fig. 30.3).

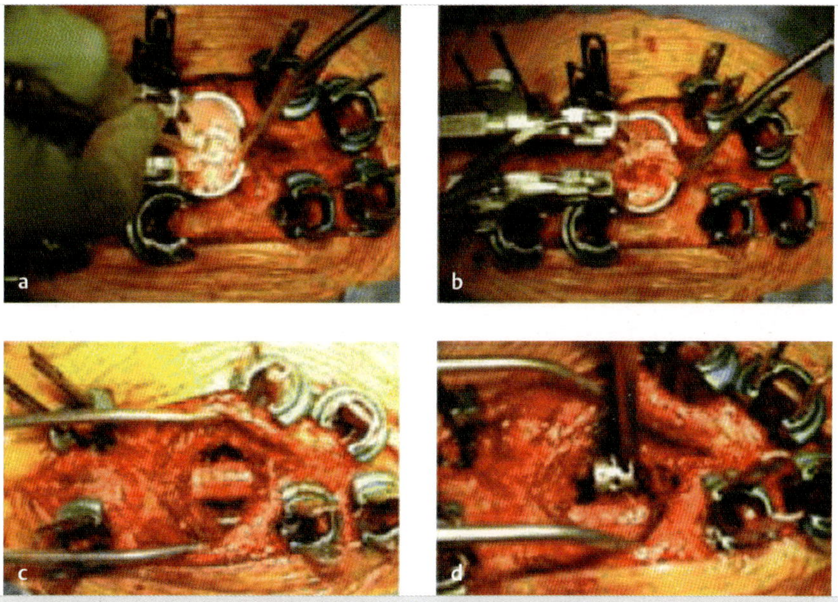

Fig. 30.3 **(a)** A laminectomy is performed and **(b)** the transverse processes are removed and a trap-door rib-head osteotomy is performed. **(c)** Optionally, the tubular retractor can be replaced with a cerebellar retractor without further opening the facia and **(d)** the cage is placed by pushing against the trap-door rib-head osteotomy.

A laminectomy is performed. The complete transverse processes, ligamentum flavum, inferior aspect of cephalad lamina, and superior aspect of the caudal lamina are removed. The rib heads are preserved. The nerve roots are ligated if this is at the thoracic spine level. Rongeurs are used to remove pedicles.

The discs at the level superior and inferior to the corpectomy level are identified with a Penfield No. 4 dissector. The transpedicular corpectomy is performed using high-speed burr, pituitary rongeurs, and 0.25-inch osteotomies. Once a unilateral corpectomy is performed, a temporary rod is placed on this side to prevent movement of the spine as the contralateral corpectomy is completed.

30.5.4 Step 4: Contralateral Transpedicular Corpectomy

The contralateral transpedicular corpectomy is completed. The intervertebral discs are removed and the end plates on the superior and inferior levels are prepared. The posterior longitudinal ligament (PLL) is separated from dura with a Woodson dissector to relieve any tension on the dura. The PLL is typically removed by cutting with a No. 15 blade superior and inferior to the corpectomy level and can be removed in one piece.

30.5.5 Step 5: Rib Head Removal

The rib head is in the way of cage insertion. It is dissected with electrocautery 3 cm lateral to the costovertebral junction and a rib-head osteotomy performed. To perform this rib-head osteotomy, a matchstick type burr is used to drill 3 cm lateral to the costovertebral junction to mobilize the rib head, which allows it to be pushed laterally. Pleural dissection is avoided.[6,7]

30.5.6 Step 6: Cage Insertion

The cage is selected and gently placed into the site of corpectomy by pushing it laterally and deep over the rib head. Once it is anterior to the plane of the spinal cord, the cage is moved medially to its final position over the ventral aspect of the spinal cord. The cage is then expanded and wedged appropriately. Fluoroscopic confirmation with anteroposterior (AP) and lateral images are performed (▶ Fig. 30.4).

Bone graft material is placed around the cage. The second rod is inserted and two crosslinks placed.

30.5.7 Step 7: Closure

Surgical drains are left in the epidural space. The fascia is closed. Figure-of-8 sutures are used to close the fascial openings. Subdermal and skin are closed.

30.6 Postoperative Care

Postoperatively, the patient is admitted to a medical-surgical ward for pain control and neurological checks. Typically, patient-controlled anesthesia (PCA) using intravenous (IV) hydromorphone or morphine is used in combination with opioid and nonopioid oral pain medications such as acetaminophen, hydrocodone-acetaminophen, or oxycodone. Nonsteroidal anti-inflammatory drugs (NSAIDs) are avoided as they can hinder bony fusion. The patient's diet is provided as per toleration and the urinary catheter is typically removed on postoperative day 1. Postoperative AP/lateral X-rays are used to confirm correct placement of implants and to exclude any unintentionally retained foreign body. Standing scoliosis X-rays are obtained prior to discharge. The patient should undergo

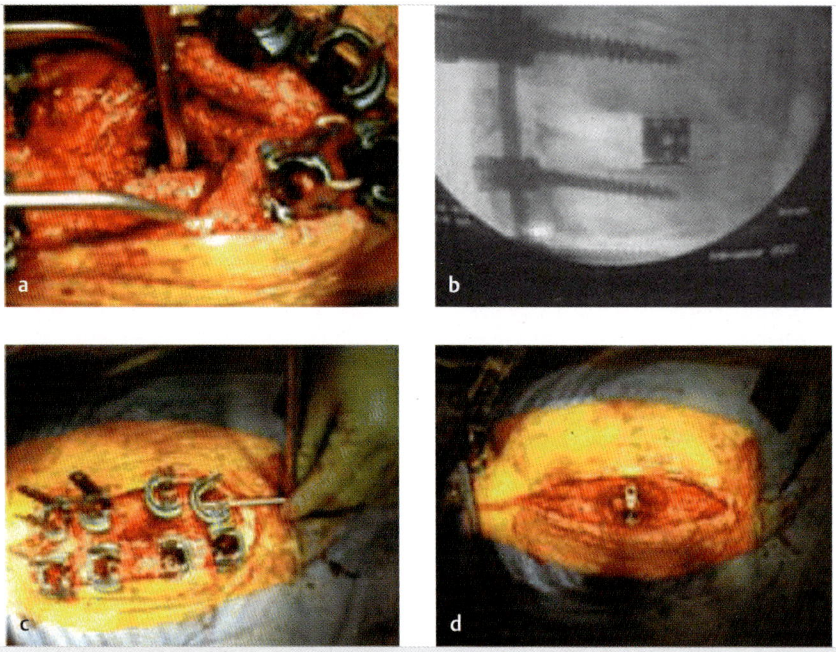

Fig. 30.4 (a) The cage is inserted past the spinal cord and (b) fluoroscopy should be performed to confirm placement of the cage. (c) The rods are inserted and set-screws are placed. (d) A crosslink is placed.

physical therapy and occupational therapy as soon as tolerated on postoperative day 1. The epidural drains can be removed when they drop below an output of 100 mL/hour starting on postoperative day 2. The patient is discharged when he/she tolerates a regular diet, bowel movements are regular, pain is controlled, and the drains have been removed.

30.7 Complications and Avoidance

Although the transpedicular corpectomy approach allows for thorough decompression and stabilization of a diseased segment, the surgical technique is not without complications. Although reports of complication rates in cases performed for osteomyelitis or an epidural abscess are limited, there are several prospective and retrospective studies in the spinal metastasis literature reporting morbidity and mortality.

For cases addressing a malignant lesion, wound infection or dehiscence is one of the most common complications seen. Although it is not unexpected to have this complication after surgery, the increased frequency may be secondary to recent chemotherapy or spinal radiotherapy which impairs wound healing. Postoperative 30-day mortality is also not negligible. Although the cause of death in some cases may be secondary to rapid systemic tumor progression, several cases involved sepsis with multiorgan failure. Street and colleagues reported a major complication rate of 26% (11 out of 42 patients) with 16.7% (7 cases) of wound infection or dehiscence. Of the 21% of cases that required reoperation, only 1 was due to hardware failure.[5] Wang and colleagues reported a 30-day major complication rate of 14.3% (20 out of 140 patients) with an 11.4% (16 cases) rate of wound infection or dehiscence; 30-day mortality was reported to be 4.3% (6 patients), and instrumentation failure was seen in 5% (7 patients) with a median failure time of 17 months.[8] Cho and Sung noted a 30-day mortality rate of 9.5% (2 patients), both due to rapid progression of primary disease. In this series, wound infection or dehiscence was seen in 9.5% (2 patients) with both reported to have had preoperative spine radiotherapy.[9] When compared to other approaches for the thoracolumbar region, the transpedicular corpectomy approach demonstrates similar complication rates compared to an anterior-only corpectomy but significantly lower complication rates compared to combined anterior-posterior approaches.[10] Other complications reported in the literature include low rates of cerebrospinal fluid (CSF) leak, postoperative hematomas, colonic perforation, and hemothorax.[11,12,13] As with any procedure, medical complications such as urinary tract infections (UTIs), pneumonia, deep vein thrombosis (DVT), and postoperative ileus are also observed complications that are best addressed with preventative measures.

Various minimally invasive techniques have also been implemented for spinal canal tumor decompression with low complication rates. For example, transpedicular corpectomy and spinal canal decompression through a tubular expandable retractor have been reported without any major complications.[14,15,16] Lau and Chou compared the open versus mini-open approach for posterior thoracic transpedicular corpectomy. There was no significant difference in complication rates in the open group compared with the mini-open group (21.4% vs. 9.5%), and no postoperative deaths were reported. For open and mini-open approaches, the overall infection rates were 17.9 and 9.5% and reoperation rates were 9.5 and 7.1%, respectively.[17] Overall implant failure rates requiring reoperation when combining patients from both groups were reported to be 1.9, 9.1, and 14.7% at 6 months, 1 year, and 2 years, respectively.[18]

In terms of complication avoidance, there are several techniques that have been recommended. Intraoperative bleeding may be minimized by considering preoperative embolization,

especially in cases involving hemorrhagic tumors such as renal cell carcinoma or melanoma.

Preoperative imaging should also be analyzed to identify significant vessels including the artery of Adamkiewicz, which much be kept intact to avoid spinal cord ischemia. Intraoperative injury to structures anterior to the spinal column, including gastrointestinal and vascular structures, may be minimized by introduction of a ribbon retractor or similar instrumentation, which acts as a firm barrier between the site of surgery and critical anterior structures. As always, excessive traction on spinal dura and nerve roots should be avoided to avoid postoperative neurological injury. In terms of preventing wound infection, standard antibiotics during and for 24 hours after surgery should be implemented. Some authors advocate for irrigation with high volumes of saline containing antibiotics or betadine at the end of decompression and fusion as a means for lower postoperative infection rates.[5,19] If a difficult closure is anticipated, there should be a low threshold for plastic surgery assisted closure with the use of flap if needed. Timing of surgery may also be important. Prior reports cite recent spine radiation as a risk factor for wound breakdown.[9] Therefore, if possible, discussion of the timing of adjunct therapy after surgery should be had with the oncologists and patient to minimize this contributing factor to postoperative wound dehiscence.

References

[1] Akeyson EW, McCutcheon IE. Single-stage posterior vertebrectomy and replacement combined with posterior instrumentation for spinal metastasis. J Neurosurg. 1996; 85(2):211–220

[2] Bilsky MH, Boland P, Lis E, Raizer JJ, Healey JH. Single-stage posterolateral transpedicle approach for spondylectomy, epidural decompression, and circumferential fusion of spinal metastases. Spine. 2000; 25(17):2240–2249, discussion 250

[3] Chou D, Wang VY, Gupta N. Transpedicular corpectomy with posterior expandable cage placement for L1 burst fracture. J Clin Neurosci. 2009; 16 (8):1069–1072

[4] Hunt T, Shen FH, Arlet V. Expandable cage placement via a posterolateral approach in lumbar spine reconstructions. Technical note. J Neurosurg Spine. 2006; 5(3):271–274

[5] Street J, Fisher C, Sparkes J, et al. Single-stage posterolateral vertebrectomy for the management of metastatic disease of the thoracic and lumbar spine: a prospective study of an evolving surgical technique. J Spinal Disord Tech. 2007; 20(7):509–520

[6] Chou D, Eltgroth M, Yang I, Lu D, Manley G. Rib head disarticulation for multilevel transpedicular thoracic corpectomies and expandable cage reconstruction. Neurol India. 2009; 57(4):469–474

[7] Chou D, Wang VY. Trap-door rib-head osteotomies for posterior placement of expandable cages after transpedicular corpectomy: an alternative to lateral extracavitary and costotransversectomy approaches. J Neurosurg Spine. 2009; 10(1):40–45

[8] Wang JC, Boland P, Mitra N, et al. Single-stage posterolateral transpedicular approach for resection of epidural metastatic spine tumors involving the vertebral body with circumferential reconstruction: results in 140 patients. Invited submission from the Joint Section Meeting on Disorders of the Spine and Peripheral Nerves, March 2004. J Neurosurg Spine. 2004; 1(3):287–298

[9] Cho DC, Sung JK. Palliative surgery for metastatic thoracic and lumbar tumors using posterolateral transpedicular approach with posterior instrumentation. Surg Neurol. 2009; 71(4):424–433

[10] Lu DC, Lau D, Lee JG, Chou D. The transpedicular approach compared with the anterior approach: an analysis of 80 thoracolumbar corpectomies. J Neurosurg Spine. 2010; 12(6):583–591

[11] Weller SJ, Rossitch E , Jr. Unilateral posterolateral decompression without stabilization for neurological palliation of symptomatic spinal metastasis in debilitated patients. J Neurosurg. 1995; 82(5):739–744

[12] Chen YJ, Hsu HC, Chen KH, Li TC, Lee TS. Transpedicular partial corpectomy without anterior vertebral reconstruction in thoracic spinal metastases. Spine. 2007; 32(22):E623–E626

[13] Chang CC, Chen YJ, Lo DF, Chen HT, Hsu HC, Lin RM. Palliative transpedicular partial corpectomy without anterior vertebral reconstruction in lower thoracic and thoracolumbar junction spinal metastases. J Orthop Surg Res. 2015; 10:113

[14] Zairi F, Arikat A, Allaoui M, Marinho P, Assaker R. Minimally invasive decompression and stabilization for the management of thoracolumbar spine metastasis. J Neurosurg Spine. 2012; 17(1):19–23

[15] Deutsch H, Boco T, Lobel J. Minimally invasive transpedicular vertebrectomy for metastatic disease to the thoracic spine. J Spinal Disord Tech. 2008; 21 (2):101–105

[16] Donnelly DJ, Abd-El-Barr MM, Lu Y. Minimally invasive muscle sparing posterior-only approach for lumbar circumferential decompression and stabilization to treat spine metastasis—technical report. World Neurosurg. 2015; 84 (5):1484–1490

[17] Lau D, Chou D. Posterior thoracic corpectomy with cage reconstruction for metastatic spinal tumors: comparing the mini-open approach to the open approach. J Neurosurg Spine. 2015; 23(2):217–227

[18] Lau D, Chou D. Minimally invasive instrumentation without fusion during posterior thoracic corpectomies: a comparison of percutaneously instrumented nonfused segments with open instrumented fused segments. J Neurosurg Spine. 2017; 27(1):35–41

[19] Cheng MT, Chang MC, Wang ST, Yu WK, Liu CL, Chen TH. Efficacy of dilute betadine solution irrigation in the prevention of postoperative infection of spinal surgery. Spine. 2005; 30(15):1689–1693

31 Techniques to Decrease the Invasiveness of Thoracic Deformity Correction

Brenton Pennicooke, Robert Nicholas Hernandez, and Michael S. Virk

Summary
This chapter summarizes techniques and technologies that can be used to minimize the invasiveness of surgery for pathologies in the thoracic spine. Given the complexity of the surgical goals, this is clearly a frontier in MISS and we can expect significant innovation to occur in these areas.

Keywords: minimally invasive thoracic spine surgery, MIS thoracic deformity correction, thoracic spine surgery, thoracic spinal deformity

31.1 Introduction

Traditional open surgical approaches to the thoracic spine for the correction of thoracic deformity include posterior techniques (posterolateral, transpedicular, costotransversectomy, lateral extracavitary) and anterior techniques (thoracotomy). An approach that allows access to both the posterior elements to achieve decompression and to the anterior vertebral column for circumferential release is required for correction of major deformities. Access to the anterior column via a posterior-only approach is commonly performed, but can result in neurologic injury as it requires reaching around the spinal cord to access the anterior column. Traditionally, thoracic deformities are corrected with extensive exposures that allow full view of and access to the bony anatomy of the vertebral column. Bony surface area is also required for arthrodesis and the longevity of the construct. However, such wide exposures are associated with high morbidity and complication rates due to blood loss, operative time, and postoperative hospital stays. The International Spine Study Group recently published a retrospective review that identified a 78% overall complication rate and 61% major complication rate associated with three-column osteotomy in patients with adult spinal deformity.[1]

Minimally invasive spine surgery (MISS) is a rapidly advancing field that has shown some benefits over traditional open approaches for the treatment of spinal pathology, particularly in the lumbar spine.[2,3,4,5] This chapter aims to describe techniques spine surgeons can employ to decrease the level of invasiveness of thoracic deformity correction with an emphasis on minimally invasive surgery (MIS) techniques.

31.2 Computer-Assisted Navigation/Robotics/Planning Software

The advent of computer-assisted navigation (CAN) has and continues to advance the field of MISS. Because of the smaller incisions and ports employed by MISS procedures, surgeons cannot rely on traditional anatomical landmarks and orientation reference points, particularly in patients with deformity. CAN facilitates precise anatomical localization when landmarks remain obscured by overlying muscle and soft tissue. Surgeons can readily identify their position and desired targets. Modular reference arrays can be attached to essentially all intraoperative instruments and calibrated for use during the procedure. Such devices include drills, pedicle probes, taps, drivers, osteotomes, and interbody device/cage introducers. Pedicle screws and cages can be sized virtually and projected over the intraoperatively acquired imaging to optimize dimensions during the planning phase as well as placement location. CAN reduces the incidence of pedicle breaches, particularly in patients with small thoracic pedicles. Thus, CAN allows surgeons to safely access and instrument the spine, as well as decompress the neural elements, through smaller incisions and ports when the surrounding anatomy cannot be directly visualized. Multiple studies have demonstrated that the use of CAN results in a lower thoracic pedicle screw breach rate compared to fluoroscopy-guided pedicle screw placement. Two meta-analyses reported the thoracic pedicle screw breach rate with the use of CAN to be 5.4 to 8.7% and the breach rate with fluoroscopic guidance to be 15.1 to 22.9%.[6,7] Moreover, CAN facilitated faster screw insertion, lower complication rate, and less intraoperative blood loss, but a longer overall operative time compared to fluoroscopy.[6] With increased repetitions leading to greater experience and smoother workflow, overall operative time generally decreases. Ultimately, experienced users will have less misplaced screws to revise intraoperatively and patients will not leave the operating room until optimal screw placement is confirmed radiographically, thus decreasing revisions for screw misplacement.

Advancements in intraoperative computed tomography (CT) scans has increased the utility and accuracy of using CAN for the placement of pedicle screws and osteotomies using minimally invasive techniques. The intraoperative CT with CAN increases pedicle screw accuracy to 99% compared to 94.1% accuracy with free-hand techniques.[8,9] Additionally, intraoperative CT allows for the merger of previously acquired imaging studies, magnetic resonance imaging (MRI) or vascular imaging, for a more detailed and nuanced assessment of spinal anatomy. For example, the intraoperative CT can be merged with an MRI to localize specific areas of neural element compression, which require a direct decompression, or to identify vascular structures. The integration of CAN with robotic pedicle screw placement and associated planning software has allowed for further technological advancements in minimally invasive techniques. Planning software is used for preoperative planning of screw placement and osteotomies; such planning can be used in a predictive fashion to estimate correction based on the size and location of osteotomies. It can also facilitate more accurate rod placement by putting pedicle screw tulip heads in the optimal alignment. It may be possible to save considerable time intraoperatively by well-planned rod contouring and passing through the use of software, particularly for long constructs. Most recently, CAN is being integrated with augmented reality (AR),

which is a technology that superimposes a computer-generated image on a user's view of the real world. AR provides the surgeon with real-time evaluation of deep bony spine structure prior to any incision being made.[10,11] Though it has not been extensively utilized in the operating room, there is potential for AR to be used for intraoperative planning of MISS procedures in the future.

31.3 Minimally Invasive Approaches to Three-Column Osteotomies and Expandable Cages

Posterior vertebral osteotomies can provide a significant amount of deformity correction in the sagittal and coronal planes and are, therefore, a mainstay technique for deformity surgeons. However, using MIS techniques for osteotomies can be challenging and does not allow for the same degree of deformity correction as open osteotomies.[12] The advent of expandable cages has augmented the ability to achieve a correction through a small corridor to the anterior column. Corridors to the anterior column include direct anterior approach, anterolateral (retropleural) approach, posterolateral (lateral extracavitary or costotransversectomy) approach, and posterior (transpedicular) approach; and each utilizes either expandable retractors or thoracoscopic techniques to allow minimal violation of surrounding tissue en route to the targeted thoracic vertebra; however, each has specific advantages and disadvantages.[13]

31.3.1 Anterior (Transthoracic)

Earlier, direct anterior access to the thoracic spine for deformity correction required a large thoracotomy. This is an invasive procedure, requiring a chest tube to be placed, and is associated with a number of complications including hemothorax, pulmonary contusion, and pleural effusions.[14,15,16] Nevertheless, video-assisted thoracoscopy techniques have been developed, which minimize the size of the incision and tissue dissection needed to access this corridor. Though technically challenging with a steep learning curve,[17,18] some authors have suggested that thoracoscopic techniques have been equivalent to open thoracotomy for spinal cord decompression and instrumentation of the anterior vertebral column.[19,20]

31.3.2 Anterolateral (Retropleural)

Scheufler illustrated the use of expandable cages in a series of 38 patients who underwent a vertebrectomy for kyphoscoliosis correction[21] using an MIS anterolateral retropleural approach and a combined lateral extrapleural/extraperitoneal thoracolumbar approach to achieve 19.3 degrees of kyphotic correction, on average. These lateral approaches for a vertebrectomy with the placement of an expandable cage can utilize laterally projecting screws that engage the inferior end plate and superior end plates of the corresponding levels above and below the expandable cage, as illustrated in ▶ Fig. 31.1. Lateral trajectory screws do not provide equivalent reduction in range of motion as the traditional pedicle screws but prevent the expandable

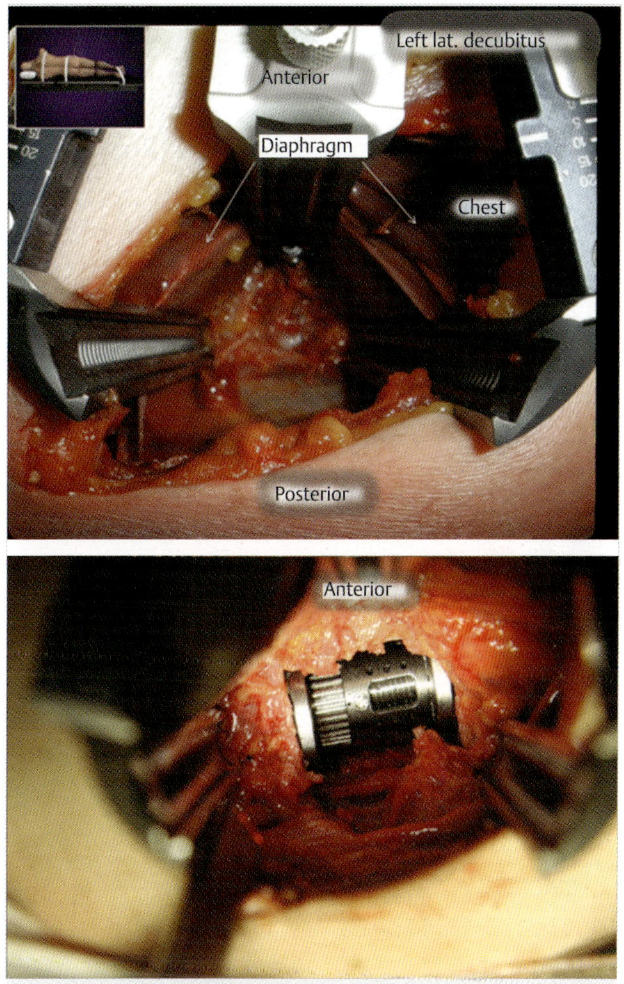

Fig. 31.1 Cadaveric photograph of a lateral approach to the lower thoracic spine (*top*) and placement of a corpectomy cage (*bottom*) for a patient in a left lateral decubitus position. (Reprinted with permission from Operative Neurosurgery, Oxford University Press.)

cage from translating laterally through the approach corridor.[22] Thus, expandable cages frequently require posterior percutaneous screw placement to augment fixation until fusion is obtained. This involves repositioning the patient from the lateral position to a supine position. Uribe et al further describes an MIS anterolateral retropleural approach in a study employing a cadaveric model and four patients.[23] These minimally invasive approaches that aim to keep the pleura intact preclude chest tube placement postoperatively. However, a high rate of pleural violation has been reported, which remains a significant limitation of this minimally invasive approach.[24]

31.3.3 Posterolateral (Lateral Extracavitary)

The use of an expandable cage for thoracic deformity correction requires a corpectomy or complete vertebrectomy. MIS techniques allow for direct lines of approach to the intended vertebra and, in certain approaches, permit a more favorable angle to the targeted vertebra than equivalent approaches during an open procedure. In a cadaveric study, it was shown that minimally

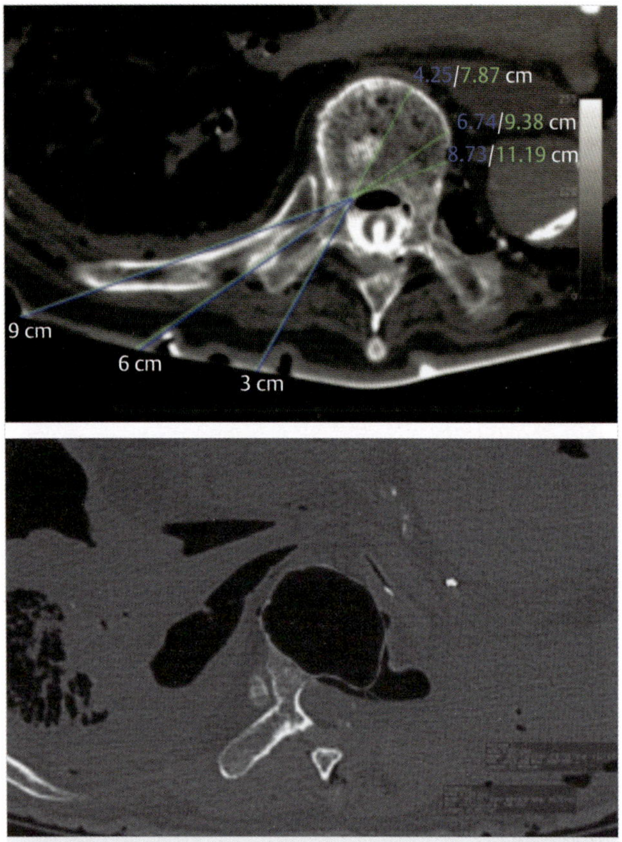

Fig. 31.2 Computed tomography (CT) with navigation showing the trajectories for a posterolateral minimally invasive corpectomy using a starting point 3, 6, and 9 cm off midline (*top*). In particular, a trajectory starting 9 cm off midline allows for a complete resection of the vertebral body to the contralateral pedicle (*bottom*). (Reprinted with permission from Clinical Spine Surgery, Wolters Kluwer Health, Inc.)

invasive corpectomy can be performed posterolaterally using a starting point 3, 6, and 9 off midline, as illustrated in ▶ Fig. 31.2.[25] Kim et al described this posterolateral approach using a minimally invasive technique in four clinical cases, reporting that they could safely remove 93% of the bone over the ventral canal and 80% of the corresponding vertebral body for implantation of an expandable cage.[26] A similar approach was utilized by Musacchio et al, who also utilized a second port for a contralateral transpedicular approach to allow for a circumferential decompression.[27]

31.3.4 Posterior (Transpedicular)

Chou et al described an MIS transpedicular vertebrectomy for the correction of focal thoracic kyphotic deformity utilizing an expandable cage during supine positioning, which eliminates the need to reposition the patient and adds the benefit of pedicle screw instrumentation. In a series of two patients with severe kyphotic deformity, Chou et al achieved 27- and 17-degree corrections of thoracic kyphosis via this technique.[28] In the technical note that precedes this publication, Chou et al described using a midline incision without taking down the fascial layer at vertebral levels, cranial and caudal to the level of the planned mini-open transpedicular corpectomy.[29] Percutaneous pedicle screws are placed at levels above and below the corpectomy levels; an expandable tubular retractor or cerebellar is placed after exposing the bony anatomy of the corpectomy level; the lamina and transverse processes are resected, leaving the rib heads intact, followed by transpedicular corpectomy, discectomy, and preparation of the end plates. As illustrated in ▶ Fig. 31.3, one rib head is then mobilized in a trap-door fashion, and an expandable cage is inserted.[29] The authors utilized this technique for long- and short-segment fusions and later compared this mini-open technique to a traditional open approach for patients with metastatic spine tumors as opposed to kyphoscoliosis correction.[30] They found that when compared to the open group, the mini-open group had significantly less blood loss and shorter hospital stay.[30] The mini-open group had fewer complications and lower infection rate, though neither reached statistical significance, while there were no differences in operative time, American Spinal Injury Association (ASIA) grade at follow-up, or need for surgical revision.[30] The amount of corrections attainable through this mini-open technique is described by Wang et al. The authors illustrate mini-open pedicle subtraction osteotomies (PSO) in seven patients, which resulted in significant deformity correction.[31,32] This case series reports lumbar Cobb angle improved from a mean of 41.2 ± 18.4 degrees to 15.4 ± 9.6 degrees, and lumbar lordosis improved from 23.1 ± 15.9 degrees to 48.6 ± 11.7 degrees.[31] Similar MIS techniques have been described for thoracic deformity corrections.[33]

31.4 Percutaneous/Transfascial Instrumentation

Percutaneous pedicle screw placement for instrumentation is a well-established technique used to minimize collateral tissue trauma. Though these techniques are easily employed for short-segment constructs, percutaneous pedicle screw placement and rod insertion can become challenging with the longer constructs required for thoracic deformity correction. One technique to overcome this challenge utilizes three incisions along the length of the instrumentation; one incision at the upper-most instrument vertebra (UIV), one at the lowest instrumented vertebra (LIV), and one at the apex of the deformity. As seen in ▶ Fig. 31.4, the use of these three segmented incisions allows for the passage of the rod through the screw heads from rostral to caudal and sequential reduction and contouring of the rod to seat within the tulips of the screws. Passing rods through the subfascial compartment becomes more difficult as the number of levels instrumented increases. Thus, placing a pre-bent/pre-contoured rod from a cranial to caudal direction helps to facilitate proper positioning of the rod in each screw head. CAN with intraoperative imaging and robotics may further help to propel intraoperative rod contouring, although this remains to be demonstrated.

31.5 Facet Joint Fusion and Arthrodesis

To perform posterior column osteotomies, facetectomies, and decortication of the facets and pars, Sarwahi et al described accessing the facets and pars using intermuscular access

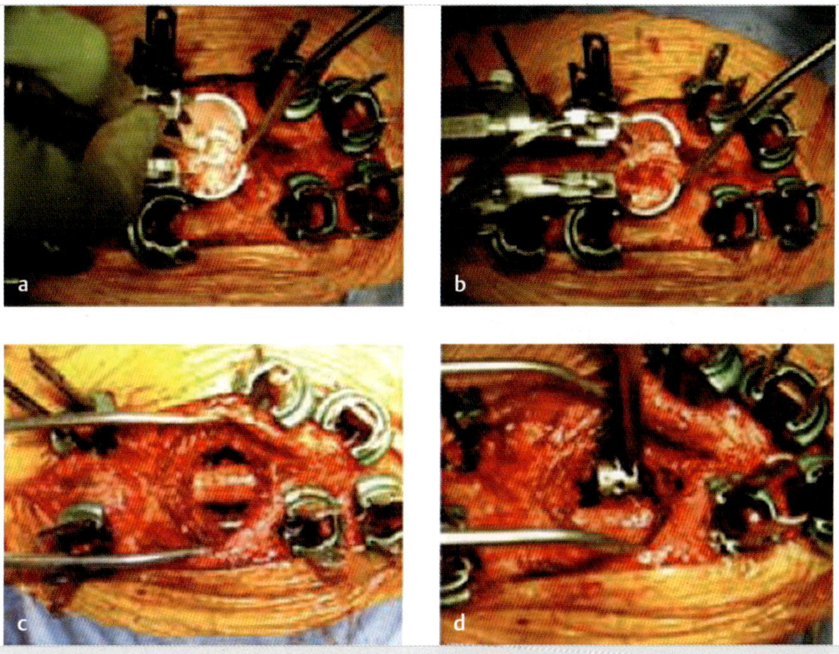

Fig. 31.3 Intraoperative photographs of the mini-open technique for transpedicular thoracic corpectomy. Using an expandable tubular retractor, a laminectomy **(a)** and trap-door rib-head osteotomy **(b)** are performed. Once completed, a circumferential view of the spinal cord is seen **(c)**. A cage can then be inserted by pushing against the trap-door rib-head osteotomy to avoid retraction on the spinal cord and pleural injury **(d)**. (Reprinted with permission from the Journal of Neurosurgery – Spine.)

corridor created by the placement of the transfascial pedicle screws.[34] A variant of this technique for osteotomies and facet joint fusion is illustrated in the chapter on minimally invasive thoracolumbar facet joint fusion. This technique entails facet decortication and insertion of bone graft by passing tubular dilators over K-wires cannulating the pedicles. After performing the facet joint decortication, the pedicle screws can then be placed using the K-wires after removal of the tubular dilators. For arthrodesis of the corresponding level with MIS techniques, the facet joint need to be decorticated and packed with bone graft. However, if the facet joints are not prepared for arthrodesis, an interbody graft must be placed to facilitate proper bony fusion of the instrumented levels.

31.6 Optical Adjuncts and Visualization

Proper visualization of the bony anatomy through a very small corridor is mandatory for all MIS techniques. There are a variety of visualization techniques which have been developed including the microscope, endoscopes, and video-assisted thoracoscopy.

31.6.1 Video-Assisted Thoracoscopic Surgery (VATS)

As stated above, access to the anterior column of the thoracic spine can facilitate realignment and correction of a thoracic deformity. Although a direct anterior approach via thoracotomy is effective, it is invasive with a considerable risk profile. Video-assisted thoracoscopy is a method to decrease the invasiveness associated with a direct anterior approach and allows the surgeon to perform anterior osteotomies, discectomies, and instrumentation through thoracoscopic ports. This approach is discussed in Chapter 21. A series published by Han et al describes using a thoracoscopic approach to perform 241 cases, which included 164 thoracic sympathectomies, 60 discectomies, 5 neurogenic tumor resections, 8 corpectomies, and spinal reconstructions, 2 anterior releases, and 2 biopsies.[35] Though the vast majority of the cases discussed in this series were sympathectomy, the series describes 10 deformity corrections using this approach and effectively illustrates how thoracoscopic technique provides full, direct access to the ventral thoracic spine.[35] The series also highlights the lower morbidity rate associated with a thoracoscopic approach compared to an open thoracotomy. Lastly, a thoracoscopic approach has an improved cosmetic result and a shorter hospital length of stay. The learning curve associated with thoracoscopic deformity correction is a potential disadvantage of the procedure. Few surgeons use a thoracoscopic approach for thoracic deformity correction, as the approach has a significant learning curve,[36] and currently, there is no comparative study showing a significant benefit over a posterolateral approach to a vertebrectomy.[37]

31.6.2 Endoscope

A transforaminal endoscopic approach in the thoracic spine has been described to treat soft thoracic disc herniations.[38] Although it has not been extensively described as an approach to correct thoracic spinal deformity, there are now several studies illustrating interbody graft placement in the lumbar spine.[39,40,41,42] Application of the technique is likely to follow in the thoracic spine.

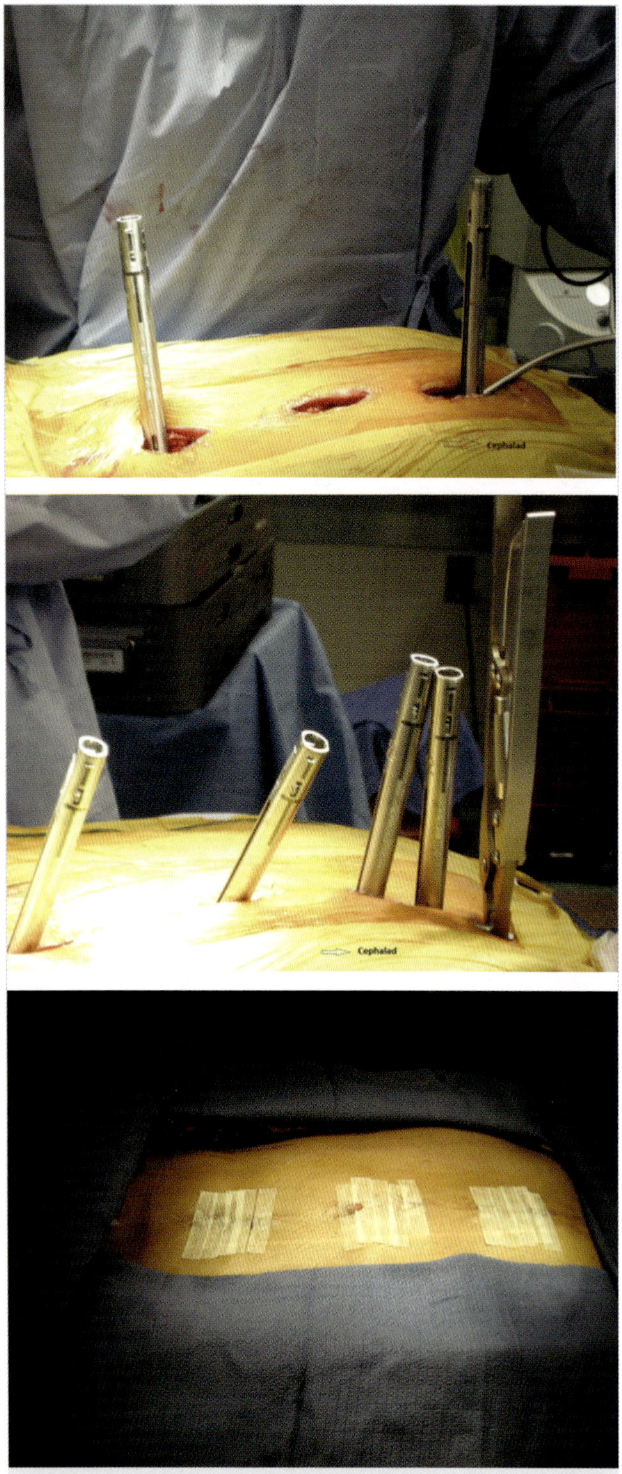

Fig. 31.4 Intraoperative photographs illustrating the minimally invasive technique to pass a rod into percutaneously placed screws. The reduction screw extenders (*top*) allow the surgeon to pass a rod into multiple screw heads using a steerable rod inserter (*center*). This minimally invasive method allows for percutaneous instrumentation of the spine through small paramedian incisions (*bottom*). (Used with permission from Sarwahi, V, Wollowick, AL, Sugarman, EP, et al. Minimally invasive scoliosis surgery: an innovative technique in patients with adolescent idiopathic scoliosis. Scoliosis 6, 16 [2011].)

31.6.3 Microscope

The use of the microscope is central to visualizing bony anatomy through long, narrow corridors characteristic of minimally invasive retractors. For example, in the thoracic spine, the corridor for a thoracic corpectomy through an anterolateral/retropleural approach typically measures 90 to 140 cm in length and with a diameter equal to the height of the vertebral body to be resected. A microscope allows for excellent visualization and illumination of the operative site.

31.7 Limitations

Although MISS has been shown to have many benefits over open approaches, it is important to be aware of the limitations of MISS. Reduced bony surface exposure limits the surface area available for arthrodesis. Fusion can be obtained across the anterior column, the facet joints, or posterolaterally, but needs careful consideration during the planning phase of the procedure. Additionally, there are limitations to the deformity correction that can be achieved using MIS techniques. Than et al published a study comparing the clinical and radiographic parameters of patients who had the greatest and least improvement in pre- and postoperative Oswestry Disability Index (ODI) scores (top 20% and bottom 20%, respectively).[43] The authors found that the top 20% group had a mean sagittal vertical axis (SVA) of 3.4 cm (vs. 6.9 cm in the bottom 20% group), a mean pelvic incidence-lumbar lordosis (PI-LL) mismatch of 10.4 degrees (vs. 19.4 degrees in the bottom 20% group), and resultant better visual analog scale (VAS) back and leg pain scores than the bottom 20% group.[43] This data corroborates the important association between sagittal correction and clinical outcome. Thus, if the global spinal parameter goals cannot be achieved using MIS techniques, the patient may benefit more from an open approach. As seen in ▶ Fig. 31.5, Mummaneni et al published a decision framework to guide on the most likely favorable outcome for the patient when using MIS techniques for deformity correction.[44] Though these papers primarily discuss patients requiring thoracolumbar and lumbar surgery, not strictly thoracic surgery, they highlight the importance of evaluating the amount of correction needed to obtain an optimal clinical outcome.

An additional limitation of MIS techniques is the learning curve associated with mastery. This well-established learning curve may dissuade surgeons from adopting MIS techniques into their armamentarium as they may be much more comfortable and facile with open techniques. Thus, it is recommended to utilize a gradual progression of complexity while integrating MIS techniques into one's surgical practice.

31.8 Conclusion

Though traditionally open surgical approaches are utilized for correction of thoracic deformity, MIS techniques are playing an increasingly important role. The ultimate goal is to achieve the same outcomes as open surgery, while reducing incision size, minimizing collateral tissue damage, decreasing blood loss/

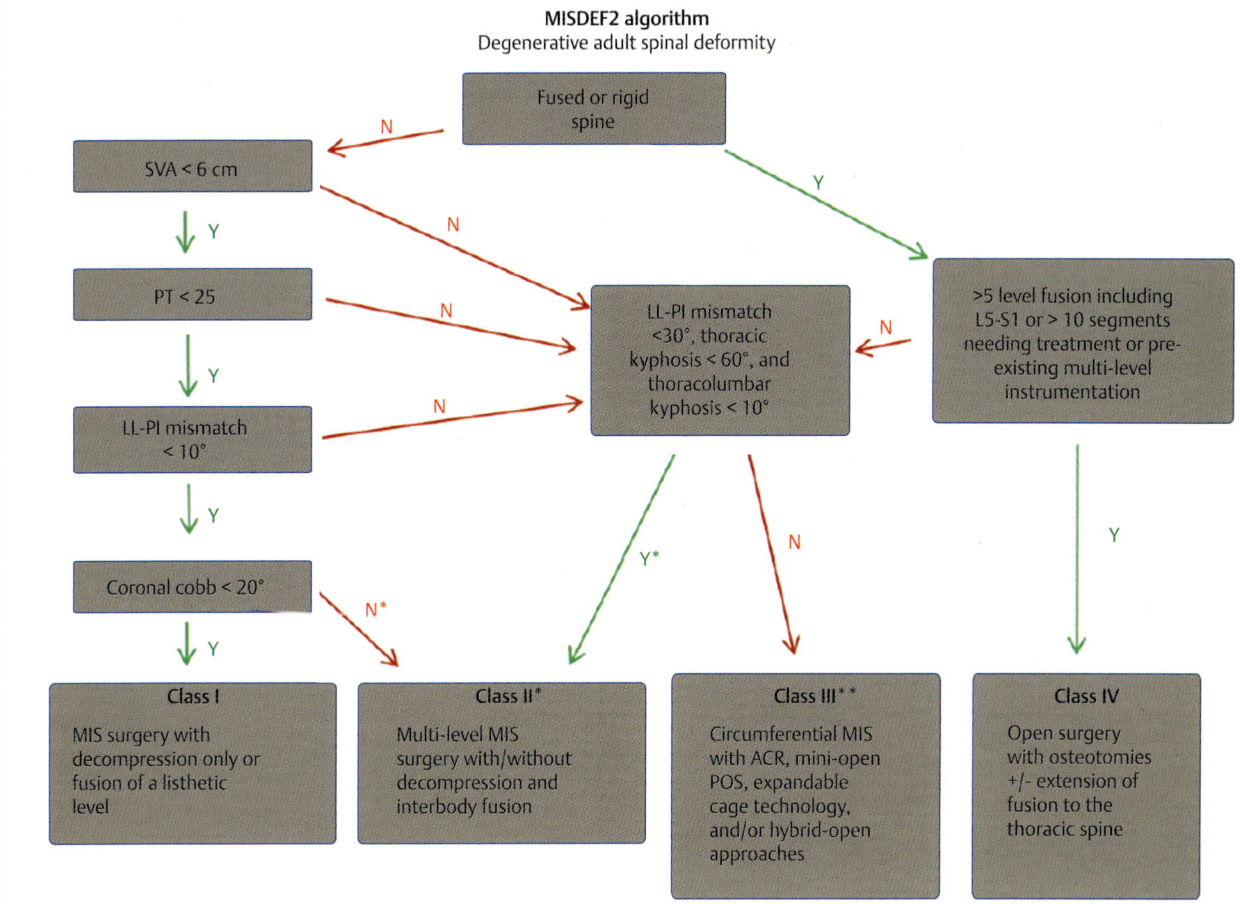

Fig. 31.5 Minimally invasive spinal deformity algorithm is a guide to assist with decision-making on which adult spinal deformity patients are candidates for minimally invasive surgical approaches. (Reprinted with permission from Neurosurgery Clinics of North America, Elsevier.)

transfusions, lowering infection rates, and promoting shorter hospital stays and earlier mobilization. However, MIS techniques are limited in the amount of correction that is achievable, particularly in the thoracic spine. Surgeons must select patients carefully and have a clear understanding of their own capabilities. There is a substantial learning curve associated with learning these techniques; thus, operative time for a given thoracic correction procedure will likely increase until the surgeon becomes more accustomed with the techniques. Nevertheless, MIS techniques for thoracic deformity correction represent a growing number of procedures that spine surgeons have in their armamentarium and will continue to proliferate as more surgeons adopt such techniques and continue to drive their evolution.

References

[1] Smith JS, Shaffrey CI, Klineberg E, et al. on behalf of the International Spine Study Group. Complication rates associated with 3-column osteotomy in 82 adult spinal deformity patients: retrospective review of a prospectively collected multicenter consecutive series with 2-year follow-up. J Neurosurg Spine. 2017; 27(4):444–457

[2] Phan K, Mobbs RJ. Minimally invasive versus open laminectomy for lumbar stenosis: a systematic review and meta-analysis. Spine. 2016; 41(2):E91–E100

[3] Phan K, Rao PJ, Kam AC, Mobbs RJ. Minimally invasive versus open transforaminal lumbar interbody fusion for treatment of degenerative lumbar disease: systematic review and meta-analysis. Eur Spine J. 2015; 24(5):1017–1030

[4] Khan NR, Clark AJ, Lee SL, Venable GT, Rossi NB, Foley KT. Surgical outcomes for minimally invasive vs open transforaminal lumbar interbody fusion: an updated systematic review and meta-analysis. Neurosurgery. 2015; 77(6):847–874, discussion 874

[5] Goldstein CL, Macwan K, Sundararajan K, Rampersaud YR. Perioperative outcomes and adverse events of minimally invasive versus open posterior lumbar fusion: meta-analysis and systematic review. J Neurosurg Spine. 2016; 24(3):416–427

[6] Meng XT, Guan XF, Zhang HL, He SS. Computer navigation versus fluoroscopy-guided navigation for thoracic pedicle screw placement: a meta-analysis. Neurosurg Rev. 2016; 39(3):385–391

[7] Shin BJ, James AR, Njoku IU, Härtl R. Pedicle screw navigation: a systematic review and meta-analysis of perforation risk for computer-navigated versus freehand insertion. J Neurosurg Spine. 2012; 17(2):113–122

[8] Silbermann J, Riese F, Allam Y, Reichert T, Koeppert H, Gutberlet M. Computer tomography assessment of pedicle screw placement in lumbar and sacral spine: comparison between free-hand and O-arm based navigation techniques. Eur Spine J. 2011; 20(6):875–881

[9] O'Brien MF, Peterson D, Casey AT, Crockard HA. A novel technique for laminoplasty augmentation of spinal canal area using titanium miniplate stabilization: a computerized morphometric analysis. Spine. 1996; 21(4):474–483, discussion 484

[10] Elmi-Terander A, Burström G, Nachabe R, et al. Pedicle screw placement using augmented reality surgical navigation with intraoperative 3D imaging: a first in-human prospective cohort study. Spine. 2019; 44(7):517–525
[11] Elmi-Terander A, Nachabe R, Skulason H, et al. Feasibility and accuracy of thoracolumbar minimally invasive pedicle screw placement with augmented reality navigation technology. Spine. 2018; 43(14):1018–1023
[12] Voyadzis J-M, Gala VC, O'Toole JE, Eichholz KM, Fessler RG. Minimally invasive posterior osteotomies. Neurosurgery. 2008; 63(3) Suppl:A:204–A-210
[13] Lall RR, Smith ZA, Wong AP, Miller D, Fessler RG. Minimally invasive thoracic corpectomy: surgical strategies for malignancy, trauma, and complex spinal pathologies. Minim Invasive Surg. 2012; 2012:213791
[14] Bohlman HH, Zdeblick TA. Anterior excision of herniated thoracic discs. J Bone Joint Surg Am. 1988; 70(7):1038–1047
[15] Sekhar LN, Jannetta PJ. Thoracic disc herniation: operative approaches and results. Neurosurgery. 1983; 12(3):303–305
[16] Sundaresan N, Shah J, Foley KM, Rosen G. An anterior surgical approach to the upper thoracic vertebrae. J Neurosurg. 1984; 61(4):686–690
[17] Dickman CA, Rosenthal D, Karahalios DG, et al. Thoracic vertebrectomy and reconstruction using a microsurgical thoracoscopic approach. Neurosurgery. 1996; 38(2):279–293
[18] Mack MJ, Regan JJ, Bobechko WP, Acuff TE. Application of thoracoscopy for diseases of the spine. Ann Thorac Surg. 1993; 56(3):736–738
[19] Rosenthal D, Marquardt G, Lorenz R, Nichtweiss M. Anterior decompression and stabilization using a microsurgical endoscopic technique for metastatic tumors of the thoracic spine. J Neurosurg. 1996; 84(4):565–572
[20] Visocchi M, Masferrer R, Sonntag VK, Dickman CA. Thoracoscopic approaches to the thoracic spine. Acta Neurochir (Wien). 1998; 140(8):737–743, discussion 743–744
[21] Scheufler KM. Technique and clinical results of minimally invasive reconstruction and stabilization of the thoracic and thoracolumbar spine with expandable cages and ventrolateral plate fixation. Neurosurgery. 2007; 61 (4):798–808, discussion 808–809
[22] Nayak AN, Gutierrez S, Billys JB, Santoni BG, Castellvi AE. Biomechanics of lateral plate and pedicle screw constructs in lumbar spines instrumented at two levels with laterally placed interbody cages. Spine J. 2013; 13(10):1331–1338
[23] Uribe JS, Dakwar E, Cardona RF, Vale FL. Minimally invasive lateral retropleural thoracolumbar approach: cadaveric feasibility study and report of 4 clinical cases. Neurosurgery. 2011; 68(1) Suppl Operative:32–39, discussion 39
[24] Kasliwal MK, Deutsch H. Minimally invasive retropleural approach for central thoracic disc herniation. Minim Invasive Neurosurg. 2011; 54(4):167–171
[25] Ogden AT, Eichholz K, O'toole J, et al. Cadaveric evaluation of minimally invasive posterolateral thoracic corpectomy: a comparison of 3 approaches. J Spinal Disord Tech. 2009; 22(7):524–529
[26] Kim DH, O'Toole JE, Ogden AT, et al. Minimally invasive posterolateral thoracic corpectomy: cadaveric feasibility study and report of four clinical cases. Neurosurgery. 2009; 64(4):746–752, discussion 752–753
[27] Musacchio M, Patel N, Bagan B, Deutsch H, Vaccaro AR, Ratliff J. Minimally invasive thoracolumbar costotransversectomy and corpectomy via a dual-tube technique: evaluation in a cadaver model. Surg Technol Int. 2007; 16:221–225
[28] Chou D, Lau D, Roy E. Feasibility of the mini-open vertebral column resection for severe thoracic kyphosis. J Clin Neurosci. 2014; 21(5):841–845
[29] Chou D, Lu DC. Mini-open transpedicular corpectomies with expandable cage reconstruction. Technical note. J Neurosurg Spine. 2011; 14(1):71–77
[30] Lau D, Chou D. Posterior thoracic corpectomy with cage reconstruction for metastatic spinal tumors: comparing the mini-open approach to the open approach. J Neurosurg Spine. 2015; 23(2):217–227
[31] Wang MY, Bordon G. Mini-open pedicle subtraction osteotomy as a treatment for severe adult spinal deformities: case series with initial clinical and radiographic outcomes. J Neurosurg Spine. 2016; 24(5):769–776
[32] Wang MY. Miniopen pedicle subtraction osteotomy: surgical technique and initial results. Neurosurg Clin N Am. 2014; 25(2):347–351
[33] Smith JS, Ogden AT, Fessler RG. Minimally invasive posterior thoracic fusion. Neurosurg Focus. 2008; 25(2):E9
[34] Sarwahi V, Wollowick AL, Sugarman EP, Horn JJ, Gambassi M, Amaral TD. Minimally invasive scoliosis surgery: an innovative technique in patients with adolescent idiopathic scoliosis. Scoliosis. 2011; 6:16
[35] Han PP, Kenny K, Dickman CA. Thoracoscopic approaches to the thoracic spine: experience with 241 surgical procedures. Neurosurgery. 2002; 51(5) Suppl:S88–S95
[36] Lonner BS, Scharf C, Antonacci D, Goldstein Y, Panagopoulos G. The learning curve associated with thoracoscopic spinal instrumentation. Spine. 2005; 30 (24):2835–2840
[37] Bess S, Boachie-Adjei O, Burton D, et al. International Spine Study Group. Pain and disability determine treatment modality for older patients with adult scoliosis, while deformity guides treatment for younger patients. Spine. 2009; 34(20):2186–2190
[38] Choi KY, Eun SS, Lee SH, Lee HY. Percutaneous endoscopic thoracic discectomy; transforaminal approach. Minim Invasive Neurosurg. 2010; 53(1):25–28
[39] Heo DH, Son SK, Eum JH, Park CK. Fully endoscopic lumbar interbody fusion using a percutaneous unilateral biportal endoscopic technique: technical note and preliminary clinical results. Neurosurg Focus. 2017; 43(2):E8
[40] Kolcun JPG, Brusko GD, Basil GW, Epstein R, Wang MY. Endoscopic transforaminal lumbar interbody fusion without general anesthesia: operative and clinical outcomes in 100 consecutive patients with a minimum 1-year follow-up. Neurosurg Focus. 2019; 46(4):E14
[41] Jacquot F, Gastambide D. Percutaneous endoscopic transforaminal lumbar interbody fusion: is it worth it? Int Orthop. 2013; 37(8):1507–1510
[42] Zhou Y, Zhang C, Wang J, et al. Endoscopic transforaminal lumbar decompression, interbody fusion and pedicle screw fixation-a report of 42 cases. Chin J Traumatol. 2008; 11(4):225–231
[43] Than KD, Park P, Fu KM, et al. International Spine Study Group. Clinical and radiographic parameters associated with best versus worst clinical outcomes in minimally invasive spinal deformity surgery. J Neurosurg Spine. 2016; 25 (1):21–25
[44] Mummaneni PV, Park P, Shaffrey CI, et al. International Spine Study Group (ISSG). The MISDEF2 algorithm: an updated algorithm for patient selection in minimally invasive deformity surgery. J Neurosurg Spine. 2019; 32(2):221–228

32 Unilateral Lumbar Approach for Over-the-Top Bilateral Decompression

Franziska C. Heider, Andreas Korge, and H. Michael Mayer

Summary

The main goal is a bilateral microsurgical decompression of the cauda equina using a unilateral over-the-top approach. The challenge is to achieve decompression with minimal iatrogenic trauma to anatomical structures in the approach region and in the target area.

Keywords: spinal canal disorders, narrowing of the spinal canal, surgical decompression, microsurgery, minimally invasive surgery, over-the-top bilateral decompression, crossover technique

32.1 Introduction

In the history of surgery, reducing iatrogenic tissue trauma has always been regarded as one of the basic principles. In the last two decades, minimally invasive surgery (MIS) techniques for spine surgery have been developed and increasingly used for degenerative conditions, as the usage of new surgical devices and techniques has envolved.[1,2] However, MIS in spine surgery must achieve the same or better results than conventional treatment but with less morbidity.

After the adoption of microscope-assisted techniques in neurosurgery in 1977/1978, more and more procedures for lumbar spinal decompression using bilateral approaches with mono- to multisegmental laminotomy were used on an increasingly widespread scale.[3,4] In 1997, Spetzger et al[2,5] modified the microscope-assisted technique and first described the unilateral approach to only one side (laminotomy) for bilateral decompression of the lumbar spine in a study detailing clinical experiences, as well as providing anatomical considerations.[2,5] One year later, Young et al[6] and McCulloch[7] followed with studies that showed bilateral decompression of the lumbar spinal canal is practical via a unilateral laminotomy performing an ipsilateral and contralateral "over-the-top" bilateral decompression of both the spinal canal and nerve root canals.[2,6,7]

The minimally invasive unilateral lumbar approach for "over-the-top" bilateral decompression allows excellent decompression of bilateral lumbar spinal canal stenosis with clearance of the contralateral recess and neuroforamen.[2,4,8] This is also refered to as unilateral laminotomy for bilateral decompression (ULBD). The main advantages of this technique are the diminished "access trauma" to the paravertebral muscles and to the facet joints. In particular, the inferior facet contralateral to the approach side as well as its outer capsular surroundings can be preserved completely.[9] Especially in cases of central spinal or foraminal stenosis associated with degenerative lumbar scoliosis, decompression can be performed from the convex side, thus preserving the stability of the heavily loaded facet joint on the concave side.[9,10] The surgical goal of this minimally invasive, unilateral approach and technique is to decrease the amount of access damage as well as the trauma to the tissue on the way to the spinal canal (skin, muscles, facet joints, and lamina). In cases of bi- or multisegmental spinal canal narrowing/stenosis, the authors recommend to perform the so-called "Slalom" technique.[9] This is an enlargement as well as improvement of the described MIS technique for selective multisegmental decompression through multiple microsurgical approaches with alternating approach sides. The spinal canal is reached through approaches with alternating the sides (e.g., left–right–left) to balance the tissue trauma on the way to the spine.[9,11]

32.2 Indications

The unilateral lumbar approach is the authors' preferred approach for the treatment of a variety of degenerative spinal disorders including lumbar spinal stenosis, foraminal narrowing, and facet joint cysts. This technique is performed in patients presenting primarily with neurogenic claudication, leg or buttock symptoms, heaviness in the legs with or without radicular symptoms, with or without neurological deficits, and comparable magnetic resonance imaging (MRI) findings.[2,4,9]

As regards patient selection, in general there are no limitations regarding age, number of affected segments, or extent of narrowing.

Overall, the range of indications for the technique described here can be defined as follows:

a) Lumbar central stenosis.
b) Lumbar lateral recess spinal stenosis.
c) Lumbar foraminal stenosis.
d) Epidural lipomatosis.
e) Thecal sac compression due to facet joint cysts.

32.3 Contraindications

The unilateral lumbar approach is contraindicated in the following situations:

a) Major contraindications for general anesthesia and surgery.
b) Grade II spondylolisthesis and worse.
c) Significant lateral and/or vertical instability, and scoliosis.
d) Significant translational instability with dynamic canal narrowing.
e) Dominant/significant mechanical back pain.

> The unilateral "over-the-top" approach for bilateral decompression is a key technique in spinal microsurgery for spinal stenosis. This decompression technique minimizes the potential instability associated with similar open procedures. For multisegmental lumbar decompression, the authors recommend the crossover "Slalom technique" with multiple skin incisions to minimize postoperative instability. As described elsewhere in this book, there are excellent surgical training opportunities using simulation and models that allow surgeons to gain experience.

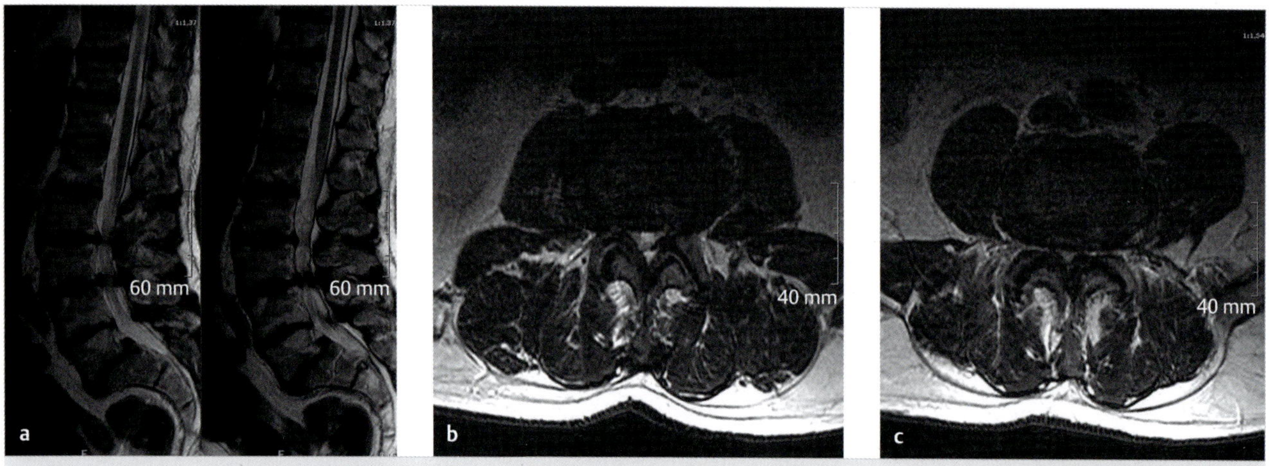

Fig. 32.1 **(a)** T2-weighted sagittal magnetic resonance imaging (MRI) of a severe two-level spinal canal stenosis at the levels L2/L3 and L3/L4. **(b, c)** T2-weighted axial MRI of a severe spinal canal stenosis at the level L2/L3 **(b)** and L3/L4 **(c)**.

32.4 Preoperative Planning

The preoperative evaluation and planning procedures are of particular importance in guaranteeing successful surgery, as well as excellent clinical outcome. Preoperative imaging provides vital information on the anatomical as well as the pathoanatomical structure and positioning of the spine, including malpositioning in all three dimensions—sagittal, frontal, and horizontal—and the topographical anatomy of the target area.

Preoperative imaging studies include mandatory standard X-rays in the anteroposterior (AP) and lateral views in a standing position, as well as functional X-rays with the patient in a lateral position (flexion–extension views). AP X-rays provide information on the curvature of the spine and on the configuration as well as size of the interlaminar window for entry toward the spinal canal. Flexion–extension views reveal the existence of possible vertical instability, as well as translational segmental slipping.

MRI is also obligatory for the preoperative planning stage. It is the diagnostic tool of choice for evaluating the neural structures including the situation within the central spinal and nerve root canals. It provides the most comprehensive information about soft-tissue structures, which may limit the size of the spinal canal such as discogenic pathologies, bulging yellow ligaments, and canal-narrowing synovial cysts. T1- and T2-weighted sagittal and T2-weighted axial images are most freuquently used in this regard (▶ Fig. 32.1a–c). The additional contributation of contrast medium can be used to differentiate between remaining scar-tissue formation following prior surgery and primary pathologies.

With the widespread availability of MRI and due to the poor resolution of soft-tissue structures and its radiation emissions, computed tomography (CT) scan has lost much of its importance in the diagnosis of lumbar spinal stenosis. Only in cases of impossibility of MRI (e.g., patients with a pacemaker), CT scan is used.

In conclusion, a standard preoperative assessment is mandatory, including information on medical history and comorbidities, operative as well as anesthetic risks, current medication, and any blood laboratory abnormalities.

32.5 Patient Positioning

No specific patient preparation is required the day before surgery. If necesssary, shaving of the surgical area is performed.

General anesthesia and complete relaxation are reqired for the operation. Venous and arterial lines are placed to ensure continuous intraoperative anesthetic monitoring. The use of a urinary catheter is not necessary in mono- or bisegmental decompression cases. If the planned surgey time is estimated to be over 3 hours, a urinary catheter is mandatory. Cell-saving procedures, as well as blood transfusion, are not routinely required.

Usually, single dose of preoperative antibiotic prophylaxis is administrated approximately 20 minutes before skin incision with a second shot after 2 hours in longer operative procedure. Routinely, prolonged antibiotic therapy is not recommended.

In order to minimize preoperative complications, the authors refer to the World Health Organization Surgical Safety Checklist for all surgical interventions.

The patient is placed in a so-called knee-thorax position with hips and knees flexed at 90 degrees, and shoulders in 90 degrees abduction and 90 degrees external rotation (attention: avoid overextension of the shoulders) (▶ Fig. 32.2). Hyperflexion of the hip and knee joint should be avoided to prevent restriction of venous blood flow from the legs with the accompanying major risk of deep venous thrombosis. Furthermore, the authors recommend to avoid overextension and hyperabduction of the shoulders to minimize the risk of brachial plexus irritations. Elbow (nervus ulnaris) and wrist joint (nervus medianus), as well as the shins are positioned on gel pads to avoid pressure sores. The abdomen should "hang" freely without any compression to maximally lower the pressure in the epidural veins. A support bracket is placed on the buttocks (▶ Fig. 32.2). On the side opposite of the surgeon, a separate lateral support is placed at the trochanteric region to secure the patient while the operating table is tilted during the over-the-top decompression procedure (▶ Fig. 32.3).

In cases of difficulty in correctly obtaining this described knee-thorax positioning (e.g., restricted knee/hip flexion, severe peripheral arterial disease), a prone position using a frame is recommended.

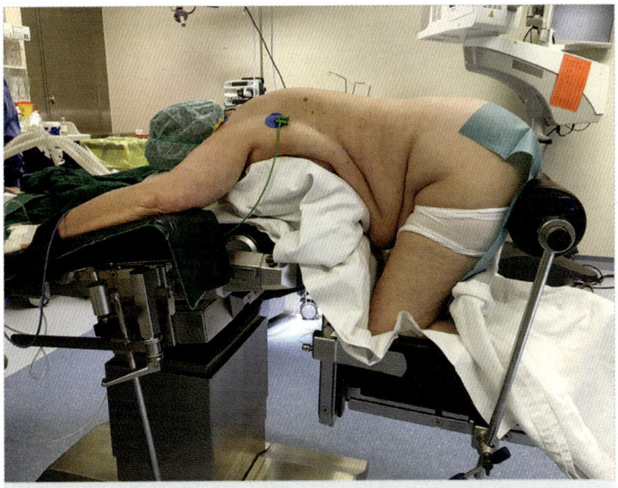

Fig. 32.2 Positioning of the patient in knee-thorax position with no pressure on the abdomen.

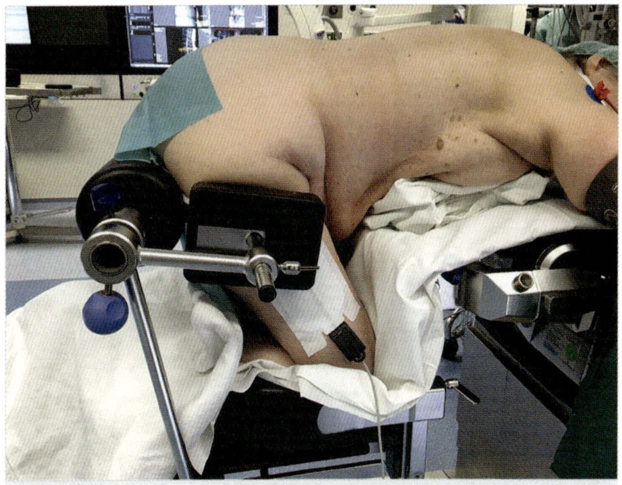

Fig. 32.3 Additional lateral support against the trochanteric region in preparation for the over-the-top decompression.

After final positioning, the operating table can be adjusted at the level of the lumbar spine in order to compensate for lumbar lordosis and provide an open interlaminar access corridor.

To obtain an optimal visualization of the spine, the operating table should have enough clearance available for the C-arm to rotate freely in both planes.

32.6 Surgical Steps

The main steps of this minimally invasive technique include:

a) A unilateral over-the-top appraoch for bilateral decompression.
b) This decompression technique minimizes the potential possible instability associated with similar open procedures by reducing iatrogenic destabilization.[2,4,9]
c) For multisegmental lumbar decompression, the authors recommend the crossover "Slalom technique" with multiple skin incisions to minimize postoperative instability[9,11] (▶ Fig. 32.4).

The projection of the target disc space and the corresponding interlaminar window on the skin level is then marked under fluoroscopic control using sterile cannulas (▶ Fig. 32.5a, b). Cannula placement is usually performed contralaterally to the approach side in order to avoid hematoma at the access corridor. In the case of bi- or multilevel surgery, separate cannula placement for each segment is helpful and recommended (▶ Fig. 32.5c). If there is a fixed lordosis, sometimes two segments can be reached through one 20-mm skin incision.[9,11]

Subsequently, the skin incision line is marked slightly about 5 mm paramedian to the midline, about 20 mm in the craniocaudal direction. In cases of multilevel decompression, separate "Slalom" incision lines should be marked.

The decision regarding which side to choose for access is based preoperatively on the anatomical situation of the spine in the frontal plane, as well as on the clinical symptoms of the patient. In cases of deformity in the frontal plane, an approach from the convex side is preferred, due to the fact that the corresponding segment is rotated toward the convexity.[4] Thus, the heavily loaded facet joint on the concave side can be protected preserving the stability of the spine.

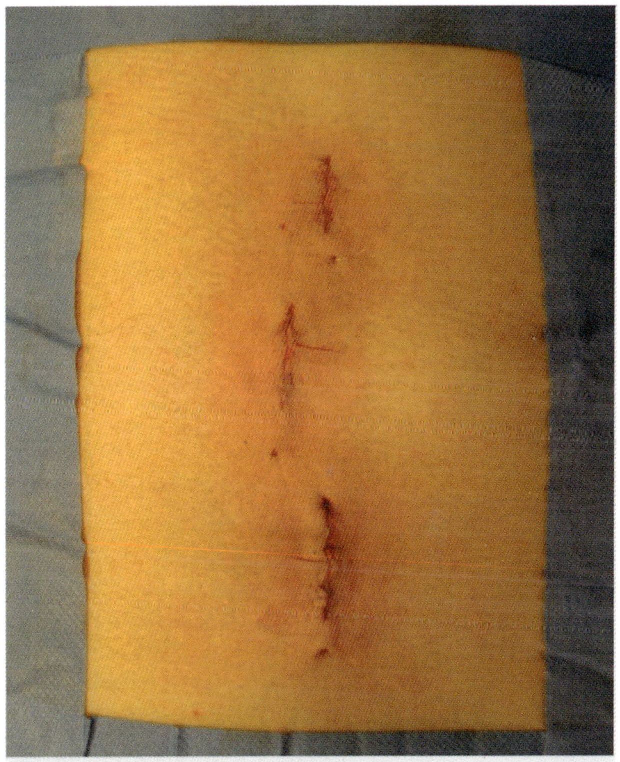

Fig. 32.4 "Slalom technique" incisions.

32.6.1 Incision

Surgery is performed skin-to-skin with the help of a surgical microscope (e.g., Zeiss N 700, Zeiss, Oberkochen, Germany) with variable 400 mm focus length to optimize visualization and illumination.[9,11] The authors prefer to begin the surgery with the microscope already in place (▶ Fig. 32.6a, b).

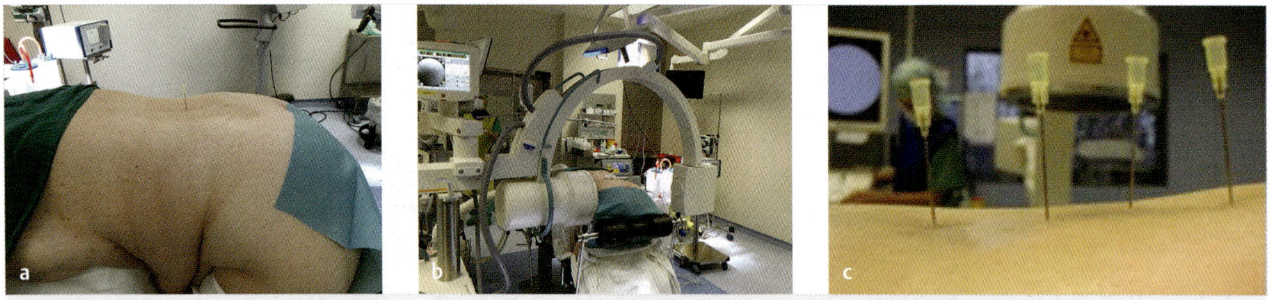

Fig. 32.5 (a) Preoperative localization of the index segment using a sterile cannula. **(b)** Fluoroscopic control of the correct cannula placement. **(c)** Preoperative localization of multilevel surgery.

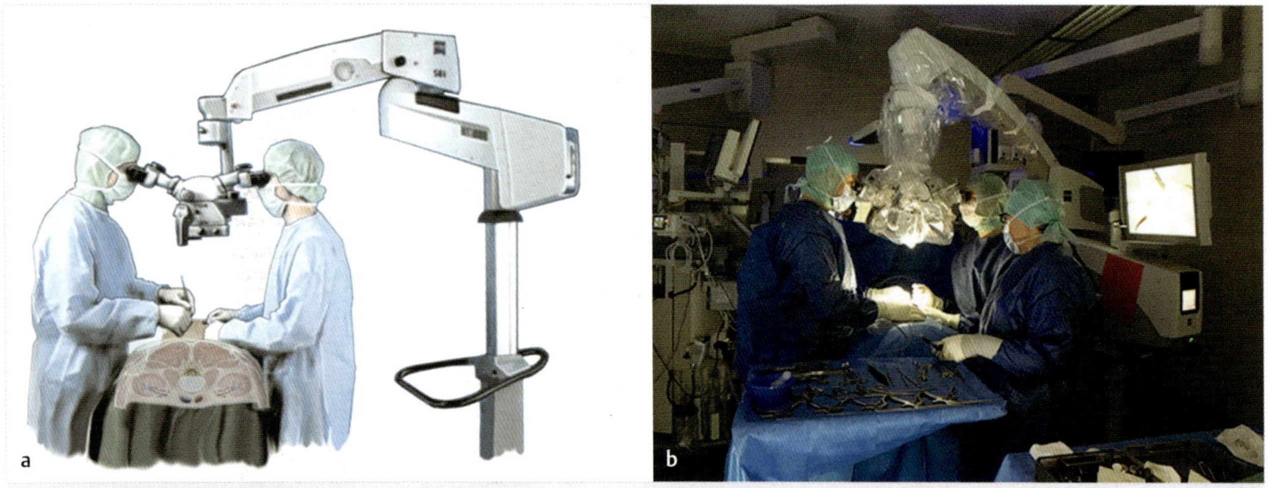

Fig. 32.6 (a, b) Operating room setup. (Used with permission from Mayer and Heider with permission.)[9,11]

After a 20-mm skin incision and sharp dissection of the subcutaneous tissue, the dorsolumbar fascia is opened about 5 mm paramedian, and the paravertebral muscles are bluntly and gently retracted from the lamina and the interlaminar window. Care has to be taken not to incise bigger attachments of the muscles to the spinous process. Small attachments of the rotators are cut from the inferior lateral part of the superior lamina to expose the interlaminar window, the adjacant superior and inferior hemilaminae, as well as the facet joint contour. An articulated or solid frame speculum retractor or a microspeculum (e.g., Piccolino, Medicon, Tuttlingen, Germany) is inserted and the interlaminar window is cleaned completely of soft tissue. Then, the level of exposure is checked under fluoroscopic control (▶ Fig. 32.7a, b).

32.6.2 Technique

The first step of decompression is to undercut the proximal lamina with a high-speed drill to expose the attachment/insertion zone of the yellow ligament, medially and cranially. Then the spinal canal is opened cranially, and the yellow ligament is removed on the ipsilateral side, starting in the midline and then toward lateral cranial and finally along the lateral recess to expose the thecal sac, the lateral border of the dura, and the exiting nerve root until it leaves the spinal canal around the caudal pedicle without any compression (▶ Fig. 32.8). In cases of a hypertrophic facet joint, the inferior facet should be thinned out medially with a small diamond burr by sparing osteoclastic facetotomy. The cranial rim of the caudal lamina is undercut 2 to 3 mm. Thus, the ipsilateral decompression is complete.

For decompression of the contralateral central canal and lateral recess, the operating table is tilted approximately 20 degrees away from the surgeon to the contralateral side and the assistant who fixes and guides the speculum tilts it as well to the ipsilateral side (surgeon's side) (▶ Fig. 32.9). The surgical microscope is adjusted to give a sufficiently oblique view to the contralateral part of the spinal canal (▶ Fig. 32.9). The anterior part of the interspinous ligament, the base of the spinous process, and the yellow ligament are removed under direct visual control of the thecal sac. The proximal lamina is undercut as is the superior facet on the contralateral side. If necessary and for safety reasons, the dura can be gently retracted medially with a nerve hook. Initially, the central part is completely decompressed. Contralateral lateral recess decompression includes osteoclastic thinning of the medial parts of the superior facet. Exposure and decompression of the exiting nerve root is completed by subarticular undercutting until the nerve root passes the contralateral inferior pedicle.

Hemostasis is achieved with repeated irrigation with saline solution, bipolar coagulation, or the use of hemostatic/sealing agents (e.g., Floseal, Baxter International Inc, Deerfield, Illinois). The table is tilted into the neutral position and the speculum is removed.

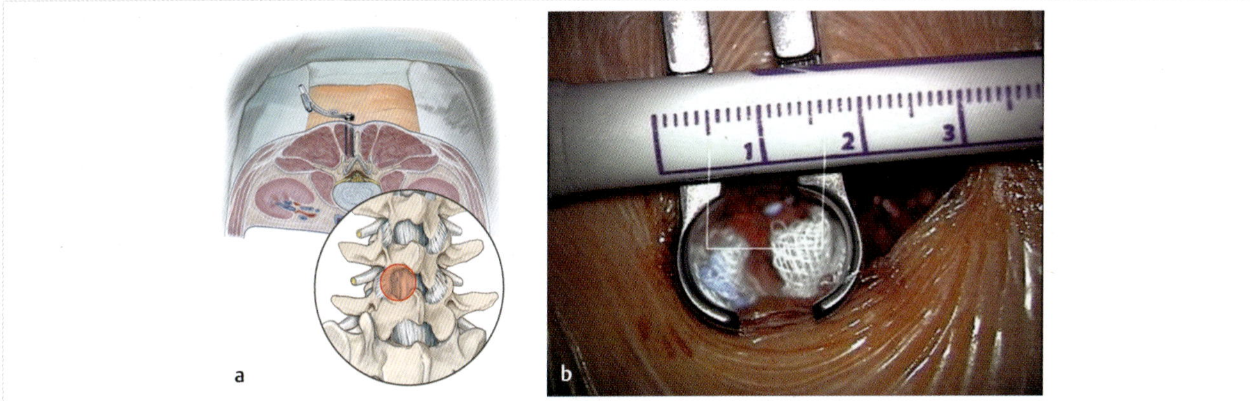

Fig. 32.7 (a) Graphic presentation of the interlaminar approach window. (Used with permission from Mayer and Heider.)[9,11] (b) Interlaminar approach window with a minispeculum.

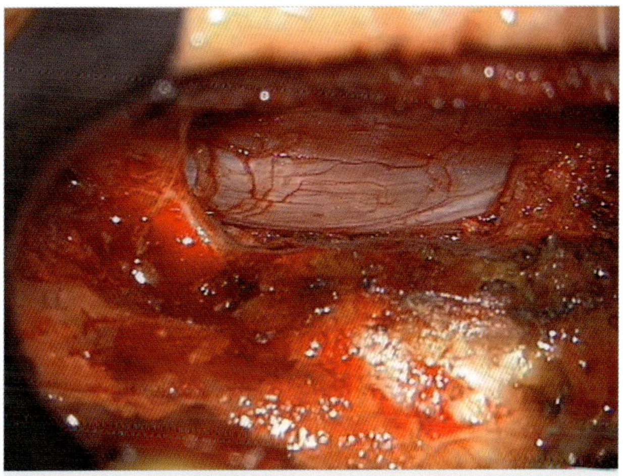

Fig. 32.8 Ipsilateral complete decompression with relieved nerve root.

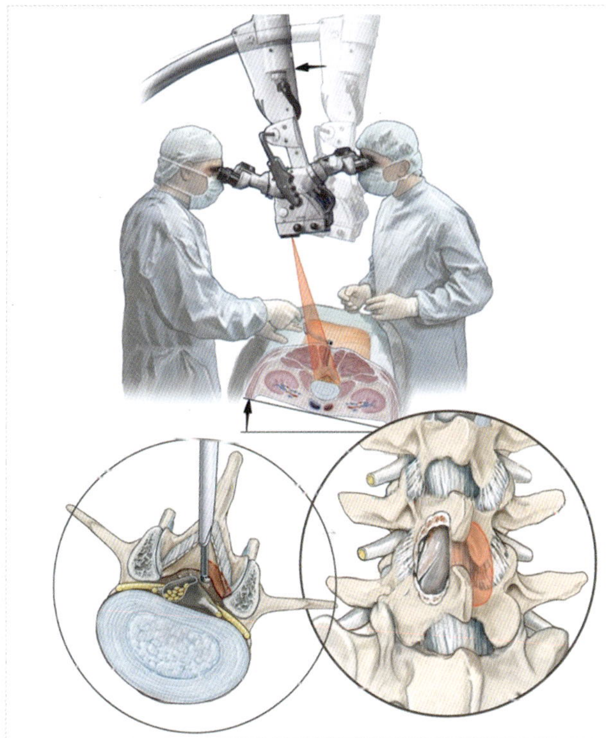

Fig. 32.9 Decompression of the contralateral side. (Used with permission from Mayer and Heider.)[9,11]

32.6.3 Closure

Before closure, a final check for complete decompression of the neural structures as well as meticulous hemostasis should be performed. To ensure a sufficient and adequate decompression, the authors recommend to check the neural structures as well as the exiting nerve roots using a ball tip nerve hook, which should be turned easily cranial, caudal, medial, lateral as well as above and below the pedicles.

The use of a subfascial drain (without sucction/vacuum) is rarely indicated, except in case there was unsual bleeding intraoperatively. The number of treated levels does not determine wether a drain is necessary or not. After closure of the fascia and adaptation sutures of the subcutaneous tissue, the skin is closed by resorbable intracutaneous running suture.

We do not use any local anesthetics in the muscle. To summarize, to recap, as well as to amplify this minimally approach and surgical technique we prepared the ▸ Video 32.1 for self-study.

32.7 Postoperative Care

The patient is generally extubated immediately after surgery. In normal cases, as well as independently of the number of levels that have been decompressed, mobilization training can be started within 4 to 6 hours following surgery. After first successful mobilization, physiotherapy is initiated and intensified without any restrictions concerning different mobility patterns such as sitting, standing, or walking. This early mobilization also reduces the need for thrombosis prophylaxis. Generally, thrombembolic prophylaxis with fractionated heparin is performed until the patient has regained full mobilization.

Drain removal is carried out within 24 to 48 hours of surgery. Sterile adhesive plastic is placed over the operated area for 72 hours. For wound healing, no further wound covering is necessary. Prolonged antibiotic therapy is not recommended.

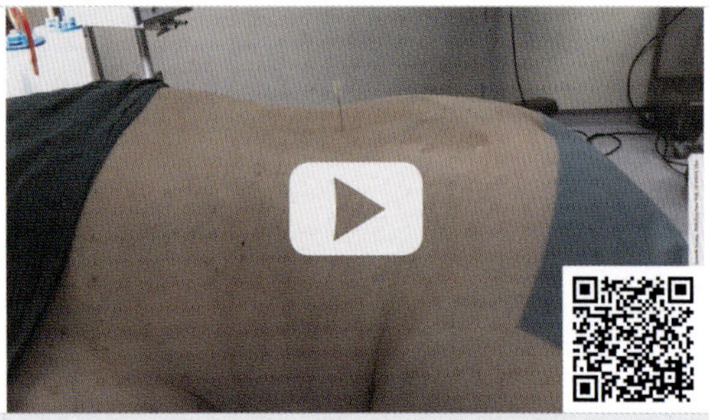

Video 32.1 Unilateral lumbar approach.

However, depending on the patient's complaints, the number of treated levels (over two levels), and if translational immobile displacements or degenerative deformities are present, temporary soft bracing may be applied for the following 4 weeks.

We do not use a Foley cathether in single and up to three level fusions and if we do, we remove them at postanesthesia care unit (PACU) at the latest.

32.8 Complication Avoidance

The following potential complications, hazards, and pitfalls can occur during the surgical steps of the unilateral lumbar approach:

a) **Incidental dural tears with subsequent cerebrospinal fluid (CSF) leakage:**
   Incidental dural tears are the most common complications during decompressive procedures in spinal stenoses, as well as when using the minimally invasive unilateral approach. According to the literature, dural tears with subsequent CSF leakage occur in 8 to 13% for primary decompressive surgery, independent of the approach.[12] Especially in the old patient population, the dura is usually very thin and frequently more adherent to the surrunding structures, resulting in the risk of increased vulnerability. In cases of an incidental durotomy, immediate repair of the dura by suturing, clipping, patching (e.g., TachoSil, Nycomed Pharma, GmbH, Konstanz, Germany), and/or surface sealing (e.g., fibrin glue) is recommended to avoid the development of a pseudomeningocele or persisting CSF fistulas. In case a dural tear occurs intraoperatively on the contralateral approach side, the approach has to be enlarged to perform a proper suture; an additional contralateral approach may be required.

b) **Epidural hematoma:**
   The occurence of postoperative epidural hematoma is relatively frequent with a reported incidence of 58%, the most cases being asymptomatic.[4,13] Thus, meticulous hemostasis check is recommended and very important to avoid postoperative epidural hematoma, due to the fact that postoperative hematomas can cause severe pain and immobility. Therefore, the authors prefer to use hemostatic agents such as Floseal (Baxter International Inc, Deerfield, Illinois). These agents help to reduce the risk of epidural hematoma.

c) **Nerve root injury:**
   Nerve root injury is a very rare complication, reported in only 1 to 2% of the literature.[14] The over-the-top decompression might in particular lead to a possible temporary compression of the cauda equina if the entrance corridor of the decompression route is too narrow due to insufficient preparation/undercutting.[4]

d) **Incomplete/insufficient decompression:**
   This complication can occur during the learning curve of the minimally invasive approach due to the fact that the unilateral lumbar approach has a steep learning curve, as with all advanced surgical techniques. If the surgeon is familiar with the microanatomy of the lumbar spine and with this approach, an incomplete decompression is very rare.

e) **Wrong-level decompression.**

f) **Potential delayed complications:**
   1. Epidural scar formation.
   2. Arachnoiditis.
   3. Segment instability/destabilization of the adjacant segment due to extensive decompression procedures.

32.9 Tips and Tricks

a) In cases with equal bilateral stenosis and symptoms, a right-sided approach is recommended for a right-handed surgeon, due to the fact that the most work is performed with the surgeon's right hand. Conversely, a left-sided approach is used by a left-handed surgeon.[2]

b) Accurate preoperative evaluation of the anatomical landmarks guarantees a successful surgery. At the levels L1/2, L2/3, and L3/L4, the lamina is less wide compared with the levels L4/L5 and L5/S1. In addition, the facet joints are oriented more sagittally and the pars is thinner in the cranial levels, which makes it more vulnerable to potential iatrogenic injury.[2]

c) For three, four, or more levels, the "Slalom" technique with separate skin incisions is the method of choice.[9,11]

d) Patient selection: Patients with up to grade I spondylolisthesis and no other signs of instability are suitable candidates for this approach. However, patients with overt instability with motion, with significant scoliosis, or with lateral listhesis should be considered for stabilization surgery.

32.10 Conclusion

The minimally invasive unilateral lumbar approach for over-the-top bilateral decompression has less impact on the paraspinal muscles compared with the open conventional surgeries.[2,4,9,11] Furthermore, in a recent biomechanical study, the described minimally invasive unilateral technique was shown to produce significantly less instability than traditional midline laminectomy.[15] The clinical results based on Oswestry Disability Index of the unilateral approaches are as effective as open decompression procedures, and better in terms of pain relief and use of analgesic.[16] MIS can potentially avoid more invasive fusion surgery and will allow treatment of patients, especially the elderly, who were previously not considered surgical candidates.[8]

The unilateral lumbar approach for over-the-top bilateral decompression offers particular advantages especially for high-risk patients, such as the obese and elderly.[17]

Minimally invasive unilateral approaches for over-the-top bilateral decompression showed a steep learning curve. However,

adoption of a workflow, and training in simulation laboratories and cadaver will help to get familiar and be more comfortable with this MIS approach.

In summary, the described MIS technique revealed similar or better clinical outcomes than classical open techniques for the treatment of lumbar degenerative diseases, with same significant benefits for the patients. These include decreased pain, less disruption of the normal anatomy, shorter duration of hospitalization, less disability, and less expenses.

With the extension of the MIS techniques and the development of specific instruments, the role of MIS is becoming clearer and the complication rate has continuously decreased.

References

[1] Oppenheimer JH, DeCastro I, McDonnell DE. Minimally invasive spine technology and minimally invasive spine surgery: a historical review. Neurosurg Focus. 2009; 27(3):E9

[2] Boukebir MA, Berlin CD, Navarro-Ramirez R, et al. Ten-step minimally invasive spine lumbar decompression and dural repair through tubular retractors. Oper Neurosurg (Hagerstown). 2017; 13(2):232–245

[3] Aryanpur J, Ducker T. Multilevel lumbar laminotomies: an alternative to laminectomy in the treatment of lumbar stenosis. Neurosurgery. 1990; 26 (3):429–432, discussion 433

[4] Härtl R, Korge A. Minimally Invasive Spine Surgery: Techniques, Evidence, and Controversies. Davos-Platz, Switzerland: AO Spine; 2012

[5] Spetzger U, Bertalanffy H, Reinges MH, Gilsbach JM. Unilateral laminotomy for bilateral decompression of lumbar spinal stenosis. Part II: Clinical experiences. Acta Neurochir (Wien). 1997; 139(5):397–403

[6] Young S, Veerapen R, O'Laoire SA. Relief of lumbar canal stenosis using multilevel subarticular fenestrations as an alternative to wide laminectomy: preliminary report. Neurosurgery. 1988; 23(5):628–633

[7] McCulloch JA. Essentials of Spinal Microsurgery. Philadelphia, PA: Liooincott Raven; 1998

[8] Alimi M, Hofstetter CP, Pyo SY, Paulo D, Härtl R. Minimally invasive laminectomy for lumbar spinal stenosis in patients with and without preoperative spondylolisthesis: clinical outcome and reoperation rates. J Neurosurg Spine. 2015; 22(4):339–352

[9] Mayer HM, Heider F. "Slalom": Microsurgical Cross-Over Decompression for Multilevel Degenerative Lumbar Stenosis. BioMed Research International. 2016,9074257,6 pages

[10] Papavero L, Thiel M, Fritzsche E, Kunze C, Westphal M, Kothe R. Lumbar spinal stenosis: prognostic factors for bilateral microsurgical decompression using a unilateral approach. Neurosurgery. 2009; 65(6) Suppl:182–187, n187

[11] Mayer HM, Heider F. [Selective, microsurgical cross-over decompression of multisegmental degenerative lumbar spinal stenoses: the "Slalom" technique]. Oper Orthop Traumatol. 2013; 25(1):47–62

[12] Tafazal SI, Sell PJ. Incidental durotomy in lumbar spine surgery: incidence and management. Eur Spine J. 2005; 14(3):287–290

[13] Sokolowski MJ, Garvey TA, Perl J , II, et al. Prospective study of postoperative lumbar epidural hematoma: incidence and risk factors. Spine. 2008; 33 (1):108–113

[14] Fourney DR, Dettori JR, Norvell DC, Dekutoski MB. Does minimal access tubular assisted spine surgery increase or decrease complications in spinal decompression or fusion? Spine. 2010; 35(9) Suppl:S57–S65

[15] Smith ZA, Vastardis GA, Carandang G, et al. Biomechanical effects of a unilateral approach to minimally invasive lumbar decompression. PLoS One. 2014; 9(3):e92611

[16] Mobbs RJ, Li J, Sivabalan P, Raley D, Rao PJ. Outcomes after decompressive laminectomy for lumbar spinal stenosis: comparison between minimally invasive unilateral laminectomy for bilateral decompression and open laminectomy: clinical article. J Neurosurg Spine. 2014; 21(2):179–186

[17] Marcus JD, James AR, Härtl R. Minimally invasive surgical treatment options for lumbar disc herniations and stenosis. Semin Spine Surg. 2011; 23(1):20–26

33 Far-Lateral Lumbar Discectomies

Eric H. Elowitz

Summary

Herniated lumbar discs are a major cause of pain and disability frequently affecting younger age patients. Although the most common location of herniated discs is within the spinal canal, in either the paracentral or central space, some disc herniations are more lateral and occur in the foraminal or extraforaminal region. These disc herniations can present with severe pain, often with a dysesthetic quality due to compression of the dorsal root ganglion. Spine surgeons are generally very comfortable with the interlaminar surgical approach for paracentral disc herniations. To approach the far-lateral disc herniations, an extraforaminal approach is the most direct method and avoids an iatrogenic destabilization of the spine. The minimally invasive tubular extraforaminal approach, as described, involves docking of the dilators and tubular working channel on the lateral pars. The pars and inferior facet are drilled exposing the ligamentum flavum. The ligament is opened at the most rostral region adjacent to the upper pedicle exposing the Kambin's triangle region. This minimally invasive approach takes advantage of the anatomy of the pars interarticularis and ligamentum flavum and can be performed in a safe and reproducible manner.

Keywords: extraforaminal, far-lateral herniated disc, herniated lumbar disc, microdiscectomy

33.1 Introduction

Herniated lumbar discs are a major source of radicular symptoms. Approximately, 90% of disc herniations occur within the spinal canal affecting the paracentral and central compartments, typically compressing the traversing nerve root or thecal sac.[1] A distinct minority of disc herniations and pathologies occur within the neural foramen or extraforaminal space.[1,2] These herniations can compress the exiting nerve root, frequently at the level of the dorsal root ganglion.[3] Mechanical nerve root compression caused by these "far-lateral" disc herniations can cause extreme pain and disability for patients. The anatomy of this region was described by Parviz Kambin,[4] and is delineated by the exiting nerve root, superior end plate of the caudal vertebral body, and the traversing nerve root or thecal sac. This "Kambin's triangle" is a critical anatomic area of the spine and a source of clinical pathology.

Lumbar microdiscectomies are a common surgery on the spine and are often performed in younger age patients.[5] The interlaminar anatomy and approach are well known to spinal surgeons. The use of minimally invasive tubular retractors have become quite commonplace for these disc pathologies.[6,7] However, far-lateral pathologies pose specific challenges due to the anatomy and less frequent need for approach. Traditional open approaches to the foraminal and extraforaminal regions require either a midline or paramedian incision. These open exposures can be quite extensive in order to reach laterally beyond the vertebral pars interarticularis and facet joint in order to obtain adequate visualization of the far-lateral herniated disc.[8,9,10] The adaptation of minimally invasive approaches using tubular retractor systems is particularly well suited to approaching Kambin's triangle and the extraforaminal space.[11,12]

In order to safely perform a minimally invasive far-lateral microdiscectomy, knowledge of the neural and bony anatomy is required. Fluoroscopic assistance is necessary for placement of the tubular retractor in order to ensure appropriate visualization and exposure of the exiting nerve root and herniated disc. The minimal bony drilling required does not result in joint destabilization. In general, the minimally invasive tubular approach has multiple advantages over the more traditional open approach to the extraforaminal region.[13,14,15,16] There is minimal tissue trauma, decreased surgical site infections, early mobilization, and short hospital stays. As this approach is generally not as familiar to spinal surgeons, a review of this anatomically based approach is useful.

33.2 Indications

The indications for a minimally invasive far-lateral microdiscectomy are the same as a more conventional approach. When evaluating patients for surgery, the majority of patients will have significant radicular pain. The pain distribution should correlate with the magnetic resonance imaging (MRI) findings of disc herniation. The exiting nerve roots are affected by pathology in Kambin's triangle and extraforaminal space such that the L4 nerve root is symptomatic due to a far-lateral herniation at L4–L5 and the L3 nerve root at L3–L4. Patients may experience a combination of pain, numbness, or weakness. Dysesthetic pain syndromes, often with allodynia, are also more frequent with pathology in this location due to involvement of the dorsal root ganglion. Some patients may complain of a burning sensation, similar to a sunburn, and find any fabric or touch against the skin very distressing. Motor weakness is also a possibility and a thorough neurologic examination, including reflexes, should be performed in all patients.

In most patients with herniated discs, a conservative, nonsurgical approach is generally recommended initially.[5] Treatment options include physical therapy, transforaminal steroid injections, and nonsteroidal anti-inflammatory medications. In patients with herniated discs and persistent radicular symptoms despite adequate conservative measures, surgery has been shown to be beneficial.[17] The presence of motor weakness may prompt surgery on an earlier basis.[18]

Once the decision for a surgical microdiscectomy has been made, the choice of approach to the spine is critical. In patients with far-lateral disc herniations, the extraforaminal approach to Kambin's triangle is most direct and expedient.[4,11] Alternatively, some patients will have disc herniations within the neural foramen directly underlying the pars interarticularis and either a standard interlaminar or extraforaminal approach can be considered. In foraminal discs compressing the exiting nerve root, it is the author's preference to utilize the extraforaminal approach as this requires less bone removal and has a lower risk of pars injury and potential destabilization.

In operative cases, review of the lumbar MRI scan is critical in determining the nature of the surgical approach; T2-weighted MRI is especially helpful in this regard. Both the sagittal and axial images need to be considered. On the lateral sagittal images, particular attention should be focused on evaluating the neural foramina and potential compression of the exiting nerve root. In normal, nonpathologic levels, the neural foramen should be well visualized with the nerve root and surrounding fat. However, with foraminal pathology, the fat plane can be obliterated and the nerve root compressed superiorly against the pedicle. Axial imaging is also helpful and can also demonstrate the exact location of the disc herniation and extent of foraminal and/or extraforaminal involvement.

33.3 Contraindications

A thorough understanding of the anatomy of the Kambin's triangle region is necessary for a safe far-lateral minimally invasive microdiscectomy. An evaluation of the MRI scans is critical prior to surgery. Some patients, particularly older individuals, will have significant facet arthropathy, which can limit the exposure to the extraforaminal space. Additional drilling of the lower vertebra superior articulating process may be necessary in these patients and can provide particular surgical challenges with the minimally invasive approach. Additionally, prior extraforaminal surgery can distort the tissue planes with scar tissue and epidural fibrosis increasing the risk of nerve injury or cerebrospinal fluid (CSF) leakage. It is the author's experience that prior midline surgery, such as a laminectomy, is not a contraindication to the minimally invasive tubular extraforaminal approach. Indeed, this is an excellent option for patients who have had prior midline open operations and present with far-lateral disc herniations.

33.4 Preoperative Planning

As in all surgeries, preoperative planning is critical to a successful outcome. A correlation between the patient's symptoms and MRI findings is necessary in order to determine the symptomatic pathology and disc level (▶ Fig. 33.1). However, in the majority of patients, the link between the herniated disc and radicular symptoms is clear-cut. Although not generally required, an electromyography (EMG)/nerve conduction study can be helpful in less straightforward patient presentations. Intraoperative three-dimensional navigation can also be helpful if available.

In patients where the disc herniation is either foraminal or far-lateral, the extraforaminal approach is well suited for nerve decompression. There are occasional patients who may have both a paracentral as well as a far-lateral disc herniation and may require an "in and out" technique utilizing both an interlaminar and an extraforaminal approach; this would require two separate docking points, but still can be performed using minimally invasive techniques. An evaluation of the facet pathology preoperatively can also be helpful as it will alert the surgeon to the degree of bone drilling required.

33.5 Patient Positioning

Once in the operating room, successful general endotracheal anesthesia is given. Prophylactic antibiotics are administered within 1 hour of incision. The procedure is performed in the prone position. The use of a classic knee-chest position or other positioning frames do afford the benefit of significant hip flexion, which may help open the intervertebral space. The arms are placed upward on arm boards and the face and eyes are carefully padded (▶ Fig. 33.2). Sequential compression boots are used during the procedure.

Intraoperative fluoroscopy is necessary for appropriate placement of the tubular retractor. A lateral fluoroscopic image is used. It is the author's practice not to use anteroposterior (AP) imaging. Prior to prepping and draping of the patient, fluoroscopy is adjusted such that a straight lateral image is obtained. The incision can then be mapped out approaching the foramen, pars, and appropriate disc level. As in all lumbar surgeries, care should be taken for adequate counting of the correct level as some patients will have transitional anatomy. A correlation between the fluoroscopic image and preoperative studies is necessary.

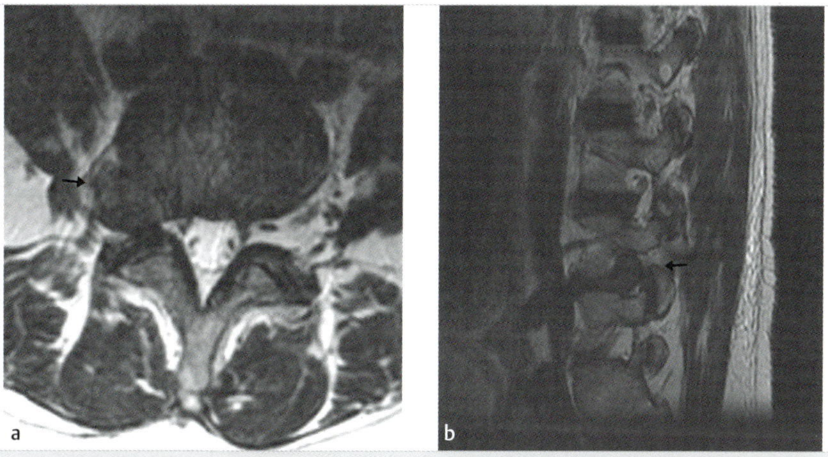

Fig. 33.1 Magnetic resonance image of a right L4/L5 far-lateral herniated disc, T2-weighted. **(a)** Axial slice; **(b)** sagittal slice with obliteration of the foramen.

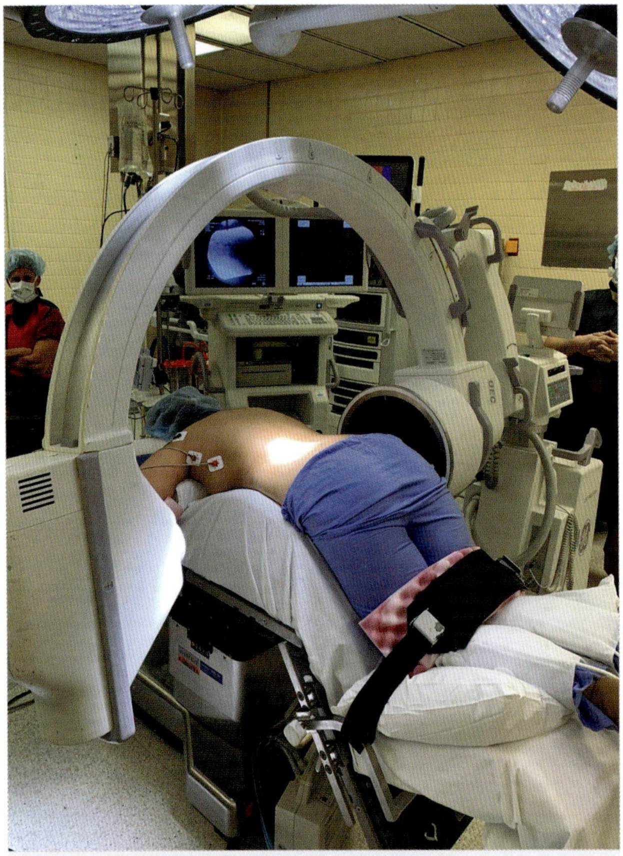

Fig. 33.2 Patient positioned prone with the arms upward on boards. Intraoperative fluoroscopy is used for localization.

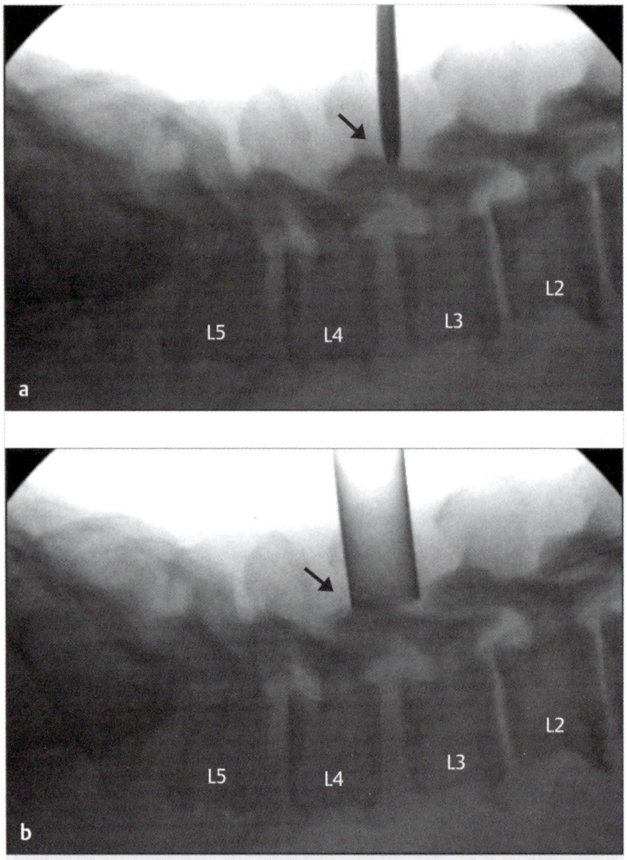

Fig. 33.3 Intraoperative lumbar fluoroscopic lateral images. **(a)** The initial dilator (arrow) docks on the lateral aspect of the pars interarticularis directly above the neural foramen. **(b)** The 18-mm tubular retractor is docked at the pars interarticularis. (Used with permission from Virk MS, Elowitz E. A minimally invasive approach to the lumbar neural foramen and extraforaminal compartment: modified surgical technique. J Spine 2014:4:203–208.)

33.6 Surgical Steps

33.6.1 Incision

The incision for a tubular extraforaminal approach is slightly lateral compared to that for an interlaminar approach. An incision is performed 2 cm from the midline just superior to the foramen and pars; often this is just a few millimeters rostral to the disc space itself. Lateral fluoroscopy is used to localize the incision and trajectory to the lateral foramen. As in other tubular minimally invasive procedures, the exact localization of the incision is critical.

33.6.2 Technique

1. Using a Bovie cautery, the subcutaneous tissues are dissected down to the fascia. A small window of fascia can be opened using a Bovie cautery. In larger patients, who have more subcutaneous lipomatous tissue, a scalpel can be used to open the fascia under fluoroscopic guidance.
2. As with other tubular procedures, a series of dilators are used to sequentially dilate the muscle and fascia until the working channel is placed. Using the initial dilator, the lateral pars interarticularis is targeted and becomes the center of interest for the working channel (▶ Fig. 33.3 and ▶ Fig. 33.4). The lateral pars interarticularis can be palpated using the small dilator and the lateral aspect cleared of tissue using a scraping technique. Great care must be taken to avoid plunging laterally into the foramen itself as this could damage the dorsal root ganglion. In patients who have marked facet arthropathy, the pars may be somewhat obscured by bony overgrowth; however, the lateral pars can still be determined by palpation. Fluoroscopy is required to assure that the small dilator is over the foramen, which is slightly rostral to the disc space itself. Although some authors have suggested docking at the junction of the transverse process (see ▶ Fig. 33.7, for example) and then redirecting the retractor more caudally, it is this author's experience that initial targeting of the lateral pars provides excellent anatomic positioning for the dilating tubes and retractor. This minimizes the need to redirect the working channel.
3. Additional dilating tubes are then inserted until the 18-mm working channel is placed and attached to a table-mounted holding arm. The dilating tubes are removed and an operative microscope is then brought into the field. The remainder of the surgery is performed using a microscope. Residual muscle and fascia are removed using Bovie cautery from the lateral pars and superior lateral aspect of the inferior facet.

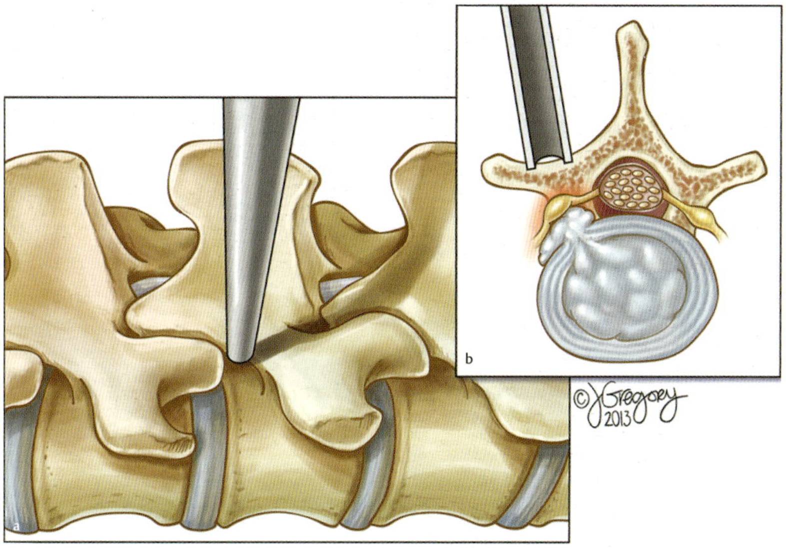

Fig. 33.4 Location of the initial dilator and later, the tubular retractor at the lateral pars. **(a)** Initial dilator is targeted at the lateral pars interarticularis, lateral view. **(b)** Axial view of dilator position. Dorsal root ganglion, exiting nerve root, and herniated disc are illustrated. (Used with permission from Jill K Gregory, CMI, from Virk MS, Elowitz E. A minimally invasive approach to the lumbar neural foramen and extraforaminal compartment: modified surgical technique. J Spine 2014:4:203–208.)

4. Frequently, an artery over the pars is identified and should be cauterized and sharply cut. A high-speed drill is then used to resect the lateral aspect of the pars exposing the ligamentum flavum. The superior-lateral aspect of the inferior facet joint is also drilled, but to a minimum degree to avoid instability. It is necessary to drill the lateral pars interarticularis to the rostral level of the pedicle (▶ Fig. 33.5). The ligamentum flavum is visualized deep to the pars interarticularis and seen extending laterally into the extraforaminal space. The ligament itself does not insert on the pedicle above, which is at the rostral aspect of the foramen. Taking advantage of this anatomy, a ball tip probe or Kerrison rongeur is used to open and then resect the ligamentum flavum in a caudal direction. By removing the ligament deep and lateral to the pars interarticularis, Kambin's triangle is exposed.
5. The exiting nerve root is identified just inferior to the pedicle (▶ Fig. 33.6). An instrument can be used to palpate the inferior, lateral, and medial aspects of the pedicle. Identifying the pedicle is extremely helpful as an internal landmark. Once the pedicle and exiting nerve root are identified, the disc space is inferior in Kambin's triangle. Great care must be taken to avoid over-manipulation of the nerve root as this is the location of the dorsal root ganglion. When dissecting laterally, care must be taken to identify the segmental artery as this can cause bleeding if inadvertently injured.[19]
6. Evaluation of preoperative MRI scan is very helpful to know the location of the disc herniation. Disc herniations can be within the foramen or extend further into the extraforaminal region. Most far-lateral and foraminal herniated discs are located just inferior to the nerve root displacing the nerve superiorly. In patients who have more laterally displaced disc herniations, the nerve root can be traced along its course until the herniation is identified. Some patients have extruded disc herniations, which can be readily identified and removed using pituitary rongeurs. Other disc herniations can be contained within the annulus and a #11 blade is used to incise the annulus within Kambin's triangle prior to disc removal. A nerve root retractor can be gently used to protect the nerve root, but care must be taken not to over-retract or compress the nerve at this sensitive location.

One of the most concerning complications of the far-lateral approach is injury to the dorsal root ganglion and nerve root, which can result in significant dysesthetic pain. Meticulous microsurgical technique and avoidance of unnecessary nerve manipulation are key. In addition to the steps mentioned in this chapter, the editors find that navigation can be helpful, especially in the learning curve for this procedure.

33.6.3 Closure

Once the disc extrusion has been removed, the nerve root is inspected to ensure that there is no residual compression or additional free disc fragments. A ball-tip probe can be passed deep to the nerve to sweep out any additional extruded disc materials. Hemostasis can be obtained using thrombin Gelfoam if there is any evidence of epidural bleeding. The wound is then irrigated using antibiotic saline. The retractor is slowly removed and bipolar cautery used to control any muscle bleeding. A single suture is placed in the fascia. The skin is closed using a running subcuticular suture and Steri-Strips are placed.

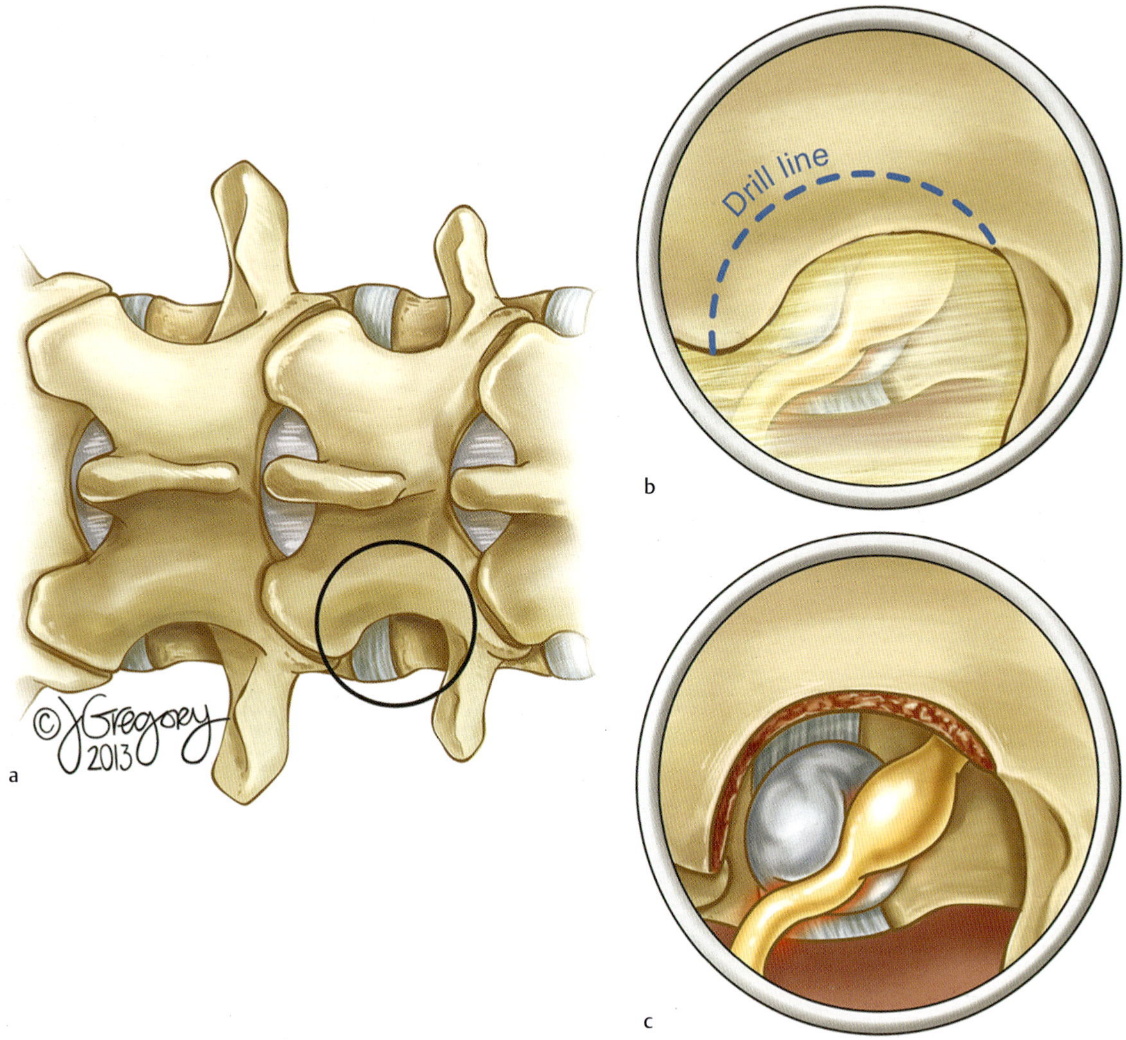

Fig. 33.5 Approach to Kambin's triangle region using tubular retractor. **(a)** Dorsal view of lumbar spine with location of 18-mm tubular retractor shown. **(b)** Microscopic view through tube with outline of bone to be drilled at the lateral pars interarticularis. **(c)** Exiting nerve root and far-lateral herniated disc are illustrated, after the lateral pars is drilled and ligamentum flavum is opened. (Used with permission from Jill K Gregory, CMI, from Virk MS, Elowitz E. A minimally invasive approach to the lumbar neural foramen and extraforaminal compartment: modified surgical technique. J Spine 2014:4:203–208.)

Patients are discharged home on the same day of the procedure. No postoperative antibiotics are administered. Oral analgesia, including oxycodone, Tylenol, and a muscle relaxant are generally prescribed to be used as needed.

33.7 Postoperative Care

Patients are instructed to refrain from strenuous activity for approximately 6 weeks. This is thought to allow time for any annular disruptions to heal. Lifting is limited to no more than 10 pounds and bending is discouraged. Most patients return to full activity after about 6 weeks and no further limitations are advised.

33.8 Complication Avoidance

One of the most concerning complications of the far-lateral approach is injury to the dorsal root ganglion and nerve root, which can result in significant dysesthetic pain.[20] Although this can occur even with minimal nerve root manipulation, it is the author's experience that more aggressive nerve retraction can lead to injury and persistent allopathic pain. Patients may complain of a severe burning sensation in the leg. Gabapentin, often at high doses, can be useful in patients who have significant dysesthetic pain following surgery. In order to avoid this complication, special care must be given to avoid injury to the dorsal root ganglion. Insertion of the small dilator at the beginning of the

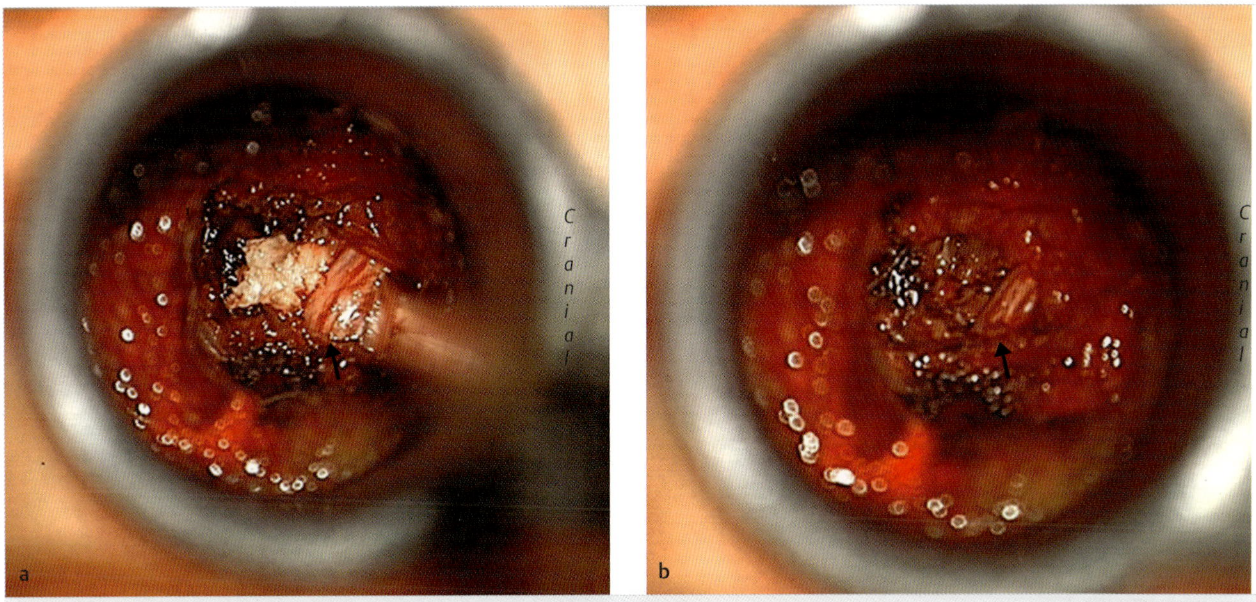

Fig. 33.6 Microscope-assisted intraoperative view through tubular retractor of right-sided extraforaminal approach. Cranial is to the left as marked. **(a)** Exiting nerve compressed from far-lateral herniated disc. Black arrow points to the exiting nerve with disc fragment lying caudally to the nerve. **(b)** Exiting nerve root shown following resection of disc herniation.

procedure deep into the foramen can cause a crush injury of the nerve. Lateral fluoroscopy is important at this stage of the operation in order to maintain the initial dilator posterior to the foramen.

Intraoperative bleeding from the radicular artery is another potential complication. If the artery is injured, it can retract back past the edge of the dilator making control difficult. An angled bipolar tip, which extends beyond the lip of the retractor, can be used. However, being cognizant of the location of the artery and cauterizing it prior to injury will prevent bleeding.

Careful inspection of the foramen and extraforaminal space is also required prior to wound closure in order to prevent retained disc fragments, which is another potential risk of the surgery. As with all surgery for herniated discs, recurrent disc herniation is a distinct risk. In cases where an annulotomy is performed using a knife, limiting the degree of annular resection may decrease the risk of disc herniation recurrence. It is the author's preference to create either a small square window, or possibly just a linear incision, in order to minimize annular disruption.

33.9 Tips and Tricks

The extraforaminal discectomy offers unique challenges to the spinal surgeon. As the pathologies in this location are less common than standard paracentral disc herniations, most surgeons have less experience in the far-lateral approach. As with all minimally invasive surgery, attention to detail is particularly critical for a successful outcome. Proper visualization on fluoroscopy is important; spending additional time prior to incision will add to the safety and reproducibility of this surgery. Focusing on the lateral pars as the center of attention for the working channel is very helpful. Even in patients with facet overgrowth, the pars interarticularis itself is rarely hypertrophied. In these degenerative cases, aggressive drilling of the superior-lateral portion of the inferior facet can be very helpful in order to expose the more normal pars interarticularis structure and foramen.

Placement of the working channel, as in all tubular surgery, is critical. Having the lateral pars at about the medial position of the working channel is optimal. Once the lateral pars is drilled, finding the junction of the pedicle and ligamentum flavum is key. As the ligamentum flavum does not insert on the pedicle, this is an ideal starting point for ligament resection and exposure of Kambin's triangle.

Frameless navigation may play a role in future as an adjunct to the extraforaminal approach. Intraoperative computed tomography (CT) imaging is becoming more routine at many centers. Using a navigation platform may be helpful in planning the incision as well as the trajectory of tube placement. ▶ Fig. 33.7 demonstrates the navigation window being used to localize the extraforaminal approach for a right L4/L5 far-lateral herniated disc.

33.10 Conclusion

Far-lateral and foraminal disc herniations can cause significant radicular symptoms due to nerve root and dorsal root ganglion compression. Although many patients can be successfully treated nonoperatively, surgery can be very beneficial for a subset of patients. The far-lateral space can be accessed safely and reproducibly using minimally invasive tubular retractors and microsurgery. A keen appreciation for the anatomy of this area is necessary for successful surgery. The extraforaminal technique affords excellent visualization to the Kambin's triangle

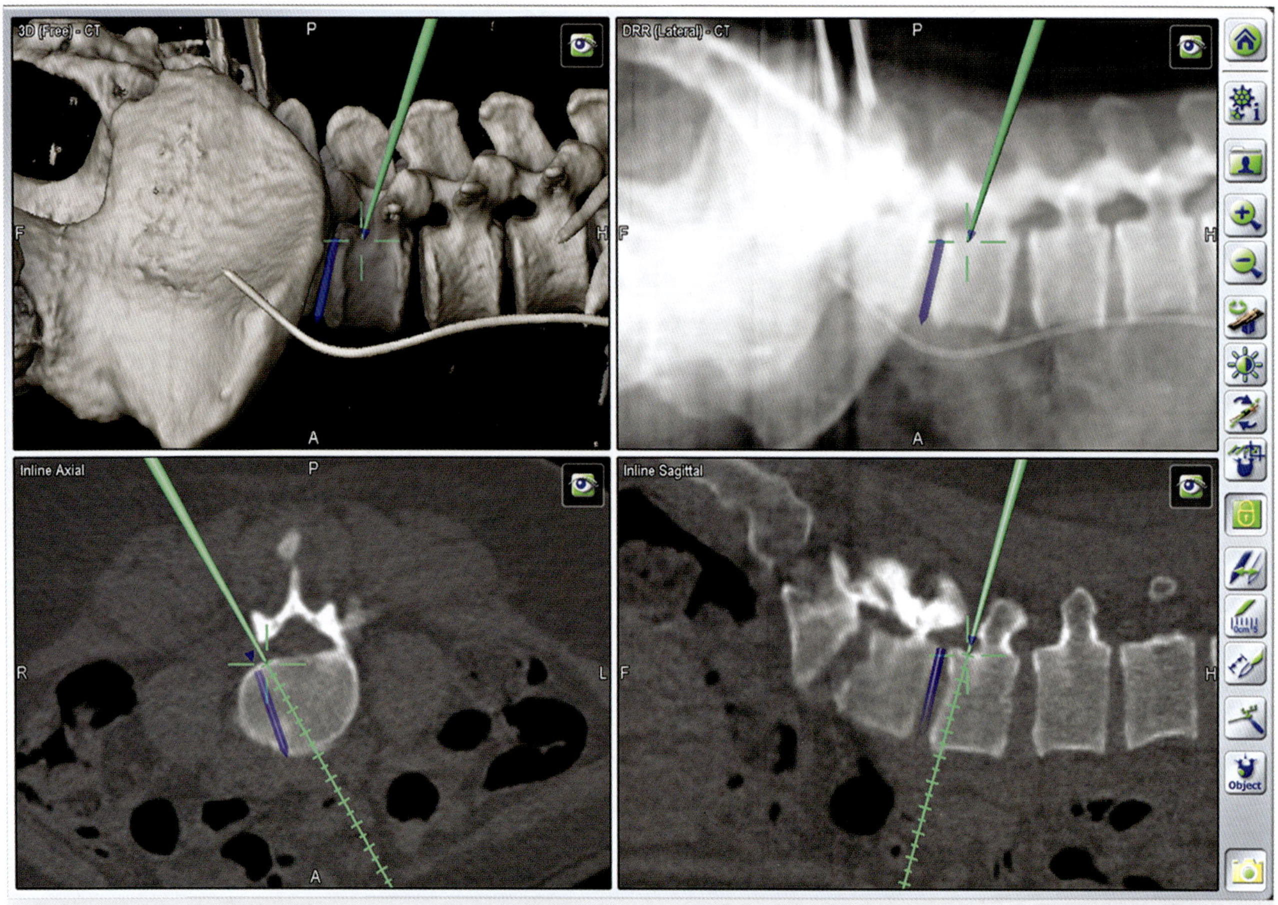

Fig. 33.7 Navigation window for surgical localization of right L4/L5 far-lateral herniated disc following performance of an intraoperative computed tomography (CT) scan. The L4/L5 disc space has been marked by a blue line and the navigation probe is being used through the tubular retractor to confirm the position at the extraforaminal space.

region encompassing the exiting nerve root, foramen, and disc. The described technique of docking on the lateral pars interarticularis and drilling the lateral pars exposes the ligamentum flavum as it extends laterally through the foramen. As the superior ligamentum flavum does not insert on the pedicle, this area is ideal to start resection of the ligament for exposure to the nerve and herniated disc. During the performance of the surgery, great care must be taken to avoid injury to the dorsal root ganglion or inadvertent disruption of radicular artery. The minimally invasive technique, compared to the more traditional open approach, can be performed quickly with far less muscle trauma and a quicker recovery for patients.

References

[1] Ebeling U, Reulen HJ. Are there typical localisations of lumbar disc herniations? A prospective study. Acta Neurochir (Wien). 1992; 117(3–4):143–148

[2] Epstein NE. Foraminal and far lateral lumbar disc herniations: surgical alternatives and outcome measures. Spinal Cord. 2002; 40(10):491–500

[3] Ohmori K, Kanamori M, Kawaguchi Y, Ishihara H, Kimura T. Clinical features of extraforaminal lumbar disc herniation based on the radiographic location of the dorsal root ganglion. Spine. 2001; 26(6):662–666

[4] Kambin P, Brager MD. Percutaneous posterolateral discectomy: anatomy and mechanism. Clin Orthop Relat Res. 1987(223):145–154

[5] Weinstein JN, Tosteson TD, Lurie JD, et al. Surgical vs nonoperative treatment for lumbar disc herniation: the Spine Patient Outcomes Research Trial (SPORT): a randomized trial. JAMA. 2006; 296(20):2441–2450

[6] Moliterno JA, Knopman J, Parikh K, et al. Results and risk factors for recurrence following single-level tubular lumbar microdiscectomy. J Neurosurg Spine. 2010; 12(6):680–686

[7] Arts MP, Brand R, van den Akker ME, et al. Tubular discectomy vs conventional microdiscectomy for the treatment of lumbar disc herniation: 2-year results of a double-blind randomized controlled trial. Neurosurgery. 2011; 69 (1):135–144, discussion 144

[8] Chang SB, Lee SH, Ahn Y, Kim JM. Risk factor for unsatisfactory outcome after lumbar foraminal and far lateral microdecompression. Spine. 2006; 31 (10):1163–1167

[9] Marquardt G, Bruder M, Theuss S, Setzer M, Seifert V. Ultra-long-term outcome of surgically treated far-lateral, extraforaminal lumbar disc herniations: a single-center series. Eur Spine J. 2012; 21(4):660–665

[10] Epstein NE. Different surgical approaches to far lateral lumbar disc herniations. J Spinal Disord. 1995; 8(5):383–394

[11] Virk MS, Elowitz E. A minimally invasive approach to the lumbar neural foramen and extraforaminal compartment: modified surgical technique. J Spine. 2014; 4:203–208

[12] Voyadzis JM, Gala VC, Sandhu FA, Fessler RG. Minimally invasive approach for far lateral disc herniations: results from 20 patients. Minim Invasive Neurosurg. 2010; 53(3):122–126

[13] Ee WW, Lau WL, Yeo W, Von Bing Y, Yue WM. Does minimally invasive surgery have a lower risk of surgical site infections compared with open spinal surgery? Clin Orthop Relat Res. 2014; 472(6):1718–1724

[14] O'Toole JE, Eichholz KM, Fessler RG. Surgical site infection rates after minimally invasive spinal surgery. J Neurosurg Spine. 2009; 11(4):471–476
[15] Park P, Upadhyaya C, Garton HJ, Foley KT. The impact of minimally invasive spine surgery on perioperative complications in overweight or obese patients. Neurosurgery. 2008; 62(3):693–699, discussion 693–699
[16] Kawaguchi Y, Matsui H, Tsuji H. Back muscle injury after posterior lumbar spine surgery: a histologic and enzymatic analysis. Spine. 1996; 21(8):941–944
[17] Lurie JD, Tosteson TD, Tosteson AN, et al. Surgical versus nonoperative treatment for lumbar disc herniation: eight-year results for the spine patient outcomes research trial. Spine. 2014; 39(1):3–16
[18] Wahezi SE, Lederman A, Elowitz EH, Singh JR. Conservative versus operative management for lumbosacral radiculopathy with motor deficit. PM R. 2015; 7(7):770–776
[19] Ahn Y, Kim JU, Lee BH, et al. Postoperative retroperitoneal hematoma following transforaminal percutaneous endoscopic lumbar discectomy. J Neurosurg Spine. 2009; 10(6):595–602
[20] Choi I, Ahn JO, So WS, Lee SJ, Choi IJ, Kim H. Exiting root injury in transforaminal endoscopic discectomy: preoperative image considerations for safety. Eur Spine J. 2013; 22(11):2481–2487

34 Percutaneous Full-Endoscopic Interlaminar Approach for Lumbar Pathologies: Disc Herniation and Lumbar Spinal Stenosis

Javier Quillo-Olvera and Jin-Sung Luke Kim

Summary

Recently, full-endoscopic techniques have emerged as a minimally invasive option for treating several spine diseases, demonstrating safety and effectiveness. The development of new endoscopic devices has allowed overcoming the anatomical barriers that prevented to reach the pathology. Among full-endoscopic procedures, the percutaneous endoscopic interlaminar approach for treating disc herniations and central or lateral recess stenosis is a very effective option. The procedure-related advantages include less iatrogenic impact for paravertebral soft tissue and facet joints. This chapter describes the technique for discectomy and lumbar decompression by using the aforementioned approach. Technical advice to avoid complications and tips for getting encouraging outcomes are also included in this chapter.

Keywords: central stenosis, endoscopic decompression, interlaminar approach, lateral recess stenosis, lumbar spinal stenosis, lumbar disc herniations, minimally invasive spine surgery, percutaneous endoscopy

34.1 Introduction

For the past two decades, full-endoscopic techniques have proven to be highly accurate and effective for lumbar disc herniations, achieving at least the same result as conventional surgery.[1,2,3,4] The interlaminar endoscopic approach is preferred for axillary type and migrated disc fragments,[5] especially in L5–S1, where transforaminal endoscopic technique can be technically demanding because of the high iliac crest, a large L5 transverse process, a large facet joint, or a narrowed disc space and foramen.[6] This approach allows focal neurologic decompression. More recently, the interlaminar endoscopic approach has been used to treat lumbar spinal stenosis (LSS).[1,7,8] The percutaneous endoscopic interlaminar approach has allowed the expansion of endoscopic surgical indications. LSS is one of the most common indications for lumbar spine surgery. In 2007, more than 37,500 surgeries for spinal stenosis were performed in Medicare patients in the United States alone, and the total cost was almost $1.65 billion.[9] The prevalence of LSS increases with age, and is estimated to be 9% in the general population and up to 47% in people over the age of 60.[10] Surgical decompression is the most common spine procedure performed in patients older than 65 years of age.[11,12] The hypertrophy of the ligamentum flavum, facet joints degeneration, and bulging disc lead to central or lateral narrowing of the spinal canal. The reduced space available for neural and vascular elements in the lumbar spine produces a clinical syndrome characterized by radiated leg pain with or without low back pain, which is exacerbated while standing/walking (claudication). The pain is absent when seated and improves when bending forward or with a wide-based gait.[13,14] The North American Spine Society defines LSS as "a clinical syndrome of the buttock or lower extremity pain, which may occur with or without back pain, associated with diminished space available for the neural and vascular elements in the lumbar spine."[12] The surgery is recommended after all conservative means fail.[15] The so-called decompressive lumbar laminectomy introduced by Henk Verbiest in 1954 was adopted as an alternative treatment for LSS.[16] However, the complications rate reported with open laminectomy in patients older than 75 years was 18%,[17,18] including a high prevalence of iatrogenic instability,[19,20] and mortality increased fourfold in patients older than 80 years.[21] The efficient decompression of neural structures while preserving most of the stabilizing components of the spine such as muscles, ligaments, facet joints, and bone is an advantage associated with the endoscopic interlaminar approach.[2] Moreover, a smaller skin incision with no need of muscular and neural retraction, the use of epidural anesthesia leading a complete communication between the surgeon and the patient to prevent a neural injury during whole procedure, a lower incidence of intraoperative complications and postoperative epidural fibrosis, shorter hospital stay, and faster return to normal daily activities are some of the advantages associated with this approach.[1,7,22] The abovementioned is especially important in elderly patients with several comorbidities and LSS; hence, the endoscopic interlaminar approach is a safe and feasible alternative to treat LSS. The development of new surgical tools, such as the endoscopic bone drill, flexible forceps, and new optic devices, has allowed overcoming the anatomical barriers to decompress the lumbar spinal canal. In this chapter, we present the percutaneous endoscopic interlaminar technique for discectomy and LSS.

34.2 Indications

The use of percutaneous endoscopic interlaminar approach is adequate in the following situations:

- Sequestered or nonsequestered disc herniation within the spinal canal.[1,3,6] The axillary type is more suitable for this approach.[23,24]
- Calcified disc herniations.[6,25]
- Upward and downward migrated disc herniations of up to 8 mm can be removed. This will depend on the vertical distance between the lower border of the L5 lamina and the upper border of the S1 lamina. In these cases, an endoscopic drill to enlarge the interlaminar window is necessary.[6,23,26]
- Recurrent disc herniation.[3]
- Intracanal L4–L5 disc herniations can be approached.[27,28]
- LSS can be classified into three categories according to the narrowing zone as follows: Central stenosis, lateral recess stenosis, and foraminal stenosis.[29,30] The percutaneous

endoscopic interlaminar approach for spinal decompression is more suitable for central and lateral recess stenosis. In our institution, the clinical criteria are neurogenic intermittent claudication and radiculopathy, which are refractory to conservative treatment for at least 12 weeks. The radiological criteria are monosegmental central or lateral recess stenosis on computed tomography (CT) and magnetic resonance imaging (MRI).[8]

34.3 Contraindications

Extraforaminal nerve entrapment is an absolute contraindication. However, foraminal stenosis is a relative contraindication. It depends on the surgeon's skills. Undercutting the inferior and superior articular process can release the traversing and exiting nerves through a highly addressed interlaminar contralateral endoscopic approach. segmental instability; degenerative spondylolisthesis of more than Meyerding Grade I; multidirectional rotation slide; scoliosis of more than 20 degrees; and coexisting pathological conditions such as neoplasms or infections.[8,31]

34.4 Preoperative Planning

The general workout consists of dynamic radiographs (flexion and extension) to exclude segmental instability.[32,33] The North American Spine Society suggests MRI as the best noninvasive imaging modality to evaluate the spinal canal anatomy in patients with radicular symptoms.[34]

For patients in whom there is a contraindication for MRI, the use of Myelo-CT or conventional myelography has been proposed for the diagnosis of LSS.[35] Information obtained from imaging studies are as follow: location of the herniated disc regarding traversing nerve root (axillary or shoulder type), interlaminar window area, diagnosis of central LSS or lateral recess stenosis, and the type of surgical target (bony element, soft tissue, or both).[36,37] The patient's symptoms will determine the side of decompression or if it will be unilateral or bilateral.

34.5 Patient Positioning

The procedure is performed under either general or regional anesthesia. Others like epidural or regional anesthesia could be used depending on the case complexity. The patient is positioned prone on a Jackson table with a Wilson frame. The operation table is adjustable to enable a kyphotic positioning for maximizing the interlaminar space[3,8,33] (▶ Fig. 34.1a).

34.6 Surgical Steps

34.6.1 Operating Room Setup

The optimal operating room setup is as follow: The patient is located at the center of the operating room (placed in prone position), and the surgeon should make the approach ipsilateral to the patient's symptoms side. If the patient does not have a dominant side of symptoms, the surgeon should stand on the left side of the patient to use his right hand (dominant hand) for working. Scrub nurse should stand along with the surgeon on the left side, and the assistant on the right side to the surgeon. The endoscopy and C-arm monitors are positioned in front of the surgeon. Next to the surgeon's right foot, the radiofrequency (RF) pedal is placed. Lastly, anesthesiology team is located cephalic to the patient (▶ Fig. 34.1b).

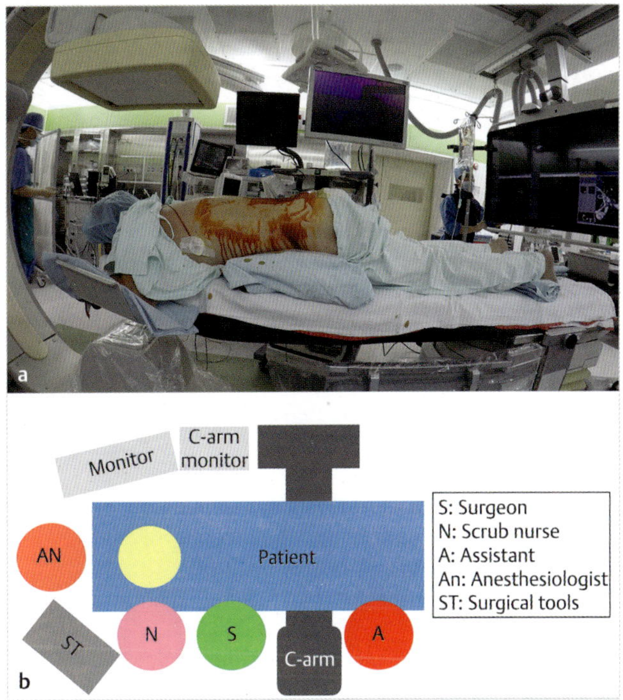

Fig. 34.1 (a) Patient positioning. (b) Operating room setup.

34.6.2 Surgical Tools

All surgical procedures for lumbar stenosis are performed with a complete endoscopic instrument set: Vertebris stenosis (RIWOspine GmbH, Knittlingen, Germany) (▶ Fig. 34.2) and Ilessys Delta® (Joimax GmbH, Raumfabrik 33A, Amalienbadstraße, 76227 Karlsruhe, Germany) (▶ Fig. 34.3). In the case of lumbar disc herniation, the endoscopic instrument set of Vertebris Lumbar is used. The characteristics of each system are summarized in ▶ Table 34.1. Two different endoscopic drill systems with different burrs are used to enlarge the interlaminar window, and remove bony structures or osteophytes: ART1 (RIWOspine GmbH, Knittlingen, Germany) and Shrill® (Joimax GmbH, Raumfabrik 33A, Amalienbadstraße, 76227 Karlsruhe, Germany). An endoscopic bipolar RF coagulator (Elliquence LLC, Baldwin, New York, USA) is useful for hemostasis and soft-tissue clearance in the surgical field, which is continuously irrigated with antibiotic-containing saline solution during whole procedure.

34.6.3 Surgical Approach

True anteroposterior (AP) and lateral intraoperative C-arm images should be used to mark the index level. The radiological landmarks recognized are the following: the inferior margin of the upper lamina and the spinous process. The entry point is planned on the midpoint between the spinous process and the lateral extension of the interlaminar window at the level of the

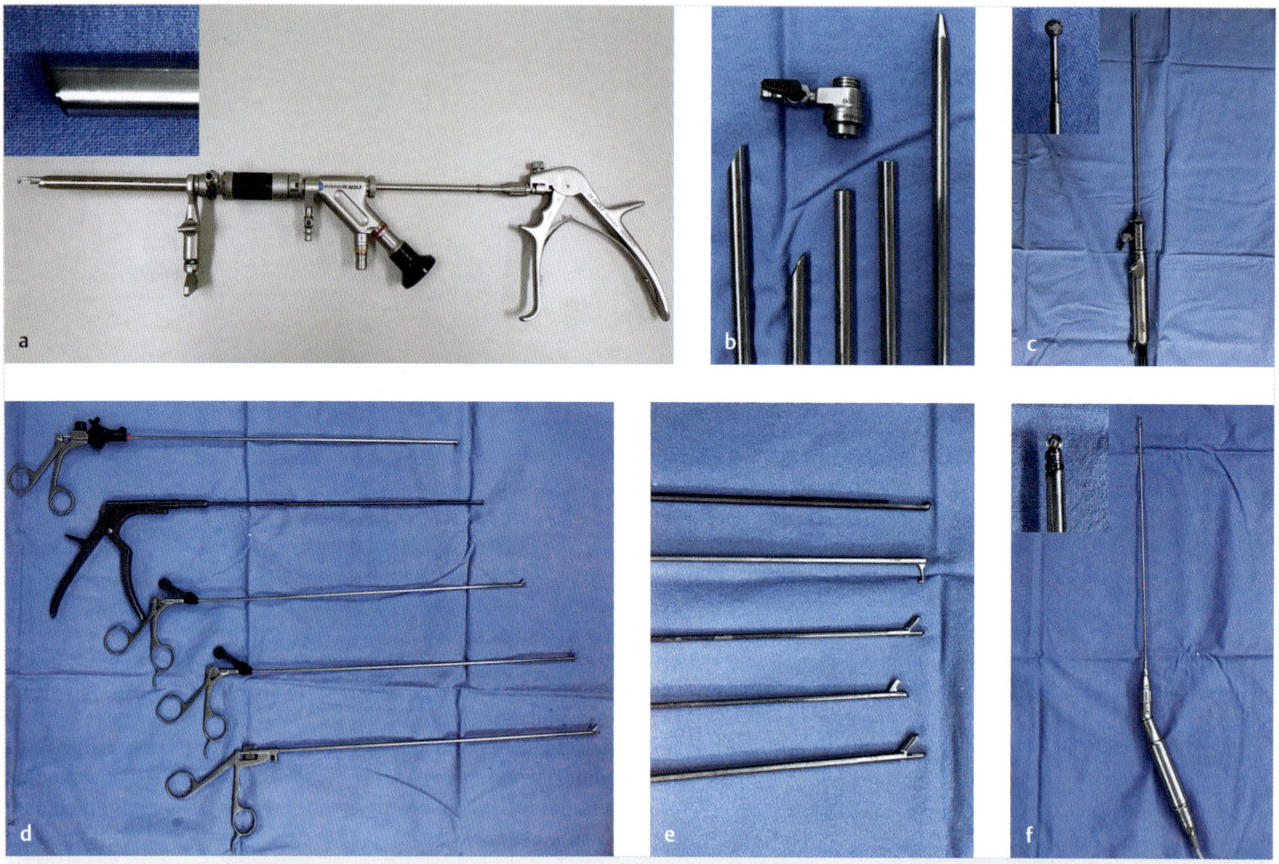

Fig. 34.2 Wolf® spinal endoscopic system: (a) 20-degree endoscope; (b) obturator and working cannulas; (c, f) endoscopic drill; (d, e) different types of rongeurs and nerve hook.

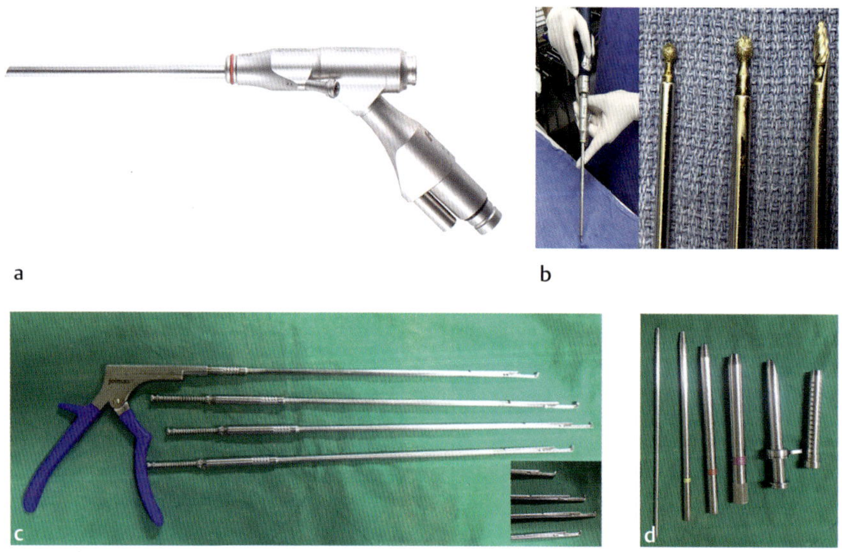

Fig. 34.3 Joimax® spinal endoscopic system: (a) 15-degree endoscope; (b) should change for the proper shrill system. (c) Kerrison rongeur with different types of tips; (d) obturator and working cannulas.

caudal margin of the upper lamina. Then the skin is infiltrated with approximately 2 or 3 mL of 1% lidocaine, and a paramedian skin incision of approximately 10 mm long is made; cutting the thick muscle fascia may facilitate the next step. Blunt insertion of serial dilator toward the target point is done under lateral projection of the C-arm. The working cannula is inserted through the final dilator with the beveled opening directed medially toward the ligamentum flavum, and the endoscope is passed through it (▶ Fig. 34.4).

Table 34.1 Characteristics of two different endoscopes used for percutaneous endoscopic interlaminar approach

	RIWOspine system	Joimax® system
Length (mm)	177	125
Total length (mm)	255	205
Out diameter (mm)	9.3	10
Working channel diameter (mm)	5.6	6
Operative angle (°)	20	15
Weight (g)	240	300

34.6.4 Endoscopic Interlaminar Approach for Discectomy

After general considerations such as operating room setup, patient positioning, and anesthesia, the use of prophylactic antibiotics for infection is recommended. An intraoperative C-arm AP and lateral views are useful for planning the entry point, which is made usually close to the midline for reaching the spinal canal with the least possible bone resection and the least disruption of the facet joint (▶ Video 34.1, Time 00:17). A 10-mm skin incision is made, and the fascia is also opened to facilitate the entrance of working instruments. The tissue is sequentially dilated and the beveled working cannula is inserted through the last dilator. The endoscopic system is inserted into the working cannula to perform discectomy under direct endoscopic vision (▶ Video 34.1, Time 00:25). Continuous irrigation with saline solution starts

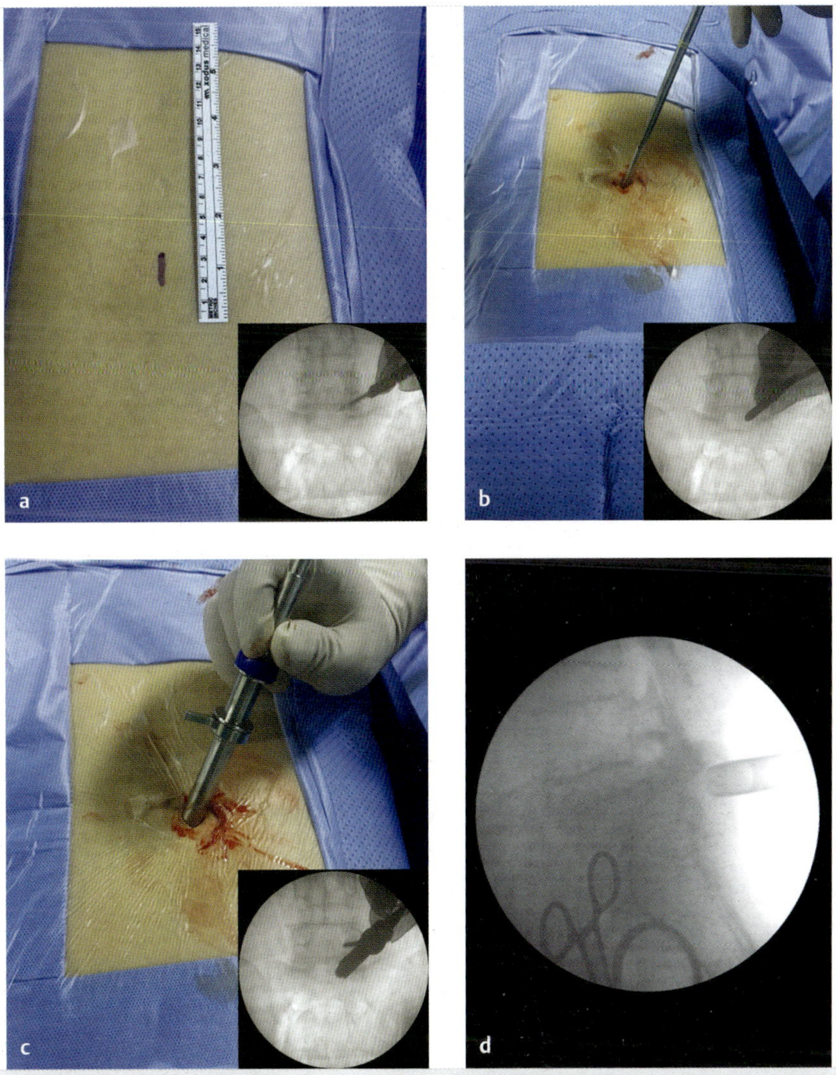

Fig. 34.4 Interlaminar endoscopic approach. **(a)** Paramedian skin incision located at the level of inferior margin of upper lamina. **(b)** Sequential dilation of paravertebral soft tissue. **(c)** Docked of working channel in the interlaminar space. **(d)** Intraoperative C-arm image on lateral view showing the proper location of working channel.

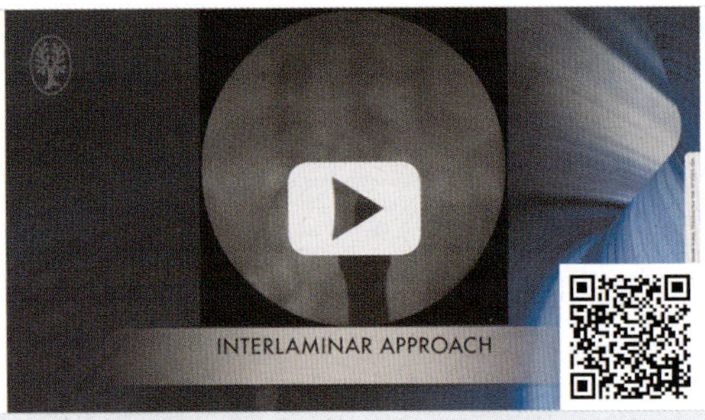

Video 34.1 Full-endoscopic lumbar interlaminar discectomy.

now. The tissue adjacent to the outer layer of the ligamentum flavum is cleared by the use of RF probe and endoscopic forceps (▶ Video 34.1, Time 00:29). The bone landmarks need to be recognized (upper and lower edge of the caudal and cephalic laminae, and the medial facet). When the interlaminar space is not very wide or the working cannula does not advance through this, the bone can be drilled enough to access the spinal canal using an endoscopic drill (▶ Video 34.1, Time 00:55). The ligamentum flavum is removed with a micropunch until the epidural space is observed (▶ Video 34.1, Time 01:40). The positive pressure of the continuous irrigation displaces the neural elements below the ligamentum flavum, which decreases the risk of neural element injury during flavectomy. The inner layer of the ligamentum flavum is removed to allow the passage of the endoscopic system. Afterwards, the traversing nerve root is observed, and the axillary space is reached (▶ Video 34.1, Time 02:10). When this space is enough to mobilize and remove the herniated disc, the surgeon can use the endoscopic forceps; otherwise when the space is limited in an axillary disc herniation, the beveled working cannula can be advanced to the spinal canal and rotated to retract with the bevel the dural sac medially and remove the axillary disc herniation (▶ Video 34.1, Time 02:09). In the case the herniated disc is located in the shoulder, a medial facetectomy should be done using the endoscopic drill to reach the fragment. The endoscopic nerve hook is used to explore the ventral epidural space and confirm that there is no residual disc (▶ Video 34.1, Time 02:33). Finally, the annular defect is sealed using an RF probe to reduce the risk of recurrence. The use of a drain after the surgery is not usually necessary for discectomies due to the minimal bleeding. When adequate hemostasis has been confirmed, the endoscope can be removed and the skin incision can be closed with a single suture (▶ Fig. 34.5). ▶ Table 34.2 summarizes the 10 steps of the technique.

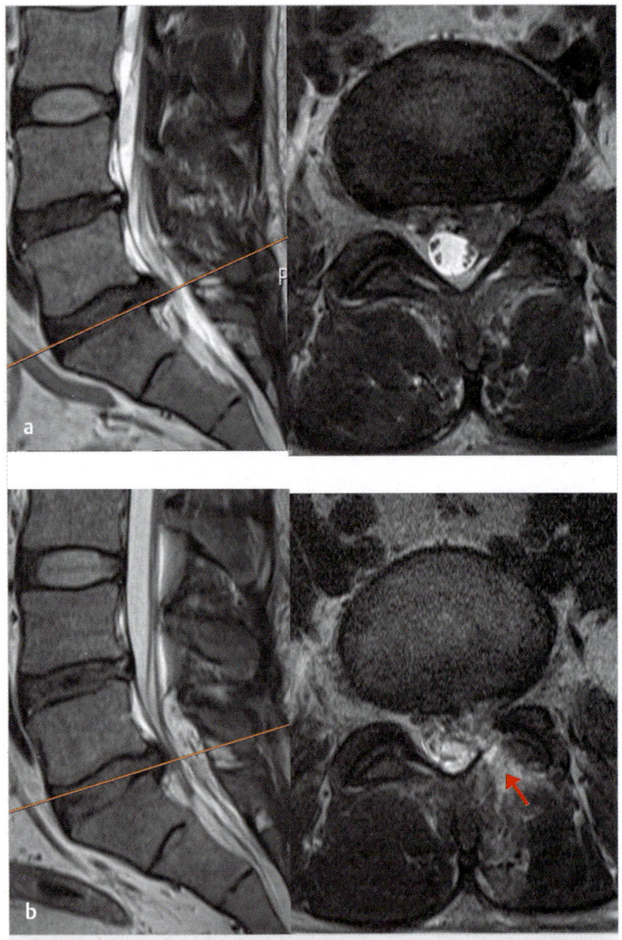

Fig. 34.5 **(a)** Superior panel: preoperative lumbar MRI showing a left-side L5-S1 subarticular disc herniation. **(b)** Inferior panel: postoperative lumbar MRI. The *red arrow* points to the interlaminar window and the small piece of flavum removed to get into the epidural space.

34.6.5 Ipsilateral Endoscopic Interlaminar Decompression

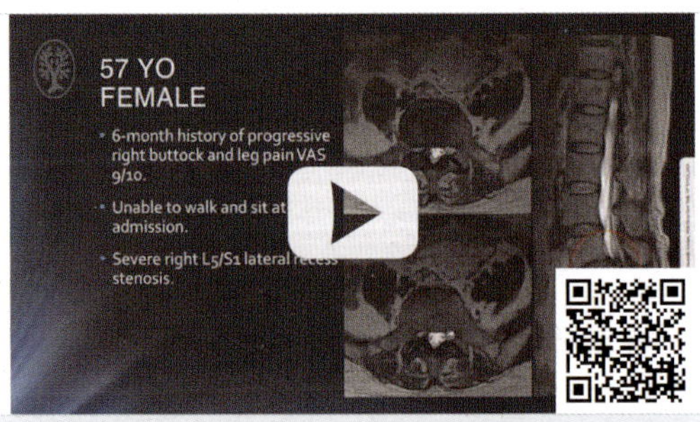

Video 34.2 Full-endoscopic interlaminar decompression for lumbar spinal stenosis.

Decompression is performed under gravity-operated continuous irrigation of saline, and direct endoscopic visual control. The continuous flow of saline helps to maintain a clear view through the endoscope and contributes to hemostasis. RF probe is used initially to clear the fat tissue overlaying the interlaminar space. The junction of the spinous process and cranial lamina is recognized (▶ Fig. 34.5a) and is used as a starting point for bone drilling (▶ Video 34.2, Time 00:52). Laminotomy is carried out from medial to lateral with the endoscopic drill and endo-Kerrison punch until the ligamentum flavum attachment is observed. A partial medial facetectomy is necessary to decompress the ipsilateral lateral recess (▶ Video 34.2, Time 01:29). The endpoint of the facetectomy is the medial margin of the superior articular process (SAP), which is drilled and removed with an endoscopic Kerrison punch (▶ Video 34.2, Time 01:43). The ligamentum flavum is left intact to protect the dura until the bone decompression is completed. The ligamentum flavum is lastly removed with the aid of endoscopic forceps (▶ Video 34.2, Time 02:16 and ▶ Fig. 34.6c).

Table 34.2 10 steps of percutaneous endoscopic interlaminar discectomy

1.	Locate the interlaminar space of the index level by using intraoperative C-arm AP and lateral views
2.	Make a 10-mm skin incision next to the spinous process of the index level
3.	Introduce the obturator and feel the bony landmarks: The inferior edge of the cranial lamina, superior edge of the caudal lamina, the spinolaminar junction medially, and the facet joint laterally
4.	Dilate paravertebral soft tissue sequentially with the sequential dilators, and dock the beveled working cannula through the last dilator. Then, introduce the endoscope with continuous irrigation system opened
5.	Clean the overlying soft tissue over the ligamentum flavum using bipolar coagulation of the RF probe and endoscopic forceps until the outer layer of ligamentum flavum is observed. Subsequently, remove the outer layer
6.	If necessary, enlarge the interlaminar window by using an endoscopic drill
7.	Use your endoscopic dissector to longitudinally split the inner layer of ligamentum flavum and to observe the epidural space. After that, you can use the endoscopic Kerrison punch to complete the flavectomy
8.	Clean the epidural fat tissue and vessels with RF probe until the neural elements are visible. Recognize the traversing nerve root laterally and the axillary space
9.	Advance the working cannula until the epidural space is reached and rotate it. The bevel can retract the dural sac medially and enlarge the axillary space. Use the endoscopic dissector to manipulate the extruded fragment and release the nerve root from adhesions. Remove the fragment with the endoscopic forceps and seal the annular fissure with the RF probe
10.	Confirm meticulous hemostasis and remove the endoscopic tools. Close the skin with a single suture

Abbreviations: AP, anteroposterior; RF, radiofrequency.

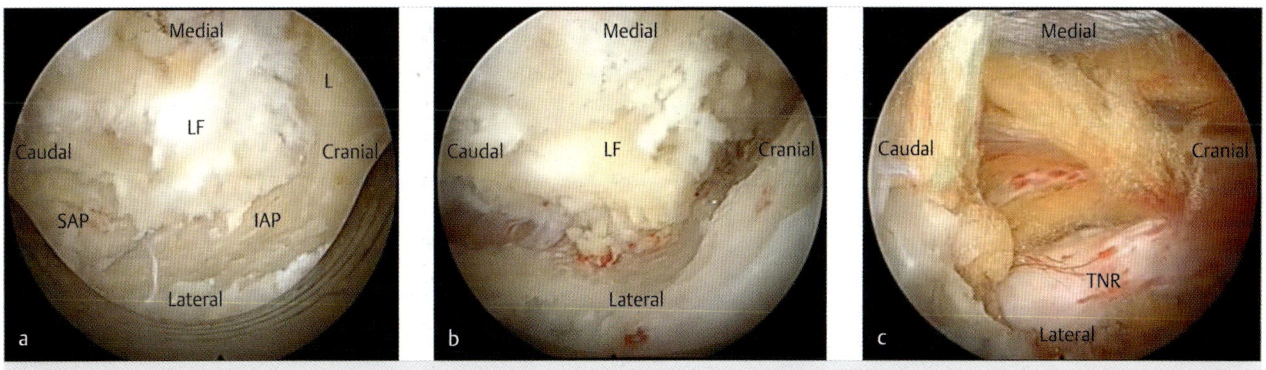

Fig. 34.6 Endoscopic view of a right interlaminar L5-S1 approach. **(a)** The image shows the bone elements and ligamentum flavum intact before laminotomy and flavectomy. **(b)** Interlaminar space enlarged after laminotomy and before flavectomy. **(c)** Traversing nerve root after lateral recess decompression. LF, ligamentum flavum; L, lamina; SAP, superior articular process; IAP, inferior articular process; TNR, traversing nerve root.

34.6.6 Contralateral Interlaminar Endoscopic Decompression

After adequate decompression of the ipsilateral side, the working cannula and endoscope are directed toward the contralateral side, which is decompressed dorsal to the dura by using the over-the-top technique. While the dural sac and contralateral nerve root are protected with the ligamentum flavum, the bone decompression using the under-cutting technique is done until the medial and ventral aspects of the contralateral facet joint are reached. The ventral margin of the contralateral SAP is observed and removed under direct endoscopic visualization by using the drill and endoscopic Kerrison punch, releasing the contralateral lateral recess. After removal of the overhanging lamina and bilateral lateral recess decompression has been achieved, we proceed to remove the exposed ligamentum flavum using endoscopic forceps. The decompression concludes when the dural sac and the bilateral traversing nerve roots are released from compression (▶ Fig. 34.7). Hemostasis is done using the RF probe; this device is especially used for those vessels located over the dura or in the epidural fat. Bleeding control is sometimes necessary for the ventral epidural vessels when the surgeon explores the traversing nerve root with the endoscopic nerve hook when feeling the nerve. ▶ Table 34.3 summarizes the 10 steps of the laminectomy technique.

34.6.7 Closure

In the cases of endoscopic decompression because of stenosis where an extensive bone drilling was performed, a drain is left postoperatively and removed one day after surgery. Finally, the skin is closed with a single suture (▶ Fig. 34.8).

34.7 Postoperative Care

Common postoperative indications are informed to patients undergoing endoscopic interlaminar approach for discectomy or decompression. Postoperative pain associated with full-endoscopic techniques is low. Therefore, oral analgesia 7 days after surgery is usually enough. Early mobilization out of bed, 2 hours after the procedure, depending on the severity of the case, is highly encouraged. As previously commented, LSS is prevalent after 65 years and patients have other comorbidities. Immediate postoperative mobilization decreases the risk of complications such as thrombosis, pneumonia, ileus, etc. The

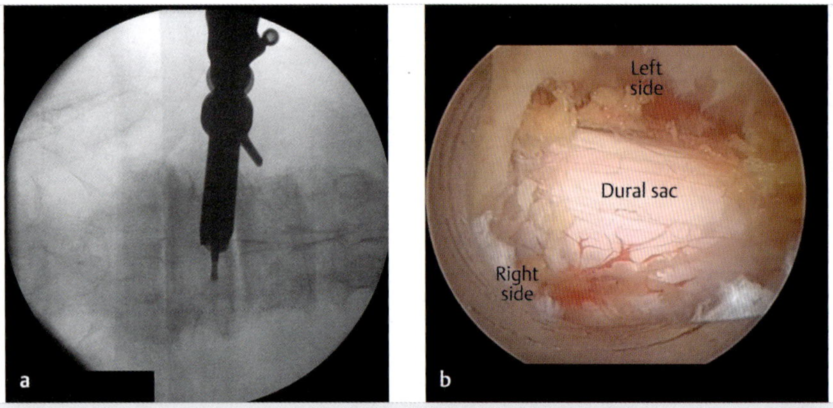

Fig. 34.7 Contralateral endoscopic decompression via interlaminar approach. **(a)** Intraoperative C-arm image showing the surgical tools crossing the midline. **(b)** Endoscopic view of bilateral decompression, both sides of dural sac can be observed.

Table 34.3 10 steps of percutaneous endoscopic interlaminar decompression for lumbar stenosis

1. Determine the radiological landmarks with intraoperative C-arm and make the incision
2. Feel the interlaminar space with the obturator; then dilate sequentially the paravertebral soft tissue with dilators
3. Locate the working channel with the beveled ending facing medially in the interlaminar space
4. Clean your surgical field by using the endoscopic RF probe and observe the landmarks: Inferior border of the cranial lamina, facet joint, and superior border of the caudal lamina
5. Make the laminotomy by using the endoscopic drill and Kerrison rongeur. Start with the cranial lamina from medial to lateral until the ligamentum flavum attachment is observed; repeat the same procedure with the caudal lamina
6. Ipsilateral recess decompression. Make a medial facetectomy until the superior articular process and the lateral attachment of ligamentum flavum are observed
7. Make the ipsilateral flavectomy after the bone removal. Observe the ipsilateral traversing nerve root
8. Contralateral decompression. Identify the base of the spinous process and undercut it. Once you have enlarged the sublaminar space, remove the ventral portion of the contralateral superior articular process
9. Conclude the contralateral flavectomy and release the contralateral traversing nerve root
10. Confirm a proper hemostasia, place an epidural drain, and close the skin incision with a single suture

Abbreviation: RF, radiofrequency.

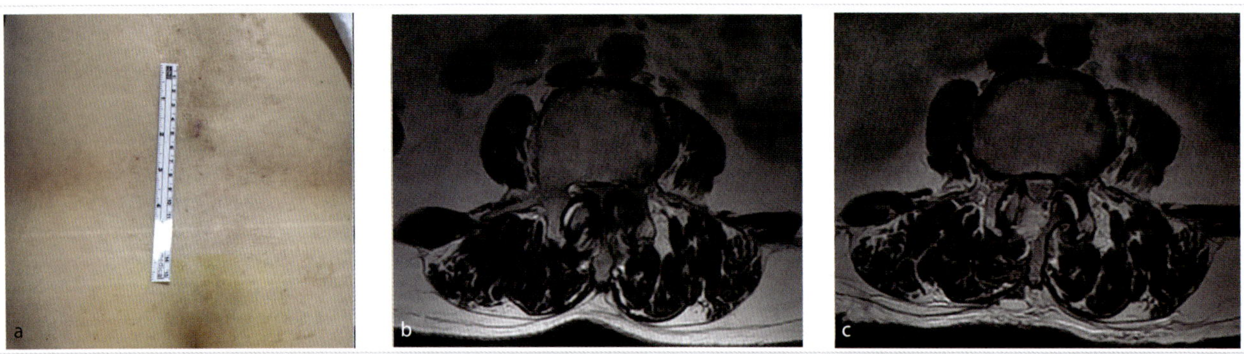

Fig. 34.8 Radiological outcomes after L3-4 interlaminar endoscopic decompression. **(a)** Preoperative T2-weighted MRI on axial view shows central stenosis. **(b)** Immediate postoperative MRI shows enough decompression. **(c)** Postoperative skin incision.

drain is removed one day after surgery in the morning, and the patient's discharge is evaluated. During hospital discharge, postoperative indications are given to all patients with the aim to decrease pain at home and back muscle spasm. The patient is seen 12 days after surgery in the outpatient clinic to remove the single skin suture and assess reincorporation to normal activities. Rehabilitation is considered just for patients with motor deficits. A postoperative MRI 1 day after surgery may be required to evaluate the radiological results of decompression.

The endoscopic approach for lumbar decompression is a logical next step for those who master the tubular decompression. We are still in the early stages of endoscopic decompression surgery and can expect significant advances in techniques and training strategies that will allow surgeons to incorporate these into their practice.

34.8 Complication Avoidance

The rate of complications related to endoscopic discectomy via interlaminar approach is low. Ruetten reported no operation-related complications in more than 1,500 full-endoscopic interlaminar discectomies.[3] However, recurrence is the most important complication associated with percutaneous endoscopic interlaminar discectomy.[6,38,39] The overall rate of recurrence is 10.3%, which can decrease to 5.5% with annular sealing after fragmentectomy or sequestrectomy.[40] Also, we recommend do not enlarge the annular fissure with microforceps or endoscopic punches. By using the endoscopic dissector, you can manipulate the disc fragment before removing it. Incomplete decompression because of residual fragment results in persistent radicular pain without a pain-free interval after the procedure. It is associated with high-canal compromise (more than 40% occupation of the spinal canal by disc herniation) and high-grade migrations (in case of high-grade upward migration, the extent of migration is located above the half of the infrapedicle level and in case of high-grade downward migration, the extent of the migration is located below the suprapedicle level).[23] For that reason, recognizing the endpoint of surgery is very important. That point can be evaluated by mobilizing the neural structures without restriction and exploring the shoulder and axillary areas with the endoscopic nerve hook.[41] Although the nerve root injury has a low incidence, it can occur. Sometimes, inflammatory changes within the spinal canal can cause adhesions between the neural elements and ligamentum flavum. During flavectomy, this should be kept in mind so as not to injure any neural element. Any blind maneuver should not be done inside the spinal canal during a bleeding. First, a gentle and correct hemostasis with the RF probe must be performed.[41] Dural tears and cerebrospinal leakage during endoscopic interlaminar discectomy are not common but possible complications. Avoiding aggressive maneuvers to expose the neural tissue and carefully using endoscopic disc forceps during discectomy in cases where the disc fragment has firm adhesions to dura are safer.[41] Percutaneous endoscopic interlaminar decompression is a feasible procedure for central and lateral recess stenosis of the lumbar spine. Surgeons are familiar with anatomy seen through a posterior approach because of similarity of the technique with open laminectomy. If a complication occurs during surgery, it could be converted to open surgery easily. A proper approach consists of a good landing of the working cannula in the interlaminar window; the sagittal and coronal angles for approaching the interlaminar space depend on the stenotic pathological target (central, lateral recess, or both). It could avoid insufficient decompression. Ligamentum flavum should be left intact until bone removal is done. It may protect the neural structures while the surgeon performs the bone resection. Early exposure of the dural sac with not enough decompression increase the risk of dura and nerve injury, or increased epidural pressure. The central and lateral dorsal surfaces of the dural sac should be seen after decompression to ensure proper central and lateral recess decompression. During lateral recess decompression, an excessive medial facetectomy with the endo-drill and Kerrison punch should be avoided since this could lead iatrogenic instability.[3,8,23,42,43]

34.9 Tips and Tricks

- Misplacement of the working cannula during the exposure of ligamentum flavum and the failure to recognize the anatomical landmarks during the discectomy are potential causes for conversion to open surgery.
- Preoperative planning and the knowledge of the exact location of the disc herniation are mandatory before performing the endoscopic interlaminar discectomy.
- The extent of decompression should be checked by using intraoperative fluoroscopy in AP and lateral views. It could be possible identifying the surgical tools crossing the midline.
- Perform the procedure step by step as follows: First the ipsilateral laminotomy and medial facetectomy. Then the contralateral laminotomy and the undercutting of the contralateral recess. Finally, perform complete flavectomy.
- Preserve the tissues covering the dura and nerves as much as possible. Less manipulation of the neural elements reduces the risk of injuring them.
- Use the beveled ending of the working cannula as a retractor. Rotate the operating sheath, and beveled opening protects the neural structures during bone removal or flavectomy.
- The endpoint of medial facetectomy is when the traversing nerve root can be visualized easily.
- The surgeon should be aware of blind spots under endoscopic view, especially during the use of drills, forceps, or Kerrison punches into the epidural space. Some maneuvers with the endoscope during these steps such as tilting or rotating the endoscope helps to identify the blind areas beyond the surgical tools and therefore reduces the risk of incidental durotomy or neural injury.
- When bleeding obscures the surgical field try increasing the pressure of the saline irrigation until the source is detected; then use the RF probe to coagulate the vessel. Avoid blind maneuvers.
- Avoid the use of RF probe with high intensity around neural structures in order to prevent postoperative dysesthesia.
- After recognizing the traversing nerve root, perform the lysis of adhesions before retracting it with the endoscopic nerve hook. This decreases the risk of neural damage.

34.10 Conclusion

The percutaneous endoscopic interlaminar discectomy is a highly effective procedure with a low rate of complications. This technique needs deep knowledge of anatomical structures surrounding the neural elements, which will be visualized directly under endoscopic view. The same approach can be used for decompression of neural structures in the setting of LSS (central and lateral recess). The procedure is a safe and effective option with the advantages associated with minimally invasive procedures in the spine. Therefore, it is a recommended option for

surgeons with experience in endoscopic spine surgery for treating this pathology.

References

[1] Ruetten S, Komp M, Merk H, Godolias G. Full-endoscopic interlaminar and transforaminal lumbar discectomy versus conventional microsurgical technique: a prospective, randomized, controlled study. Spine. 2008; 33(9):931–939

[2] Casimiro M. Short-term outcome comparison between full-endoscopic interlaminar approach and open minimally invasive microsurgical technique for treatment of lumbar disc herniation. World Neurosurg. 2017; 108:894–900.e1

[3] Ruetten S. The full-endoscopic interlaminar approach for lumbar disc herniations. In: Mayer HM, ed. Minimally Invasive Spine Surgery: A Surgical Manual. Berlin, Heidelberg: Springer-Verlag; 2006:346–355

[4] Birkenmaier C, Komp M, Leu HF, Wegener B, Ruetten S. The current state of endoscopic disc surgery: review of controlled studies comparing full-endoscopic procedures for disc herniations to standard procedures. Pain Physician. 2013; 16(4):335–344

[5] Choi KC, Kim JS, Ryu KS, Kang BU, Ahn Y, Lee SH. Percutaneous endoscopic lumbar discectomy for L5-S1 disc herniation: transforaminal versus interlaminar approach. Pain Physician. 2013; 16(6):547–556

[6] Choi G, Lee SH, Raiturker PP, Lee S, Chae YS. Percutaneous endoscopic interlaminar discectomy for intracanalicular disc herniations at L5-S1 using a rigid working channel endoscope. Neurosurgery. 2006; 58(1) Suppl:ONS59–ONS68, discussion ONS59–ONS68

[7] Nellensteijn J, Ostelo R, Bartels R, Peul W, van Royen B, van Tulder M. Transforaminal endoscopic surgery for symptomatic lumbar disc herniations: a systematic review of the literature. Eur Spine J. 2010; 19(2):181–204

[8] Ahn Y. Percutaneous endoscopic decompression for lumbar spinal stenosis. Expert Rev Med Devices. 2014; 11(6):605–616

[9] Bagley C, MacAllister M, Dosselman L, Moreno J, Aoun SG, El Ahmadieh TY. Current concepts and recent advances in understanding and managing lumbar spine stenosis. F1000Res. 2019; 8:F1000 Faculty Rev-137

[10] Kalichman L, Cole R, Kim DH, et al. Spinal stenosis prevalence and association with symptoms: the Framingham Study. Spine J. 2009; 9(7):545–550

[11] Gibson JN, Waddell G. Surgery for degenerative lumbar spondylosis: updated Cochrane Review. Spine. 2005; 30(20):2312–2320

[12] Deyo RA, Gray DT, Kreuter W, Mirza S, Martin BI. United States trends in lumbar fusion surgery for degenerative conditions. Spine. 2005; 30(12):1441–1445, discussion 1446–1447

[13] Watters WC , III, Baisden J, Gilbert TJ, et al. North American Spine Society. Degenerative lumbar spinal stenosis: an evidence-based clinical guideline for the diagnosis and treatment of degenerative lumbar spinal stenosis. Spine J. 2008; 8(2):305–310

[14] de Schepper EI, Overdevest GM, Suri P, et al. Diagnosis of lumbar spinal stenosis: an updated systematic review of the accuracy of diagnostic tests. Spine. 2013; 38(8):E469–E481

[15] Zaina F, Tomkins-Lane C, Carragee E, Negrini S. Surgical versus nonsurgical treatment for lumbar spinal stenosis. Spine. 2016; 41(14):E857–E868

[16] Verbiest H. A radicular syndrome from developmental narrowing of the lumbar vertebral canal. J Bone Joint Surg Br. 1954; 36-B(2):230–237

[17] Deyo RA, Cherkin DC, Loeser JD, Bigos SJ, Ciol MA. Morbidity and mortality in association with operations on the lumbar spine. The influence of age, diagnosis, and procedure. J Bone Joint Surg Am. 1992; 74(4):536–543

[18] Carreon LY, Puno RM, Dimar JR , II, Glassman SD, Johnson JR. Perioperative complications of posterior lumbar decompression and arthrodesis in older adults. J Bone Joint Surg Am. 2003; 85(11):2089–2092

[19] Johnsson KE, Willner S, Johnsson K. Postoperative instability after decompression for lumbar spinal stenosis. Spine. 1986; 11(2):107–110

[20] Lee CK. Lumbar spinal instability (olisthesis) after extensive posterior spinal decompression. Spine. 1983; 8(4):429–433

[21] Jansson KA, Blomqvist P, Granath F, Németh G. Spinal stenosis surgery in Sweden 1987–1999. Eur Spine J. 2003; 12(5):535–541

[22] Mayer HM, Brock M. Percutaneous endoscopic discectomy: surgical technique and preliminary results compared to microsurgical discectomy. J Neurosurg. 1993; 78(2):216–225

[23] Choi KC, Lee DC, Shim HK, Shin SH, Park CK. A strategy of percutaneous endoscopic lumbar discectomy for migrated disc herniation. World Neurosurg. 2017; 99:259–266

[24] Dezawa A, Sairyo K. New minimally invasive discectomy technique through the interlaminar space using a percutaneous endoscope. Asian J Endosc Surg. 2011; 4(2):94–98

[25] Dabo X, Ziqiang C, Yinchuan Z, et al. The clinical results of percutaneous endoscopic interlaminar discectomy (PEID) in the treatment of calcified lumbar disc herniation: a case-control study. Pain Physician. 2016; 19(2):69–76

[26] Ruetten S, Komp M, Merk H, Godolias G. Use of newly developed instruments and endoscopes: full-endoscopic resection of lumbar disc herniations via the interlaminar and lateral transforaminal approach. J Neurosurg Spine. 2007; 6 (6):521–530

[27] Nakamura JI, Yoshihara K. Initial clinical outcomes of percutaneous full-endoscopic lumbar discectomy using an interlaminar approach at the L4–L5. Pain Physician. 2017; 20(4):E507–E512

[28] Koga H, Inanami H. Minimal laminectomy using the interlaminar approach for percutaneous endoscopic lumbar discectomy. Mini-invasive Surg. 2017; 1:56–62

[29] Speciale AC, Pietrobon R, Urban CW, et al. Observer variability in assessing lumbar spinal stenosis severity on magnetic resonance imaging and its relation to cross-sectional spinal canal area. Spine. 2002; 27(10):1082–1086

[30] Andreisek G, Imhof M, Wertli M, et al. Lumbar Spinal Stenosis Outcome Study Working Group Zurich. A systematic review of semiquantitative and qualitative radiologic criteria for the diagnosis of lumbar spinal stenosis. AJR Am J Roentgenol. 2013; 201(5):W735–W746

[31] Lee CW, Yoon KJ, Jun JH. Percutaneous endoscopic laminotomy with flavectomy by uniportal, unilateral approach for the lumbar canal or lateral recess stenosis. World Neurosurg. 2018; 113:e129–e137–; [Epub ahead of print]

[32] Kim HS, Paudel B, Jang JS, et al. Percutaneous full endoscopic bilateral lumbar decompression of spinal stenosis through uniportal-contralateral approach: techniques and preliminary results. World Neurosurg. 2017; 103:201–209

[33] Birjandian Z, Emerson S, Telfeian AE, Hofstetter CP. Interlaminar endoscopic lateral recess decompression-surgical technique and early clinical results. J Spine Surg. 2017; 3(2):123–132

[34] Kreiner DS, Shaffer WO, Baisden JL, et al. North American Spine Society. An evidence-based clinical guideline for the diagnosis and treatment of degenerative lumbar spinal stenosis (update). Spine J. 2013; 13(7):734–743

[35] Bartynski WS, Lin L. Lumbar root compression in the lateral recess: MR imaging, conventional myelography, and CT myelography comparison with surgical confirmation. AJNR Am J Neuroradiol. 2003; 24(3):348–360

[36] Choi G, Deshpande K, Asawasaksakul A, Lee SH. New era of percutaneous endoscopic lumbar surgery: lumbar stenosis decompression—a technical report. J Spine. 2014; 3(5):182

[37] Passacantilli E, Lenzi J, Caporlingua F, et al. Endoscopic interlaminar approach for intracanal L5-S1 disc herniation: classification of disc prolapse in relation to learning curve and surgical outcome. Asian J Endosc Surg. 2015; 8(4):445–453

[38] Ruetten S, Komp M, Godolias G. A new full-endoscopic technique for the interlaminar operation of lumbar disc herniations using 6-mm endoscopes: prospective 2-year results of 331 patients. Minim Invasive Neurosurg. 2006; 49(2):80–87

[39] Chen HT, Tsai CH, Chao SC, et al. Endoscopic discectomy of L5-S1 disc herniation via an interlaminar approach: prospective controlled study under local and general anesthesia. Surg Neurol Int. 2011; 2:93

[40] Kim HS, Park JY. Comparative assessment of different percutaneous endoscopic interlaminar lumbar discectomy (PEID) techniques. Pain Physician. 2013; 16(4):359–367

[41] Xie TH, Zeng JC, Li ZH, et al. Complications of lumbar disc herniation following full-endoscopic interlaminar lumbar discectomy: a large, single-center, retrospective study. Pain Physician. 2017; 20(3):E379–E387

[42] Ruetten S, Komp M, Merk H, Godolias G. Surgical treatment for lumbar lateral recess stenosis with the full-endoscopic interlaminar approach versus conventional microsurgical technique: a prospective, randomized, controlled study. J Neurosurg Spine. 2009; 10(5):476–485

[43] Komp M, Hahn P, Merk H, Godolias G, Ruetten S. Bilateral operation of lumbar degenerative central spinal stenosis in full-endoscopic interlaminar technique with unilateral approach: prospective 2-year results of 74 patients. J Spinal Disord Tech. 2011; 24(5):281–287

35 Transforaminal Approach for Endoscopic Decompression

Ralf Wagner

Summary
The transforaminal approach for endoscopic decompression gives different options for accessing a disc herniation or spinal stenosis. Different techniques should be chosen depending on the pathology. Diverse tools and instruments allow approaching the spinal canal in almost any possible direction, only limited by neural structures or anatomic borders, such as the retroperitoneal organs. Small changes in entry point and needle angulation make a difference in clinical outcome. Thorough preparation of the surgery is essential to avoid complications. The endoscopic surgeon should choose the approach with the least bone destruction to guarantee a safe and fast procedure. The key to success in endoscopic decompression surgery for degenerative lumbar spine disease is to work on the bone, not in the disc.

Keywords: endoscopic decompression, migrated disc, foraminal stenosis, lumbar stenosis, disc herniation, transforaminal approach, intracanal technique, transpedicular technique

35.1 Introduction

In a lumbar motion segment, the neuroforamen consists of the superior articular facet (or superior articulating process = SAP, see ▶ Fig. 35.1), lower and upper pedicle, posterior wall of the cranial and caudal vertebra, the disc, the interarticular portion, and the flaval ligament. The posterior intervertebral disc, covered by the lateral expansion of the posterior longitudinal ligament, provides a major part of the ventral border of the neuroforamen. The joint capsule of the articular facet and the ligamentum flavum contribute as major components of its dorsal limitation.[1] Loss of the disc space leads to a subluxation and spondylophyte formation of the facet joint, changes in biomechanical forces, and hypertrophy of the ligamentum flavum. The loss of disc height in the intervertebral space and apposition of bone and ligamentous structures result in a narrowing of neural structures in the spinal canal or the neuroforamen.[2,3]

Spinal stenosis is a wide term for different entities that decrease the available space for the neural structures in the spinal canal. Lateral spinal root stenosis occurs in 8 to 11% of surgical cases of lumbar degenerative disease. Lumbar spondylolysis, hypertrophy of the superior facet joints, hypertrophy of the ligamentum flavum, disc bulge, protrusion, and osteophyte formation can lead to an impingement of the exiting nerve root[4,5] (▶ Fig. 35.1). According to Postacchini three different forms of degenerative lumbar spinal stenosis can be identified.[6] The term central stenosis includes: (a) stenosis of the central part of the spinal canal, which also often involves the lateral recess; (b) lateral recess stenosis, which often affects the course of the traversing nerve root; and (c) foraminal stenosis leading to compression of the exiting nerve.

The intervertebral foramen and its elliptical shape are responsible for many of its relational problems. The vertical diameter of the foramen varies from 12 to 19 mm. A complete disc collapse rarely contributes to nerve compression; however, the sagittal diameter may be as little as 7 mm. Especially in L4/L5 and L5/S1, the tolerance for pathological alterations is limited.[1] Dynamic changes in the lumbar neuroforaminal dimensions were observed in positional magnetic resonance imaging (MRI) of young adults, showing an increase in flexion and decrease in extension of all motion segments except L5/S1. Lumbar angular motion showed an effect at L3/L4 and L4/L5 foraminal width only.[7]

Transforaminal ligaments are frequently found in the intervertebral foramen, often limiting the space of the exiting nerve root.[8,9] The dorsal root ganglion (DRG) may measure over 6 mm and is often located in the neuroforaminal space at the level of L5/S1. Width of pedicles and DRG increase from L1 to L5. The DRG is found more lateral while going from L1 to L5.[10] Kikuchi et al determined the location of the DRG at L5 to be 19.2% intraspinal, 72.8% intraforaminal, and 8% extraforaminal, also potentially limiting the transforaminal approach at the level of L5/S1 and effecting the postoperative course.[11] Dynamic linear movement of the DRG of up to 5 mm with increasing movement

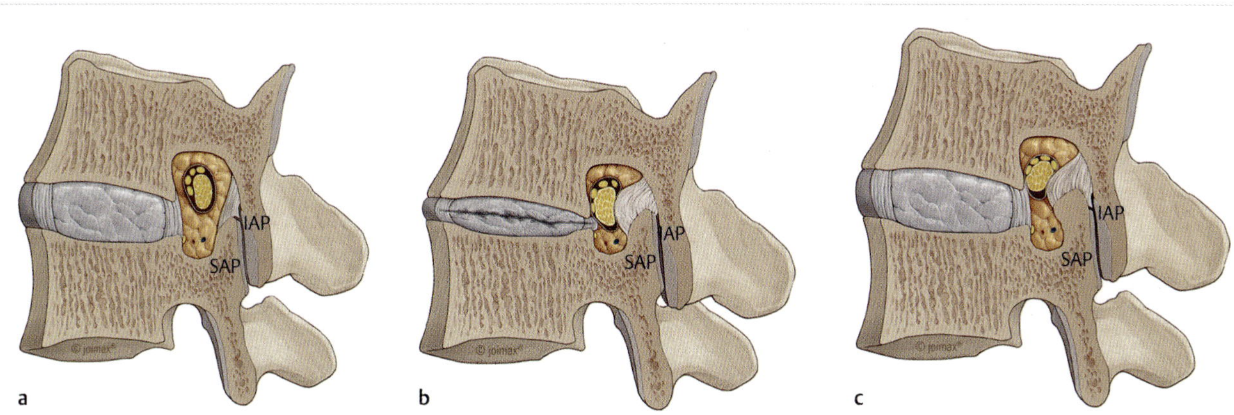

Fig. 35.1 **(a)** Physiological foramen intervertebrale; **(b)** loss of disc height with hypertrophy of ligamentum flavum and narrowing; **(c)** Processus articularis stenosis, facet subluxation, and nerve impingement. IAP, inferior articular process; SAP, superior articular process.

during hip flexion of 30 degrees was observed in cadaver studies by Smith et al.[12]

The foraminal ligaments might limit distal displacement of the exiting nerve roots.[13] A central or lateral recess stenosis leads to an anterior shifting of the traversing nerve root, which needs to be evaluated before surgery. Disc herniations may also displace the traversing nerve root laterally and therefore increase the risk of injury. Highly migrated disc herniations as well as hidden zone pathologies require a clear and structured preoperative planning.[14,15]

The endoscopic approach highly depends on the location of the pathology. Preoperative evaluation of the patient's anatomy and radiological and clinical findings have to be considered altogether to find the appropriate endoscopic approach to the lumbar spine.

35.2 Indications

The transforaminal endoscopic approach is used for disc herniations in all areas of the lumbar spine, lateral recess stenosis, central spinal stenosis, foraminal stenosis as well as extraforaminal pathologies (▸ Fig. 35.2). This approach can be advantageous for recurrent disc herniations after microdiscectomy, adjacent level disease after fusion, facet joint cysts, discitis as well as resection of displaced bone fragments after fusion or arthroplasty.

35.3 Contraindications

Although there is no clear contraindication, some clinical findings make the surgery far more difficult: nerve root anomalies, such as low exiting nerve root or doubled nerve root; high iliac crest for level L5/S1; primary or secondary spinal stenosis in combination with hypertrophic facet joints; severe spinal deformity; and severe spondylolisthesis (Grade II Meyerding or higher).

35.4 Preoperative Planning

The physical examination of the patient helps in localizing the affected nerve root. The neurological examination and the nerve root tension sign are obligatory to further locate the compressed nerve root. In multiple degenerative lumbar pathologies, facet joint blocks or radicular blocks are used to further define the symptomatic level. The imaging diagnosis consists of (i) plain X-ray films in standing posture to detect a high iliac crest or sclolio-sis, (ii) flexion and extension X-ray to rule out instability, and (iii) MRI scans of the lumbar spine. A computed tomography (CT) scan might be useful to determine calcifications in chronic lesions. The clinical symptoms of the patient should have a correlate on the imaging diagnostics. In disc herniations, the exact location of the traversing nerve root, sequester size, and spinal canal anatomy should be evaluated preoperatively. In case of stenosis, the extent of compression determines the amount of bone removal.

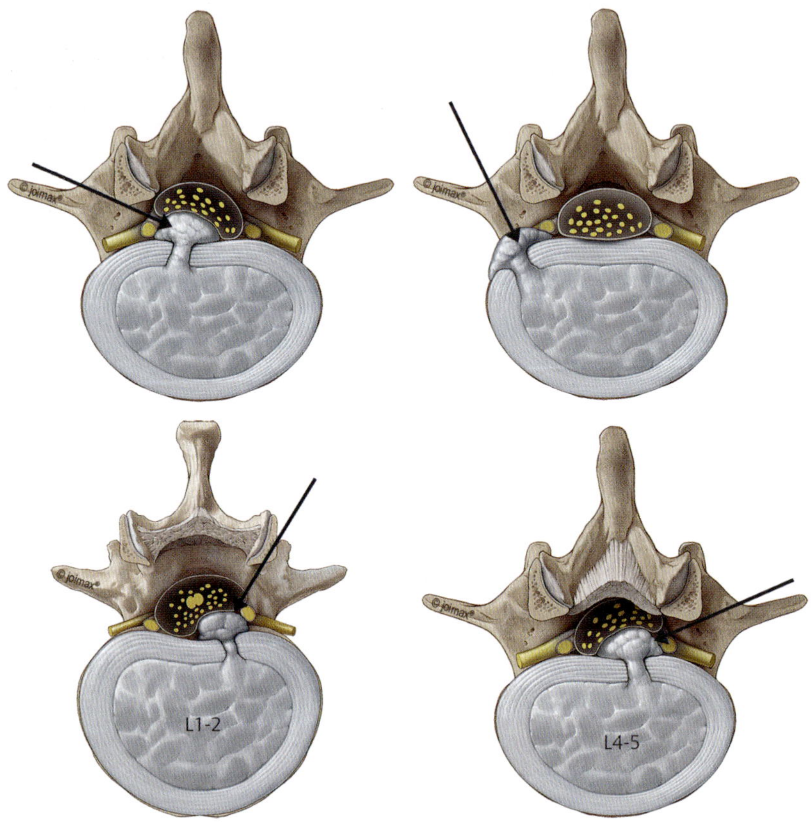

Fig. 35.2 Pathology determined approaches.

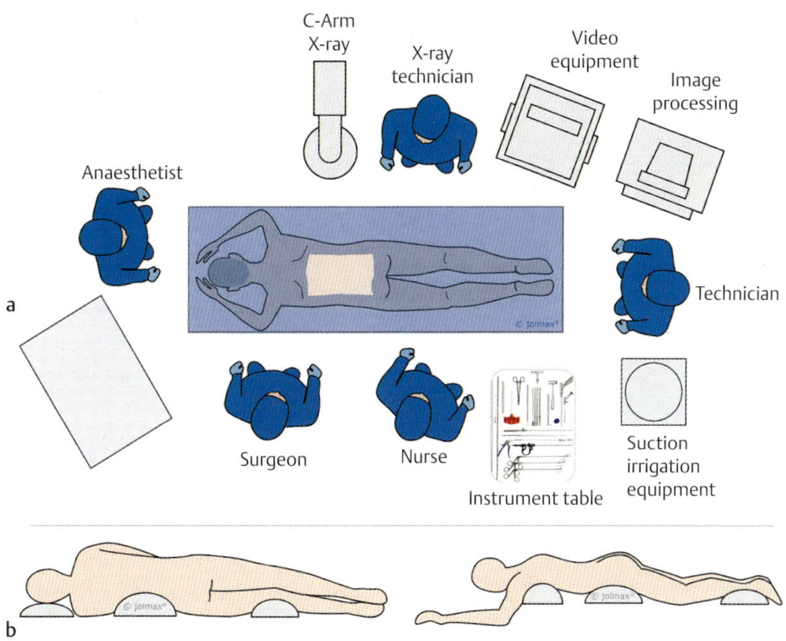

Fig. 35.3 **(a)** Operating room (OR) setup; **(b)** lateral and prone patient positions.

35.5 Patient Positioning

The patient can be posititioned in the prone or lateral position (▶ Fig. 35.3). Advantages of the prone position are an easier orientation for the surgeon, the possibility of bilateral surgery, and combined interlaminar and transforaminal surgery. The degree of required side bending or delordosing is less in prone position. The abdominal pressure on the epidural veins should be avoided by correct patient positioning. The lateral position has advantages in obese patients, in patients with deformity, and in surgeries under local anesthesia. The table can be angled to achieve changes of the iliac crest position and to open up the neuroforamina, without putting pressure on the epidural veins. Testing of the straight leg sign in patients under local anesthesia is possible. The lordosis can be straightened by hip and knee flexion of the patient in lateral position.

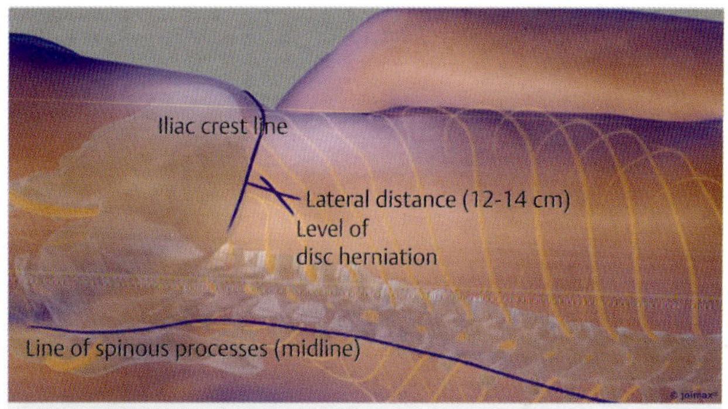

Fig. 35.4 Lateral patient position and marking.

35.6 Surgical Technique

The procedure is performed under local or general anesthesia. The author prefers general anesthesia with short acting muscle relaxants. The correct disc level is identified with lateral and anteroposterior (AP) C-arm imaging. Disc level, iliac crest, midline, and trajectory of entry as well as the lateral facet joint line are marked on the skin (▶ Fig. 35.4). The pathology determines the trajectory and the volume of bone removal for the transforaminal procedure.

35.6.1 Surgical Steps

1. **Needle insertion, needle placement, and skin incision:**
   The needle insertion is performed under lateral X-ray. The needle tip first touches the superior articular process (SAP), then it is advanced to the neuroforamen. After AP and lateral X-ray control of the needle placement, a K-wire is inserted and then the skin incision is made. In case of foraminal or lateral recess stenosis a Jamshidi needle is docked on the bone of the SAP (▶ Fig. 35.5). *Refer to B. Different approaches section for other approaches.*
2. **Dilation of soft tissue:**
   Soft tissue is gradually displaced using sequential dilators increasing in diamenter.
3. **Widening of foramen with coronary reamers or bone drills:**
   The neuroforamen is widened with coronary reamers with increasing diameters and side-cutting blunt bone drills. They also resect most of the yellow ligament. The medial pedicular line must not be crossed.
4. **Insertion of working tube:**
   The working tube is inserted with its lip first placed caudally (▶ Fig. 35.6a), then turned into the direction of the exiting nerve root (▶ Fig. 35.6).

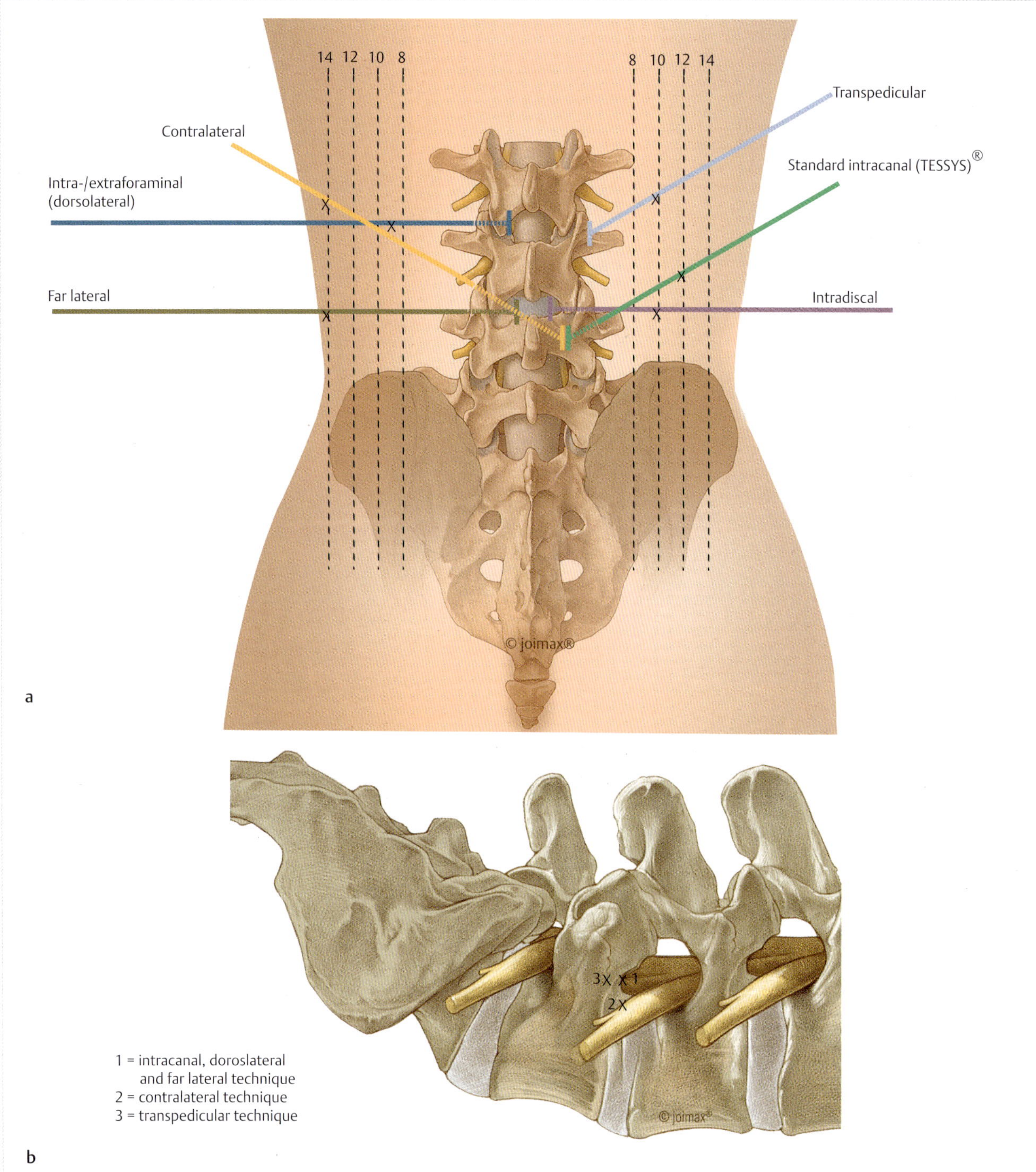

Fig. 35.5 (a) Skin entry points and trajectories of different approaches; **(b)** needle target points.

5. **Identifying the SAP and pedicle, arch of Wagner:**
   A clear understanding of cranial/caudal and medial orientations of the endoscope (joimax®) is necessary to identify the pedicle and superior facet (▶ Fig. 35.6c and ▶ Fig. 35.7).
6. **Preparation of epidural space:**
   The lateral recess is prepared from caudal to cranial. The site of disc herniation is identified (▶ Fig. 35.6d).
7. **Resection of disc herniation:**
   The disc herniation is resected. In cases of a contained disc, the posterior ligament has to be incised.
8. **Control of decompression:**
   The nerve root should be visualized and then decompressed starting at the lower pedicle to the site of the exiting nerve root.

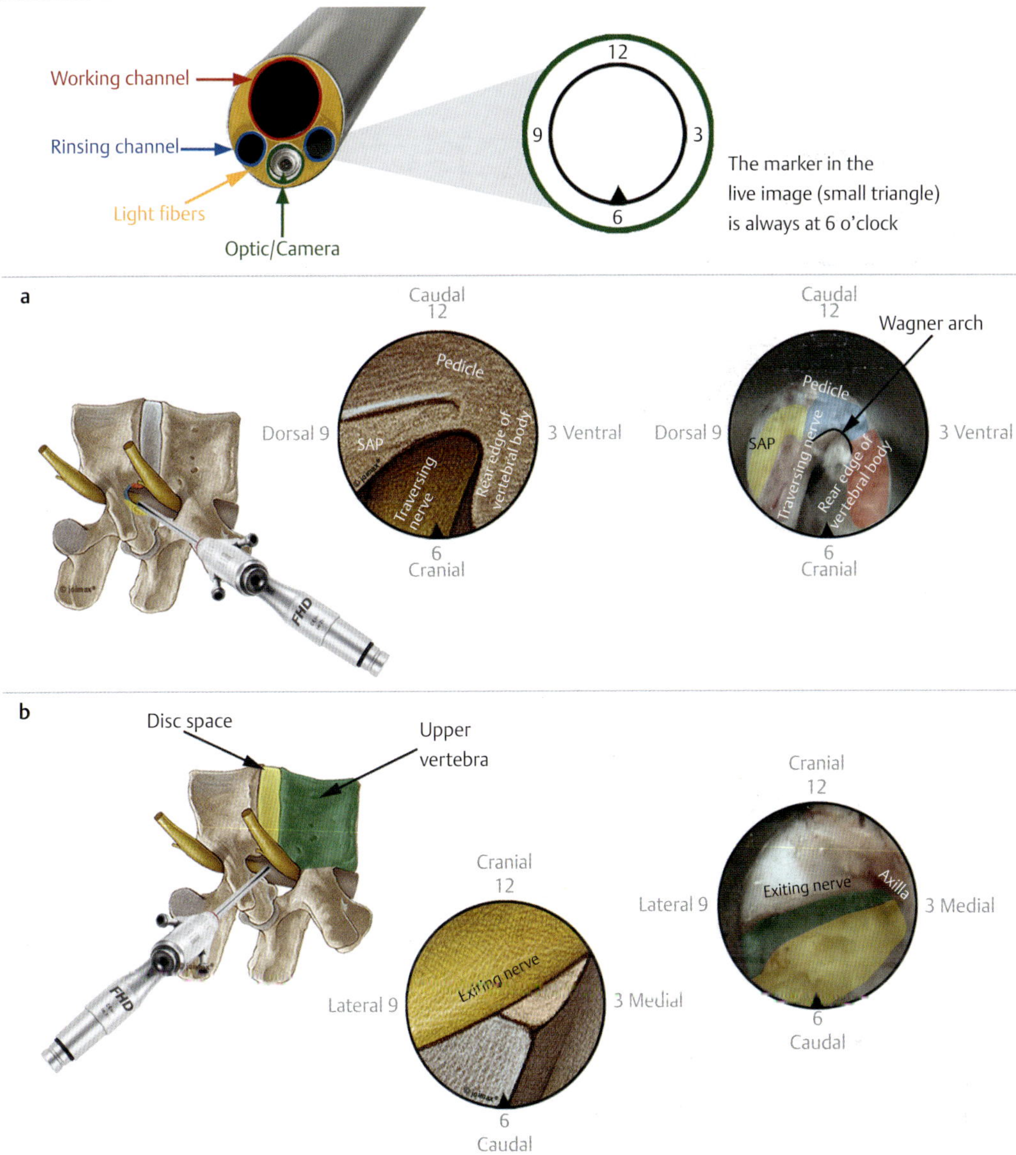

Fig. 35.6 Endoscopic view of surgical site: different views and orientations of endoscope. **(a)** Caudal view to lateral recess, **(b)** cranial foraminal view.

(Continued)

9. **Removal of instruments and skin closure:**
   The instruments are removed and the skin is closed.

35.6.2 Different Approaches

1. **The intracanal technique (outside-in):**
   The intracanal technique (standard TESSYS®) is accomplished with a needle angulation of approximately 45 to 60 degrees in the lateral C-arm beam aiming at the lateral recess in craniocaudal direction. The goal is to directly address the lateral recess for caudally sequestrated disc herniations or pathologies of the lateral recess (▶ Video 35.1).
   Schubert and Hoogland described the combination of foraminoplasty with endoscopic transforaminal nucleotomy with excellent or good results in 95.3% with a low complication rate.[16] Lee et al classified the migrated disc herniations into four zones and recommended an epiduroscopic or intracanal technique for far migrated disc hernations only. Further they described the necessity to combine it with foraminoplasty to obtain access for the endoscope and forceps. Back in 2007, they described the direct approach to the epidural space as dangerous and recommended to start the procedure from the disc.[17] This point of view has changed over the past years. The intracanal technique shows a clear advantage for decompression and removal of bone and ligamentous structures of the lumbar spinal canal and neuroforamen. In a degenerative spine and elderly patients, injury of the posterior ligament and disc should be avoided. This procedure is similar to the existing tubular or micorsurgical techniques.

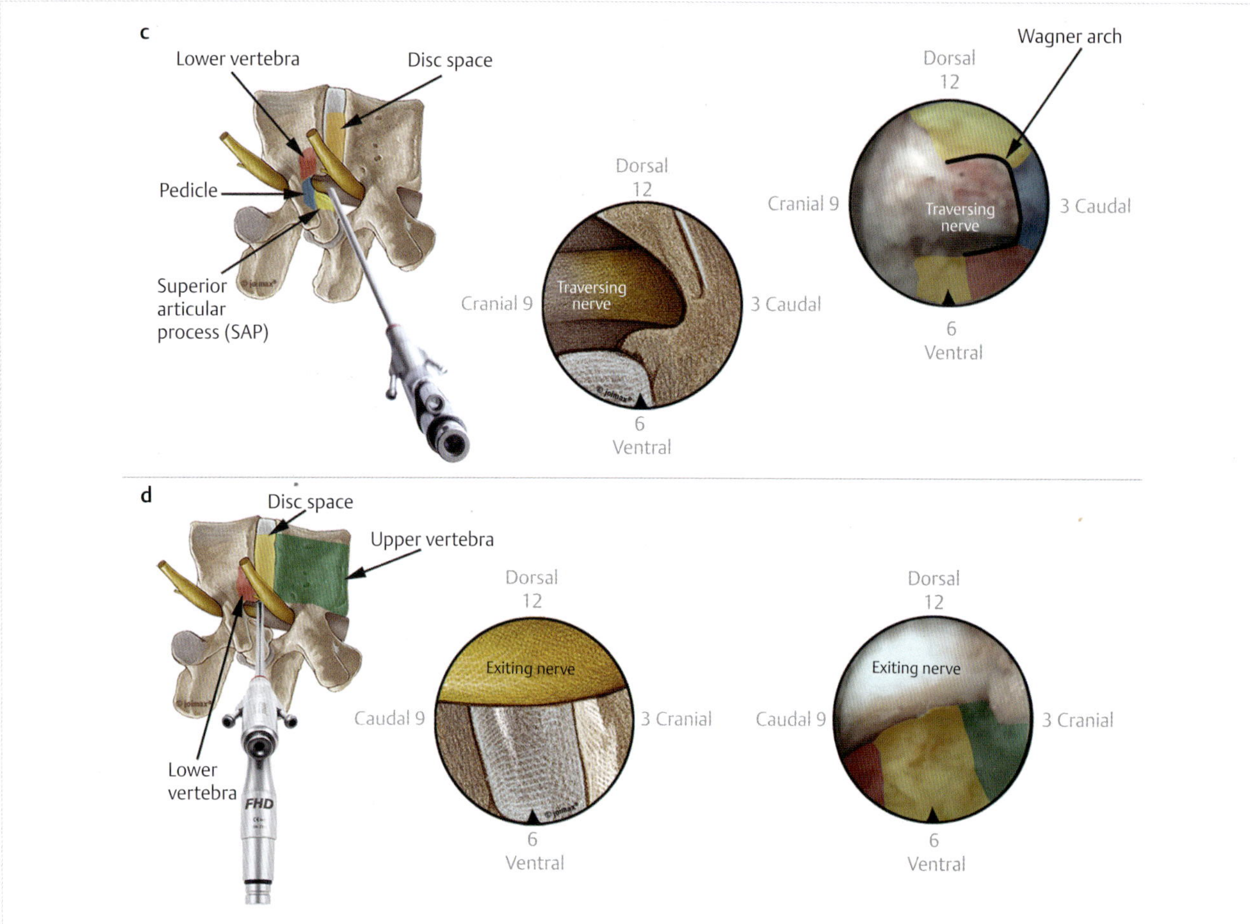

Fig. 35.6 *(Continued)* **(c)** horizontal view, and **(d)** extraforaminal view.

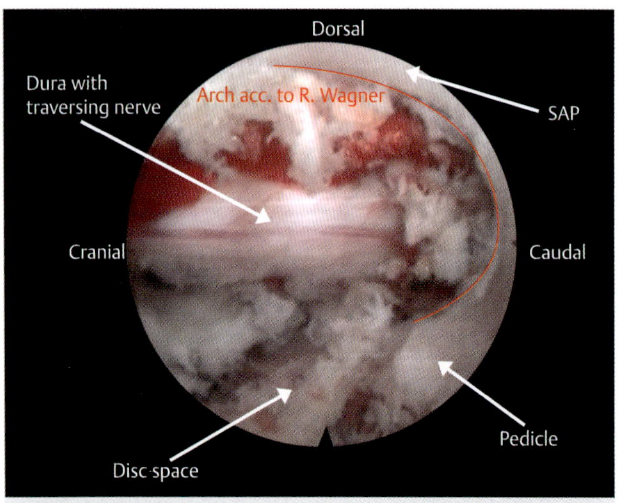

Fig. 35.7 Arch of Wagner.

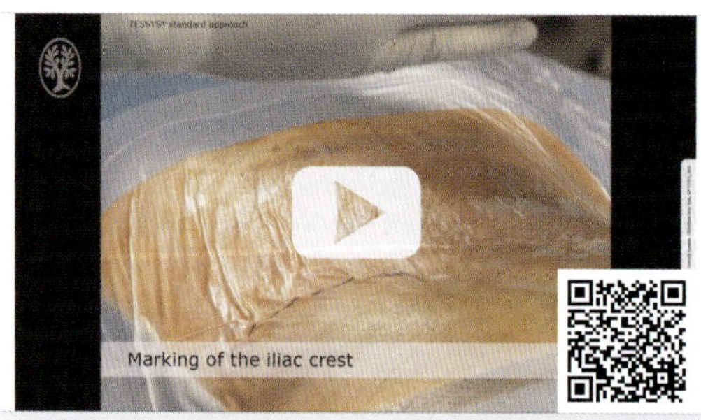

Video 35.1 First steps for the endoscopic approach with TESSYS.

The Jamshidi needle is a powerful tool to achieve a posterior positioning of the instruments. The approach tools, reamer and bone drill, are very efficient and allow an X-ray controlled decompression of the foramen and lateral recess. Basically, the first steps of the transforaminal approach create the space for the working tube and the endoscope. To advance to the pathology, bone has to be removed. The most important point of this technique is to stop at the medial pedicular line during the reaming maneuver.

2. **The intradiscal technique (inside-out):**
   The intradiscal technique is accomplished with a more horizontal placement of the needle in the lateral X-ray, in cases of contained and medial disc herniations. The approach is more parallel to the disc space and uses the disc as a safe starting point. The idea is to undermine the pathology from anterior and therefore also create a rather indirect decompression. Especially for contained disc herniations without migration, this technique is useful to decompress the spinal canal anterior to the posterior ligament[18] (▶ Video 35.2).

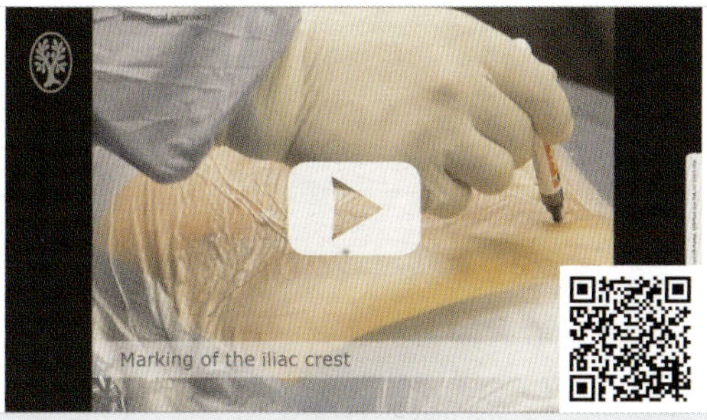

Video 35.2 First steps for the intradiscal endoscopic approach.

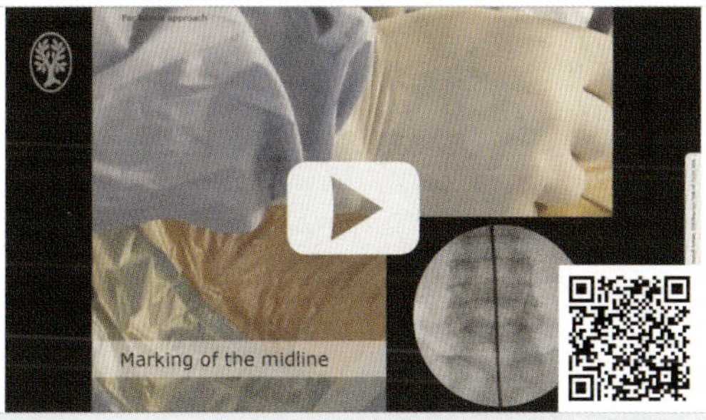

Video 35.3 First steps for the far lateral endoscopic approach.

3. **The far-lateral approach:**
   The far-lateral approach is used in central spinal pathologies and was described as an alternative for microsurgery. The entry point is 13 to 18 cm off the midline and uses the posterior facet line projection for prevention of peritoneal perforation. In 2005, Ruetten et al described this approach for disc herniations inside the spinal canal with a high success and low complication rates.[19] The study by Hang et al revealed a rather high percentage of dysesthesia of 19.7%.[20] Keep in mind that the Kambin's triangle gets smaller the further lateral the approach is—with a possible elevation compromising the exiting nerve root. Therefore, a more posterior starting point on the bone should be chosen to avoid exiting nerve damage. At the higher levels of the lumbar spine, the approach is at higher risk of damaging retroperitoneal organs. A preoperative evaluation of the MRI scans and control of kidneys, vessels, and bowel are therefore mandatory (▶ Video 35.3).
4. **The transpedicular approach:**
   The transpedicular approach is used as an alternative for hidden zone pathologies and highly migrated disc herniations. Krzok et al described the technique as a new method to directly target highly migrated discs by reaming a small canal through the lateral wall of the pedicle. The surgery starts at the lateral border of the pedicle. A Jamshidi needle is necessary for the first needle placement. The risks include missing the pathology, fracturing the pedicle or transverse process, and damaging the traversing nerve[15] (▶ Video 35.4).
5. **The contralateral transforaminal approach:**
   The contralateral transforaminal approach is used in contralateral caudally sequestered disc herniations. The entry point for this technique is further lateral than in the ipsilateral technique. It is used for highly migrated disc herniations in the axilla of the contralateral side or hidden zone pathology. The endoscope is introduced through the epidural space to access the migrated disc fragment.[21,22] This approach has a higher incidence of bleeding and often requires an anterior decompression of the caudal vertebral body to gain enough space. This might result in prolonged operation time[21] (▶ Video 35.5).

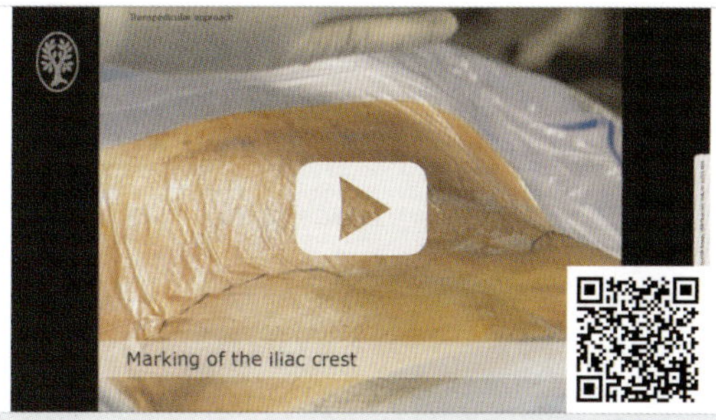

Video 35.4 First steps for the transpedicular endoscopic approach.

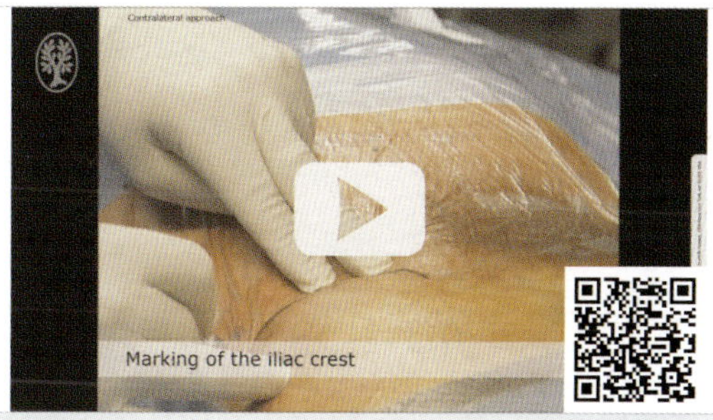

Video 35.5 First steps for the contralateral endoscopic approach.

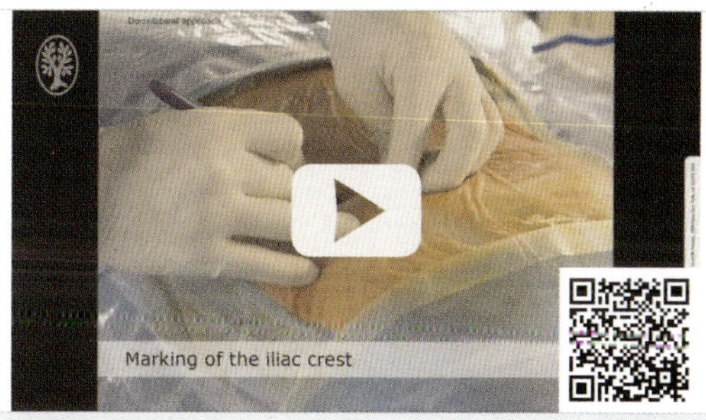

Video 35.6 First steps for the dorsolateral endoscopic approach.

6. **The dorsolateral approach:**
   The dorsolateral approach is used for the decompression of the neuroforamen. The ideal approach is almost horizontal to the disc space, entering the disc at the pedicle center line. Therefore, the approach is closer to the midline at approximately 8 to 10 cm. The endoscope is pulled out of the foramen to target the extraforaminal pathology. The possibility of exiting nerve or ganglion compression must be considered.[23] Another option is to prepare the traversing nerve root and follow it with a turning maneuver to the extraforaminal space (▶ Video 35.6).

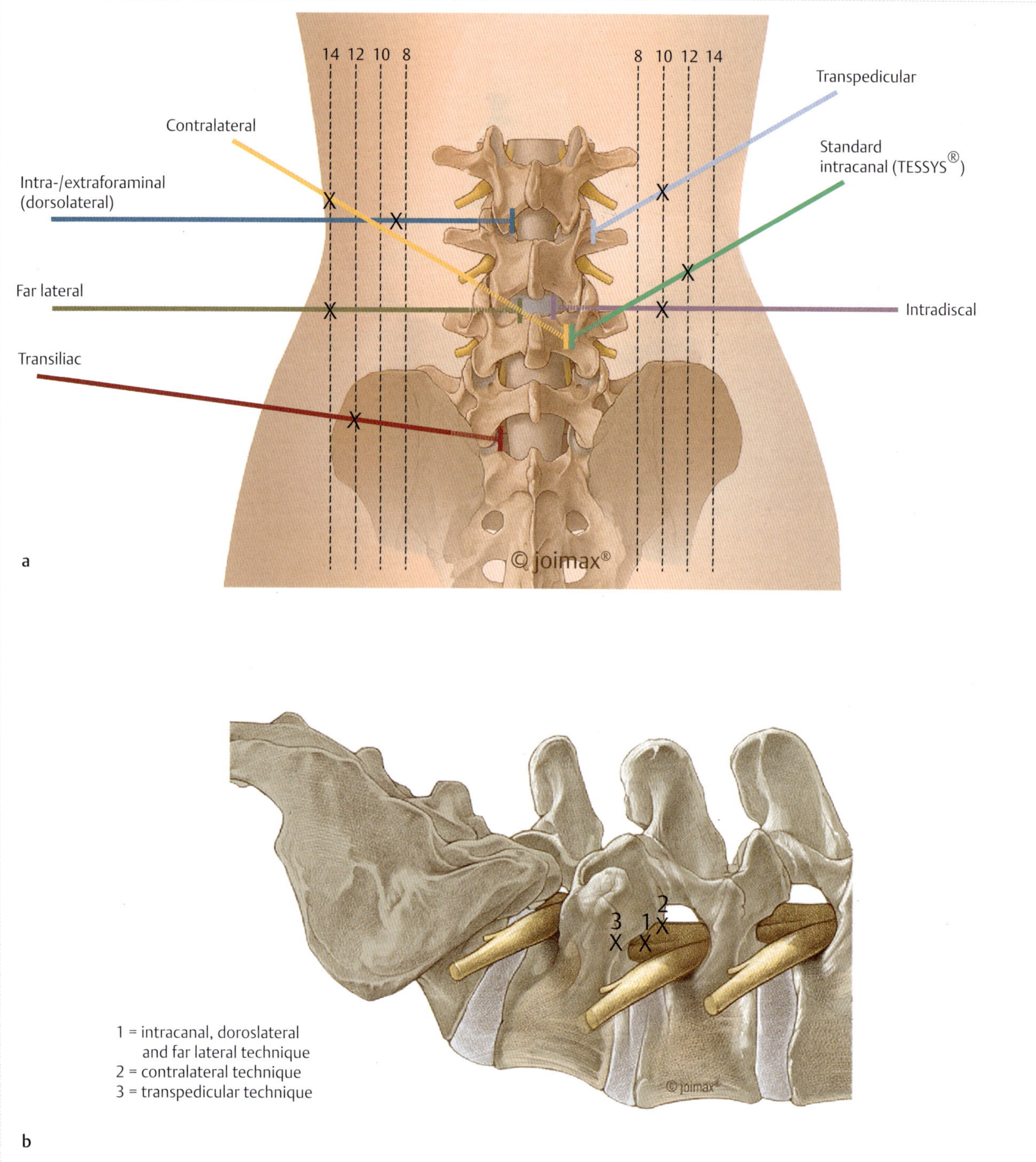

Fig. 35.8 (a, b) Trajectories of various approaches.

7. **The transiliac approach:**
The transiliac approach is used as a possible access to the disc space L5/S1 in patients with high iliac crest. This approach is a rescue option for transforaminal surgery of the L4/L5 and L5/S1 level in select cases with a deep location of the disc space. A canal is drilled through the os ilium. The following steps are similar to the known procedure of transforaminal endoscopy. Osman et al showed in a cadaver study that no damage to important structures occurred in any of their cases.[24] In a later clinical study, they described the approach as safe with minimal blood loss and operation time.[25] Choi et al described the transiliac approach as an alternative in select cases with a high iliac crest (▶ Fig. 35.7 and ▶ Fig. 35.8).[26]

35.7 Postoperative Care

Walking is encouraged a few hours after surgery. Nonsteroidal anti-rheumatics (NSAR) are prescribed for 1 week after surgery and sutures are removed after 2 weeks. Stabilizing orthesis and walking only are recommended for 3 weeks. After L5/S1 disc surgery, long sitting should be avoided for the first 2 weeks. Isometric physiotherapy can be started at 2 weeks, movements only with own body weight at 4 weeks, and muscle strengthening therapy at 6 weeks after surgery.

35.8 Complication Avoidance

35.8.1 Exiting Nerve Root Injury

The exiting nerve root is the most fragile and important structure that can be injured. Potential iatrogenic damage could happen at the beginning of the surgery during needle advancement or reaming. The risk of exiting nerve root injury is higher with an anterior shift or far-lateral approach, since the Kambin's triangle is reduced. Therefore, the needle should be advanced under constant AP and lateral X-ray control. A centered X-ray image and an initially posterior position of the needle tip are necessary. Once the tip of the needle hits the SAP, the needle is slightly withdrawn and slid into the foramen. In cases of stenosis, the use of a Jamshidi needle allows to dock on the bone and therefore guarantees a fixed tip and correct entry point. A more caudal entry point may be useful to avoid exiting nerve root damage.[27]

35.8.2 Dura or Traversing Nerve Root Damage

The first steps of the endoscopic approach bear the risk of damaging the dura and/or traversing nerve root. Khan et al showed that the incidence of dural tear in primary lumbar surgery was found to be 7.6%, compared to 15.9% in revision surgery.[28] Ahn et al showed that the undiagnosed dural tears showed an unfavorable outcome with neurologic sequelae.[29] Especially in stenotic pathologies, the traversing nerve root is shifted anteriorly and has a potential danger to be in the center of the working area. A subtle preparation of the bone, SAP, and pedicle as well as the anterior caudal recess should be performed to identify the caudal part of the traversing nerve root. From this point on, the nerve root should always be in the surgeon's sight. In case of dural damage, in most cases a 2-day bed rest is sufficient. In patients with relevant neurological deficit or symptomatic liquid loss, the damage should be repaired with a conventional microsurgical approach.

35.8.3 Intraoperative Bleeding and Postoperative Hematoma

In case of intraoperative epidural bleeding, the bipolar probe can be applied, the irrigation pressure raised, the blood pressure lowered, and the adrenaline/noradrenaline added to the saline irrigation. Be aware that there is also a risk of retroperitoneal hematoma, attributed to abnormal vascular distribution around the foraminal area.[30] The author experienced one case with postoperative bleeding oozing through the psoas muscle into the retroperitoneal cavity, which had to be revised in an open surgery. Another complication is the postoperative epidural hematoma, which rarely requires revision surgery.

35.8.4 Infection

Compared to open lumbar surgery, the risk for spondylodiscitis is far lower. The main risk factors include diabetes, immunosuppression, prolonged operation time, and inadequate sterilization. The infection rate reported by six surgeons was as low as 0.2%, leading to back pain and immobility of the lumbar spine as a common symptom.[31,32]

35.8.5 Incomplete Decompression or Reherniation

Incomplete decompression may result in persisting clinical symptoms after endoscopic decompression surgery and is often due to technical difficulties during the surgery or lacking anatomical knowledge. The incidence of reherniation largely depends on the technical skills of the surgeon and is comparable to the open technique.[33,34]

35.9 Tips and Tricks

Evaluation of the preoperative MRI and anticipation of potential problems are essential. The key to address degenerative pathologies is the amount of bone removal in the spinal canal. Lumbar stenosis is often associated with secondary shortening of the pedicles and hypertrophic facet joints. This leads to an anterior placement of the needle, which makes an adequate decompression almost impossible. The use of a Jamshidi needle is very helpful in maintaining a posterior position and therefore avoiding anteriorly misplaced starting tools. Keep in mind that the spinal stenosis might cause an anterior shift of the traversing nerve root.

During surgery several different endoscopically controlled decompression methods are used to achieve mobility of the endoscope in the spinal canal (▶ Fig. 35.7 and ▶ Fig. 35.9).

35.9.1 Posterior Decompression

To achieve posterior decompression, the endoscope has to be pulled out of the foramen. Next the anterior part of the SAP is partly removed with a drill to enlarge the size of the foramen in posterior direction.

35.9.2 Anterocaudal Decompression

Bone is removed at the cranial part of the lower pedicle as well as the posterior wall of the caudal vertebral body using a high-speed drill. More space in the lateral recess is gained and the pedicle is elongated in anterior direction.

35.9.3 Central Decompression

The central part of spinal canal can be freed up after achieving posterior and anterocaudal decompression. The endoscope has to be advanced inside the spinal canal underneath the dural sac.

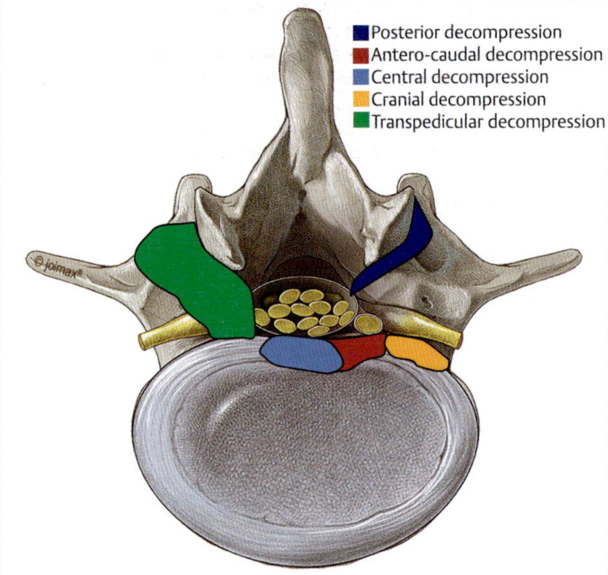

Fig. 35.9 Decompression sites.

35.9.4 Cranial Decompression

The cranial decompression is important for the removal of lateral osteophytes in the neuroforamen. The endoscope has to be pulled out of the foramen and turned toward cranial.

35.9.5 Extraforaminal Decompression

The extraforaminal area is part of far-lateral pathologies, such as disc herniations or osteophyte formation. The endoscope is turned 180 degrees and then pulled out of the foramen.

35.10 Conclusion

A broad variety of transforaminal endoscopic approaches have been developed within the past years. In the past, the inside-out technique was promoted; nowadays, it is mainly used for contained disc herniations and medial spinal pathologies. The endoscopic transforaminal intracanal approach is the key to success in transforaminal decompression of spinal stenosis or migrated disc surgery. In stenosis of the central spinal canal, lateral recess, and/or foramen, a disc-saving approach and decompression avoid further instabilities or recurrent disc herniations. This technique has the advantage of placing the working tube exactly at the pathology of the spinal canal with little or no harm to the disc. The use of rigid or angled drills allows endoscopic decompression of the foramen and spinal canal under direct visual control. The far-lateral approach allows a medial working target area, but has a higher risk of exiting nerve root injury. In case of pathologies in the hidden zone or highly migrated disc herniations, the transpedicular approach is a promising method for resecting sequester. Surgery time might be reduced significantly. The approach should be based on an accurate review of the preoperative MRI, clinical findings, and individual skills of the surgeon.

References

[1] Park WW, Bono CM, Garfin SR. Applied anatomy of the spine. In: Herkowitz HN, Garfin SR, Eismont FJ, et al, eds. The Spine. 5th ed. Philadelphia, PA: Saunders-Elsevier; 2007

[2] Epstein NE, Epstein JA, Carras R, Hyman RA. Far lateral lumbar disc herniations and associated structural abnormalities. An evaluation in 60 patients of the comparative value of CT, MRI, and myelo-CT in diagnosis and management. Spine. 1990; 15(6):534–539

[3] Jenis LG, An HS, Gordin R. Foraminal stenosis of the lumbar spine: a review of 65 surgical cases. Am J Orthop. 2001; 30(3):205–211

[4] Hasegawa T, An HS, Haughton VM, Nowicki BH. Lumbar foraminal stenosis: critical heights of the intervertebral discs and foramina. A cryomicrotome study in cadavera. J Bone Joint Surg Am. 1995; 77(1):32–38

[5] Shenouda EF, Gill SS. Laminal fenestration for the treatment of lumbar nerve root foraminal stenosis. Br J Neurosurg. 2002; 16(5):494–496, discussion 497

[6] Postacchini F. Surgical management of lumbar spinal stenosis. Spine. 1999; 24(10):1043–1047

[7] Ren Z, Liu A, Yang K, Wang D, Buser Z, Wang JC. Evaluation of changes in lumbar neuroforaminal dimensions in symptomatic young adults using positional MRI. Eur Spine J. 2017; 26(8):1999–2006

[8] Golub BS, Silverman B. Transforaminal ligaments of the lumbar spine. J Bone Joint Surg Am. 1969; 51(5):947–956

[9] Park HK, Rudrappa S, Dujovny M, Diaz FG. Intervertebral foraminal ligaments of the lumbar spine: anatomy and biomechanics. Childs Nerv Syst. 2001; 17 (4–5):275–282

[10] Silverstein MP, Romrell LJ, Benzel EC, Thompson N, Griffith S, Lieberman IH. Lumbar dorsal root Ganglia location: an anatomic and MRI assessment. Int J Spine Surg. 2015; 9:3

[11] Kikuchi S, Sato K, Konno S, Hasue M. Anatomic and radiographic study of dorsal root ganglia. Spine. 1994; 19(1):6–11

[12] Smith SA, Massie JB, Chesnut R, Garfin SR. Straight leg raising. Anatomical effects on the spinal nerve root without and with fusion. Spine. 1993; 18 (8):992–999

[13] Grimes PF, Massie JB, Garfin SR. Anatomic and biomechanical analysis of the lower lumbar foraminal ligaments. Spine. 2000; 25(16):2009–2014

[14] Reinshagen C, Redjal N, Molcanyi M, Rieger B. Surgical approaches to the lumbar hidden zone: current strategies and future directions. EBioMedicine. 2015; 2(9):1005–1007

[15] Krzok G, Telfeian AE, Wagner R, Iprenburg M. Transpedicular lumbar endoscopic surgery for highly migrated disc extrusions: preliminary series and surgical technique. World Neurosurg. 2016; 95:299–303

[16] Schubert M, Hoogland T. Endoscopic transforaminal nucleotomy with foraminoplasty for lumbar disc herniation. Oper Orthop Traumatol. 2005; 17 (6):641–661

[17] Lee S, Kim SK, Lee SH, et al. Percutaneous endoscopic lumbar discectomy for migrated disc herniation: classification of disc migration and surgical approaches. Eur Spine J. 2007; 16(3):431–437

[18] Yeung AT. The evolution of percutaneous spinal endoscopy and discectomy: state of the art. Mt Sinai J Med. 2000; 67(4):327–332

[19] Ruetten S,. Komp M, Godolias G. An extreme lateral access for the surgery of lumbar disc herniations inside the spinal canal using the full-endoscopic uniportal transforaminal approach–technique and prospective results of 463 patients. Spine. 2005; 30(22):2570–2578

[20] Han J, Han I. Extreme lateral endoscopic transforaminal lumbar discectomy for lumbar disc herniation in young patients. The Nerve. 2016; 2(2):26–32

[21] Liu C, Chu L, Yong HC, Chen L, Deng ZL. Percutaneous endoscopic lumbar discectomy for highly migrated lumbar disc herniation. Pain Physician. 2017; 20 (1):E75–E84

[22] Yeom KS, Choi YS. Full endoscopic contralateral transforaminal discectomy for distally migrated lumbar disc herniation. J Orthop Sci. 2011; 16(3):263–269

[23] Liao Z, Chen W, Wang CH. Transforaminal percutaneous endoscopic surgery for far lateral lumbar intervertebral disc herniation. Orthopedics. 2014; 37 (8):e717–e727

[24] Osman SG, Marsolais EB. Endoscopic transiliac approach to L5-S1 disc and foramen. A cadaver study. Spine. 1997; 22(11):1259–1263

[25] Osman SG, Sherlekar S, Malik A, et al. Endoscopic trans-iliac approach to L5-S1 disc and foramen—a report on clinical experience. Int J Spine Surg. 2014; 8:8

[26] Choi G, Kim JS, Lokhande P, Lee SH. Percutaneous endoscopic lumbar discectomy by transiliac approach: a case report. Spine. 2009; 34(12):E443–E446

[27] Ahn Y. Transforaminal percutaneous endoscopic lumbar discectomy: technical tips to prevent complications. Expert Rev Med Devices. 2012; 9(4):361–366

[28] Khan MH, Rihn J, Steele G, et al. Postoperative management protocol for incidental dural tears during degenerative lumbar spine surgery: a review of 3,183 consecutive degenerative lumbar cases. Spine. 2006; 31(22):2609–2613

[29] Ahn Y, Lee HY, Lee SH, Lee JH. Dural tears in percutaneous endoscopic lumbar discectomy. Eur Spine J. 2011; 20(1):58–64

[30] Ahn Y, Kim JU, Lee BH, et al. Postoperative retroperitoneal hematoma following transforaminal percutaneous endoscopic lumbar discectomy. J Neurosurg Spine. 2009; 10(6):595–602

[31] Zhu B, Jiang Y, et al. Complicatons of percutaneous endoscopic lumbar discectomy: experiences and literature review. J Spine. 2017; 6(6):402

[32] Ahn Y, Lee SH. Postoperative spondylodiscitis following transforaminal endoscopic discectomy: clinical characteristics and preventive strategies. Br J Neurosurg. 2012; 26:482–486

[33] Kim DH, Choi G, Lee SH. Complications in Percutaneous Endoscopic Lumbar Discectomy: Endoscopic Spine Procedures. NY, USA: Thieme Medical Publishers; 2011:253–267

[34] Gadjradj PS, Rubinstein SM, Peul WC, Depauw PR, Vleggeert-Lankamp CL, Seiger A, et al. Full endoscopic versus open discectomy for sciatica: randomised controlled non-inferiority trial. BMJ. 2022:376:e065846

36 Endoscopic Interlaminar Lumbar Laminectomy

Christoph Hofstetter

Summary

The endoscopic interlaminar lumbar laminectomy is becoming the least invasive option to decompress the lumbar spine from a dorsal approach. This technique represents another option in the MIS armamentarium. In this chapter, the reader will obtain extremely valuable information from the expert on how to perform this type of surgery safely, efficiently, some tips and tricks, and also how to avoid complications.

Keywords: ILELL, endoscopic spine surgery, endoscopic lumbar decompression, lumbar spine decompression

36.1 Introduction

Symptomatic lumbar spinal stenosis is a common diagnosis in the elderly population. Pathophysiological processes that lead to spinal stenosis include thickening of the interspinous ligaments and overgrowth of the facet joints. This leads to narrowing of the spinal canal and eventually compression of neural elements with subsequent signs of neural claudication. The feasibility of a unilateral laminotomy for bilateral access to the spinal canal was first demonstrated by Spetzger et al.[1,2] This cadaveric study demonstrated that a unilateral approach allowed for bilateral over-the-top decompression of the thecal sac by resection of the ipsilateral facet, the median portion of the lamina arch, the contralateral facet, and the yellow ligament. A case series of 29 patients by the same authors demonstrated feasibility, safety, and favorable clinical outcomes.[1,2] Concurrent development of microendoscopic tubular systems by Foley et al provided a minimally invasive surgical corridor to the spinal canal without detachment of paraspinal muscles.[3] Tubular retractors have been used in combination with an operative microscope to achieve bilateral decompression in the setting of lumbar spinal stenosis. A thorough step-by-step description of a minimally invasive lumbar decompression has been recently published.[4] This technique has been adapted for a working channel endoscope, to allow for decompression of central and lateral recess stenosis in the lumbar spine.[5,6,7] A prospective randomized controlled study on a total of 161 patients demonstrated favorable functional outcomes at 2-year follow-up with endoscopic technique compared to minimally invasive technique.[6]

36.2 Patient Selection

Case selection: Approach and bony decompression can be challenging in cases with severe spondylotic changes with facet hypertrophy or scoliosis. If these cases are addressed with endoscopic technique, attention to planning the surgical corridor and nonambiguous identification of anatomical landmarks is critical in order to maintain a smooth workflow. Moreover, cases with scoliosis and stable spondylosis require more extensive decompression to allow for sufficient decompression of neural structures during more extensive motion. However, once spondylolisthesis leads to symptomatic foraminal compression of the exiting nerve roots surgical reconstruction of the spinal segment via an arthrodesis procedure should be considered.

> In the opinion of the editors, the unilateral tubular "over-the-top" decompression for lumbar spinal stenosis is one of the key competences for a successful minimally invasive surgery (MIS) spine surgeon. Whether or not endoscopic surgery will be able to surpass tubular approaches will depend on its ability to perform this task with the same efficiency and with less patient morbidity. This will need to be established in the upcoming years.

36.3 Indications

Endoscopic interlaminar lumbar laminectomy allows for central and bilateral lateral recess decompression in patients presenting with primarily leg or buttock symptoms with neurogenic claudication. Surgical indications are consistent with open or minimally invasive laminectomies.[8] Similar to minimally invasive lumbar decompression, decompression of the neural elements is achieved primarily at the level of the disc–facet joint complex; thus, degenerative lumbar spinal stenosis is an appropriate indication for this procedure. In contrast, endoscopic interlaminar decompression may be less effective to achieve sufficient decompression in cases of epidural hematomas, lipomatosis, or phlegma as these pathologies are typically not confined to the disc–facet joint complex but often expand rostrocaudally beyond these structures. Endoscopic interlaminar laminectomy may be combined with resection of synovial cysts, discectomies, and contralateral foraminotomies. Endoscopic technique is in particular advantageous compared to open and MIS technique for spinal decompression in obese patients. A thick subcutaneous fat pannus neither requires additional exposure nor affects the lengths of working corridor or quality of visualization. Grade I spondylolisthesis is not a contraindication as long as there is no dynamic instability on flexion and extension X-rays or vertical foraminal stenosis. Contraindications to endoscopic laminectomies include grade II spondylolisthesis, isthmic spondylolysis, significant lateral listhesis, and significant scoliosis (SVA >6 cm, lumbar lordosis-pelvic incidence [LL-PI] mismatch >10 degrees, Coronal Cobb >20).[9]

36.4 Surgical Technique

36.4.1 Approach

An optimal rostrocaudal approach angle for interlaminar lumbar laminectomies is of extreme importance. Precise determination of his angle enlarges the interlaminar window and greatly reduces the need for bony removal and thereby the operative time. Moreover, an optimized approach angle helps to spare the pars interarticularis, as the spinal canal is approached

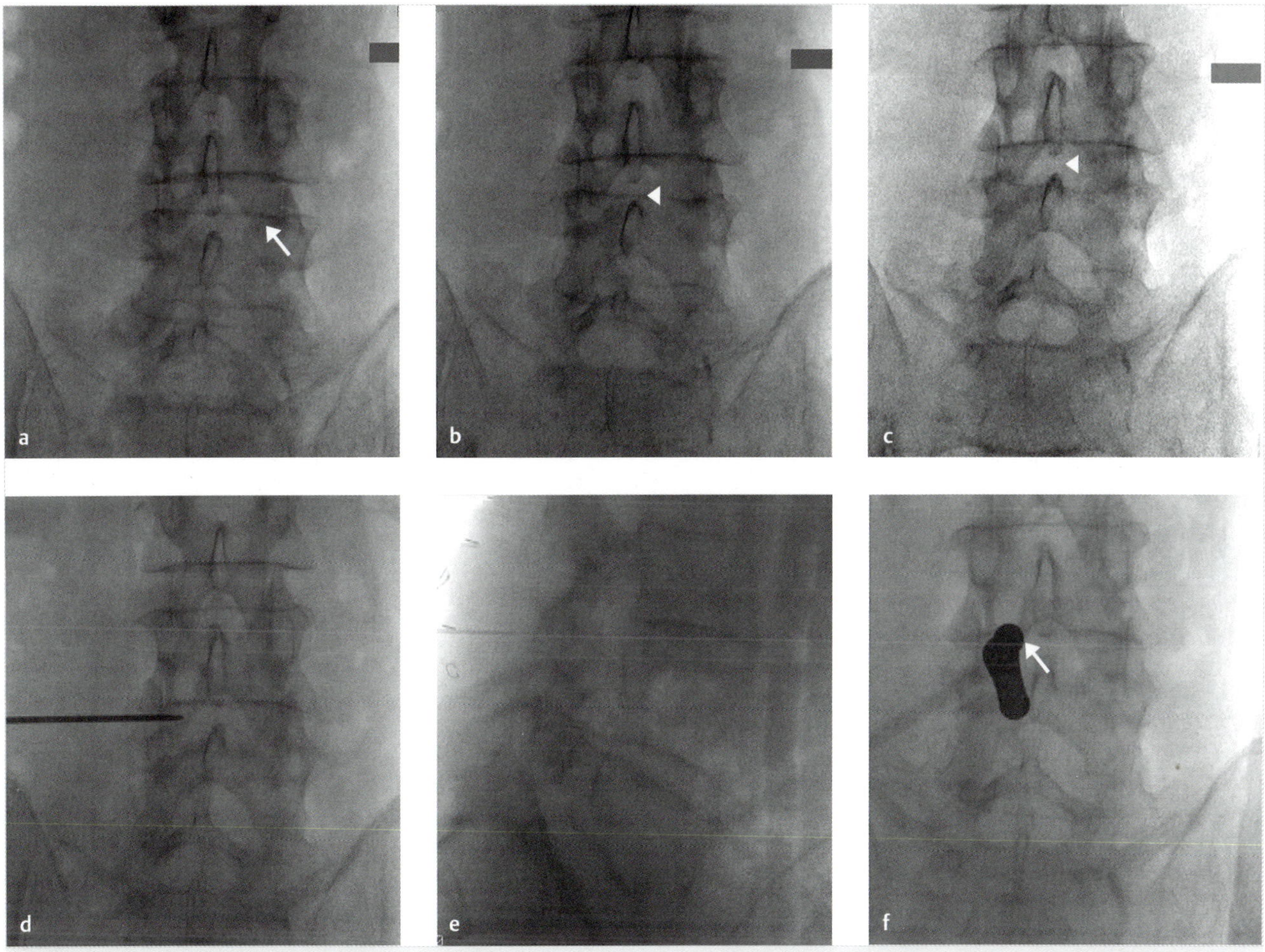

Fig. 36.1 Anteroposterior (AP) fluoroscopic intraoperative images for approach planning. First an AP end plate view of the superior end plate of the caudal level is obtained (L3/L4, *arrow*) **(a)**. The addition of kyphosis of the rostrocaudal X-ray beam angle moves the projection of the interspinous process space toward the disc space (*arrowhead*) **(b)**. An ideal rostrocaudal trajectory has been determined (*arrowhead*) **(c)**. The skin incision is marked at the tip of the radiopaque object **(d)**. A lateral X-ray may be obtained to confirm the level **(e)**. Once the working tube is brought into place, an AP X-ray confirms the location of the working tube at the inferior margin of the lamina (*arrow*) **(f)**.

via the inferior portion of the lamina. An optimal approach angle needs to provide access to spinal canal spanning from the tip of the superior articular process (SAP) to the mid-portion of the pedicle of the caudal segment—this constitutes the goal for the rostrocaudal decompression. For intraoperative determination of the rostrocaudal approach angle, an end plate view of the caudal vertebral body is obtained on anteroposterior (AP) fluoroscopy (▶ Fig. 36.1a). Based on this, angle addition of approximately 10 to 15 degrees of kyphosis is typically required in the lower lumbar levels. The goal is to center the gap between spinous processes over the projection of the disc space (▶ Fig. 36.1a–c). In the lower thoracic and upper lumbar spinal segments, less rostrocaudal angulation should be used. At these levels, spinal stenosis is often caused by overgrowth of the sagittally oriented facet joints. Choosing a too steep rostrocaudal approach angle may interfere with decompression of the caudal aspect of stenosis since the endoscope is deflected by caudal lamina. The incision is marked where the disc space crosses the medial aspect of the facet joint (▶ Fig. 36.1d). A small vertical skin incision is made using an 11-blade. Serial dilators are then advanced with small rostrocaudal movements along the AP trajectory of the fluoroscopy until the medial aspect of the facet joint and the inferior margin of the lamina can be palpated. Beveled dilators may be used to strip muscles off the lamina in order to facilitate the transition from palpation to visualization. Attention should be paid to staying in solid contact with the edge of the lamina. At L5/S1, the dilators may rest on the yellow ligament. In these cases, lateral fluoroscopic images may help to confirm appropriate depth (▶ Fig. 36.1e). Blind penetration of the yellow ligament is not advised as it could lead to damage of neural structures. Following the serial dilation, the working tube is placed with the bevel facing medially (Fig. 36.1f). At this point the endoscope is brought in.

36.4.2 Identify Bony Landmarks

Using the bipolar cautery and micropunches, the inferior edge of the lamina to the base of the spinous process and the medial aspect of the facet joint extending to the caudal tip of the inferior articular process are exposed (▶ Fig. 36.2a). Thoroughly stripping off muscle tissue with the beveled retractor system greatly facilitates this step. Also, the tip of the tubular retractor may be used like a Cobb elevator to both palpate the bony landmarks as well as to assist with retraction of soft tissue during

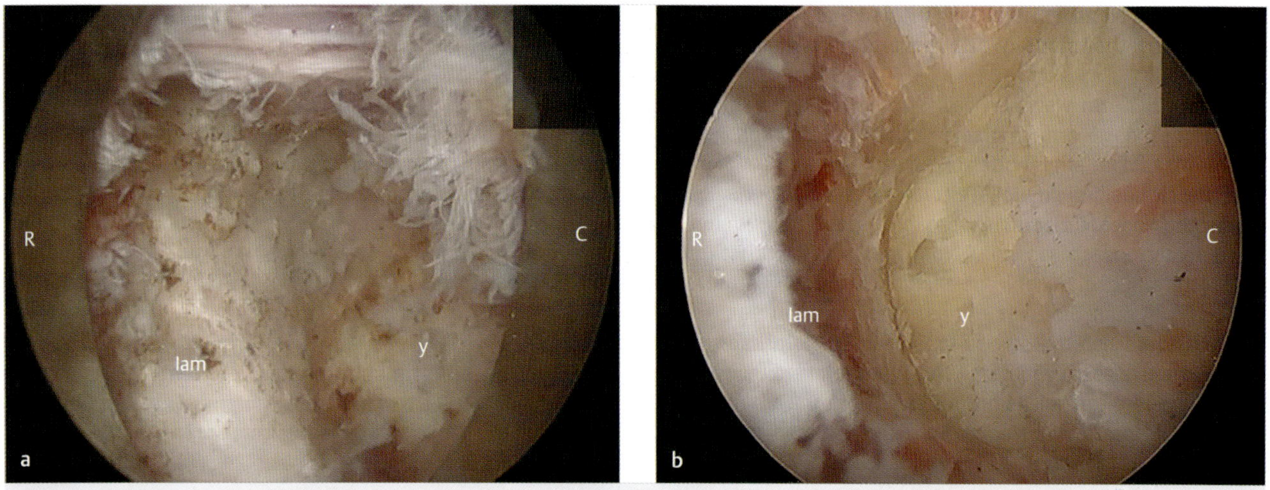

Fig. 36.2 As an initial anatomical landmark, the inferior edge of the lamina is exposed (lam) **(a)**. Often the yellow ligament (y) may be seen too. Following resection of the inferior edge of the lamina, the bony insertion of the yellow ligament can be nonambiguously identified **(b)**.

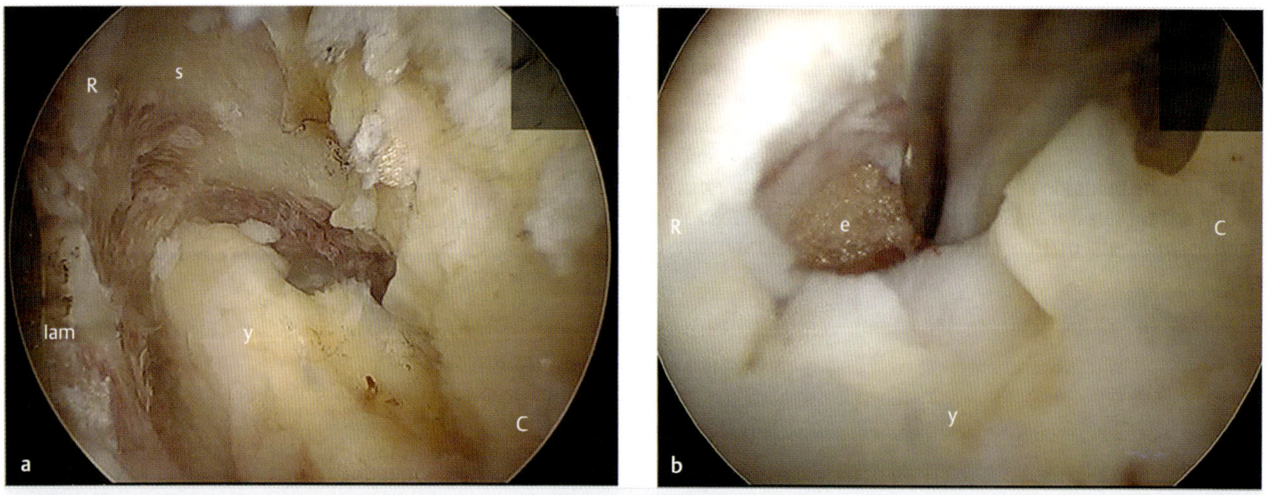

Fig. 36.3 The inferior edge of the lamina (lam) and base of the spinous process (s) are resected **(a)**. Using a micropunch, the yellow ligament (y) is opened. Note the ample epidural space and epidural fat (e) **(b)**.

exposure of bony landmarks. Once the bony landmarks are exposed, an AP X-ray is obtained to confirm appropriate position of the endoscope. Then the superficial layer of the yellow ligament is resected using a micropunch. The goal is to unambiguously identify the attachment of the yellow ligament. In patients with severe facet hypertrophy or scoliosis, identification of the bony attachment of the yellow ligament constitutes one of the most reliable anatomical landmarks. The laminar attachment of the yellow ligaments is followed medially toward the base of the spinous process and caudally toward the tip of the descending articular process. Determination of the ligament attachment may be facilitated by drilling along the inferior portion of the lamina or medial aspect of the facet joint with a diamond drill bit (▸ Fig. 36.2b).

36.4.3 Laminectomy

Using a diamond drill bit or side-biting drill bit, the central decompression is initiated along the inferior aspect of the lamina. Drilling is performed along the insertion of the yellow ligament and lamina is resected until the yellow ligament thins out. Then the base of the spinous process is undercut along the insertion of the yellow ligament (▸ Fig. 36.3a). Undercutting of the base of the spinous process is particularly important at the lower lumbar segments where the spinal canal is wide. In the upper lumbar spine, minimal undercutting of the spinous process typically suffices to achieve contralateral decompression of the thecal sac. Once the spinous process is undercut, the contralateral laminectomy is continued by undercutting the contralateral lamina along the attachment of the yellow ligament. At this point the steepness of the contralateral lamina can be determined and additional undercutting of the spinous process may be performed if necessary. This concludes the central bony decompression.

36.4.4 Resection of the Yellow Ligament

Resection of the yellow ligament is initiated using a micropunch. The punch is oriented normal to the fibers of the

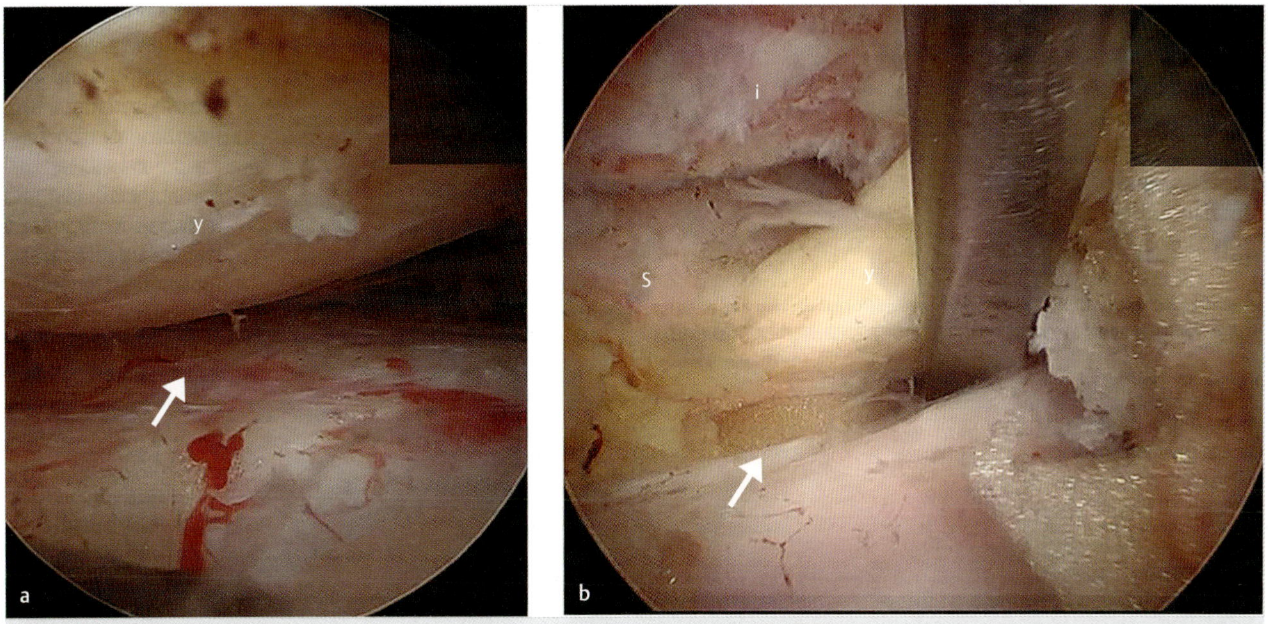

Fig. 36.4 The inside of the *yellow* ligament (y) covering the contralateral medial facet is seen **(a)**. The *arrow* indicates the traversing nerve root. Partial resection of the *yellow* ligament exposes the facet join consisting of the superior articulate process (S) and the inferior articulate process (i) **(b)**. Again the traversing nerve root is marked with an arrow (*arrow*).

ligament and slowly advanced with a rotational movement (▶ Fig. 36.3b). Just prior to transgressing the ligament, a greyish blue discoloration of the ligament can be observed. Once the yellow ligament is opened, inflow of irrigation fluid immediately retracts the epidural fat and thecal sac. Close approximation of the dura sac to the yellow ligament is only seen in revision cases or cases with extremely severe bony stenosis, or large disc herniations. In these cases, like in traditional surgery, a more medial entry can be chosen, and yellow ligament resected along the midline raphe until the dura is visualized. Prior to resection of the yellow ligament, cauterization of the inside of the yellow ligament with the bipolar cautery can avoid cumbersome bleeding. Likewise, epidural fat and vessels should be cauterized prior to resection. A meticulous exposure of the dura of the thecal sac is required for nonambiguous identification of the lateral margins of the neural elements.

36.4.5 Contralateral Medial Facetectomy

Blood vessels of the contralateral yellow ligamentum and epidural fat tissue are thoroughly coagulated using the bipolar cautery. Typically, the inside of the contralateral facet joint can be seen (▶ Fig. 36.4a). Yellow ligament is resected using micropunches and Kerrison rongeurs. Protected side-cutting drill bits are utilized to undercut the contralateral facet joint. The medial facetectomy is carried out spanning from the tip of the SAP to the mid-portion of the caudal pedicle. The joint space is typically seen (▶ Fig. 36.4b). Using a blunt dissector, the contralateral foramen, disc, and pedicle may be palpated and then visualized. A bony decompression of the contralateral foramen can be performed if indicated.

36.4.6 Contralateral Decompression of Neural Elements

The lateral margin of the neural structures is identified. A meticulous exposure of the thecal sac with removal of epidural fat, vessels, and fascial layers greatly facilitates this step (▶ Fig. 36.5a). Visualization of the traversing L5 nerve root at L4/L5 and the S1 traversing nerve root at L5/S1 needs to be accomplished. Once visualized, a blunt dissector is used to gently medialize the lateral margin of the neural structures (thecal sac or traversing nerve root). In case of tethering, there should be a high suspicion for incomplete decompression with the traversing nerve root trapped still within an incompletely decompressed lateral recess. This is commonly encountered at L4/L5. In these cases, further decompression needs to be carried out in the rostral aspect of the lateral recess until the shoulder of the traversing nerve root is identified and decompressed. Residual lateral recess stenosis is then decompressed along the traversing nerve using Kerrison rongeurs and side-biting drill bits. Adequate decompression of neural structures should extend from tip of the SAP to the mid-portion of the caudal pedicle (▶ Fig. 36.5b). Appearance of perineural fat tissue provides additional confirmation of sufficient decompression.

36.4.7 Ipsilateral Medial Facetectomy

Residual yellow ligament in the lateral recess is resected using Kerrison rongeurs and up-angled micropunches. Prior coagulation of the inside of the yellow ligament helps to minimize hemorrhage. The ipsilateral medial facetectomy is carried out utilizing a diamond drill bit or side-biting drill bit. Turning the endoscope 180 degrees and using a large diamond drill bit facilitate undercutting of the ipsilateral lateral recess in order to

minimize resection of the inferior articular process. Maximum medial decompression of the SAP without further resection of the descending articular process can be facilitated by gently retracting the inferior articular process with the working sleeve. This maneuver should only be carried out very gently and avoided in patients with osteoporosis as it can fracture the inferior articular process.

36.4.8 Ipsilateral Decompression of Neural Elements

The ipsilateral margin of the thecal sac is identified. Additional bone is resected as necessary. Using a small side-biting drill bit, the medial facet is trimmed along the thecal sac/traversing nerve root. Decompression should extend from the tip of the SAP to the mid-portion of the caudal pedicle (▶ Fig. 36.6a). Similar to the contralateral decompression, the lateral margin of neural elements should be gently mobilized using a blunt dissector. In case of tethering, there should be a high level of suspicion for an incompletely decompressed lateral recess. In particular at L4/L5 and L5/S1 the traversing nerve root should be nonambiguously identified, which is most easily accomplished in the rostral aspect of the decompression (at or above the tip of the SAP). Adequate compression of neural structures using Kerrison rongeurs or a small side-biting drill bit should span from tip of the SAP to the mid-portion of the caudal pedicle (▶ Fig. 36.6b).

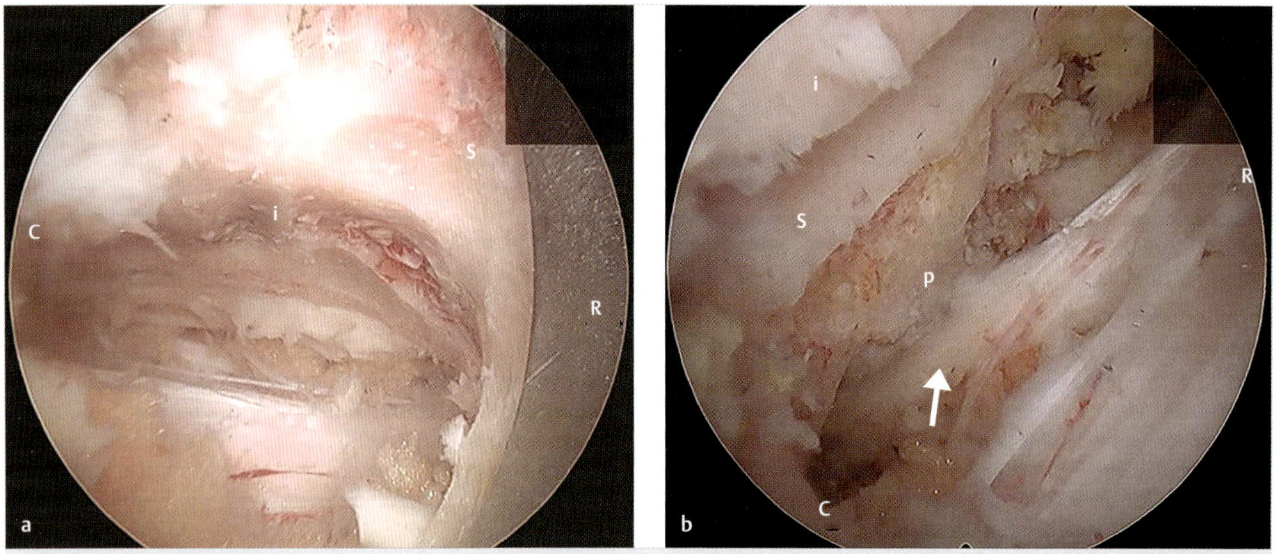

Fig. 36.5 Following undercutting of the spinous process (s), the contralateral interior articular process (i) forming the lateral recess becomes visible **(a)**. Following decompression of the medial aspect of the superior articulate process (S), the contralateral pedicle (p) and traversing nerve root (*arrow*) can be inspected **(b)**.

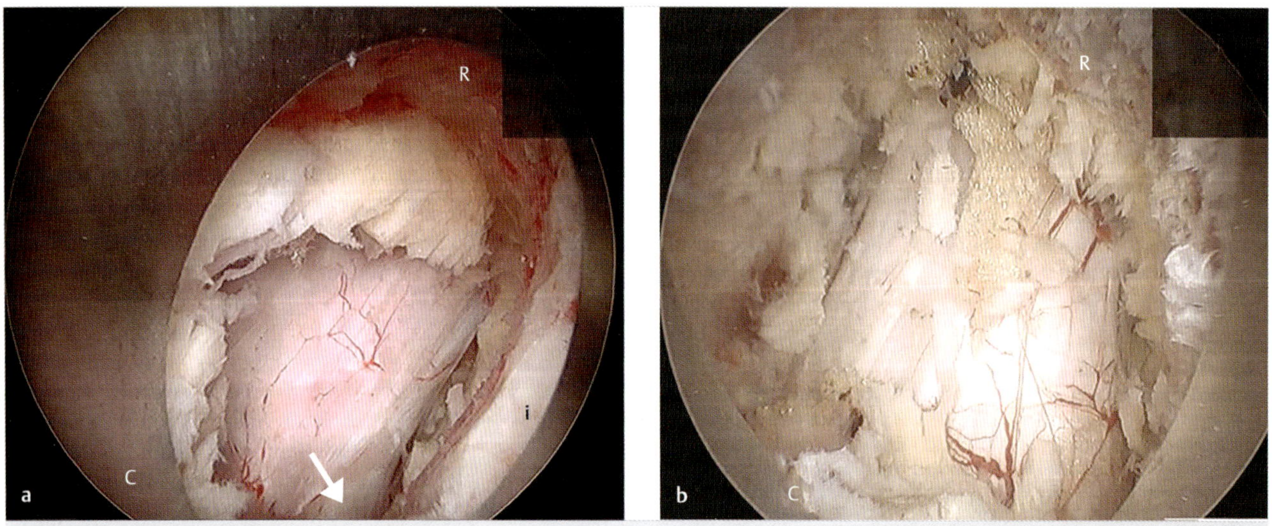

Fig. 36.6 Decompression of the ipsilateral lateral recess is completed and the ipsilateral traversing nerve root is unroofed (*arrow*) **(a)**. At the completion of the laminectomy, the entire thecal sac including bilateral traversing nerve roots are decompressed **(b)**.

36.4.9 Caudal Laminectomy

At this point, additional resection of the caudal lamina may be accomplished using the high-speed drill and/or Kerrison rongeurs. This is particularly necessary in cases with spondylolisthesis in order to create additional space for the neural elements.

36.4.10 Hemostasis and Closure

Meticulous hemostasis is achieved using the bipolar cautery and thrombin. The wound is closed in layers.

36.5 Tips and Tricks

Choice of endoscopic approach: Patients with unilateral lateral recess stenosis may also be candidates for a trans-superior articular process (trans-SAP) approach for lateral recess decompression. In particular, in patients with previous posterior surgery a trans-SAP approach avoids the scar tissue from the previous surgical corridor and allows for ventral and dorsal recompression of the traversing nerve root within the lateral recess.

Choice of appropriate endoscope: Small diameter (iLESSYS pro [Joimax] or interlaminar endoscope [Wolf]) versus large diameter endoscope (iLESSYS delta, [Joimax] or central stenosis endoscope [Wolf]). In patients with a congenitally narrow spinal canal or in the upper lumbar spinal segments, the use of a smaller endoscope makes visualization easier, since the remaining ipsilateral facet joint may block the view obtained with the larger endoscopes. Visualization can still be obtained via rotation of the endoscope to allow for visualization. However, this adds another dimension of difficulty to the procedure. Also, the larger endoscope makes initial docking of the endoscope more difficult since the approach corridor may be blocked by the overgrown facet joint. Thus, it is difficult to define initial bony landmarks. However, the smaller interlaminar endoscopes are not as efficient in removal of bone and yellow ligament and surgeries take more time.

36.6 Complications and Avoidance

a) Inability to identify anatomical landmarks:
   1. Repeat AP and lateral X-rays to confirm appropriate position and level.
   2. Check anatomical landmarks.

b) Bone bleeding: Bleeding from small capillaries close to the articular surface may be difficult to control. Precise targeting with the bipolar cautery as well as physical pressure onto the area of bleeding helps to stop bleeding.

c) Bleeding from the yellow ligament: Use the bipolar cautery first and then resect yellow ligament.

d) In rare cases, sacral nerve roots are already partially formed at L5/S1. The correct plane for contralateral approach may be difficult to find. Adherence to the lamina/yellow ligament/dura planes allows for unambiguous identification of the correct working corridor.

References

[1] Spetzger U, Bertalanffy H, Naujokat C, von Keyserlingk DG, Gilsbach JM. Unilateral laminotomy for bilateral decompression of lumbar spinal stenosis. Part I: Anatomical and surgical considerations. Acta Neurochir (Wien). 1997; 139(5):392–396

[2] Spetzger U, Bertalanffy H, Reinges MH, Gilsbach JM. Unilateral laminotomy for bilateral decompression of lumbar spinal stenosis. Part II: Clinical experiences. Acta Neurochir (Wien). 1997; 139(5):397–403

[3] Foley KT, Smith MM, Rampersaud YR. Microendoscopic approach to far-lateral lumbar disc herniation. Neurosurg Focus. 1999; 7(5):e5

[4] Boukebir MA, Berlin CD, Navarro-Ramirez R, et al. Ten-step minimally invasive spine lumbar decompression and dural repair through tubular retractors. Oper Neurosurg (Hagerstown). 2017; 13(2):232–245

[5] Komp M, Hahn P, Oezdemir S, et al. Bilateral spinal decompression of lumbar central stenosis with the full-endoscopic interlaminar versus microsurgical laminotomy technique: a prospective, randomized, controlled study. Pain Physician. 2015; 18(1):61–70

[6] Ruetten S, Komp M, Merk H, Godolias G. Surgical treatment for lumbar lateral recess stenosis with the full-endoscopic interlaminar approach versus conventional microsurgical technique: a prospective, randomized, controlled study. J Neurosurg Spine. 2009; 10(5):476–485

[7] Wagner R, Telfeian AE, Kzrok G, Iprenburg M. Fully-endoscopic lumbar laminectomy for central and lateral recess stenosis: technical note. Interdiscip Neurosurg. 2018; 13:6–9

[8] Härtl, R, Korge A. AOSpine: Minimally Invasive Spine Surgery—Technique, Evidence, and Controversies. Davos-platz, Stuttgart, Germany: Thieme; 2012

[9] Mummaneni PV, Shaffrey CI, Lenke LG, et al. Minimally Invasive Surgery Section of the International Spine Study Group. The minimally invasive spinal deformity surgery algorithm: a reproducible rational framework for decision making in minimally invasive spinal deformity surgery. Neurosurg Focus. 2014; 36(5):E6

37 LLIF T12/L1-L2

Cristiano Magalhães Menezes and Érica Godinho Menezes

Summary
The lateral transpsoas approach to the T12/L1-L2 (thoracolumbar junction) level requires careful management of the diaphragm, the pleura and the 11th and 12th ribs. In this chapter, the authors describe these steps with a couple of cases and a very comprehensive video, sharing their experience and the complication avoidance tips and tricks.

Keywords: XLIF, MIS thoracolumbar, corpectomy, thoracic disc herniation

37.1 Introduction

The lateral lumbar interbody fusion (LLIF) procedure described by Ozgur et al[1] to address different conditions in lumbar spine, has become increasingly popular to achieve fusion due to the advantages of smaller incisions, decreased blood loss, and shorter hospital stays.[2,3,4,5] The development of the technique permitted not only interbody fusion but also indirect decompression neural elements, corpectomies, restoration of vertebral height, alignment, and stabilization, especially in thoracic and thoracolumbar segments, where lumbar plexus is not a concern.[3,4,5]

There are multiple indications for LLIF in thoracolumbar region including traumatic and degenerative conditions.[2,3,4] It is part of any multilevel surgery, starting at lower lumbar levels, as in scoliosis surgery, or targeting the thoracolumbar junction, as in a corpectomy to treat a fracture.

The thoracolumbar junction (T11L1) challenges the spine surgeon's anatomy knowledge, especially the diaphragm anatomy, which separates the thoracic and abdominal cavities.[2,6,7,8] Dealing with this complex anatomic region, using a minimally disruptive anterolateral corridor for T12L1 cases, is the key to decreasing morbidity of open thoracophrenolumbotomies. For this, it is crucial to keep dissection out of the pleural cavity, using an extracavitary approach, mastering the specific anatomy of the region to mobilize the thoracic diaphragm in a reproducible and safe manner.[2] A retropleural approach is used when a plane between the parietal pleura and inner surface of the rib inferior to the access incision is created with the diaphragm and pleura retracted and dissected anteriorly.[6] This enables the approach to the spine, vertebral body, and disc spaces as well as ventral dural sac for decompression from a lateral trajectory.

In this chapter, we describe the technique for minimally invasive lateral retropleural approach at T12/L1 using the LLIF tubular expandable retractor, the potential pitfalls, and expected outcomes.

37.2 Indications

There are many potential indications for a retropleural LLIF approach at the thoracolumbar junction, including degenerative, deformity, trauma, tumor, and infection of the spine.

Over the past decade, less invasive surgical approaches for neural decompression and fusion have been popularized and recently applied for the treatment of degenerative conditions. Single degenerative disc disease at T12L1 and thoracolumbar disc herniation with conus medullaris compression are examples of these indications (▶ Fig. 37.1). More commonly, T12L1 multiple-level LLIF surgery for adult spinal deformity is an attempt to achieve sagittal and coronal alignment with decreased morbidity. The lateral approach may be used as part of a minimally invasive anterior-only or anterior-posterior procedure for the management of degenerative scoliosis, or may be combining it with an open posterior fusion with or without osteotomies.[3,9,10]

In traumatic fractures, this approach can be used in association with percutaneous short segment posterior fixation or with modern lateral or anterior plates to perform a thoracolumbar corpectomy.[11] The same can be done for corpectomies due to spinal tumors (▶ Fig. 37.2), aiming at palliation, stabilization, spinal cord decompression, pain control, and overall quality of life improvement.[12] It is also possible that through lateral access surgery, the spinal canal can be reached for certain tumor resections. An example of an infectious case that can be approached laterally is a thoracolumbar discitis case where this can be safely approached through a mini-open lateral approach.

37.3 Contraindications

Relative contraindications include: anomalous vascular anatomy, such as lateralized vessels (deformity cases with vertebral rotation) or the presence of the artery of Adamkiewicz on the surgical corridor; vascular disease; retroperitoneal or retropleural scar due to prior surgery; intense pleural inflammatory

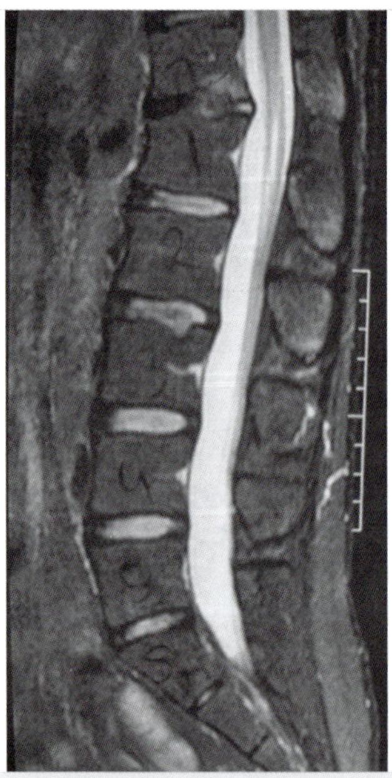

Fig. 37.1 Single-level degenerative disc disease at T12L1 with Modic 1 changes.

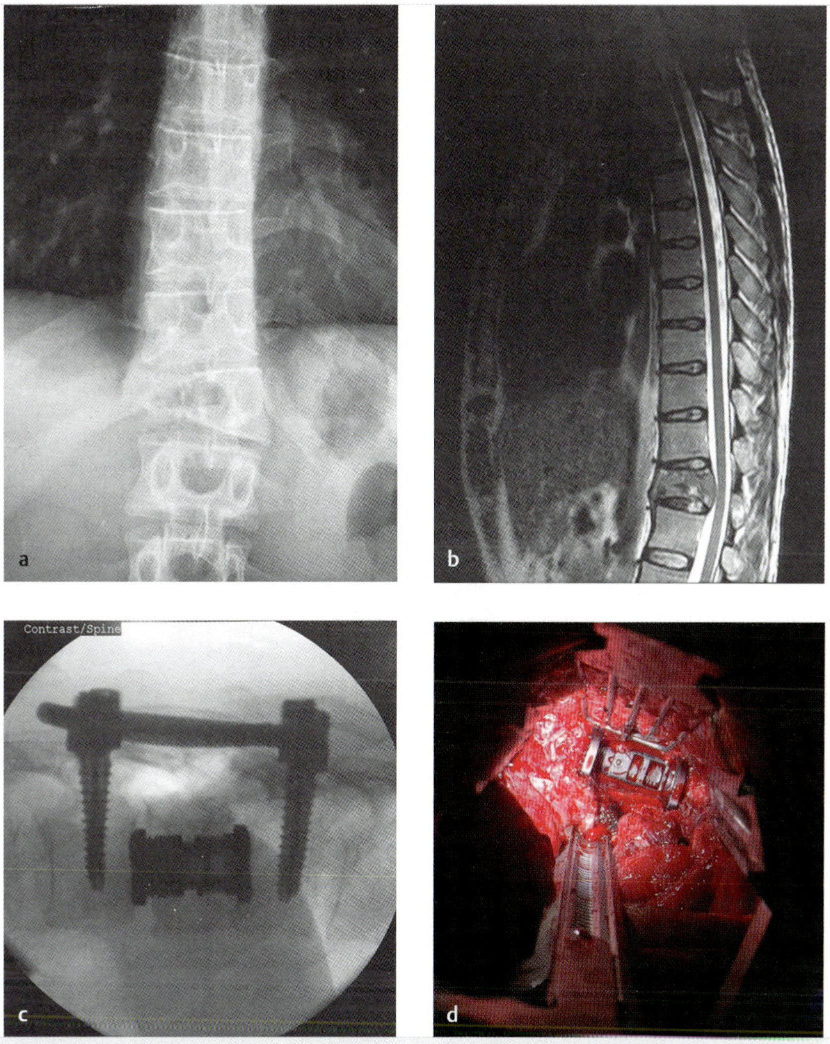

Fig. 37.2 Pathologic fracture due a plasmacytoma at T12. **(a)** Anteroposterior X-ray; **(b)** sagittal magnetic resonance imaging (MRI), T2-weighted image; **(c)** intraoperative fluoroscopic image; **(d)** expandable cage positioned after corpectomy.

reaction due to infection (spondylodiscitis); when posterior direct decompression is required; when potential bony structures could limit the access (large osteophytes); morbid obesity; and thoracic or pulmonary anomalies.

Thus, it is mandatory to evaluate the spine orientation and rotation effects on vascular and visceral structures in order to determine if a safe working channel can be achieved.

37.4 Preoperative Planning

It is important to identify patients suitable for a lateral LLIF approach to the thoracolumbar junction based on the patient's pathology and anatomy, as well as on surgeon's proficiency. Patient selection, with special attention to patient's medical history and those potential contraindications to the anterior approach to spine, as well as correct evaluation of anteroposterior (AP) and lateral X-ray and axial magnetic resonance imaging (MRI), is critical.

The operating room (OR) setup for a lateral procedure must be planned to optimize the efficiency and workflow. The surgical bed is oriented in order to fit the patient properly and still have enough room to place the fluoroscopy monitor and neuromonitoring machine directed toward the surgeon and the OR personnel. Ensuring a clear path for C-arm travel into the room and to the ventral side of the patient is recommended. A mayo stand is placed toward the feet of the bed, allowing access to the scrub nurse, and avoiding interfering with the C-arm or surgeon. If the bed needs to be reversed, move the headpiece to the caudal part of the bed and reposition the arm board in line with the axilla on the ventral side of the patient (▶ Fig. 37.3).

Dual lumen intubation can be used to reduce lung size on the operative side, but it is not routinely necessary. It can be achieved by reducing the insufflation tidal volume and increasing the respiration rate to keep the patient oxygenated during anesthesia.

37.5 Patient Positioning

After intubation and general anesthesia, with the back facing the surgeon and in lateral decubitus, the patient is placed

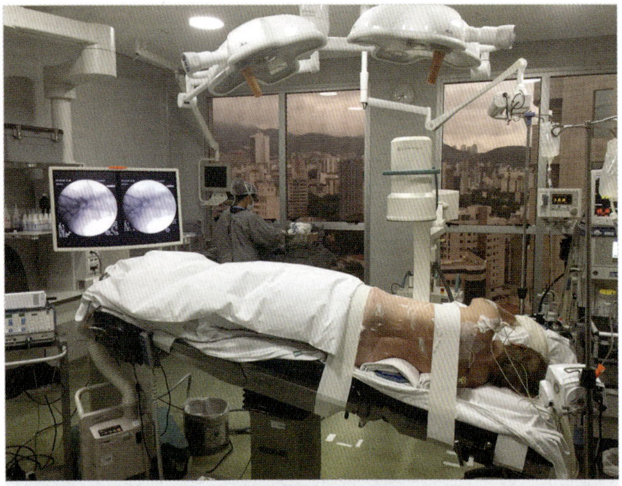

Fig. 37.3 In the operating room, the setup for lateral procedure must be planned to optimize the efficiency and workflow. The surgical bed is oriented in order to fit the patient properly.

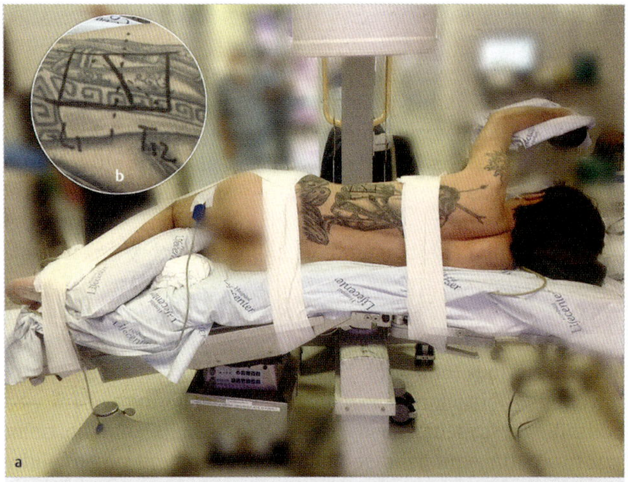

Fig. 37.4 (a) Patient positioning: Tape over the padded osseous prominences. Do not break the table. (b) Markings for skin incision.

approximately 4 to 6 inches from the posterior edge of the bed. The head of the patient needs to be supported and should face the anesthesiologist to ensure adequate access to the face and the endotracheal tube. Place an axillary roll under the patient's downside axilla while maintaining space for the C-arm to enter the sterile field. Padding to protect the patient's nipple, peroneal nerve, and lateral malleolus of the ankle is also recommended.

Now, the torso of the patient is adjusted approximating the spine until a true AP fluoroscopy is achieved. The surgeon needs to instruct the C-arm technician to take AP shots, adjusting the patient until true images can be achieved (both the pedicles and a single linear end plate can be seen above and below the vertebrae at the area of interest). Once this has been achieved, hold the patient in this position while ensuring the C-arm is clear of chest taping site. At the level of patient's chest, tape from the anterior side of the bed, taping around the chest, over padded nipple, adhering tape directly to the patient's skin on the lateral aspect of the chest, while holding the patient in true AP of the operative level. Adhere the tape to the posterior rail of bed, continuing under to meet the tape at its origin. Without tearing the tape, repeat one more loop. Secure the patient's arms to an arm board. Use pads between under the lateral downside to protect the shoulders (▶ Fig. 37.3). With the aid of an assistant, adhere tape in front of the bed, below the break on anterior side of the patient. Pull the tape up and over the crest, adhering it directly to the skin just below the iliac crest. Without tearing the tape, continue under the bed to go around the patient and repeat until completing one more loop around the patient. Adhere a new piece of tape just below the iliac crest, pulling across the lateral thigh, over the padded knee, and under the anterior side of the bed, emerging at the patient's foot. Continue pulling tape over the padded ankle, cross over the padded knee, then under the anterior section of bed, emerging posteriorly at level of the patient's hip (before the break), and continue the tape until it overlaps the initial starting point of this piece of tape. Retractor attachment (flexible arm) should be placed at the posterior side of the patient in line with his/her scapula (▶ Fig. 37.4a).

37.6 Surgical Steps

37.6.1 Incision

The planned incision is marked over the skin to guide the surgeon to make an optimal incision that allows for access to the T12L1 disc space (▶ Fig. 37.4b):

1. Obtain a true lateral image of the operative disc space. With a targeting instrument on skin, mark the border of anterior longitudinal ligament (ALL), posterior longitudinal ligament (PLL), and an extended line anterior to the disc space.
2. Place a K-wire along the rib closest to the disc space and mark along it. Mark for incision along the rib or between the ribs centered over the disc space biased 20% posteriorly. Note that the rib will need to be resected if it is found overlying the disc space. Perform the skin incision and dissect tissue until the rib or intercostal space is exposed (▶ Fig. 37.5). At this point it is extremely important to review the diaphragm anatomy.

The diaphragm is a musculotendinous sheet extending between the thoracic and abdominal cavities. Its attachments include sternal or anterior, costal or lateral, and lumbar or posterior attachments. The sternal attachment is not part of this approach. The costal and lumbar attachments are crucial. The lateral costal attachment is in the medial aspect of 9th and 10th ribs, and the posterolateral attachments are in the 11th and 12th ribs. Posteriorly, the diaphragm has two arcuate ligaments on each side. The lateral arcuate ligament spans the *quadratus lumborum*, whereas the medial arcuate ligament spans the origin of the psoas muscle. The intervening point of attachment is on the transverse process of L1.[7] For a more extensive revision, the authors recommend to check our references for this topic.[6,7,8]

37.6.2 Technique

1. Safely access the retropleural space and place initial dilator by the location of incision. Usually for T12/L1 disc space, the incision will be at or between the 9th and 11th ribs. To reach the T12L1 disc, one must keep the extracoelomic space, developing

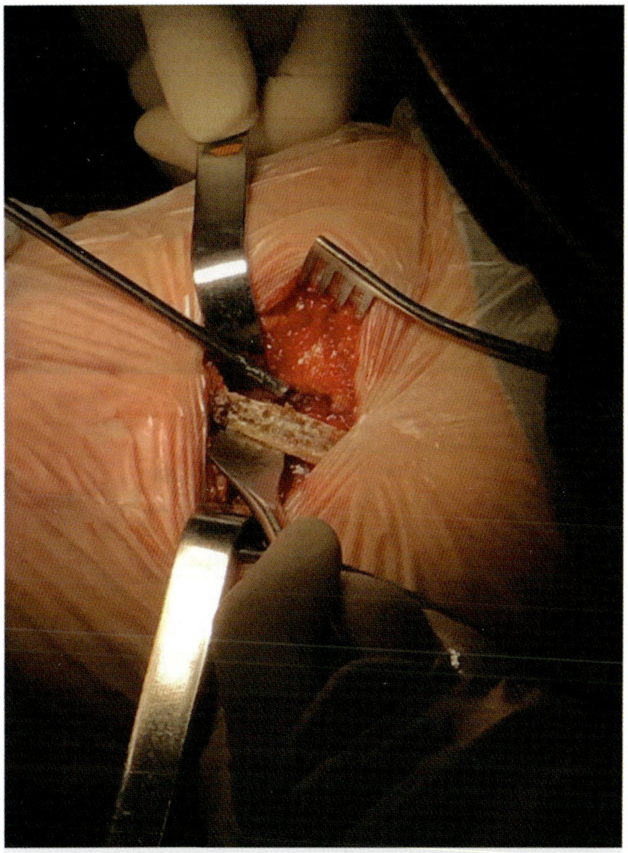

Fig. 37.5 Rib preparation.

the plane retropleuraly by mobilizing the diaphragm from its posterior costal and lumbar insertions. Initially, dissect the muscle layer away from the rib overlying the targeted disc space, skeletonizing the rib on its proximal surface.

2. Use elevators to carefully release the parietal pleura and diaphragm from the underside of the rib. Preserve the neurovascular bundle and protect it throughout the procedure. Remove a 3- to 5-cm section of the rib that impedes access to the targeting disc space. Bias this cut more posteriorly to aid in retropleural dissection. Use the finger to release the parietal pleura by placing it inside of the posterior section of the remaining rib and sweeping it in cranial and caudal direction as the finger moves down the rib toward the spine (▶ Fig. 37.6). Once at the spine, palpate the L1 transverse process to locate the arcuate ligament and release it to gain access to the spine in the retroperitoneal space. Guide the dilator down to the surface of the psoas using your finger in the posterior incision to reflect diaphragm and abdominal contents away from the dilator. After docking of initial dilator and neuromonitoring, insert the K-wire 30 mm into the disc space confirming location at its posterior one-third. Use fluoroscopy to confirm initial dilator placement over the targeted disc space.
3. Once adequate position over the T12L1 disc is confirmed, the goal is to keep the retractor deployed coaxial to the disc space allowing proper discectomy and implant placement. For this purpose, it is important to measure blade length from the initial dilator (add 10 mm from skin level to determine blade length). Wet dilators with saline while inserting each one to ensure no soft tissue damage, splitting psoas

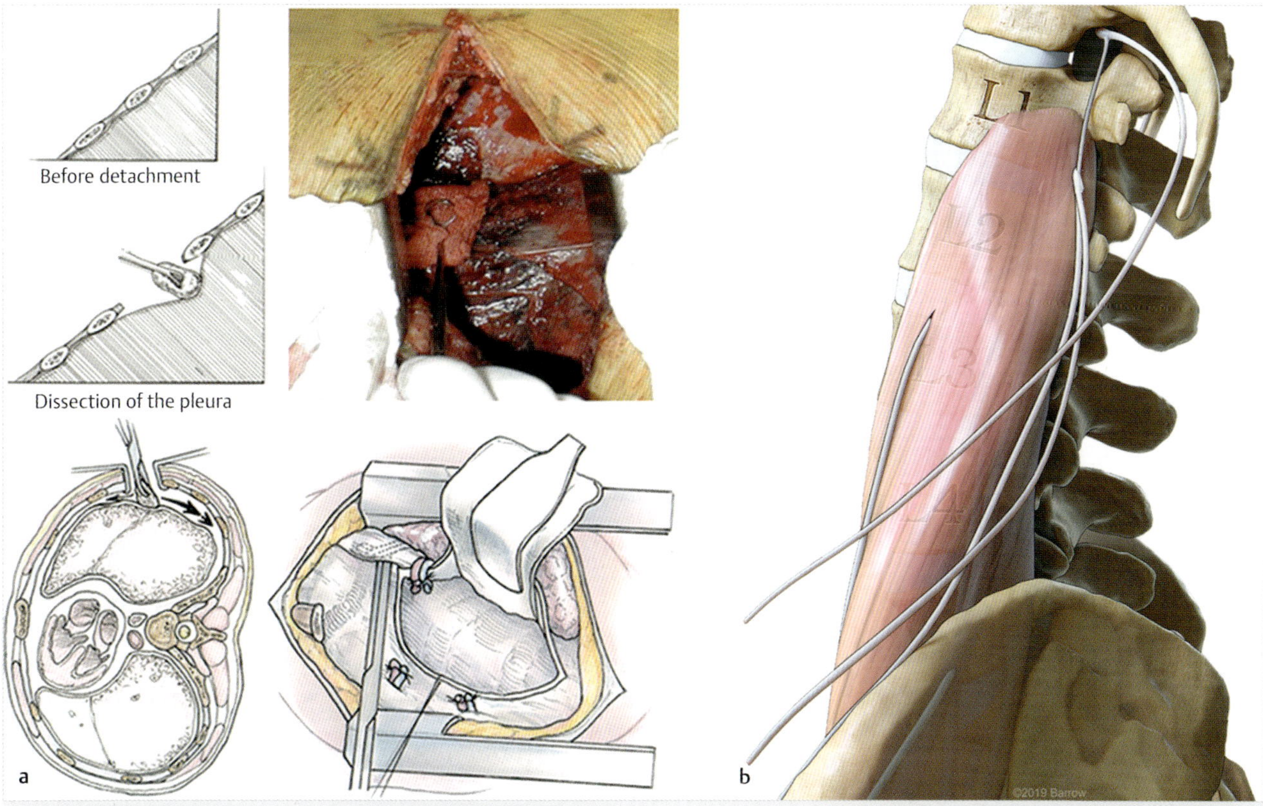

Fig. 37.6 Illustrations of the retropleural exposure **(a)** and the lateral view of the spine at T12-L1, note the absence of psoas at that level and also the location of the lumbar plexus **(b)**. (Reproduced from (a) Open lateral transthoracic approach. In: Fessler R, Sekhar L, eds. Atlas of Neurosurgical Techniques: Spine and Peripheral Nerves. 2nd ed. Thieme; 2016. (b) Major Sensory and Motor Nerves Relative to the Disc Space. In: Tumialán L, ed. Minimally Invasive Spine Surgery: A Primer. 1st Edition. New York: Thieme; 2020.)

Table 37.1 10 steps to disc preparation (▶ Video 37.1)

Step	Procedure
1	Annulotomy
2	Discectomy (Pituitary Rongeur)
3	Cobb
4	Discectomy (Pituitary Rongeur)
5	Broach
6	Discectomy (Pituitary Rongeur)
7	Stirrup curette
8	Trial cage
9	End plate preparation (Rasp)
10	Implant

Notes: Use lateral fluoroscopy when guiding Cobb, Broach, and Stirrup Curette in disc space to redirect instruments away from entering into end plate. Use trials under AP and lateral fluoroscopy to confirm appropriate implant size.
To the reader: All of these steps are better illustrated in the ▶ Video 37.1.

muscle and dilating the muscle fibers between dilator and lateral surface of the disc. Insert retractor properly guided by AP initial skin marking to guide the rotation to line up with the disc space. Retractor handles are used for bisecting the anterior aspect of the extended AP disc space skin marking.

4. Attach retractor to articulating arm using the anterior attachment point. While using one hand to apply downward pressure, and second hand to grasp the handles, squeeze until one click is heard. Insert the lights halfway down the cranial blade and bend back to secure. If retractor moves, insert screw shim down cephalad or caudal blade. Open the retractor using one hand to apply downward pressure, and second hand to grasp the thumbwheel on the side of retractor; rotate until four clicks are heard. Use shim to retract any tissue coming into the field. Dissect the remaining thin layer of muscle at the spine with laparoscopic peanut or bipolar cautery. Insert intradiscal shim to fixate retractor to spine. Confirm position with fluoroscopy.
5. The goal now is to clean the disc corridor and end plates for interbody spacer implantation. Pay special attention to perform a complete discectomy and end plate preparation. Do not violate the end plate during discectomy and protect the neural elements posteriorly located inside the foramen and spinal canal. Follow the 10 steps to disc preparation (▶ Table 37.1).

37.6.3 Closure

1. Remove the retractor (and intradiscal shim if used) under direct visualization, maintaining hemostasis of the surgical field. Perform a bubble test if desired: Submerge retropleural space in saline and have anesthesia insulate the lung. If no bubbles are present, the parietal pleura is intact and a chest tube is not needed. Insert a red rubber catheter into the chest and submerge the open end in a saline filled emesis basin. Reapproximate intercostal muscles under direct vision. Perform layered closure of serratus muscles up to the dermal layer under direct visualization.
2. Suture is run in 1-cm intervals (maximally), with at least 1 cm bit of fascia in each throw, leaving a red rubber catheter in the cavity secured with a purse string closure method. Fill the lung with anesthesia with a “valsalva” and watch for any air that evacuates the cavity by watching the bubbles in the emesis basin. Once the bubbles stop, pull the catheter and close the purse string (▶ Fig. 37.7).

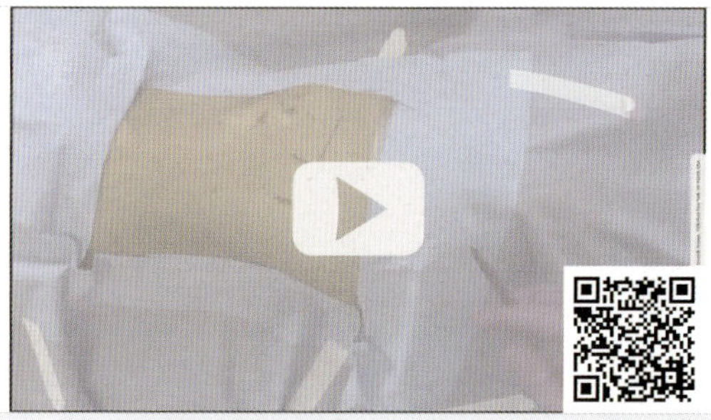

Video 37.1 LLIF step-by-step technique.

37.7 Postoperative Care

Usually, the patient is transferred to a recovery room, where an X-ray check of the thorax is desired. If a single-level LLIF is performed at T12L1 level, no intensive care unit (ICU) is required and the patient is admitted in an ambulatory basis. Postoperative analgesics are administered as necessary and oral feeding allowed. Ambulation is encouraged few hours after surgery, on the same day. Hospital stay under 23 hours is desired.

37.8 Complication Avoidance

a) Step-by-step observation in LLIF T12L1 mitigates the chances of complications. In the preoperative planning, patient selection and correct evaluation of X-ray and axial MRI must be part of this care. Visualization of fluoroscopic images during surgery prevents implant misplacement. So make sure C-arm is accessible without any interference such as cassette risers or bed rail. If the patient is positioned too far posterior on the bed, lateral edge of bed to may interfere with viewing the anatomy in the C-arm images.
b) An axillary roll is mandatory to avoid brachial plexus injury. Safely secure the patient in position with tapes. If the patient moves during surgery, visceral or vascular injuries may occur due to the lack of orthogonal orientation. Vascular and visceral damages are very rare, and may be avoided with proper orientation during surgery.
c) Check pre- and intraoperative images to identify transitional anatomy, such as rudimentary 12th rib that may confuse the surgeon about the right level.
d) Damage of neurovascular bundle of the 12th rib due to improper use of eletrocautery during initial dissection, for example, can cause pseudohernia or denervation of rectus muscle, if 12th intercostal (subcostal nerve) is the first rami of lumbar plexus.
e) Damage to pleural structures with inadvertent thorax violation must be avoided with proper knowledge of thoracolumbar anatomy while mobilizing the diaphragm and pleura, and retracting and dissecting anteriorly.
f) Pseudoarthosis, nerve injury, and subsidence are precluded with proper surgical technique.

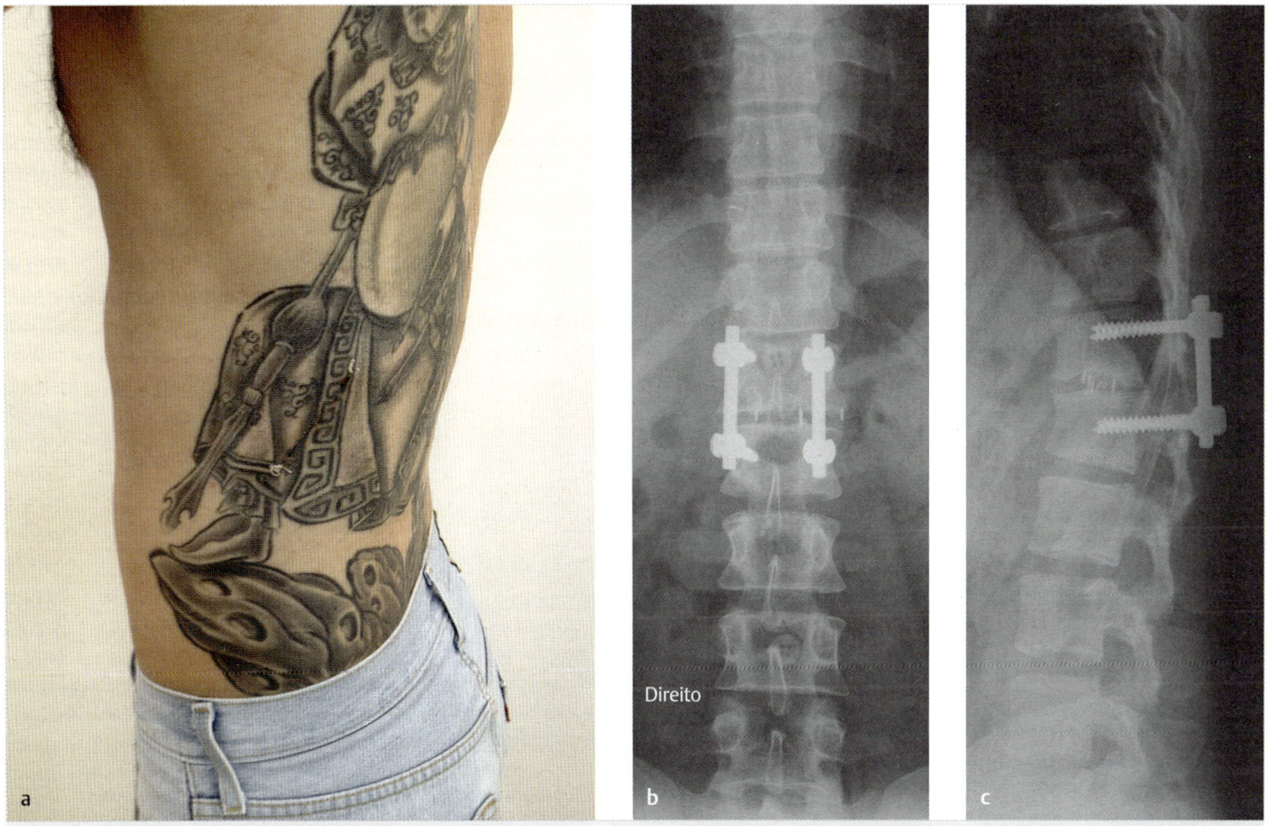

Fig. 37.7 (a) Postoperative skin incision appearance; **(b, c)** Anteroposterior (AP) and lateral X-rays of a single-level T12L1 extreme lateral interbody fusion (XLIF).

37.9 Tips and Tricks

One simple way to choose the most appropriate approach in the thoracolumbar junction is to consider ribs as markers of the underlying anatomy: Once your incision for LLIF stays under the 12th rib, a standard LLIF approach is used to gain access to the retroperitoneal space. If the incision is marked in between the 11th and 12th ribs, a transdiaphragmatic retroperitoneal approach is performed. Access the retroperitoneum with the posterior incision inferior to the 12th rib. Confirm access by palpating anatomical landmarks (underside of 12th rib, underside of the diaphragm, and transverse process). Use your finger to sweep the tissue away from the underside of the diaphragm and the abdominal wall. Incise the diaphragm over your finger to ensure that there is only diaphragm between your finger and the retroperitoneum. Guide the dilator down to the surface of the psoas using your finger in the posterior incision to reflect the diaphragm and abdominal contents away from the dilator. If the incision is marked at or superior to the 11th rib, a retropleural technique can be used to access the spine, as previously described in this chapter.

37.10 Conclusion

The MIS lateral retropleural access for the thoracolumbar junction is safe and feasible technique to perform an LLIF at T12L1, as well as corpectomy and ventral decompression of the spinal canal. The three key points for success of this operation are: (1) preoperative planning; (2) gaining access to the retropleural plane, with anterior mobilization of the diaphragm releasing its main attachments from the 12th rib and transverse process of L1; and (3) performing an orthogonal operation to adequately perform a complete discectomy and end plate preparation for final cage implantation.

References

[1] Ozgur BM, Aryan HE, Pimenta L, Taylor WR. Extreme lateral interbody fusion (XLIF): a novel surgical technique for anterior lumbar interbody fusion. Spine J. 2006; 6(4):435–443

[2] Sun JC, Wang JR, Luo T, et al. Surgical incision and approach in thoracolumbar extreme lateral interbody fusion surgery: an anatomic study of the diaphragmatic attachments. Spine. 2016; 41(4):E186–E190

[3] Dakwar E, Cardona RF, Smith DA, Uribe JS. Early outcomes and safety of the minimally invasive, lateral retroperitoneal transpsoas approach for adult degenerative scoliosis. Neurosurg Focus. 2010; 28(3):E8

[4] Smith WD, Dakwar E, Le TV, Christian G, Serrano S, Uribe JS. Minimally invasive surgery for traumatic spinal pathologies: a mini-open, lateral approach in the thoracic and lumbar spine. Spine. 2010; 35(26) Suppl:S338–S346

[5] Uribe JS, Dakwar E, Le TV, Christian G, Serrano S, Smith WD. Minimally invasive surgery treatment for thoracic spine tumor removal: a mini-open, lateral approach. Spine. 2010; 35(26) Suppl:S347–S354

[6] Uribe JS, Dakwar E, Cardona RF, Vale FL. Minimally invasive lateral retropleural thoracolumbar approach: cadaveric feasibility study and report of 4 clinical cases. Neurosurgery. 2011; 68(1) Suppl Operative:32–39, discussion 39

[7] Dakwar E, Ahmadian A, Uribe JS. The anatomical relationship of the diaphragm to the thoracolumbar junction during the minimally invasive lateral extracoelomic (retropleural/retroperitoneal) approach. J Neurosurg Spine. 2012; 16(4):359–364

[8] Baaj AA, Papadimitriou K, Amin AG, Kretzer RM, Wolinsky JP, Gokaslan ZL. Surgical anatomy of the diaphragm in the anterolateral approach to the spine: a cadaveric study. J Spinal Disord Tech. 2014; 27(4):220–223

[9] Mundis GM, Akbarnia BA, Phillips FM. Adult deformity correction through minimally invasive lateral approach techniques. Spine. 2010; 35(26) Suppl: S312–S321

[10] Isaacs RE, Hyde J, Goodrich JA, Rodgers WB, Phillips FM. A prospective, nonrandomized, multicenter evaluation of extreme lateral interbody fusion for the treatment of adult degenerative scoliosis: perioperative outcomes and complications. Spine. 2010; 35(26) Suppl:S322–S330

[11] Smith WD, Dakwar E, Le TV, Christian G, Serrano S, Uribe JS. Minimally invasive surgery for traumatic spinal pathologies: a mini-open, lateral approach in the thoracic and lumbar spine. Spine. 2010; 35 26 Suppl:S338–S346

[12] Uribe JS, Dakwar E, Le TV, Christian G, Serrano S, Smith WD. Minimally invasive surgery treatment for thoracic spine tumor removal: a mini-open, lateral approach. Spine. 2010; 35 26 Suppl:S347–S354

38 LLIF L2/3/4/5

Frank M. Phillips and Sravisht Iyer

Summary
The extreme lateral interbody fusion (XLIF) or lateral lumbar interbody fusion (LLIF) is a minimally invasive approach to fusion in the lumbar spine. LLIF can treat foraminal stenosis, moderate lateral recess stenosis, and degenerative scoliosis. Safely performing LLIF requires paying close attention to the neurovascular anatomy, identifying the lumbar plexus using EMG, and minimizing table break and retractor time. Close adherence to these principles can help minimize complications.

Keywords: lateral lumbar interbody fusion, psoas anatomy, EMG monitoring, patient positioning, lateral technique

38.1 Introduction

First described in 2006, lateral lumbar interbody fusion (LLIF) was developed as a minimally invasive, lateral, retroperitoneal trans-psoas approach to the lumbar spine.[1] Since that time, the LLIF procedure has since been widely adopted as a method for placing anterior lumbar interbody devices in the lumbar spine.[2] This chapter discusses the most common indications and contraindications for this procedure. We also discuss surgical techniques, postoperative care, and tips and tricks that have been learned through the authors' experience.

38.2 Indications

The United States Food and Drug Administration has only approved LLIF for one- and two-level lumbar fusions with supplemental posterior fixation.[2] However, clinically, the LLIF is frequently utilized, with or without posterior fixation (i.e., stand-alone),for multilevel pathology (e.g., in adult spinal deformity). Commonly practiced indications for LLIF include various lumbar degenerative pathologies (degenerative scoliosis, spinal stenosis, degenerative disc disease, adjacent segment degeneration) and adult spinal deformity (ASD).[2]

For lumbar degenerative disease, the LLIF has enjoyed success in achieving indirect neural decompression via disc space distraction in patients with mild to moderate lateral recess and central canal stenosis and/or moderate to severe foraminal stenosis.[3] There is also considerable evidence to suggest that LLIF may be effective in treating patients with low-grade (Grade I/II) degenerative spondylolisthesis as well as degenerative scoliosis.[4,5,6]

LLIF aims to restore lumbar disc height via the use of an interbody biomechanical cage device. Compared to posterior approaches, LLIF allows for placement of a substantially larger interbody cage without the need for entry into the spinal canal or neuroforamen. This avoids the need for neural manipulation and retraction. Placement of these larger cages provides direct restoration of the foraminal height and indirect decompression of the spinal canal via stretching of the posterior longitudinal ligament (PLL) and unbuckling of the ligamentum flavum; increases in foraminal, central, and lateral recess area have been demonstrated on postoperative imaging.[7,8,9,10] LLIF in patients with foraminal stenosis has been shown to improve health-related quality of life (HRQOL) scores at up to 1-year follow-up.[6,8,10,11]

One recent systematic review found that LLIF was similar to posterior and anterior interbody approaches in success rates for addressing foraminal stenosis.[3] There is considerably more debate regarding the ability of LLIF to treat central canal stenosis.[12,13,14] Although some authors have suggested that indirect decompression can result in improved outcomes,[5,14] the limits of this technique are not yet well defined. The LLIF may not be an appropriate option to provide indirect decompression in patients with severe central stenosis, significant facet hypertrophy and ankylosis, bony stenosis (congenital stenosis), or calcified discs.

The ability to restore disc height and lordosis makes LLIF an attractive operation for patients presenting with ASD. In this population, LLIF has been associated with excellent (40–75%) correction of coronal deformity with more modest increases in lumbar lordosis.[6,15] The addition of an anterior column release (ACR) via transection of the anterior longitudinal ligament (ALL) and placement of hyperlordotic cages can restore lumbar lordosis via the lateral approach.[16,17,18]

38.3 Contraindications

Any aberrant neurovascular anatomy that limits safe access to the disc space is a contraindication to LLIF. Several authors have described the anatomy of the psoas muscle and lumbar plexus with respect to the lateral approach.[19,20] The "safe zone" for approach is between the lumbar plexus (posterior) and abdominal vessels (anterior). At L4–L5 in particular, this safe zone narrows as the lumbar plexus moves more anteriorly and the vascular structures are more posterior on the disc space (▶ Fig. 38.1). The access corridor at L4–L5 is generally narrower on the right hand side due to the vascular structures being more posterior.[19] Despite these anatomic concerns, there is a robust body of literature supporting safety and efficacy of the LLIF using real-time, directional neural monitoring at the L4–L5 level.[21,22,23]

Another important consideration with establishing access to the disc space is pelvic morphology; a high pelvic brim may not allow for access to the L4–L5 disc space (▶ Fig. 38.2). Other contraindications to LLIF include retroperitoneal scarring (due to prior retroperitoneal surgery, abdominal radiation, diverticulitis, etc.) and comorbidities that preclude fusion surgery (e.g., poor bone quality).

38.4 Preoperative Planning

Preoperative considerations for LLIF include: the side of approach, implant selection, implant sizing, and whether to add posterior instrumentation (▶ Table 38.1). If L4–L5 is planned, the orientation of the L4–L5 disc space usually determines the side of approach. Obliquity of the L4–L5 disc space (e.g., in patients with degenerative scoliosis) can make the level accessible from one side only. In practice, we typically add posterior

instrumentation for multilevel LLIF, patients with spondylolisthesis or spinal deformity, patients requiring anterior column (ALL) release, and patients at higher high risk for subsidence (e.g., poor bone quality). There is data to suggest that standalone LLIF may be sufficient in patients with low-grade degenerative spondylolisthesis.[5] It is also important to closely assess the cross-sectional anatomy on magnetic resonance imaging (MRI) with particular attention being paid to the psoas muscle, the location of the vasculature, and the lumbar plexus. Louie et al recently described specific psoas morphology that may make lateral approaches more challenging in the lower lumbar spine.[24]

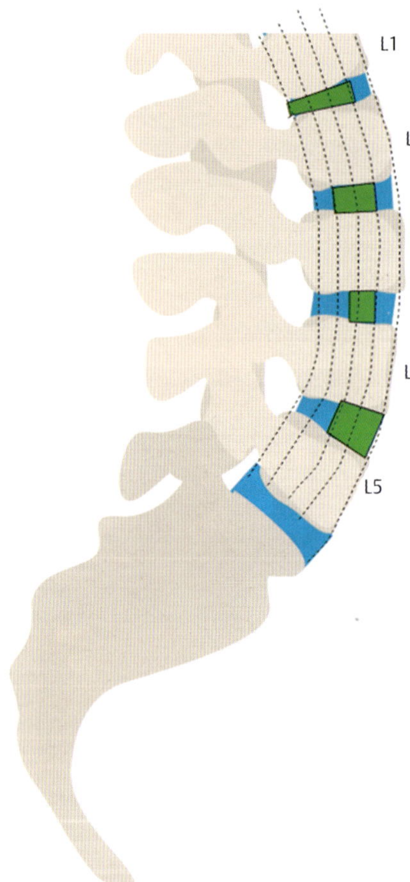

Fig. 38.1 Illustration of the safe zones relative to the neurovascular anatomy in the lumbar spine. Please note that the safe zone moves more anterior in the lower lumbar spine.

38.5 Patient Positioning

Patient positioning is a critical component of the LLIF procedure. Appropriate positioning requires a bendable, radiolucent surgical table. It is important to ensure that the fluoroscopy C-arm can rotate freely without being impeded by the base of the table.

Neuromonitoring leads (free-run electromyography [EMG]) are placed following induction of anesthesia while the patient is still supine. Because neuromonitoring is used during the approach, it is important that the anesthesiologist only use short-acting paralytics during induction.

Next, the patient is turned to lateral decubitus position with the iliac crest positioned at the level of the break in the table (▶ Fig. 38.3). It is often helpful to slightly break the table to facilitate access to L4–L5 above the iliac crest and L1–L2 below the rib cage. It is important to ensure that all "down" surfaces (axilla, peroneal nerve, ulnar nerve) are appropriately padded. The arms are flexed approximately 90 degrees at the shoulder and elbow and supported on an arm board. A pillow or stack of blankets is typically placed between the arms.

The hips and knees are then flexed to relax the psoas muscle and lumbar plexus. The patient is then secured to the bed with tape. We secure the torso with tape just below the iliac crest (over the greater trochanter) and just below the ribs. Tape is then run from the greater trochanter to the knees and brought around the table to the ankle and past the knee in a figure-of-

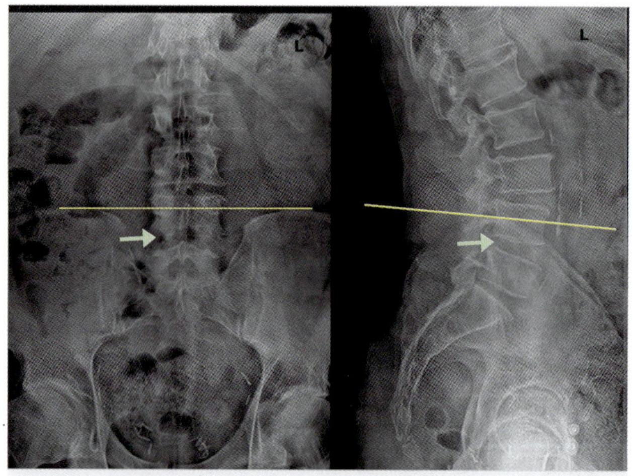

Fig. 38.2 Example of a patient with a high pelvic brim. Approaching the L4–L5 disc space would likely be not feasible via the lateral approach in this patient.

Table 38.1 Ideal case, advantage, and radiologic goals of regular and hyperlordotic cages for an XLIF at L4–L5

XLIF L4–L5 Cages	XLIF L4–L5 Ideal case	XLIF L4–L5 Advantages	XLIF L4–L5 Radiologic goal degrees (max-min)
Regular	Degenerative disc disease or spondylolisthesis without sagittal imbalance	Excellent indirect decompression, large surface area for fusion	0–10 degrees[25]
Hyperlordotic	Adult spinal deformity with PI-LL mismatch (use age-adjusted alignment), especially in patients with high pelvic incidence (majority of the lordosis should be at L4–S1); typically paired with ALL release	Sagittal correction without osteotomy; reduced EBL, fewer levels of fusion required[26]	10–25 degrees[25]

Abbreviations: ALL, anterior longitudinal ligament; EBL, estimated blood loss; PI-LL, pelvic incidence minus lumbar lordosis; XLIF, extreme lateral interbody fusion.

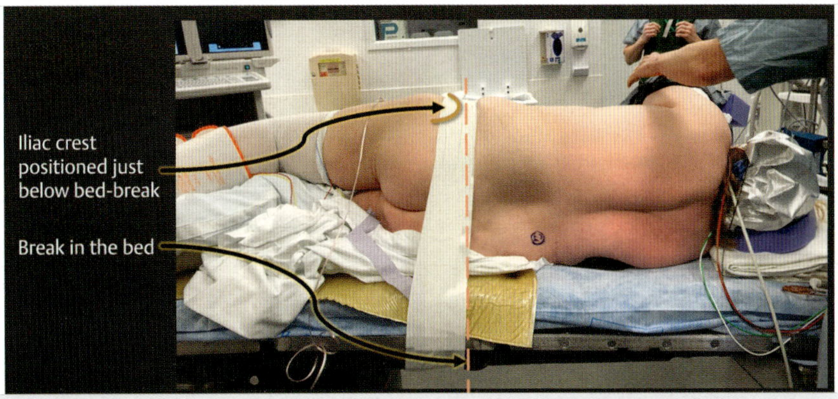

Fig. 38.3 Appropriate positioning for a patient. Note that the Iliac crest is positioned just below the table break.

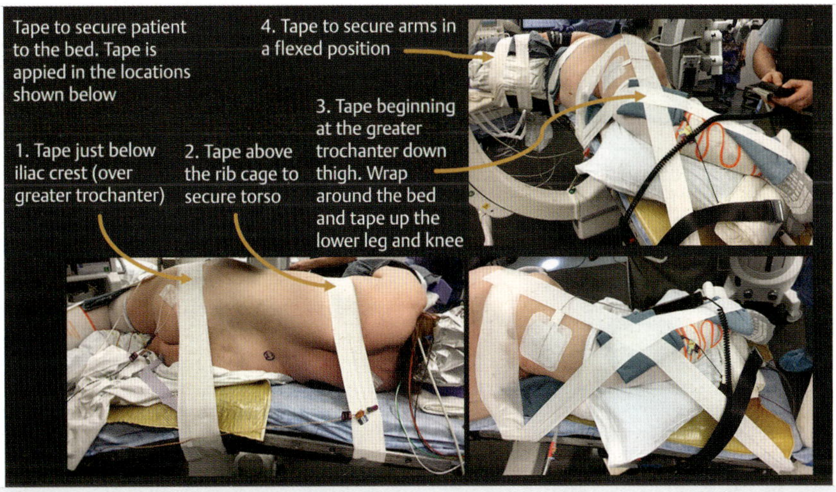

Fig. 38.4 Tape is applied to secure the patient to the bed in the locations shown above. Please note that caution must be applied when taping the knee to ensure there is no undue pressure on the fibular head.

eight fashion (▶ Fig. 38.4). We routinely also secure the arms with a roll of tape.

With the patient secured to the table, the bed is bent so that the head tilts down. This is done in conjunction with reverse Trendelenburg to keep the spine roughly parallel to the floor. The net effect of this maneuver is to tilt the pelvis away from the spine and allow for easier access to the disc spaces, particularly at L4–L5. An excessive break in the bed can cause neuropraxic injury to the lumbar plexus; therefore, we recommend bending the table just enough to tension the skin and allow for access to the disc space in question.

A twitch test is performed to ensure that muscle relaxants and paralytics are appropriately reversed before proceeding.

At this point, fluoroscopy is typically brought in to obtain an anteroposterior (AP) view of the spine. The C-arm base is brought in from the patients' front (i.e., abdomen) side while the surgeon typically operates from the back (i.e., dorsal) side.

To ensure that the surgeon is oriented in an "up-down" position and working vertically across the disc space, the bed is adjusted to match the fluoroscopy machine, that is, the bed is rotated so that a perfect AP is obtained with the C-arm parallel to the floor (▶ Fig. 38.5). Once the perfect AP is obtained, the C-arm is rotated 90 degrees to obtain a perfect lateral view of the disc in question. Again, the bed is adjusted so that a perfect lateral view is obtained with the C-arm perpendicular to the floor (▶ Fig. 38.6).

With the C-arm in place for the lateral imaging, we mark the disc spaces being addressed during the procedure. This is useful particularly at the L4–L5 level to ensure that the disc space is clear of the ipsilateral pelvic brim. If this is not the case, more break may be necessary to tilt the pelvis further away from the spine.

The attachment for the table-mounted retractor is applied at this time. Although it may be placed on either side of the table (patients' front or back), we usually place it on the patients' front side.

The patient is then prepared and draped widely. We usually attempt to extend the sterile field to include the entire torso. Dorsally, we drape across the midline of the spine. Ventrally, we drape well past the anterior edge of the vertebral body. If percutaneous pedicle screws are planned from the lateral procedure, it is important to drape even wider dorsally.

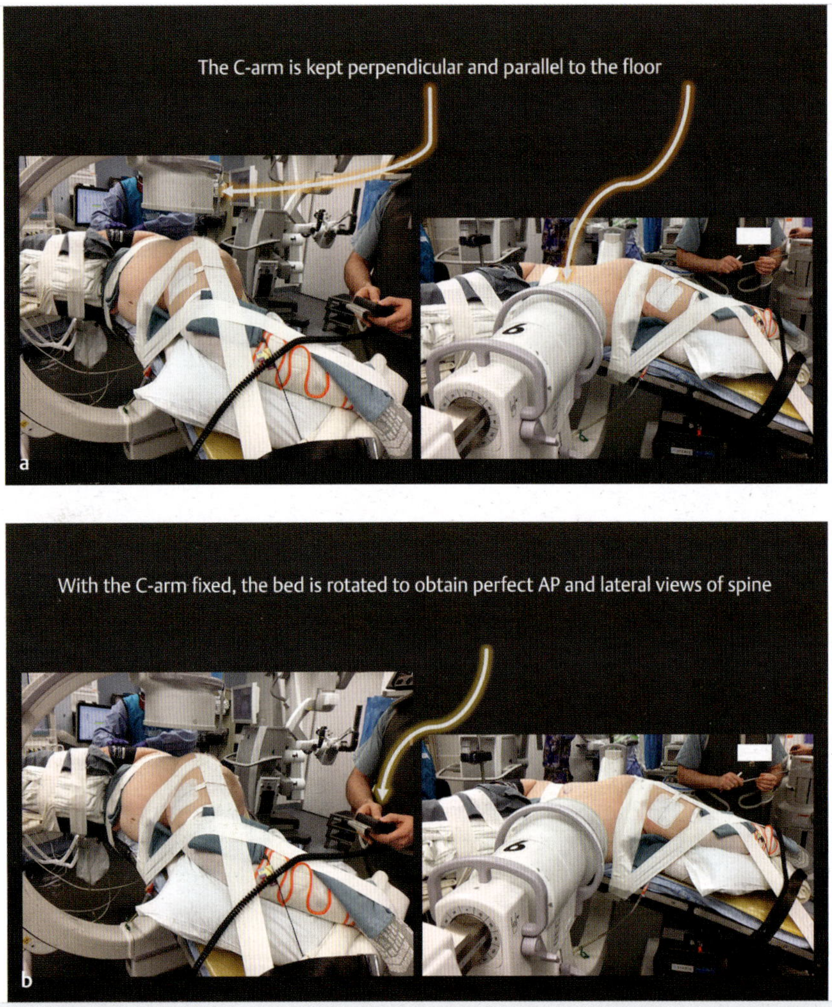

Fig. 38.5 Once the patient is positioned, fluoroscopy is brought in perfectly perpendicular and parallel to the floor **(a)** and the bed is rotated to obtain perfect anteroposterior (AP) and lateral images **(b)**.

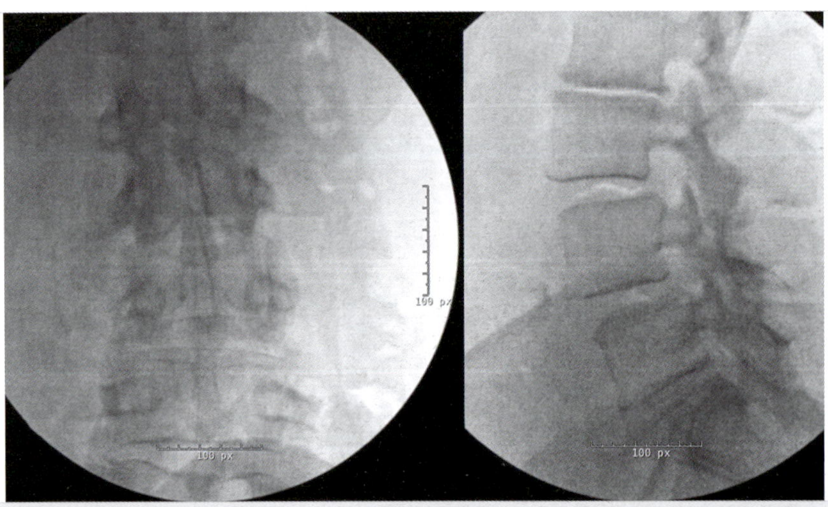

Fig. 38.6 Example of a perfect anteroposterior (AP) and lateral image prior to beginning the procedure. Note that the spinous process is centered between the pedicles on the AP view and the pedicles are perfectly overlapped with crisp end plates on the lateral view.

The lateral approach for discectomy and cage implantation is one of the key techniques for any minimally invasive surgery (MIS) surgeon. Careful planning has to be done preoperatively in terms of the individual patient anatomy to make sure that a given patient is a good candidate for the procedure. At the same time the goals have to be established for indirect decompression and deformity correction. Based on these goals, the final approach and the implant and surgical technique have to be chosen. Other chapters in this book address this particular process.

Early experience with prone transpsoas technique (PTP) suggests it is not only feasible but offers some advantages, as it allows for single-position surgery maximizing both anterior and posterior column access and corrective techniques. Although the first case series look promising, long-term follow-up and multicenter studies of this technique are still ongoing.

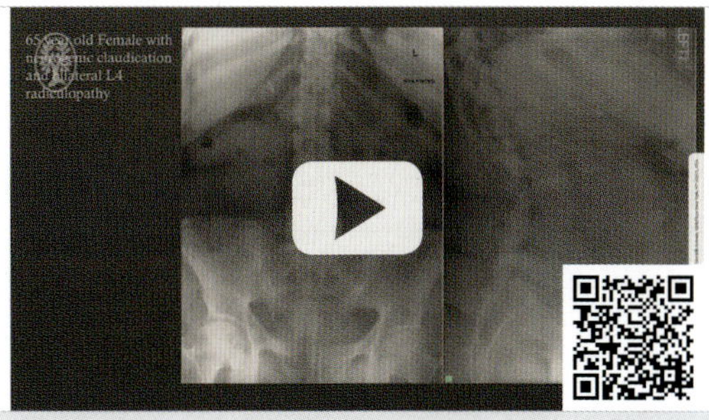

Video 38.1 Lateral lumbar interbody fusion L2/L3/L4/L5.

38.6 Surgical Steps

38.6.1 Incision Placement

Following a standard surgical preparation, the table-mounted retractor is first attached to the table. We then begin by bringing in the C-arm to a lateral position. At this time, appropriate landmarks are marked on the skin. These include: the line of the disc space, the anterior border of the vertebral body, the posterior border of the vertebral body, and the posterior third of the vertebral body. We use a two-incision approach with an accessory incision used to place a finger in the retroperitoneal space to safely escort the dilators placed from laterally to the psoas muscle. A single-incision approach may also be utilized. If an accessory incision is planned, the line of the disc space is traced back to the lateral edge of the paraspinal musculature and a second approximately 2-cm incision is marked. If a two-level approach is planned, we attempt to make a single incision between the two disc spaces if feasible.

38.6.2 Exposure

We begin by working through the accessory incision first. A knife is used to incise the skin followed by Bovie electrocautery to the level of the retroperitoneal fascia. A large curved hemostat is then used to come through the retroperitoneal fascia. Once the retroperitoneal space is entered, the hemostat is spread widely to allow for widening of the opening into the retroperitoneal space. We then use our index finger and palpate the psoas muscle and transverse processes to confirm we are in the retroperitoneal space.

Next, the lateral incisions are utilized to access the disc space. In general, the incision is centered over the middle of the disc. A knife and electrocautery are used to dissect down to the level of the external oblique fascia. We prefer to use a curved hemostat to spread through the abdominal muscles to avoid the risk of injury to the abdominal wall innervation and paresis and hernia. When spreading with the hemostat, we will usually have a finger in the retroperitoneal space to direct the tip of the hemostat appropriately.

Once we have confirmed and established entry to the retroperitoneal space, the initial dilator is introduced via the lateral incision and advanced to the psoas muscle. Neuromonitoring is performed via an electrode attached to the dilator. A finger in the accessory incision is used to "guide" the dilator to the appropriate position but not through the psoas. Lateral fluoroscopy is used to fine tune positioning on the disc space (▶ Video 38.1).

Once the dilator is in an appropriate position, it is advanced through the psoas using neuromonitoring to ensure the lumbar plexus is a safe distance away. Positioning is once again confirmed on lateral fluoroscopy. A guidewire is placed through the dilator into the disc space. Sequential dilators are then passed through the psoas with directional EMG stimulation. Low stimulation thresholds with the dilators (usually in the posterior direction) suggest that a more anterior docking position may be required.

A self-retaining retractor is then passed over these dilators. Again, neuromonitoring is utilized to ensure the lumbar plexus is a safe distance away from the retractor. Lateral fluoroscopy is obtained at this time to confirm positioning of the retractor over the disc space. The retractor is provisionally expanded and attached to the table-mounted arm. At this time, biplanar fluoroscopy is obtained. Once appropriate retractor positioning is confirmed, the self-retaining retractor can be opened. We aim to complete each level within 20 minutes of opening the retractor blades as prolonged operative time has been associated with an increased rate of neurologic complications.[27,28]

After opening the retractor, an EMG probe is also within the field to confirm there are no nerves running across the field. At this time, peanuts and bipolar dissection are utilized to expose the intervertebral disc and establish access to the disc space.

38.6.3 Disc Space Preparation

We utilize a disc knife to make our annulotomy. The fluoroscopy is positioned to obtain an AP view of the spine. We then utilize a Cobb to release the disc from the superior and inferior end plates. A mallet is used at the contralateral annulus to complete this release. We utilize fluoroscopy periodically as the Cobb is being advanced across the disc space and adjust our trajectory to avoid any end plate violations (▶ Video 38.1).

A series of pituitary rongeurs and curettes are then utilized to remove disc material and prepare the end plates. Trials are then inserted into the disc space. All instruments are inserted into the disc space under direct visualization. We are also careful to pay meticulous attention to our trajectory to ensure the trials are inserted straight "up and down"; an oblique working angle risks

placing the trials too anterior or posterior across the disc. We obtain biplanar fluoroscopy with our final trial to check for positioning of the implant within the disc space. The trials are also used to gauge the implant length across the disc space.

Once an appropriate size and height is identified, the implant can then be loaded with bone graft and/or biologic material and malleted into position under fluoroscopic guidance. We choose the largest possible implant footprint to minimize the risk of subsidence.[29]

38.6.4 Closure

Closure is performed in layers to minimize the risk of hernia. The abdominal musculature is closed with a 0-vicryl suture followed by closure of the fascia. We typically close the skin with a subcuticular dissolvable suture and use a surgical glue.

38.7 Postoperative Care

In a high-functioning patient with limited comorbidities, LLIF can be performed as an ambulatory procedure. We treat patients with a pre- and postoperative multimodal analgesia protocol consisting of local anesthesia, acetaminophen, neuromodulatory agents (Lyrica or Gabapentin), and narcotics (tramadol/hydrocodone).[30]

Following surgery, patients are typically mobilized from bed to chair on postoperative day 0. We do not routinely use bracing. Patients are asked to perform no heavy lifting, bending, or twisting for 6 weeks.

38.8 Complications and Avoidance

One recent systematic review found that the most common complication associated with LLIF was thigh pain (26.51%) followed by hypoesthesia (17.13%) and motor (usually hip flexion) weakness (14.11%).[31] The prevalence and severity of these deficits decreases with longer term follow-up; the reported rates of persistent neurologic complications vary but generally range from 0 to 5% (most commonly thigh motor or sensory loss).[27,28,31] These complications are more common at the L4–L5 levels due to a narrower corridor for retractor placement. Thigh pain and neurologic injuries following lateral lumbar fusion are likely due to dissection through the psoas muscle belly in conjunction with neuropraxic injury following retractor placement. We have found that adhering to best practices can greatly reduce the rate of complications; these include: minimal table break, identifying the lumbar plexus using EMG, avoiding multiple punctures through the psoas while docking the dilators, ensuring excellent hemostasis, minimizing retractor expansion, and psoas dilatation times under 20 minutes. There is a substantial learning curve associated with lateral procedures and complication rates gradually decrease over time.[2,27,28,29]

Besides approach-related complications, other significant complications with LLIF are generally rare and comparable to the complication rates reported for other interbody fusion techniques.[32] Vascular injury represents a potentially serious complication but is, thankfully, a rare occurrence with rates estimated at 0.1 to 0.81%.[31] These injuries can be avoided using direct visualization during disc preparation, trialing, and implant placement.

Wound complications are also relatively rare with infection rates generally < 1%. Psoas hematoma has been reported in 1.08%.[31] We routinely use hemostatic agents such as thrombin-based gels to achieve hemostasis following implant placement.

Implant subsidence and pseudarthrosis are postprocedural complications that can negatively impact patient outcomes. In cases with significant implant subsidence, patients may have recurrent symptoms and require revision surgery. We have found that implant subsidence can be avoided by placing the widest possible interbody graft. Interbody cages that are at least 22 mm in the anterior/posterior dimension are preferred.[29] The addition of percutaneous screws posteriorly can also provide additional mechanical stability.

38.9 Tips and Tricks

a) When positioning the patient, it is best to ensure the patient as close to the surgeon's side of the bed as safely possible. This allows the surgeon to more comfortably reach and visualize the spine during the procedure. If the patient is positioned in the center of the bed, the surgeon often needs to bend forward to visualize the spine.
b) After a perfect AP and lateral image is obtained and the spine is centered on both planes. This makes it faster for the fluoroscopy technician to rotate from an AP to lateral image during the procedure and saves retractor time.
c) When obtaining a lateral image to start our procedure, we have the fluoroscopy technician push the C-arm boom all the way forward. This allows the technician to retract the boom when the surgeon requires room to work (make incision, dissect, place probe, etc.) and quickly return to the correct position when fluoroscopic confirmation is required (e.g., dilator position on the disc) without moving the C-arm base.
d) We find the bipolar cautery is most effective for safely exposing the disc. This technique provides hemostasis and most effectively clears the psoas fibers of the disc space. In addition, we are alerted to any proximity to the neurovascular structures as we use free-run EMG during the case.
e) Long instruments (long sucker tip, long bipolar, etc.) are critical to successfully performing this procedure as the spine is usually > 10 cm away from the skin.
f) During disc prep, it is safest to "backhand" the pituitary rongeur as this grabs disc material more posteriorly; this prevents the surgeon from inadvertently grasping vascular structures anteriorly.
g) When trialing implants, we become suspicious of an accidental anterior column release (ACR) when large trials are placed easily in the disc space. For example, if an 8-mm height trial is initially difficult to pass but then feels "loose" and subsequent trials pass easily, an ACR should be suspected. In these cases, we often place an interbody cage that provides a moderate fit (as opposed to a tight fit) and roughly matches the adjacent disc heights. If an ACR is suspected, we add pedicle screws for additional stability.

h) We place the final implant over "sleds" to protect the end plates and minimize extravasation of bone graft material outside the disc space during cage impaction.

38.10 Conclusion

Lateral lumbar interbody fusion is a safe and effective minimally invasive approach to interbody fusions. LLIF in the lumbar spine can be used to treat foraminal stenosis, moderate cases of lateral recess stenosis, and degenerative scoliosis and can help restore sagittal balance when paired with an anterior column release. Safely performing LLIF requires a close review of the preoperative imaging to ensure the patients' anatomy allows for safe lateral access to the disc space. Adhering to good LLIF principles (minimal table break, identifying the lumbar plexus using EMG, and minimizing retractor expansion and psoas dilatation times under 20 minutes) can help surgeons minimize complications.

References

[1] Ozgur BM, Aryan HE, Pimenta L, Taylor WR. Extreme lateral interbody fusion (XLIF): a novel surgical technique for anterior lumbar interbody fusion. Spine J. 2006; 6(4):435–443

[2] Kwon B, Kim DH. Lateral lumbar interbody fusion: indications, outcomes, and complications. J Am Acad Orthop Surg. 2016; 24(2):96–105

[3] Lang G, Perrech M, Navarro-Ramirez R, et al. Potential and limitations of neural decompression in extreme lateral interbody fusion—a systematic review. World Neurosurg. 2017; 101:99–113

[4] Ahmadian A, Verma S, Mundis GM , Jr, Oskouian RJ , Jr, Smith DA, Uribe JS. Minimally invasive lateral retroperitoneal transpsoas interbody fusion for L4–5 spondylolisthesis: clinical outcomes. J Neurosurg Spine. 2013; 19 (3):314–320

[5] Campbell PG, Nunley PD, Cavanaugh D, et al. Short-term outcomes of lateral lumbar interbody fusion without decompression for the treatment of symptomatic degenerative spondylolisthesis at L4–5. Neurosurg Focus. 2018; 44 (1):E6

[6] Phillips FM, Isaacs RE, Rodgers WB, et al. Adult degenerative scoliosis treated with XLIF: clinical and radiographical results of a prospective multicenter study with 24-month follow-up. Spine. 2013; 38(21):1853–1861

[7] Oliveira L, Marchi L, Coutinho E, Pimenta L. A radiographic assessment of the ability of the extreme lateral interbody fusion procedure to indirectly decompress the neural elements. Spine. 2010; 35(26) Suppl:S331–S337

[8] Kepler CK, Sharma AK, Huang RC, et al. Indirect foraminal decompression after lateral transpsoas interbody fusion. J Neurosurg Spine. 2012; 16 (4):329–333

[9] Caputo AM, Michael KW, Chapman TM, et al. Extreme lateral interbody fusion for the treatment of adult degenerative scoliosis. J Clin Neurosci. 2013; 20 (11):1558–1563

[10] Lee YS, Park SW, Kim YB. Direct lateral lumbar interbody fusion: clinical and radiological outcomes. J Korean Neurosurg Soc. 2014; 55(5):248–254

[11] Malham GM, Parker RM, Goss B, Blecher CM, Ballok ZE. Indirect foraminal decompression is independent of metabolically active facet arthropathy in extreme lateral interbody fusion. Spine. 2014; 39(22):E1303–E1310

[12] Kim SJ, Lee YS, Kim YB, Park SW, Hung VT. Clinical and radiological outcomes of a new cage for direct lateral lumbar interbody fusion. Korean J Spine. 2014; 11(3):145–151

[13] Nemani VM, Aichmair A, Taher F, et al. Rate of revision surgery after stand-alone lateral lumbar interbody fusion for lumbar spinal stenosis. Spine. 2014; 39(5):E326–E331

[14] Alimi M, Hofstetter CP, Cong GT, et al. Radiological and clinical outcomes following extreme lateral interbody fusion. J Neurosurg Spine. 2014; 20(6):623–635

[15] Anand N, Baron EM, Khandehroo B, Kahwaty S. Long-term 2- to 5-year clinical and functional outcomes of minimally invasive surgery for adult scoliosis. Spine. 2013; 38(18):1566–1575

[16] Demirkiran G, Theologis AA, Pekmezci M, Ames C, Deviren V. Adult spinal deformity correction with multi-level anterior column releases: description of a new surgical technique and literature review. Clin Spine Surg. 2016; 29 (4):141–149

[17] Theologis AA, Mundis GM , Jr, Nguyen S, et al. for the International Spine Study Group. Utility of multilevel lateral interbody fusion of the thoracolumbar coronal curve apex in adult deformity surgery in combination with open posterior instrumentation and L5-S1 interbody fusion: a case-matched evaluation of 32 patients. J Neurosurg Spine. 2017; 26(2):208–219

[18] Mundis GM, Akbarnia BA, Phillips FM. Adult deformity correction through minimally invasive lateral approach techniques. Spine. 2010; 35(26) Suppl: S312–S321

[19] Kepler CK, Bogner EA, Herzog RJ, Huang RC. Anatomy of the psoas muscle and lumbar plexus with respect to the surgical approach for lateral transpsoas interbody fusion. Eur Spine J. 2011; 20(4):550–556

[20] Hu W-K, He S-S, Zhang S-C, et al. An MRI study of psoas major and abdominal large vessels with respect to the X/DLIF approach. Eur Spine J. 2011; 20 (4):557–562

[21] Uribe JS. Neural anatomy, neuromonitoring and related complications in extreme lateral interbody fusion: video lecture. Eur Spine J. 2015; 24 Suppl 3:445–446

[22] Uribe JS, Vale FL, Dakwar E. Electromyographic monitoring and its anatomical implications in minimally invasive spine surgery. Spine. 2010; 35(26) Suppl: S368–S374

[23] Tohmeh AG, Rodgers WB, Peterson MD. Dynamically evoked, discrete-threshold electromyography in the extreme lateral interbody fusion approach. J Neurosurg Spine. 2011; 14(1):31–37

[24] Louie PK, Narain AS, Hijji FY, et al. Radiographic analysis of psoas morphology and its association with neurovascular structures at L4–5 with reference to lateral approaches. Spine. 2017; 42(24):E1386–E1392

[25] Uribe JS, Smith DA, Dakwar E, et al. Lordosis restoration after anterior longitudinal ligament release and placement of lateral hyperlordotic interbody cages during the minimally invasive lateral transpsoas approach: a radiographic study in cadavers. J Neurosurg Spine. 2012; 17(5):476–485

[26] Uribe JS, Beckman J, Mummaneni PV, et al. MIS-ISSG Group. Does MIS surgery allow for shorter constructs in the surgical treatment of adult spinal deformity? Neurosurgery. 2017; 80(3):489–497

[27] Lykissas MG, Aichmair A, Hughes AP, et al. Nerve injury after lateral lumbar interbody fusion: a review of 919 treated levels with identification of risk factors. Spine J. 2014; 14(5):749–758

[28] Aichmair A, Lykissas MG, Girardi FP, et al. An institutional six-year trend analysis of the neurological outcome after lateral lumbar interbody fusion: a 6-year trend analysis of a single institution. Spine. 2013; 38(23):E1483–E1490

[29] Marchi L, Abdala N, Oliveira L, Amaral R, Coutinho E, Pimenta L. Radiographic and clinical evaluation of cage subsidence after stand-alone lateral interbody fusion. J Neurosurg Spine. 2013; 19(1):110–118

[30] Singh K, Bohl DD, Ahn J, et al. Multimodal analgesia versus intravenous patient-controlled analgesia for minimally invasive transforaminal lumbar interbody fusion procedures. Spine. 2017; 42(15):1145–1150

[31] Hijji FY, Narain AS, Bohl DD, et al. Lateral lumbar interbody fusion: a systematic review of complication rates. Spine J. 2017; 17(10):1412–1419

[32] Teng I, Han J, Phan K, Mobbs R. A meta-analysis comparing ALIF, PLIF, TLIF and LLIF. J Clin Neurosci. 2017; 44:11–17

39 Translumbar Surgery Comparison: Four Surgeons and Regions

Luiz Pimenta, Khai Lam†, Massimo Balsano, and Masato Tanaka

39.1 How I Do It

Summary

This chapter will provide the reader with the "step sequence" from four different surgeons around the world, performing translumbar surgery (LLIF). The format presented here includes "classic" case example images, patient positioning tips, and surgical details (approach, incision, tricks, closure) displayed in columns and simultaneously presented in a side-by-side format to facilitate their comparison. After going through this chapter, the readers should be able to reinforce, adopt, or change their practice based on the sequence and/or tricks presented by the authors.

Keywords: lateral lumbar surgery, transpsoas surgery, XLIF, extreme lateral interbody fusion, lateral approach, lateral interbody fusion

Region: America *Dr. Luiz Pimenta*	Region: Europe/UK *Dr. Khai Lam*
Step 1: Preoperative planning	**Step 1: Preoperative planning**
• Anteroposterior (AP) and lateral X-ray with measurement of spinopelvic parameters and global spinal alignment. • Flexion/extension X-ray to determine need for posterior fixation. • Computed tomography (CT). • Magnetic resonance imaging (MRI)—evaluate psoas anatomy and location of the lumbar plexus. • Neuromonitoring (IOM) is mandatory. 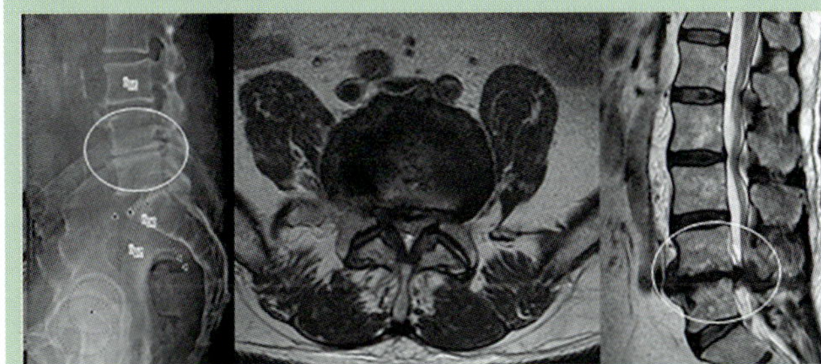	• Standing AP and lateral X-ray with measurement of spinopelvic parameters and global spinal alignment. • CT. • MRI—evaluate psoas anatomy and location of the lumbar plexus. • IOM. 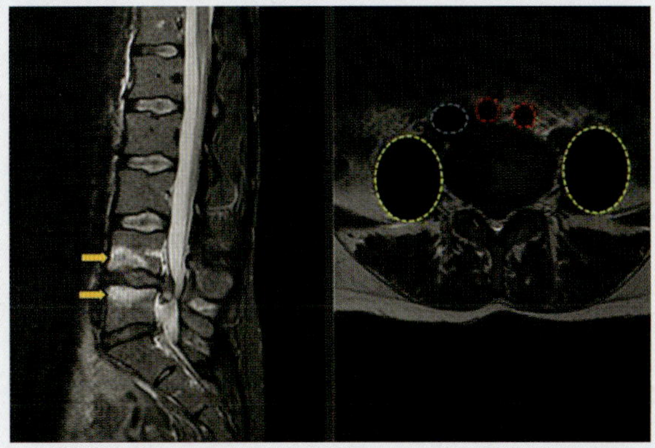
Step 2: Patient positioning	**Step 2: Patient positioning**
• Radiolucent table, can be bent to increase space between iliac crest and ribs. • Lateral decubitus with padding between the knees. • Securely tape patient: Below iliac crest (A), thoracic region (B), from greater trochanter over knee to table (C), from knee over ankle to table (D). • True 90-degree lateral position: AP image at 0 degree shows spinous processes in midline and lateral image at 90 degrees shows pedicles and end plates are aligned. • Notice the 1,2,3 of the picture, highlighting the "single vertebral body image" pattern of a "true" lateral (*left*) view and the perfect round circles observed on a "true" AP view (*right*). 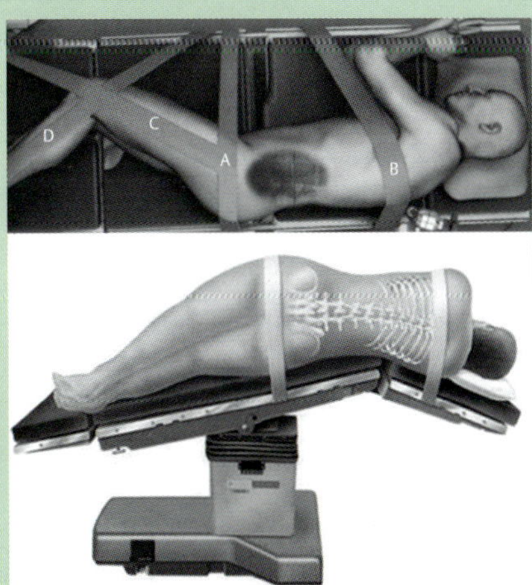 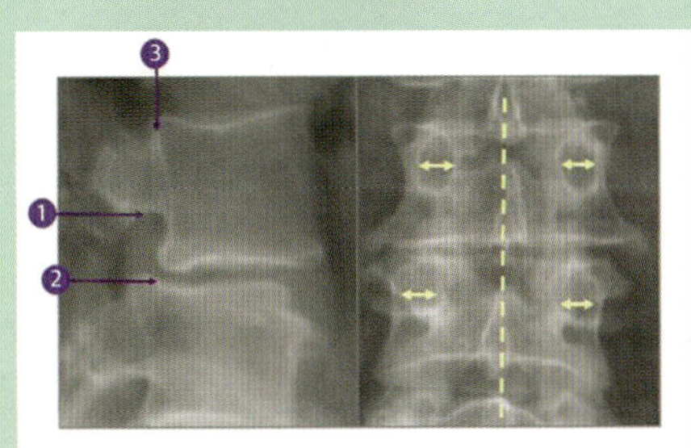	• Breakable Allen table, can be flexed to open space between iliac crest and ribs; avoid over-flexion (typically 20–30 degrees) to prevent excess traction on psoas and neural plexus. • Lateral decubitus with hips and knees flexed to 30 degrees, ipsilateral leg placed on top of a rectangular bolster. • Securely tape patient: Upper torso (1), "figure of 8" tape to secure pelvis and legs (2,3). • Obtain a true lateral fluoroscopic image: Pedicles and end plates are perfectly aligned (Refer to the Step 2 of Dr. Luiz Pimenta). 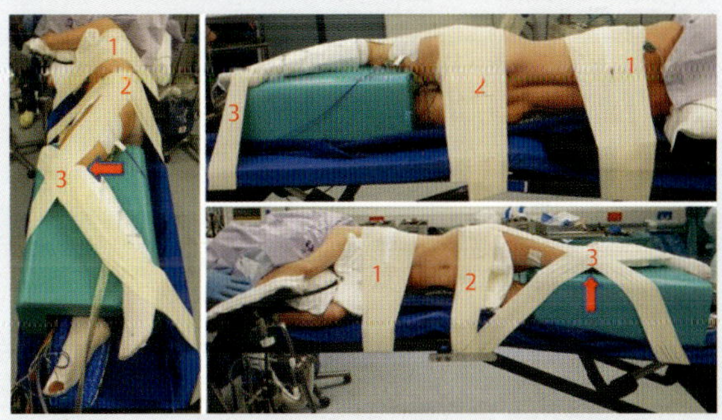

Region: Europe

Dr. Massimo Balsano

Step 1: Preoperative planning

- AP and lateral X-ray.
- Flexion/extension X-ray.
- MRI—evaluate psoas anatomy and location of the lumbar plexus
- IOM.

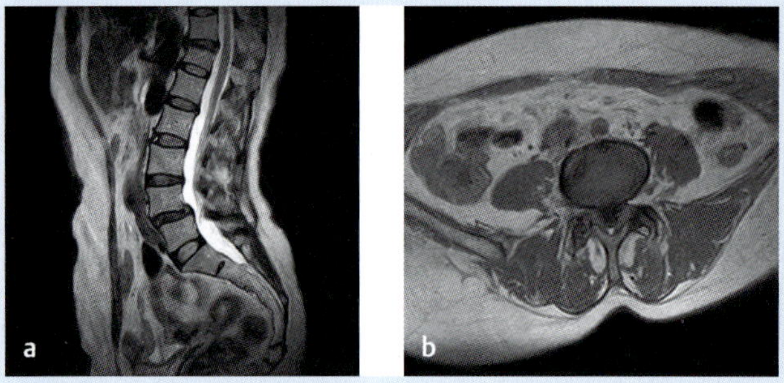

Region: Asia

Dr. Masato Tanaka

Step 1: Preoperative planning

- Evaluate location of iliac crest relative to L4–L5 disc space on lateral X-ray.
- High rising psoas is a contraindication.
- Evaluate vascular anatomy on MRI.
- IOM.

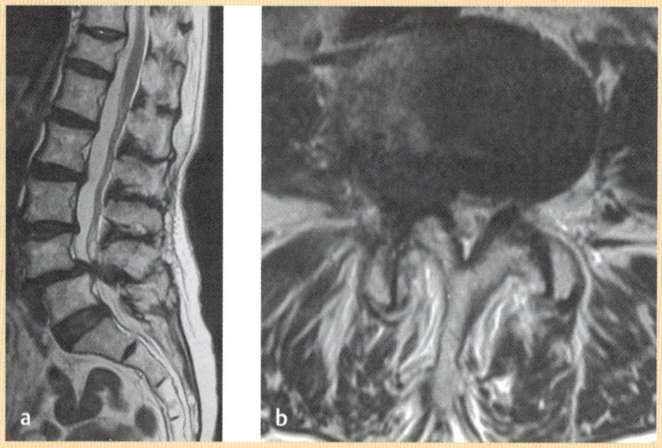

Region: Europe

Step 2: Patient positioning

- Radiolucent table; can break table at the level of iliac crest to open the space between crest and ribs.
- If necessary break table to access L4–L5; increase the degree of knee flexion to relieve stretch on the lumbar plexus.
- Lateral decubitus with secure patient taping.

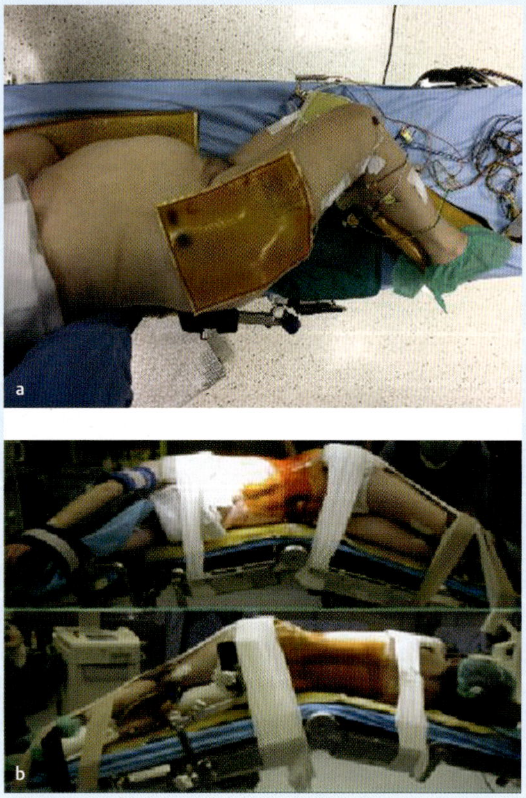

Region: Asia

Step 2: Patient positioning

- Radiolucent table; can break table by 15 degrees to access L4–L5; high rising psoas is a contraindication.
- Lateral decubitus, true lateral position which also enables percutaneous pedicle screw insertion.
- Legs slightly flexed to loosen psoas and lumbar plexus and secured with tape.

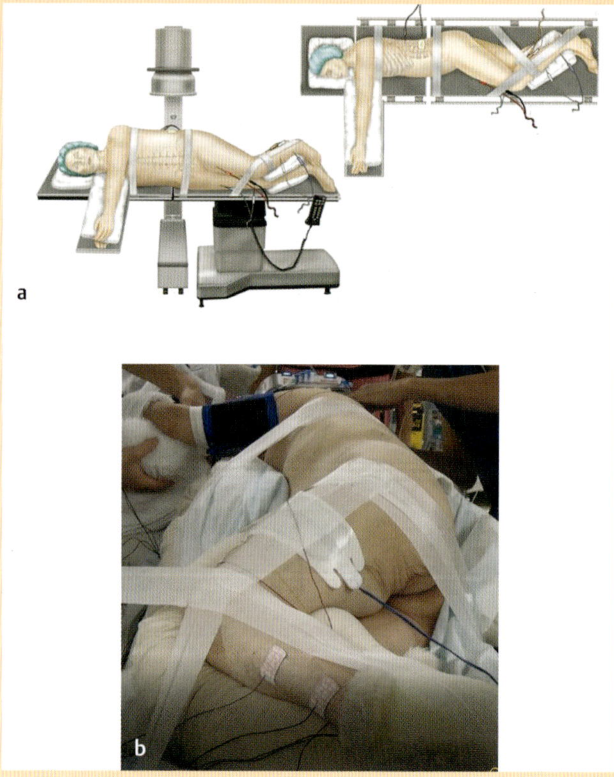

Region: America

Dr. Luiz Pimenta

Step 3: Incision

- Two K-wires identify the center of the target disc space using lateral fluoroscopy.
- One line drawn in the AP direction in line with the disc space.
- One line drawn in the superior-inferior direction crossing center of the vertebral bodies adjacent to the disc space.
- A single skin incision made at the intersection of these two lines.

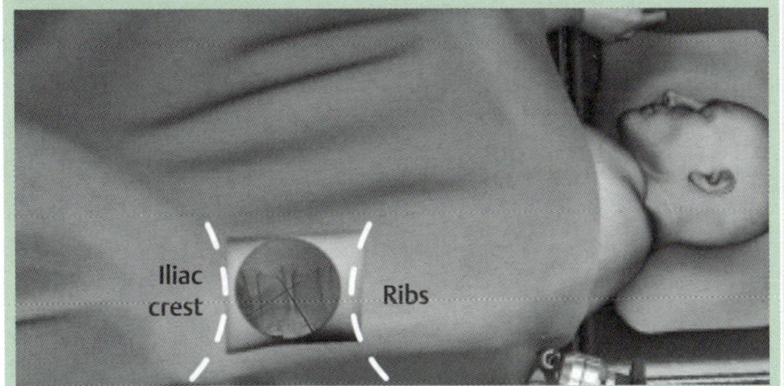

Step 4: Approach

- Lateral abdominal layers identified and opened (external and internal obliques, transversus abdominis, transversalis fascia) until retroperitoneal fat is encountered.
- Index finger dissects through the retroperitoneal fat, sweeping finger deep and up toward skin to open the space above the psoas muscle.
- A second incision is made in the fascia through which index finger guides first dilator onto the psoas (single skin incision, two fascial incisions).

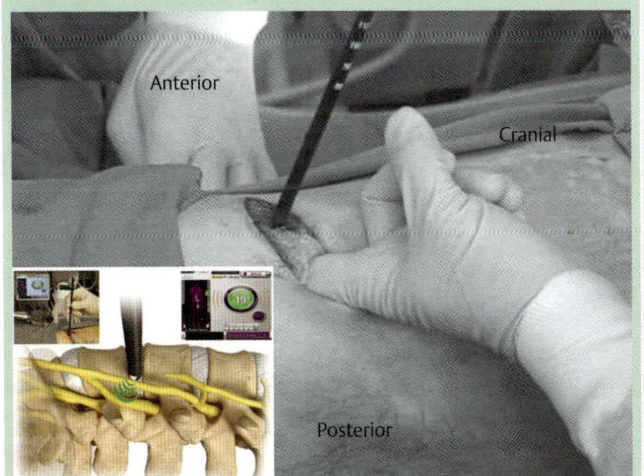

Region: Europe/UK

Dr. Khai Lam

Step 3: Incision

- A radio-opaque cross is placed over the target disc space and a 4 cm oblique skin mark is made in line with the disc 0.5 cm anterior to center of the disc.

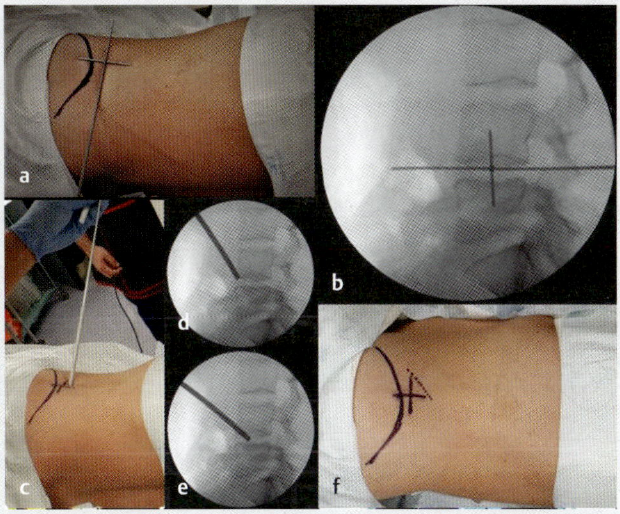

Step 4: Approach

- External and internal obliques and transversus abdominis are identified and sharply dissected with scissors.
- Langenbeck retractors used to retract in the direction of the muscle fibers until the transversalis fascia is identified (*green arrow*, figure "a" and "b") and sharply punctured using scissors to access the retroperitoneal space.
- Peanut swabs on a 22-cm Roberts artery forceps used to gently sweep the retroperitoneal sac anteriorly to reveal psoas.
- The retroperitoneal space is further enlarged by index finger sweeping ("c" *blue arrow*).
- Index finger palpates psoas and the first dilator is passed posterior to the finger atop the psoas.

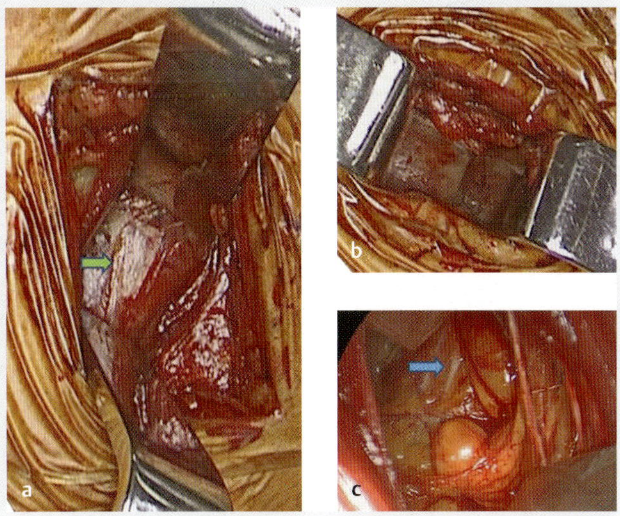

Region: Europe

Dr. Massimo Balsano

Step 3: Incision

- A metal cross is used to localize the middle third of the disc space.
- A transverse incision of 4 cm is sufficient for one level.

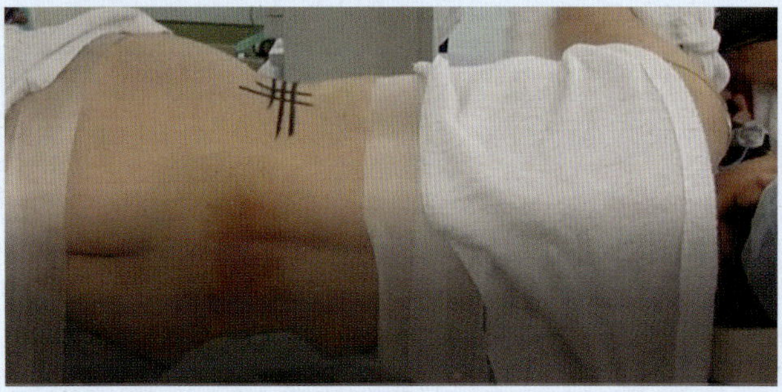

Step 4: Approach

- Blunt scissors are used to dissect through subcutaneous tissue until external oblique muscle is identified.
- The muscles are then gently divided along their natural course using a Langenbeck retractor in sequence.
- Index finger touches the "spaghetti bag" psoas muscle and sweeps the peritoneum anteriorly.
- Blunt scissors are used to split the lateral fibers of the psoas and the first dilator is inserted with electromyography (EMG) monitoring.

Region: Asia

Dr. Masato Tanaka

Step 3: Incision

- Lateral X-ray used to mark location, orientation, and anterior and posterior margins of L4–L5.
- Target site for docking indicated by line perpendicular to disc space at the posterior third.
- 4 cm oblique skin incision.

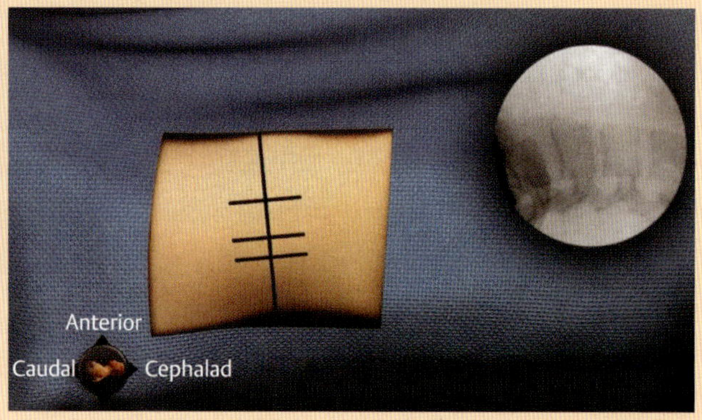

Step 4: Approach

- External and internal oblique and transversalis muscles divided along the fibers; avoid cutting the fibers.
- Monopolar is not used to avoid iliohypogastric and ilioinguinal injury.
- Once in retroperitoneal space, index fingers follow internal abdominal wall posteriorly down to psoas muscle.
- First dilator placed on lateral border of psoas and EMG used to identify lumbar plexus.

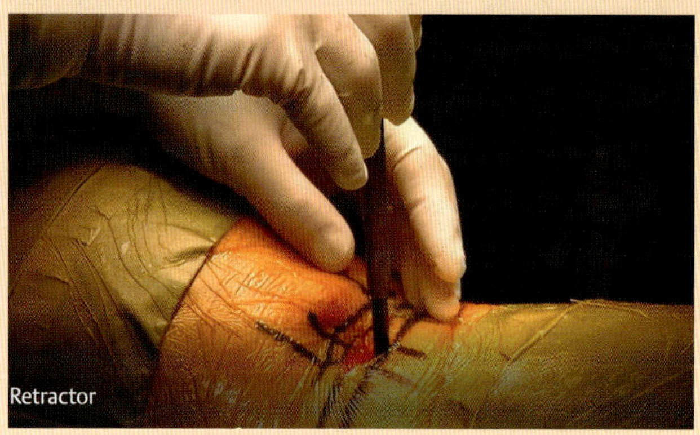

Region: America

Dr. Luiz Pimenta

Step 5: Dilator and retractor docking

- Sequentially, enlarging dilators are passed through the psoas using evoked EMG.
- Rotate each dilator to identify the position and proximity of the dilator relative to the lumbar plexus.
- AP and lateral X-ray confirms dilator placement.
- An expandable retractor is passed over the dilators with EMG monitoring and attached to a table mount.
- Ensure no neural elements traversing the disc space prior to shim placement.

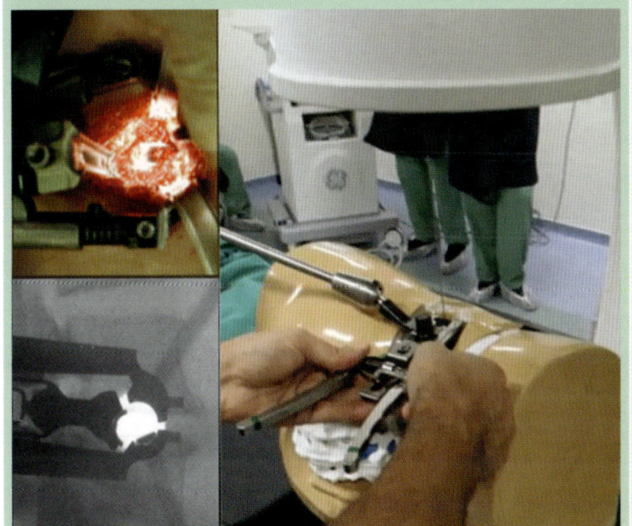

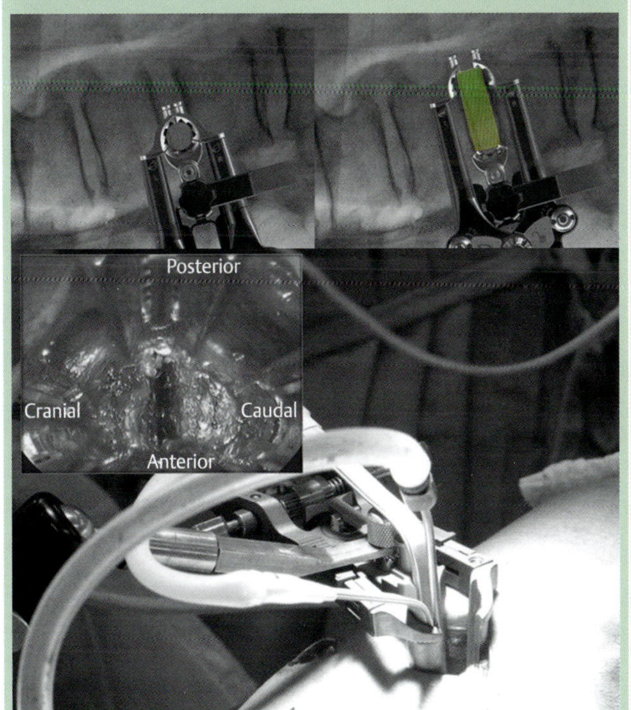

Region: Europe/UK

Dr. Khai Lam

Step 5: Dilator and retractor docking

- A long forceps holds the first dilator while it is passed through the psoas using fluoroscopy and EMG onto the mid-point of the target disc.
- Position the dilator as posterior as possible before inserting the guidewire (superior a & b).
- AP and lateral X-ray confirms placement.
- Rotate the dilator by 360 degrees using EMG.
- Sequential dilators are passed using EMG followed by retractor placement "en face" to the AP gantry of the fluoroscope.
- X-ray confirms placement and the retractor expanded two to three clicks in the cranial-caudal and AP directions (lower a & b).
- Direct EMG stimulation is performed in all four corners of the field followed by shim insertion and attachment to the table mount.
- The guidewire is removed.

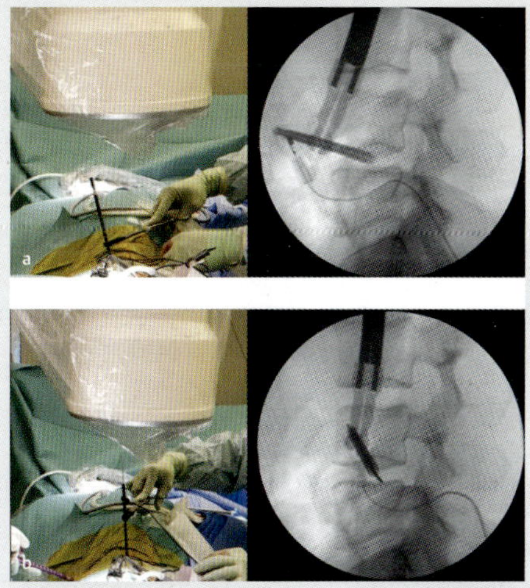

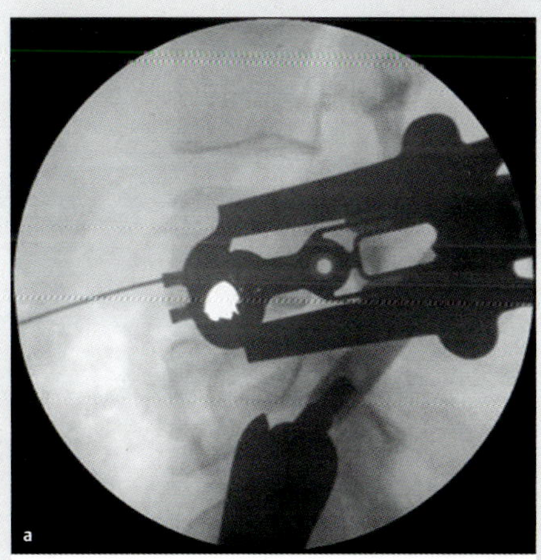

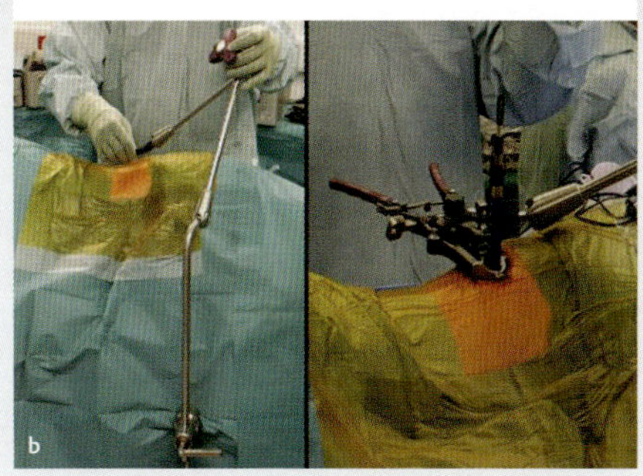

Region: Europe

Dr. Massimo Balsano

Step 5: Dilator and retractor docking

- Fluoroscopy confirms correct placement of the first dilator followed by guidewire placement into the disc space.
- Three dilators and the retractor are sequentially introduced under motor evoked EMG.
- The retractor must be docked anterior to neural structures—rotate the dilators to identify their position relative to the neural elements.
- Visual inspection and direct EMG stimulation of the field to ensure no neural elements traverse the working channel.
- The posterior intradiscal shim is inserted and the retractor is fixed to the table mount.
- No longer than 30 to 40 minutes of open retractor time is suggested to decrease risk of lumbar plexus injury.

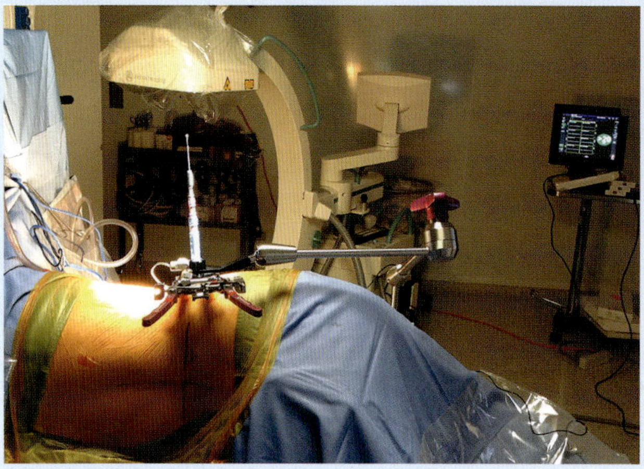

Region: Asia

Dr. Masato Tanaka

Step 5: Dilator and retractor docking

- First dilator passed through psoas under EMG monitoring.
- Sequential dilation to 22 mm.
- Retractor inserted and confirmed with X-ray.
- Retractor secured to the flexible arm attached to table and intradiscal shim is delivered.

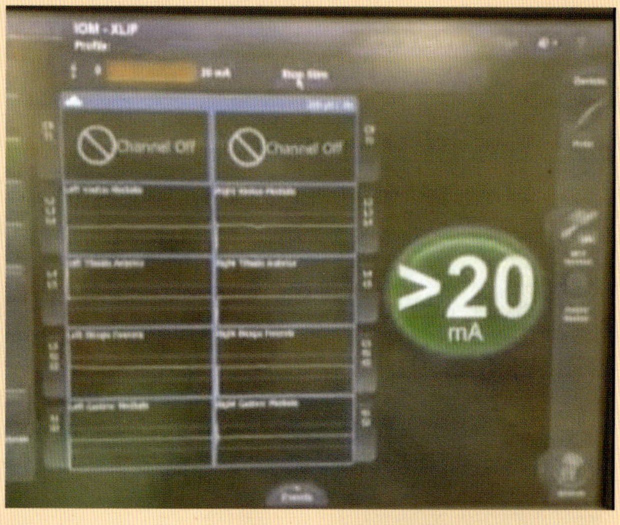

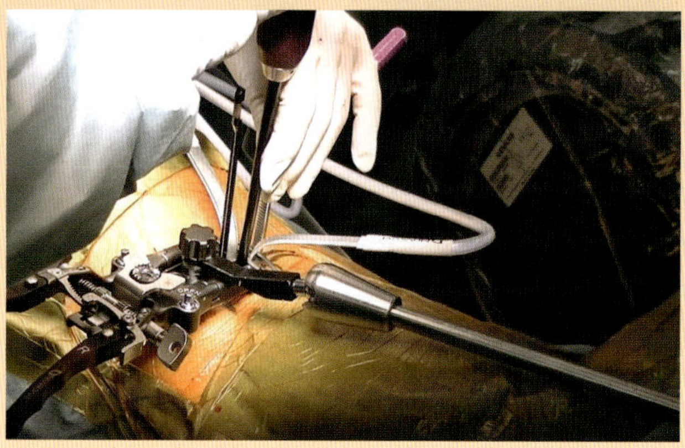

Region: America

Dr. Luiz Pimenta

Step 6: Discectomy

- The annulus is incised and a pituitary rongeur is used to remove the nucleus pulposus.
- A Cobb elevator is passed along both end plates and used to disrupt the contralateral annulus to enable parallel end plate distraction.
- Meticulous removal of all disc material and end plate cartilage necessary for adequate end plate preparation.
- Cautious preservation of the ALL and PLL is key to maintain the principle of ligamentotaxis and indirect neural decompress.

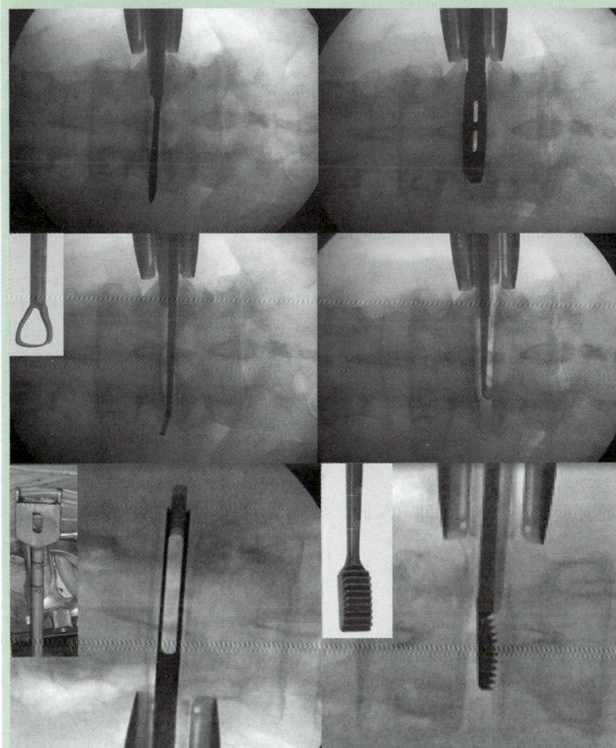

Region: Europe/UK

Dr. Khai Lam

Step 6: Discectomy

- Annulus is incised and radical direct lateral channel discectomy is performed.
- Cobb elevator is advanced along both end plates just beyond contralateral annulus under fluoroscopy until resistance is broken.
- Take care to avoid severing the ALL.
- Remove disc material and prepare end plates, taking care to avoid damaging end plates.
- A scraping sensation and audible noise and/or end plate bleeding are useful guides to confirm adequate end plate preparation.

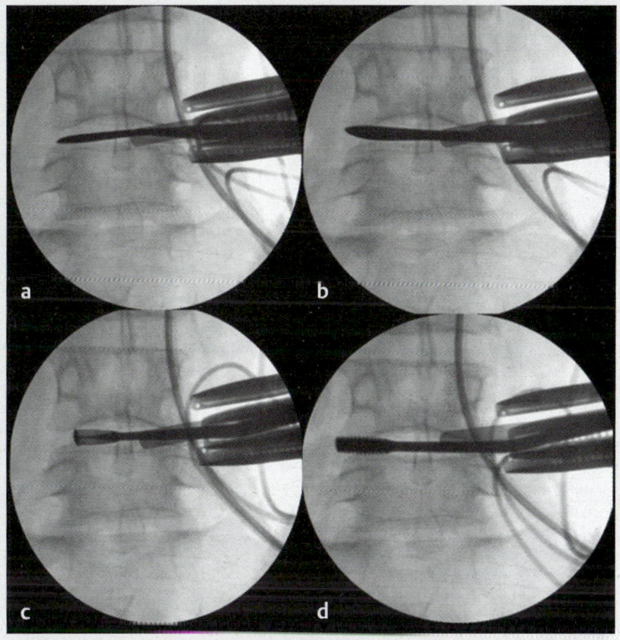

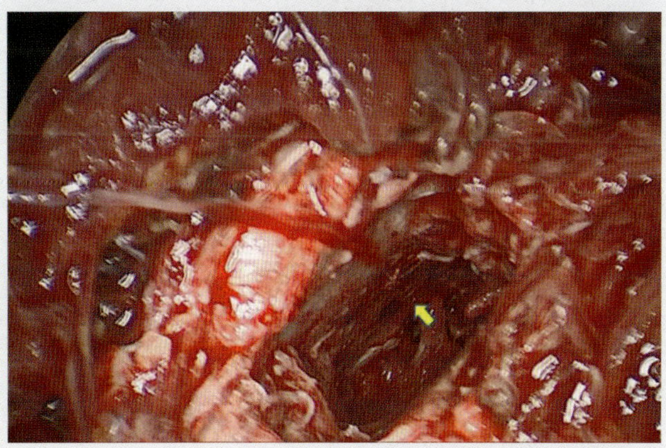

Region: Europe

Dr. Massimo Balsano

Step 6: Discectomy

- Annulus incised followed by discectomy and careful end plate preparation.
- Obtaining true AP and lateral fluoroscopic images is mandatory to protect from incorrect trajectory of instruments during discectomy, avoids vascular injury anteriorly and neural injury posteriorly. Notice on (a) the position of the blades and how there is no muscle or nerves in proximity to the retractor and on (b) how the retractor and shim are aligned with the end plate on the AP X-rays.
- Work parallel to end plates to prevent unintended end plate violation to decrease the risk of cage subsidence.

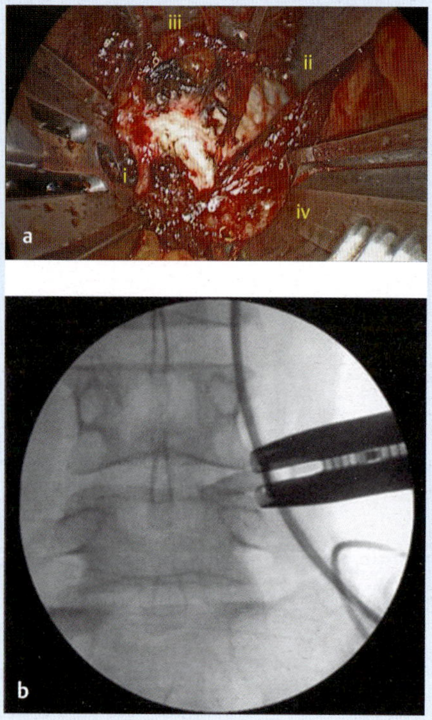

Region: Asia

Dr. Masato Tanaka

Step 6: Discectomy

- Annulus incised and thorough discectomy performed using Kerrison and pituitary rongeurs and ring curettes.
- Cobb elevator passed along both end plates and through the contralateral annulus using a mallet.

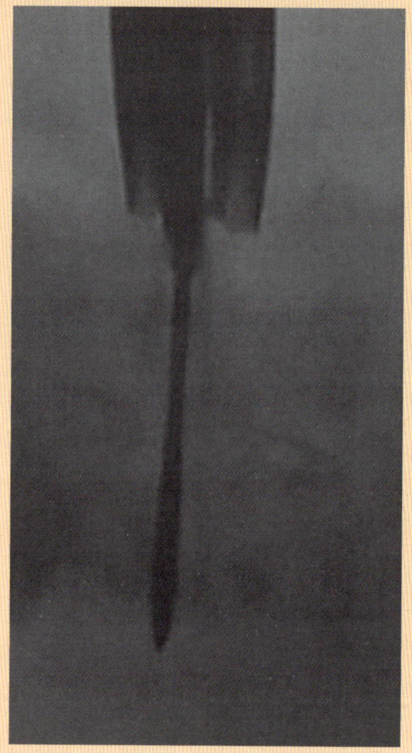

Region: America

Dr. Luiz Pimenta

Step 7: Cage insertion

- Implant trials are inserted under fluoroscopy to determine proper height and length.
- Final implant should bridge the apophyseal ring bilaterally to enhance biomechanical support and allow stand-alone constructs.
- Ideal position is with the central markings of cage aligned with the spinous process in AP view and between the anterior and middle thirds of the disc space in lateral view.
- This position favors restoration of focal lordosis, discal/foraminal height, ligamentotaxis, and resultant indirect decompression.
- We use synthetic bone graft rather than autologous bone harvested from iliac crest to avoid morbidity of harvest.

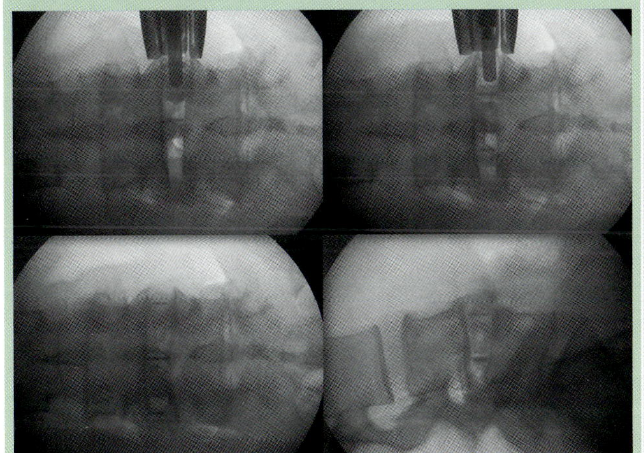

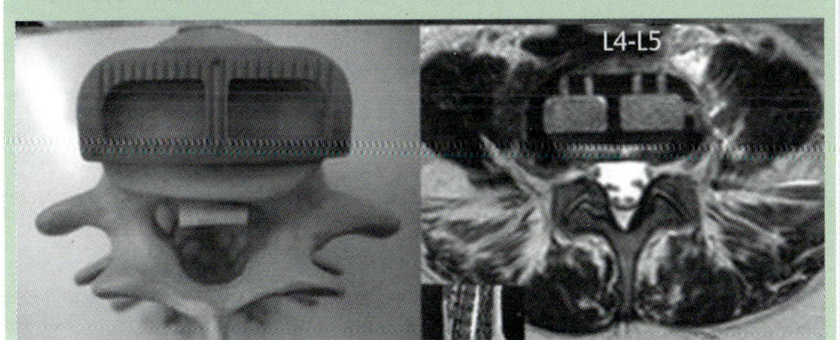

Region: Europe/UK

Dr. Khai Lam

Step 7: Cage insertion

- Trial spacers are sequentially inserted into the disc space under fluoroscopy until a comfortably fitting spacer is achieved.
- Final position of the spacer should be seated in the posterior third of the disc space with maximal AP end plate coverage to ensure optimal area for fusion and indirect neural decompression.
- A titanium cage filled with allograft or autograft is implanted under fluoroscopy.
- Typically, 10-degree lordotic, 10-mm height, 22-mm width, 45- to 50-mm long cage is used.
- We prefer silicate tricalcium phosphate bone graft substitute or BMP for revision cases.

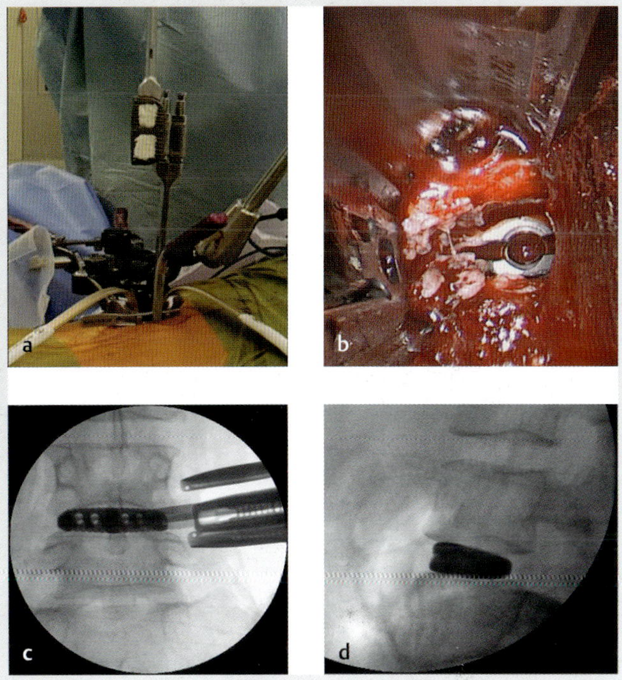

Region: Europe

Dr. Massimo Balsano

Step 7: Cage insertion

- Use increasing size trials to achieve proper size in which only a moderate amount of force is able to remove the trial without use of a slap hammer.
- Tall implants may strain the ALL, PLL, and end plates—the choice of cage height is essential in this procedure.
- Aim to restore the disc height to physiologic levels, estimated by the height of the levels above and below the index level.
- We always use a 22-mm width polyetheretherketone (PEEK) cage and aim to cover bilateral apophyseal rings.

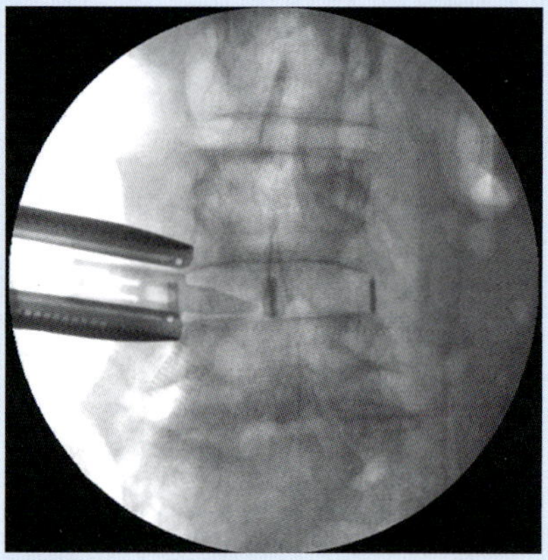

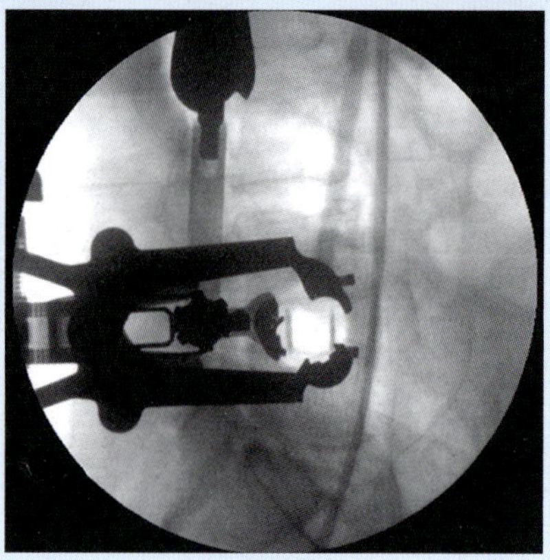

Region: Asia

Dr. Masato Tanaka

Step 7: Cage insertion

- Disc space distracted with trials until adequate disc height is obtained.
- Tightness of fit and preop disc height measurement are key to choosing correct cage height.
- X-ray used to confirm appropriate cage size and location.
- Two sliders inserted to avoid end plate violation, and mallet used to insert cage under fluoroscopy.
- Iliac autograft inserted into cage; when allograft is used, prefer hydroxyapatite or demineralized bone material.

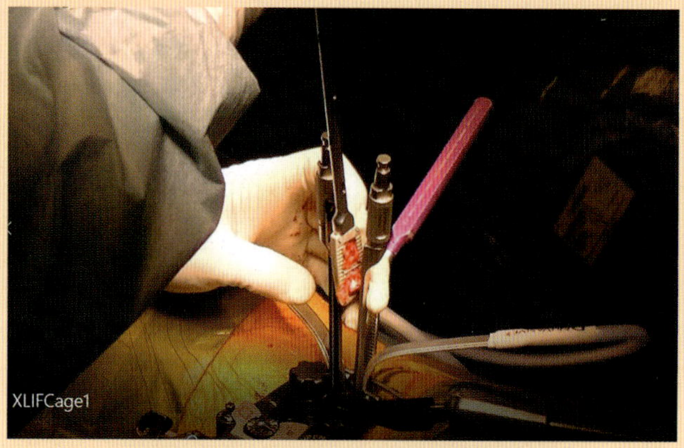

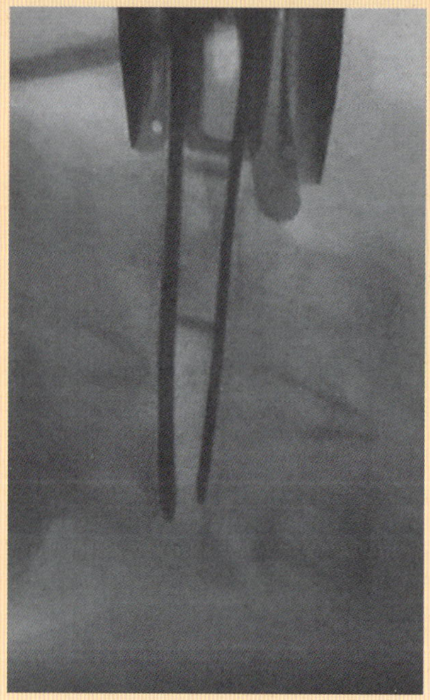

Region: America
Dr. Luiz Pimenta

Step 8: Posterior fixation

- Can perform stand-alone LLIF without posterior fixation, with unilateral posterior fixation in lateral decubitus, or with bilateral posterior fixation.
- For unstable spondylolisthesis, bilateral posterior instrumentation is highly recommend to safeguard primary fusion achieved via cage insertion.

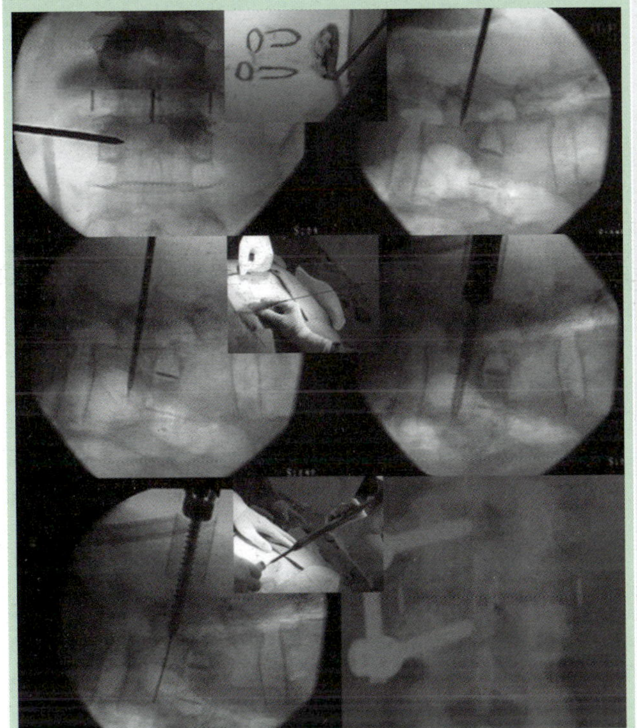

Step 9: Closure

- Remove shim.
- Retractor is closed and slowly removed to observe the psoas closure and confirm hemostasis.
- Standard closure.
- No drain required.

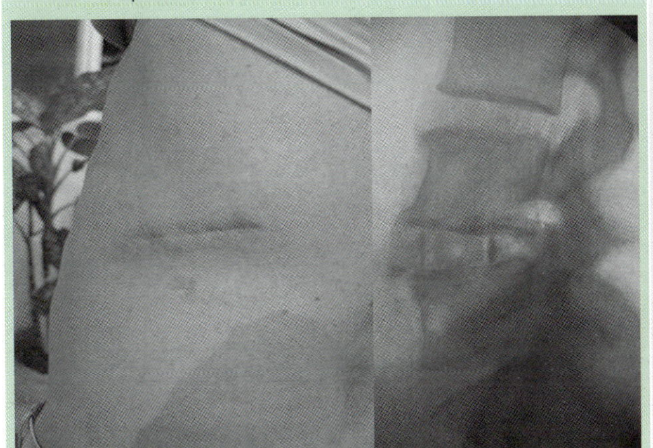

Region: Europe/UK
Dr. Khai Lam

Step 8: Posterior fixation

- Stand-alone LLIF cage is not recommended.
- We prefer pedicle screw fixation in all cases to ensure biomechanical stability; use four-hole lateral plate in frail patients to decrease general anesthesia time.
- Patient positioned prone.
- Two bilateral 3 to 4 cm incisions; Wiltse mini-open approach; pedicle screw insertion under fluoroscopy or computer-assisted navigation.
- Lordotic titanium rods.
- Compression followed by final tightening.

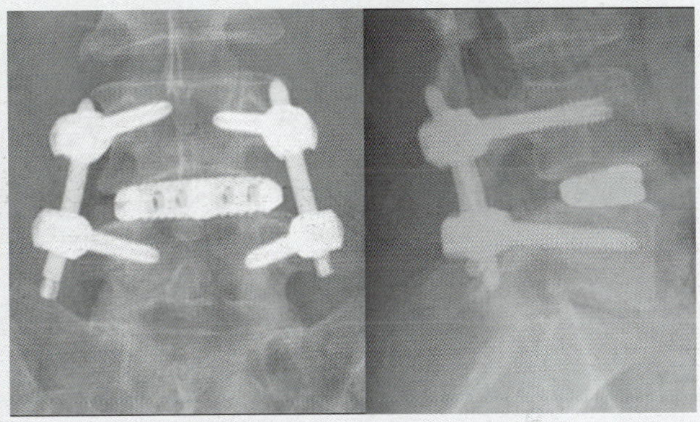

Step 9: Closure

- Shim is withdrawn and the retractor is removed with the blades closed.
- It is important to keep shim-to-shim time under 30 minutes as studies show this reduces incidence of neuropraxia.
- Psoas and abdominal wall muscles visualized for any bleeding.
- External oblique fascia closed primarily.

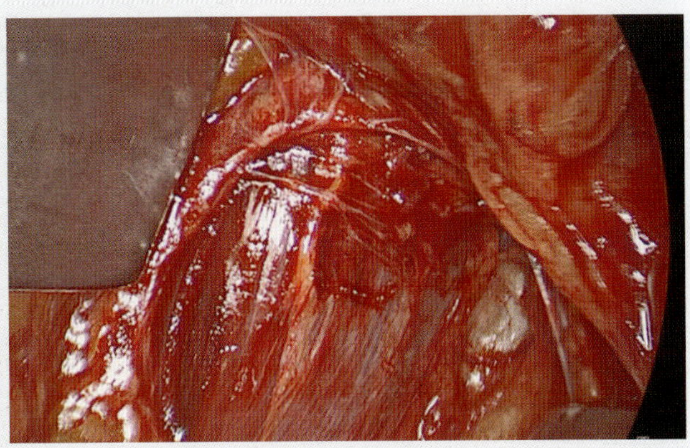

Region: Europe

Dr. Massimo Balsano

Step 8: Posterior fixation

- We prefer to add posterior pedicle fixation.
- Patient kept in the lateral decubitus position.
- Unilateral pedicle screws and rod inserted on side facing upwards percutaneously under fluoroscopy.

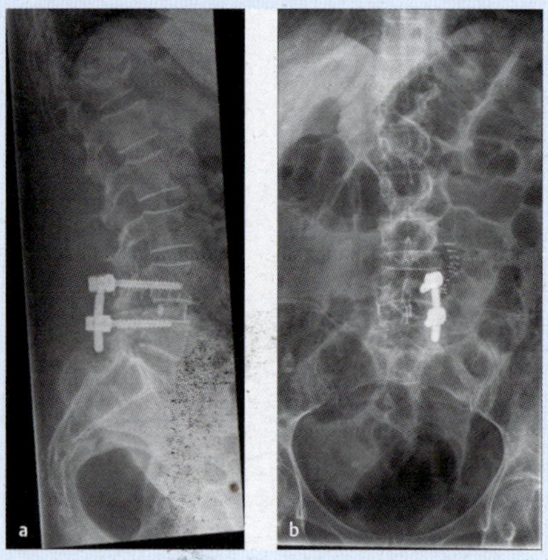

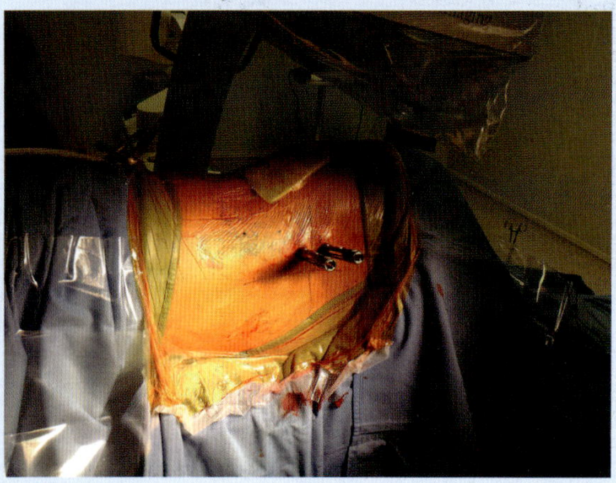

Step 9: Closure

- Retractor is slowly removed and the muscles are inspected for bleeding.
- Retraction time of no greater than 30 to 40 minutes is suggested.
- Standard closure.

Region: Asia

Dr. Masato Tanaka

Step 8: Posterior fixation

- In the same lateral position, percutaneous pedicle screws and rods are placed under fluoroscopy.
- Compression is performed to facilitate lordosis.

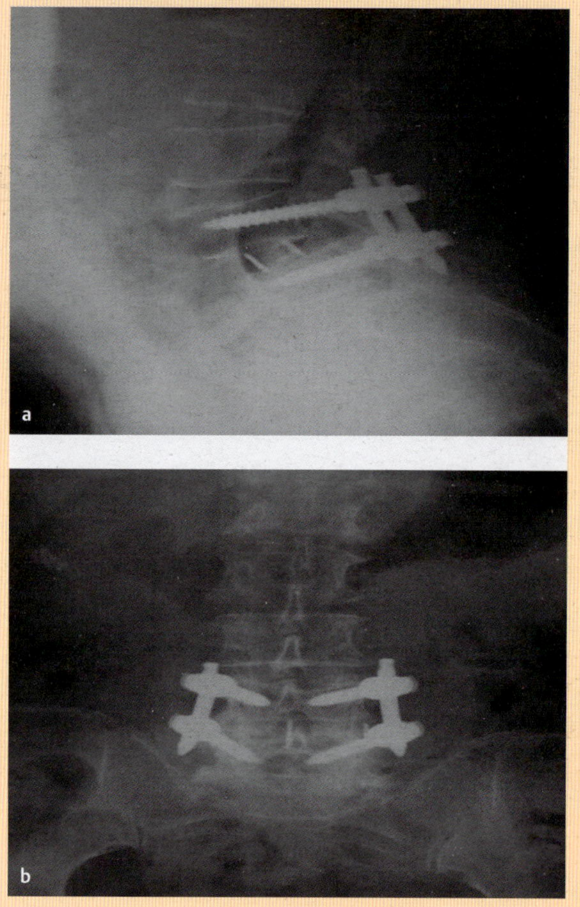

Step 9: Closure

After retractor removal, only the external oblique and transversalis fascia are closed. Then the skin is approximated using non-absorbable sutures in a subcuticular fashion.

Region: America *Dr. Luiz Pimenta*	Region: Europe/UK *Dr. Khai Lam*
Step 10: Postoperative care	**Step 10: Postoperative care**
• Patients encouraged to walk the same day. • Majority discharged on the following day. • No need for lumbar brace. • Transient hip flexion weakness should be expected and patients must be aware of this prior to surgery.	• Patients are mobilized as soon as possible postop. • Typical length of stay is 2 to 3 days. • Do not routinely use bracing. • All patients are counseled that anterior thigh pain with or without mild dysesthesias may occur not uncommonly after surgery, but this improves or resolves over time. • Transient mild weakness of the psoas (approach related) and/or quadriceps muscle (L4 nerve root traction) is not uncommon; avoid these by reducing psoas muscle retraction time and using EMG.
Tips and tricks	**Tips and tricks**
• Painful dysesthesias and motor disturbances are rare, but possible, and such symptoms should prompt a CT scan to rule out psoas hematoma. • Contralateral release of the annulus is critical to facilitate parallel distraction of the disc space, achieve proper coronal alignment, and place a large implant that spans the apophyseal ring. • If the ALL must be resected for deformity correction, the ALL and remaining annulus are released and a paddle distractor is used inside the disc space to confirm adequate release. • Implantation of wider cages has been shown to maximize end plate support with lower incidences of cage subsidence.	• High riding iliac crest or a deep-seated pelvis make lateral access challenging. • Prefer to access the spine from the left side to avoid injury to IVC. • Anterior position of the psoas typically occurs in hyperlordotic spine or with transitional anatomy; in this case, the lumbar plexus is stretched and lies more anteriorly and therefore precludes safe positioning of the retractor. • It is acceptable to use a longer incision when surgeon first embarks on the procedure and subsequently evolve to smaller incision as experience is gained. • It is easier to access disc space utilizing a slightly anterior to posterior directed trajectory. • Tip of first dilator should be placed slightly obliquely in an anterior to posterior direction at an angle of 15 to 20 degrees before gradual verticalization of the dilators as guidewire is inserted; this maneuver helps to create a cuff of psoas anterior to L4 nerve root. • A larger Cobb or trial spacer may be used to enlarge a collapsed disc space. • Keeping knees gently flexed over a pillow or motorized bed allows some tension to be taken off psoas when lying in bed postop.

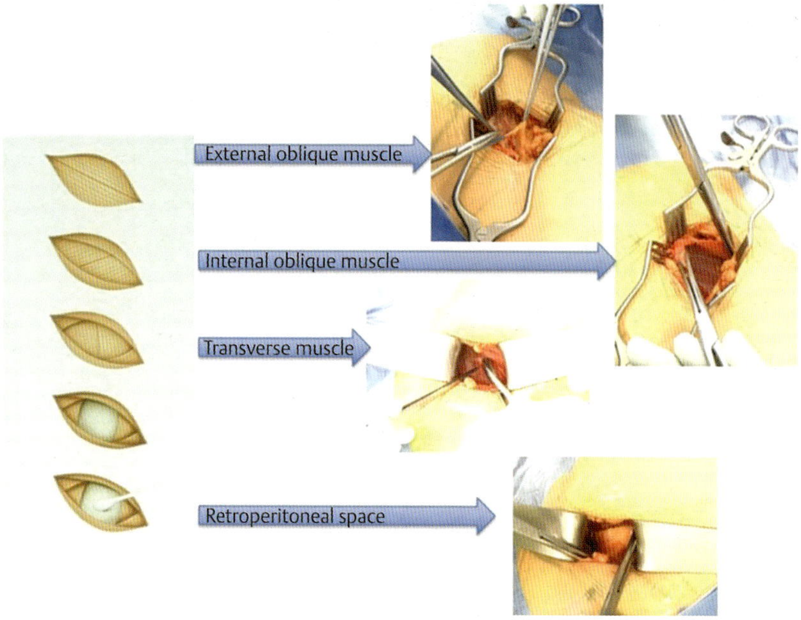

Fig. 40.3 Blunt muscle-splitting approach with dilation of the fibers of the different muscle layers.

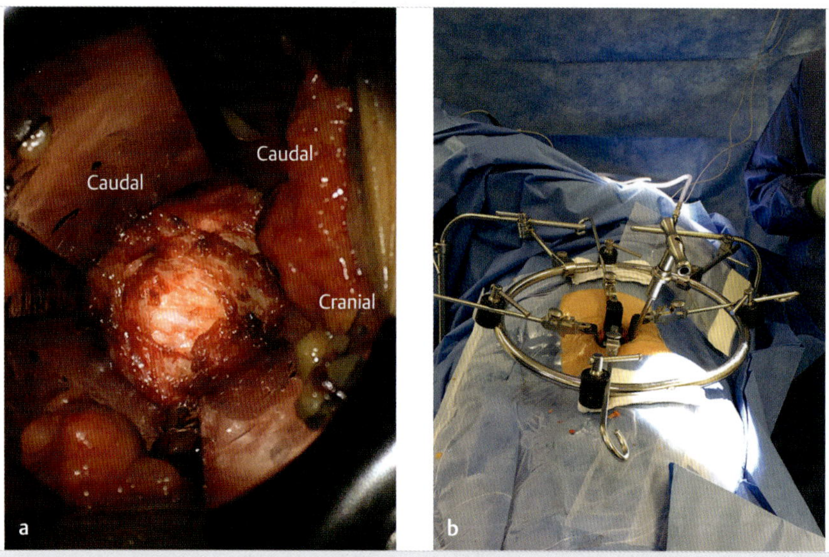

Fig. 40.4 **(a)** Exposure of the disc space. **(b)** Synframe (Synthes, Solothurn, Switzerland) in place.

4. **Discectomy and preparation of graft bed:**
The annulus fibrosis is incised in a rectangular way and the nucleus pulposus is removed (▶ Fig. 40.5a). The cartilaginous end plates are carefully removed with curettes, rongeurs, or custom-made shavers. Special care has to be taken to preserve the subchondral bone, especially in patients with poor bone quality to prevent subsidence. Depending on the type of interbody cage used, trial implants are inserted to determine the appropriate size, height, and angle (▶ Fig. 40.5b).
The type of anterior fusion is optional once the target area is exposed. All types of grafting techniques are possible (autologous bone graft; cages [PEEK, titanium] combined with allograft, femoral ring allografts, bone morphogenetic proteins [BMP], etc.) (▶ Fig. 40.6a–c).
Before implantation of the cage, the contralateral part of the intervertebral space is filled with cancellous bone, allograft, or BMP.
Implantation of the cage is performed under fluoroscopic control. If oval cages are implanted (e.g., Oracle), the tip of the cage is inserted obliquely into the intervertebral space while the direction of insertion is then changed to achieve a placement parallel to the posterior border of the disc space (▶ Fig. 40.7).[9]

40.6.3 Closure

The fusion area is covered with Surgicel (Tabotamp, Ethicon, Germany). The muscle layers are closed with absorbable sutures; the skin is closed with an intracutaneous suture.

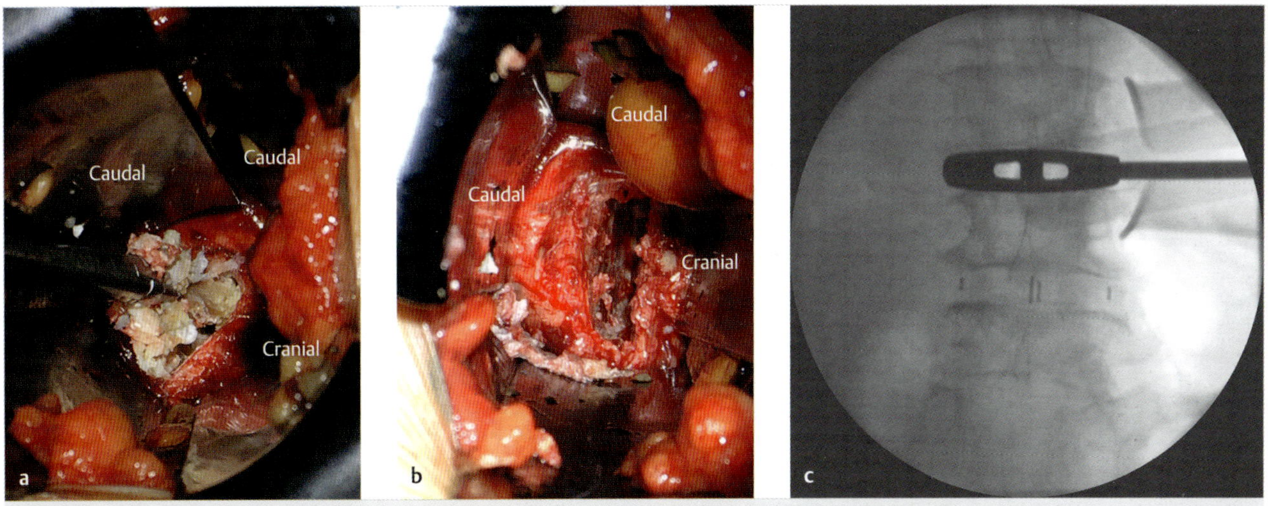

Fig. 40.5 **(a)** Removal of the disc after incision of the annulus fibrosis. **(b)** Disc space prepared for cage implantation. **(c)** Anteroposterior (AP) X-ray: Oracle cage trial (Synthes, Solothurn, Switzerland) in place at L3–L4. Oracle cage already implanted at L4–L5.

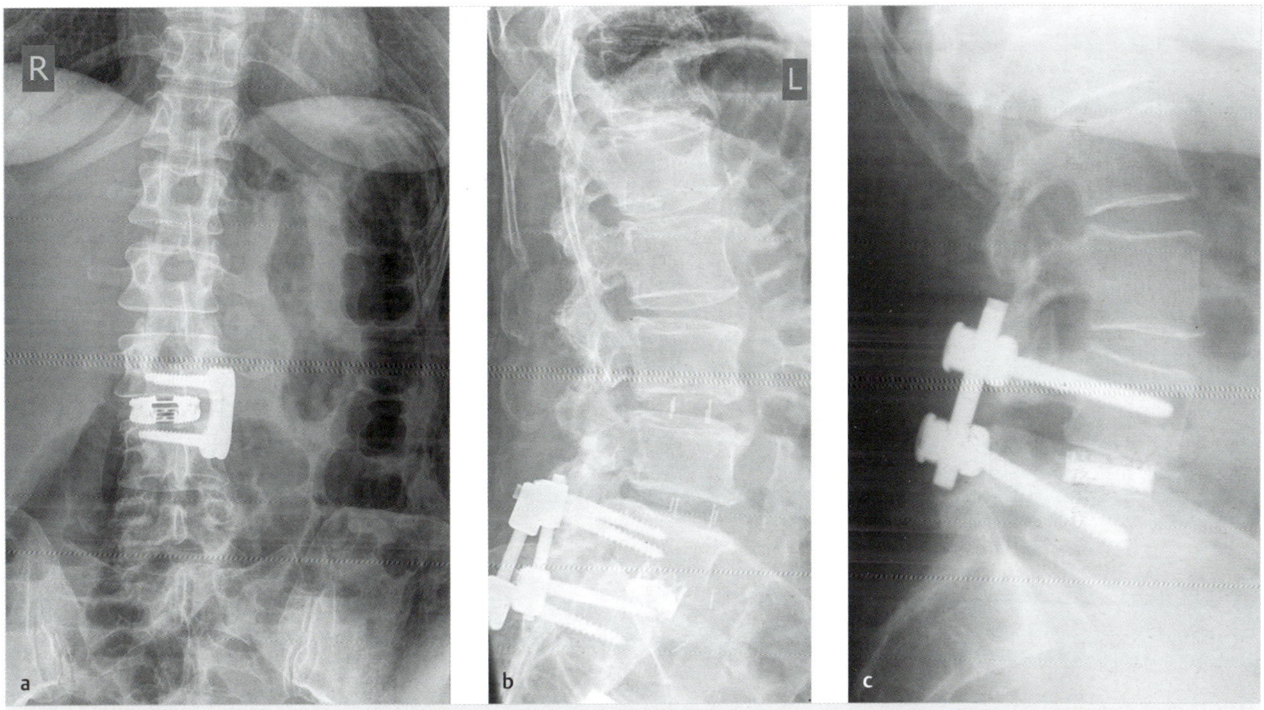

Fig. 40.6 Different types of interbody fusion (examples). **(a)** Syncage + ATB plate (Synthes Solothurn, Switzerland) for stand-alone fusion L3–L4. **(b)** Oracle multisegmental (L3-4-5) in segments adjacent to a previous fusion. **(c)** Harms cage + pedicle screws at L4–L5.

40.7 Postoperative Care

No drains are necessary. In most of the patients, OLIF is combined with posterior instrumentation. Patients are mobilized 6 hours postop. Thromboembolic prophylaxis is performed with fractionated heparin until full mobilization (usually around day 1 or 2).

Patients are discharged from the hospital between the 3rd and 5th day. We recommend a semi-rigid brace (Softec-lumbo, Bauerfeind) for 10 to 12 weeks.

40.8 Complication Avoidance/Tips and Tricks

There are a number of potential complications, pitfalls, and hazards at various steps of the operation:

a) Wrong positioning of the patient:
   When positioning the patient, special attention must be paid to the parallel orientation of the disc space borders in order to get a good approach to the disc space for cage insertion.

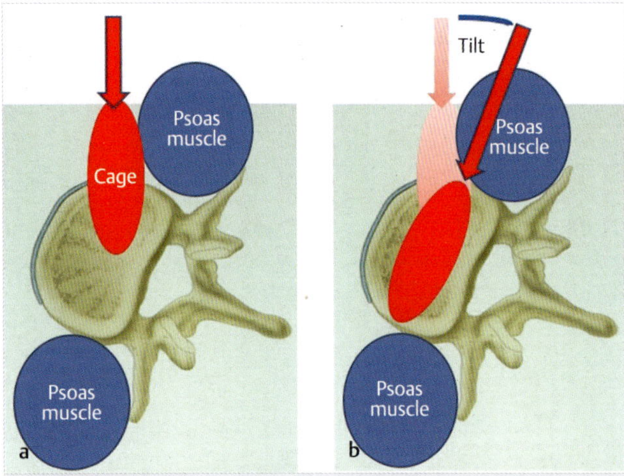

Fig. 40.7 Implantation principle of an oval-type cage. **(a)** Step 1: Vertical insertion into the disc space. **(b)** Step 2: Posterior tilt during implantation to achieve position parallel to posterior border of the disc space. This is associated with a minimum and short-term pressure on the psoas muscle.

b) High muscle tension due to insufficient relaxation of the patient:
The patient has to be completely relaxed to avoid pressure injury to the muscles.

c) Common iliac artery:
In patients with severe arteriosclerosis, the common iliac artery might kink laterally and thus reach into the approach corridor. It is not a problem to retract the vessel. However, if there are calcifications, the retraction should be very gentle in order to avoid lesions to the calcified wall of the vessel.

d) Genitofemoral nerve:
This nerve courses on the medial surface of the psoas muscle. It should not be injured by bipolar coagulation and pressure on it due to the retractor blade should be avoided. Lesion of this nerve can cause paresthesia, pain, and discomfort projecting into the groin and medial thigh.

40.9 Conclusion

The approach can be performed with optical aids such as a headlamp, loupe, surgical microscope, or "open" videoendoscopy. The skin incision is small (4 cm). The lateral abdominal wall function is preserved due to the muscle-splitting approach. The anterior-lateral circumference of the lumbar spine is exposed by blunt dissection medial to the psoas muscle. The exposure facilitates different types of interbody fusion techniques (e.g., iliac crest autografts, homografts [bank bone] as well as autografts or homografts augmented by allografts [e.g., PEEK, titanium cages]).

There are a number of other advantages:

a) The surgical approach to the lumbar spine is well known to spine surgeons. The learning curve usually is short.
b) The approach requires only one assistant (costs!).
c) No access surgeon required (costs!).
d) No neuromonitoring required.[10]
e) Low blood loss (< 100 mL).
f) Low complication rates.[11,12]
g) Good clinical results.[6]

The main disadvantages are:

a) Approach limited to L2–L5; however, recent publications have described a modified oblique approach to L5–S1.[13]
b) Additional posterior instrumentation (pedicle screw systems or other MIS systems) might be necessary.

References

[1] Greenough CG, Taylor LJ, Fraser RD. Anterior lumbar fusion: results, assessment techniques and prognostic factors. Eur Spine J. 1994; 3(4):225–230

[2] Grob D, Scheier HJG, Dvorak J, Siegrist H, Rubeli M, Joller R. Circumferential fusion of the lumbar and lumbosacral spine. Arch Orthop Trauma Surg. 1991; 111(1):20–25

[3] Obenchain TG. Laparoscopic lumbar discectomy: case report. J Laparoendosc Surg. 1991; 1(3):145–149

[4] Mayer HM. A new microsurgical technique for minimally invasive anterior lumbar interbody fusion. Spine. 1997; 22(6):691–699, discussion 700

[5] Li JX, Phan K, Mobbs R. Oblique lumbar interbody fusion: technical aspects, operative outcomes, and complications. World Neurosurg. 2017; 98:113–123

[6] Mobbs RJ, Phan K, Malham G, Seex K, Rao PJ. Lumbar interbody fusion: techniques, indications and comparison of interbody fusion options including PLIF, TLIF, MI-TLIF, OLIF/ATP, LLIF and ALIF. J Spine Surg. 2015; 1(1):2–18

[7] Mayer HM. Microsurgical approaches for anterior interbody fusion of the lumbar spine: In: McCulloch JA, Young PA, eds. Essentials of Spinal Microsurgery. Philadelphia: Lippincott-Raven; 1998:633–649

[8] Mehren C. Minimally invasive anterior oblique lumbar interbody fusion (OLIF) (2016): https://www.oot-esj.com/en/product/152971/Minimally_invasive_anterior_oblique_lumbar_interbody_fusion_%28OLIF%29

[9] Zairi F, Sunna TP, Westwick HJ, et al. Mini-open oblique lumbar interbody fusion (OLIF) approach for multi-level discectomy and fusion involving L5-S1: preliminary experience. Orthop Traumatol Surg Res. 2017; 103(2):295–299

[10] Lee H-J, Ryu K-S, Hur J-W, Seong J-H, Cho H-J, Kim J-S. Safety of lateral interbody fusion surgery without intraoperative monitoring. Turk Neurosurg. 2018; 28(3):428–43-3

[11] Silvestre C, Mac-Thiong J-M, Hilmi R, Roussouly P. Complications and morbidities of mini-open anterior retroperitoneal lumbar interbody fusion: oblique lumbar interbody fusion in 179 patients. Asian Spine J. 2012; 6(2):89–97

[12] Mehren C, Mayer HM, Zandanell C, Siepe CJ, Korge A. The oblique anterolateral approach to the lumbar spine provides access to the lumbar spine with few early complications. Clin Orthop Relat Res. 2016; 474(9):2020–2027

[13] Wakita H, Shiga Y, Ohtori S, et al. Less invasive corrective surgery using oblique lateral interbody fusion (OLIF) including L5-S1 fusion for severe lumbar kyphoscoliosis due to L4 compression fracture in a patient with Parkinson's disease: a case report. BMC Res Notes. 2015; 8:126

41 Maximum Access Surgery Posterior Lumbar Interbody Fusion

Joel Martin, Laura Hein, Pavan S. Upadhyayula, Vincent Cheung, and William Taylor

Summary

This chapter describes a brief history of the minimally invasive posterior lumbar interbody fusion (PLIF) procedure and illustrates the maximum access surgery posterior lumbar interbody fusion (MAS PLIF) technique with additional tips from the authors.

Keywords: maximum access surgery posterior lumbar interbody fusion (MAS PLIF), minimally invasive posterior lumbar interbody fusion (MIS PLIF), minimally invasive spinal surgery, spondylolisthesis, lumbar stenosis, degenerative disc disease

41.1 Introduction

The maximum access surgery posterior lumbar interbody fusion (MAS PLIF) has been developed as an alternative to minimally invasive lateral or posterior approaches. MAS PLIF uses a well-known medialized approach, resulting in less lateral retraction and dissection of the muscles, as opposed to open PLIF, where wide dissection is required for fusion cage placement and pedicle fixation in treating spinal pathologies. Minimally invasive PLIF may confer several advantages, including smaller incision, reduced scarring, reduced blood loss, decreased need for transfusion, shorter hospital stay, faster recovery time and return to ambulation, as well as reduced facet joint manipulation.[1,2,3,4,5] We also propose that decrease in subsidence would be an added benefit, as cages are placed laterally along the cortical bone. Finally, there is increasing economic data that suggests both direct and indirect cost-savings in favor of minimally invasive surgery (MIS) fusion as compared to open fusion.[2]

41.2 Indications

Similar to other minimally invasive procedures, MAS PLIF is applicable to many general deformity and degenerative conditions, including degenerative disc disease, lumbar stenosis, recurrent disc herniation, and Grades 1 and 2 spondylolistheses. An ideal patient has mid- to low-grade spondylolisthesis in the lower lumbar spine without severe osteoporosis, and bilateral symptoms without significant deformity. The most common surgical levels remain L4–L5 and/or L5–S1, but it is appropriate for all levels in the lower lumbar spine. It has the advantage of being a single-position surgery, combing bilateral decompression along with interbody fusion. The main drawbacks include difficulties in treating high-grade spondylolisthesis or significant hyperlordosis in the lower lumbar spine, both of which can complicate the surgery. MAS PLIF does require a change in pedicle screw instrumentation, namely, through the use of cortical bone screws with an alternative trajectory. MAS PLIF is relatively easy to learn, and it is also well-suited for navigation systems that can provide teaching and/or training tools. The cortical bone screws compare very favorably in biomechanical testing with pedicle fixation and are important in maintaining the medialized approach that provides much of the benefit.

41.3 Contraindications

One primary contraindication is multiple prior posterior procedures with significant scar tissue. Often in this case, a TLIF and/or lateral approach to avoid scar tissue may be a more appropriate choice. High-grade spondylolisthesis or spondylosis can be completed but should not be your initial case series.

41.4 Preoperative Planning

As with any surgical procedure, a complete history and physical examination should be completed. Preoperative radiographs can include anteroposterior and lateral views to determine sagittal alignment, disc space height, and often full-length films to evaluate for scoliosis. In suitable patients, flexion and extension views can provide further information of instability. Magnetic resonance imaging (MRI) can be performed to evaluate for canal or foraminal stenosis. In select patients with specific contraindications (aging pacemaker, metallic implant) a computed tomography (CT) myelogram may be used. Perhaps most importantly, a thin-slice CT scan for evaluation of soft tissue and bony architecture can be obtained for preoperative planning. Using preoperative imaging, the site of decompression and fusion should be determined and a plan for instrumentation should be discussed. Intraoperative neuromonitoring with electromyography (EMG) is a useful adjunct and may offer some protection of neural structures. For this purpose, discussion with the anesthesiologist to avoid long-acting muscle relaxants during induction and maintenance is important.

41.5 Patient Positioning

The patient is positioned on a radiolucent operating table in the prone position that allows for fluoroscopy and/or navigation. A bedrail on the table is necessary in order to attach an articulating arm (▶ Fig. 41.1). After draping the patient in the usual manner, adjust the table so that the C-arm provides an anteroposterior (AP) image when the orbital angle is at 90 degrees. Adjust the cranial/caudal angle of the C-arm to obtain a true AP image of the targeted vertebra, and a true lateral image when the orbital angle is at 0 degree.

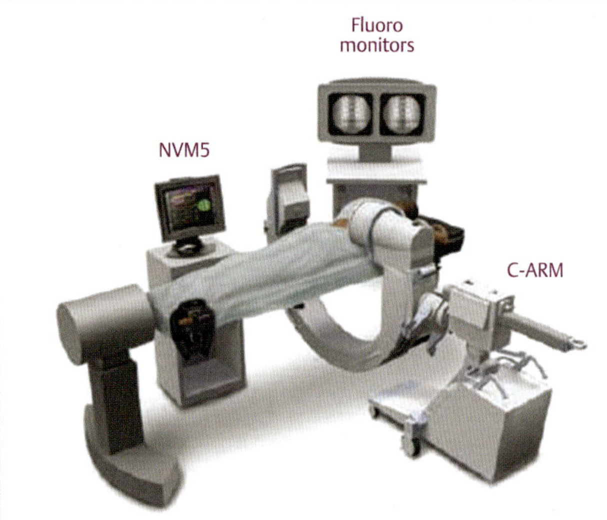

Fig. 41.1 Positioning and setup. Basic operating room setup for maximum access surgery posterior lumbar interbody fusion (MAS PLIF), including neuromonitoring unit, fluoroscopy monitors, and C-arm. (Used with permission from NuVasive, Inc. Mas Plif Surgical Technique. San Diego, CA: Nuvasive, Inc; 2013, 2.)

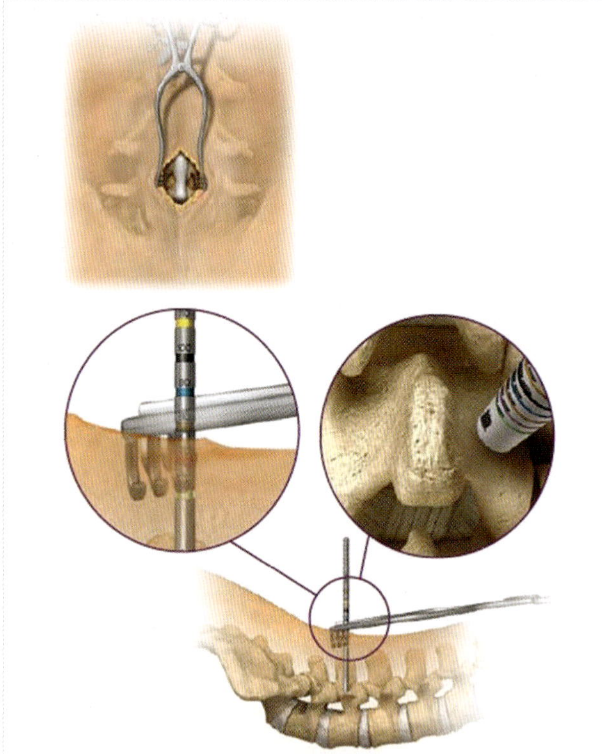

Fig. 41.2 Exposure. Dissect bilaterally down the spinous process to the lamina. Place the distal end of the blade measurement tool on the pars and select the appropriate retractor blade length using the scale on the blade measurement tool. (Used with permission from NuVasive, Inc. Mas Plif Surgical Technique. San Diego, CA: Nuvasive, Inc; 2013, 4.)

41.6 Surgical Technique

a) Incision:
   1. Locate the affected level by using fluoroscopy in the AP and lateral views. Using the targeting tool, obtain a true AP image to identify and mark the starting location.
   2. The incision is localized by extending a midline marker from the inferior one-third of the cranial spinous process down to the middle of the caudal spinous process, as defined by the targeting tool.

b) Technique:
   1. Exposure:
      i) Dissect bilaterally down the spinous process to the lamina and elevate muscles laterally to the facet capsule (▶ Fig. 41.2). Place the distal end of the blade measurement tool on the pars and select the appropriate retractor blade length using the scale on the blade measurement tool.
      ii) Use the blade attachment handle to retract the muscle and place the blades directly over the facet capsule (▶ Fig. 41.3). Insert light cable tips and attach the other end of the light cable to a light source. Attach the articulating arm to the retractor body, and lock the articulating arm.
   2. Identify shank entry points:
      i) Visualize and identify the superior-most lateral edge of the pars and move 3 to 5 mm medial for shank entry points (▶ Fig. 41.4).
      ii) The starting point of S1 screws will be superior and medial to the S1 foramen, and the trajectory will be parallel to the sacral end plate at a slight 10 degrees medial to lateral trajectory. This trajectory is also commonly used for the inferior shank placement.

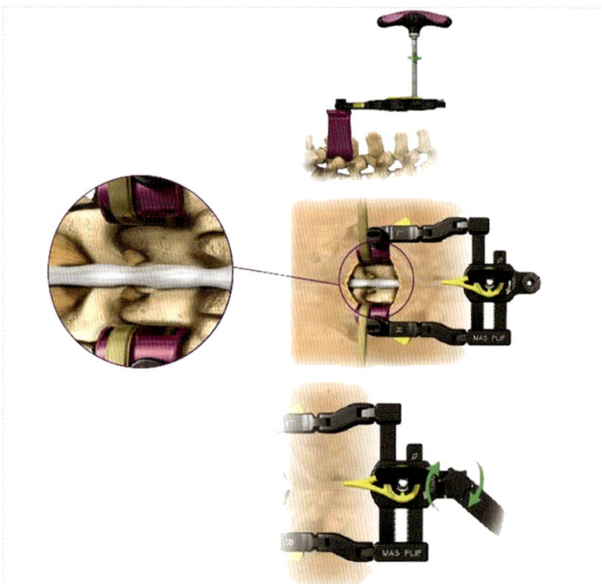

Fig. 41.3 Exposure. Place the retractor T-handle onto the hex bolt and turn to hold exposure. Attach light cables. Attach and lock the articulating arm to the retractor body. (Used with permission from NuVasive, Inc. Mas Plif Surgical Technique. San Diego, CA: Nuvasive, Inc; 2013, 6.)

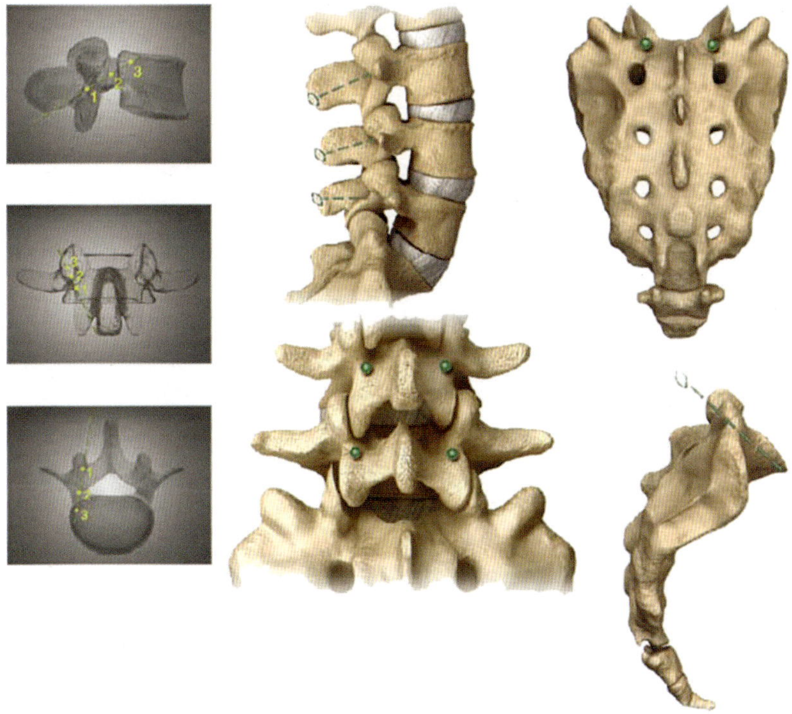

Fig. 41.4 Shank entry points. Using a Penfield, visualize and identify the superior-most lateral edge of the pars and move 3 to 5 mm medial for shank entry points. The starting point of S1 screws will be superior and medial to the S1 foramen. The trajectory will be parallel to the sacral end plate at a slight 10 degrees medial to lateral trajectory. (Used with permission from NuVasive, Inc. Mas Plif Surgical Technique. San Diego, CA: Nuvasive, Inc; 2013, 7–8.)

3. Pilot hole preparation:
   i) Starting with the cephalad level, perforate the proximal cortex using a high-speed burr. Cephalad shanks should be placed in a medial to lateral and inferior to superior trajectory.
   ii) Under lateral fluoroscopy, drill through the pedicle in a medial to lateral and inferior to superior trajectory to the posterior, superior-most aspect of the vertebral body. Ensure that the drill guide insulator is properly attached. Attach the stimulation clip onto the drill and activate the stimulation to obtain dynamic monitoring readings while drilling.
   iii) Use a ball tip probe to inspect the pilot hole for perforations.
   iv) Under lateral fluoroscopy, tap through the pedicle to the posterior, superior-most aspect of the vertebral body. Ensure that the tap insulator is properly attached and attach the stimulation clip onto the tap and activate the stimulation to obtain dynamic monitoring readings while tapping.
4. Shank insertion:
   i) Use a ball tip probe for inspection and measure for appropriate shank length. Insert the shank head into the distal tip of the shank driver (▶ Fig. 41.5).
   ii) Introduce the screw shank into the pilot hole and advance until the distal end of the shank tip reaches the posterior, superior-most aspect of the vertebral body. Release the shank driver and ensure that the shank driver insulator is properly attached. Attach the stimulation clip onto the shank driver and activate the stimulation to obtain dynamic monitoring readings while driving in the screw.
5. Decompression:
   i) Perform bilateral decompression, removing the inferior articular processes and superior two-thirds of the superior articular processes (▶ Fig. 41.6).
6. Disc removal and sizing:
   i) Make an ipsilateral annulotomy and perform a conventional discectomy. Using the paddle sizers, sequentially distract the disc space prior to trial placement (▶ Fig. 41.6). Insert the final trial size on the ipsilateral side. Repeat disc prep and sizing sequence on the contralateral side. Once the contralateral disc space is prepared, use the paddle shavers to prepare the end plates.
7. Interbody grafting:
   i) Place the appropriate size implant onto the Inserter. Prior to implant placement, pack the anterior third of the disc space with graft material. Insert the contralateral implant. Once the implant is in its final orientation, ensure the markings on the inserter are in the proper orientation.
   ii) Use the paddle shaver to prepare the end plates and pack the center of the disc space with graft material using the bone graft funnel (▶ Fig. 41.7). Insert the ipsilateral implant and ensure the markings on the inserter are in the proper orientation.

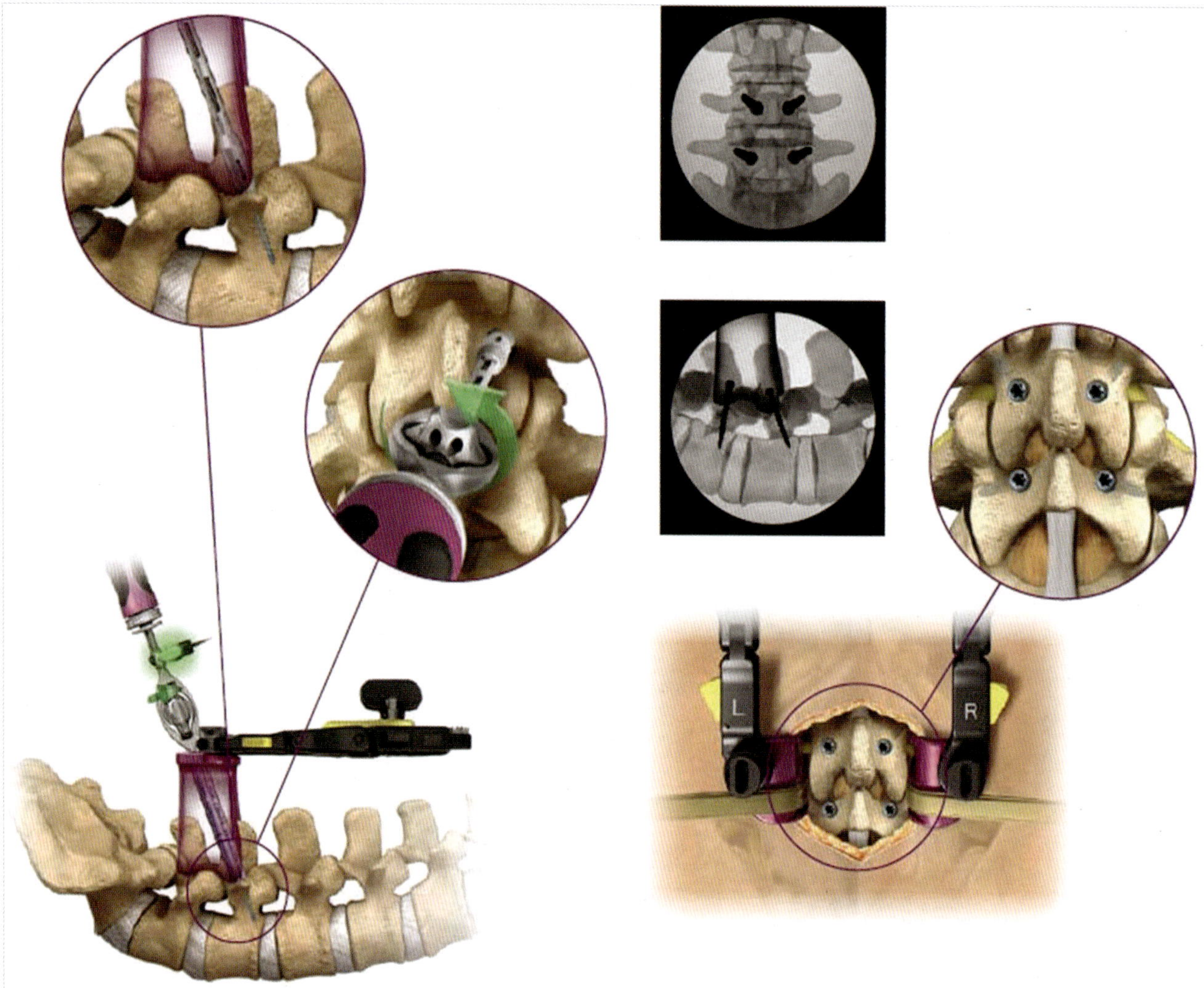

Fig. 41.5 Shank insertion. Introduce the screw shank into the pilot hole and advance the distal end of the shank tip until it reaches the posterior, superior-most aspect of the vertebral body. Attach the stimulation clip onto the shank driver and activate it to obtain dynamic monitoring readings while driving in screw. (Used with permission from NuVasive, Inc. Mas Plif Surgical Technique. San Diego, CA: Nuvasive, Inc; 2013, 14–15.)

8. Screw head attachment:
   i) With the head inserter fully threaded into the screw head, align with the long axis of the screw shank and attach by applying downward force. Rotate the head inserter in a 360 degrees orbital motion while applying downward force to facilitate screw head engagement.
   ii) Release the head inserter from the tulip and repeat the previously described process to attach the other tulip heads.
9. Rod insertion:
   i) Use the head adjuster to position the tulips in the proper orientation and select the desired rod length and place in tulips. Load up to four lock screws directly from the caddy (▶ Fig. 41.8).
10. Final tightening:
   i) Place the counter-torque over the superior tulip and tighten until the T-handle breaks free and repeat on remaining screws (▶ Fig. 41.8).

c) Closure:
   1. Closure is very standard and is one of the advantages of working through well-known anatomy, with incisions and closure of the dorsal fascia subcutaneous layers and skin closure. A drain can often be avoided, as the patient is often discharged within 24 hours.

41.7 Postoperative Care

Postoperative care in MAS PLIF should prioritize neurological and vascular assessments, wound care, pain management, progressive mobility, and pulmonary rehabilitation. Initially, following transfer from the operating suite, patients will recover in the postanesthesia recovery unit. To establish baseline function, neurologic assessment of motor and sensory function at and below the level of operation should be performed every 4 to 8 hours. In the immediate postoperative window, patients may require intravenous (IV) pain medications. Once tolerated,

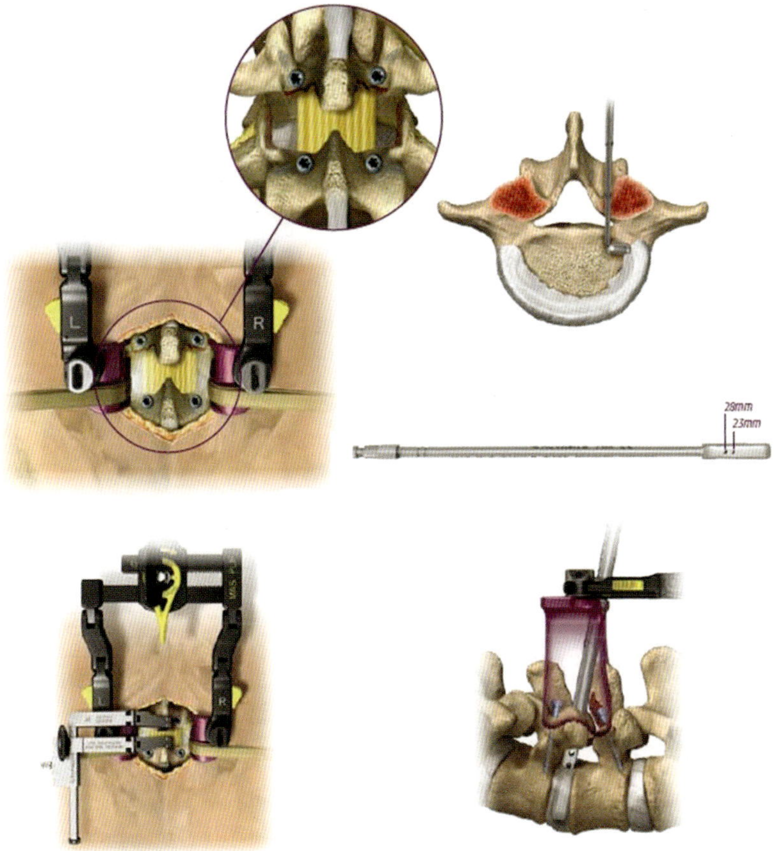

Fig. 41.6 Decompression, disc removal, and sizing. Perform bilateral decompression, removing the inferior articular processes and superior two-thirds of the superior articular processes. Make an ipsilateral annulotomy and perform a conventional discectomy. Using the paddle sizers, sequentially distract the disc space prior to trial placement. (Used with permission from NuVasive, Inc. Mas Plif Surgical Technique. San Diego, CA: Nuvasive, Inc; 2013, 16–17.)

they should be transitioned to oral medications. Coordination with physical and occupational therapies to encourage ambulation and activity without excessive bending, lifting, and twisting should begin promptly after surgery. Taken together, mobility and pain control are two key factors determining a patient's readiness for discharge. Patients should expect to be discharged from the hospital 1 to 2 days post-operation. The wound should be covered with gauze and kept dry and clean. Patients can shower after the procedure but should avoid submerging the wound under water for 4 to 8 weeks. A soft or rigid lumbar support brace, although not medically indicated, may be issued for patient comfort.

41.8 Complications and Avoidance

Accurately classifying the risk profile associated with MAS PLIF requires understanding complication rates for open and minimally invasive posterior fusion techniques. In a 1-year study of 51 patients, open PLIF demonstrated a fusion rate of 88% with clinical improvement in 82% of cases.[6] In hopes of achieving higher union rates, PLIF was combined with posterolateral instrumentation to achieve circumferential fusion.[7] Although PLIF is already noted to have high rates of dural tears (5.4–10%) and of neurologic injury (9–16%),[8] this combined technique was noted to have even higher rates of neurologic injury due to excessive retraction of the thecal sac. Open transforaminal lumbar interbody fusion (TLIF) was created to achieve circumferential fusion without excessive retraction of the thecal sac noted in the combined posterior and posterolateral approach. A meta-analysis combining two randomized controlled trials (RCTs) with multiple observational trials demonstrated a beneficial effect of TLIF on arthrodesis rates, Oswestry Disability Index (ODI), and visual analog scale (VAS) leg pain. PLIF was shown to decrease rates of blood loss and operative time with no inter-group differences in other complications such as hospital length of stay, rate of durotomy, and readmission.[9] Moreover, in comparison to open lumbar fusion, multiple studies have shown that minimally invasive lumbar interbody fusion has been associated with decreased estimated blood loss and decreased hospital length of stay.[2,10,11]

Given the elective nature of this surgery, MAS PLIF should continue the trend for decreasing intraoperative blood loss, surgical site infection, and hospital length of stay while providing similar-to-lower complication rates. Another key consideration is avoiding nerve root retraction. A helpful approach involves wide lateral decompressions providing greater access around traversing nerve roots. Creating a large operative window should also help improve on nonunion rates. Current MIS posterior fusion techniques have nonunion rates ranging from 0 to

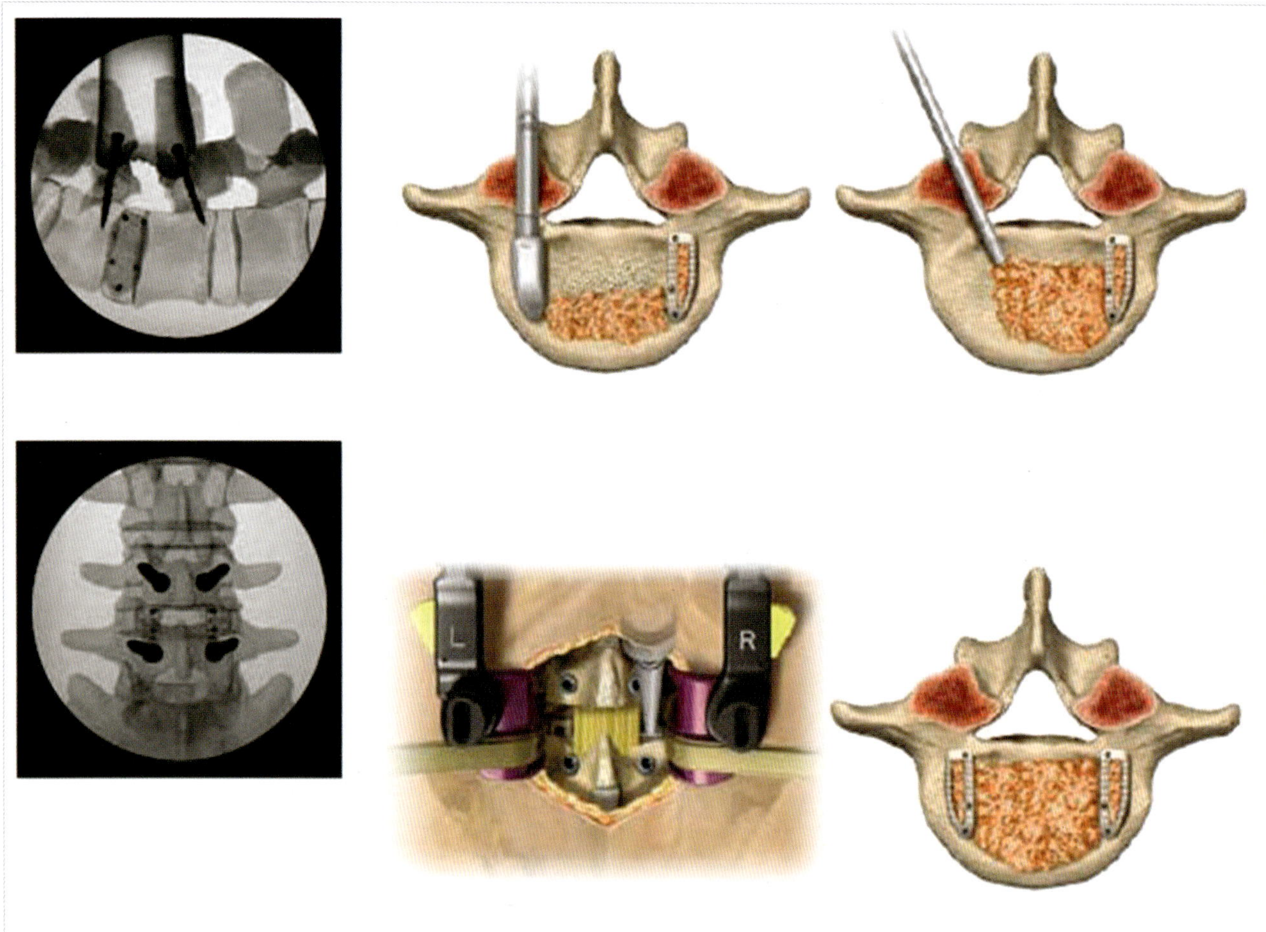

Fig. 41.7 Interbody grafting. Use the paddle shaver to prepare the end plates and pack the center of the disc space with graft material using the bone graft funnel. Insert the ipsilateral implant. (Used with permission from NuVasive, Inc. Mas Plif Surgical Technique. San Diego, CA: Nuvasive, Inc; 2013, 20.)

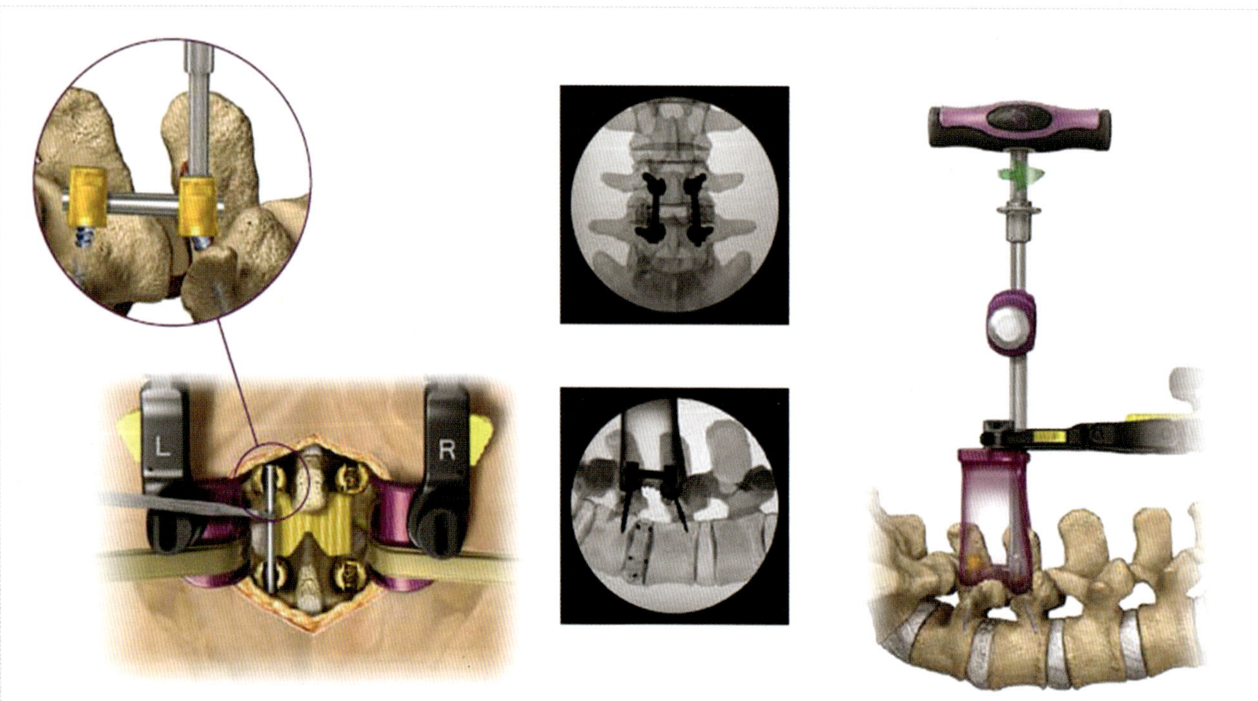

Fig. 41.8 Rod insertion and final tightening. Select the desired rod length and place in tulips. Place the counter-torque over the superior tulip, and place the lock screw final tightener and tighten until the T-handle breaks free and repeat on remaining screws. (Used with permission from NuVasive, Inc. Mas Plif Surgical Technique. San Diego, CA: Nuvasive, Inc; 2013, 25–26.)

16.7%.[2] A larger decompression and bilateral access is thought to lower the incidence of retraction-related neuropraxia while improving fusion outcomes.

41.9 Tips and Tricks

a) Positioning and planning:
 1. Patient positioning and operating room setup are critical. Make adjustments so that you are able to obtain both AP and lateral images if navigation is used, and place the reference array in a location that will not interfere with positioning of cortical bone screws, which often take more of an acute trajectory than pedicle screws.
 2. Care must be taken to ensure that a direct AP image is obtained, as the placement of the incision is critical, and hyperlordosis of the lower lumbar spine can make it difficult to place the incision properly. Ensure the location in AP X-ray; but the lateral fluoroscopy is also very helpful in ensuring the appropriate superior and inferior locations.
 3. This procedure is extremely well-suited to navigation and we routinely use intraoperative CT scan for our screw trajectories and postoperative films as both a teaching and a learning tool, although not required. The starting point for superior shank placement can be visualized along the medial aspect of the pars. Occasionally, a chisel will be needed to remove overhanging bone from the superior level for entry point of the shank screw placement. Navigation will greatly aid in quick learning and will reduce misplacement of screws.
 4. We routinely reserve this procedure for a patient with low-grade spondylolisthesis and with bilateral symptoms of radiculopathy and/or lumbar stenosis at L5/1. We often use this procedure at L4/5 and above when TLIF or LLIF are not adequate options for TLIF and lateral lumbar interbody fusions to maintain lordosis and prevent subsidence are more difficult.

b) Surgical technique:
 1. A light source is helpful both in maintaining this small exposure and with visualization. A head light can be used if preferred along with a lighting source that is deployed in the retractor blades.
 2. For the cephalad shank, it is important to avoid the adjacent facet capsule and make the entry point slightly inferior.
 3. Cortical bone is routinely placed prior to decompression but can be performed at any stage through decompression and interbody fixation.
 4. For S1 screws, it is advised to under-tap with the 5.5-mm tap and utilize 6.5-mm diameter screws.
 5. Lateral fluoroscopy should be used at an average angle of 15 degrees medial to lateral to take an image, aiming for the posterior, superior-most aspect of the targeted vertebral body.
 6. It is important to tape line-to-line to prevent the creation of microfractures, which can occur when the pilot hole is under-tapped.
 7. MAS PLIF interbody implants are lordotic; it is therefore important to trial for a precise height measurement.
 8. To remove cartilaginous end plates prior to implant placement, use a paddle shaver one size smaller than the measured trial.
 9. Decompression can be tailored to the patient's symptoms, but the goal of decreasing nerve retraction is important in avoiding neuropraxia and postoperative scarring.
 10. Interbodies are designed to be placed in a far-lateral position. Implant placement is along the cortical margin at the periphery of the interbody space rather than a midline location that would encourage retraction.
 11. With a wide decompression, lordotic implants, and thorough packing of the disc space with decompression harvested bone and/or allograft is easily completed. Distraction of the screws, with complete removal of the facet joint, is possible but interbody distraction is routinely adequate for these procedures.
 12. Use navigation or intraoperative CT scan to allow for any correction with fusion. Given the interbody distraction, place the screws before posterior compression to decrease errors. Navigation is particularly helpful both at the initial placement of fixation, and during the procedure to ensure proper location of all fixational devices. However, performing this procedure with AP and lateral fluoroscopy is routinely done.

41.10 Conclusions

The MAS PLIF combines posterior fusion with interbody fusion and offers the benefits of open PLIF. Compared with open PLIF, the use of minimally invasive PLIF may confer several advantages, including smaller incision, reduced scarring, reduced blood loss, reduced needs for transfusion, reduced length of time spent in the hospital, faster recovery time, reduced time to ambulation, reduced facet joint manipulation, as well as potential cost-savings.[1,2,3,4,5] In general, an ideal patient is a mid- to low-grade spondylolisthesis in the lower lumbar spine without severe osteoporosis and bilateral symptoms without significant deformity. Similar to other minimally invasive procedures, MAS PLIF is applicable to many general deformity and degenerative conditions including degenerative disc disease, lumbar stenosis, recurrent disc herniation, and low-grade spondylolisthesis.

References

[1] Nuvasive, I., MAS PLIF-Maximum Access Surgery Posterior Lateral Interbody Fusion. 2017

[2] Goldstein CL, Phillips FM, Rampersaud YR. Comparative effectiveness and economic evaluations of open versus minimally invasive posterior or transforaminal lumbar interbody fusion: a systematic review. Spine. 2016; 41 Suppl 8:S74–S89

[3] Khanna N, Deol G, Poulter G, Ahuja A. Medialized, muscle-splitting approach for posterior lumbar interbody fusion: technique and multicenter perioperative results. Spine. 2016; 41 Suppl 8:S90–S96

[4] Park Y, Ha JW. Comparison of one-level posterior lumbar interbody fusion performed with a minimally invasive approach or a traditional open approach. Spine. 2007; 32(5):537–543

[5] Gautschi OP, Garbossa D, Tessitore E, et al. Maximal access surgery for posterior lumbar interbody fusion with divergent, cortical bone trajectory pedicle screws: a good option to minimize spine access and maximize the field for nerve decompression. J Neurosurg Sci. 2017; 61(3):335–341

[6] Tullberg T, Brandt B, Rydberg J, Fritzell P. Fusion rate after posterior lumbar interbody fusion with carbon fiber implant: 1-year follow-up of 51 patients. Eur Spine J. 1996; 5(3):178–182

[7] Heary RF, Bono CM. Circumferential fusion for spondylolisthesis in the lumbar spine. Neurosurg Focus. 2002; 13(1):E3

[8] DiPaola CP, Molinari RW. Posterior lumbar interbody fusion. J Am Acad Orthop Surg. 2008; 16(3):130–139

[9] Levin JM, Tanenbaum JE, Steinmetz MP, Mroz TE, Overley SC. Posterolateral fusion (PLF) versus transforaminal lumbar interbody fusion (TLIF) for spondylolisthesis: a systematic review and meta-analysis. Spine J. 2018; 18 (6):1088–1098

[10] Lau D, Lee JG, Han SJ, Lu DC, Chou D. Complications and perioperative factors associated with learning the technique of minimally invasive transforaminal lumbar interbody fusion (TLIF). J Clin Neurosci. 2011; 18(5):624–627

[11] Lee LY, Idris Z, Beng TB, et al. Outcomes of minimally invasive surgery compared to open posterior lumbar instrumentation and fusion. Asian J Neurosurg. 2017; 12(4):620–637

42 MIS-TLIF with Total Navigation and Expandable Interbody Cages

Rodrigo Navarro-Ramirez, Sertac Kirnaz, and Roger Härtl

Summary

The MIS-TLIF is one of the best techniques to treat single level pathologies that require instrumentation and interbody fusion. This technique reduces hospital stay, blood loss, and recovery time, and is especially useful in obese patients. In this chapter, we go through the key steps of the technique and how to integrate total navigation into the procedure.

Keywords: interbody fusion, spinal fusion, pseudoarthrosis, spondylolisthesis, tubular surgery, expandable cage

42.1 Introduction

The transforaminal lumbar interbody fusion (TLIF) surgical technique is a versatile technique to treat different lumbar disorders such as spondylolisthesis, stenosis, and instability.[1] The TLIF technique relies on a single posterior approach to achieve a 360-degree stabilization and spinal canal and neural foramina decompression. Also, it can reduce listhesis, restoring and maintaining lumbar lordosis especially today with the availability of expandable cages. The TLIF far-lateral surgical corridor is ideal to avoid dural and nerve root manipulation/retraction, which decreases the incidence of the intraoperative durotomy and postoperative radiculitis in comparison with PLIF.[2]

The minimally invasive transforaminal lumbar interbody fusion (MIS-TLIF) is a modification of the original technique, performed through a paramedian transmuscular corridor.[3] The MIS-TLIF approach decreases collateral muscle damage and detachment, preserving ligaments and facet joint integrity most of the times.[4] In addition, MIS-TLIF has shown to decrease the estimated blood loss (EBL), hospital stay, and postoperative pain when compared to conventional approaches, while maintaining similar clinical and radiographical outcomes.[5,6,7]

Minimally invasive techniques depend on an indirect localization of anatomical structures using X-rays, fluoroscopy, or intraoperative computed tomography (CT) (iCT) scanners. However, reducing radiation exposure is still a challenge. Some authors have reported that there is significantly longer patient fluoroscopic exposure in the MIS-TLIF group compared with the open TLIF.[8,9] More recently, we have been able to adapt the MIS-TLIF technique using a portable iCT scanner, Airo (Brainlab AG, Feldkirchen, Germany), combined with state-of-the-art computer navigation, not only for navigated instrumentation but also for intraoperative planning throughout the procedure, inserting the cage and eliminating the need for fluoroscopy. Moreover, our group published this modification in a "total navigation" modality, which can reduce staff radiation exposure to 0 by navigation/augmented reality, real time over iCT obtained images that can be acquired while the surgical staff is protected or outside the operating room (OR).[10] With the iCT-CAS and image-guided navigation, real-time and virtual intraoperative imaging of screws and their planned trajectory is feasible. This helps surgeon's orientation during instrumentation and also helps to predict cage placement and size.[10]

The purpose of this chapter is to describe our latest experience in navigated MIS-TLIF procedure. More details about the alternatives on how to perform an MIS-TLIF procedure will be included in Chapter 43.

42.2 Patient Selection: Indications and Contraindications

a) **Indications:**
   1. Central stenosis, with lateral recess and foraminal stenosis.
   2. Radicular symptoms due to foraminal or lateral recess radicular compression.
   3. Primary degenerative disc disease (DDD) causing discogenic low back pain for 12 to 16 weeks that do not respond to conservative therapy.
   4. Segmental instability causing low back pain with or without nerve root compression:
      a) Idiopathic or traumatic grade I or II spondylolisthesis.
      b) De novo or iatrogenic biomechanical instability, including pseudoarthrosis.
      c) Bilateral facet joint cysts with unilateral nerve compression.

b) **Relative contraindications:**
   1. Severe deformity and/or severe sagittal and coronal imbalance of the lumbar spine.
   2. Multilevel disease (more than two).
   3. Systemic and local infection.
   4. Tumors—either local or metastatic lesions.
   5. Severe osteoporosis.
   6. Previous surgery with extensive epidural scarring on magnetic resonance imaging (MRI).
   7. Grade III or IV spondylolisthesis.
   8. Acute spinal end-plate fracture.

42.3 Preoperative Planning

a) Patient's previous history and physical examination are key.
b) Diagnostic testing and imaging studies: Imaging information (e.g., MRI, CT scan, and flexion/extension X-rays) should be sufficient to determine the appropriate level or levels requiring surgery, as well as the characteristics of the pathology (e.g., calcified disc, migrated disc, synovial joint cyst, etc.).

Recommended routine preoperative investigations are:

a) Full body standing anteroposterior (AP) and lateral X-rays including the pelvis and femoral heads are mandatory.
b) For all our patients, we measure: SVA, PI-LL, Cobb angle, and C2 plum line.
c) Flexion/extension X-rays are extremely useful in cases of spondylolisthesis. They provide basic information about important parameters concerning sagittal balance and coronal balance, which are clinical outcomes prognostic factors.
d) MRI provides accurate information regarding the perineural structures, for example, disc, muscle, scars, fibrotic tissue, etc.

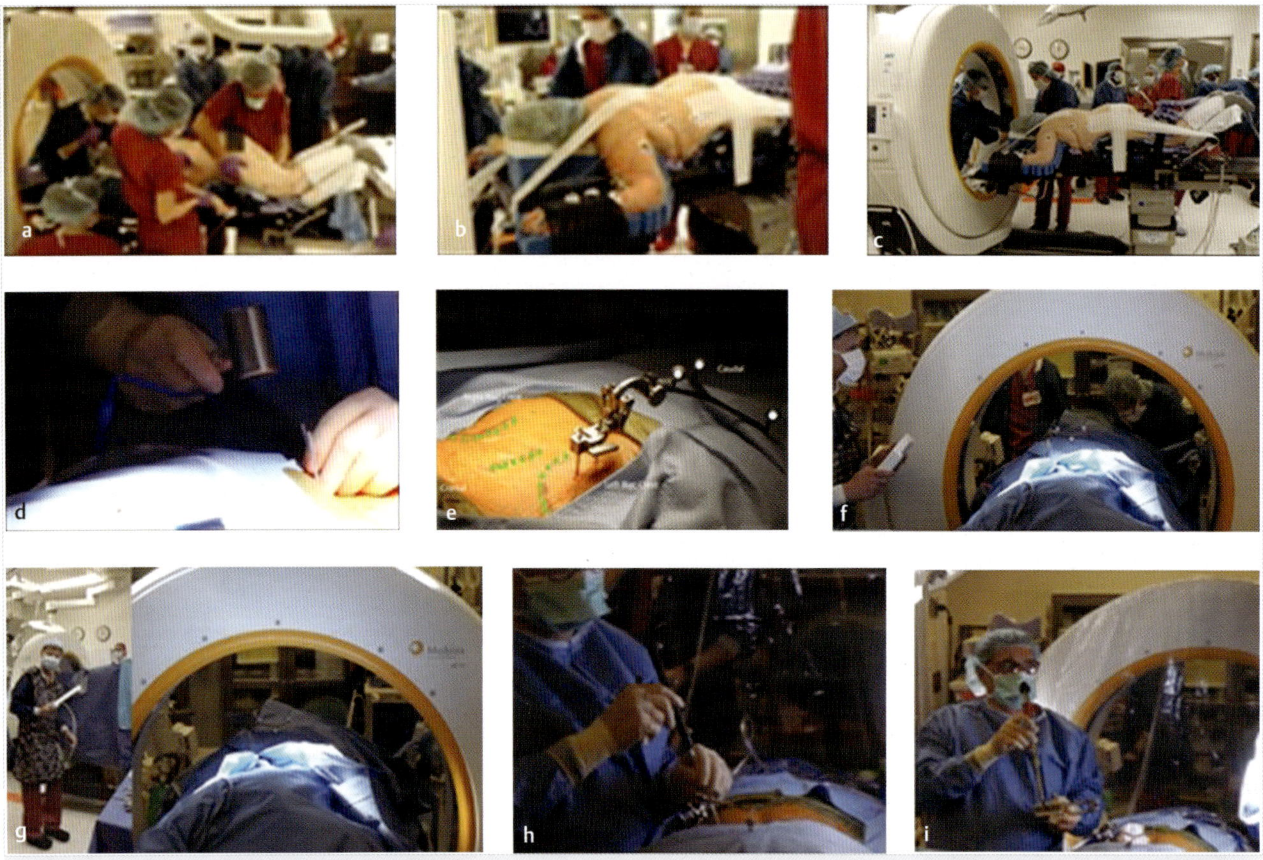

Fig. 42.1 **(a)** Patient is positioned prone and all the bony prominences are covered and padded. **(b)** Patient is taped down to the frame to prevent shifting. **(c)** The final position and orientation of the gantry and the table. **(d)** Steinmann pins are inserted into the superior iliac crest ideally deep enough to reach but not perforate the ventral cortex of the iliac crest. **(e)** Final position of the reference array (aiming medially and inferiorly. Preferably, contralateral to the side of the facetectomy/cage insertion site. **(f)** The patient is covered with two sterile half sheets and the technician makes sure the area to scan is visible. **(g)** The technician leaves the operating room (OR) and the patient is hold on apnea while everyone leaves the room and the scan is obtained. **(h)** The incision is then navigated and planned. **(i)** The tools to be used are then registered and calibrated (▶ Video 42.1).

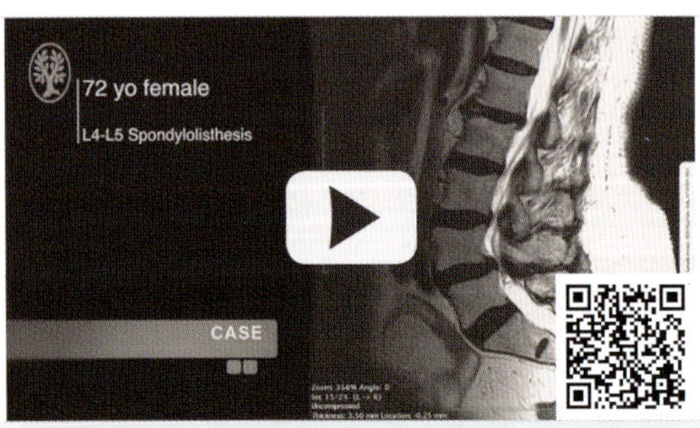

Video 42.1 Total navigation MIS TLIF.

e) CT scans are especially important in those pathologies where either bone structures or calcification of soft tissue is expected. For example, bony foraminal spurs, stenotic calcified foramens, calcified discs, and calcified facet joint cysts. Also, they are useful to predict the pedicle dimensions.

42.4 Patient Positioning

a) After endotracheal general anesthesia, all pertinent monitoring extensions, such as the intubation tube, Bovie, and suction, are positioned through the gantry of the Airo (▶ Fig. 42.1a–c).

b) The patient is taped down and fixed to the table to ensure immobilization of skin and soft tissue especially in overweight patients. This helps to prevent shift during intraoperative navigation (▶ Fig. 42.1a–c).

c) The posterior midline and iliac crests are marked, and then the patient is scrubbed and draped in regular fashion (▶ Fig. 42.1d–e).

d) The patient reference array is fixed to the left iliac crest using two Steinmann pins. Two sterile half sheets are used to cover the surgical site, leaving exposed only the reference array (▶ Fig. 42.1d–f).

e) First scan: All the staff leave the OR, including the radiology technician, who brings the Airo touch screen outside the door to control the scan. Therefore, not wearing lead aprons is possible for the surgical staff (▶ Fig. 42.1g).

f) When the scan is complete, the images are automatically transferred to the Brainlab Curve navigation system (Brainlab Curve, Brainlab AG, Feldkirchen, Germany) (▶ Fig. 42.1h).

g) After registration, data is transferred to the navigation unit. Confirmation of the anatomical landmarks to confirm accuracy is performed and the trajectory to reach the pedicles is identified and marked over the skin/ioban using a marking pen (▶ Fig. 42.1i).

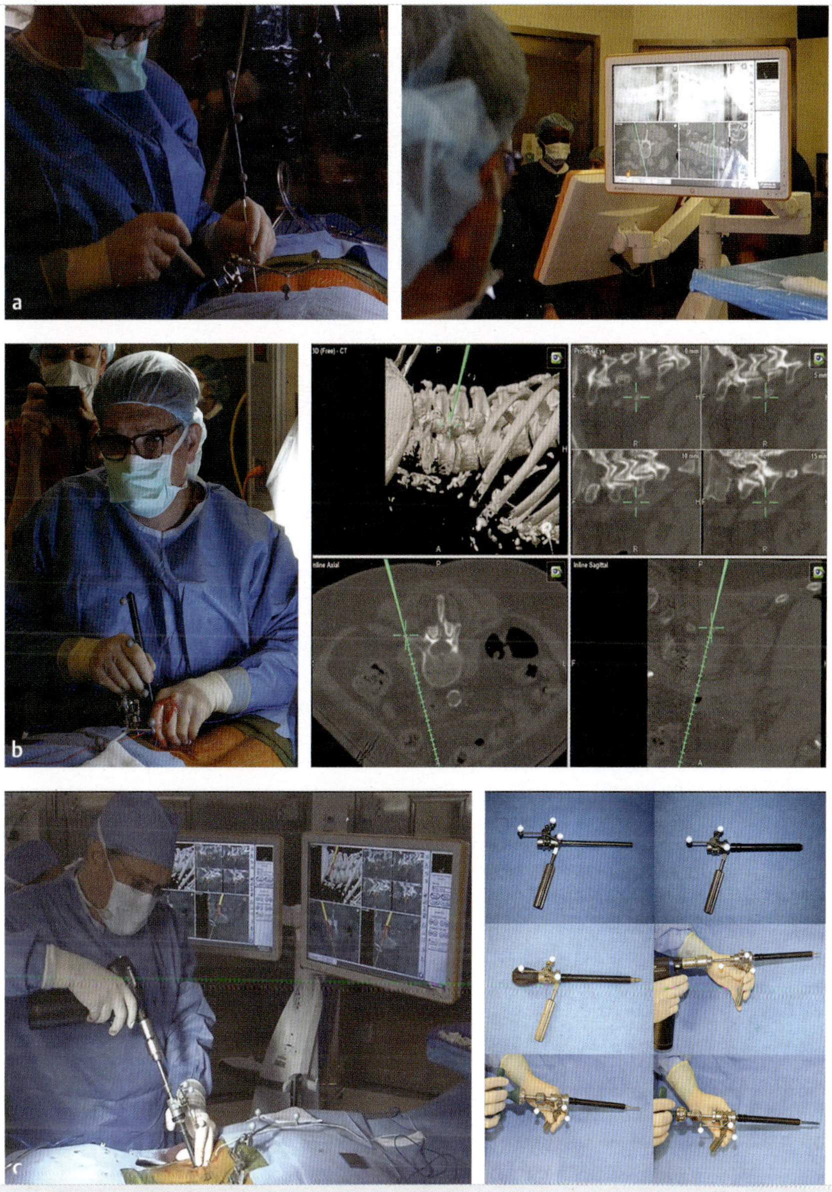

Fig. 42.2 For those systems that still use a navigated guide tube after the first scan is obtained. **(a)** The incision is planned and navigated. **(b)** The anatomical landmarks are used to confirm accuracy; in this case the transverse process is recommended. **(c)** A navigated guide tube is used to drill, tap, and introduce the "headless" screw.

42.5 Surgical Technique

We use total navigation in every step of our MIS-TLIF surgery, i.e., total navigation, to increase accuracy of our implants and better plan our surgical steps.

The side of the approach is ipsilateral to the more painful side or the side with the most significant compression identified on the preoperative CT scan:

a) Skin incision is marked using navigation guidance to identify the site of incision and the proper trajectory of the screws, which help in obtaining the best exposure with the smallest possible access. The goal of navigated planning is also to prevent "fighting the fascia"; this means to be able to angle the screw handle while cannulating the pedicles (▶ Fig. 42.2a).

b) Manual verification: After skin incision has been made, accuracy is confirmed using the Brainlab Pointer over a transverse process previously identified with the tip of the surgeon's finger (▶ Fig. 42.2b).

c) The navigated screw and screw driver are calibrated using the Brainlab Instrument Calibration Matrix (ICM4) and the Brainlab starlink array. This eliminates the need for K-wires (▶ Fig. 42.1i).

   1. In case self-tapping screws are not available, a navigated guide tube can be calibrated. This modality allows navigating only one instrument, which simplifies the workflow of the procedure, in the sequence of: point, drill, tap, and then insert the screw (▶ Fig. 42.2c). Headless screws are inserted through the navigated tube guide bilaterally as planned (▶ Fig. 42.2c).

d) Using a long electrode probe, we use electrical neurostimulation (8 mA) to test for any breach of the pedicle walls, and then insert the screws. Navigation helps in planning the size and length of the screw. We usually place the screws first trying to be as gentle as possible to decrease anatomical shifting and navigation inaccuracies. The average time for iCT NAV setup and pedicle screw insertion was 12 minutes for a single-level MIS-TLIF, preserving a screw accuracy of 99%[11] (▶ Fig. 42.3 and ▶ Fig. 42.4).
e) Autologous bone graft is harvested from the iliac crest under the navigation guidance. This graft is added to the facet joint that will be resected to later be packed inside the "prepared" interbody space (▶ Fig. 42.5).
f) With the assistance of the pointer, the tubular retractor scope of vision is predicted; usually third medial fascial incision is made (Right Screws #1, Left Screws #2). A 21-mm tubular retractor tube is positioned toward the facet joint to be removed. We aim to land over the top of the working zone, which includes the pars and the inferior laminar border of the upper level and the superior articular process of the lower level, forming the facet joint. Then the tube is fixed in position (▶ Fig. 42.6a). The bony anatomy is then reconfirmed with the pointer and the tubular retractor is adjusted as needed (▶ Fig. 42.6b). Using a combination of high-speed drill and Kerrison rongeurs, the inferior articular process is removed, followed by removal of the inferior vertebra superior articular process, both forming the facet joint of interest (▶ Fig. 42.6c–f). If central canal or contralateral decompression is planned, the tube must be tilted away from the surgeon and angled medially to undercut the spinous process and contralateral lamina (▶ Fig. 42.7a–c).
g) Once the entire facet (IAP/SAP) has been removed, the dural sac disc, and exiting nerve root are identified. We proceed to perform the discectomy, using a combination of shavers, ring curettes, and rongeurs without violating the end plate

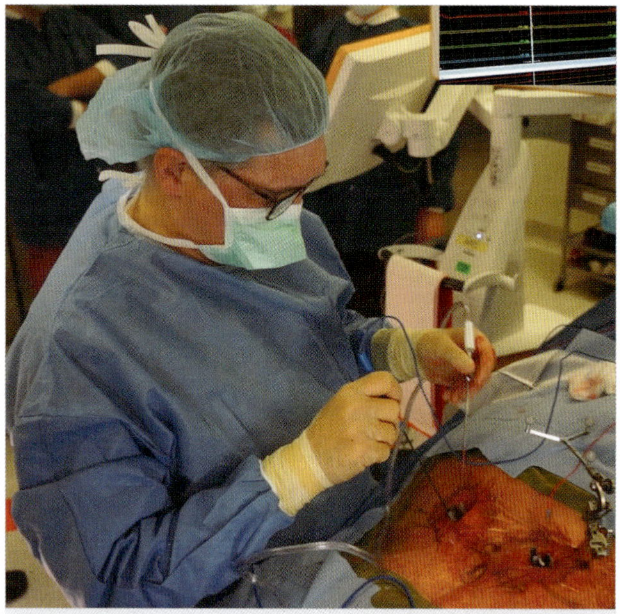

Fig. 42.3 Image showing that every screw after it is implanted is tested for any potential breach signals present on stimulation over 8 mAmps, which are considered concerning and may be revised depending on the surgeon's decision.

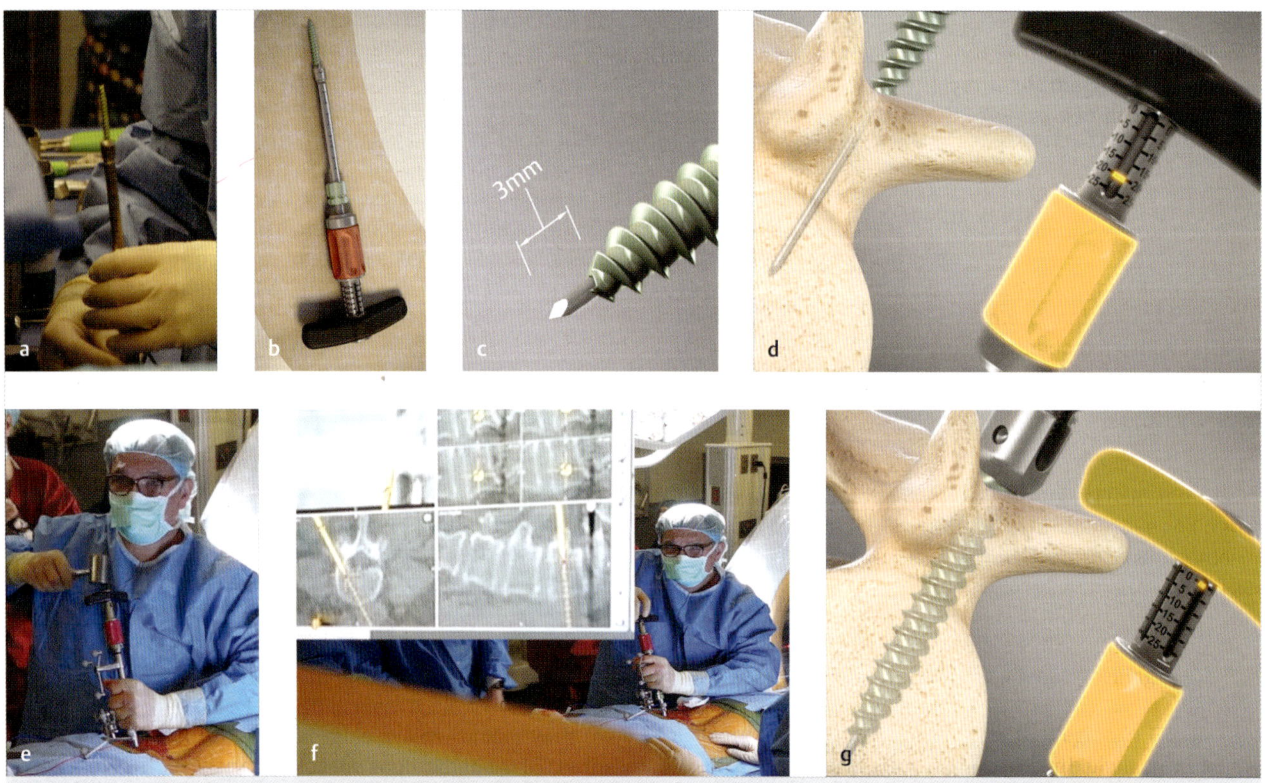

Fig. 42.4 (a–g) The new pedicle screws are equipped with reference arrays, and come with a safe small 3-mm K-wire that allows the screw to attach to the bone, preventing shifting and making its insertion safe (▶ Video 42.1).

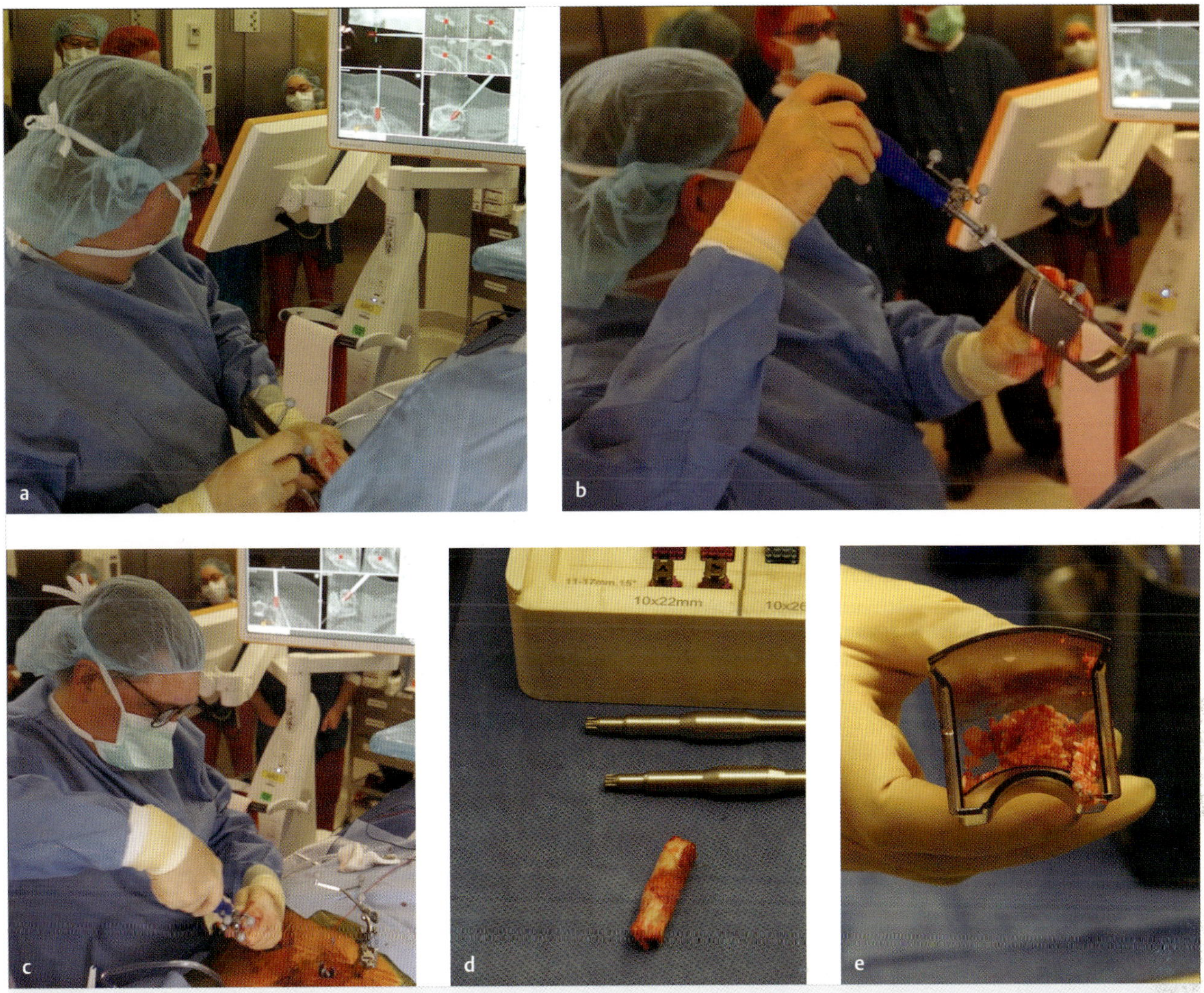

Fig. 42.5 (a–e) Bone harvesting obtained from the iliac crest on the contralateral side of the reference array; a 4-cm column of bone is obtained and the bone graft is later morselized using a bone mill (▶ Video 42.1).

(▶ Fig. 42.7a–c). A series of trials are used to open disc space enough to be able to insert a collapsed expandable cage (▶ Fig. 42.7a). Although identification of the disc space is easy in most of the cases, it could be difficult when the disc space is collapsed. Here the navigation is helpful to identify with precision the intervertebral disc space before the shavers are inserted. We believe this prevents end plate violations on those more severely degenerated cases.

h) The disc space is filled with the graft material (bone chips, bone enhancers, autologous bone graft). We normally use the collected local bone from the resected facet joint and expand by using autologous bone graft harvested from the iliac crest under the guidance of navigation (▶ Fig. 42.5). Other alternatives are the use morselized bone chips mixed with synthetic bone graft materials (Actifuse®, Apatech, Hertfordshire, UK; DBX®, Synthes Spine, Westchester, PA) followed by the cage containing graft materials. We use expandable titanium cages. The size and orientation of the cage are determined by navigation. Once the cage is in place, we back fill the hollow expandable cage with Actifuse mixed with bone from the facet joint.

i) A final intraoperative CT scan is performed to confirm adequate positioning of the cage and screws, leaving the navigation reference in place in case we need to do further adjustment of the instruments or decompression (▶ Fig. 42.8 and ▶ Fig. 42.9). At this point, we can use the navigation system to predict the appropriate length of the rod using a pointer on the screen (▶ Fig. 42.10). After this, the rods are inserted and fixed in place.

j) The wound is generously irrigated and washed after meticulous hemostasis is performed. Local anesthesia is used to infiltrate the muscle after removal of the tubular retractor. The fascia and the subcutaneous tissue are closed with absorbable sutures and the skin is properly approximated.

42.6 Postoperative Care

a) Foley catheter should be removed as soon as possible.
b) The patient is allowed to walk few steps the same night with the aid of a physiotherapist.
c) If a dural tear was identified during surgery, the patient will remain flat in bed for 24 hours.

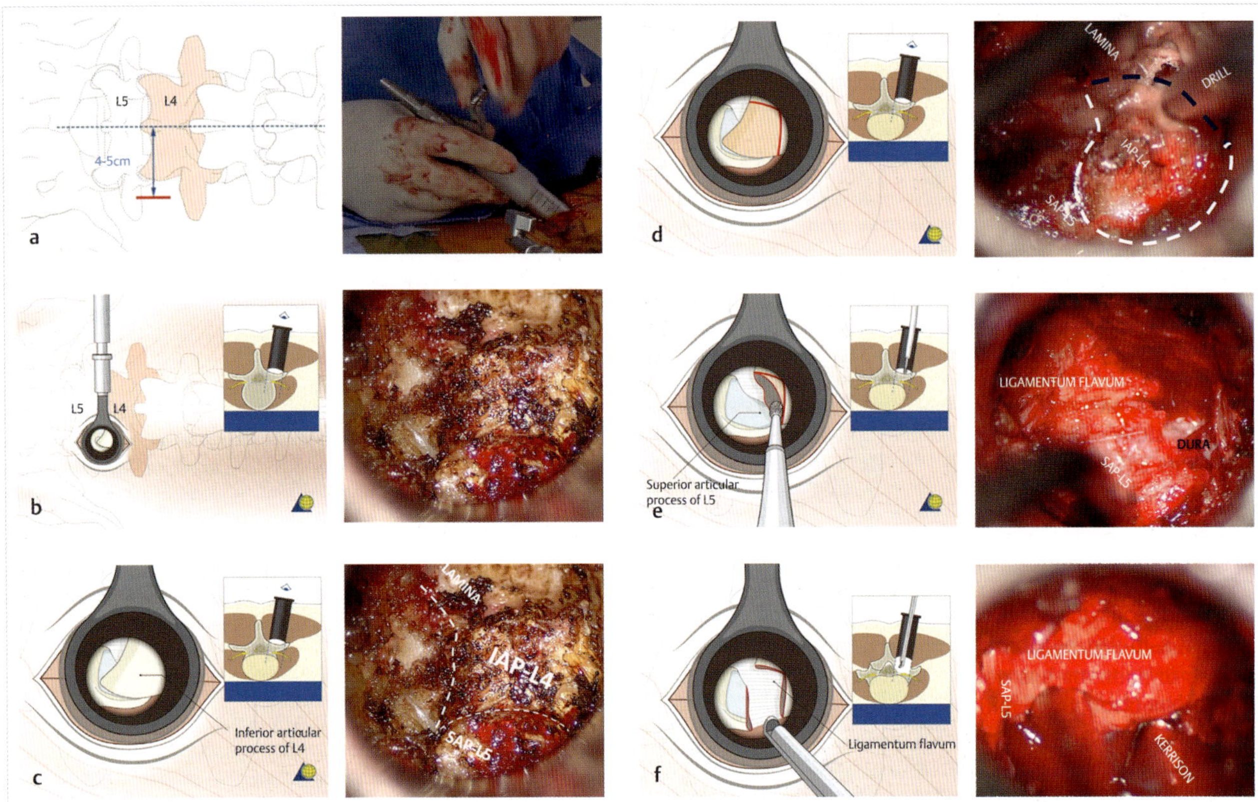

Fig. 42.6 **(a)** Incision is planned 4 to 5 cm from midline. **(b)** The tube is inserted and wanding of the soft tissue is performed. **(c)** The inferior facet of the indexed level is exposed using monopolar. **(d)** The inferior facet of the indexed level is then removed cutting it and detaching it from the lamina as a whole piece to be used later as graft. **(e)** The roof of the foramen is then drilled and the facetectomy is completed using the match stick drill tip. **(f)** Complete removal of the bone and exposure of the disc space and exiting nerve root are performed using a 2- to 3-mm Kerrison rongeur (▶ Video 42.1). (Copyright by AOSpine International, Switzerland.)

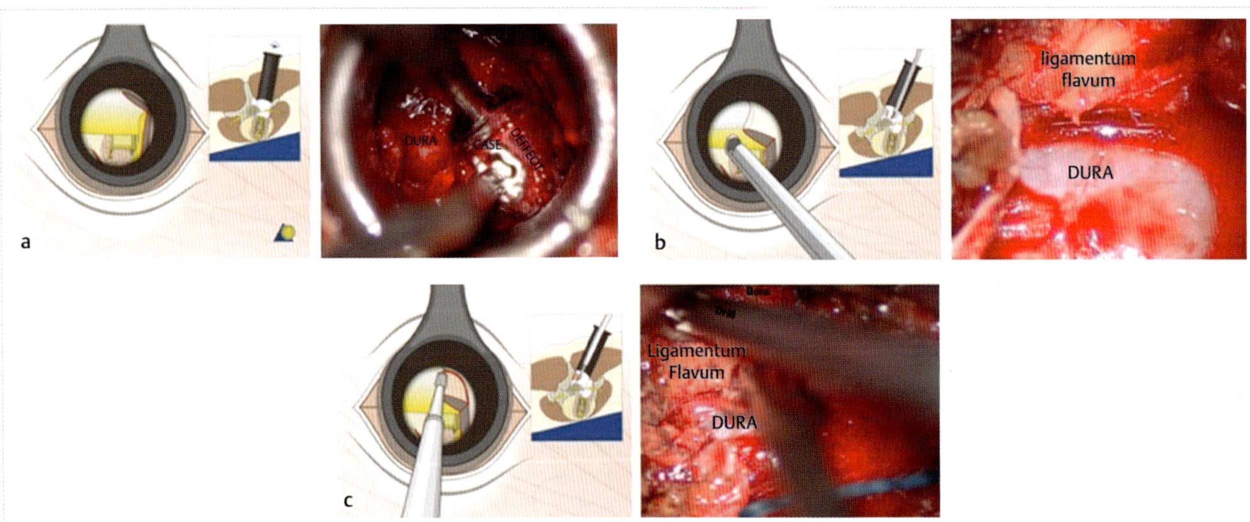

Fig. 42.7 Cage insertion and contralateral decompression: **(a)** The cage is inserted and then expanded once in position after pieces of bone graft are inserted into the well-prepared disc space. **(b)** The covering dura above the central canal is removed. **(c)** The contralateral lateral recess is decompressed using the undercutting technique, always over the remaining ligamentum flavum to prevent dural lacerations. (Copyright by AOSpine International, Switzerland.)

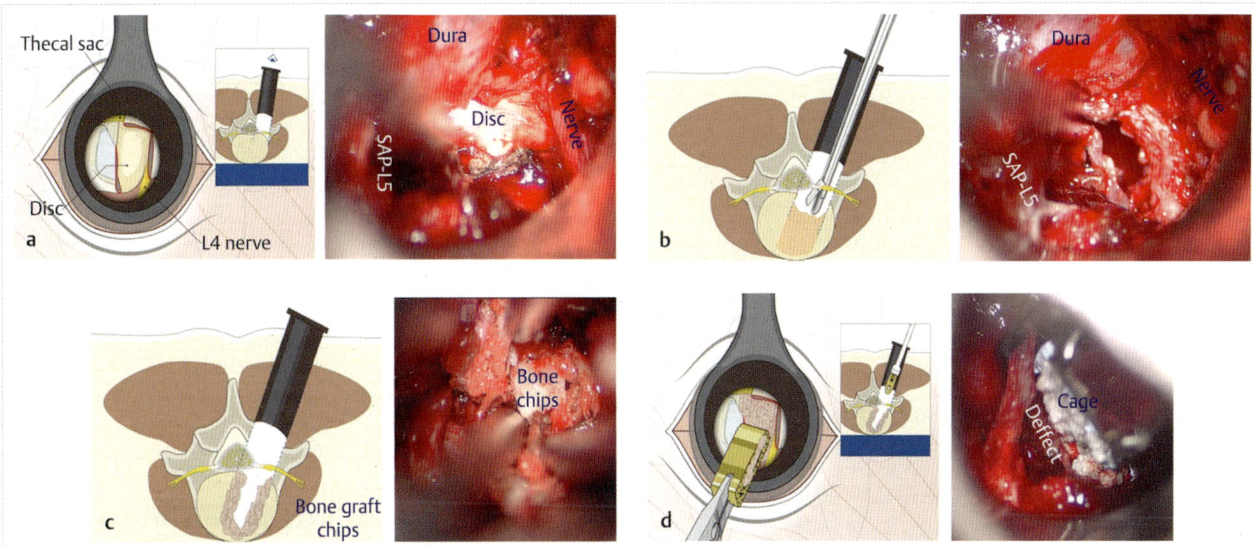

Fig. 42.8 **(a)** After the key anatomical structures (disc, nerve) are clearly identified **(b)** the disc is removed and the endplates prepared in standard fashion. **(c)** The disc defect is filled out with morselized bone graft and **(d)** the expandable cage is inserted. (Copyright by AOSpine International, Switzerland.)

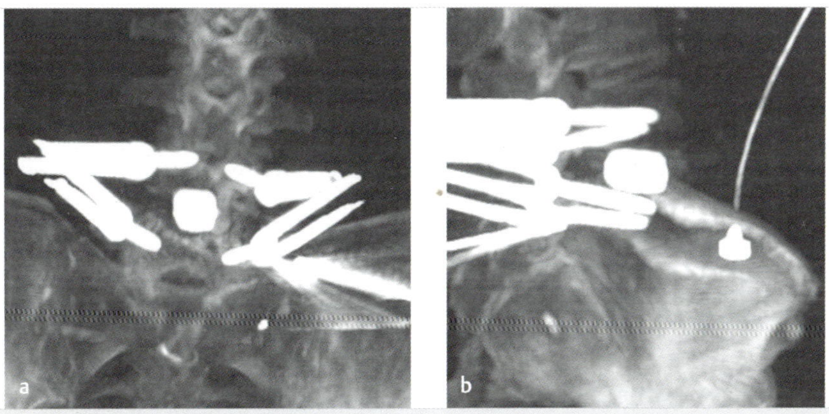

Fig. 42.9 **(a, b)** Intraoperative images of the 3D iCT reconstruction are shown.

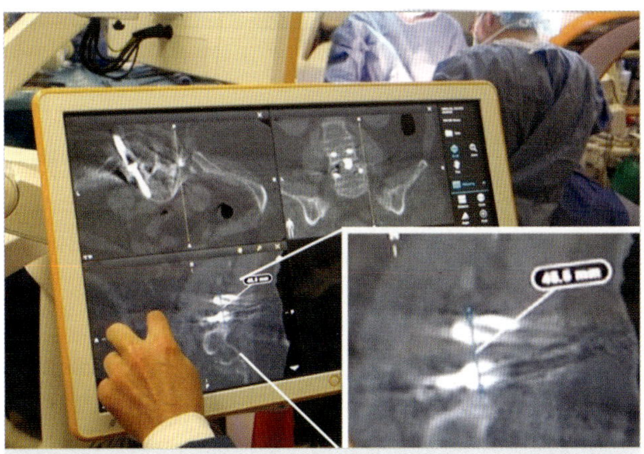

Fig. 42.10 Use of the navigation system to predict the appropriate length of the rod by using a pointer on the screen.

d) No additional immobilization or brace is required.
e) Standing AP and lateral X-rays are ordered the next day after surgery.
f) The patient is discharged normally within the first 24 hours of hospital stay and scheduled for follow-up appointment at 2 weeks post-op and at any given time if symptomatic.
g) We recommend muscle relaxants for the first week after surgery to decrease muscle spasms.
h) At 2 weeks, the patients are allowed to walk, do elliptical, recumbent stationary bike, or swimming.
i) Physical therapy with specific goals; strength, core training at 6 weeks postoperative.
j) The patient is advised to avoid carrying anything heavier than 8 to 10 pounds and to avoid high impact exercise for 3 months after surgery.
k) Routine clinical assessment (Oswestry Disability Index [ODI] and visual pain analog scale [VAS]) should be performed at every follow-up appointment.

l) Optional CT/MRI after surgery is performed only if pseudoarthrosis, failure, or any specific complication is suspected.

42.7 Complications and Avoidance

a) Poor bone quality should be treated 2 to 4 months before surgery, especially in the elderly.
b) Perform meticulous hemostasis using bipolar, thrombin-soaked gel foam or any other hemostatis agent. Symptomatic epidural hematoma is rare (1.4%) but possible.
c) Avoid retraction of the neural structures to decrease the chances of nerve injury.
d) Pseudoarthrosis and implant failure:
   1. Use of bone morphogenetic proteins (BMP) for MIS-TLIF is still "off-label" and the side effects including bone growth or nerve inflammation must be explained to the patient.
   2. Complete intervertebral disc removal and careful end plate preparation are critical to achieve high-quality interbody fusion and to prevent subsidence.
e) Cerebrospinal fluid (CSF) leaks:
   1. If a CSF leak is identified during surgery, this can be addressed intraoperatively using a Scanlan set as we previously described (▸ Video 13.1, pp. 114).[7]

42.8 Conclusion

MIS-TLIF with "total navigation" and expandable interbody cages improves the workflow of the conventional TLIF procedure; the tailored access to the spine is translated into smaller but more effective surgical corridors. iCT-CAS benefits are well documented in the literature, but there is an individual learning curve for each surgeon. In this regard, it is also helpful to identify the anatomy and master the surgical technique. MIS-TLIF using total navigation iCT is feasible, safe, and the steps have been displayed in this chapter.

References

[1] Hari A, Krishna M, Rajagandhi S, Rajakumar DV. Minimally invasive transforaminal lumbar interbody fusion-indications and clinical experience. Neurol India. 2016; 64(3):444–454

[2] Harms J RH. Die operative Behandlung der Spondylolisthese durch dorsale Aufrichtung und ventrale Verblockung. 2008

[3] Wiltse LL, Bateman JG, Hutchinson RH, Nelson WE. The paraspinal sacrospinalis-splitting approach to the lumbar spine. J Bone Joint Surg Am. 1968; 50 (5):919–926

[4] Holly LT, Schwender JD, Rouben DP, Foley KT. Minimally invasive transforaminal lumbar interbody fusion: indications, technique, and complications. Neurosurg Focus. 2006; 20(3):E6

[5] Khan NR, Clark AJ, Lee SL, Venable GT, Rossi NB, Foley KT. Surgical outcomes for minimally invasive vs open transforaminal lumbar interbody fusion: an updated systematic review and meta-analysis. Neurosurgery. 2015; 77 (6):847–874, discussion 874

[6] Schwender JD, Holly LT, Rouben DP, Foley KT. Minimally invasive transforaminal lumbar interbody fusion (TLIF): technical feasibility and initial results. J Spinal Disord Tech. 2005; 18 Suppl:S1–S6

[7] Boukebir MA, Berlin CD, Navarro-Ramirez R, et al.. Ten-step minimally invasive spine lumbar decompression and dural repair through tubular retractors. Oper Neurosurg (Hagerstown). 2017; 13(2):232–245

[8] Parker SL, Adogwa O, Bydon A, Cheng J, McGirt MJ. Cost-effectiveness of minimally invasive versus open transforaminal lumbar interbody fusion for degenerative spondylolisthesis associated low-back and leg pain over two years. World Neurosurg. 2012; 78(1–2):178–184

[9] Singh K, Nandyala SV, Marquez-Lara A, et al. A perioperative cost analysis comparing single-level minimally invasive and open transforaminal lumbar interbody fusion. Spine J. 2014; 14(8):1694–1701

[10] Lian X,, Navarro-Ramirez R, Berlin C, et al. Total 3D Airo® navigation for minimally invasive transforaminal lumbar interbody fusion. Biomed Res Int. 2016; 2016:5027340

[11] Navarro-Ramirez R, Lang G, Lian X, et al. Total navigation in spine surgery; a concise guide to eliminate fluoroscopy using a portable intraoperative computed tomography 3-dimensional navigation system. World Neurosurg. 2017; 100:325–335

43 MIS-TLIF Comparison: Four Surgeons and Regions

Seang-Beng Tan, Kevin Foley, Nestor Taboada, and Guiseppe Barbagallo

43.1 How I Do It

Summary

The goal of this chapter is to summarize in a concise fashion the variability among different leading surgeons around the globe performing a MIS-TLIF for a low grade L4–L5 spondylolisthesis case.

Here, we highlight the MIS-TLIF technique by dividing it into various "steps": Incision planning, screw insertion, facetectomy, disc/cage insertion, and rod placement/closure. To date, there is no consensus about the order of these steps, but we know that certain order is preferred by some authors, and we would like to offer the readers some more options to create a successful technique on their own.

Authors from different geographical areas around the globe sent in their case descriptions in the following format:

- General description of the patient.
- Incision planning: Some authors use navigation (see Chapter 39), while others use X-ray to identify the pedicles. If a single level is treated, separate incisions (4) or connecting incisions, pedicle to pedicle, can be made (2).
- Screw insertion: Can vary from single step, K-wire, navigated insertion.
- Facetectomy: This can be performed with osteotomes or with the aid of a high-speed drill bit.
- Disc/cage: Some authors use banana cages and bullet cages for sagittal balance and coronal balance improvement. Also, graft before the cage or graft inside and after the cage, fibrillar hemostatics around the cage or expandable cages are used (see Chapter 39).
- Rod placement and closure: Although there is not much variability in this step, it is worth noticing that some authors perform unilateral or bilateral facetectomies and place one rod before the other to achieve better compression or distraction, depending upon the case and step of the procedure.

Keywords: transforaminal fusion, interbody fusion, lumbar fusion, expandable cage

Region: Asia

Dr. Seang-Beng Tan

Step 1: Representative case, initial setup, and incision planning

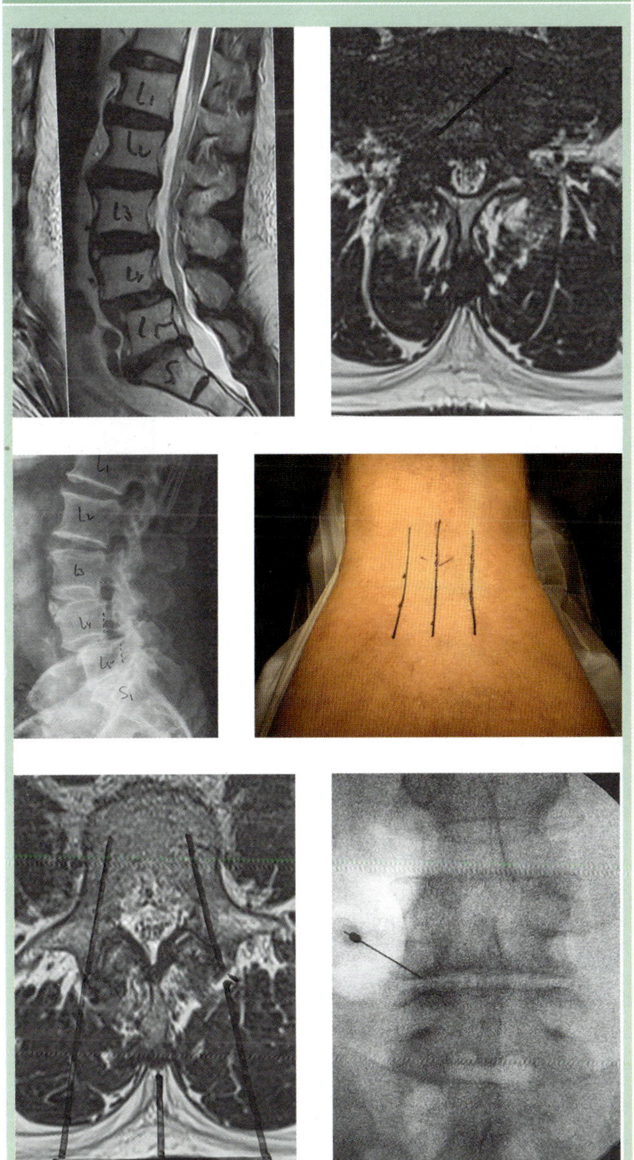

- A vertical line is drawn over the spinous processes. Then two subsequent lines parallel to the first are drawn, typically 3.5 to 4 cm, on either side of the initial line.
- The actual distance of the two lines from the midline depends upon the size of the patient and can be measured from the preoperative magnetic resonance imaging (MRI) or computed tomography (CT).
- A spinal needle is then placed on the ipsilateral side of the intended facetectomy, starting from the outer line and angled toward the facet joint. An anteroposterior (AP) fluoro-shot is taken.
- An incision, approximately 3 cm long, centered over the spinal needle is made and it is deepened down to the fascia.

Region: North America

Dr. Kevin Foley

Step 1: Representative case, initial setup, and incision planning

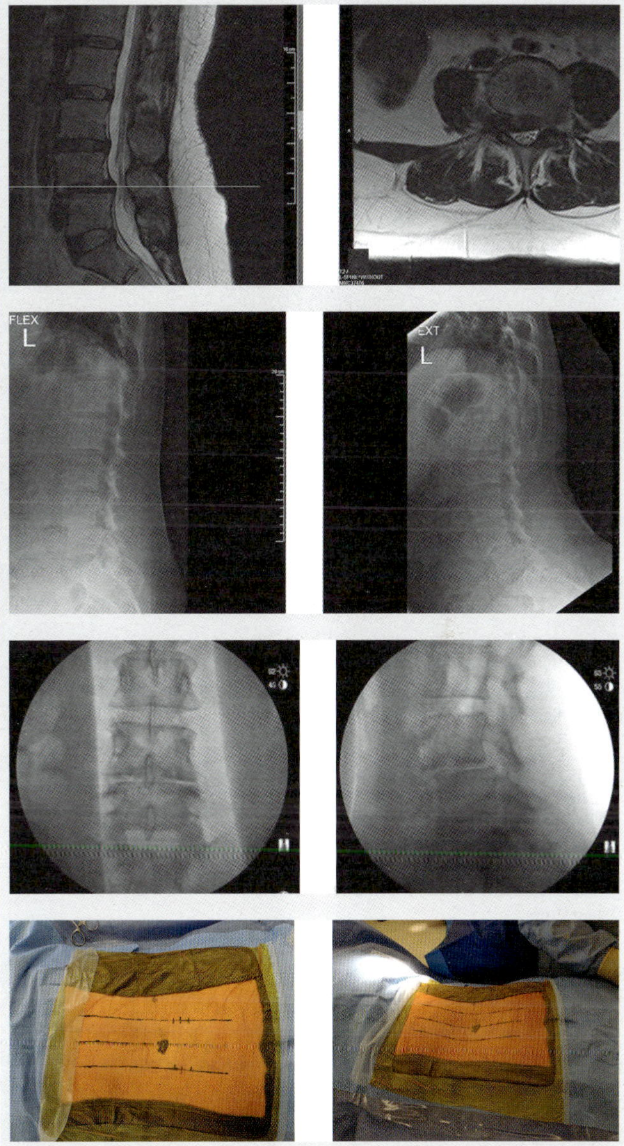

- MRI and X rays of the representative case.
- Patients are placed in the prone position on a flat-top Jackson table with gel chest rolls.
- The C-arm fluoroscope is then brought into AP position to capture the appropriate fluoroscopic image, which produces a "true AP" view of each vertebral body.
- A lateral fluoroscopic image is also taken, and the C-arm coordinates recorded for a "true lateral" image for each level.
- A lateral fluoroscopic image is also taken, and the C-arm coordinates recorded for a "true lateral" image for each level.
- In obese patients in whom the spinous processes cannot be easily palpated, the midline can be confirmed with an AP fluoroscopic image. Using lateral fluoroscopy, a 22-gauge spinal needle is inserted through one of the paramedian lines to localize the incision; the needle should be directed slightly medially, approximately 20 to 30 degrees.

Region: Latin America

Dr. Nestor Taboada

Step 1: Representative case, initial setup, and incision planning

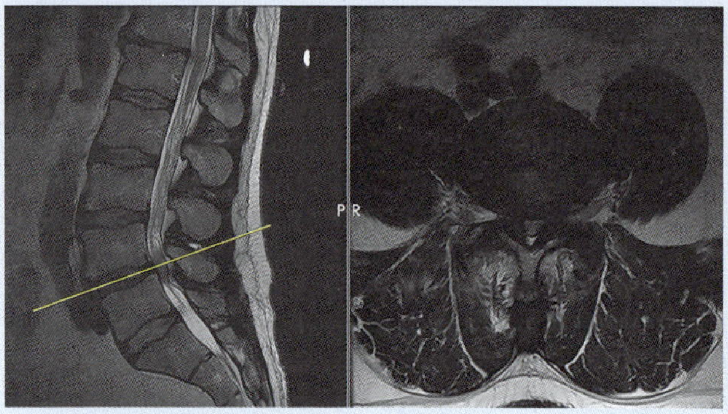

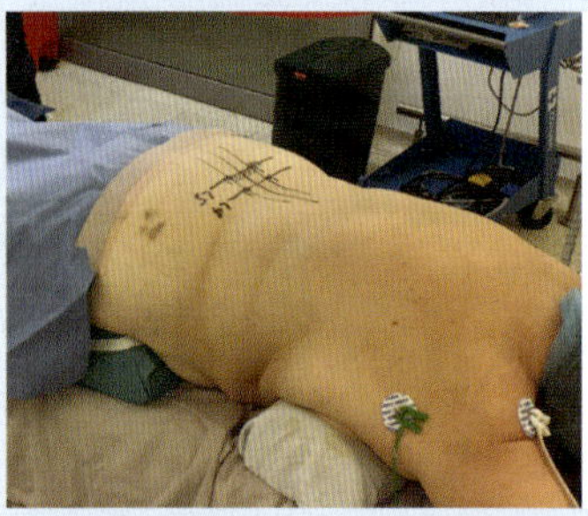

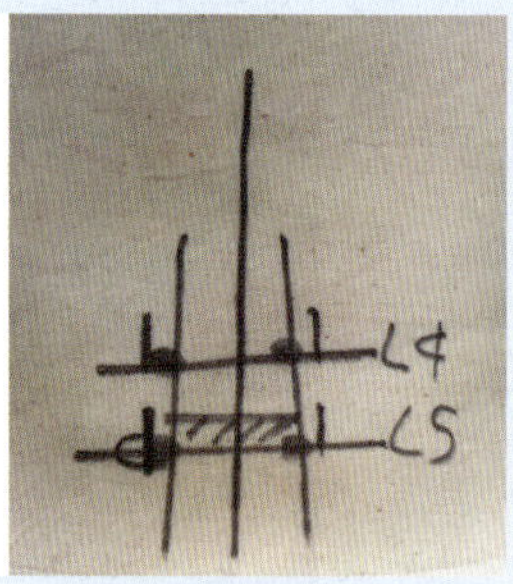

- With the image intensifier, the midline is marked on the skin as both L4L5 pedicles, the disc space, and the tip of L5 transverse process on the side where the cage will be inserted.
- To properly visualize the pedicles, the end plates must not be superimposed, and the spinous process must be centered. In some cases, it is necessary to rotate the table slightly until these parameters are achieved. It is always preferable to keep the C-arm at "zero or neutral" so that the surgeon does not lose the "feeling" during the placement of the screws and the cage.
- The initial AP views (two on average) allow the identification and marking of L4L5 pedicles, spinous process, and end plate. If the patient has a rotational deformity which requires the table to be moved, the views can increase (double).
- About 1-cm lateral to the mark of the pedicles, which corresponds on average to 3 to 4 cm off the midline, skin is infiltrated with 2 mL of xylocaine with epinephrine at the three points of introduction of screws and 5 mL of xylocaine with epinephrine at the site where decompression will be performed and the cage will be inserted. The skin incision at L5 level, where the cage will be introduced and decompression will happen, is approximately 2 cm long.
- The scalpel incisions of the skin and then fascia allow adequate introduction of dilators and retractor. Using the previously placed K-wire and cannula in the L5 pedicle, the dilators are introduced, turning them constantly in a clockwise direction, to separate as much muscle as possible, supported on the pedicle and the facet complex.

Region: Europe

Dr. Guiseppe Barbagallo

Step 1: Representative case, initial setup, and incision planning

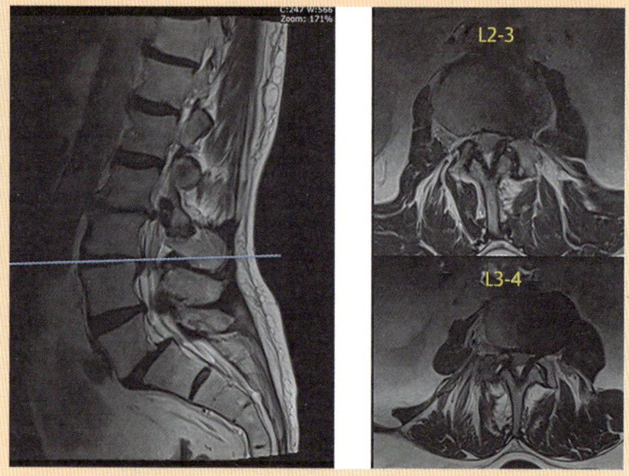

- We start the fluoroscopy-guided surgical procedure on the contralateral side.
- Under AP fluoroscopic control, a K-wire or a knife is placed in line with the outer border of the ipsilateral pedicles, about 2 cm laterally, to mark the skin incision and entry point.

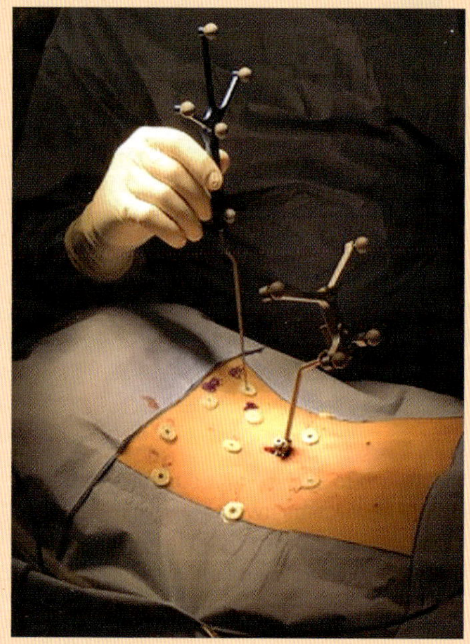

- Percutaneous instruments and screws will follow a lateral to medial trajectory. Such technique allows achieving better triangulation of the screws, with their tips aiming toward the vertebral body midline, thus increasing the biomechanical efficiency of the implant.
- In cases of navigation-guided surgery, percutaneous screw trajectory is checked by navigating the projection of passive navigation probe, and skin incisions are marked accordingly.
- We prefer to use small multiple skin incisions to insert the percutaneous screws; however, a single, longer skin incision can also be used. Skin and prevertebral fascia are separately incised and, in cases of copious bleeding from soft tissues, hemostasis is obtained with bipolar forceps.

Region: Asia

Dr. Seang-Beng Tan

Step 2: Facetectomy

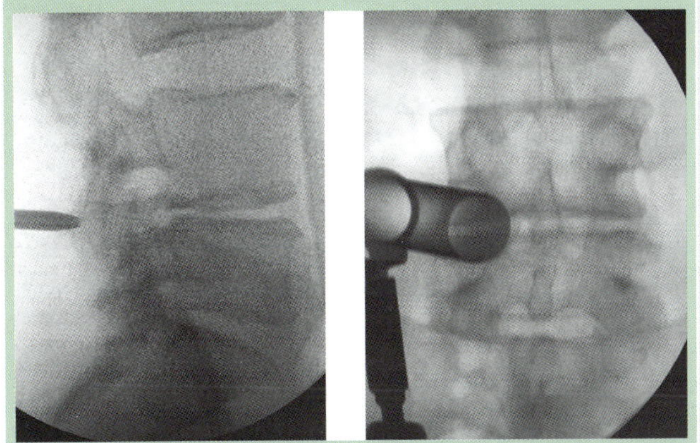

- With the muscles split using the hemostat, a blunt trochar is then placed directly over the facet joint.
- While wanding the trochar, it is also used as a feeler to confirm that the outer edge of the facet joint is palpable.
- Finally, a 20 mm tube is placed over the dilator and locked into position.
- The operating table is now tilted 20 to 30 degrees away from the surgeon.
- A right-angled osteotome is then used to osteotomize the lateral facet.

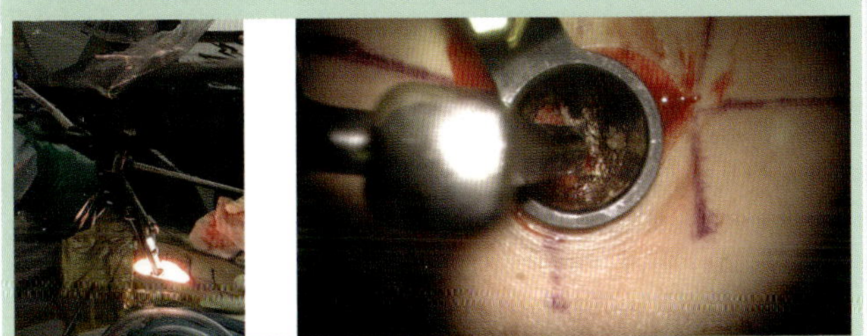

- The starting point of the osteotomy should be in the middle of the tube, assuming that the tube had been previously centered over the disc space. The lateral facet is then removed using large pituitary rongeurs and used for bone graft.

Region: North America

Dr. Kevin Foley

Step 2: Screw placement

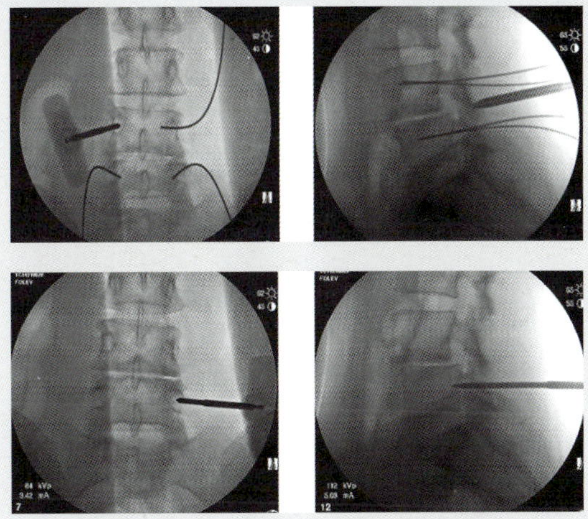

- Under fluoroscopic guidance, pedicle access needles are used to cannulate and safely traverse the pedicles. Although this step may be done using AP views alone, we prefer to use lateral views as well.
- A true AP fluoroscopic image is obtained to confirm the medial-lateral coordinate for the entry point (the needle tip is adjusted as necessary to achieve this).
- For a left pedicle, the ideal entry point is at the 9 o'clock position, whereas for a right pedicle the ideal entry is at the 3 o'clock position. Once the entry point is confirmed on AP, the needle is directed 20 to 30 degrees medially and malleted to penetrate the bony cortex and advanced into the pedicle to just proximal to the vertical midline of the pedicle.
- Once the access needle is in proper position, the inner trochar is removed and a K-wire is inserted through the needle and into the vertebral body. The access needle is then removed, making sure the K-wire remains in place. The proximal end of the K-wire is then attached to the drape using a hemostat. The same sequence is then repeated for the remaining pedicles.

Region: Latin America

Dr. Nestor Taboada

Step 2: Screw placement

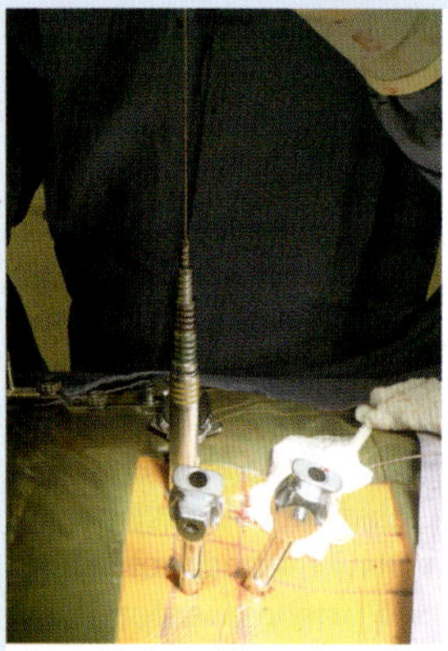

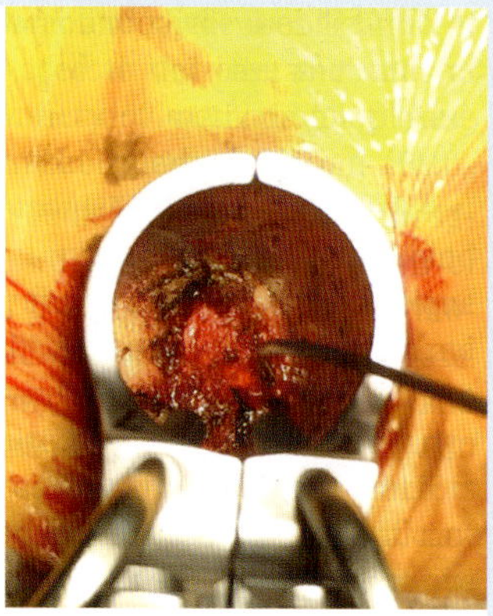

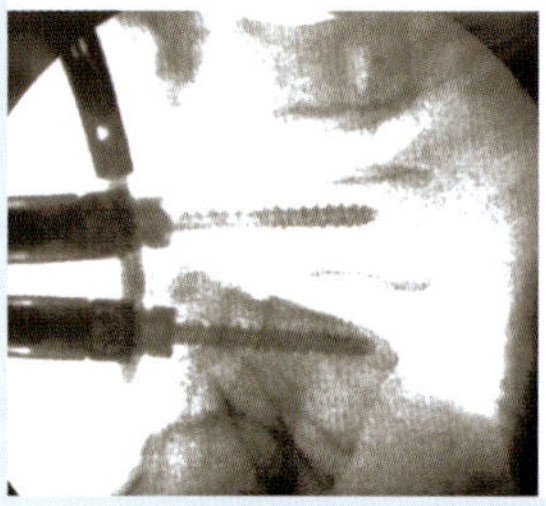

- In our service, the four pedicles are cannulated with Jamshidi needles, through which the K-wires are introduced.
- On the contralateral side of where the TLIF is to be made, the two cannulated screws with their respective work sleeves are placed.
- On the TLIF (facetectomy) side, the K-wire of L4 is fixed to the operative field and the dilators are inserted through the K-wire of L5. Finally, the retractor is positioned to perform the decompression and placement of the cage. During the introduction of the Jamshidi needles, the surgeon and his assistant position two needles at the time, first L4 bilaterally and when the midpoint of the pedicle is reached, it is confirmed with a lateral view to determine that needles are already in the vertebral body and continue the introduction of the needle avoiding violating medial or lateral wall. The same process is done at the same time in L5 and in this way the number of views is decreased. Once the pedicles are cannulated, decompression is performed (next step).

Region: Europe

Dr. Guiseppe Barbagallo

Step 2: Screw placement

- A Jamshidi needle, followed by a K-wire, is inserted into the pedicle according to the standard technique; cannulated screws are then inserted over K-wires under navigation or fluoroscopic guidance.

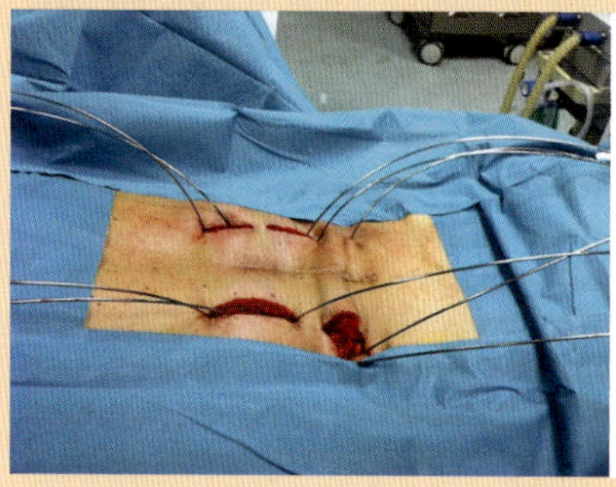

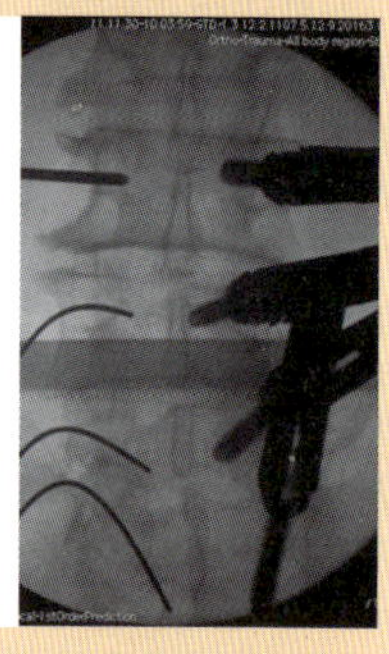

- K-wires must always be meticulously checked during screw insertion, particularly in osteoporotic patients, because impingement of the screw's tip on the K-wire can push the wire anteriorly and cause breakage of anterior vertebral wall.
- Fluoroscopic check during this step is advised. On the contralateral side (i.e., the side selected for facetectomy and TLIF), after identifying the pedicles as described above, a single skin incision linking together the pedicles above and below the index disc level for the m-open TLIF is performed.
- A Jamshidi needle is then inserted into the first pedicle, and through it a K-wire is passed and left in place.
- The wire is bent down and secured with a towel clip. The same technique is applied to the other pedicle before positioning a tubular retractor, either fixed or expandable, which is then secured to the table with a self-retaining articulated arm.

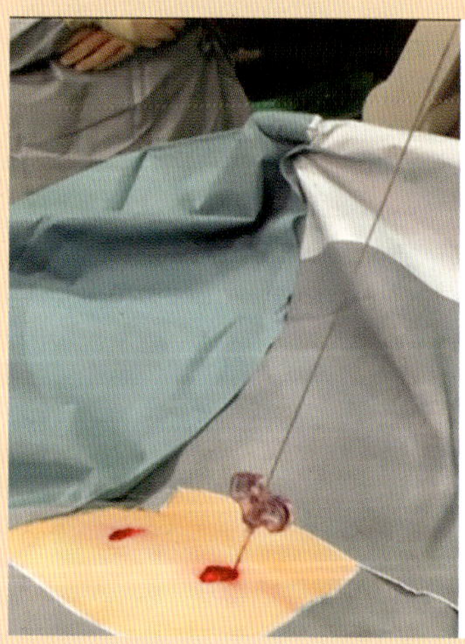

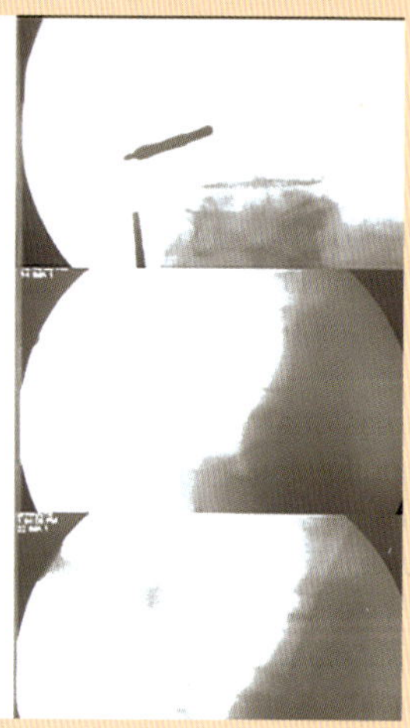

Region: Asia

Dr. Seang-Beng Tan

Step 3: Discectomy

- At this point in time, the facet capsule would have to be removed first.
- If the disc space cannot be entered, then the location is marked with a right-angled osteotome, and a lateral fluoro-shot is taken with the osteotome in position.

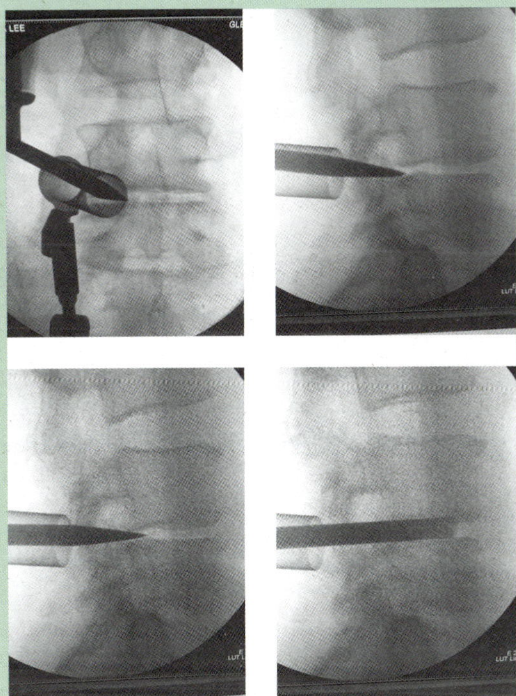

Region: North America

Dr. Kevin Foley

Step 3: Facetectomy

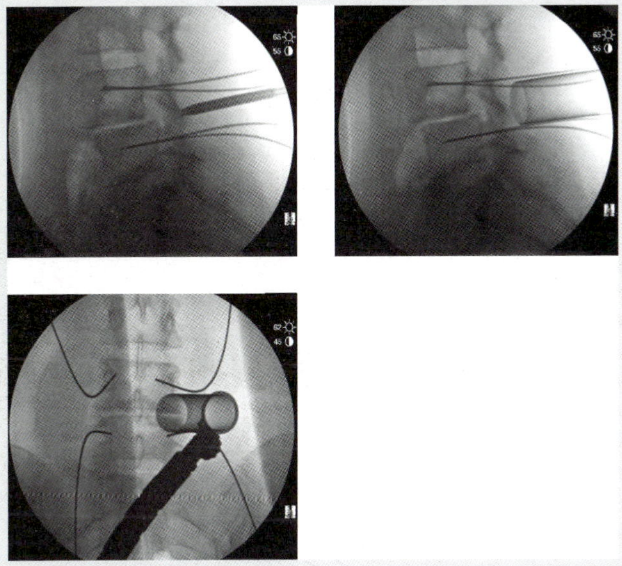

- After infiltrating local anesthetic into the subfascial musculature, a K-wire and sequential tubular dilators are inserted through one of the previously created 2.5-cm skin incisions. The side of placement of the tubular retractor is dictated by the side of the patient's leg pain.
- A 22-mm-diameter tubular retractor of appropriate length is inserted over the final dilator, after which the dilators are removed.

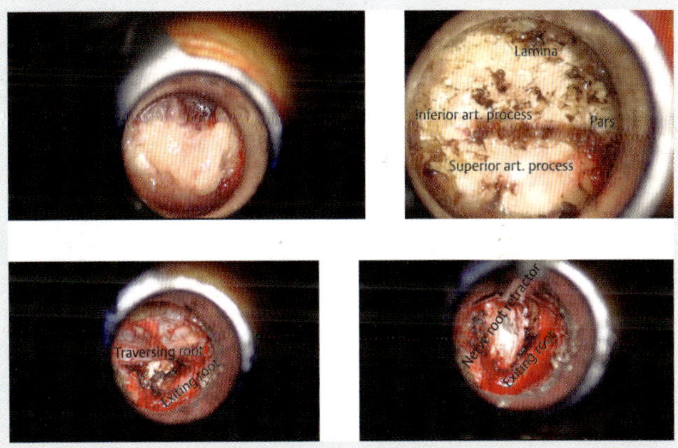

- For a typical unilateral decompression, we dock the tube over the facet complex. If we are planning a bilateral decompression, we dock the tube as far medially as possible, against the base of the spinous process (this facilitates performing an "over the top" approach to the contralateral portion of the decompression).
- The ideal position of the 22-mm tube under lateral fluoroscopy should be between the pedicles and pointing toward the disc space.
- Following soft-tissue removal, the facet joint line should be visible between the lamina and the inferior articular process medially, and the superior articular process laterally. If necessary, the 22-mm tube can be moved by inserting the largest dilator and "wanding" the tube in the appropriate direction to gain access to adjacent anatomy.
- The microscope is now utilized to proceed with the decompression within the 22-mm tube. Residual soft tissue overlying the bone at the base of the tubular retractor is removed with a combination of monopolar cautery and pituitary rongeurs.
- Short and long ball–hook probes can then be used to confirm that the nerve roots have been fully decompressed. An ideal TLIF exposure includes resection of enough of the facet complex to leave significant space lateral to the dural sac at the level of the disc space.

Region: Latin America

Dr. Nestor Taboada

Step 3: Facetectomy

- Once the facet complex is identified, it must be determined if only the external facet is to be resected to introduce the TLIF cage, or if it is necessary to also resect the internal facet to release the L5 root and/or over the top.

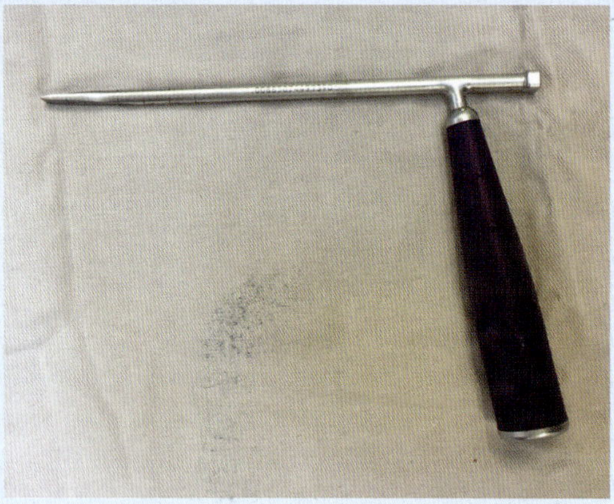

- It is recommended to use a 90-degree osteotome that does not obstruct the tubular vision. The first cut is directed vertical and intra-articular, reaching the base of the pedicle; the second cut is perpendicular to the first one at the base of the external facet, trying not to exceed in depth the union with the transverse process. Then with the same osteotome, the external facet is released.
- Using a high-speed drill with a small tip (3 mm), the remaining external facet and part of the internal facet are drilled, allowing a 1-cm square window. It is preferable to identify the disc by resecting the capsular ligament and identifying the fat surrounding the emerging root, in this case L4, and in this triangle, perform the discectomy.

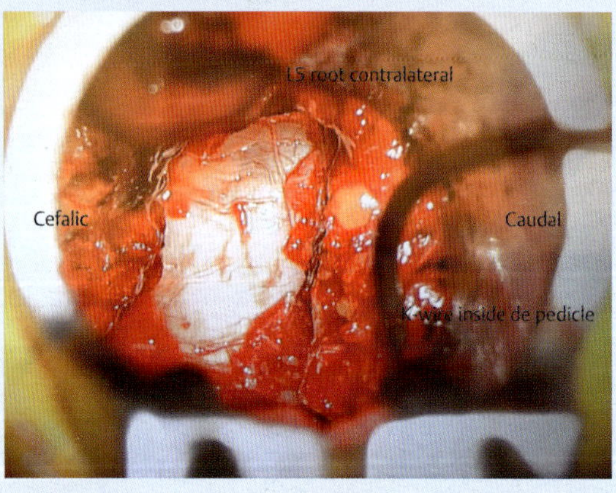

- In patients with severe spinal stenosis associated with listhesis, once the internal capsule is milled, the L5 root exposed, and the foramen is extended, the tube is tilted, visualizing the ipsilateral lamina that is completely drilled from superior to inferior, avoiding a tunnel decompression (the ligamentum flavum must be preserved).
- The base of the spinous process and the internal border of the contralateral lamina over ligamentum flavum are drilled until a dome is visualized which is the contralateral facet that must be drilled. At this point, if the ligamentum flavum has been resected, reject the dural sac rostral in order to visualize the contralateral L5 root. With angulated Kerrison, resect the roof of the contralateral L5 foramen; unlike what it seems it is more comfortable to resect the contralateral foramen roof of L5 root.
- Using the tip of the bayonet dissector positioned over the foramen, AP fluoroscopy is taken to verify that the contralateral foramen has been reached. This means we have completed our "over the top" approach.

Region: Europe

Dr. Guiseppe Barbagallo

Step 3: Facetectomy

- TLIF is usually performed on the side where worse radicular symptoms are reported or, in cases with bilateral symptoms, on the side where the compressive disease is more severe on imaging. In multilevel cases, when two adjacent TLIFs from the same side are planned, single skin and fascia incisions, including all the three pedicles and the two intervening disc spaces, are made; other pedicle screws can be inserted through additional, smaller skin incisions.
- When both the pedicles are identified and K-wires left inside each vertebral body, as described previously, a tubular retractor is positioned over the facet joint covering the index disc space. Under AP fluoroscopy, sequential dilating tubes are inserted to progressively and bluntly split the paraspinal muscles over the index facet joint. An expandable tubular retractor, held in place by an articulated-arm clamp, is then docked over it and secured to the table. The articulated-arm clamp must be oriented and fixed, avoiding superimposition of its projection over the disc space on fluoroscopic images. Its medial-lateral and cranial-caudal position is checked with AP fluoroscopy.
- The microscope is then brought in place.
- If required for further safety, particularly during the initial learning curve, after stripping the muscles off the facet joint, and slightly angulating the microscope, it is possible to see the K-wires entering the cranial and caudal pedicles on the inner surface of the tubular retractor's blades.
- A high-speed drill and/or Kerrison rongeur are used to perform the facetectomy. We use 5 or 6 mm spherical cutting burr to remove the external cortical bone of the facets and the cancellous bone. A diamond burr is used for the inner cortical surface, close to the neural structures. After removing the facet joint, the ipsilateral lamina, and the base of the spinous process (in cases requiring medial decompression), the ligamentum flavum is exposed and dissected off the dura; its resection is completed with Kerrison rongeurs. Small bony fragments can be harvested and used to fill the intervertebral cage(s).

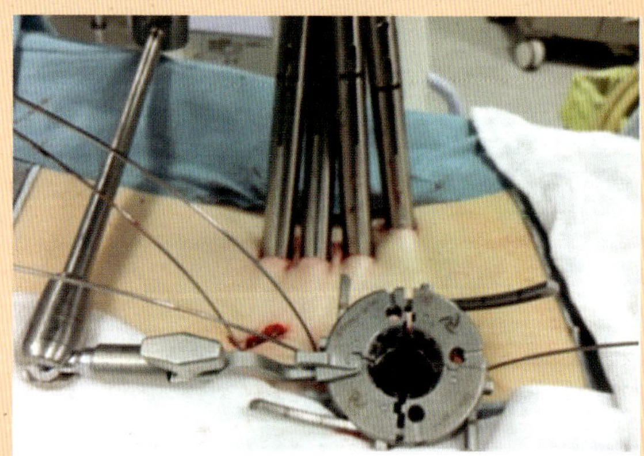

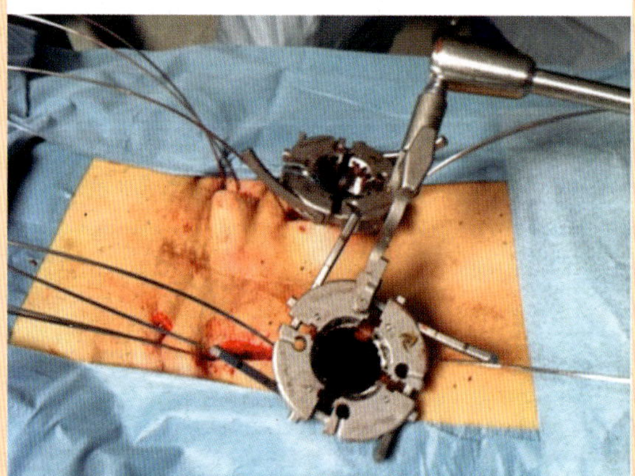

Region: Asia

Dr. Seang-Beng Tan

Step 4: Cage insertion

- Once the disc is exposed, an annulotomy is done with a scalpel.
- Having done so, the osteotome can be rotated 90 degrees, thereby distracting the disc space.
- The length of the cage in general is measured preoperatively on the MRI or CT, but the most commonly used length would be 23 or 27 mm.
- A funnel is inserted into the disc space and bone grafting is performed.

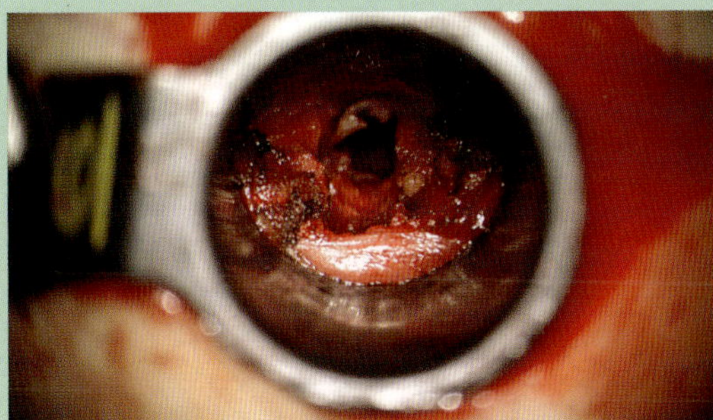

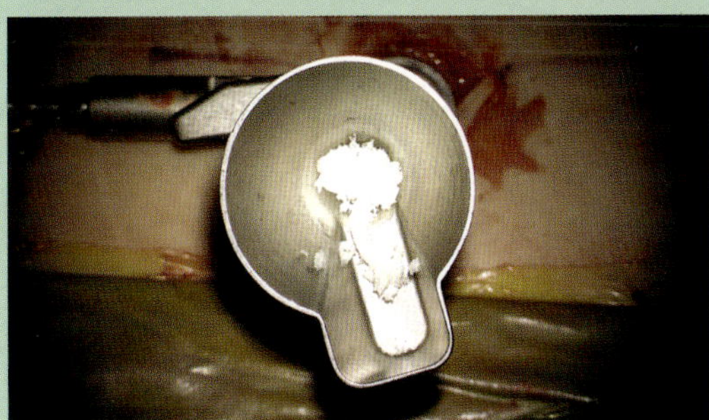

Region: North America

Dr. Kevin Foley

Step 4: Discectomy and cage insertion

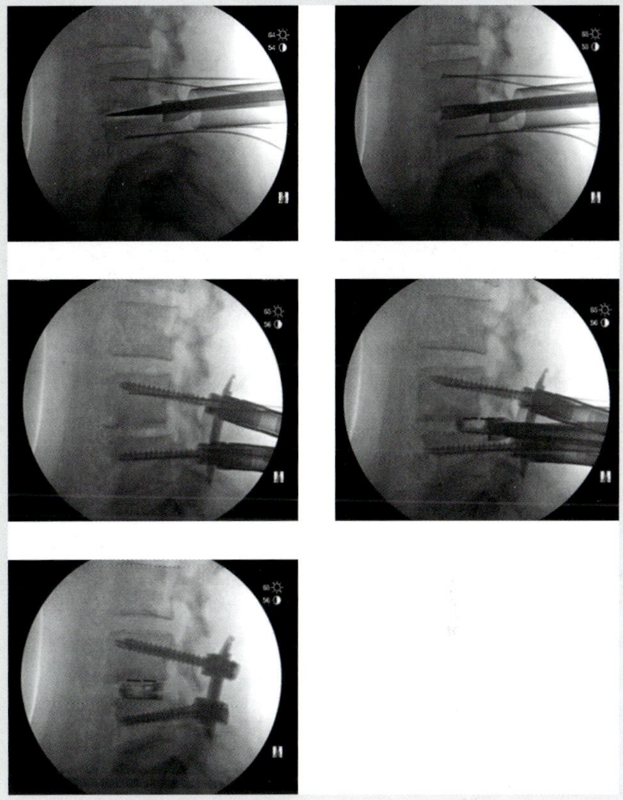

- The identification of the exiting and traversing nerve roots will yield the safe entry zone for discectomy.
- A bayoneted 15-blade is then used to perform a large annulotomy. Disc material can be retrieved with pituitary rongeurs.
- We start with a disc osteotome to begin the distraction process. Once adequate interbody height has been restored, we proceed with the next step (contralateral screw-rod fixation) to maintain the distraction.
- Trials are used to determine the proper dimensions of the chosen interbody fusion device.
- The harvested autograft bone dust is packed into the expandable device.
- The combined autograft and cancellous allograft bone is placed into the disc space and packed contralaterally and ipsilaterally, leaving a channel for placement of the interbody fusion device.
- The provisionally tightened set screw on the contralateral screw-rod construct is loosened so that the interbody implant can be expanded with minimal resistance. Following this expansion, the set screw is fully tightened.

Region: Latin America

Dr. Nestor Taboada

Step 4: Discectomy and cage insertion

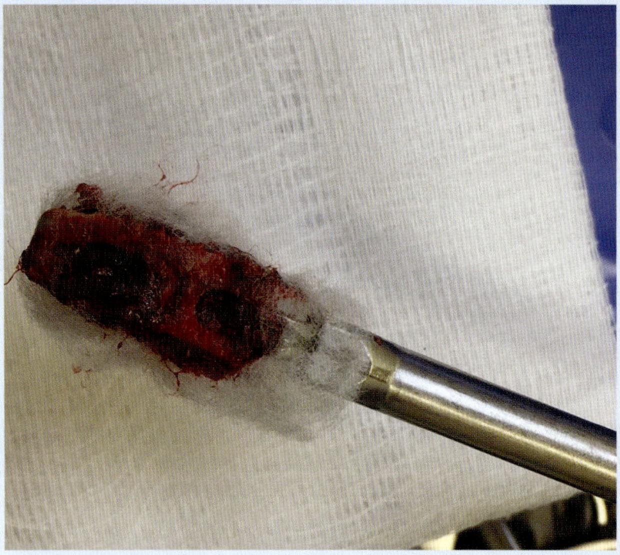

- First, we coagulate the vessels over the disc in the safety triangle using bipolar cautery (intensity of 8). With the scalpel, a box annulotomy of approximately 1 cm is performed, and with straight and 30-degree alligator forceps, the initial discectomy is performed.
- The interspace is filled with autologous bone taken from the remains of the facet complex and ipsilateral lamina combined with bone matrix and blood taken from the vertebral body at the time of cannulation with the Jamshidi needles.

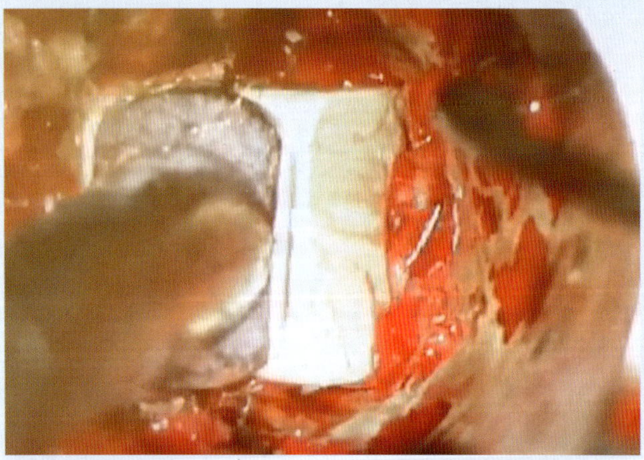

- Once the cage is inserted, medial facetectomy and "over the top" approach can be performed if necessary.
- Leaving the internal facet intact until the positioning of the cage avoids the contact of the implant with the L5 root and the dural sac, and thus possible tears or direct injuries of these structures can be avoided.
- Bullet-type cages are preferred as they are more comfortable to position in the TLIF; when you use banana-type cages.
- Once the cage is positioned, in a lateral view evaluate the depth of the cage and in an AP view evaluate that it is as medial as possible; in other words, the tantalum lines should be seen at the level of the spinous process.

Region: Europe

Dr. Guiseppe Barbagallo

Step 4: Discectomy and cage insertion

- After dissection of the epidural plexus, the dural sac is gently retracted.
- In this phase, it is important to maintain the visual control of the nerve root axilla and avoid excessive traction, which can cause a dural tear.
- The posterior longitudinal ligament and the annulus are incised to gain access to the disc space.
- Disc fragments are initially removed with punches; then spreaders and shavers of progressively increasing size are used to fragment the disc and remove the cartilaginous end plates.
- A proper end plate preparation is essential to enhance chances of fusion. After completing the discectomy, a cage trial is inserted and fluoroscopically checked. Banana-shaped cages are used to obtain a better restoration of segmental lordosis.
- Conversely, bullet cages are preferred in cases of coronal imbalance.
- During disc preparation and cage insertion, if necessary, the contralateral screws and rod can be used to apply some intervertebral distraction and facilitate both the access to and the maneuvers within the disc space as well as cage insertion.

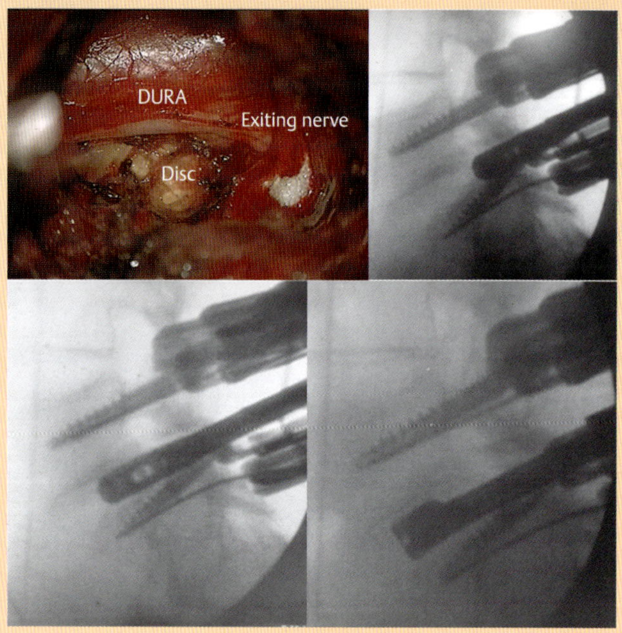

Region: Asia

Dr. Seang-Beng Tan

Step 5: Screw + rod placement

- Bilateral K-wires are inserted inside the pedicles using the percutaneous fluoroscopy technique (AP/LAT or Bullseye) (*top images* a and b). Cannulated screws are inserted over the K-wires (*lower image* a).

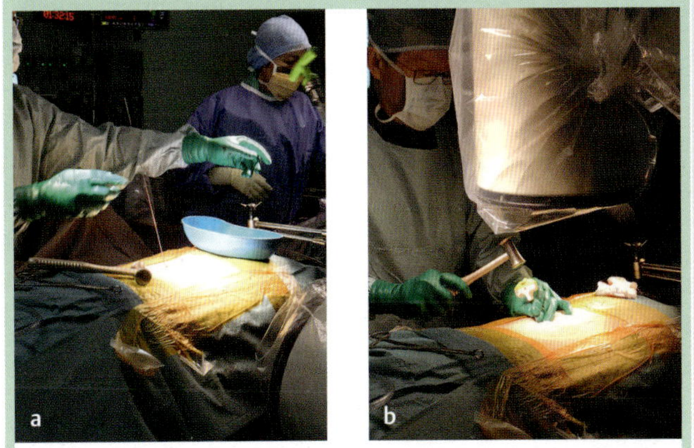

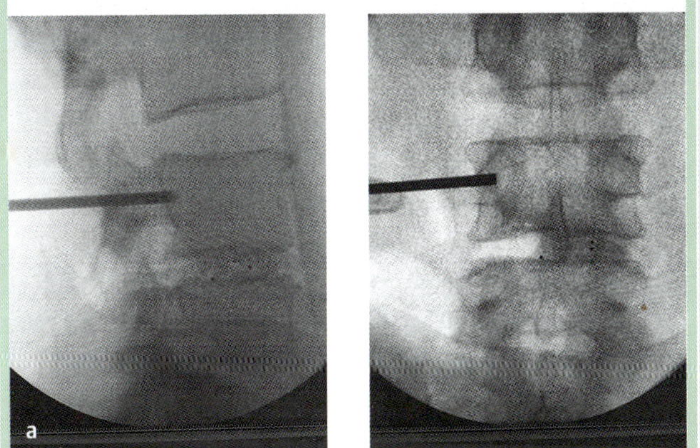

- For multiple-level fixation, intraoperative cone CT imaging with computer navigation–assisted pedicle screws, or preoperative CT imaging with intraoperative robot-assisted pedicle screws may be helpful in reducing radiation exposure to the surgical team.
- The rod length is predicted with the aid of special tools from the set.
- The rod is guided down and secured in place with two caps, leaving them loose enough to hold the rod but allowing rod sliding to allow compression.
- Compression of the screws is done especially when banana cages are used in order to create segmental lordosis and to favor graft compression.

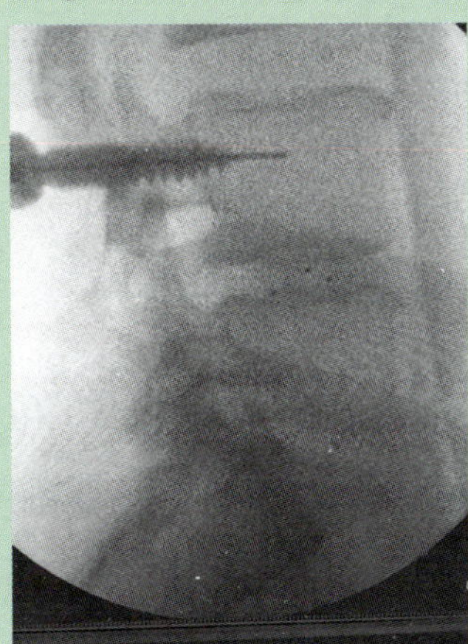

Region: North America

Dr. Kevin Foley

Step 5: Rod placement and closure

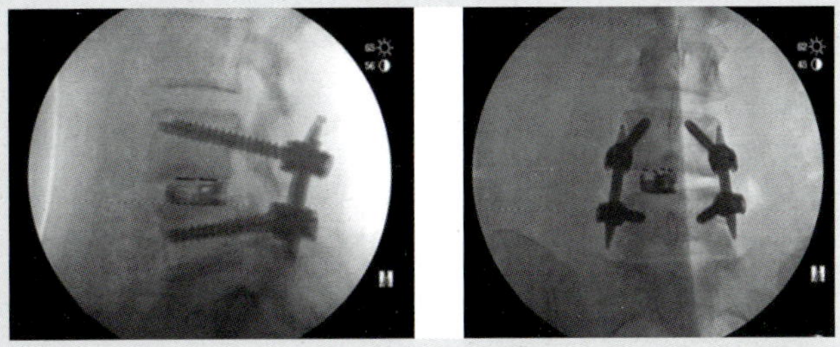

- The tubular retractor is removed after hemostasis has been confirmed; bipolar cautery and thrombin-soaked absorbable gelatin sponge are used as necessary. Following this, the microscope can be taken out of the field.
- An ipsilateral, percutaneous pedicle screw-rod construct is then placed and the K-wires are removed.
- Final lateral and AP fluoroscopic images are obtained to confirm proper hardware placement, and the C-arm is removed from the field.

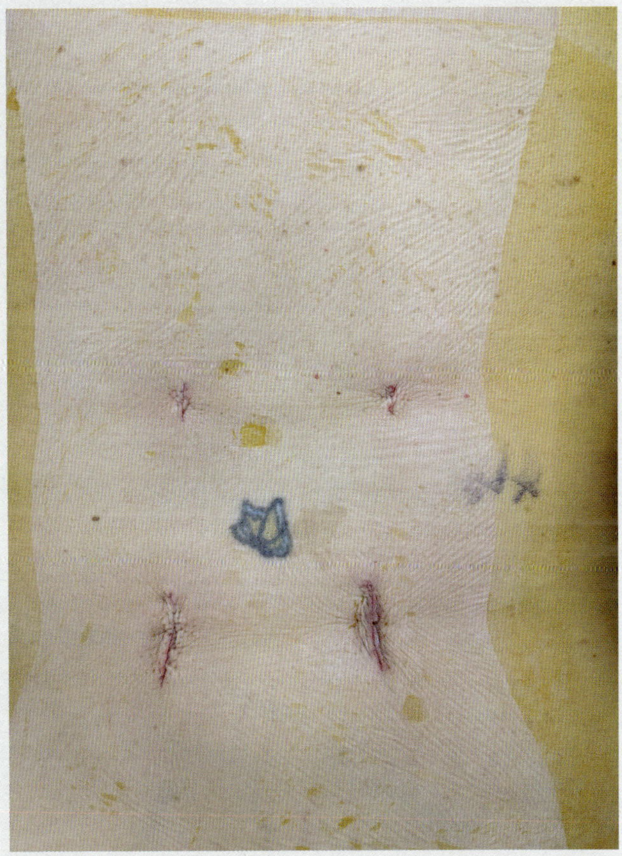

- The fascia is closed with 2–0 absorbable sutures. The subcutaneous tissues are reapproximated with 3–0 absorbable sutures. The skin is reapproximated with Steri-Strips and dressed. Drain is unnecessary.

Region: Latin America *Dr. Nestor Taboada*	Region: Europe *Dr. Guiseppe Barbagallo*
Step 5: Rod placement and closure	**Step 5: Rod placement and closure**
• When an "over the top" approach is performed, an *Absorbable Hemostat* (Surgicel Fibrillar/SNOW) is very useful to control layer bleeding (▶ Video 43.1). • Before closing, the wounds are washed with 0.9% saline solution and the muscle plane is infiltrated with xylocaine without epinephrine at 1%, since the passing of the percutaneous bar can generate bruises along the way that can be painful in the postoperative period. • The first percutaneously introduced rod to which compression is given is ipsilateral to the cage, then compression is applied to the contralateral rod and a final lateral image is obtained to verify compression. 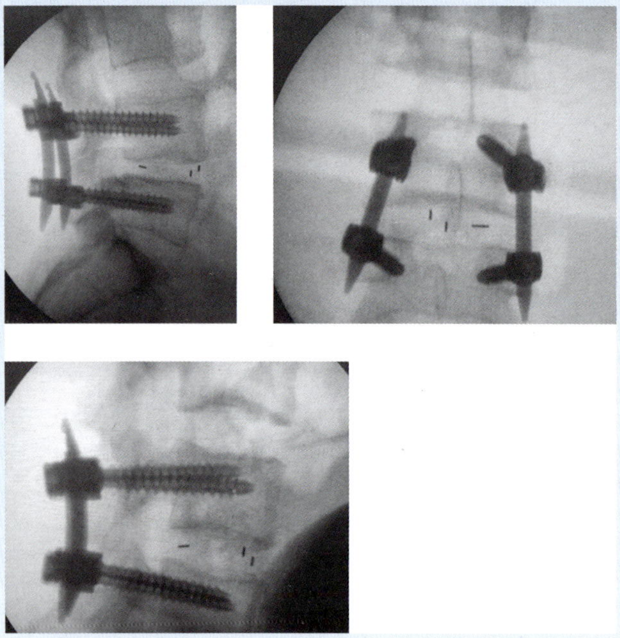	• Rods are curved according to physiological spinal curvature at the targeted levels. Rods are inserted through the screw extensions, starting from the caudal or cranial end according to the case. • The correct length, shape, and position of the rod are checked fluoroscopically, both in AP and lateral views. • Screw extenders are removed, and final AP and lateral fluoroscopic images are obtained. Deep fascia and subcutaneous layers are sutured with 2–0 absorbable stitches. Metal clips are applied to the skin. 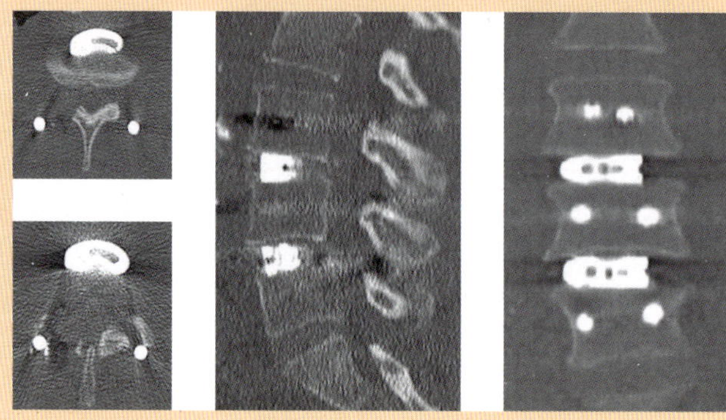

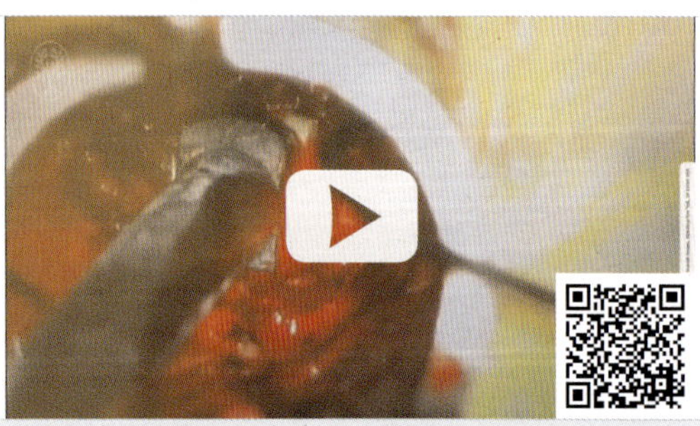

Video 43.1 MIS TLIF cage insertion with K-wire through the retractor.

Region: Asia

Dr. Seang-Beng Tan

Step 6: Final intraoperative X-ray and postoperative care

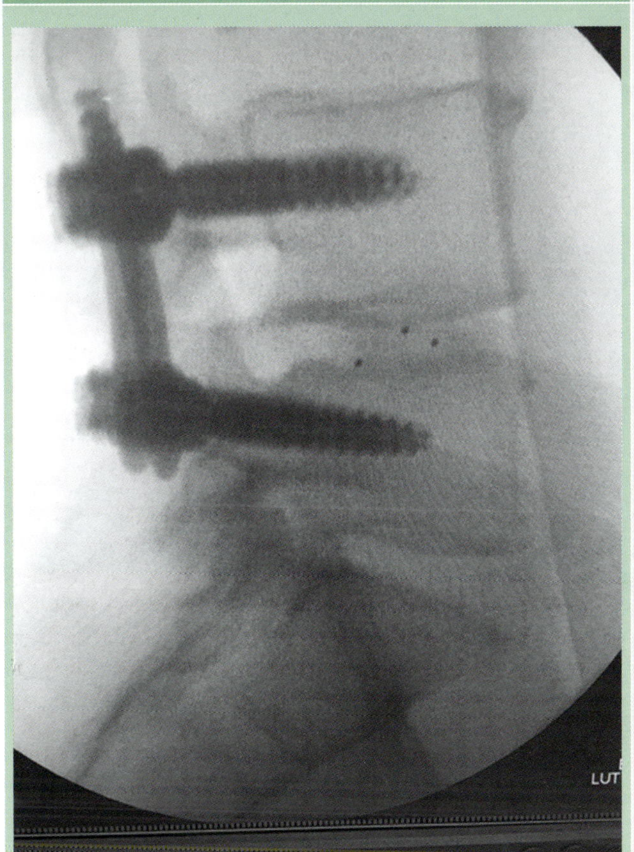

- Postoperative care
  - 3 hours prior to surgery, patients are loaded with analgesics typically using a combination of an NSAID such as diclofenac or cox-2 inhibitor such as celecoxib, and pregabalin. In general, in order to enhance recovery after anesthesia, the use of intraoperative and postoperative narcotics are minimized.
  - Patients are often mobilized after 4 to 6 hours from completion of the surgery. The patients are given a brace and allowed to sit for meals and walk with assistance 6 hours after surgery. Typical length of stay following a single-level MIS-TLIF ranges from 1 to 3 days. Postoperative pain control is typically with a combination of an NSAID for the first week only, with additional pregabalin and/or tramadol.

Region: North America

Dr. Kevin Foley

Step 6: Postoperative care and tips and tricks from the masters

- Postoperative pain control is achieved with muscle relaxants, oral analgesics, and intravenous narcotics.
- Patients are encouraged to mobilize as soon as reasonably possible; we find that early mobilization leads to quicker recovery and helps facilitate the discharge of selected patients on the same day as surgery.
- When out of bed, patients are instructed to wear a lumbar corset for added support.
- Postoperative follow up entails a wound check at 1-week, then 1-month, 3-month, 6-month, 1-year, and 2-year follow-up with X rays to ensure progressive fusion.
- Patients are encouraged to walk to tolerance in the early post-operative period.
- Aquatic therapy is initiated at the 1-month mark and office based physical therapy is prescribed at 3 months.
- Obtain true AP and lateral fluoroscopic images.
- Beveled-tip trochars can be used to move the distal ends of pedicle needles in bone.
- When withdrawing a pedicle access needle, make sure the K-wire does not get pulled out inadvertently; this is most likely if excessive force is applied as the needle exits the bone.
- Dock the tubular retractor at the base of the spinous process if planning a bilateral decompression via a unilateral approach.
- A discosteotome can be used to enter a collapsed disc space.
- Placement of a contralateral screw rod-construct can maintain disc space distraction and deformity reduction while allowing removal of the interbody distractor and additional disc space preparation. This also allows additional bone to be packed into the interbody space for fusion.

44 Percutaneous Pedicle Screw Fixation and MISS SI Joint Fusion

Greg Anderson

Summary
The appropiate radiological identification of the pedicles and sacroilliac joint is key in every lumbosacral instrumentation case. This chapter provides the reader with detailed images about how to perform a transpedicular and sacroiliac instrumentation in a safe and efficient way.

Keywords: SI joint fusion, SI joint, SI instrumentation, percutaneous pedicle screws, percutaneous technique, pedicle screws

44.1 Introduction

Posterior instrumentation techniques performed via a standard open approach with a midline lumbar incision and subperiosteal muscle dissection are associated with iatrogenic soft-tissue and muscle injury. As early as 1984, Magerl described thoracic and lumbar percutaneous skeletal fixation.[1] Atraumatic instrumentation techniques have now become established as reliable, and are regularly performed as the method of choice for many spine surgeons practicing minimally invasive spine surgery (MISS) for the treatment of a wide range of spinal disorders.

44.2 Indications

Pedicle screws are utilized to correct deformity, stabilize segmental instability, and support interbody implants. When compared to open techniques, minimally invasive spine procedures utilizing percutaneous pedicle screws require less soft tissue dissection, reduce postoperative pain, reduce intraoperative blood loss, and shorten hospitalization.[2,3,4]

44.3 Contraindications

The only absolute contraindications to the use of percutaneous pedicle screws are the presence of pedicles that are too small to accommodate the available implants or inadequate intraoperative images (usually fluoroscopy) to guide the procedure. Scenarios that can lead to problems with intraoperative imaging can include broken or poor-quality imaging equipment, severe obesity, overlying gastrointestinal (GI) contrast, or severe osteoporosis.

A relative contraindication may exist for the use of percutaneous fixation in a complex case by an inexperienced surgeon. The placement of percutaneous pedicle fixation has a well-defined learning curve and thus less experienced surgeons should apply this technique to simple cases initially. As the surgeon gains experience with percutaneous fixation, more challenging cases can be approached in this fashion. Factors that can make a case more challenging include: morbid obesity, significant spinal deformity, severe osteoporosis, major spinal instability, or a long surgical construct.

44.4 Technique

44.4.1 Step 1: Preoperative Planning

It is important to review the advanced imaging studies, including computed tomography (CT) and/or magnetic resonance imaging (MRI), prior to the procedure to understand the size and number of implants required for the procedure and the anatomy of the spine in the region of surgery. Additionally, it is useful to note the lumbosacral junction anatomy when performing lower lumbar surgery as lumbosacral dysmorphisms may exist that could impact the difficulty of surgery.

44.4.2 Step 2: Set Up and Positioning

The key to successful minimally invasive spine techniques is maintaining high levels of precision and attention to detail in each step of the procedure, beginning with positioning. Placement of the chest pad along the sternum (just below the sternal notch) and the hip pads just below the anterior superior iliac spine allows the abdomen to be decompressed, minimizing epidural bleeding during surgery. The surgeon should also ensure that the patient is properly aligned on the bed, eliminating an iatrogenic rotation and/or side bending of the spine. Draping should be wide to allow appropriate trajectories for minimally invasive Wiltse approaches, especially in obese patients.

44.4.3 Step 3: Localization

After sterile prep and draping of the surgical site and C-arm, the C-arm is brought into the surgical field. The surgical levels are identified using reproducible fluoroscopic landmarks, such as the lumbosacral junction. In some cases, prior implants can be used as useful surgical landmarks. A spinal needle placed under fluoroscopic guidance can be used to define the ability of a proposed surgical incision to reach a particular region of the spinal anatomy prior to committing to a specific incision.

The authors find it useful to mark out the location of the pedicles on a "true" anteroposterior (AP) image of the vertebra. A true AP image is obtained by aligning the C-arm so that there is perfect overlap of the anterior and posterior margins of the superior end plate (end plate projects as a single radiolucent line). When using the true AP view, the pedicles will be located just caudal to the superior end plate and the spinous process will be centered between the pedicles. Subpar alignment of the vertebra on fluoroscopic images should not be accepted, as this can lead to the inaccurate placement of instrumentation (▶ Fig. 44.1).

Using the true AP view, the authors will mark out each vertebral level in the construct prior to making any incisions. A K-wire is laid over the skin and adjusted until it is seen to bisect the pedicles of a particular level. Next, a transverse line is drawn over the midline of the pedicles. The authors prefer to

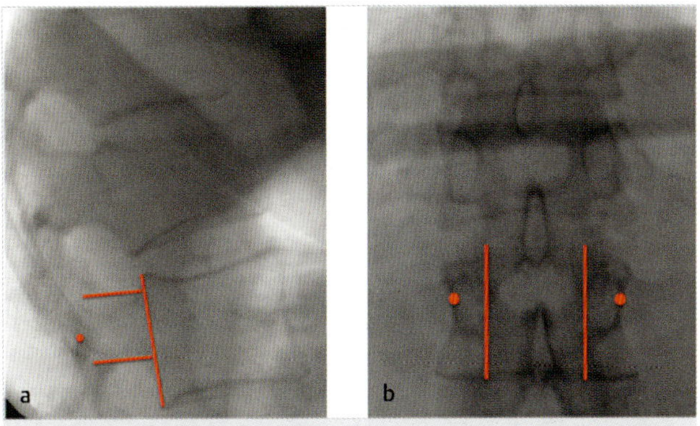

Fig. 44.1 Lateral (a) and anteroposterior (AP) (b) fluoroscopic images. On the lateral, perfect overlap of the superior and inferior end plates, creating an outline of the vertebral body and pedicles, is obtained. On the AP, the pedicles are at the upper and outer corners of the vertebra and symmetric in appearance. The superior and inferior end plates are overlapped and the spinous process is in midline. (Reproduced from Positioning. In: Vialle L, ed. AOSpine Masters Series, Volume 6: Thoracolumbar Spine Trauma. 1st Edition. New York: Thieme; 2015.)

write the level of each line and the sagittal angle of the C-arm neck to each pedicle line (i.e., L3, + 10 degrees of sagittal plane angle on the true AP view). Next, vertical lines are drawn over the lateral boarders of each pedicle. Next, the optimal location of the skin incision(s) can be determined. Generally speaking, the authors use paramedian incisions, positioned about 2 cm lateral to the lateral boarder of the pedicle. In some situations, a single incision can be utilized to reach multiple pedicles due to the lordosis of the spine (▶ Fig. 44.2). Obese patients will require a more lateral incision to reach the pedicle as their soft tissue envelope is thicker, creating a longer distance at the medical to lateral trajectory to reach the spine (▶ Fig. 44.3). In contrast, a very thin patient or an upper lumbar instrumentation site (e.g., L1) may require a small distance (10 mm) between the incision and the lateral boarder of the pedicle.

44.4.4 Step 4: Approach

After making the skin incision, the two layers of fascia must be incised. Remember that when working lateral, you will encounter both the thicker lumbodorsal fascia as well as the thinner epimysium covering the erector spinae muscles. It is crucial to adequately release the fascia so that the implants can be placed in the correct trajectory without applying undue force. This may require undercutting of the fascia relative to the skin incision, which can be accomplished using curved scissors. It is also useful to use digital palpation to feel the facet joint and transverse process prior to placing the Jamshidi needle.

44.4.5 Step 5: Pedicle Preparation and Pedicle Screw Placement

With the C-arm aligned on the true AP view of a particular level, the Jamshidi needle can be docked at the base of the transverse process as medial as possible. The goal is to position the tip of the needle at the 9 o'clock (left side) and 3 o'clock (right side) position of the pedicle shadow as seen on the true AP view (▶ Fig. 44.4). If the needle tip is malpositioned, it

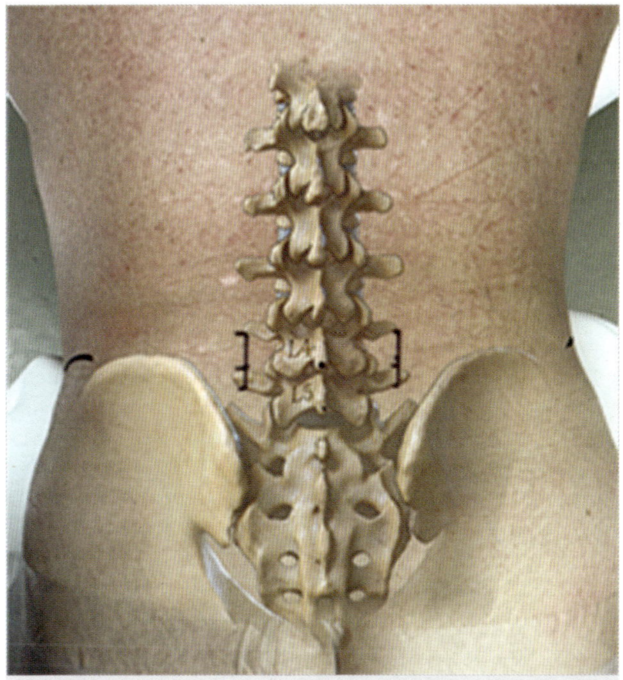

Fig. 44.2 Artist's depiction of spine superimposed on photograph of proposed skin incision demonstrating the proximity of the requisite anatomy relative to the entry point for percutaneous pedicle screw trajectory. (Reproduced from Phase I: Incision, Docking Minimal Access Ports and Pedicle Screw Placement. In: Tumialán L, ed. Minimally Invasive Spine Surgery: A Primer. 1st Edition. New York: Thieme; 2020.)

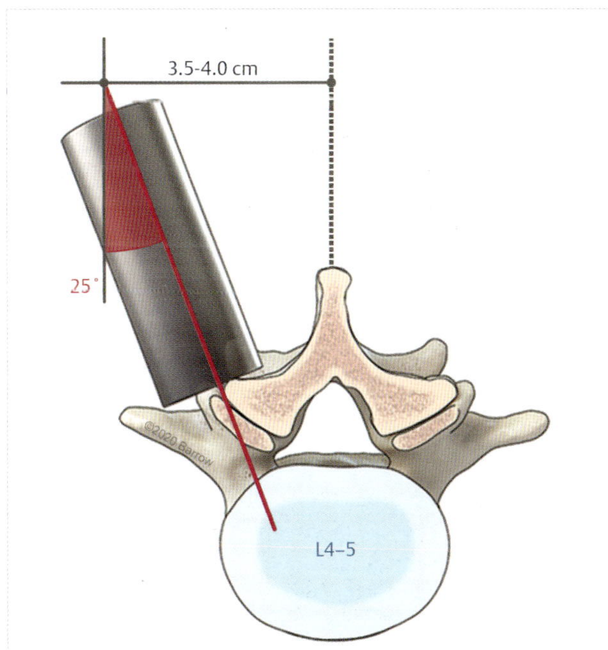

Fig. 44.3 The larger angles at L5 and S1 mandate a more lateral starting point to ensure the trajectory of the access port is parallel or nearly parallel to the pedicle angle. Therefore, at L4–5 and L5–S1, 4.0 cm is preferred, whereas 3.5 cm is preferred in patients with a lower body mass index. (Reproduced from Phase I: Incision, Docking Minimal Access Ports and Pedicle Screw Placement. In: Tumialán L, ed. Minimally Invasive Spine Surgery: A Primer. 1st Edition. New York: Thieme; 2020.)

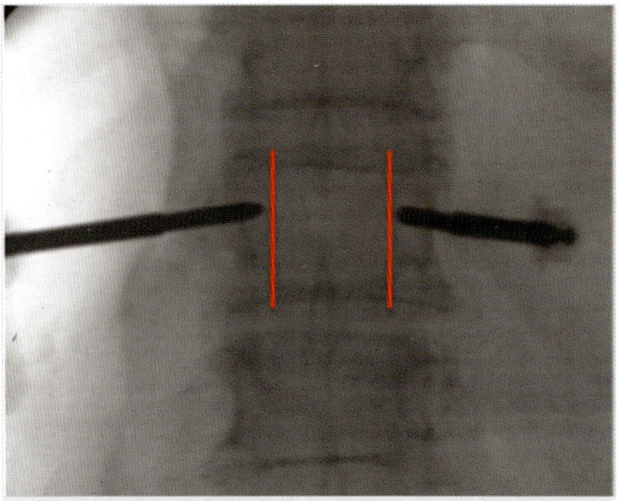

Fig. 44.4 Left pedicles start at approximately 9 o'clock at lateral border of pedicle. Right pedicles start at approximately 3 o'clock at lateral border of pedicle. Ensure appropriate medial angulation and proper sagittal trajectory for the level. The *red line* is the limit. After advancing 2.5 cm, you should make sure you have not passed that *red line* (medial border of the pedicle) at this point. You switch to lateral view. (Reproduced from Screw Placement. In: Vialle L, ed. AOSpine Masters Series, Volume 6: Thoracolumbar Spine Trauma. 1st Edition. New York: Thieme; 2015.)

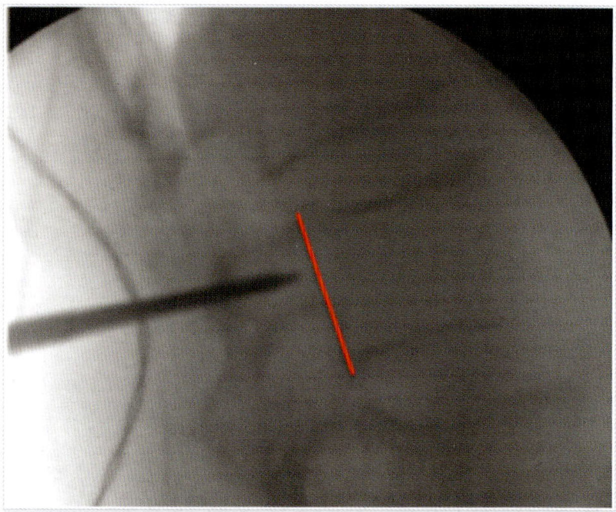

Fig. 44.5 Lateral view indicates too much convergence, while the needle tip is still inside the pedicle. The needle should not be further advanced. On the AP, the tip of the needle is touching the medial border of the pedicle "shade," and on the lateral, the needle has not reached the posterior wall of the vertebral body. In this case, the needle has to be pulled back and angled laterally in order to place the K-wire/screw safely. (Reproduced from Screw Placement. In: Vialle L, ed. AOSpine Masters Series, Volume 6: Thoracolumbar Spine Trauma. 1st Edition. New York: Thieme; 2015.)

should be adjusted to achieve this position prior to penetrating the bony surface. After the tip has been properly positioned, the cortex of the bone is penetrated with a gentle tap of the mallet on the upper portion of the Jamshidi needle. Next, the position is rechecked fluoroscopically to ensure the Jamshidi needle remains on target to the pedicle. The needle should be held so that the tip is pointing toward the center of the pedicle. By adjusting the amount of angulation of the needle, the needle can be directed more or less aggressively directed toward the center of the pedicle. This allows the surgeon to "steer" the needle into position based on imaging taken during pedicle penetration. After the bone is initially penetrated, a mark (using a marking pen) is placed on the needle shaft about 20 mm above the skin edge. This is used to follow the depth of penetration of the needle into the bone. As the needle is inserted deeper into the pedicle, the surgeon will know that the tip of the needle has reached the pedicle–vertebral body junction when the needle shaft mark reaches the skin edge. At this point, a fluoroscopic image can be utilized to assess the position of the tip of the needle. The needle tip should still lie within the pedicle shadow about three-fourths of the distance from lateral to medial across the pedicle. Crossing the medial wall prior to the 20 mm of needle advancement would suggest a medial pedicle breach, and reposition of the needle should be immediately pursued. Although not required in each case, lateral C-arm imaging is useful to confirm the depth of needle penetration (▶ Fig. 44.5).

Assuming the pedicle is safely traversed by the Jamshidi needle, the needle is impacted another 10 to 15 mm into the bone of the vertebral body and then the guidewire is placed. The surgeon should take note of the "crunchy" feel of the cancellous bone as the guidewire is advanced into the vertebral body. Ensure that the anterior boarder of the vertebral body is not penetrated, especially in osteoporotic bone, due to the risk of vascular or visceral injury. In some cases, it can be useful to clamp the guidewires to the drapes to reduce the risk of migration as the remainder of the pedicles in the construct are prepared for screw insertion.

Following guidewire placement, some surgeons prefer to tap the pedicles using a cannulated tap (▶ Fig. 44.6). It is important that the guidewires are secured manually at all times, as surgeon pass instruments over the guidewires, to prevent guidewire migration. The lateral fluoroscopic view is useful to follow the depth of tapping.

Next, a cannulated pedicle screw can be inserted over the guidewire. Lateral fluoroscopic imaging is helpful to follow the depth of screw placement during this maneuver (▶ Fig. 44.7). When the pedicle screw has traversed the pedicle, the guidewire can be withdrawn to reduce the risk of wire migration or breakage. These steps are then repeated for all pedicles within the planned construct.

A slight modification of this technique is used for the S1 pedicle screws. On the true AP view of the sacrum, the S1 pedicles project as an upside-down "fishhook." The Jamshidi needle tip is docked about 10 mm lateral to the medial edge of the pedicle boarder and targeted parallel to the sacral ala. The Jamshidi tip should be about three-fourths of the distance between the docking point and the medial wall of the pedicle when 20 mm of needle advancement has been achieved.

When indicated, iliac fixation can be obtained percutaneously using an S2-Alar-Iliac (S2AI) technique. A 2 to 3 cm midline incision is made approximately over the L5–S1 disc space with a small parasagittal fascial incision. The true AP image of the sacrum is used (same as for S1 pedicle screw) to identify the S1 and S2 foramina. The Jamshidi needle is docked lateral to

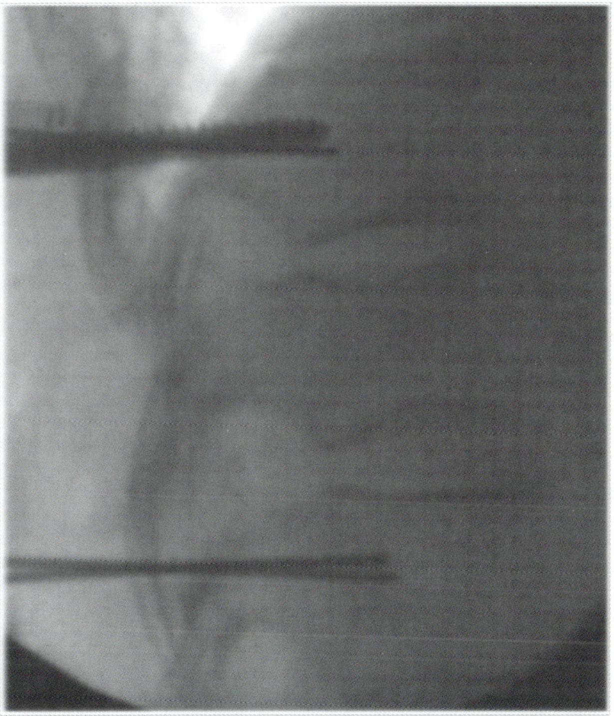

Fig. 44.6 Tapping of pedicle path using cannulated tap over previously placed guidewire. (Reproduced from: Screw Placement. In: Vialle L, ed. AOSpine Masters Series, Volume 6: Thoracolumbar Spine Trauma. 1st Edition. New York: Thieme; 2015.)

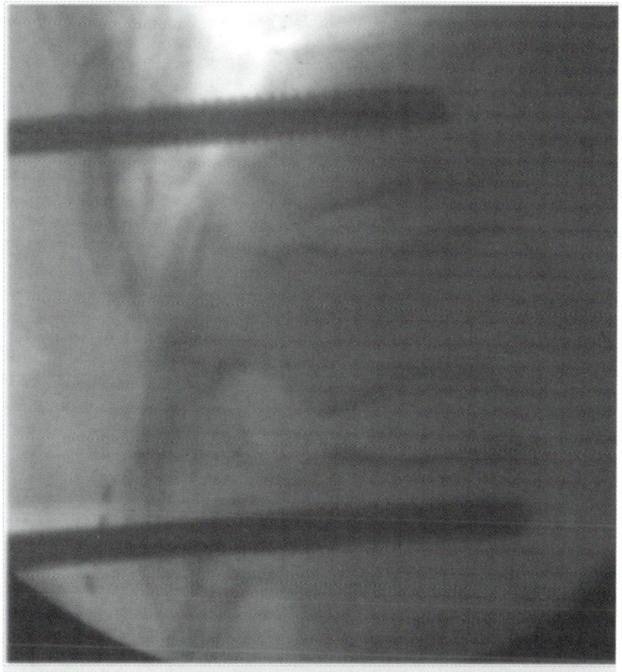

Fig. 44.7 The pedicle/Schanz screw is placed over the guidewire. Prior to any further advancement of this pedicle screw, the guidewire should be removed. (Reproduced from Screw Placement. In: Vialle L, ed. AOSpine Masters Series, Volume 6: Thoracolumbar Spine Trauma. 1st Edition. New York: Thieme; 2015.)

the foramina about midway between the S1 and S2 foraminal openings. Next, the C-arm is adjusted to the "teardrop" view by angulating about 30 degrees lateral until the "teardrop" of the ilium can be visualized just cranial to the superior acetabulum of the hip. The surgeon can palpate the ipsilateral greater trochanter through the surgical drapes as an aiming point. Next, the needle is advanced, ensuring that the tip of the needle remains within the teardrop (▶ Fig. 44.8). After about 40 mm of advancement, the authors switch to an AP view of the ipsilateral pelvis to ensure that the needle is cranial to the sciatic notch. Next, a guidewire is placed, and tapping and screw insertion are achieved in a similar fashion to a pedicle screw.

44.4.6 Step 6: Placement of Rods

MIS pedicle screw systems may vary on the exact technique used to place rods. However, it is common to have instruments that are used to determine rod length from the position of the pedicle screws in the construct. The rods of appropriate size are chosen and any contouring that may be required to accommodate the desired sagittal plane alignment of the construct is performed. Next, the rods may be inserted through the pedicle screws of the construct. Commonly, some kind of rod handle is utilized to facilitate rod passage. After the rods have been successfully passed, capturing each screw in the construct, set screws are applied to secure the construct. In some cases, reduction instrument may be helpful to ensure good seating of the rods onto the pedicle screws. Final fluoroscopic imaging is routinely used to confirm adequate rod length, alignment, and capture of each of the implants in the construct.

44.5 Complication and Avoidance

The same general list of complications that is routine in traditional open surgery also applies to percutaneous pedicle screw fixation. In addition, potentially preventable complications of percutaneous pedicle screw placement may result from a wide array of technical or judgment errors during the procedure. Careful attention to detail and use of a structured technique can help to reduce the incidence of these types of complications. Important steps include preoperative planning, the acquisition of precisely aligned images, adherence to optimal starting points and trajectories during pedicle preparation, and the use of confirmatory imaging for each critical process.

44.6 Tips and Tricks

Fluoroscopically guided percutaneous pedicle screws demonstrate comparable breach rates and pedicle fractures when compared to open pedicle screw cases. However, certain complications of open surgery are minimized with percutaneous surgery. In particular, less soft tissue trauma, lower infection rate, less intraoperative blood loss, and less postoperative pain are expected with percutaneous pedicle fixation when compared to open surgery.[5] Reported breach rates as determined by CT scan range from 9 to 20%, with severe breach (> 4 mm) rates ranging from 0.1 to 3.8%.[6,7,8,9,10] Despite upper thoracic pedicles (T1–T6) demonstrating small pedicle sizes, fluoroscopic pedicle screws technique can still be performed safely. Kwan and colleagues reviewed 260 T1–T6 percutaneous pedicle screw, reporting 12.3% perforation rate and no pedicle screw related complications.[11] Furthermore, AP-only

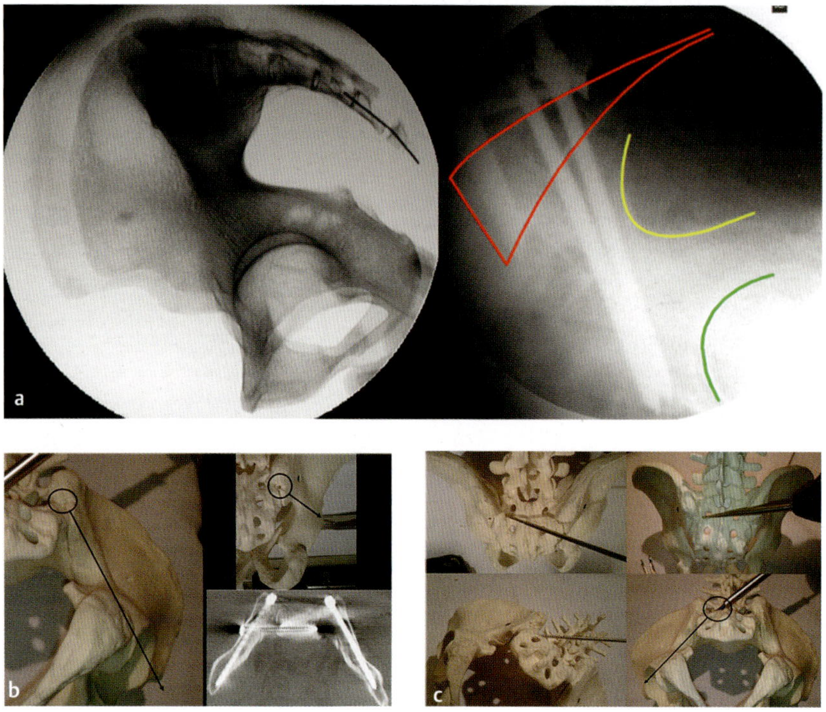

Fig. 44.8 Technique of long iliac screw place- ment. **(a)** A true lateral view, as determined by the exact overlap of the sciatic notches, is the primary view used to guide iliac screw trajectory within the column of bone above the sciatic notch and acetabulum. Iliac screws can be placed from a starting point on either **(b)** the medial aspect of the posterior ilium or **(c)** within the sacrum, inferolateral to the S1 foramen. (Reproduced from AO Spinopelvic Classification Type C Injuries: Sacral Fractures with Spinopelvic Instability. In: Vialle L, ed. AOSpine Masters Series, Volume 6: Thoracolumbar Spine Trauma. 1st Edition. New York: Thieme; 2015.)

pedicle screw techniques can demonstrate similar safety profiles to AP and lateral X-ray techniques, while minimizing operating room (OR) time and potential contamination risk of the C-arm going between AP and lateral positions. Sethi et al reported 5% breach rate with no neurologic complications in 1,806 pedicle screws using an "AP-only" fluoroscopic technique.[12]

> Percutaneous pedicle screw placement is a valuable technique that can be performed with relatively simple equipment. Key point to keep in mind is that if there is a rotational component, work level by level. Throughout the procedure, rotate the patient/table and keep the C-arm in a straight AP/lateral position. Review preoperative imaging including to identify challenging or abnormal anatomy. Pay particular attention to avoiding the cranial facet joint.

44.7 MIS SI Joint Fusion

44.7.1 Indications

Minimally invasive sacroiliac (SI) screw placement is most commonly performed either for acute SI joint/sacral injuries resulting in instability or to support SI joint fusion for treatment of persistent SI joint localized pain failing conservative management. As the discussion of SI fixation for acute traumatic injuries is outside the scope of this chapter, the remainder of the discussion will focus on SI fusion for the treatment of degenerative pathology. The most common etiologies include adjacent segment degeneration following lumbar and lumbosacral fusion, inflammatory SI arthritis, and post-traumatic SI arthritis. Prior to performing SI fusion, physicians should first rule out lumbar and hip pathology and ensure an SI joint etiology of the patient's pain. Physical examination should look for provocative tests including Gaenslen, FABER, compression, distraction, and thigh thrust testing. Although individual tests demonstrate low specificity, three or more positive signs improve diagnostic accuracy of examination findings.[13] SI joint injections should be performed prior to an SI fusion procedure. This is done both as a confirmatory diagnostic test and to attempt nonoperative care prior to surgery. At least two injections that result in at least 50 to 75% improvement in symptoms are considered diagnostic for SI joint etiology.[14,15]

44.7.2 Imaging

Preoperative X-rays of the pelvis including inlet and outlet views and CT pelvis should be reviewed for preoperative planning and evaluation of sacral dysmorphism preventing safe placement of screws. For SI fusion, the S1 and S2 corridors should be evaluated for safe screw placement. Features of sacral dysmorphism include apparent lumbosacral junction disc collinear with iliac crests on outlet X-ray, large oval-shaped foramina seen on AP and outlet views, vestigial disc spaces seen between S1 and S2 on lateral X-rays, downsloping sacral ala on outlet and lateral views, alar mammillary processes, and tongue-in-groove appearance of SI joint on inlet X-ray and CT axial imaging.[16]

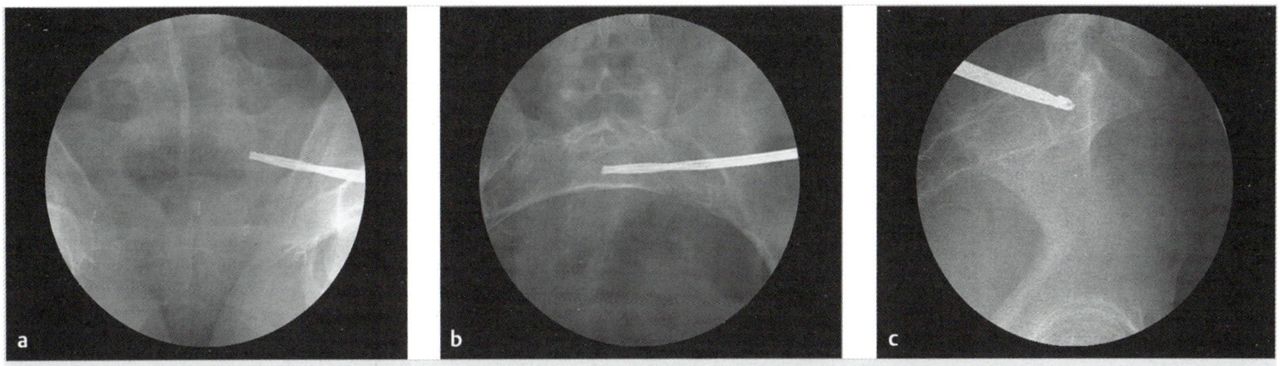

Fig. 44.9 (a) The outlet view enables visualization and avoidance of the S1 and S2 foramina. (b) The inlet view requires overlap of the S1 and S2 anterior cortices and enables the screws to be positioned as anteriorly as possible without penetrating the anterior cortex of the sacrum, which could potentially injure the L5 nerve root, the superior gluteal artery, anterior to the SI joint. These three structures are at risk of injury if the drill bit, guidewire, or screw penetrates through the ala. (c) The lateral view is essential to ensure a starting point posteroinferior to the sacral alar slope and anterosuperior to the S1 foraminal tunnel, which avoids injury to the L5 and S1 nerve roots, respectively. (Reproduced from AO Spinopelvic Classification Type B Injuries: Sacral Fractures with Posterior Pelvic But Not Spinopelvic Instability. In: Vialle L, ed. AOSpine Masters Series, Volume 6: Thoracolumbar Spine Trauma. 1st Edition. New York: Thieme; 2015.)

44.7.3 Positioning

Patients can be positioned either supine or prone, depending on surgeon's preference. Prone positioning on the open Jackson table with wide draping allows adequate access to the lateral hip. Hip and thigh pads should not obstruct access to the lateral gluteal area. For supine positioning, a radiolucent bump is placed underneath the sacrum to lift the pelvis off the table. C-arm fluoroscopy is brought in from the contralateral side.

44.7.4 Technique

1. **Step 1**
   Using lateral, AP, inlet, and outlet views, the starting point on the lateral ilium is identified. High-quality fluoroscopy is essential to safe SI screw placement.
2. **Step 2**
   Properly aligned lateral fluoroscopy will demonstrate overlapping greater sciatic notches and iliac cortical densities (▶ Fig. 44.9). It is generally recommended that the SI fixation screws are placed approximately perpendicular to the SI joint.
3. **Step 3**
   The skin incision is determined by lateral fluoroscopy. A 3 cm long skin incision is made in line with the posterior cortex of the sacral body and beginning approximately 1 cm distal to top of sacrum. In obese patients, the incision may need to be moved 1 to 2 cm dorsal to the sacral body.
4. **Step 4**
   The guidewire start point is posterior and inferior to the iliac cortical density, anterior to the sacral spinal canal, and superior to the sacral nerve root tunnel. The guidewire is then advanced anteromedially for approximately 10 mm, and then safe trajectory is confirmed with inlet and outlet views. The inlet view should show the guidewire posterior to the anterior cortex and the outlet view should show the guidewire parallel and approximately 1 cm caudad to the S1 end plate and should be advanced through the sacral ala to the lateral edge of the sacral body.
5. **Step 5**
   Although the length of implant is not as long as SI screws, good fluoroscopic percutaneous technique and knowledge of the S1 and S2 corridors are essential to avoiding foraminal implant placement and nerve injury. The appropriate screw length is measured by placing a depth gauge over the pin up to the edge of the ilium. Multiple implants exist for SI fusion and surgeons should reference each implant's technique guide for implant preparation and placement.
6. **Step 6**
   Commonly, the screw path is then tapped over the guidewire and a cannulated implant is inserted over the guidewire. X-rays are used to confirm the position of the SI implants.

44.7.5 Complications and Avoidance

Cortical breaches of guidewires or implants risks injury to visceral, vascular, and neurologic structures. Lack of attention to preoperative imaging or intraoperative fluoroscopy can lead to nerve injury and/or dural tears.

44.7.6 Tips and Tricks

The MIS SI fusion technique offers substantial benefits in estimated blood loss, surgical time, and postoperative length of stay when compared with open techniques, but provides similar clinical outcomes in regards to postoperative Oswestry Disability Index (ODI) scores.[17] When appropriately indicated, MIS SI fusions can lead to substantial reduction in opiate use, pain, disability, and improvement in physical function for up to 5 years postoperatively.[18,19,20,21] A recent systematic review found reported reoperation rates ranging from 0 to 17% with a mean of 6%.[22]

References

[1] Magerl FP. Stabilization of the lower thoracic and lumbar spine with external skeletal fixation. Clin Orthop Relat Res. 1984(189):125–141
[2] Lau D, Khan A, Terman SW, Yee T, La Marca F, Park P. Comparison of perioperative outcomes following open versus minimally invasive transforaminal lumbar interbody fusion in obese patients. Neurosurg Focus. 2013; 35(2):E10

[3] Terman SW, Yee TJ, Lau D, Khan AA, La Marca F, Park P. Minimally invasive versus open transforaminal lumbar interbody fusion: comparison of clinical outcomes among obese patients. J Neurosurg Spine. 2014; 20(6):644–652

[4] Wang J, Zhou Y, Feng Zhang Z, Qing Li C, Jie Zheng W, Liu J. Comparison of the clinical outcome in overweight or obese patients after minimally invasive versus open transforaminal lumbar interbody fusion. J Spinal Disord Tech. 2014; 27(4):202–206

[5] Kwan MK, Chiu CK, Lee CK, Chan CY. Comparison between percutaneous fluoroscopic-guided and conventional open pedicle screw placement techniques for the thoracic spine: a safety evaluation in human cadavers. Bone Joint J. 2015; 97-B(11):1555–1561

[6] Nevzati E, Marbacher S, Soleman J, et al. Accuracy of pedicle screw placement in the thoracic and lumbosacral spine using a conventional intraoperative fluoroscopy-guided technique: a national neurosurgical education and training center analysis of 1236 consecutive screws. World Neurosurg. 2014; 82 (5):866–71.e1, 2

[7] Chiu CK, Chan CYW, Kwan MK. The accuracy and safety of fluoroscopic-guided percutaneous pedicle screws in the thoracic and lumbosacral spine in the Asian population: a CT scan analysis of 1002 screws. J Orthop Surg (Hong Kong). 2017; 25(2):2309499017713938

[8] Chiu CK, Kwan MK, Chan CY, Schaefer C, Hansen-Algenstaedt N. The accuracy and safety of fluoroscopically guided percutaneous pedicle screws in the lumbosacral junction and the lumbar spine: a review of 880 screws. Bone Joint J. 2015; 97-B(8):1111–1117

[9] Hansen-Algenstaedt N, Chiu CK, Chan CY, Lee CK, Schaefer C, Kwan MK. Accuracy and safety of fluoroscopic guided percutaneous pedicle screws in thoracic and lumbosacral spine: a review of 2000 screws. Spine. 2015; 40(17): E954–E963

[10] Kwan MK, Chiu CK, Chan CY, Zamani R, Hansen-Algenstaedt N. A comparison of feasibility and safety of percutaneous fluoroscopic guided thoracic pedicle screws between Europeans and Asians: is there any difference? Eur Spine J. 2016; 25(6):1745–1753

[11] Kwan MK, Chiu CK, Chan CYW, Zamani R, Hansen-Algenstaedt N. The use of fluoroscopic guided percutaneous pedicle screws in the upper thoracic spine (T1-T6): is it safe? J Orthop Surg (Hong Kong). 2017; 25 (2):2309499017722438

[12] Sethi A, Lee A, Vaidya R. Lumbar pedicle screw placement: using only AP plane imaging. Indian J Orthop. 2012; 46(4):434–438

[13] Laslett M, Aprill CN, McDonald B, Young SB. Diagnosis of sacroiliac joint pain: validity of individual provocation tests and composites of tests. Man Ther. 2005; 10(3):207–218

[14] Soto Quijano DA, Otero Loperena E. Sacroiliac joint interventions. Phys Med Rehabil Clin N Am. 2018; 29(1):171–183

[15] Manchikanti L, Abdi S, Atluri S, et al. An update of comprehensive evidence-based guidelines for interventional techniques in chronic spinal pain. Part II: guidance and recommendations. Pain Physician. 2013; 16(2) Suppl:S49–S283

[16] Miller AN, Routt ML , Jr. Variations in sacral morphology and implications for iliosacral screw fixation. J Am Acad Orthop Surg. 2012; 20(1):8–16

[17] Ledonio CG, Polly DW , Jr, Swiontkowski MF. Minimally invasive versus open sacroiliac joint fusion: are they similarly safe and effective? Clin Orthop Relat Res. 2014; 472(6):1831–1838

[18] Rudolf L, Capobianco R. Five-year clinical and radiographic outcomes after minimally invasive sacroiliac joint fusion using triangular implants. Open Orthop J. 2014; 8:375–383

[19] Polly DW, Cher DJ, Wine KD, et al. INSITE Study Group. Randomized controlled trial of minimally invasive sacroiliac joint fusion using triangular titanium implants vs nonsurgical management for sacroiliac joint dysfunction: 12-month outcomes. Neurosurgery. 2015; 77(5):674–690, discussion 690–691

[20] Duhon BS, Bitan F, Lockstadt H, Kovalsky D, Cher D, Hillen T, SIFI Study Group. Triangular titanium implants for minimally invasive sacroiliac joint fusion: 2-year follow-up from a prospective multicenter trial. Int J Spine Surg. 2016; 10:13

[21] Sturesson B, Kools D, Pflugmacher R, Gasbarrini A, Prestamburgo D, Dengler J. Six-month outcomes from a randomized controlled trial of minimally invasive SI joint fusion with triangular titanium implants vs conservative management. Eur Spine J. 2017; 26(3):708–719

[22] Zaidi HA, Montoure AJ, Dickman CA. Surgical and clinical efficacy of sacroiliac joint fusion: a systematic review of the literature. J Neurosurg Spine. 2015; 23(1):59–66

45 Intradural Extramedullary Tumors

Hani Malone, Richard G. Fessler, and John E. O'Toole

Summary

The resection of intradural extramedullary (IDEM) spinal tumors using minimally invasive techniques has been shown to be safe and effective. Compared to traditional open surgery, minimally invasive surgery (MIS) techniques may reduce complications, morbidity, and cost, in appropriately selected patients. In this chapter, we will present a step-by-step guide on how to use an MIS approach for resection of IDEM tumors. Preoperative planning, technical details, postoperative considerations, and potential complications will be discussed. Surgical workflow will be illustrated by a video case presentation accompanying this chapter (▶ Video 45.1).

Keywords: minimally invasive spine surgery, spinal tumor, intradural, intradural extramedullary, MIS, IDEM

45.1 Introduction

The increasing availability of advanced diagnostic imaging has brought greater numbers of intradural spinal tumors to surgical attention. Nevertheless, these lesions represent a relatively rare clinical entity with an annual incidence of approximately 1 in 10,000.[1] Intradural tumors are traditionally resected using a standard midline incision, subperiosteal muscle dissection, and bilateral laminectomies. This "open" dissection has been shown to cause denervation and devascularization of the paraspinal musculature leading to significant loss of axial muscle strength.[2] By comparison, minimally invasive surgery (MIS) techniques utilize a tubular retractor system through a paramedian approach, sparing the midline ligaments, and minimizing damage to the paraspinal musculature.

The microsurgical resection of intradural spinal tumors can be technically challenging. Accordingly, the learning curve associated with performing this already difficult procedure through a tubular retractor system has led some to avoid adopting MIS techniques for intradural pathology. Nevertheless, minimally invasive approaches to spinal tumors have evolved rapidly over the past 10 to 15 years, as more surgeons become comfortable with MIS techniques and seek to avoid the morbidity associated with traditional open surgery.[3,4,5,6,7,8,9,10,11,12,13,14,15] This evolution was driven, in part, by the morbidity and significant complication rates associated with traditional surgical approaches to spinal tumors, particularly for metastatic disease.[16,17,18,19]

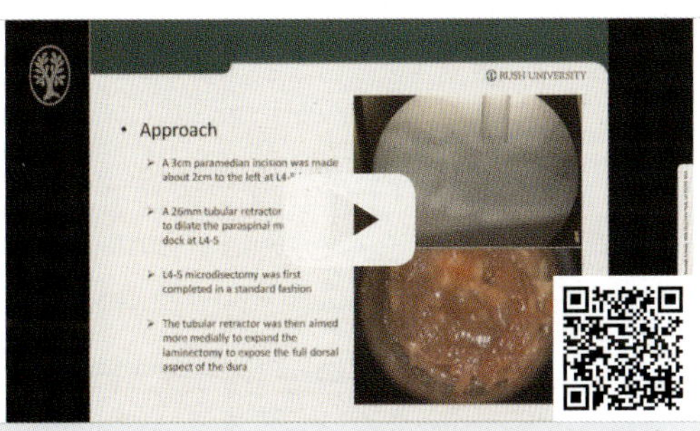

Video 45.1 Intradural extramedullary tumors.

There is a growing body of evidence that minimally invasive approaches can be used to reduce the morbidity associated with the resection of intradural spinal tumors, without compromising extent of resection or safety.[3,4,5,6,7,8,9,10,11,12,13,14,15] When properly performed, MIS techniques should aim to reduce operative time, blood loss, pain, postoperative immobilization, and length of hospital stay. These benefits should ultimately translate into faster recovery and cost reduction.

45.2 Patient Selection: Indications and Contraindications

Advances in MIS technology and surgical navigation continue to expand the indications and capabilities of minimally invasive spine surgery (MISS) for degenerative disease. This progression has led to corollary advances in MIS for intradural spinal tumors.[3,4,5,6,7,8,9,10,11,12,13,14,15] There have been successful reports of MIS resection of well-circumscribed intramedullary spinal tumors.[20,21] Likewise, the treatment of spinal vascular malformations has been shown to be safe and effective through a tubular retractor system.[22,23] Nevertheless, minimally invasive approaches to intradural spinal pathology is most commonly used for intradural extramedullary (IDEM) spinal tumors, which will be the focus of this chapter.

A traditional open approach to intradural tumors does provide a number of definitive advantages.[24], Midline approaches provide a wide exposure and large surgical corridor. This exposure may be necessary for large lesions that span multiple segments. Dural closure is also more facile when a large surgical corridor is created. However, this exposure comes at the cost of a larger excision with greater soft tissue destruction, blood loss, and recovery time.[4,5,6] Open surgical approaches also sacrifice the support provided by posterior midline structures, specifically the interspinous ligaments. Compromise of this posterior tension band may predispose patients to segmental instability and/or postoperative kyphosis, necessitating instrumented fusion. The risk of postoperative kyphosis may be particularly significant following surgery for intradural tumors.[16,25,26] By comparison, MIS techniques generally utilize a unilateral paramedian approach that preserves the posterior tension band, mitigating the risk of postoperative instability and kyphosis.[16]

The fundamental advantages of MISS for degenerative disease (reduced soft tissue destruction, blood loss, mobilization, and hospital stay) have been reproducible in series of patients with intradural tumors.[3,4,5,6,7,8,9,10,11,12,13,14,15] There is also evidence that MIS approaches limit the risk of postoperative cerebrospinal fluid (CSF) leak following intended durotomies, which in turn reduces the risk of wound breakdown and postoperative infection.[6,7,27] This is most likely due to the relatively small amount of dead space that remains following removal of an MIS tubular retractor, compared to traditional midline approaches.

The appropriateness of an MIS approach to IDEM tumors is largely dictated by a preoperative assessment of the space required to remove the lesion. For example, tumors that lie ventral to the spinal cord are not amenable to an MIS approach. These lesions often require a larger dural opening to facilitate sectioning of the dentate ligaments and slight mobilization of the spinal cord. By comparison, dorsal and lateral intradural lesions are candidates for MIS. Good visualization of these lesions can be achieved using a tubular retractor from a contralateral paramedian approach (see ▶ Video 45.1).[3] Size is not necessarily a contraindication, as rather large lesions (up to 4 cm) can be removed with the use of expandable retractors.[3] Nevertheless, MIS approaches should be limited to intradural lesions that are one or two levels in length.[15,16]

There is a learning curve associated with all minimally invasive techniques. This may be particularly true for intradural tumors and some repetition is necessary to become facile with dural closure in a limited corridor.[27] However, as MIS for degenerative spine pathology becomes more ubiquitous and is increasingly incorporated into residency training, more neurosurgeons are likely to consider MIS approaches to IDEM pathology.

45.3 Preoperative Planning

For all patients with a known or suspected spinal tumor, clinical evaluation must begin with a detailed history and neurologic examination. Compared to patients with epidural disease or tumors of the vertebral column, those with intradural lesions are relatively less likely to present with severe radicular or axial back pain. However, these patients may develop neurologic deficits from ongoing compression of the spinal cord or nerve roots.[28] Magnetic resonance imaging (MRI) is the primary imaging modality used to evaluate intradural spinal tumors.

T1-weighted sequences with gadolinium contrast are useful to define the extent and margins of intradural pathology. Although the degree of enhancement on postcontrast sequences may vary considerably for intramedullary pathology, commonly encountered IDEM lesions, such as schwannomas, nerve sheath tumors, and meningiomas, tend to avidly enhance (▶ Fig. 45.1). T2-weighted sequences are useful for determining the nature and extent of cord deformation and/or nerve impingement, as well as cord edema and syrinx formation. For patients with pacemakers, pain pumps, or other metallic foreign bodies precluding MRI, computed tomography (CT) myelography can be used as an alternative modality.

When considering a minimally invasive approach to intradural pathology, special attention must be paid to the space required to remove the lesion. It is critical that the MIS retractor used allows for adequate visualization of the full length of the tumor. In ideal conditions, normal (nonpathologic) tissue rostral and caudal to the lesion should also be visualized to allow for accurate identification of tumor margins.[24] Inadequate visualization of IDEM tumors may lead to the piecemeal and subtotal resection of lesions that could otherwise be removed en bloc.[3,24] It is important to consider that adjustment of the tubular retractor system is limited after making a durotomy and any attempt to do so may introduce blood into the subarachnoid space and risk injury to exposed neural tissue. Some have advocated that the retractor used should be 5 to 10 mm larger than the planned length of the dural incision, in order to ensure enough length to reliably obtain a watertight dural closure.[3,24] It is also important to consider that the length of the durotomy should generally be 5 to 10 mm longer than the underlying intradural pathology to ensure adequate visualization.

When counseling patients with intradural pathology, expectations and operative goals must be frankly discussed prior to formulating a surgical plan. For intramedullary lesions, the nature of the pathology and the presence or absence of a safe dissection plane often limit extent of resection, making diagnosis the primary goal of surgery. Conversely, for IDEM tumors, surgical resection is often curative. Accordingly, careful surgical planning is critical to ensure maximal resection and definitive treatment when possible. Like all spinal tumor surgery, the primary goals for IDEM tumor surgery are pathologic diagnosis, symptomatic relief, tumor resection/source control, and decompression of the spinal cord and/or roots. The operating surgeon

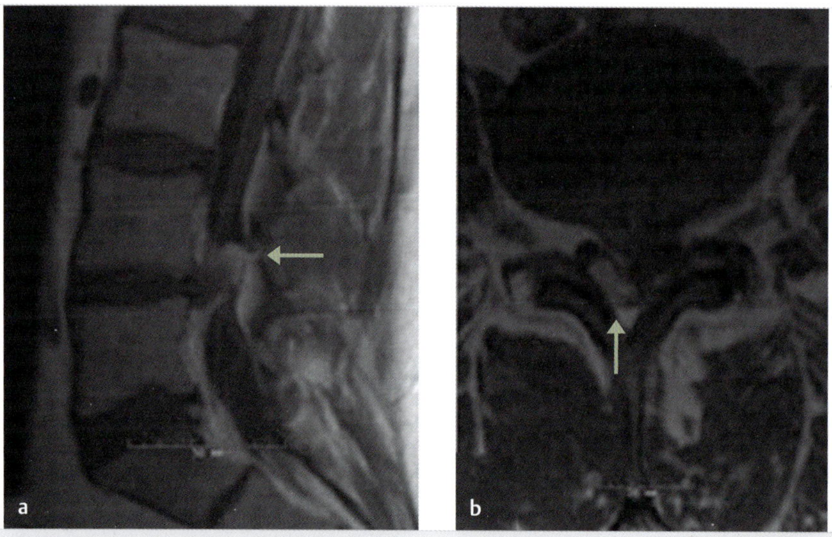

Fig. 45.1 Magnetic resonance imaging (MRI) of a patient with an intradural extramedullary lesion. The lesion enhances avidly, seen here on sagittal **(a)** and axial **(b)** T1 postcontrast images.

must be confident that these goals can be effectively addressed through an MIS approach before attempting a minimally invasive operation.

45.4 Technique

45.4.1 Patient Positioning

General anesthesia is recommended for all minimally invasive approaches to intradural pathology. We use intraoperative neurophysiologic monitoring with continuous somatosensory evoked potentials (SSEPs), electromyography (EMG), and, when indicated, motor evoked potentials and/or a stimulation probe. Open communication between the anesthesia and neuromonitoring teams is critical to achieve the appropriate balance between muscle relaxation and accurate neurophysiologic recording. Prepositioning potentials may be necessary when intradural pathology has led to significant deformation of the spinal cord, but is generally not necessary.

Following the induction of anesthesia, the patient is placed in the prone position on a standard radiolucent spine table. A Wilson frame (Mizuho OSI | Union City, CA) may be used to open the interlaminar space at lumbar levels, but at thoracic levels it may limit anteroposterior (AP) fluoroscopy and complicate localization. In the thoracic spine, we generally use a combination of standard radiolucent chest, hip, and thigh pads for this reason. With the patient positioned, fluoroscopy is used to identify the appropriate spinal level and mark the intended incision and site of dilation.

45.4.2 Navigation

Challenges to accurate localization with intraoperative fluoroscopy may be obviated with the use of surgical navigation. Recent reports have studied the utility of MRI-based navigation that is co-registered to intraoperative three-dimensional fluoroscopy images.[29,30] In these studies, the authors suggest that in addition to localizing the correct spinal level, navigation minimizes the skin incision and muscle dissection, reduces bone removal, and allows for precise dural openings.[29,30] Nevertheless, in most cases, localization can be achieved with standard fluoroscopy and the details of surgical approach can be aptly extrapolated from careful study of the relevant anatomy on preoperative imaging.

45.4.3 Surgical Technique in Steps

1. **Incision and exposure:**
   We typically approach eccentric IDEM tumors across the spinal canal from a contralateral approach for lumbar tumors and ipsilaterally for cervical and thoracic tumors. An approximately 3 cm paramedian skin incision is made several centimeters lateral to the midline. The position of the lesion in the spinal canal dictates the lateral extent of the incision, which can be measured on MRI preoperatively. An incision made too medial will prevent angulation of the tubular retractor and limit exposure of the midline and contralateral canal. Following skin incision, the opening is carried through the subcutaneous fat with monopolar cautery, achieving hemostasis and leaving the thoracolumbar fascia intact. We generally prefer to cut the fascia sharply prior to dilation, but others traverse the fascia upon dilation with the K-wire and tubular dilators.
   Dilation with the tubular retractor system then takes place in a stepwise fashion. We generally initiate dilation and localize with a K-wire, but some favor starting with the smallest dilator to mitigate the risk of passing the K-wire past the interlaminar space. The initial dilator should target the laminofacet junction. Dilators of increasing caliber are then passed over each other using a circular motion to pass deep to the fascia. Lateral fluoroscopic guidance is used to ensure the correct depth at the level of the joint (▶ Fig. 45.2).

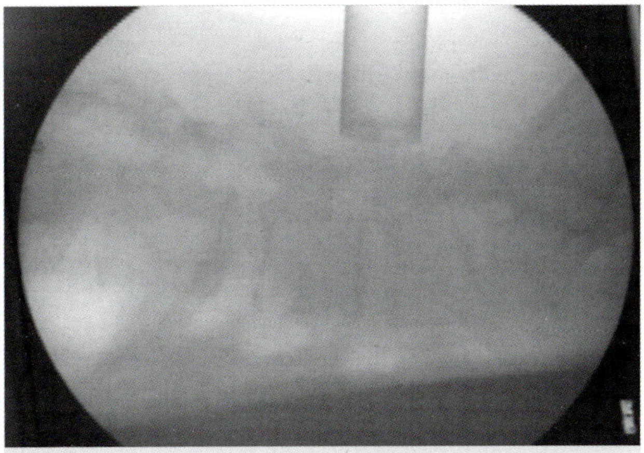

Fig. 45.2 Intraoperative lateral fluoroscopic image demonstrating dilation of the minimally invasive surgical tubular retraction system at the laminar-facet junction at L4/L5.

2. **Localization:**
   Once the planned dilator width has been achieved and the depth of dilation measured, the corresponding tubular retractor can be placed and secured to the system's table-mounted articulating arm. Fluoroscopy should be used judiciously during MIS, given the cumulative risk of radiation exposure to the operating surgeon and ancillary staff. However, optimal retractor placement is paramount to success in MIS for IDEM lesions and fluoroscopy should be used as needed until this can be confidently achieved.
   The choice of tubular retractor should be based on the location and size of the IDEM tumor, with the retractor diameter ideally at least a few millimeters larger than the length of the lesion. We have experienced using fixed diameter tubes ranging from 20 to 26 mm for intradural pathology, which are significantly larger than the standard 18-mm diameter tubes commonly used for lumbar microdiscectomy. Expandable retractors can be used for larger lesions, which are capable of providing over 4 cm of longitudinal exposure. Once the retractor is secured in place, the microscope is brought into position and focused to the depth of the operative site. We prefer a working distance of 350 mm to allow for facile passing of instruments in and out of the tubular dilator without interference from the operative microscope.
3. **Dissection:**
   At the depth of the tubular retractor, a soft tissue muscle plug is circumferentially sectioned and removed with

monopolar cautery, exposing the underlying lamina and medial facet joint. Using a high-speed burr, a standard ipsilateral hemilaminectomy is performed, exposing the underlying ligamentum flavum, which is preserved. With the ligament serving as a protective barrier to the dura, the tubular retractor is then redirected medially. The high-speed burr can then be used to undercut the spinous process. The inner cortex of the contralateral lamina is then removed with a combination of drilling and the use of a Kerrison punch until the contralateral pedicle is visualized. This approach provides access to both the ipsilateral and contralateral sides of the spinal canal, while maintaining the integrity of the spinous process, interspinous ligaments, and posterior tension band.

Next, the ligamentum flavum, which has served as a barrier to the dura during drilling, can be efficiently removed. A straight curette can be used to separate the two bellies of the ligament in the midline, establishing an epidural plane. The ligament can then be freed from its rostral and caudal laminar attachments using a ball tip probe, angled curette, and Kerrison punch, exposing the underlying dura.

4. **Tumor resection:**
   Prior to initiating the dural opening, it is important to ensure that meticulous hemostasis is achieved to prevent blood from running into the operative field and subarachnoid space. We use a long-handled no. 11 blade scalpel to initiate the durotomy in the midline, and then extend the opening rostrally and caudally using a nerve hook. The dural edges are then tacked up using 4–0 Nurolon or silk sutures.
5. Following the dural opening, tumor resection begins with careful dissection of the arachnoid layers overlying the mass and adjacent neural elements. At this stage in the operation, standard microsurgical techniques are used to remove the lesion. We most frequently utilize microscissors and Rhoton dissectors to create a plane around the mass. When addressing tumors in the thoracic and cervical spine, microdissection must free extramedullary tumors from the spinal cord and exiting nerve roots. In the lumbar spine, microsurgical technique must be similarly used to dissect the tumor free from the nerves of the cauda equina.
6. Once an IDEM tumor has been dissected from adjunct neural tissue, the size and location of the mass dictate how it can be then safely and efficiently resected. Large extramedullary lesions that deform the adjacent spinal cord, such as large thoracic meningiomas, generally have to be debulked prior to removal to avoid any additional physical stress to the spinal cord. In some cases, an ultrasonic aspirator with an MIS attachment can be used to perform debulking.
7. Importantly, the ultrasonic aspirator must be used on low power settings to minimize the risk of collateral mechanical injury to the adjacent cord. Although piecemeal tumor removal is less efficient and may increase the likelihood of subtotal resection, it is occasionally necessary to avoid cord injury and neurologic deficit.
8. Conversely, schwannomas and other nerve sheath tumors at the level of the cauda equina can often be safely removed en bloc, without internal debulking.[28] For these lesions, microsurgical dissection is used to isolate the tumor and its associated afferent and efferent fascicles from all other roots in the thecal sac (▶ Fig. 45.3). Special care should be taken to ensure that no traversing roots are adherent to the ventral side of the mass, which may be originally difficult to identify. Once isolated, direct stimulation with a unipolar probe is applied to both the afferent and efferent nerve fascicles associated with the mass.
9. In the case of schwannoma, direct stimulation will produce a motor response in only rare cases. If a motor response is recorded, it is often because the nerve stimulated was not the nerve fascicle truly associated with the tumor, but rather a traversing nerve adherent to the mass. If there is no motor response, the afferent nerve is sectioned first and then the efferent nerve. This is to prevent rostral rebounding of the tumor mass above the dural opening from rostral nerve tension. Once the afferent and efferent roots are coagulated and sectioned, the mass can be removed en bloc. While performing microsurgery, surgeons accustomed to using the operating microscope may observe fewer differences than anticipated between MIS and open approaches, as the operation is reduced to a small corridor.
10. **Closure:**
    Dural closure represents one of the more technically challenging components of MIS for intradural tumors. As with open surgery, a watertight dural closure is paramount to avoiding CSF leakage, pseudomeningocele formation,

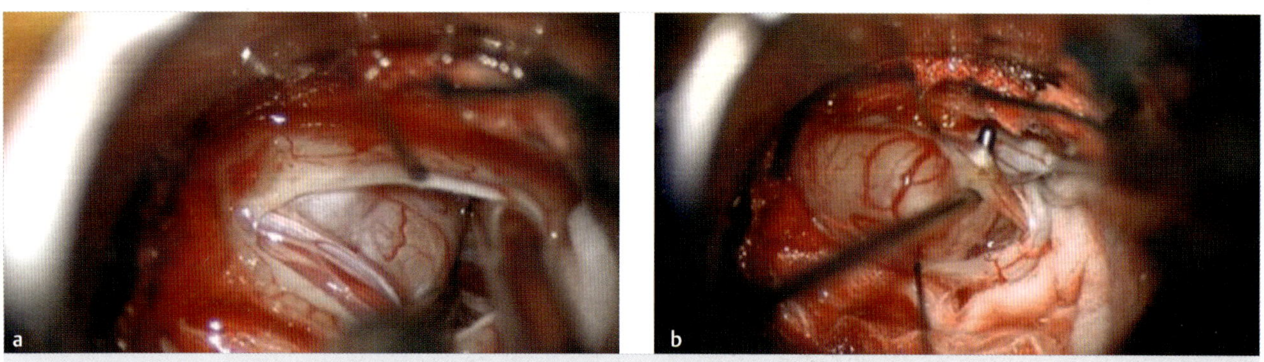

Fig. 45.3 (a, b) Microscopic view of an intradural extramedullary (IDEM) schwannoma. The tumor is first dissected free from the nerves of the cauda equina. Like most IDEM tumors in the lumbar spine, this lesion can be removed en bloc. The mass is partially herniated through the dural opening to allow for visualization and micro-dissection of the ventral tumor plane.

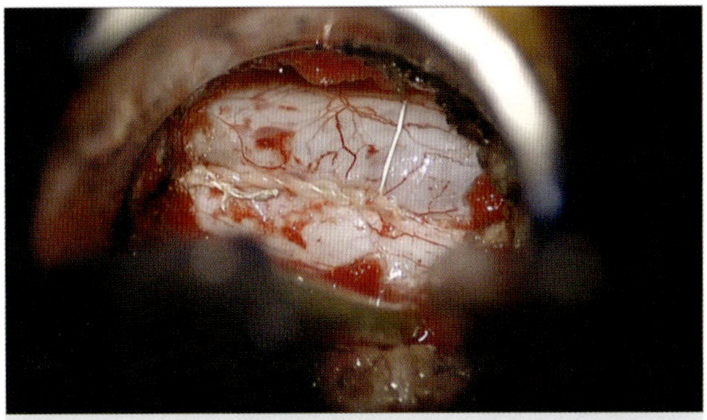

Fig. 45.4 We prefer to repair the dura with a running 6.0 tapered Gore-Tex suture, using elongated instruments adapted for use through a minimally invasive surgical tubular retractor. A Valsalva maneuver is performed at the end of the closure to evaluate for any defects.

infection, and wound breakdown in the postoperative period. Prior to closing the dura, it is again critical to ensure that hemostasis is achieved, as the drainage of CSF during surgery precipitates bleeding from stretched epidural veins. Although a number of dural closure devices have been developed,[31] we prefer to repair the dura with a running suture. With elongated instruments adapted for use through an MIS tubular retractor, dural closure can be performed in a manner similar to open techniques. We favor the facility associated with a 6.0 tapered Gore-Tex suture. Some advocate interrupted sutures or running interlocked suture lines, but we prefer a standard running suture (▶ Fig. 45.4). A Valsalva maneuver is performed at the end of the closure to evaluate for any defects in the suture line and to ensure a watertight closure. Hydrogel or fibrin-based dural sealants can be used as an adjunct to reinforce the suture line. At the conclusion of the case, the retractor system is removed slowly, taking care to identify and cauterize any sites of bleeding. The fascia and subcutaneous layers are closed with inverted 0 and 2.0 Vicryl sutures, respectively. We close the skin with topical adhesive glue.

45.5 Postoperative Care

CSF leakage is the primary postoperative concern specific to intradural spine tumor surgery. To reduce the amount of pressure on the healing durotomy closure, patients are kept flat on bed rest following surgery. Traditionally, open surgery postoperative protocols recommend that patients be kept flat and immobilized until postoperative day 2. Following MIS this may not be necessary.[27] Compared to open intradural surgery, the minimal epidural dead space following MIS reduces the risk of postoperative CSF leakage.[4,6,27] We routinely keep patients on bed rest for only a few hours on the day of surgery, and mobilize them thereafter.

45.6 Complications and Avoidance

The most common complication following surgery for IDEM spinal tumors is CSF leakage and/or pseudomengocele formation, occurring in 5.3% of patients.[4,32] Yet compared to open surgery, MIS approaches are generally protective against CSF-related complications.[9,15,16] This is due to a reduction in tissue destruction and displacement that allows for re-expansion of the paraspinal musculature upon removal of the tubular retractors. This re-expansion obliterates much of the dead space that remains following open surgery and creates a physical barrier to CSF leakage. In a retrospective series directly comparing MIS to open surgery for IDEM tumors, Wong and colleagues reported a significant difference in the number of postoperative CSF leaks between patients treated with MIS (1 patient, 3.7%) versus open approaches (3 patients, 16.7%).[6] In a study similarly comparing MIS to open surgery for IDEM lesions, Raygor et al reported that 1 of 25 (4%) MIS patients had a CSF leak or pseudomeningocele, while 3 of 26 (11.5%) patients in the open cohort experienced CSF leaks.[7] In our own retrospective study of 23 consecutive patients with an MIS dural closure following intended durotomy, we did not experience any cases of CSF leakage or symptomatic pseudomeningocele.[27] All patients were allowed full activity less than 24 hours after surgery in this study, further suggesting that prolonged bed rest after successful primary dural closure appears unnecessary after MIS.

Reports of MIS approaches to IDEM lesions have also consistently found reductions in blood loss (EBL) compared to open surgery. In the meta-analysis conducted by Pham et al, blood loss from MIS cohorts ranged from 134 to 153 mL, while EBL in open surgeries ranged from 320 to 558.8 mL.[6,7,33] In the comparative series by Wong and colleagues, three open surgery patients required blood transfusions, but no MIS patients did.[6] Similarly, in the study by Raygor et al, three patients in the open group received a blood transfusion comparted to one MIS patient.[7] This difference can be attributed to the decreased muscle cutting and soft tissue destruction caused by an MIS approach, as well as the tamponading effect of muscle re-expansion in the surgical cavity following retractor removal.

This reduction in dead space may also contribute to lower infection rates in MIS intradural surgery, as the volume of hematomas and seromas that may act as an infectious nidus is minimized. There is evidence suggesting that MIS for degenerative spinal conditions may reduce postoperative wound infections as much as 10-fold.[34] In their meta-analysis, Pham and colleagues found evidence of postoperative infection in only 1 of the 114 patients analyzed (0.88%), a significantly lower rate compared to previous studies of open surgery for IDEM lesions.[4,35]

45.7 Tips and Tricks

a) Dorsal and lateral IDEM lesions can be well visualized from a contralateral paramedian MIS approach in the lumbar spine and ipsilateral approach in the cervical and thoracic spine.
b) Adjustment of the tubular retractor system is limited after making a durotomy; thus, the retractor used should optimally be 5 mm larger than the planned length of the dural incision.
c) For IDEM lesions in the lumbar spine, make certain no traversing roots are adherent to the ventral side of the mass.
d) Direct stimulation of the efferent/afferent nerves associated with IDEM tumors will rarely produce a motor response. If a motor response is recorded, it is often because the nerve stimulated was a traversing nerve adherent to the mass. If

the lesion is truly a motor-based nerve sheath tumor, microdissection of the tumor off the rootlet with anatomic preservation of the rootlet is necessary.

e) For IDEM nerve sheath tumors, the afferent nerve is sectioned first and then the efferent nerve, to prevent rostral rebounding of the tumor mass above the dural opening.

f) A watertight dural closure is paramount to avoiding CSF leakage, pseudomeningocele formation, infection, and wound breakdown.

g) Following MIS for IDEM spinal tumor resection, most patients can be mobilized by postoperative day 1.

45.8 Conclusion

The use of minimally invasive techniques in the resection of intradural spinal tumors has been shown to be both safe and effective. There is increasing evidence from retrospective data that MIS approaches can be used to reduce the morbidity and cost of IDEM tumor resection, without compromising extent of resection or safety.[4] Neurosurgeons who have become facile using MIS retractors for degenerative disease may be well equipped to adapt MIS techniques for intradural tumors. Success is contingent upon an understanding of the proper indications and advantages/disadvantages related to these techniques. Due to the growth of MISS in residency training and an ever-increasing emphasis on cost effectiveness, more neurosurgeons are likely to adopt MIS techniques for IDEM pathology in the future.

References

[1] Kurland LT. The frequency of intracranial and intraspinal neoplasms in the resident population of Rochester, Minnesota. J Neurosurg. 1958; 15(6):627–641

[2] Sasaoka R, Nakamura H, Konishi S, et al. Objective assessment of reduced invasiveness in MED. Compared with conventional one-level laminotomy. Eur Spine J. 2006; 15(5):577–582

[3] Snyder L, Clark J, Nakaji P, Tumialán L. Minimally invasive surgical techniques for intradural extramedullary lesions of the thoracic spine. Barrow Quarterly. 2016; 26(1):20–25

[4] Pham MH, Chang KE, Liu JC, Hsieh PC. Minimally invasive surgery for intradural extramedullary spinal tumors: a comprehensive review with illustrative clinical cases. World Spinal Column J. 2016; 7(2):84–96

[5] Fontes RB, Wewel JT, O'Toole JE. Perioperative cost analysis of minimally invasive vs open resection of intradural extramedullary spinal cord tumors. Neurosurgery. 2016; 78(4):531–539

[6] Wong AP, Lall RR, Dahdaleh NS, et al. Comparison of open and minimally invasive surgery for intradural-extramedullary spine tumors. Neurosurg Focus. 2015; 39(2):E11

[7] Raygor KP, Than KD, Chou D, Mummaneni PV. Comparison of minimally invasive transspinous and open approaches for thoracolumbar intradural-extramedullary spinal tumors. Neurosurg Focus. 2015; 39(2):E12

[8] Afathi M, Peltier E, Adetchessi T, Graillon T, Dufour H, Fuentes S. Minimally invasive transmuscular approach for the treatment of benign intradural extramedullary spinal cord tumours: technical note and results. Neurochirurgie. 2015; 61(5):333–338

[9] Nzokou A, Weil AG, Shedid D. Minimally invasive removal of thoracic and lumbar spinal tumors using a nonexpandable tubular retractor. J Neurosurg Spine. 2013; 19(6):708–715

[10] Gandhi RH, German JW. Minimally invasive approach for the treatment of intradural spinal pathology. Neurosurg Focus. 2013; 35(2):E5

[11] Lee B, Hsieh PC. Minimally invasive lumbar intradural extramedullary tumor resection. Neurosurg Focus. 2012; 33 Suppl 1:1

[12] Dahlberg D, Halvorsen CM, Lied B, Helseth E. Minimally invasive microsurgical resection of primary, intradural spinal tumours using a tubular retraction system. Br J Neurosurg. 2012; 26(4):472–475

[13] Mannion RJ, Nowitzke AM, Efendy J, Wood MJ. Safety and efficacy of intradural extramedullary spinal tumor removal using a minimally invasive approach. Neurosurgery. 2011; 68(1) Suppl Operative:208–216, discussion 216

[14] Dakwar E, Smith WD, Malone KT, Uribe JS. Minimally invasive lateral extracavitary resection of foraminal neurofibromas. J Clin Neurosci. 2011; 18 (11):1510–1512

[15] Tredway TL, Santiago P, Hrubes MR, Song JK, Christie SD, Fessler RG. Minimally invasive resection of intradural-extramedullary spinal neoplasms. Neurosurgery. 2006; 58(1) Suppl:ONS52–ONS58, discussion ONS52–ONS58

[16] O'Toole JE, Eichholz KM, Fessler RG. Minimally invasive approaches to vertebral column and spinal cord tumors. Neurosurg Clin N Am. 2006; 17(4):491–506

[17] Klimo P , Jr, Kestle JR, Schmidt MH. Treatment of metastatic spinal epidural disease: a review of the literature. Neurosurg Focus. 2003; 15(5):E1

[18] Weigel B, Maghsudi M, Neumann C, Kretschmer R, Müller FJ, Nerlich M. Surgical management of symptomatic spinal metastases: postoperative outcome and quality of life. Spine. 1999; 24(21):2240–2246

[19] Ghogawala Z, Mansfield FL, Borges LF. Spinal radiation before surgical decompression adversely affects outcomes of surgery for symptomatic metastatic spinal cord compression. Spine. 2001; 26(7):818–824

[20] Haji FA, Cenic A, Crevier L, Murty N, Reddy K. Minimally invasive approach for the resection of spinal neoplasm. Spine. 2011; 36(15):E1018–E1026

[21] Ogden AT, Fessler RG. Minimally invasive resection of intramedullary ependymoma: case report. Neurosurgery. 2009; 65(6):E1203–E1204, discussion E1204

[22] On Tsang AC, Hang Tse PY, Ting Ng GH, Kit Leung GK. Minimal access microsurgical ligation of spinal dural arteriovenous fistula with tubular retractor. Surg Neurol Int. 2015; 6:99

[23] Patel NP, Birch BD, Lyons MK, DeMent SE, Elbert GA. Minimally invasive intradural spinal dural arteriovenous fistula ligation. World Neurosurg. 2013; 80 (6):e267–e270

[24] Tan LA, O'Toole JE. Tubular retractor selection in minimally invasive spinal tumor resection. J Neurosurg Spine. 2014; 20(5):596–597, author reply 597–598

[25] Fassett DR, Clark R, Brockmeyer DL, Schmidt MH. Cervical spine deformity associated with resection of spinal cord tumors. Neurosurg Focus. 2006; 20 (2):E2

[26] McGirt MJ, Chaichana KL, Atiba A, et al. Incidence of spinal deformity after resection of intramedullary spinal cord tumors in children who underwent laminectomy compared with laminoplasty. J Neurosurg Pediatr. 2008; 1 (1):57–62

[27] Tan LA, Takagi I, Straus D, O'Toole JE. Management of intended durotomy in minimally invasive intradural spine surgery: clinical article. J Neurosurg Spine. 2014; 21(2):279–285

[28] Tan LA, Kasliwal MK, Wewel J, Fontes RB, O'Toole JE. Minimally invasive surgery for synchronous, same-level lumbar intradural-extramedullary neoplasm and acute disc herniation. Neurosurg Focus. 2014; 37 Suppl 2:Video 16

[29] Stefini R, Peron S, Mandelli J, Bianchini E, Roccucci P. Intraoperative spinal navigation for the removal of intradural tumors: technical notes. Oper Neurosurg (Hagerstown). 2018;15(1):54 – 59

[30] Maduri R, Bobinski L, Duff JM. Image merge tailored access resection (IMTAR) of spinal intradural tumors. Technical report of 13 cases. World Neurosurg. 2017; 98:594–602

[31] Park P, Leveque JC, La Marca F, Sullivan SE. Dural closure using the U-clip in minimally invasive spinal tumor resection. J Spinal Disord Tech. 2010; 23 (7):486–489

[32] Hoover JM, Clarke MJ, Wetjen NM, Mandrekar J, Puffer RC, Krauss WE. Complications necessitating a return to the operating room following intradural spine surgery. World Neurosurg. 2012; 78(3–4):344–347

[33] Lu DC, Chou D, Mummaneni PV. A comparison of mini-open and open approaches for resection of thoracolumbar intradural spinal tumors. J Neurosurg Spine. 2011; 14(6):758–764

[34] O'Toole JE, Eichholz KM, Fessler RG. Surgical site infection rates after minimally invasive spinal surgery. J Neurosurg Spine. 2009; 11(4):471–476

[35] Omeis IA, Dhir M, Sciubba DM, et al. Postoperative surgical site infections in patients undergoing spinal tumor surgery: incidence and risk factors. Spine. 2011; 36(17):1410–1419

46 Three-Dimensional Navigation in Lumbar Spine to Facilitate Minimally Invasive Spine Surgery

Jang W. Yoon, Gaetano De Biase, and Eric W. Nottmeier

Summary

Three-dimensional navigation has increased both the efficiency of the spine surgeon and the accuracy and precision of spinal instrumentation. It is important to have adequate planning prior to starting image-guided lumbar spinal surgery. Navigation can be used in minimally invasive lumbar spinal surgery to accurately localize the underlying anatomy, thereby facilitating accurate skin incision and a safe trajectory to the underlying pathology. Although three-dimensional image-guided navigation offers the surgeon an excellent tool for accurate identification of the anatomy, this should only be used as an adjunct and should not replace a thorough knowledge of the spinal anatomy. The robotic spine procedure has still not hit its prime time due to various reasons including added complexity of the case, longer operative time versus the standard techniques, high cost of installation, and so on.

Keywords: image guidance, lumbar fusion, three-dimensional navigation, MIS, robotics, augmented reality

46.1 Introduction

The utilization of three-dimensional image guidance in spine surgery was first introduced in the mid-1990s.[1] In an effort to improve the accuracy and precision of spinal instrumentation such as pedicle screw placement, this technology has evolved from the traditional open fixation to two-dimensional fluoroscopy guidance with Kirschner wire (K-wire) placement and now to three-dimensional image guidance without the use of K-wires. This has increased both the efficiency of the spine surgeon and the safety of spinal instrumentation, all of which serve tremendous benefits for patients undergoing spine surgery. Nottmeier et al were able to demonstrate in a retrospective review of 220 consecutive patients undergoing posterior spinal fusion using three-dimensional image guidance, a low complication rate and high accuracy of instrumentation despite a high percentage of revision cases.[2] As a result of the introduction of three-dimensional image guidance, Tehli et al have demonstrated a 98% accuracy in pedicle screws placement using neuronavigation and intraoperative image guidance in spinal stabilization surgery.[3] An added advantage of three-dimensional image-guided navigation in minimally invasive spine surgery (MISS) is the complete elimination of radiation exposure to the surgeon and operating room (OR) staff, unlike the two-dimensional intraoperative fluoroscopy guidance with significant radiation exposure.[4]

Minimally invasive lumbar spine surgery continues to gain popularity among patients due to its shorter recovery time, better cosmetics, and an overall decreased morbidity.[5] Employing three-dimensional image guidance in minimally invasive lumbar spine surgery can help facilitate percutaneous instrumentation without the use of fluoroscopy or K-wires and can also enable the surgeon to register multiple vertebral segments at a time. This makes three-dimensional image-guided minimally invasive lumbar spine surgery a very attractive option for both the spine surgeon and for the patients. In this chapter, we review three-dimensional navigation in the lumbar spine and how it facilitates MISS.

46.2 Preoperative Planning

It is important to have adequate planning prior to starting image-guided lumbar spinal surgery. Spinal image guidance can be accomplished by point-matching registration using a preoperative computed tomography (CT) scan or images can be acquired intraoperatively. Other preoperative factors include adequate patient selection, positioning, neuromonitoring, and the right surgical tools needed for the specific surgery. Surgeon's competency and experience in image-guided minimally invasive lumbar spine surgeries is also paramount to the success of the operation.

46.3 Patient Selection: Indications and Contraindications

Navigation can be used in minimally invasive lumbar spinal surgery to accurately localize the underlying anatomy, thereby facilitating accurate skin incision and a safe trajectory to the underlying pathology. This is useful because it gives the surgeon an added layer of assurance especially when dealing with complex patients and distorted anatomy due to prior surgeries. Also, this technology can be applied to different minimally invasive approaches to the lumbar spine and for different conditions, including spinal deformity, degenerative disc disease, traumatic fractures, malignancy, and adjacent segment disease from previous spinal fusions.

There are few contraindications to the use of three-dimensional navigation in minimally invasive lumbar spine surgery; the first being unfamiliarity with this technology and its utilization, and any condition that precludes exposure to radiation like pregnancy.

46.4 Patient Positioning

46.4.1 Surgical Table Selection

Selecting the right table is critical for the success of image-guided lumbar spine surgery. Ideally, the surgical table should allow for easy patient positioning, exposure, and intraoperative imaging. The O-arm should be able to fit around the patient on the table and move up and down without any obstruction from the base of the table. The Jackson table is suitable for this purpose as it is able to conform to the patient's normal lumbar lordosis while in the prone position.

46.4.2 Sterile Draping

To avoid contamination of the surgical field, the entire O-arm has to be properly draped which can be a cumbersome task. Also, if not properly done, the drape can become lose and get caught during movement, which can cause delays and frustrations during surgery. The preferred method of draping the patient in our practice is to cover the patient in a 360-degree circumferential manner with sterile drapes (▶ Fig. 46.1). It is also important to make sure the reference arc is not covered by the drape as it has to be visible to the camera on the navigation system.

46.4.3 Registration Process

Accurate registration and image acquisition is a crucial step in the navigation process; therefor the surgeon must continuously validate and assess the accuracy of navigation throughout the surgery. A reference arc is percutaneously placed on the patient's iliac crest or spinous process during the registration process (▶ Fig. 46.2). This reference arc should be optimally placed between the camera and the surgical area where instruments are being tracked. The surgeon must be cautious not to move the reference arc after the registration process as this can result in navigation errors.

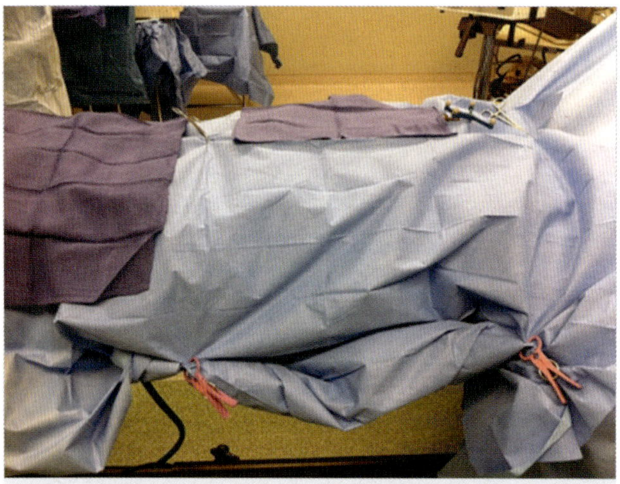

Fig. 46.1 For sterile draping technique, antibiotic irrigation solution is used to fill the surigcal cavity and split-sheet drapes is circumferentially enclosed sterily while keeping the reference arc just above the drapes. The position of the navigation camera is adjusted to ensure that the navigation arc is in line while the intraoperative cone beam computed tomography (CT) scan is obtained.

Alternatives to the reference arc exist; an example is the Stryker SpineMask tracker which can serve the same registration purpose as the reference arc and has the advantage of being minimally invasive. It is an adhesive device that can be placed on the patient's back, and offers an automatic registration process with imaging devices in the OR.

Confirming accuracy throughout the entire case is important and can be achieved by constantly touching the tip of the navigation probe on the spine and confirming the anatomy on the navigation screen. The spinous and transverse processes are suitable structures for confirming the accuracy of the navigation system. In our practice, we revalidate and recheck the accuracy of navigation after completing pedicle screw placement at each level with a known anatomic landmark (e.g., spinous process, lamina, or other boney landmarks). If any inaccuracy is detected, we obtain a new intraoperative CT scan to update the navigation images.

46.5 Surgical Technique

46.5.1 General Principles

Although three-dimensional image-guided navigation offers the surgeon an excellent tool for accurate identification of the anatomy, this should only be used as an adjunct and should not replace a thorough knowledge of the spinal anatomy. The surgeon must constantly look out for errors and should be able to identify inaccuracies when his or her anatomic knowledge of the landmark does not correlate with the navigation system.

46.5.2 Pedicle Screw Insertion Technique

In minimally invasive lumbar spine cases, navigation is used to choose the pedicle screw starting point. This is then used in the navigation computer system to plan for the size and trajectory

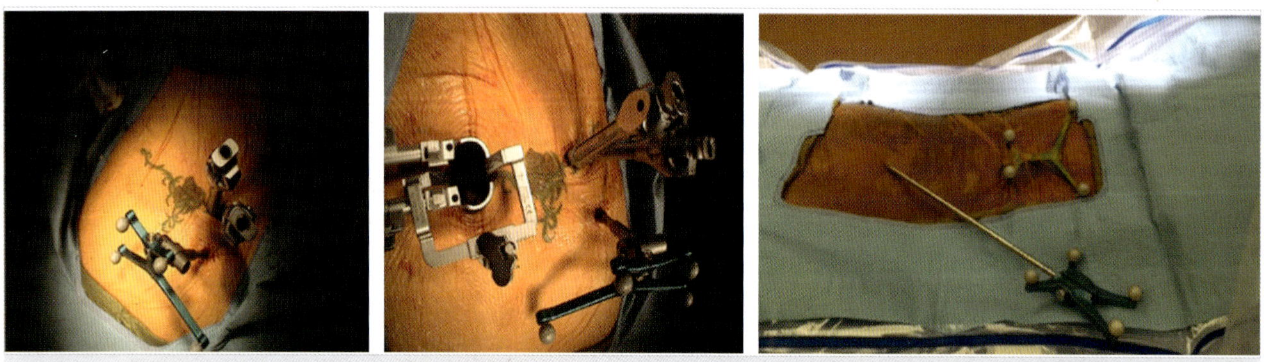

Fig. 46.2 Navigation reference arc can either be anchored to the patient's iliac crest, spinous process, or secured using strong adhesives such as Ioban. The reference is anchored to the patient's iliac crest and positioned away from surgeon's working space so that it does not interfere with the placement of spine instrumentation and surgical steps. In addition, the navigation arc is turned in line with the navigation camera. The reference arc can also be taped using Ioban. It is important for the surgeon to realize taping with Ioban can introduce inaccuracy in navigation if skin is retracted. Therefore, we typically tape the navigation arc at least 10 cm away from our planned incision and we do not use this method if spine instrumentation involves more than one level.

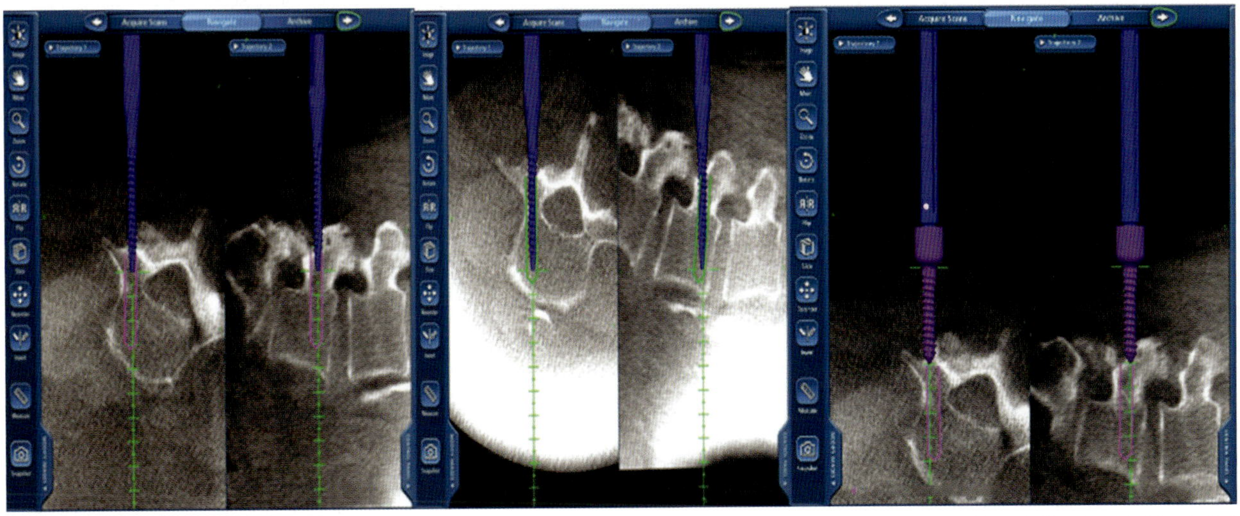

Fig. 46.3 First, the navigated probe is used to mark the location of the skin incision. A skin incision is made with a 10-blade. The navigated awl is placed on the pedicle entry point and a virtual plan for the pedicle screw is finalized. After the plan is locked into place, the awl is tapped down the pedicle thereby creating a pilot hole. The pedicle is tapped with the navigated tap. The pedicle is probed with the navigated probe as well as a ball-tip pedicle feeler to check for breach. Finally, the pedicle screw is placed using the navigated screwdriver along the virtual plan. It is important for surgeons to continually assess the tactile feel of the pedicle screw as it threads the pedicle as well as to periodically check on the navigation monitor to ensure the screw follows the intended virtual plan. This is an excellent contribution by one of the pioneers of spinal navigation. As explained, it is important to realize that three-dimensional spinal navigation encompasses not only navigation for the placement of pedicle screws, but much more: the concept of total navigation and elimination of fluoroscopy for most spinal cases, robotic surgery and also augmented reality and virtual reality for surgeon and patient education. The editors believe that stereotactic navigation technologies will significantly transform spinal surgery over the coming years.

of the of the pedicle screws, taking into account the long axis and associated bony anatomy of the pedicles. This information is then applied to the navigation images. In this method, an image-guided probe is used to determine the optimal point where the stab incision is to be made. This will allow adequate trajectory to the pedicles as determined by three-dimensional image guidance. After this point is located, a small incision is made and an image-guided awl is placed down onto the pedicle screw entry point. The intraoperative planning function of the image-guided system places a virtual plan on the tip of the instrument to enable the surgeon to determine the proper trajectory, width, and length of the screw (▶ Fig. 46.3).

46.6 Use of Robotics and Augmented Reality in Spine Surgery: Future Implications

The use of robotics in spine instrumentation has been available in the United States ever since the Mazor SpineAssist system was first introduced in 2014. Since then, the number of robotic assisted spine surgery has been on the rise and approximately 3,000 procedures have been performed in the United States in 2015.[6,7,8,9] The robotic spine procedure still has not hit its prime time due to various reasons including added complexity of the case, longer operative time versus the standard techniques, high cost of installation, and others. With the current systems available in the market, no clear advantage in the workflow, usability, interdisciplinary setups, efficacy, and cost-effectiveness has been demonstrated prospectively when compared to the standard image-guided and freehand techniques for spine instrumentation although they appear to be safe and feasible.[10,11,12,13] Currently, for pedicle screw placement, robots simply act as guides to keep the trajectory of the screws in an ideal position and a locking system in place to prevent the screw from deviating. Further modification in robotics that allows for finer tissue handling and advanced haptics for more complex manipulation are needed to make this technology widely adopted. In addition to robotic systems, there has been much interest in using head-up displays for performing surgery since the 1990s.[14,15,16] Although there has been some prior interest in using augmented reality and head-up displays in the OR, currently there are no reliable commercial head-up display visualization systems that are utilized routinely in spine surgeries. Google Glass was used successfully to project navigation images onto the surgical field in image-guided pedicle screw placement in lumbar spine, ventriculostomy, and craniotomy for supratentorial meningioma (▶ Fig. 46.4).[17,18,19] There was a decrease in time spent placing pedicle screws as well as overall improvement in operative experience for the surgeon. Considering there are 21 million image-guided surgeries performed across the United States each year or 118 million image-guided surgeries performed worldwide each year, augmented reality systems that are capable of being incorporated into currently existing navigation system can potentially have a big impact in image-guided surgeries.[20]

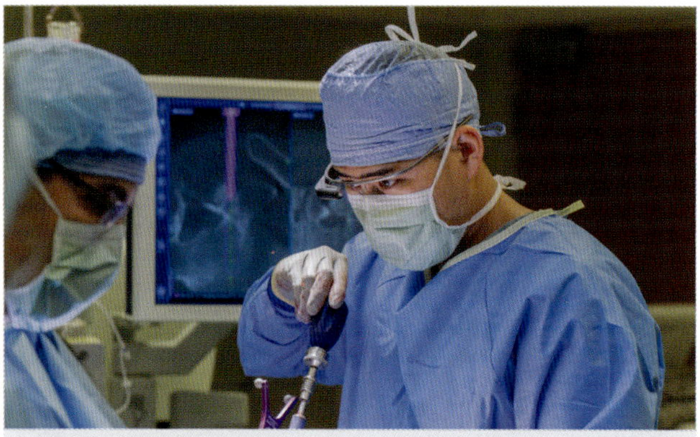

Fig. 46.4 Navigation images can be transferred via a secure WiFi network to a wearable device, in this case Google Glass, to the right upper corner of the surgeon's visual field. This eliminates the head motion that is necessary to see the navigation images during pedicle screw placement, and thus decreases the time it takes to complete the pedicle screw placement.

References

[1] Rahmathulla G, Nottmeier EW, Pirris SM, Deen HG, Pichelmann MA. Intraoperative image-guided spinal navigation: technical pitfalls and their avoidance. Neurosurg Focus. 2014; 36(3):E3

[2] Nottmeier EW, Seemer W, Young PM. Placement of thoracolumbar pedicle screws using three-dimensional image guidance: experience in a large patient cohort. J Neurosurg Spine. 2009; 10(1):33–39

[3] Tehli O, Harman F, Temiz C, et al. The use of neuronavigation and intraoperative imaging in spinal stabilization surgery. Turk Neurosurg. 2016; 26 (5):771–776

[4] Nottmeier EW, Bowman C, Nelson KL. Surgeon radiation exposure in cone beam computed tomography-based, image-guided spinal surgery. Int J Med Robot. 2012; 8(2):196–200

[5] Oppenheimer JH, DeCastro I, McDonnell DE. Minimally invasive spine technology and minimally invasive spine surgery: a historical review. Neurosurg Focus. 2009; 27(3):E9

[6] Patel V. Future of robotics in spine surgery. Spine. 2018; 43:S28

[7] Prasad S. Applications of robotics. Spine. 2018; 43(7S):S24–s25

[8] Theodore N, Ahmed AK. The history of robotics in spine surgery. Spine. 2018; 43(7S):S23

[9] Yu L, Chen X, Margalit A, Peng H, Qiu G, Qian W. Robot-assisted vs freehand pedicle screw fixation in spine surgery—a systematic review and a meta-analysis of comparative studies. Int J Med Robot. 2018; 14(3):e1892

[10] Hyun SJ, Kim KJ, Jahng TA, Kim HJ. Minimally invasive robotic versus open fluoroscopic-guided spinal instrumented fusions: a randomized controlled trial. Spine. 2017; 42(6):353–358

[11] Kim HJ, Jung WI, Chang BS, Lee CK, Kang KT, Yeom JS. A prospective, randomized, controlled trial of robot-assisted vs freehand pedicle screw fixation in spine surgery. Int J Med Robot. 2017; 13(3)

[12] Roser F, Tatagiba M, Maier G. Spinal robotics: current applications and future perspectives. Neurosurgery. 2013; 72 Suppl 1:12–18

[13] Franken RJ, Gupta SC, Banis JC , Jr, et al. Microsurgery without a microscope: laboratory evaluation of a three-dimensional on-screen microsurgery system. Microsurgery. 1995; 16(11):746–751

[14] Gupta SC, Klein SA, Barker JH, Franken R, Banis JC , Jr. Introduction of new technology to clinical practice: a guide for assessment of new VR applications. The J Med Virtual Reality. 1995:16–20

[15] Spicer MA, Apuzzo ML. Virtual reality surgery: neurosurgery and the contemporary landscape. Neurosurgery. 2003; 52(3):489–497, discussion 496–497

[16] Yoon JW, Chen RE, ReFaey K, et al. Technical feasibility and safety of image-guided parieto-occipital ventricular catheter placement with the assistance of a wearable head-up display. Int J Med Robot. 2017; 13(4)

[17] Yoon JW, Chen RE, Han PK, Si P, Freeman WD, Pirris SM. Technical feasibility and safety of an intraoperative head-up display device during spine instrumentation. Int J Med Robot. 2017; 13(3)

[18] Diaz R, Yoon J, Chen R, Quinones-Hinojosa A, Wharen R, Komotar R. Real-time video-streaming to surgical loupe mounted head-up display for navigated meningioma resection. Turk Neurosurg. 2017

[19] Macario A. What does one minute of operating room time cost? J Clin Anesth. 2010; 22(4):233–236

[20] Nottmeier EW, Fenton D. Three-dimensional image-guided placement of percutaneous pedicle screws without the use of biplanar fluoroscopy or Kirschner wires: technical note. Int J Med Robot. 2010; 6(4):483–488

47 Strategies to Minimize Invasiveness and Optimize Success: OC Fusion

Bernhard Meyer and Sandro M. Krieg

Summary
OC fusion could be one of the most complex and incapacitating procedures in spine surgery. However, true indications for OC fusion are almost unavoidable. Due to this, it is relevant to study, understand and improve our strategies to minimize invasiveness and improve outcomes. In this chapter, the authors share their experience after several publications and a thorough literature analysis about how to achieve this. In this chapter, the reader will find more information on how to avoid occipital inclusion, how to spare subaxial levels, how to avoid anterior surgery or when a transnasal approach could be better than a transoral approach all of these through a couple of case examples.

Keywords: spine, occipitocervical fusion

47.1 Introduction

47.1.1 General Considerations

The craniocervical junction (CCJ) is defined as occiput, C1 plus C2. It is a complex anatomical area, which can be affected by a range of different pathologies causing pain, myelopathy, and instability. Basis each pathology need to be taken into consideration when planning surgical treatment. Occipitocervical (OC) fusion is the treatment of choice for craniocervical instability. Most of the rotation of the spine, its flexion, and extension occur at the CCJ.[1] It is thus a procedure with considerable impact on the patients' quality of life (QOL).

In the past, several techniques were used for OC fusion, such as noninstrumented onlay graft or an onlay graft plus wire fusion and halo placement, semirigid and sublaminar-occipital wire fixation, and rigid rods with occipital plating combined with lateral mass or pedicle screws.[2,3,4,5] The latter should be regarded as today's standard of care,[6] making short constructs from C0 to C2 or C3 possible. Sparing segments is the most efficient way to reduce invasiveness of OC fusion, especially sparing the C0/C1 segment whenever possible, despite the fact that most of the cervical range of motion (ROM) happens in the atlantoaxial complex. Having the head additionally fixed in a given position has a clear negative impact on the patient's life. Because we still observe a rather liberal inclusion of the occiput into pure C1/C2 instabilities, we would primarily like to advocate a prudent use of OC fusion.

47.2 Indications for OC Fusion

As mentioned above, indications for OC fusion can be instability due to neoplastic, infectious, degenerative, inflammatory, congenital, or traumatic pathologies. Neural decompression can also require OC fusion because it may cause instability in a prior stable situation.[7]

The most common indication is still rheumatoid arthritis (RA) of the CCJ, which causes instability plus myelopathy and pain in most cases.[4,6] Especially in RA, most cases can be handled by atlantoaxial fixation alone. Moreover, the anterior decompression, formerly considered a standard, is unnecessary in almost every case, because the retrodental mass disappears usually after stabilization.[8] The strict indication for respective avoidance of anterior decompression in these procedures reduces the invasiveness of surgery even more.

Cranial settling is also not in all cases an indication for OC fusion followed by anterior decompression. One option is to distract the atlantoaxial joint with cages and fuse C1/C2 alone as popularized by Goel. If not feasible, distraction and OC fusion without anterior decompression would be second best option.

In trauma, only atlanto-occipital dislocation indicates OC fusion, a condition which is however rarely treated, because it is associated with a high rate of immediate on-site death. Any form of atlantoaxial instability even when combined (C1 ring plus C2 fracture) is nowadays not necessarily an indication to fuse the occiput. Modern screw-rod techniques make this unnecessary.

The above concepts should also be applied for tumorous, infectious, or any other indications.

Yet, revision of failed C1–C2 fixation may be an infrequent indication requiring OC fusion as presented in case 1.[4]

47.3 Risks

Bhatia and colleagues not only analyzed their own series of 100 patients who underwent OC fusion, they also performed a literature review providing comprehensive data on the largest eight series of OC fusion.[6] Follow-up of these series was between 8 and 50 months. Instrumentation failure, such as screw-rod breakage or screw loosening, averaged 4% but some series even reported up to 25%.[5,6] Yet, such high rates were only reported in older series. With the currently used technique of occipital plating and lateral mass/pedicle screws, implant failures were considerably lower. Besides this major risk, other complications, such as wound infection (4–15%), vertebral artery injury (1–4%), cerebrospinal fluid (CSF) leak (1%), and misplaced screws (4%), were reported. Due to the general state of health of most patients necessitating OC fusion, mortality rates of 1 to 8% were reported.[6]

47.4 Outcomes

Winegar et al analyzed 34 articles reporting 799 patients who underwent OC fusion due to various indications and via several techniques (graft plus wire, wire plus rod, screws, and rod).[9] In general, outcomes for OC fusion are reasonably good. Although surgical and medical adverse events sum up to around 33%, long-term outcome is usually good. Around 93% of patients show bony fusion, 82% improvement in neurology, and up to 100% improvement in pain scores.[9] On a larger scale, modern

constructs using occipital plating and lateral mass screws show superior results compared to wiring plus bone graft or wiring plus rods. Moreover, patients undergoing OC fusion due to inflammatory disease, such as RA, show better results than tumor patients.[9] Yet, it needs to be taken into account that no published series provides a level of evidence better than IV.[9]

47.5 Options for Reducing Invasiveness

In the last years, several articles were published on different decompression and fusion techniques.[10,11] In all series and analyses, constructs using plates, screws, and rods showed the best results. Not only in our opinion but also after performing an extensive literature search, there are only few published minimally invasive surgery (MIS) techniques for OC instrumentation per se using transarticular screws.[12,13]

Instead of this, as already alluded to above, the only option to reduce invasiveness, complications, recovery rates, and impact on QOL is to think "laterally," which implies (1) avoiding inclusion of the occiput whenever possible; (2) sparing subaxial segments by the use of modern constructs; (3) avoiding anterior decompression; and, if unavoidable, (4) using the endoscopic transnasal or transcervical route instead of the transoral.

As outlined above, for example, in many RA cases, fusion of the C0–C1 joint is not required pathophysiologically, which allows treating many patients by pure C1–C2 fixation. Although there are some transarticular techniques published in which C1–C2 instrumentation is done percutaneously, this technique does not allow proper preparation for bony fusion and also no distraction of the C1–C2 joint. Its indication is thus somewhat unclear to us. We advocate Harms-Goel technique for C1–C2 fusion as the default procedure. By distracting and by opening the joints on each side plus insertion of bone or cage into the joint, this technique helps to avoid anterior decompression in most cases. Moreover, in many RA cases, posterior fusion leads to shrinking of the anterior pannus within the first weeks after surgery.[8,14]

If anterior decompression is still required, the option to do it via MIS is the transnasal endoscopic route, which shows proven and distinct reduction of invasiveness, complication, and recovery rate over the traditional transoral route.

Although for many years anterior decompression of the CCJ via odontoid resection was performed transorally, peaking in the 1980s and 1990s, the considerably high morbidity of this approach led to a much stricter indication in recent years.[14,15]

According to us, it should be avoided if possible. Especially infection, dysphagia, and wound healing problems are clear arguments against the transoral route increasing the complication rates by up to 19% and above. The time for recovery is significantly longer due to the necessity of N/G tubes and/or even tracheotomies.

Thus, endoscopic transnasal odontoid resections are increasingly performed. No necessity for splitting of the soft palate, a less aggressive nasal flora, and immediate postoperative oral intake are only some of the advantages.[15] The only limitation of this approach is the rhinopalatine line, which limits the extent of resection caudally as we present in case 2 (▶ Fig. 47.1).[16,17] However, the second MIS option for anterior decompression is also presented in case 2, that is, an anterior transcervical submandibular approach for decompressions caudal to the rhinopalatine line (▶ Fig. 47.2).

47.6 Case 1

47.6.1 History

An 81-year-old female patient underwent C1–C2 fusion due to a progressive myelopathy under the assumption of RA-induced

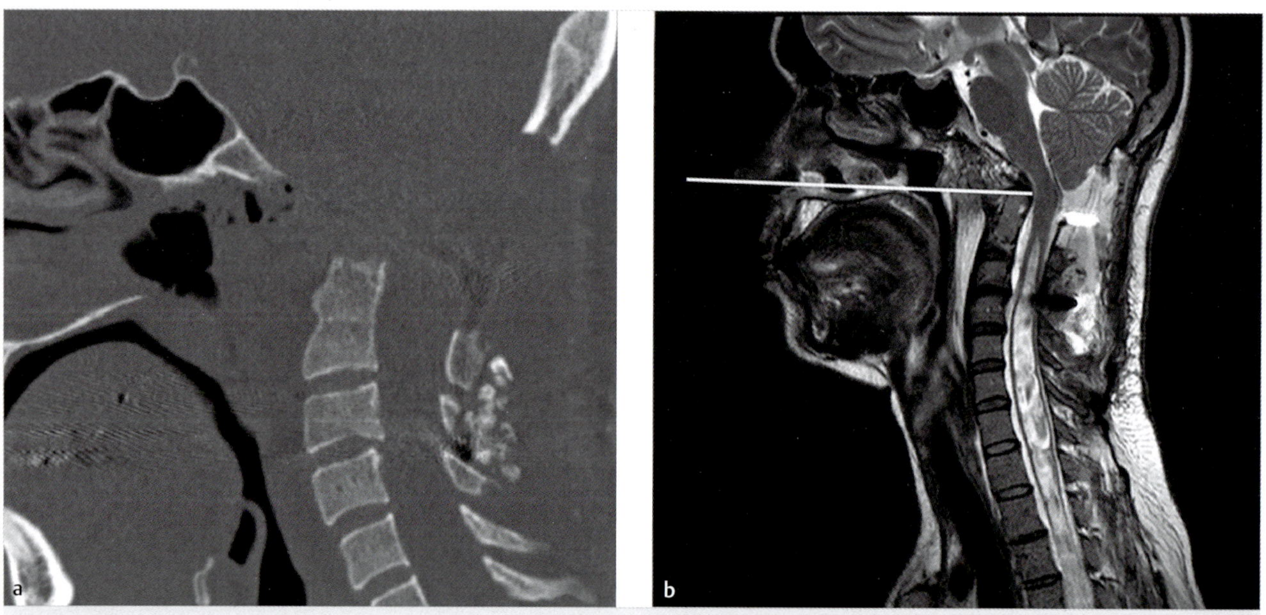

Fig. 47.1 Postoperative computed tomography (CT) and magnetic resonance imaging (MRI) scan after second surgery. This CT **(a)** and MRI **(b)** scans show the decompression of the medulla oblongata after the transnasal resection. As the white rhinopalatine line shows, the inferior extent of the endonasal odontoidectomy is limited by the nasal bone and hard palate.

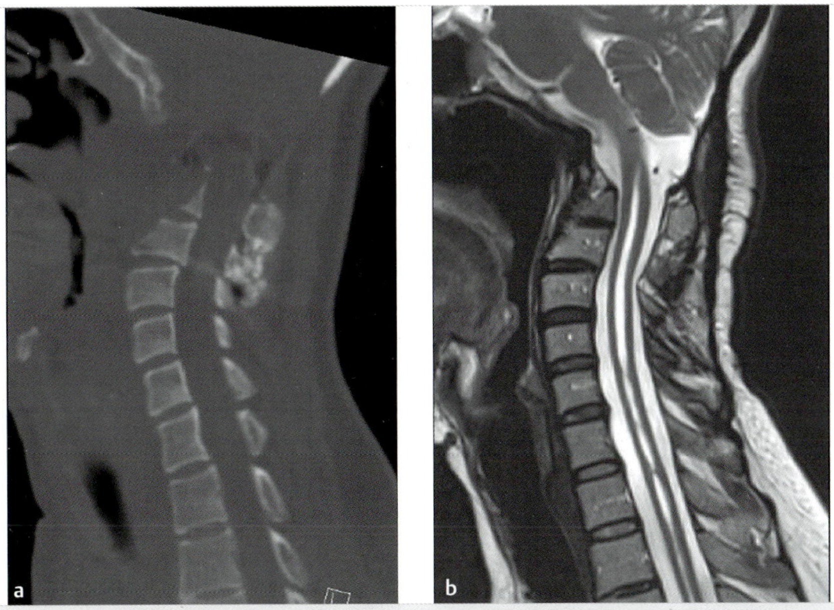

Fig. 47.2 Postoperative computed tomography (CT) and magnetic resonance imaging (MRI) scan after third surgery. This CT **(a)** and MRI **(b)** scans show the decompression of the upper cervical spinal cord after submandibular C2 resection and anterior decompression.

instability in another hospital (▶ Fig. 47.3). After instrumentation failure, she presented with increasing myelopathy and neck pain in our unit (▶ Fig. 47.4). She underwent revision surgery via occiput–C4 fusion following intraoperative distraction and posterior decompression (▶ Fig. 47.5). Neck pain improved significantly and myelopathy did not progress further.

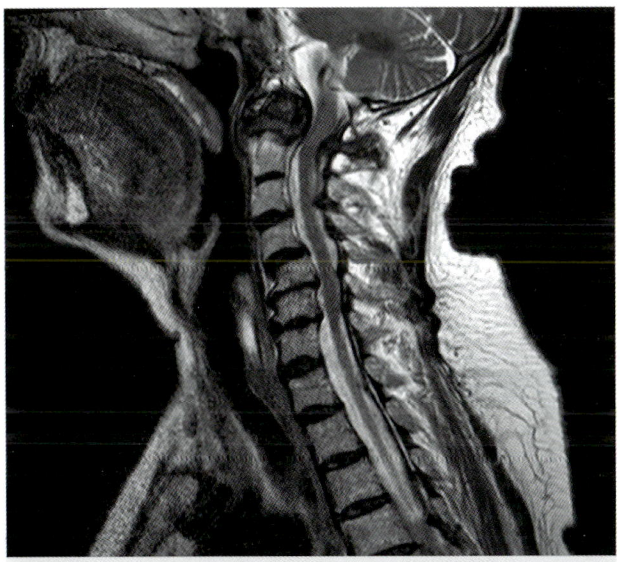

Fig. 47.3 Magnetic resonance imaging (MRI) scan prior to surgeries. This MRI scan shows the retrodental rheumatoid mass and spinal stenosis at C1 level prior to C1–C2 fusion.

47.6.2 Surgical Steps

Occipital Plate

Various occipital plate systems are available with comparable applicability. The plate is placed in the midline but caudally to the external occipital protuberance (EOP). Any placement above the EOP will cause severe healing issues of the skin. The screws are placed at the thickest part of the cranium that is runs vertically in line with the internal occipital crest. It is 10- to 15-mm thick. For preparation, the occipital bone is dissected up to the EOP. In cases of spinal canal stenosis, the posterior arch of C1 can be removed. The occipital plate is then placed in the midline and sizing and shaping should be adapted, by proper bending. The first screw is planned via setting the drill guide to 8 to 10 mm at the beginning continued by longer burr depth until the internal tabula is breeched. Preoperatively this can be measured on sagittal CT reconstructions of the midline and the level of the screw placements. The screw hole is palpated in order to verify that the internal tabula was penetrated. A cortical blunt screw of the respective length is then inserted. However, it is crucial that all screws are placed bicortically. There should still be some movement of the plate for further adjustment. The other screws are then inserted in the same way. If systems with lateral screws are used, consider that the bone is far thinner than in the midline (around 5 mm); yet all screws shall be placed bicortically.

Cervical Screws

C1 fixation requires lateral mass screws. Subperiosteal preparation of the lower lateral arch of C1 reduces the frequently known massive blood loss from the venous vertebral plexus when placing the screws. Drilling of the lower lateral arch of C1 along the screws' trajectory enables a more cranial entry point but also contributes to further reducing blood loss due to reduced retraction of the C2 root.

Transarticular screws are only an option of choice if C1–C2 distraction is not necessary. We prefer C2 pars screws since

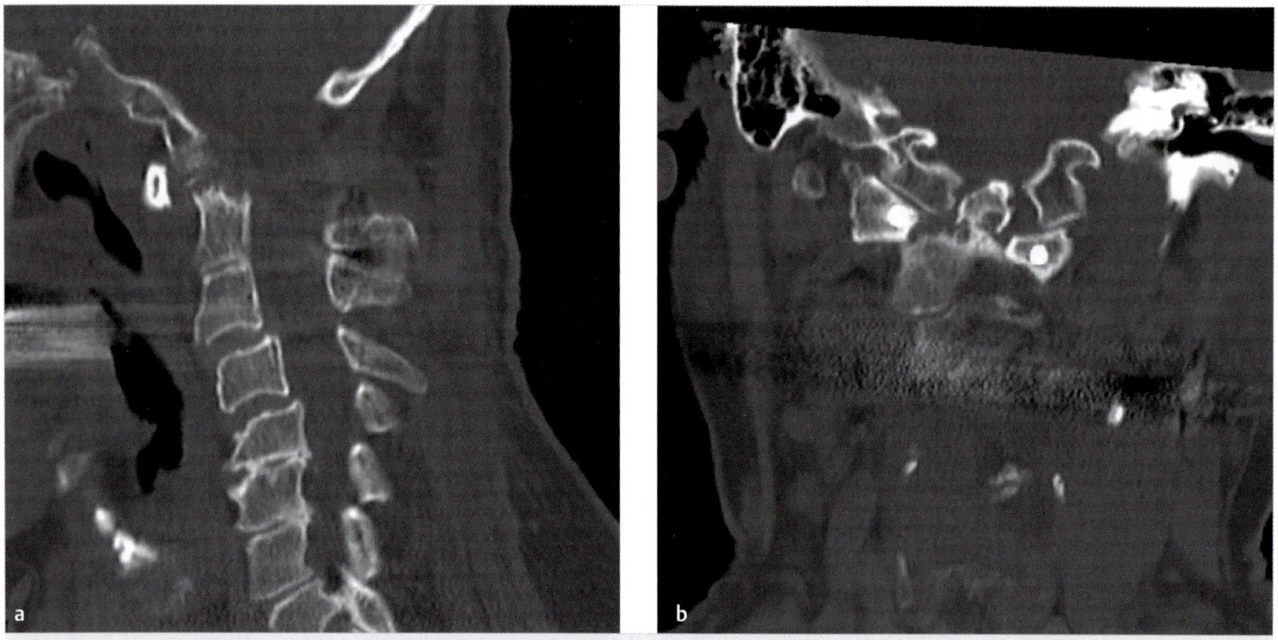

Fig. 47.4 Preoperative computed tomography (CT) scan. This CT scan shows failure C1–C2 fixation including rotation of C1–C2 and new odontoid displacement. **(a)** Sagittal and **(b)** coronal.

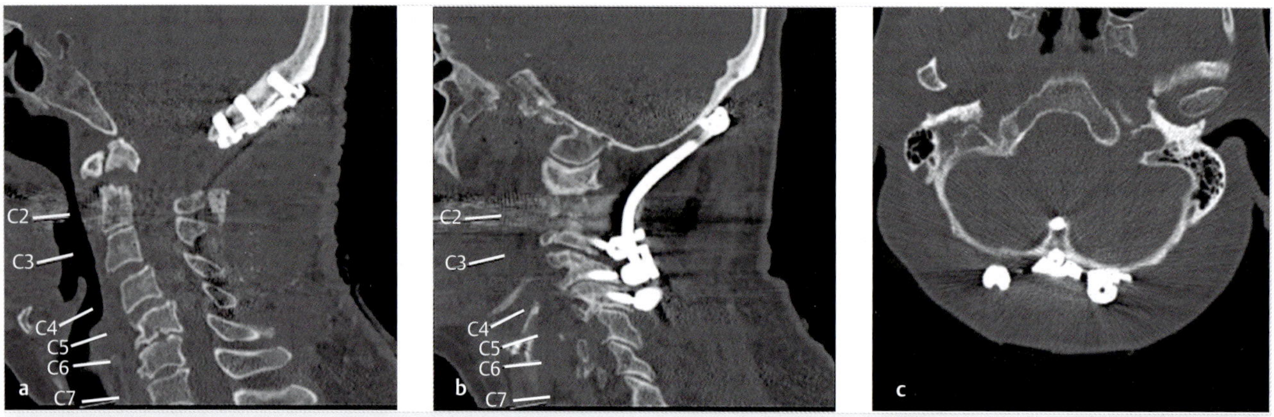

Fig. 47.5 Postoperative computed tomography (CT) scan. Postoperative CT scan showing C0 to C4 instrumentation with lateral mass screws. Distraction and decompression can be appreciated. **(a)** Midline sagittal, **(b)** paramedian sagittal showing the facet joint, and **(c)** axial.

they are low risk screws, provide firm instrumentation, and the tulips end in line with the occiput and C1 screws (▶ Fig. 47.6).

Instrumentation and Graft

The lowest level of cervical fixation should be chosen by the most caudal extent of stenosis or instability.

In terms of alignment, proper positioning in the head clamp is crucial. Optimally, horizontal gaze should be the goal. Before placing the rods, lamina facets and posterior aspects of the skull should be decorticated to provide optimal conditions for bony fusion. After the rod placement, bone grafting should be done.

Some options for grafting material are available:

a) Local bone from occipital external tabula, lamina, or spinous process.
b) Autograft (iliac crest).
c) Allograft.
d) Biomaterials.

The bone graft is placed on the decorticated dorsal areas and held in place by rod connectors or suture. Currently, the use of bone forming agents such as bone morphogenetic proteins (BMP) are off label.

47.7 Case 2

47.7.1 History

A 40-year-old female patient suffered from headache and myelopathy due to a Chiari malformation Type I with basilar

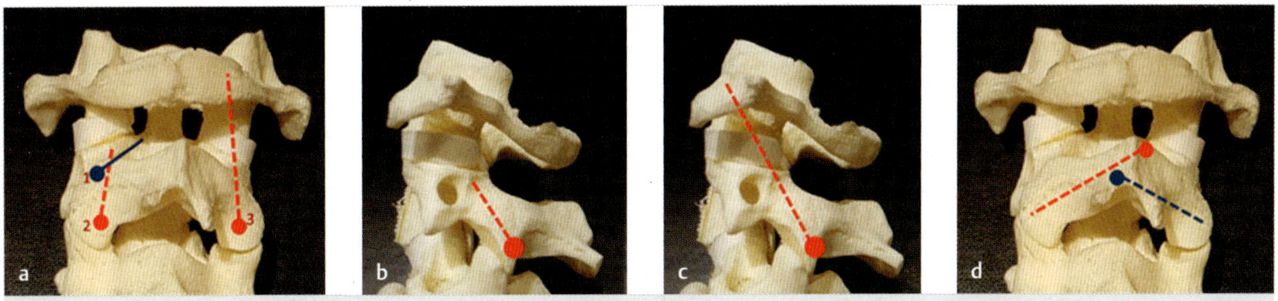

Fig. 47.6 C2 screw options. **(a)** (1) C2 pedicle screw trajectory, (2) C2 pars screw trajectory, (3) C2–C1 transarticular screw. **(b)** Lateral view of A#2 (pars screw). **(c)** Lateral view of A#3 (transarticular screw). **(d)** C2 translaminar screws. (Reproduced from Joaquim A, Riew K. Axis Screw Fixation: A Step-by-Step Review of the Surgical Techniques. Arquivos Brasileiros de Neurocirurgia: Brazilian Neurosurgery 2017; 36(02):101–107, Fig. 2.)

impression (▸ Fig. 47.7). Pain and myelopathy progressed within months. The imaging showed additional syringomyelia and assimilation of C1 to the occiput (▸ Fig. 47.8).

She then underwent C1–C3 fusion in our department with intraoperative distraction and posterior decompression via foramen magnum (plus C1) decompression and laminectomy C2 (▸ Fig. 47.9). As scheduled before the instrumentation, anterior decompression was performed due to the severe compression of the medulla oblongata via a transnasal endoscopic approach (▸ Fig. 47.3). Since the lower part of C2 still caused considerable spinal cord compression, further C2 resection was performed via a submandibular approach (▸ Fig. 47.4). The patient recovered quickly from all three surgeries. At her last visit 4 years after surgery, bony fusion was excellent and the myelopathy dissolved completely.

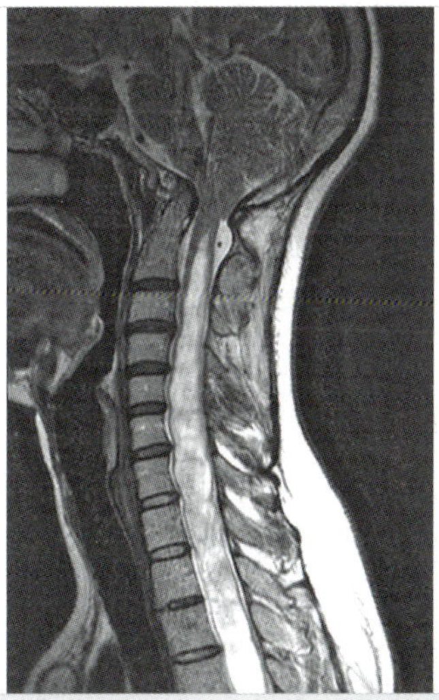

Fig. 47.7 Initial magnetic resonance imaging (MRI) scan. This MRI scan shows a Chiari malformation Type I combined with a basilar invagination causing foramen magnum stenosis and syringomyelia.

47.7.2 Surgical Steps for Transnasal Approach

The patient underwent C1–C3 instrumentation and fusion as outlined in case 1.

47.7.3 Transnasal Approach

1. Intubation:
   The transnasal endoscopic odontoid resection was scheduled. We use a four-hand binostril technique. After transoral, endotracheal intubation, patients are positioned in supine position with the head fixed in a head clamp. Midface, forehead, and nose are disinfected and draped, leaving all three free for sterile CT surface registration. After OC fusion, the navigational CT scan can then also be used for the instrumented upper cervical spine.
2. Dissection:
   The dorsal vomer is resected via a binostril approach. From the bony floor of the sphenoid sinus and the clivus in the midline to the carotid protuberance laterally, the neuronavigation guides the tip of the odontoid below soft tissue which is then incised.
3. Odontoidectomy:
   The odontoid is thinned by a high-speed 4-mm diamond drill from the tip to the base, limited caudally by the hard palate. While drilling caudally, the atlas' anterior arch is reached and drilled. When sufficient decompression is reached, pulsation of the soft tissue can be seen as the transmitted CSF pulsation.
4. Closure:
   After ensuring sufficient decompression, the local wound is covered by fibrin glue only. Usually, patients can be extubated the day of surgery but require a gastric tube for 7 days followed by regular oral diet.
   Occipitocervical fusion is one of the more invasive procedures done by spine surgeons and presents a challenge when it comes to minimally invasive spine surgery (MISS). However, this chapter outlines some techniques used by the authors to cut down on the invasiveness of the procedure. As MISS surgeons we should focus more on the challenges of addressing cervical procedures, especially those involving fusion procedures and the OC junction.

47.7.4 Tips and Tricks for the Endonasal Approach

From an equipment point of view, a considerably long angled drill and hand piece (18 cm) is required. A straight 4-mm endoscope with an irrigation shaft is sufficient. For optimal visualization of the odontoid base, a 30 degrees optic can be used. Depending on the level of medulla oblongata and spinal cord

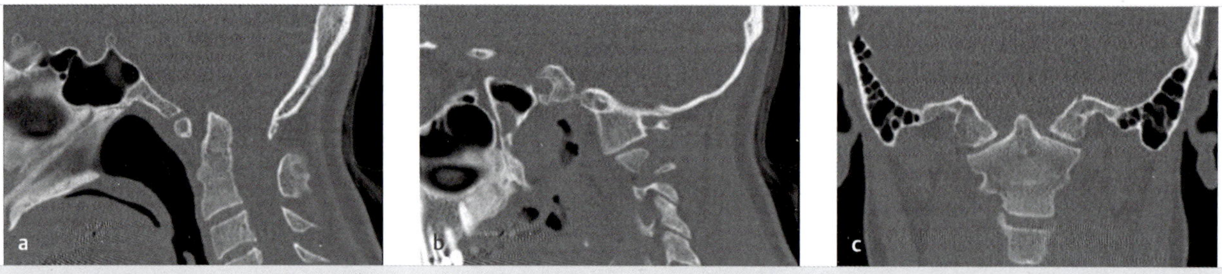

Fig. 47.8 Initial computed tomography (CT) scan. The CT scan shows the high-riding odontoid and assimilation of C1 to the occiput in sagittal midline **(a)**, sagittal paramedian **(b)**, and coronal **(c)** slices.

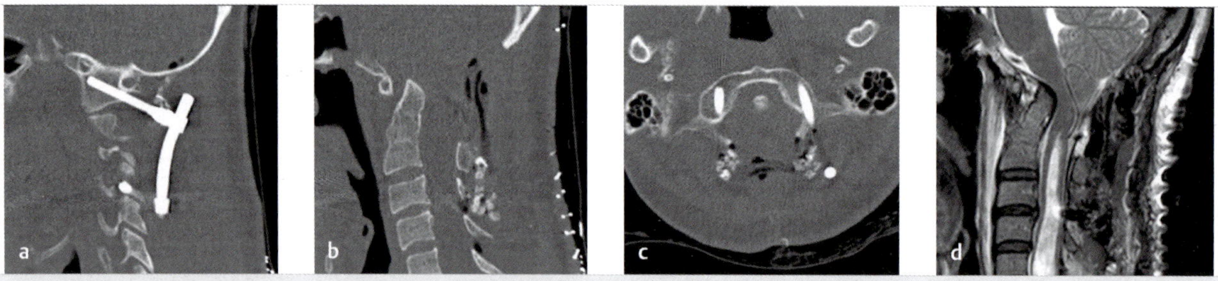

Fig. 47.9 Postoperative computed tomography (CT) and magnetic resonance imaging (MRI) scan after first surgery. This CT scan shows occipitocervical (OC) fusion via instrumentation of the assimilated C1 to C3 in sagittal paramedian **(a)**, sagittal median **(b)**, and axial slices at C1 **(c)**. The MRI scan shows considerable decompression but still persisting anterior compression of the medulla oblongata due to the odontoid **(d)**.

compression, the sphenoid sinus needs to be opened or not. The dorsal part of the nasal septum/vomer should be resected in all cases in order to allow for a binostril approach.

The same patient in this case also required a more caudal resection that was limited by the hard palate via the endonasal route. Thus, in order to avoid the transoral approach due to the abovementioned reasons, a submandibular anterior approach similar to that for a C2/C3 anterior cervical discectomy and fusion (ACDF) was used. This approach is quick and surgically straightforward, known by all spine surgeons, and therefore offers a considerably low rate of complications. As ▶ Fig. 47.7 and ▶ Fig. 47.8 show, it allows for a very caudal decompression even in patients with basilar impression.

The approach is very high and the mandible limits the cranial extent. Endonasal intubation, however, enables full closure of the jaw and therefore another 10 to 14 mm of space cranially since it allows for a more cranial retraction of the mandible.

47.8 Discussion

As mentioned above, MIS options for OC fusion lie mainly within the avoidance of some traditional concepts:

a) Limiting fusions to C1 instead of occiput if possible.
b) Reducing the necessity of anterior decompression by distraction and posterior decompression.
c) Using transnasal endoscopic or transcervical anterior decompression if needed.

The odontoid process is one of the most difficult spinal areas to reach. The transoral route is still commonly used. However, the transnasal approach became more popular in recent years[17] and it has several advantages which need to be detailed:

a) It can be used with standard equipment by a neurosurgical team without the necessity of an access surgeon.
b) In combination with neuronavigation and possibly intraoperative imaging, the extent of decompression can be estimated very well.
c) Complications arising from the soft tissue defect are rare compared to the transoral approach.[18]
d) Opening of the pharynx is not required thus avoiding the bacterial flora of the oral cavity.[19]
e) Especially in patients with a higher prevalence of swallowing problems, splitting of the soft palate with consequent velopharyngeal incompetence is not required.[20]
f) Time to extubation (3.5 d transoral vs. 0.43 d transnasal) and time to feeding (5.2 d transoral vs. 3.86 d transnasal) are low.[18]

This approach is limited to midline decompression and any process lower than the rhinopalatine line cannot be resected, thus requiring an additional submandibular approach as outlined in case 2. Yet, especially in cases of basilar impression, the odontoid is considerably high.[16]

47.9 Conclusion

Although there is no reasonable approach to make OC fusion itself less invasive, there are several ways to treat the pathologies requiring OC fusion less invasively, mostly by segment-sparing instrumentations, such as C1–C2, avoiding anterior decompression and, if indicated, endoscopic transnasal decompression.

References

[1] Wolfla CE. Anatomical, biomechanical, and practical considerations in posterior occipitocervical instrumentation. Spine J. 2006; 6(6) Suppl:225S–232S

[2] Newman P, Sweetnam R. Occipito-cervical fusion: an operative technique and its indications. J Bone Joint Surg Br. 1969; 51(3):423–431

[3] Itoh T, Tsuji H, Katoh Y, Yonezawa T, Kitagawa H. Occipito-cervical fusion reinforced by Luque's segmental spinal instrumentation for rheumatoid diseases. Spine. 1988; 13(11):1234–1238

[4] Nockels RP, Shaffrey CI, Kanter AS, Azeem S, York JE. Occipitocervical fusion with rigid internal fixation: long-term follow-up data in 69 patients. J Neurosurg Spine. 2007; 7(2):117–123

[5] Vale FL, Oliver M, Cahill DW. Rigid occipitocervical fusion. J Neurosurg. 1999; 91(2) Suppl:144–150

[6] Bhatia R, Desouza RM, Bull J, Casey AT. Rigid occipitocervical fixation: indications, outcomes, and complications in the modern era. J Neurosurg Spine. 2013; 18(4):333–339

[7] Klekamp J. Chiari I malformation with and without basilar invagination: a comparative study. Neurosurg Focus. 2015; 38(4):E12

[8] Landi A, Marotta N, Morselli C, Marongiu A, Delfini R. Pannus regression after posterior decompression and occipito-cervical fixation in occipito-atlanto-axial instability due to rheumatoid arthritis: case report and literature review. Clin Neurol Neurosurg. 2013; 115(2):111–116

[9] Winegar CD, Lawrence JP, Friel BC, et al. A systematic review of occipital cervical fusion: techniques and outcomes. J Neurosurg Spine. 2010; 13(1):5–16

[10] Kukreja S, Ambekar S, Sin AH, Nanda A. Occipitocervical fusion surgery: review of operative techniques and results. J Neurol Surg B Skull Base. 2015; 76(5):331–339

[11] Morales-Valero SF, Serchi E, Zoli M, Mazzatenta D, Van Gompel JJ. Endoscopic endonasal approach for craniovertebral junction pathology: a review of the literature. Neurosurg Focus. 2015; 38(4):E15

[12] Gonzalez LF, Crawford NR, Chamberlain RH, et al. Craniovertebral junction fixation with transarticular screws: biomechanical analysis of a novel technique. J Neurosurg. 2003; 98(2) Suppl:202–209

[13] Grob D. Transarticular screw fixation for atlanto-occipital dislocation. Spine. 2001; 26(6):703–707

[14] Chieng LO, Madhavan K, Vanni S. Pooled data analysis on anterior versus posterior approach for rheumatoid arthritis at the craniovertebral junction. Neurosurg Focus. 2015; 38(4):E18

[15] Choi D, Crockard HA. Evolution of transoral surgery: three decades of change in patients, pathologies, and indications. Neurosurgery. 2013; 73(2):296–303, discussion 303–304

[16] La Corte E, Aldana PR, Ferroli P, et al. The rhinopalatine line as a reliable predictor of the inferior extent of endonasal odontoidectomies. Neurosurg Focus. 2015; 38(4):E16

[17] Liu JK, Patel J, Goldstein IM, Eloy JA. Endoscopic endonasal transclival transodontoid approach for ventral decompression of the craniovertebral junction: operative technique and nuances. Neurosurg Focus. 2015; 38(4):E17

[18] Komotar R J, Starke R M, Raper D MS, Anand V K, Schwartz T H. Endonasal endoscopic versus transoral microscopic odontoid resection. Innovative Neurosurg. 2013; 1(1):37–47

[19] Baird CJ, Conway JE, Sciubba DM, Prevedello DM, Quiñones-Hinojosa A, Kassam AB. Radiographic and anatomic basis of endoscopic anterior craniocervical decompression: a comparison of endonasal, transoral, and transcervical approaches. Neurosurgery. 2009; 65(6) Suppl:158–163, discussion 63–64

[20] Nayak JV, Gardner PA, Vescan AD, Carrau RL, Kassam AB, Snyderman CH. Experience with the expanded endonasal approach for resection of the odontoid process in rheumatoid disease. Am J Rhinol. 2007; 21(5):601–606

48 Strategies to Minimize Invasiveness and Optimize Success: Cervical Front/Back Surgery for Deformity Correction

Lee A. Tan and K. Daniel Riew

Summary

Surgical treatment of cervical spine deformity can be challenging. In this chapter, we provide a detailed narrative review of preoperative evaluation, surgical planning, and surgical techniques for cervical deformity correction with an illustrative case. Various strategies for minimizing surgical invasiveness and complication avoidance in cervical deformity surgery were also discussed.

Keywords: cervical spine deformity, anterior osteotomy, Smith-Petersen osteotomy, pedicle subtraction osteotomy, complication avoidance

48.1 Introduction

Cervical spine deformities can have significant negative impact on patients' quality of life. Many different surgical techniques exist for operative treatment of cervical spine deformities, including anterior cervical discectomy and fusion (ACDF), cervical corpectomy, anterior osteotomy with bilateral uncinate resection (ATO), posterior cervical instrumentation and fusion with or without laminectomy, Smith-Petersen osteotomy (SPO), and pedicle subtraction osteotomy (PSO). For flexible cervical deformities, anterior or posterior approach alone may be adequate for deformity correction. However, rigid cervical deformity correction often requires a multistage surgery utilizing a combination of anterior and posterior techniques.

In this chapter, we provide an illustrative case to demonstrate the decision algorithm for selecting the appropriate and least invasive approach for cervical spine deformity correction that minimizes surgical morbidity and optimizes clinical outcome.

48.2 Surgical Planning for Cervical Spine Deformity

An essential part of any successful surgery requires a sound surgical plan based on clear understanding of the pathology and well-defined goals of surgery. In the setting of cervical spine deformity, the surgeon must consider how much correction of the deformity is required and if any neural decompression is needed. The main goals for cervical spine deformity surgery should include adequate deformity correction in order to restore horizontal gaze and lessen spinal cord tension, and decompress the neural elements if needed, achieving a biomechanically sound construct with meticulous arthrodesis technique to minimize the risk of pseudarthrosis and other surgical complications. Several important factors must be considered preoperatively, including: (1) presence of any spinal cord or nerve root compression, (2) flexibility of the deformity, (3) presence of bony fusion, (4) location of the deformity, (5) prior cervical surgery, (6) degenerative changes at adjacent spinal levels, and lastly (7) the patient's general health status and medical comorbidities.

Preoperative dynamic X-rays, magnetic resonance imaging (MRI), and computed tomography (CT) of the cervical spine must be carefully studied. If significant ventral compression of the spinal cord is present, then an anterior approach usually needs to be included in the overall treatment strategy to ensure adequate spinal cord decompression. However, if an indirect decompression can be achieved via deformity correction, the posterior-only approach may be adequate. Furthermore, if the structural integrity of the anterior spinal column is compromised, such as in the setting of infection or neoplasm, then the anterior approach is usually necessary to address the anterior pathology and reconstruct the anterior spinal column.

The flexibility of the deformity is also an important factor in determining the overall treatment strategy and can be assessed on dynamic cervical X-rays. If the deformity is flexible and corrects on extension, then a posterior-only approach may be possible to obtain adequate deformity correction. If the deformity is stiff, then thin-cut CT should be obtained to evaluate for presence and location of possible existing bony fusion. If the facet joints are not fused, then anterior-only correction may be possible, although some surgeons may still prefer backing up the construct posteriorly if the anterior instrumentation spans more than three levels (anterior-posterior). If the facet joints *and* the anterior spinal column are fused, then posterior release may need to be performed prior to anterior correction, followed by posterior instrumentation and fusion with or without additional osteotomy (posterior-anterior-posterior), depending on the extent of correction needed.

The location of kyphotic deformity is also an important factor in formulating the overall treatment plan. A focal kyphotic deformity in the mid-cervical spine usually can be corrected via anterior corpectomy; a severe focal kyphotic deformity at the cevicothoracic junction can be treated with either a C7 or T1 PSO. In patients with cervical spinal deformity and concurrent severe thoracic kyphosis, additional osteotomies in the thoracic spine may be required to obtain the necessary correction.

If the patient had prior cervical spine surgery, prior operative reports should be obtained and reviewed to gain information regarding the type of surgery performed, the specific instrumentation used, and any pertinent intraoperative findings. Prior fusion mass should be assessed with CT to check for pseudoarthrosis. If a prior anterior cervical approach is used, it is preferable to go through the contralateral side to avoid scar tissues; however, otolaryngology consultation must be obtained preoperatively to confirm vocal cord motility bilaterally. If the recurrent or superior laryngeal nerve has been injured or ear, nose, and throat (ENT) evaluation is unable to be obtained for any reason, then the ipsilateral side should be used to avoid

possible bilateral recurrent laryngeal nerve injuries. If a prior posterior cervical spine surgery was performed, the wound should be inspected for the integrity of soft tissues. If the muscles are dehisced and there is a large cavity in the center of the wound or poor soft tissue coverage, then wound-related complications are much more common. Dehisced muscles have to be mobilized from their lateral position and reattached in the midline. If the surgeon does not have experience with such techniques, a plastic surgery consultation should be obtained.

To formulate a sound surgical plan, the desired amount of correction must be calculated to determine the specific surgical techniques required. Although there is no universally accepted "normal values" for cervical alignment parameters, current limited literature suggests that T1 slope minus C2–C7 lordosis < 15 degrees, C2–C7 sagittal vertical axis (SVA) < 40 mm, and chin-brow vertical angle (CBVA) between −10 degrees and + 20 degrees are generally acceptable ranges.[1,2,3,4] Of course, each patient is unique and the optimal surgical correction needs to be determined on individual basis. As a general rule, the amount of lordosis (kyphosis correction) obtained is about 5 degrees for a single-level ACDF, 10 degrees for an SPO, 17 degrees for an ATO, and up to 35 degrees for a C7 PSO.[5,6]

48.3 Surgical Technique to Minimize Invasiveness

Anterior cervical surgery is already a relatively minimally invasive approach. One can perform even an eight-level anterior operation from C2 to T3 through a cosmetically pleasing single or double transverse incisions. To minimize trauma to the trachea and esophagus, we dissect as though we are performing two levels more than what is required (e.g., to perform a C3–C7 operation, we dissect to expose C2 to T1). When this exposure wide, less retraction force is required and therefore, less trauma to the midline structures. We also move the retractor to expose one to two levels at a time so that the retraction time is minimized at each level. We work as quickly as possible and make every attempt to keep the retraction time to less than 3 hours. If the retraction time is greater than 3.5 to 4 hours, we usually keep the patient intubated at least overnight and check a cuff leak test prior to extubating.

In contrast to the anterior exposure, the posterior exposure for a circumferential procedure for a deformity correction would hardly qualify as a "minimally invasive" procedure. However, much can be done to minimize the exposure. We utilize a muscle-sparing approach to the posterior cervical spine. This involves finding the avascular and amuscular midline, which is more difficult than it sounds. As someone so aptly put it, "the midline is rarely in the middle and there is no line." The easiest way to find this is to palpate the C7 spinous process and cut down to it. Then, we carefully dissect cranially from that point under the microscope. The spinous processes are palpated repeatedly to maintain a midline dissection. Deep to the fascia, we use blunt dissection with the index finger to separate the two halves. If that proves ineffective, we use monopolar electrocautery or Metzenbaum scissors. Meticulous dissection helps to optimize healing, prevent bleeding, and decrease postoperative pain associated with the procedure. If the exposure has been done correctly, the muscles should still be enveloped in their fascia and there should be minimal bleeding. After exposing the spinous processes, we use electrocautery, without power, as a dissector to identify and widen the raphe between the two halves of the interspinalis muscle, which connects one spinous process to the next. Note that there is no interspinous ligament in the cervical spine. The interspinalis muscle is found in its place. We then cut each half of the bifid spinous process with a bone cutter, leaving the muscle attached to each side. If the spinous process is not bifid, we cut a thin sliver of bone on each side of the monofid process. During the closure, we will place sutures lateral to these bony fragments, so that the closure is bone-to-bone, instead of muscle-to-muscle. This helps to minimize muscle trauma during closure and also helps to prevent dehiscence.

We continue the deep dissection with an electrocautery set to 20, minimizing the burn and lightly dissecting the muscles subperiosteally off the lamina. There is minimal bleeding until one gets just lateral to the beginning of the lateral mass, where there are bony bleeders. These can be controlled with bone wax. The dissection stops at the lateral border of the lateral mass because further laterally, there is a venous plexus that bleeds profusely.

Just as important as the dissection is the closure. We place a deep drain and leave hemostatic agents superficial to the drain, so long as the lamina is intact to protect the cord. If there has been a laminectomy, one cannot leave hemostatic agents in the wound, as they will expand and cause cord compression. We then put in approximately 500 mg of vancomycin powder and sprinkle another 500 mg at every layer during closure. We typically use 120–150 pop-off sutures (placed every 7–10 mm) to close the wound. This leaves no dead space in which fluid, which can be a nidus for an infection, can accumulate. We have not had an infection in the posterior cervical spine in the last 2,000 + cases. The first layer of closure is the bone-to-bone spinous process re-approximation. Then, if the dissection was done correctly, the fascial covering of the muscles should be undisturbed and this fascia is used to close the wound. It takes three to four layers to close this layer. The next layer is the supraspinous and nuchal ligament complex. Above that, the fat layer is closed with 2–0 pop-off sutures with no dead space. We close the skin with subcuticular sutures to enhance cosmesis.

48.4 Case Illustration

48.4.1 Presentation

A 20-year-old male patient presented with progressive gait imbalance and worsening right upper extremity weakness. His pertinent past medical history included achondroplasia and multiple craniospinal surgeries including suboccipital craniectomy with C1–C2 laminectomies, and spinal fusion from C5 to L4. Physical examination was remarkable for diffuse right arm weakness (4/5), as well as overt myelopathic signs including hyperreflexia in bilateral upper and lower extremities, positive Hoffmann's reflex bilaterally, clonus, and unsteady gait.

48.4.2 Imaging Studies

The cervical spine X-rays revealed a kyphotic cervical deformity with C2–C7 kyphosis measuring 36.1 degrees; the apex of the kyphosis was located at C2–C3 and C3–C4 above the prior fused

levels (▶ Fig. 48.1). Dynamic cervical X-rays showed that the deformity was rigid without any movement on flexion and extension (▶ Fig. 48.2). The MRI of the cervical spine demonstrated severe cervical stenosis and anterior cord compression at C2–C3 and C3–C4 (▶ Fig. 48.3). The C2–C7 SVA was measured to be 37.2 mm. Given the patient's worsening neurological status, surgical correction of the fixed cervical deformity with spinal cord decompression was deemed the most appropriate management strategy.

Since the kyphotic deformity in this patient was rigid and not flexible on flexion/extension X-rays, anterior cervical osteotomies were planned at C2–C3, C3–C4 along with C4–C5 ACDF for anterior column release, along with posterior cervical spine decompression, instrumentation, and fusion from C2 to C5 with connection to the prior posterior spinal instrumentations. The rationale of utilizing anterior osteotomy for anterior column release in this case is that it obviates the need for a more invasive, and more biomechanically unstable, multilevel anterior cervical corpectomy; it also reduces the need for challenging and more invasive posterior osteotomies such as cervical SPO and PSO.

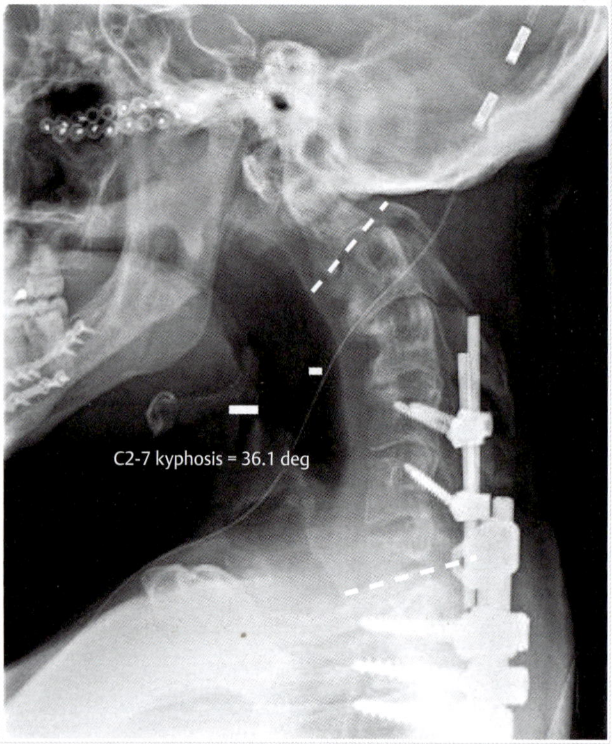

Fig. 48.1 The cervical spine X-rays revealed a kyphotic cervical deformity with C2–C7 kyphosis measuring 36.1 degrees; the apex of the kyphosis is located at C2–C3 and C3–C4 above the prior fused levels.

Of note, one important surgical pearl during the anterior part of this case is to use stand-alone anterior cervical cages with only a single screw holding the cage anterior osteotomy sites. This strategy allows additional kyphosis correction during the posterior stage, where additional cervical lordosis can be obtained via the anterior osteotomy sites with neck extension during the posterior approach. Furthermore, the course of both vertebral arteries must be carefully studied on preoperative imaging, given that soft tissue dissection during anterior osteotomy would extend lateral to the uncinate process. Any aberrant course of the vertebral arteries must be carefully noted to minimize the risk of inadvertent vertebral artery injuries while performing uncinate resection during an anterior cervical osteotomy.

Strategies to reduce the invasiveness of complex front/back cervical deformity correction procedures include meticulous surgical planning in order to define the goal of the surgery and avoid overtreatment, the preference of anterior versus posterior surgery if possible, and muscle-sparing dissection for the posterior approach.

48.4.3 Surgical Technique

1. The patient was brought into the operating room and underwent general endotracheal anesthesia. During the initial positioning, the patient's head can be suspended in the air in cases of severe rigid cervical kyphotic deformities. In this situation, we recommend using folded sheets to support the head at the beginning of the case. The sheets can be taken away by the anesthesia team as each level of anterior osteotomy is completed to facilitate kyphosis correction. Cervical traction with Gardner-Wells tongs with 15 pounds of traction can also be applied to facilitate intubation and initial approach to the kyphotic anterior cervical spine.
2. After successful intubation, the anterior neck was prepped and draped in the usual fashion. The microscope was draped and brought into the field to be used throughout the procedure. A standard, left side Smith-Robinson approach was used to expose the anterior cervical spine from C2 to C5.

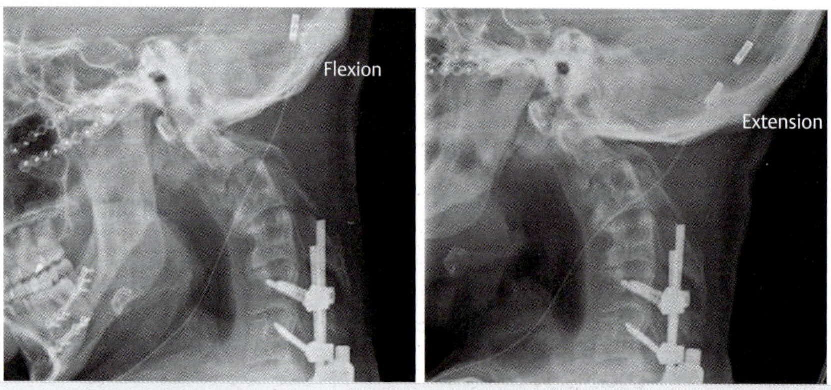

Fig. 48.2 Dynamic cervical X-rays demonstrated that the deformity was rigid with no movement on flexion and extension.

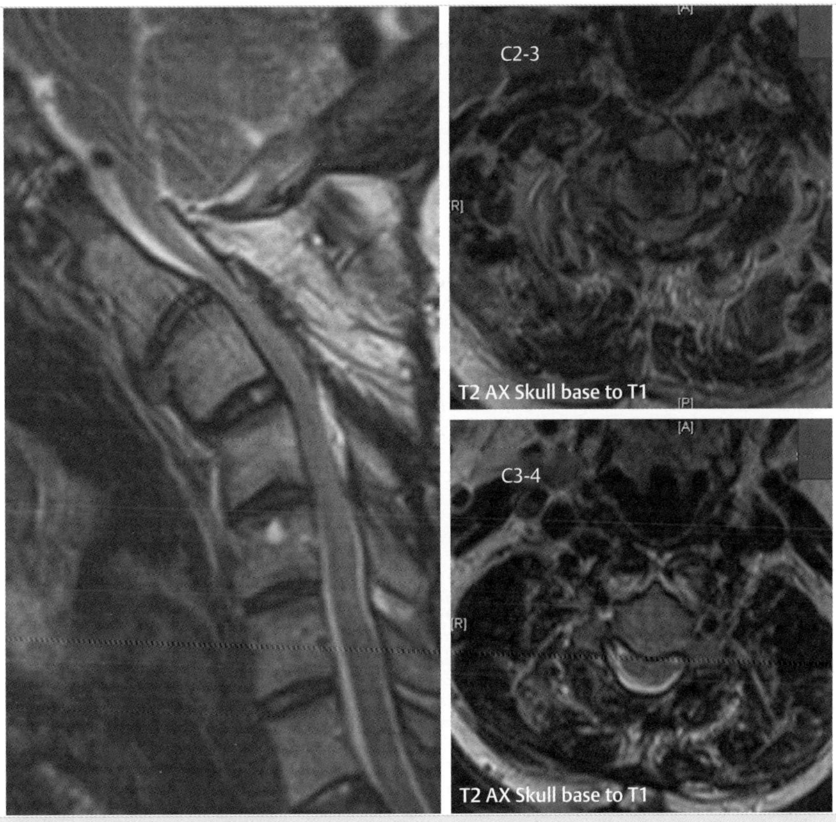

Fig. 48.3 Magnetic resonance imaging (MRI) of the cervical spine demonstrated severe cervical stenosis and anterior cord compression at C2–C3 and C3–C4.

The longus colli muscles were detached and elevated laterally with a bipolar cautery, and a table-mounted anterior cervical retractor was used to maintain the exposure. Next, a Penfield #2 dissector was used for blunt dissection lateral to the uncinate processes bilaterally.

3. Anterior osteotomy was then begun with a high-speed burr with 3-mm match-stick tip to complete the bony resection in the disc space similar to a typical ACDF. The high-speed burr was kept perpendicular to the cervical spine to recreate the same space as the previous disc, therefore minimizing the risk of iatrogenic coronal plane deformity. In patients with mixed coronal and kyphotic deformities, the asymmetrical bony resection can be performed to produce correction in both the coronal and sagittal planes. The bony resection was extended posteriorly to the posterior longitudinal ligament (PLL). The PLL was then thinned with the high-speed burr and then removed with Kerrison rongeurs. The anterior dura at this level was completely visualized to ensure adequate anterior decompression. Caspar pins were then inserted at C2 and C3 to facilitate distraction of the disc space. The pins were placed perpendicular to the anterior plane of the kyphotic cervical spine, which resulted in a divergent alignment of the pins. This pin arrangement can help to produce lordosis as the pins are distracted after the anterior osteotomy is completed.
4. Next, the uncinate process resection was begun. Iatrogenic vertebral artery injury is a potential complication during the bony resection of the lateral uncinate process. Therefore, this portion of the procedure must be performed with extreme caution and with meticulous surgical technique. To minimize the risk of this potential complication, a Penfield #2 dissector was used to mark the lateral border of the uncinate processes and to protect the vertebral artery during the lateral bony resection (▶ Fig. 48.4). When a thin shell of bone from the lateral uncinate process is left, it is broken off easily with a microcurette pushing from lateral to medial, away from the vertebral arteries. Then anterior foraminotomies were then performed bilaterally to prevent nerve root compression during neck extension at the level of anterior osteotomy.
5. After completion of bilateral uncinate resection and bilateral foraminotomies, kyphosis correction was begun by removing the sheets under the head one at a time by the anesthesia team, applying a steady downward force on the forehead through the sterile drapes by the attending surgeon. Caspar pins were distracted by the assistant at the same time to further facilitate kyphosis correction. A Cobb elevator can also be inserted into the osteotomy site and gently rotated to distract the disc space while simultaneously distracting along the Caspar pins, if needed. In addition, vertebral body spreaders along with sequentially larger disc space sizers can also be helpful in kyphosis correction. Once the correction of kyphosis gets to the point where the occiput touches the operating table, the correction is complete. If the correction is still inadequate, the anesthesiologist can place a rolled sheet under the shoulders to provide further cervical lordosis. The cervical traction was then increased to 25 pounds to maintain the correction.

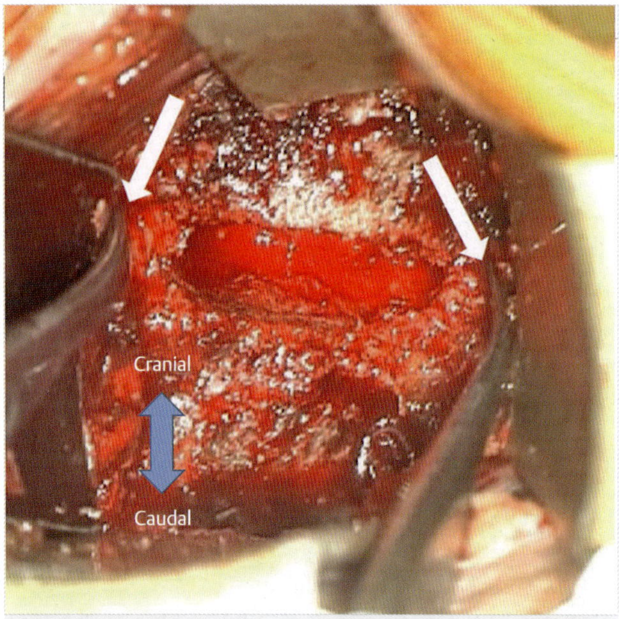

Fig. 48.4 An intraoperative photograph demonstrating use of a Penfield #2 dissector (*arrows*) to mark the lateral border of the uncinate processes and to protect the vertebral artery during the lateral bony resection.

6. In this case, an 8 × 14 × 12 mm Solitaire-C cage (Zimmer Biomet, Warsaw, IN, USA) was secured in the C2–C3 disc space with only the cranial screw, which allowed further kyphosis correction during the posterior stage of the procedure (▶ Fig. 48.5). Anterior cervical osteotomy was also performed at C3–C4 in the same manner as described above, followed by a standard ACDF at C4–C5 to complete the anterior portion of the procedure.
7. The patient was then turned prone on to a Jackson frame, and the head was secured in Gardner-Wells tongs with bivector cervical traction. Care was taken to pad all prominences. Poster cervical and upper thoracic regions were sterilely prepped and draped in the usual manner.
8. A midline incision utilizing the old incision was made. The posterior cervical spine was dissected subperiosteally where the lamina was still intact and exposed from C1 down to T4. The existing connectors and rods in the cervical and spine were removed. Smith-Petersen osteotomies were performed at C2–C3, C3–C4 with partial resection of facets using a high-speed burr. The neck was extended further using bivector cervical traction after the bilateral partial facet resections at C2–C3 and C3–C4.
9. New instrumentation was then placed from C2 to T2 in the standard fashion, and connected to the previous thoracolumbar construct while maximizing cervical lordosis. Posterior decompression from C1 to C3 was also performed using microsurgical technique and a microscope. To prevent adherence and soft tissue scarring from compressing the spine cord, a cross-link was placed between C2 and C3; in addition, another cross-link was placed at C6 to provide additional stability against torsion. Intraoperative fluoroscopy was used to confirm adequate deformity correction and proper position of the instrumentation.

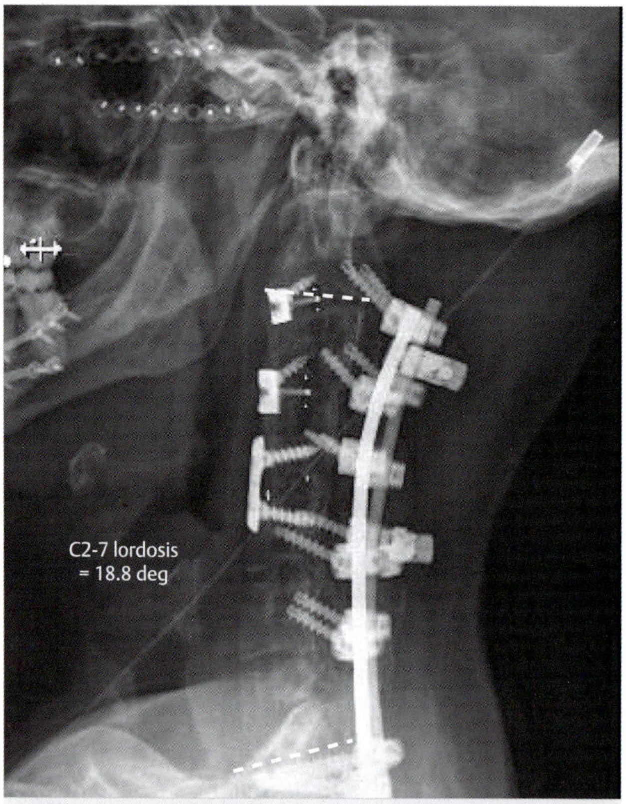

Fig. 48.5 Lateral cervical X-ray demonstrating placement of two Solitaire-C cages (Zimmer Biomet, Warsaw, IN, USA) at C2–C3 and C3–C4 disc spaces with only the cranial screws in place; this allowed further kyphosis correction through the anterior osteotomy site during the posterior stage of the procedure by extending the neck.

10. Finally, the bony surfaces were thoroughly decorticated and allograft was placed to optimize fusion. A surgical drain was used and the wound was closed carefully in a multilayered fashion to minimize the risk of surgical site infection. Vancomycin powder was also placed in the wound prior to closure.

48.4.4 Clinical Outcome and Follow-up

The patient tolerated the procedure well with stable neurological examination postoperatively. Follow-up cervical X-rays demonstrated excellent kyphosis correction with a postoperative C2–C7 lordosis of 18.8 degrees, which equated to a 54.9 degrees increase in cervical lordosis. The C2–C7 SVA improved from 37.2 to 0 mm postoperatively. The patient remained neurologically stable at the 2-year follow-up visit.

48.5 Conclusion

Complex cervical spine deformity can be challenging to treat. However, careful preoperative planning with clearly identified surgical goals can help to minimize surgical complications and achieve optimal clinical outcome.

References

[1] Ames CP, Smith JS, Eastlack R, et al. International Spine Study Group. Reliability assessment of a novel cervical spine deformity classification system. J Neurosurg Spine. 2015; 23(6):673–683

[2] Iyer S, Lenke LG, Nemani VM, et al. Variations in occipitocervical and cervicothoracic alignment parameters based on age: a prospective study of asymptomatic volunteers using full-body radiographs. Spine. 2016; 41(23):1837–1844

[3] Suk K-S, Kim K-T, Lee S-H, Kim J-M. Significance of chin-brow vertical angle in correction of kyphotic deformity of ankylosing spondylitis patients. Spine. 2003; 28(17):2001–2005

[4] Song K, Su X, Zhang Y, et al. Optimal chin-brow vertical angle for sagittal visual fields in ankylosing spondylitis kyphosis. Eur Spine J. 2016; 25(8):2596–2604

[5] Gillis CC, Kaszuba MC, Traynelis VC. Cervical radiographic parameters in 1- and 2-level anterior cervical discectomy and fusion. J Neurosurg Spine. 2016; 25(4):421–429

[6] Kim HJ, Piyaskulkaew C, Riew KD. Comparison of Smith-Petersen osteotomy versus pedicle subtraction osteotomy versus anterior-posterior osteotomy types for the correction of cervical spine deformities. Spine. 2015; 40 (3):143–146

49 MIS Cervical Pedicle Screws—Percutaneous-Assisted Technique

Marcus Richter and Philipp Hartung

Summary

Although lateral mass screws are still the most commonly used technique for posterior instrumentation of the subaxial cervical spine, they have several significant drawbacks in terms of biomechanical stability and reduction possibilities. Pedicle screws, which are standard for thoracic and lumbar stabilizations, show significantly improved stability and reduction performance in the cervical spine. However, they are still used rarely due to difficult placement and potential risks due to misplacement. The application of a minimal invasive technique with percutaneous-assisted placement of cannulated pedicle screws through tubes allows for a significantly reduced misplacement risk, comparable to thoracic and lumbar pedicle screws, a better reduction possibilities, and a significantly reduced implant failure rate compared to lateral mass screws.

The use of spinal navigation for the placement of the cervical pedicle screws allows for further reduction of the approach size and reduces the rate of screw misplacement.[2]

Keywords: cervical spine, minimally invasive spine surgery, pedicle screw fixation, percutaneous-assisted technique, posterior instrumentation, spinal navigation

49.1 Introduction

Pedicle screw instrumentation is the gold standard in the lumbar and thoracic spine, but it is still uncommon in the cervical spine. The small dimensions of the cervical pedicle and the proximity of vascular and neural structures may explain this. The mainly used posterior screw technique in the cervical spine, i.e., lateral mass screw fixation, results in a biomechanical stability clearly below the stability achieved with pedicle screws[1,2] and there are also complications due to the placement of lateral mass screws documented in the literature. The incidence of lateral mass fractures is 6 to 7% and injury or irritation of the posterior root is found in 4 to 10% depending on the used technique.[3] Nevertheless, there are potential risks of iatrogenic damage to neural or vascular structures[1,4] when using cervical pedicle screws.

Due to the advantages of cervical and high thoracic pedicle screws over other instrumentation techniques, the interest of spine surgeons in this technique was increasing rapidly.[5,6] As a result of improved biomechanical stability of pedicle screws compared to lateral mass screws, pedicle screws allow for shorter instrumentations with improved reduction capacities. Although excellent results with very low screw misplacement rates were published by Abumi et al,[4] demonstrating 7% misplacement rate out of 669 cervical pedicle screws when using a conventional screw insertion technique without a computer-assisted surgery (CAS) system, this data may not be applicable to many other spine surgeons with significantly less experience in cervical pedicle screws.

In 1993, CAS systems were developed for the installation of pedicle screws in the lumbar spine[7,8] based on reports of misplacement rates of between 5 and 40% using conventional techniques.[9] In vitro studies showed that misplacement rates of pedicle screws can be significantly reduced when using spinal navigation.[10] In vivo studies confirmed these results.[11] As in vitro studies have shown that cervical pedicle screws can be safely applied using spinal navigation,[12,13] we started using spinal navigation intraoperatively for pedicle screws of the cervical and cervicothoracic spine. Meanwhile several systematic reviews have shown that the malplacement rate of pedicle screws is significantly lower when using spinal navigation, and there is no difference in the malplacement rates between cervical, thoracic, and lumbar spine.[14]

We decided to use a drill to prepare the pedicles due to the reduced friction of a rotating drill compared to a pedicle awl. The results of our in vitro study[12] showed that this technique is suitable for cervical pedicle instrumentation. In our clinical study,[15] we had a pedicle perforation rate of 3% in the spinal navigation group without any screw-related complications. Also, the low pedicle perforation rate in the conventional group of 8.6% without any screw-related complication shows that cervical pedicles can be applied safely without spinal navigation when using the described technique with cannulated screws and percutaneous application at C3–C6. Preoperative planning and determination of the pedicle angles are mandatory for cervical pedicle screw placement without spinal navigation. The entrance point can be defined well with anatomical landmarks and the pedicle can be identified in the lateral image intensifier view but it is very difficult for the surgeon to define the exact angle of the drill guide. Especially if the angle is too low, there is a high risk of injury to the vertebral artery. Therefore, intraoperatively the use of an angle-measurement device is also mandatory. Nevertheless, the use of spinal navigation reduces the risk of screw malplacement and should be used, if available.

Pedicle widths of C3 averages 4.9 mm in males and 4.5 mm in females, the minimum reported width being 3.0 mm. C4 averages 4.7 mm in males and 4.6 mm in females, with the minimum reported width of 3.1 mm.[14,16] The pedicle widths in C5 and C6 are slightly larger. These anatomic data show that some pedicles may not be suitable for pedicle screws. Therefore, pedicle width should be measured preoperatively using computed tomography (CT). Although the risk associated with pedicle screws C3–C6 is obviously higher compared to C7 and high thoracic pedicle screws, the use of spinal navigation for C7 and high thoracic pedicle screws may also be beneficial, as the quality of the intraoperative image intensifier picture in this region is usually rather poor due to the shoulders of the patient.

Although spinal navigation is a useful and fascinating tool for spine surgery, anyone using such a system should be aware of possible errors. As the system can crash at any time during the operation due to hardware, software, or human failure, every

surgeon using the system should be experienced in the operation without the use of spinal navigation. Furthermore, the surgeon should never rely on the virtual information from spinal navigation without his or her own verification if the surgical reality matches the virtual reality shown on the screen of the spinal navigation system. The surgeon must ensure that the correct vertebrae are instrumented via image intensifier control or other techniques. Although registration of the instrumented vertebrae is possible in all cases, it can be difficult especially in C3 and C4, as these vertebrae have very small spinous processes and in many patients, the posterior surface of the vertebrae, which is used for the surface matching, is quite similar. Therefore, it is possible to achieve an acceptable registration on C3 with the surface data of C4 or vice versa. This problem underlines the mandatory need for the surgeon to verify that he/she is working on the correct vertebra. Another error may result from the reference clamp, which is attached to the vertebra on which the surgeon will be working. In the middle of the cervical spine, the small dimensions of the spinous processes make it difficult to achieve a stable fixation of the reference clamp, especially as most of the reference clamps available for the different spinal navigation systems were initially designed for the lumbar and thoracic spine.

49.2 Indications

In general, this technique can be used for all patients requiring a posterior cervical stabilization. Indications are instabilities, degenerative changes, and tumor involvement. The following indications have to be taken into consideration:

a) Instabilities due to rheumatoid arthritis.
b) Instabilities due to neoplasia with/without spinal cord compression.
c) Spondylodiscitis of the cervical spine.
d) Traumatic instabilities, especially in patients with ancylosing spondylitis.
e) Cervical spondylotic myelopathy, especially multisegmental or significant posterior stenosis, also in mono- and bisegmental cases.
f) Pathologies of the sagittal profile of the cervical spine requiring corrective surgery.
g) Congenital instabilities.
h) Posterior stabilization of the cervical spine in patients with severe osteoporosis.

49.3 Contraindications

a) Poor health prohibiting general anesthesia.
b) Small pedicle dimensions with a pedicle width below the screw diameter or anatomical variations of the vertebral artery.

49.4 Preoperative Planning

Clinical assessment including neurological status should be done.

The following imaging studies are needed:

a) X-ray in anteroposterior (AP) and lateral projection.
b) Extension/flexion in lateral projection X-rays if instability is suspected.
c) CT/angio-CT with multiplanar reconstructions.
d) Magnetic resonance imaging (MRI)/angio-MRI if spinal cord compression is suspected or in tumor cases.

Preoperative screw planning is done based on the CT and multiplanar reconstructions in the axis of the pedicles with determination of the vertebral artery course and planning of angulation and length of the screws (▶ Fig. 49.1a–c). If pedicle screws are not possible due to anatomical reasons, lateral mass screws are the alternative in C3–C7. In C2, translaminar screws are a viable alternative to pedicle screws.

49.5 Patient Positioning

General endotracheal anesthesia with muscle relaxation is mandatory. Once the patient is in supine position, disinfection of the pin sites is done and the Mayfield clamp is fixed to the occiput in the standard technique and location. Positioning of the head without using a Mayfield head holder may also be possible but is not recommended as the possibilities of reduction and fixation in reduced position are limited with the head over an unsteady surface. Then the patient is then flipped to the prone position over a gel-filled mattress; support of the thorax and pelvis is done using foam pillows. The arms are fixed

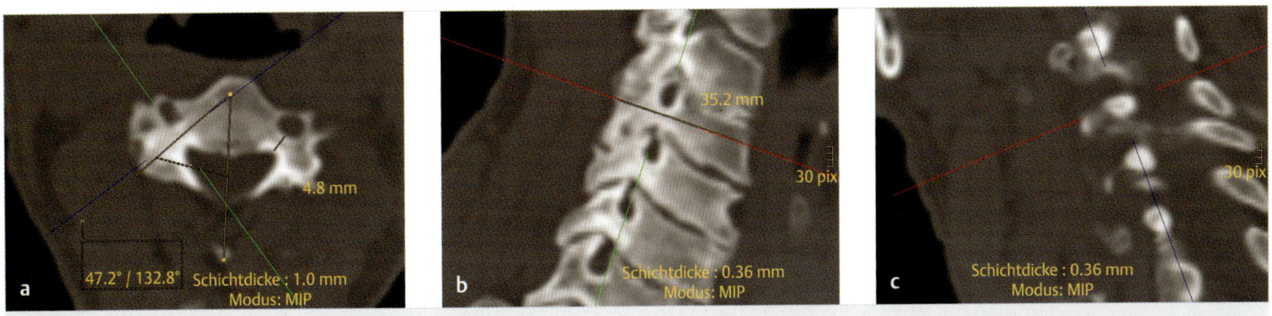

Fig. 49.1 (a–c) Preoperative computed tomography (CT) with multiplanar reconstructions in the axis of the pedicles at C4 with determination of the vertebral artery course and planning of the angulation (47.2 degrees) and the length (35.2 mm) of the screws. The width (4.8 mm) of both pedicles is adequate for placing pedicle screws on both sides.

with adhesive tapes. In our center, we also use pulley systems and 2.5 kg traction on each side (▶ Fig. 49.2).

Prior to surgery, shaving of the surgical area is performed using a clipper.

Perioperative antibiotic prophylaxis is given once 20 to 30 minutes prior to the skin incision.

49.6 Surgical Steps

49.6.1 Incision

After prepping and draping with the image intensifier in the lateral view, a midline incision is done from the upper instrumented vertebra to the lower instrumented vertebra. After subcutaneous preparation, incision of the fascia in the midline and subperiosteal exposure of the posterior aspect of the instrumented area are carried out. It is important to stay exactly in the midline to reduce blood loss and muscle trauma. The preparation can be done using an electrocautery knife. To reduce further blood loss and tissue trauma, the use of a harmonic scalpel is beneficial.

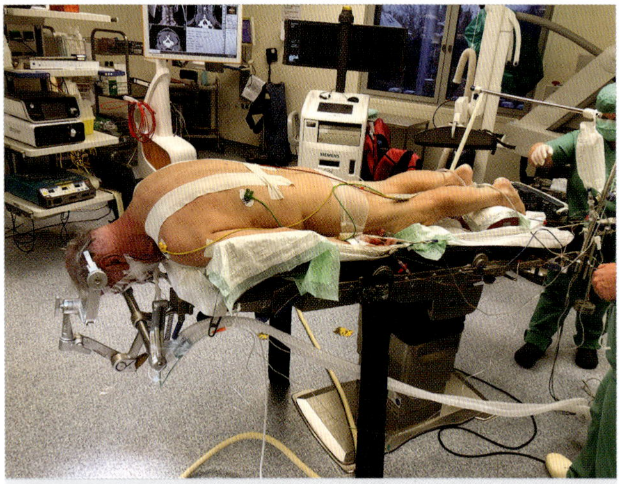

Fig. 49.2 Patient in prone position on a gel-filled mattress; support of the thorax and pelvis is done with foam pillows. The arms are fixed by adhesive tapes and continuously pulled with a pulley system of 2.5 kg each side.

49.6.2 Technique (▶ Video 49.1)

The short incision, percutaneous-assisted screw placement method for pedicle screw fixation is less invasive due to the reduced approach morbidity:

Step 1

Before describing the various surgical steps, the trajectory and insertion point of the pedicle screws must be explained. They differ significantly between C2, C3–C6, and C7. The entry point for pedicle screws in C3–C6 is very lateral and just below the facet joint of the adjacent cranial segment (▶ Fig. 49.3). Due to the high convergence (40–60 degrees) a percutaneous-assisted approach allows for a significantly shorter midline incision and a correct convergence of the screw. If the entrance point is correct, but the convergence is reduced, the risk of a vertebral artery injury is increased.

In C7, the convergence is less (25–45 degrees) and there is normally no vertebral artery which could be injured (▶ Fig. 49.4).

The C2 pedicles usually have a width of > 5 mm and less convergence (10–35 degrees) and a 10 to 20% ascending screw trajectory (▶ Fig. 49.5).

Step 2

For minimal invasive instrumentation, a cannular system for percutaneous-assisted screw placement is needed because otherwise due to the recommended screw angulation the incision needed would have to be longer for open screw placement.

After preparation and draping of the surgical field, the insertion point for the trocar system is determined. This is done by holding the trocar lateral to the neck and looking for the correct screw

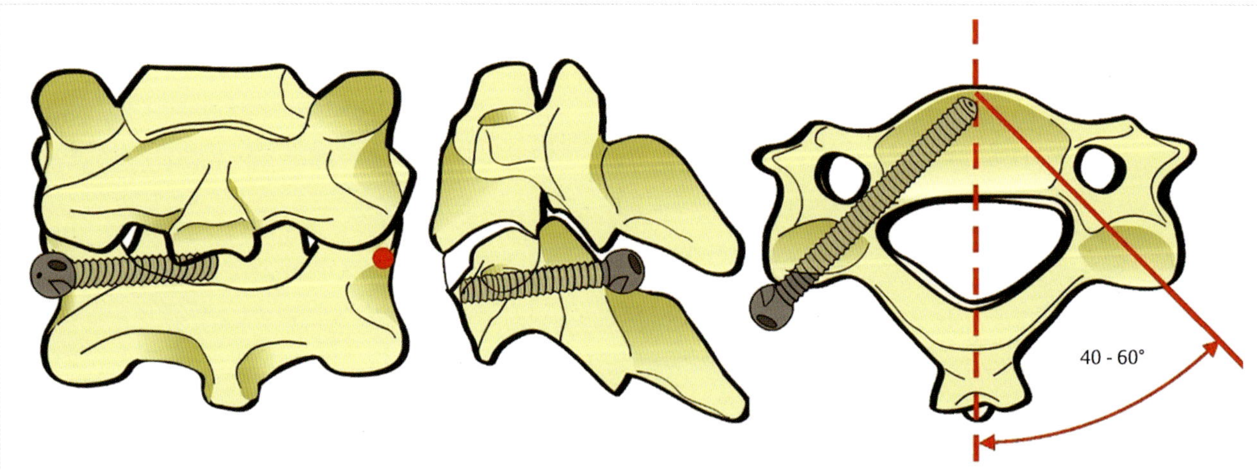

Fig. 49.3 The entry points for pedicle screws in C3–C6 are far lateral, just below the facet joint of the adjacent cranial segment. The average convergence is between 40 and 60 degrees.

direction in the lateral X-ray view. Then a stab incision is made and the trocar system is introduced percutaneously to the screw insertion point. If spinal navigation is not used, it is mandatory to measure the angle of every pedicle planned to instrument preoperatively and intraoperatively. A sterile angle measurement device must be used to achieve the correct angle during pedicle preparation and screw placement (▶ Fig. 49.6a, b).

Step 3

Then the hole for the pedicle screw is prepared with a drill guide through the trocar system with a drill under X-ray control in the lateral view (▶ Fig. 49.7a). The advantage of the drill compared to a pedicle awl is the better feeling of bony resistance as a result of reduced friction of the rotation drill (sliding friction vs. sticking friction) and reduced ap-forces during preparation of the pedicle hole, which is beneficial especially in instabilities. Then a blunt K-wire is inserted through the drill guide, the drill guide is removed and a cannulated screw is inserted over the K-wire through the trocar system (▶ Fig. 49.7b).

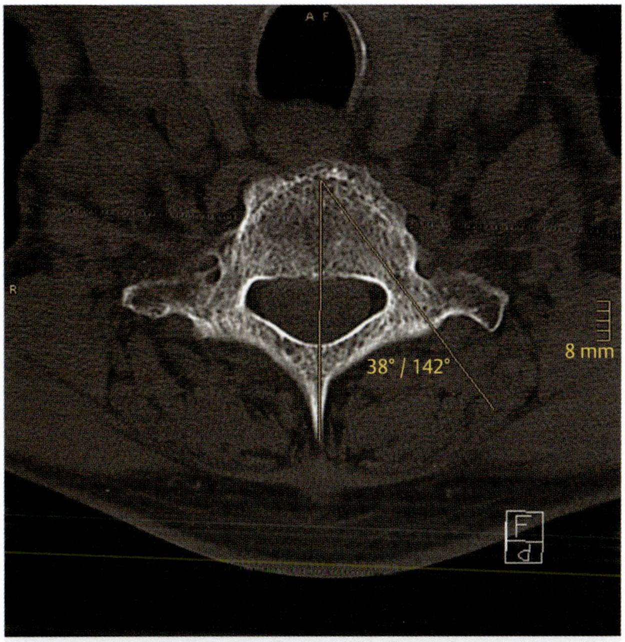

Fig. 49.4 In C7, the convergence is on average around 25 to 45 degrees. In this patient, it is 38 degrees. As shown in the picture, there is usually no vertebral artery which could be injured.

Step 4

When using noncannulated screws, you have to be careful not to perforate the pedicle laterally. A lateral pedicle perforation has a high risk of a vertebral artery injury. Therefore, for safety reasons the use of a K-wire and cannulated screws is strongly recommended.

Cervical pedicle screws can be placed with adequate accuracy in the minimal invasive technique as described above. Nevertheless, there are potential risks of iatrogenic damage to the vertebral artery or reduced screw anchorage due to screw misplacement. The use of spinal navigation is recommended for cervical pedicle screw placement, because the rate of misplaced screws is significantly reduced.[14,15]

Multisegment posterior cervical spinal instrumentation and complex thoracolumbar deformity correction are the frontiers for minimally invasive spine surgery (MISS). In this chapter, we learn about a hybrid technique where a reduced midline incision is performed for decompression and rod placement and separate stab incisions are placed for the placement of cervical pedicle screws. The choice of pedicle screws instead of lateral mass screws increases the biomechanical stability and allows reduction of screw density. The use of intraoperative three-dimensional navigation seems to make a lot of sense in this setting, especially if a true intraoperative CT scan is used with excellent image quality and autoregistration.

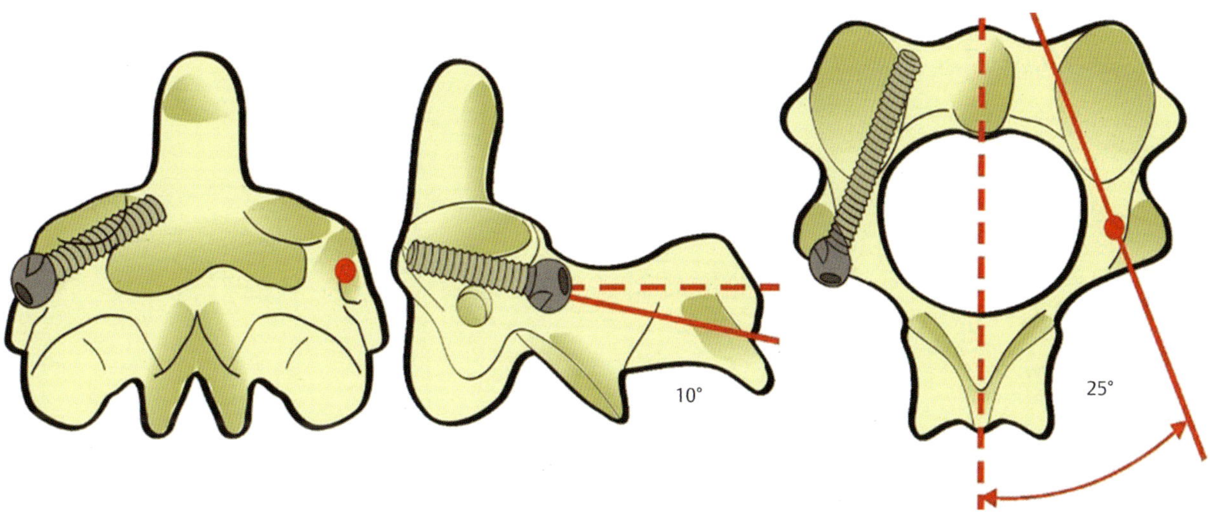

Fig. 49.5 The C2 pedicles usually have a width of >5 mm and less convergence (10–35 degrees) and a 10 to 20% ascending screw trajectory.

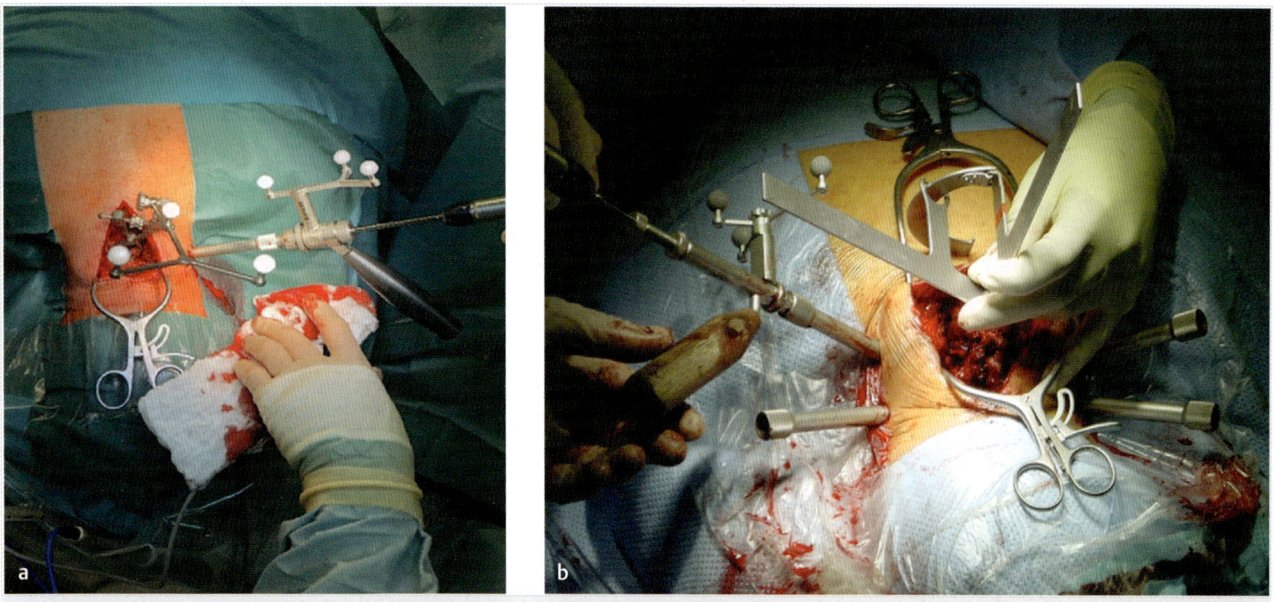

Fig. 49.6 **(a)** Intraoperative setup with the navigated drill guide in the trocar system, which is introduced percutaneously over a tab incision to the screw insertion point. **(b)** Intraoperative setup with placing of the drill guide through the trocar percutaneously to the screw insertion point without the use of spinal navigation. It is mandatory to measure the angle of every pedicle planned to instrument preoperatively with a sterile angle measurement device intraoperatively. The device should be used during the pedicle preparation and the screw placement to achieve the correct angulation.

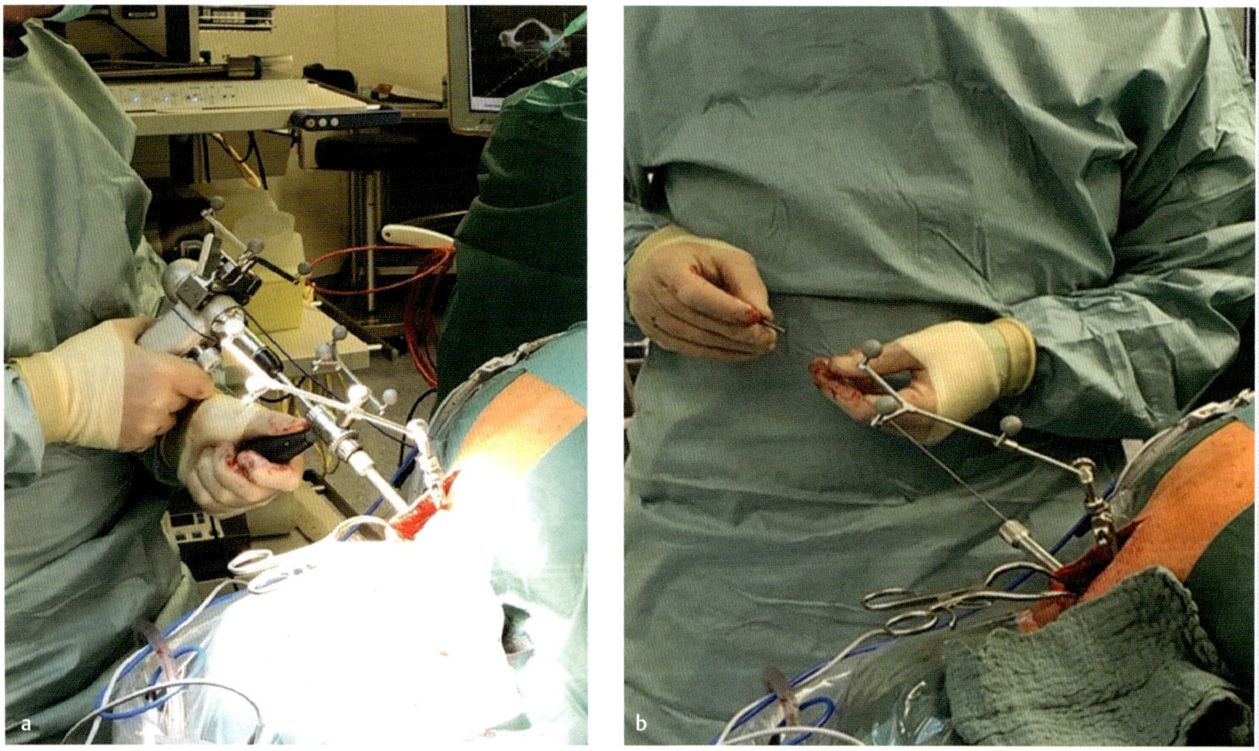

Fig. 49.7 **(a)** The corridor for the pedicle screw is prepared with a navigated drill guide and a navigated drill through the trocar system. Additional X-ray control in the lateral view is recommended. **(b)** After removing the drill guide, a blunt K-wire is inserted through the drill guide. Finally, a cannulated screw is inserted over the K-wire through the trocar system.

49.6.3 Spinal Navigation

In 1993, spinal navigation systems were first presented for the installation of pedicle screws in the lumbar spine based on reports of misplacement rates between 5 and 40% using conventional techniques. In vitro studies showed that misplacement rates of lumbar pedicle screws could be significantly reduced when using spinal navigation. In vivo studies confirmed these results. As in vitro and in vivo studies have shown that cervical pedicle screws can be safely applied using a spinal navigation system,[12,13,14,15] this technique should also be described, although spinal navigation is not mandatory for placement of cervical pedicle screws.

The CAS system is positioned on the right side of the patient once the posterior aspect of the spine has been approached. The monitor with the touch screen is positioned so that the surgeon has a good view and can easily reach the draped touch screen. To ensure a good line of sight, the camera is positioned over the legs of the patient. The surgeon stands or sits (preferred) at the head of the patient.

After the posterior approach is done, the dynamic reference clamp (DRB) is fixed to the spinous process of first vertebra which is planned for pedicle screws. The DRB should not be fixed at the Mayfield clamp, because in the mobile cervical spine there is too much movement possible between the head fixed with the Mayfield clamp and the instrumented vertebra. Especially for cervical pedicle screws, the accuracy should be as high as possible to prevent screw malpositioning.

Next, registration of the vertebra is performed using the surface matching algorithm, where a predicted accuracy of < 1.0 mm is acceptable. If the predicted accuracy is >1.0 mm, a repeated registration procedure should be done until an accuracy of < 1.0 mm is achieved. After registration of the vertebra, verification has to be done to ensure that the virtual reality of the spinal navigation system corresponds with the surgical reality. This is easily done by tapping with the pointer at points on the posterior surface of the vertebra which are easy to find and clearly identifiable and then confirming if the position of the pointer shown by the spinal navigation system corresponds to the pointer position in the sites. If verification is accurate, the navigated instrumentation can begin. If verification is inaccurate, the whole registration procedure must be repeated.

The spinal navigation system can be used to find the ideal position for the stab incision for percutaneous-assisted screw placement. The pointer with offset setting of 4 to 8 cm (depending on the individual thickness of the fat/muscle layer above the spine) is used to identify the optimal position for the stab incision (▶ Fig. 49.8a). After the stab incision is done, the calibrated trocar system is introduced, the screw is planned (▶ Fig. 49.8b, c), and the screw trajectory is drilled with the navigated drill guide and the navigated drill machine (▶ Fig. 49.8d, e). After that the K-wire is placed (▶ Fig. 49.9a). Finally, a cannulated screw is inserted over the K-wire through the trocar system (▶ Fig. 49.9b).

The steps described are repeated for every vertebra which is planned for pedicle screws. For accuracy reasons it is important

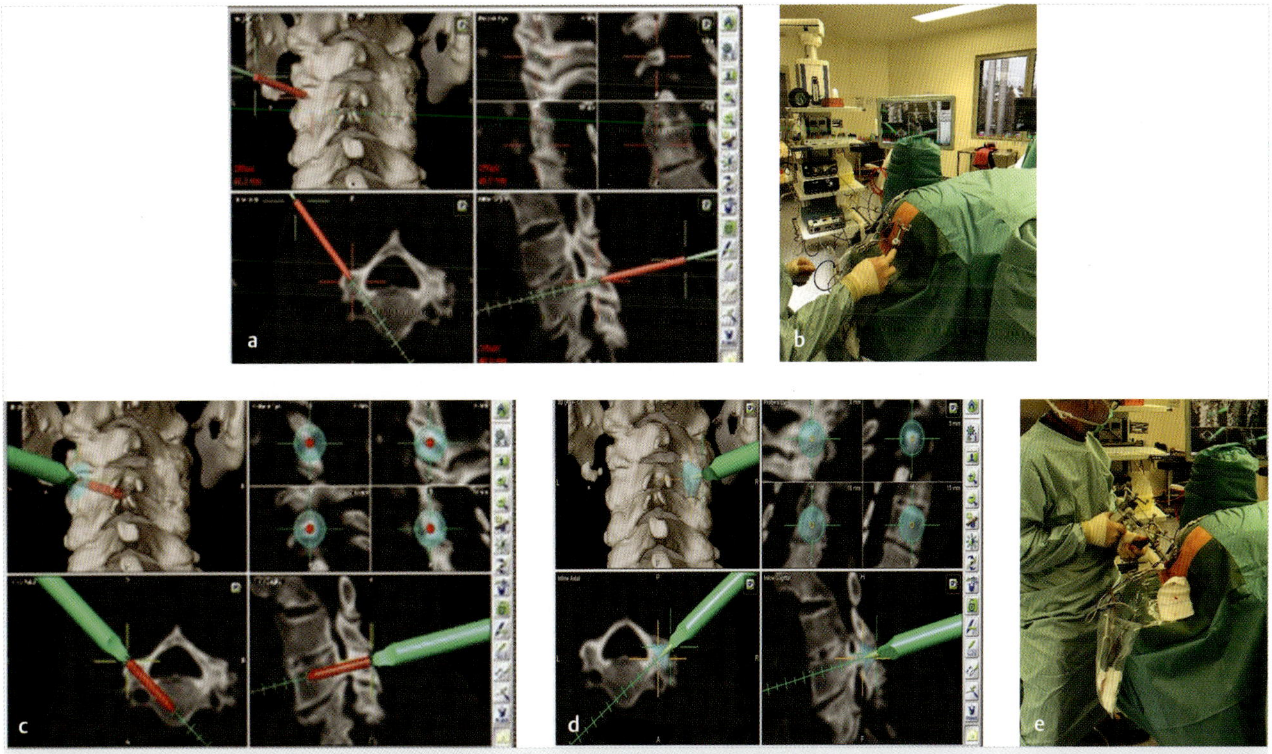

Fig. 49.8 **(a)** Intraoperative screenshot of the navigation system while the correct position for the stab incision for the percutaneous screw placement is determined using the pointer in offset setting. **(b, c)** Intraoperative screenshot of navigated screw planning after percutaneous-assisted placement of the precalibrated and verified drill guide through the trocar. **(d, e)** Intraoperative screenshot of the screw trajectory, which is getting drilled with the navigated drill guide and the navigated drill machine.

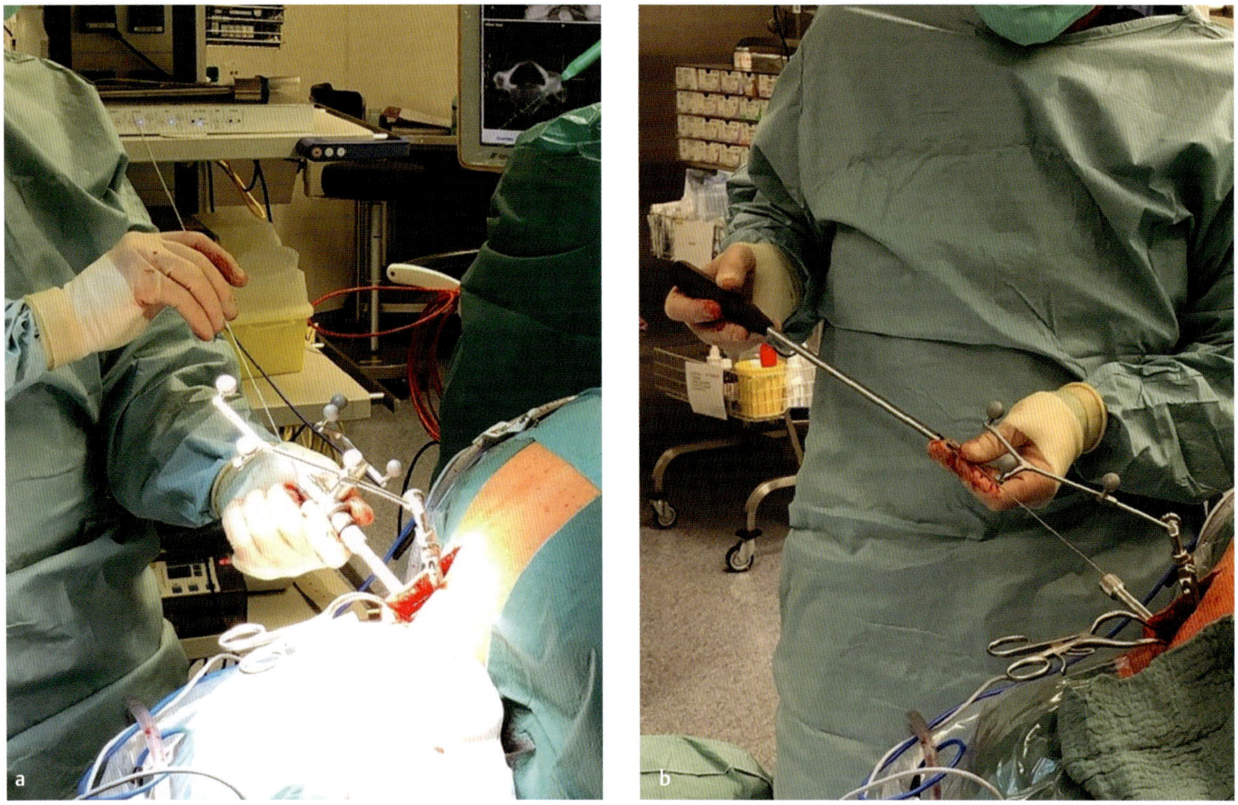

Fig. 49.9 (a, b) After placing the K-wire, a cannulated screw is inserted over the K-wire through the trocar system.

to place the DRB always at the spinous process of the vertebra, which is actually instrumented to achieve the highest possible accuracy. For adjacent vertebra, the same trocar system can be used. In all other cases a new stab incision and the placement of an additional trocar on each side is necessary.

After the pedicle screw implantation, the necessary surgical procedures due to the pathology can be performed. Before the final instrumentation with the rods it is possible to gain reduction with the pedicle screw system. It must be pointed out that the fixation of the Mayfield clamp to the operating table has to be loosened first.

49.6.4 Closure

Wound closure is done over a subfascial drain. Skin closure should be done with interrupted sutures. The cannulas can be removed either before or after wound closure of the midline incision (▶ Fig. 49.10). The stab incisions are closed with subcutaneous suture and skin suture. After turning the patient, the Mayfield clamp is removed and sterile draping of the pin sites should be done (▶ Fig. 49.11a–e).

49.7 Postoperative Care

Due to the excellent biomechanical stability of the pedicle screws no postoperative collar is needed. The drain can be removed 2 days postoperatively; skin sutures are removed 14 days postoperatively. X-ray controls are recommended before discharge and after 3 and 12 months.

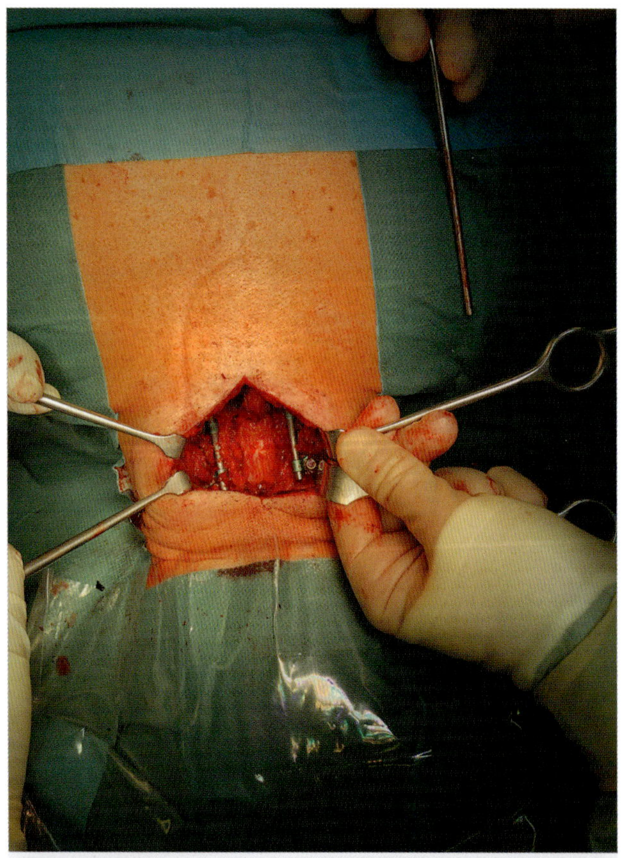

Fig. 49.10 Intraoperative site before wound closure after instrumentation, decompression, and posterolateral fusion are completed. Note the cannulas are removed already.

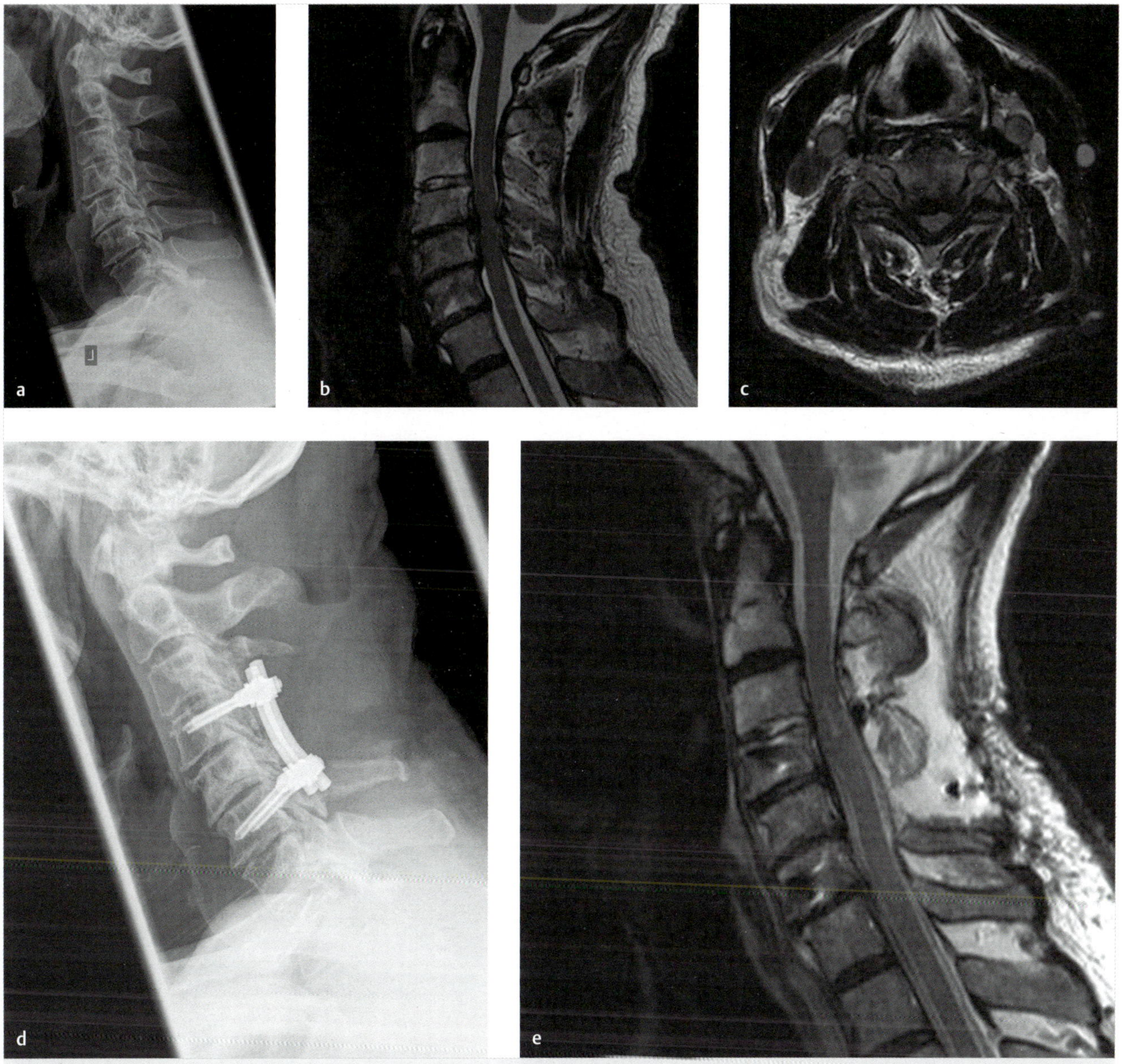

Fig. 49.11 (a) The presented case: A 74-year-old male patient with cervical spondylotic myelopathy (CSM). Preoperative lateral X-ray. (b, c) The magnetic resonance imaging (MRI) is showing cervical spondylosis with compression of the spinal cord in C3–C5. (d) In the postoperative lateral X-ray, the correct positioning of the implants is documented. (e) The postoperative MRI demonstrates the sufficient decompression. Note the posterior shift of the spinal cord, which is conducting the indirect anterior decompression of the spinal cord.

49.8 Complication Avoidance

The main complications of cervical pedicle screws are related to placement of screws in vertebra with unsuitable anatomy for pedicle screws, especially when the pedicle dimensions are not matching the diameter of the used screws.

Vertebral artery injury, reported in approximately < 1% of patients, may lead to arteriovenous fistula, occlusion, narrowing, or dissection of the vertebral artery, which may remain asymptomatic or lead to transient ischemic attacks, stroke, or death.[4,17,18] The best strategy to reduce the risk of vertebral artery injury is thorough preoperative planning with preoperative CT (▶ Fig. 49.1a–c) and exclusion of the patients with pedicle dimensions which are unsuitable for cervical pedicle screws on one or both sides.[6]

If there are any doubts concerning the course of the vertebral artery an angio-CT or angio-MRI should be done.

In case of an injury of the vertebral artery on one side, the screw on this side should be inserted to stop the bleeding. A repair of the vertebral artery in this location is not possible. If the vertebral artery was injured on the side of the first screw, a lateral mass screw should be chosen for the other side which makes an injury of the vertebral artery impossible.

Other possible complications are typical complications of spine stabilization such as wound healing problems or infections. Due to the minimal invasive approach, these complications are

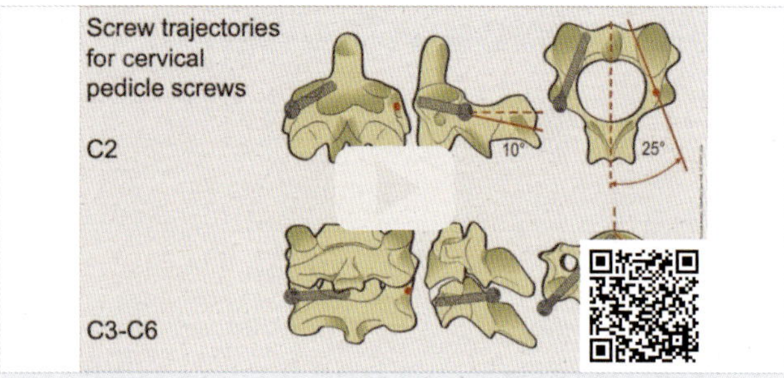

Video 49.1 Pedicle screws cervical MIS.

less frequent as compared to traditional approaches. In case of wound healing disturbances, early revision with debridement and perhaps vacuum suction helps to avoid deep infections. In case of deep infection of the implant site early revision is also beneficial. Implant removal is not necessary but placement of local antibiotics, such as Septopal chains, is recommended.

49.9 Tips and Tricks

a) Thorough preoperative planning using CT with multiplanar reconstruction should be done to ensure that cervical pedicle screws are possible. If pedicle screws are not possible without increased risk for vertebral artery injury use lateral mass screws.
b) More anterolateral fixation of the sterile drapes to ensure that placement of the cannulas for the percutaneous-assisted placement of the pedicle screws is possible.
c) If possible, use spinal navigation for placement of the pedicle screws.
d) If you are in doubt that the vertebral artery could be injured on one side, place the screw on this side and use lateral mass screws without the risk of vertebral artery injury on the opposite side.
e) In case of possible vertebral artery injury intraoperatively, postoperative angiography is mandatory to rule out a fistula or pseudoaneurysm, which could be treated by endovascular techniques.
f) When not using spinal navigation, preoperative measurement of the angle of all pedicles planned to instrument and intraoperative sterile angle measurement device to ensure a correct angle of the pedicle screw.

49.10 Conclusion

a) Cervical pedicle screws allow the highest biomechanical stability and the best reduction capabilities compared to all other techniques.
b) Percutaneous-assisted cervical pedicle screw placement in combination with a reduced midline incision reduces the approach related morbidity and makes the correct screw placement easier.
c) Computer navigation is not needed for screw placement, but reduces the risk of screw misplacement.

References

[1] Jones EL, Heller JG, Silcox DH, Hutton WC. Cervical pedicle screws versus lateral mass screws: anatomic feasibility and biomechanical comparison. Spine. 1997; 22(9):977–982
[2] Kotani Y, Cunningham BW, Abumi K, McAfee PC. Biomechanical analysis of cervical stabilization systems: an assessment of transpedicular screw fixation in the cervical spine. Spine. 1994; 19(22):2529–2539
[3] Choueka J, Spivak JM, Kummer FJ, Steger T. Flexion failure of posterior cervical lateral mass screws: influence of insertion technique and position. Spine. 1996; 21(4):462–468
[4] Abumi K, Shono Y, Ito M, Taneichi H, Kotani Y, Kaneda K. Complications of pedicle screw fixation in reconstructive surgery of the cervical spine. Spine. 2000; 25(8):962–969
[5] Abumi K, Shono Y, Kotani Y, Kaneda K. Indirect posterior reduction and fusion of the traumatic herniated disc by using a cervical pedicle screw system. J Neurosurg. 2000; 92(1) Suppl:30–37
[6] Abumi K, Kaneda K. Pedicle screw fixation for nontraumatic lesions of the cervical spine. Spine. 1997; 22(16):1853–1863
[7] Nolte L, Zamorano L, Arm E, et al. Image-guided computer-assisted spine surgery: a pilot study on pedicle screw fixation. Stereotact Funct Neurosurg. 1996; 66(1–3):108–117
[8] Amiot LP, Labelle H, DeGuise JA, Sati M, Brodeur P, Rivard CH. Computer-assisted pedicle screw fixation: a feasibility study. Spine. 1995; 20(10):1208–1212
[9] Vaccaro AR, Rizzolo SJ, Balderston RA, et al. Placement of pedicle screws in the thoracic spine. Part II: an anatomical and radiographic assessment. J Bone Joint Surg Am. 1995; 77(8):1200–1206
[10] Nolte LP, Zamorano L, Visarius H, et al. Clinical evaluation of a system for precision enhancement in spine surgery. Clin Biomech (Bristol, Avon). 1995; 10 (6):293–303
[11] Laine T, Schlenzka D, Mäkitalo K, Tallroth K, Nolte LP, Visarius H. Improved accuracy of pedicle screw insertion with computer-assisted surgery: a prospective clinical trial of 30 patients. Spine. 1997; 22(11):1254–1258
[12] Richter M, Amiot LP, Neller S, Kluger P, Puhl W. Computer-assisted surgery in posterior instrumentation of the cervical spine: an in-vitro feasibility study. Eur Spine J. 2000; 9 Suppl 1:S65–S70
[13] Ludwig SC, Kowalski JM, Edwards CC , II, Heller JG. Cervical pedicle screws: comparative accuracy of two insertion techniques. Spine. 2000; 25 (20):2675–2681
[14] Shin BJ, James AR, Njoku IU, Härtl R. Pedicle screw navigation: a systematic review and meta-analysis of perforation risk for computer-navigated versus freehand insertion. J Neurosurg Spine. 2012; 17(2):113–122
[15] Richter M, Cakir B, Schmidt R. Cervical pedicle screws: conventional versus computer-assisted placement of cannulated screws. Spine. 2005; 30(20):2280–2287
[16] Ebraheim NA, Xu R, Knight T, Yeasting RA. Morphometric evaluation of lower cervical pedicle and its projection. Spine. 1997; 22(1):1–6
[17] Wright NM, Lauryssen C, American Association of Neurological Surgeons/ Congress of Neurological Surgeons. Vertebral artery injury in C1–2 transarticular screw fixation: results of a survey of the AANS/CNS section on disorders of the spine and peripheral nerves. J Neurosurg. 1998; 88(4):634–640
[18] Uehara M, Takahashi J, Ikegami S, et al. Screw perforation features in 129 consecutive patients performed computer-guided cervical pedicle screw insertion. Eur Spine J. 2014; 23(10):2189–2195

50 Treatment of Degenerative Lumbar Scoliosis with Minimally Invasive Multilevel LLIF in Combination with Lateral ALIF

James E. Dowdell, Giuseppe Barbagallo, and Sheeraz Qureshi

Summary

Adult degenerative lumbar scoliosis (ADLS) contributes to significant disability and decrease in quality of life. Minimally invasive spine surgery has seen many advancements over recent years. New surgical techniques allow for spine deformity correction in a minimally invasive fashion. Here we present a case of ADLS that was treated with a combined lateral lumbar interbody fusion (LLIF) and lateral position anterior lumbar interbody fusion (ALIF) with posterior percutaneous fixation.

Keywords: lateral ALIF, MIS XLIF, MIS deformity, degenerative scoliosis, adult deformity

50.1 Introduction

Adult degenerative lumbar scoliosis (ADLS) is a progressive condition characterized by asymmetrical intervertebral disc degeneration, facet hypertrophy, loss of lumbar lordosis, and deformity in the coronal and sagittal planes.[1,2] The prevalence of degenerative scoliosis ranges from 6 to 68% in the elderly population.[1,2,3] The etiology of this condition is thought to be multifactorial. One theory is that this condition arises from asymmetric load applied to the lumbar spine over time, while another theory implicates osteoporosis because ADLS is most common in the elderly female population (over 50 years of age). ADLS frequently presents as an isolated lumbar curve, unlike adult idiopathic scoliosis. There is a rotatory deformity present at the apex of the lumbar curve and there is frequently lateral subluxation of the vertebral body as well.[3]

Increased attention has been paid to the impact of degenerative scoliosis on the aging population with the increasing focus of quality of life outcome measures. ADLS contributes to significant pain and disability for patients. Frequently, nonoperative treatment fails in symptomatic patients. Unlike adolescent idiopathic scoliosis (AIS), degenerative scoliosis can progress at a rate of 3 degrees per year.[2,3] Historically, ADLS has been treated nonoperatively secondary to perioperative morbidity, high incidence of neurological deficit, rigidity of deformity, and difficulty of the surgery. However, with the advent of new fusion techniques, treatment for degenerative scoliosis is now commonplace.[1,2,3]

50.2 Preoperative Presentation

Most patients with ADLS present with a chief complaint of pain. The pain can be both axial or radicular in nature. The axial back pain is activity related and is the result of muscular fatigue. Often this pain is relieved with rest and is exacerbated by prolonged upright standing. Patients will also frequently complain of pain overlying muscular insertions around the iliac crest, spinous processes, and sacrum. Radicular pain and neurogenic claudication will often impact the patient simultaneously. Overgrowth of facets and ligamentum hypertrophy can produce symptoms of neurogenic claudication. Radicular pain can be the result of direct compression of the nerve root by a disc herniation, traction of the nerve root on the convexity of the deformity, or compression of the nerve root on the concavity of the deformity. Due to the unstable nature of the spine, the radicular pain associated with the deformity will often be worse with standing or walking.[3] Cosmetic deformity is generally well tolerated in the elderly population, but this can be a presenting sign as well.

50.3 Imaging Studies

All patients who are undergoing preoperative workup for surgical correction for ADLS should have either an anteroposterior (AP) and a lateral scoliosis radiograph or an EOS radiograph if available. EOS imaging will expose the patient to less radiation and are often higher quality and easier to interpret and thus is the imaging modality of choice in our practice. There are a variety of radiographic measurements that will be calculated on these imaging studies. Cobb angles will be measured on the AP radiograph to assess the deformity in the coronal plane, and sagittal parameters are measured on the lateral radiograph.[4] In our practice, these parameters are measured easily with the assistance of a surgical planning software called Surgimap.[5] Pelvic tilt (PT), pelvic incidence (PI), lumbar lordosis (LL), PI-LL mismatch, and the sagittal vertical axis (SVA) are all measured automatically with Surgimap. Bending films may be utilized to assess both the flexibility of the curve and the compensatory ability of adjacent levels. However, bending films are more commonly used in AIS as patients with degenerative lumbar scoliosis frequently have very stiff deformities.[3]

Advanced imaging is useful to evaluate bony anatomy, the intervertebral discs, and ligamentum flavum. This allows for evaluation of central, lateral recess, and foraminal stenosis in addition to any disc herniation. A lumbar CT scan is useful for assessment of bony anatomy and in most cases it will be obtained. A lumbar MRI is somewhat difficult to interpret in the setting of a degenerative lumbar scoliosis secondary to the obliquity of the vertebral body and the three-dimensional nature of the deformity. MRI is still useful for evaluation of stenosis, assessment of ligamentum hypertrophy, and disc herniation and should be obtained prior to any planned surgical intervention.[3]

50.4 Indications for Surgery

Proper indications for surgery will increase the chance for a successful outcome. There are multiple potential surgical options for treatment of adult degenerative lumbar scoliosis. Very infrequently will an isolated decompression be performed secondary

to the risk of rapid decompensation and destabilization of the degenerative curve.[3] Depending on the preoperative symptoms of the patient, an instrumented fusion with or without decompression can be performed. Traditional posterolateral spinal fusion in the setting of degenerative scoliosis has a high rate of pseudoarthrosis without the use of interbody devices.[1,2,3]

Interbody devices have been used to decrease the rates of pseudoarthrosis.[6] There are a variety of methods for placing interbody devices: Posterior lumbar interbody fusion (PLIF), anterior lumbar interbody fusion (ALIF), lateral lumbar interbody fusion (LLIF), oblique lateral interbody fusion (OLIF), and transforaminal lumbar interbody fusion (TLIF); each has unique advantages and disadvantages. PLIF often does an inadequate job of restoring lumbar lordosis and carries the risk of injury to nerve roots secondary to excessive retraction.[6] TLIF, similar to PLIF, often does not adequately restore lumbar lordosis.[6] ALIF is suitable for the L4–L5 and L5–S1 levels, but carries significant risk at more cephalad lumbar levels secondary to extensive peritoneal retraction and risk of superior mesenteric artery thrombosis.[6] The use of ALIF in the setting of degenerative lumbar scoliosis has the advantage of offering extensive correction of lumbar lordosis and lower pseudoarthrosis rates secondary to maximal fusion surface area for fusion.[6] However, due to ALIF being limited to lower lumbar levels it is most useful as an adjunct to other interbody techniques in degenerative scoliosis. LLIF is useful for access to the interbody disc space from T12–L1 down to L4–L5 and allows for the correction of both sagittal and coronal deformities, but is not useful in the setting of severe central canal stenosis or lateral recess stenosis.[6] OLIF allows for access to the L5–S1 level from the lateral position by accessing the disc space anterior to the psoas musculature and this option also allows for correction of significant sagittal and coronal deformities.[6] OLIF is contraindicated in the setting of severe central canal stenosis.

There are no consensus guidelines to develop a surgical plan in the setting of symptomatic degenerative lumbar scoliosis, but there is a recent publication that can help guide decision-making when choosing minimally invasive spine deformity correction.[7] Patients presenting with adult degenerative lumbar scoliosis will often have many medical comorbidities including obesity, anemia, diabetes, and osteoporosis. These conditions favor the use of minimally invasive techniques such as LLIF and ALIF/OLIF by preventing extensive dissection and stripping of paraspinal musculature.[8] Patients tend to have quicker in-hospital recoveries with MIS techniques.

50.5 Case Presentation

A 61-year-old female presented with axial back pain for the past several years, which had significantly worsened over the last 1 to 2 years. The patient has significant walking intolerance and must stop after walking about two city blocks. She is also presenting with bilateral buttocks pain that is claudicatory in nature. The patient denies any medical comorbidities and she has no smoking history. Over the past 2 years, the patient has attempted nonsteroidal anti-inflammatory drugs (NSAIDs), physical therapy, acupuncture, and epidural steroid injections (ESI) with initial relief. However, nonoperative modalities were no longer helping the patient with her pain. The patient had a normal neurological examination with palpable pedal pulses. Her only symptomatic finding on physical examination is pain with back extension.

The patient had obtained full-length EOS imaging, which showed an LL of 29 degrees and a PI of 56 degrees for a PI-LL mismatch of 27 degrees (▶ Fig. 50.1a, b). The patient was sent for a lumbar MRI, which showed multilevel foraminal stenosis as well as lateral recess/central canal stenosis which was moderate at L4–L5 and L5–S1 (▶ Fig. 50.2, ▶ Fig. 50.3, ▶ Fig. 50.4,

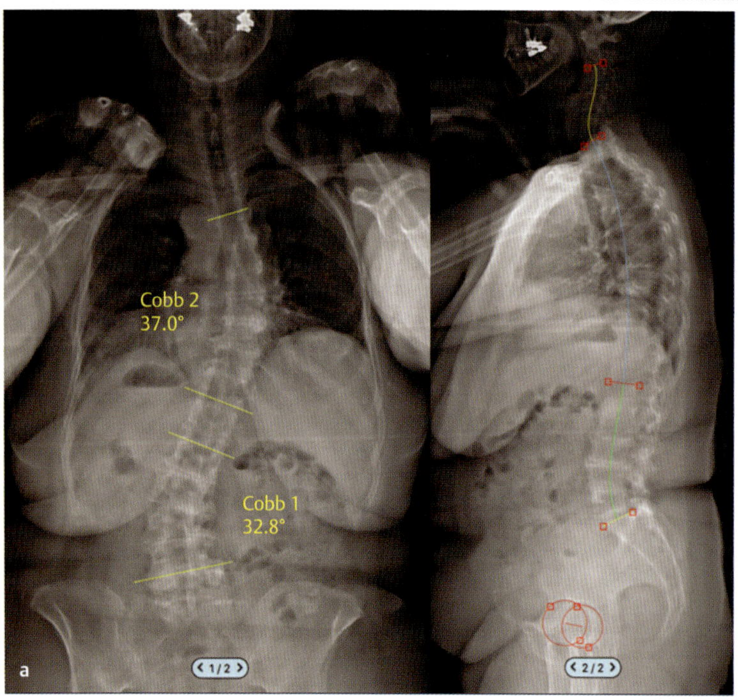

b

Parameter	Value
Pelvic incidence	56
Pelvic tilt	25
Lumbar lordosis	28
L4-S1 lordosis	29
SVA	4.5 cm

Fig. 50.1 **(a)** EOS radiographs with measurement for pelvic parameters and Cobb angles. **(b)** Sagittal parameter measurements.

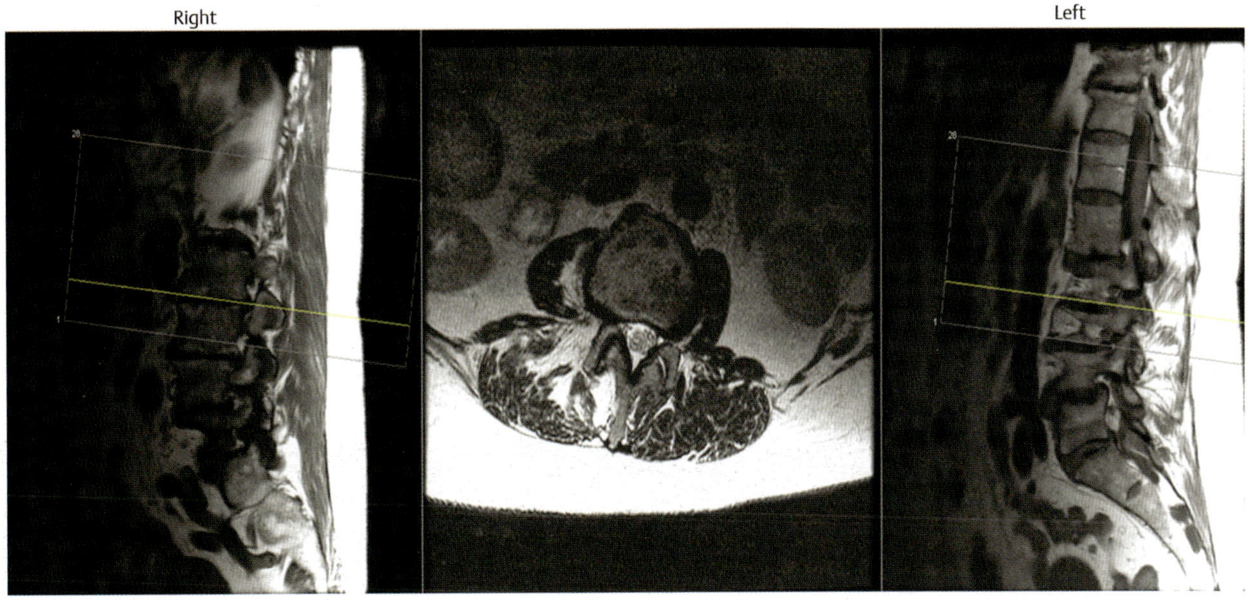

Fig. 50.2 Magnetic resonance imaging (MRI) of L2–L3.

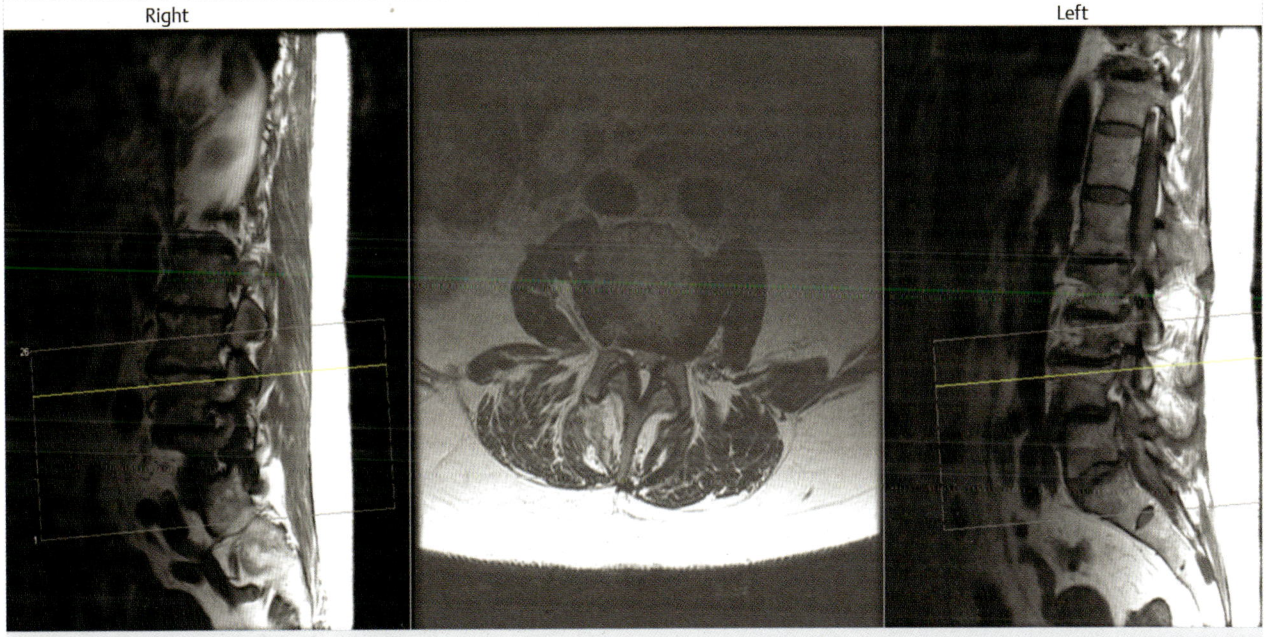

Fig. 50.3 Magnetic resonance imaging (MRI) of L3–L4.

▶ Fig. 50.5). The goals of treatment for this patient include a restoration of age-adjusted pelvic parameters through hyperlordotic interbody cages and indirect decompression of foraminal stenosis through minimally invasive techniques to minimize morbidity and allow quicker recovery.

50.6 Applied Anatomy of the Lateral Approach to the Spine

The lateral abdominal wall comprises the superficial anatomy of the lateral approach to the lumbar spine. The layers that must be dissected to reach the retroperitoneum are in the order: skin, subcutaneous tissue, fascia, external oblique muscle, internal oblique muscle, and transversalis muscle. The psoas muscle overlies the lateral lumbar spine in the retroperitoneum (▶ Fig. 50.6a). The lumbosacral plexus, genitofemoral nerve, and lateral femoral cutaneous nerve are located within the psoas muscle. In general, the lumbosacral plexus becomes more ventrolateral as you progress distally in the lumbar spine, but there is great variability between different individuals as shown by Moro et al in a cadaveric study[9] (▶ Fig. 50.6b). The aorta and inferior vena cava (IVC) run anterior to the lumbar spine with the IVC on the right and the aorta on the left.

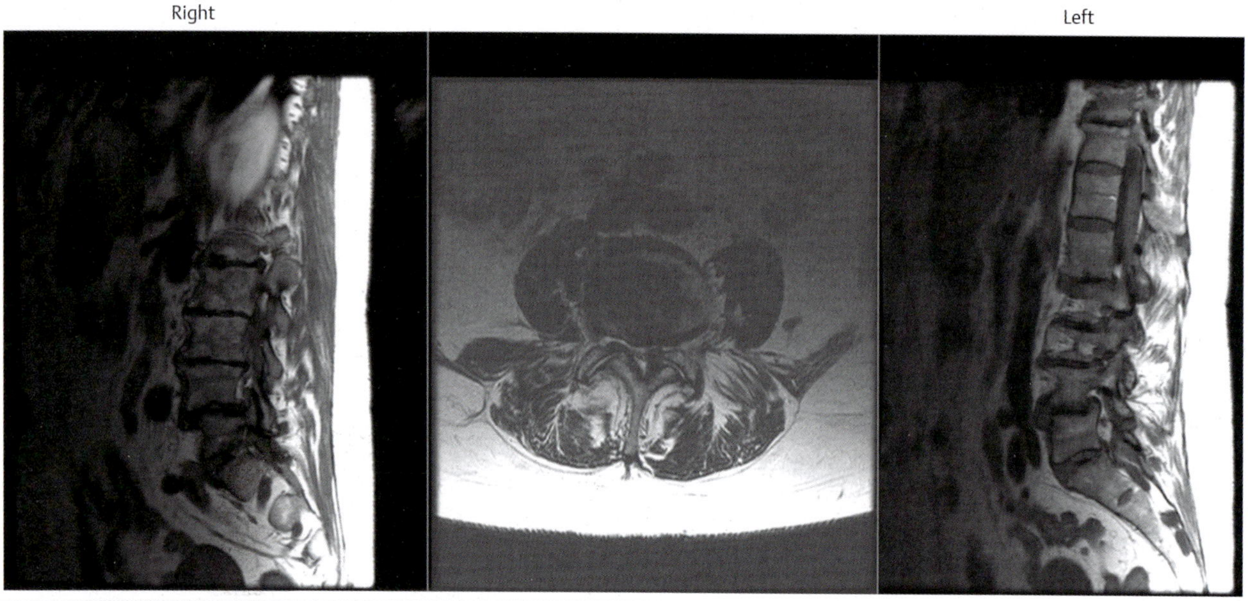

Fig. 50.4 Magnetic resonance imaging (MRI) of L4–L5.

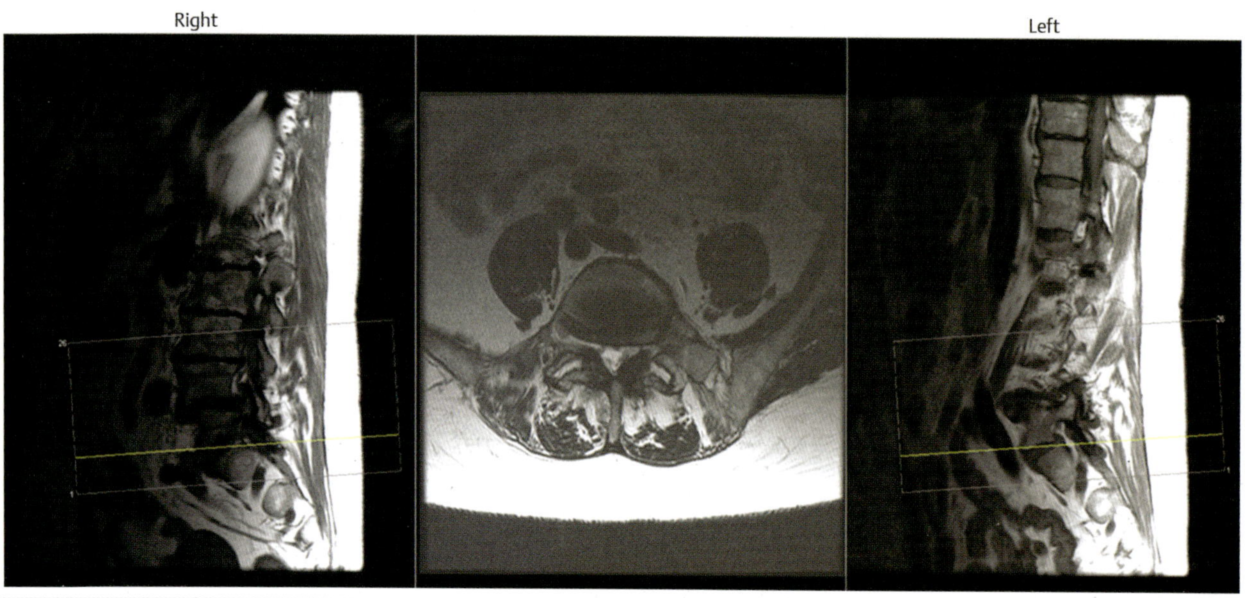

Fig. 50.5 Magnetic resonance imaging (MRI) of L5–S1.

50.7 Surgical Procedure

50.7.1 Preoperative

Initial preoperative plan should include a plan on which side should be utilized for approach and a thorough evaluation of radiographs to assess the ribs and the iliac crest levels which are accessible from a lateral approach. The laterality of approach is surgeon dependent; some surgeons prefer to approach from the left due to the anterior position of the vascular structures from this side. Other considerations include the convexity of the curve for approach. Some surgeons approach from the convex side of the curve to facilitate intradiscal work, while other surgeons prefer approaching from the concave side to facilitate approaching several levels through the same incision.[9,10] Our preference is to approach from the convex side of the deformity for the ease of intradiscal use and make multiple small incisions if needed. It is important to discuss the operative plan with the anesthetist prior to surgery as neuromonitoring is essential to this approach due to the proximity to the lumbar plexus.

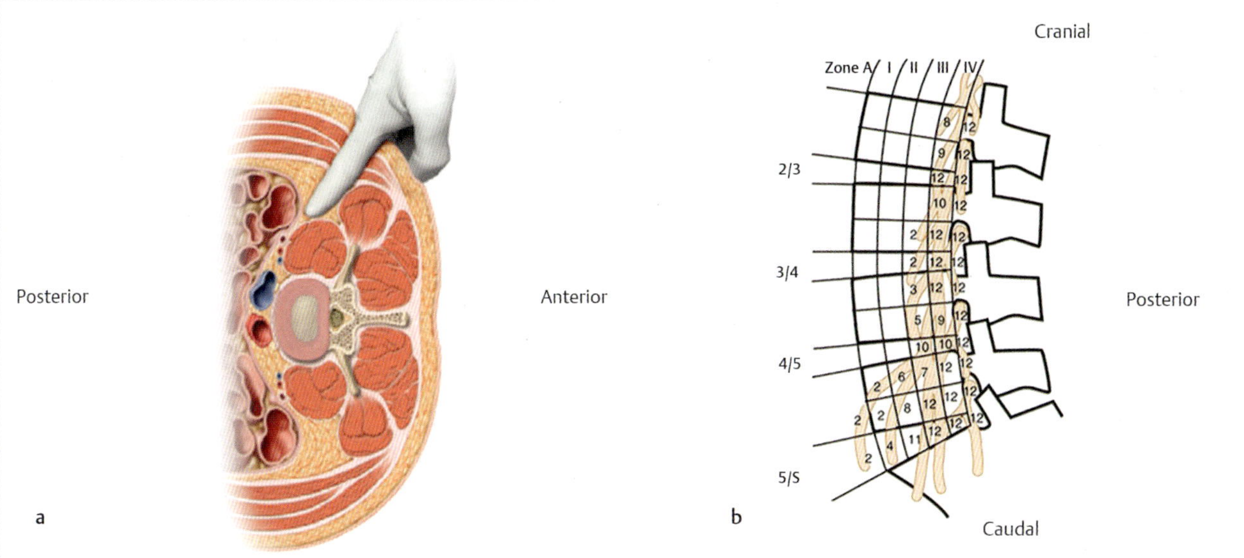

Fig. 50.6 **(a)** Applied anatomy of the lateral approach to the lumbar spine. (Reprinted from NuVasive XLIF Guide. NuVasive, San Diego, CA. 2019; p. 8, Fig. 12, with permission from NuVasive.) **(b)** Location of lumbosacral plexus during lateral surgery. (Reprinted from Lu YI, Wong JM, and Chi JH. Schmidek and Sweet: Operative Neurosurgical Techniques. Elsevier. 2012; pp. 1963–1972, with permission from Elsevier.)

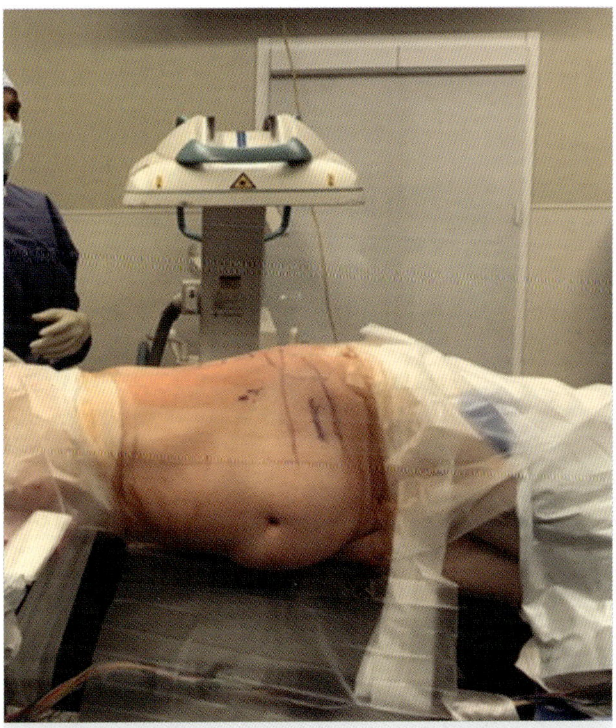

Fig. 50.7 Patient is placed in lateral position with the use of a Wilson frame and taped into a secure position.

50.7.2 Positioning, X-Ray, and Equipment

Positioning for lateral interbody fusion is of the utmost importance and is what allows facilitation of minimally invasive techniques to be performed. Patients are placed in the true lateral position. Some surgeons will position on a regular operating room (OR) table with the iliac crest just proximal to the table break, allowing for flexion of the table and easier access to the interbody space. Our preference is to position the patient in the lateral position on a Wilson frame in the maximally closed position to facilitate more efficient flipping for percutaneous pedicle screw placement as there is no need to switch operating tables. In addition, the Wilson frame also allows for the lateral bending necessary to facilitate easier access to the disc space (▶ Fig. 50.7). The hips are flexed to around 30 degrees to take pressure of the psoas muscle. The patient is then taped to the OR table to prevent any motion during the procedure. This tape is placed overlying the greater trochanter and overlying the chest in a horizontal fashion (▶ Fig. 50.7).

Our C-arm is positioned to come in from the posterior of the patient for easy access to lateral and AP radiographs (▶ Fig. 50.7). We use a Ziehm Vision intraoperative CT scanner as we will navigate our percutaneous screws and sometimes navigate the first level of the lateral interbody, but any standard C-arm can be used for localization. The navigation computer—we use Stryker NAV3i—should be positioned at the foot of the table (▶ Fig. 50.8a). We position a Stryker SpineMask tracker on the patient to allow for a noninvasive method for registration of intraoperative images (▶ Fig. 50.8b). The remainder of the equipment needed for this procedure include neuromonitoring, retractor arm attached to the bed, and hyperlordotic interbody cages.

50.8 Surgical Steps

50.8.1 Localizing the Incision

There are two options for localizing the incision for lateral interbody fusion. We have used each successfully in the past. There are limitations to either method.

1. The first method involves obtaining a perfect lateral radiograph of the lumbar spine. The end plates of the vertebrae should be parallel. A guidewire is then used to mark the

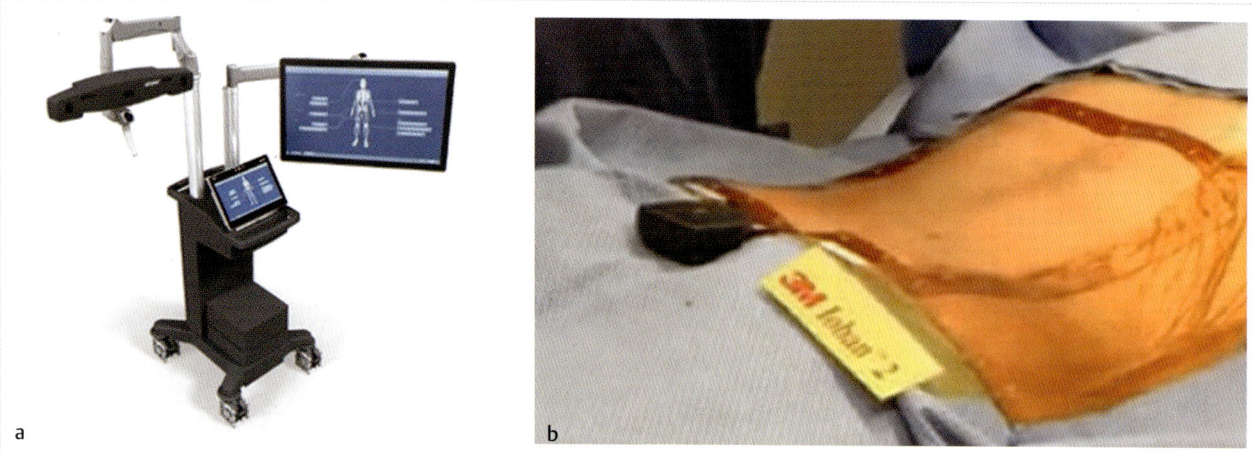

Fig. 50.8 **(a)** Stryker Navigation Software (NAV3i). (Used with permission from Stryker Spine.) **(b)** SpineMask.

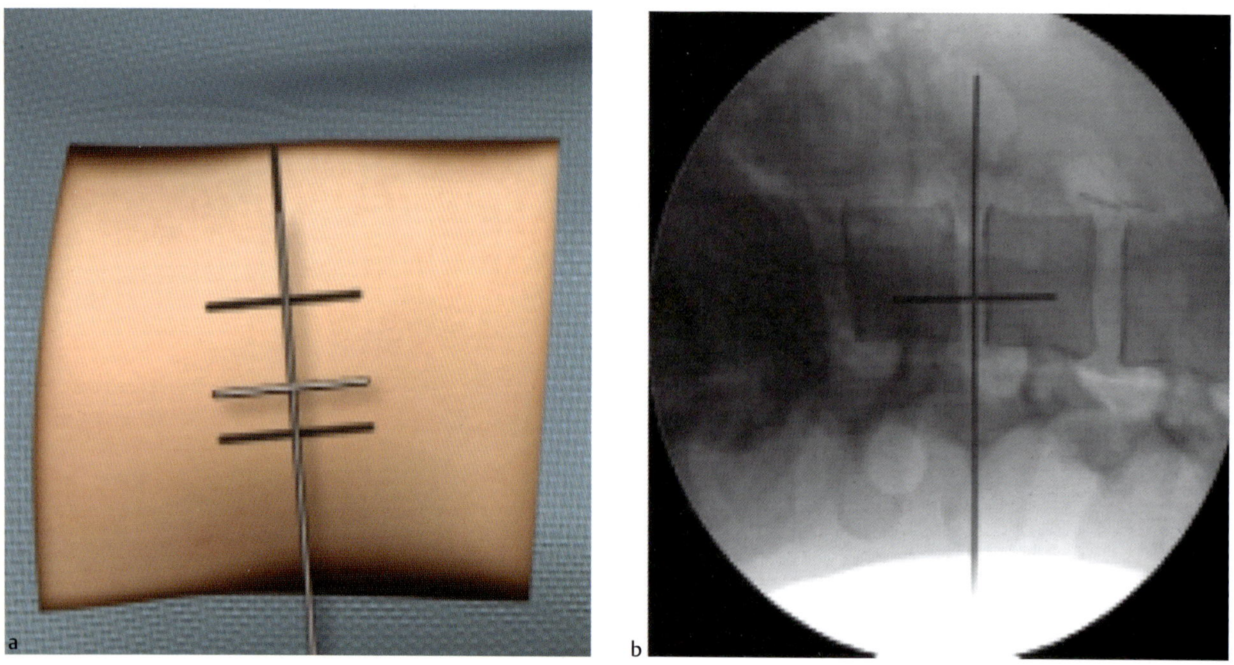

Fig. 50.9 **(a)** Marking the lateral incision. **(b)** True lateral radiograph of lumbar spine. (Reprinted from NuVasive XLIF Guide. NuVasive, San Diego, CA. 2019; p. 7, Fig. 8, with permission from NuVasive.)

incision between the anterior and posterior borders of the involved disc in a parallel fashion (▶ Fig. 50.9a). This should be repeated for all the levels involved. The main drawback to this method is radiation exposure to the operative staff.

2. The second method involves navigation. An intraoperative CT scan is obtained with the three-dimensional C-arm. These images are then uploaded to the navigation system, which are correlated with preoperative images and allows for real-time visualization of radiographs without the need for constant radiation (▶ Fig. 50.10). The drawback to this method is that all incisions would have to be marked out prior to the first interbody being placed for maximal accuracy.

50.8.2 Approach

There are two options for the approach to the lumbar spine from the lateral position. A one-incision or two-incision technique can be utilized. Our preference is for a one-incision technique, which entails making an incision in line with our prior marking and dissecting through the external oblique, internal oblique, and transversalis to reach the retroperitoneum. Care should be taken to avoid electrocautery once the transversalis muscle layer has been reached to avoid accidental injury to the peritoneum. Blunt dissection is carried down to the level of the psoas. Two reference points to ensure you are in the retroperitoneum include the

feeling of striations that correlate with the psoas musculature and the presence of retroperitoneal fat; both features should be identified prior to proceeding to the next step of surgery.

Alternatively, a two-incision technique can be utilized. A posteriorly based incision about 5 cm posterior to the standard transverse incision is made and carried down to the level of the retroperitoneum. The standard transverse incision is then made and carried down to the fascia. A finger is passed from the posterior incision and pushed up from underneath the abdominal musculature, which allows for identification of the retroperitoneal space before dissection of the external oblique, internal oblique, and tranversalis.

50.8.3 Dilator Tubes/Retractor Docking

A small dilator is placed trans-psoas into the disc space (▶ Fig. 50.11a). Some surgeons will prefer to dock on top of the psoas muscle to allow for dissection of the psoas under direct visualization. This is surgeon's preference. The position of the dilator will vary level by level, but generally for most levels care should be taken to be at the midpoint of the disc (▶ Fig. 50.11b). Neuromonitoring is performed to evaluate the distance of the lumbar plexus from the dilator. Sequential dilation is then performed with neuromonitoring performed after placement of every dilator. After the last dilator is placed, a member of the operative team will then attach the retractor arm to the operating table. A retractor is placed over the last dilator and connected to the retractor arm. The retractor should be positioned slightly posterior to the midline of the disc space to allow it to open anteriorly (▶ Fig. 50.12a). At this point any remaining soft tissue present over the lateral disc space can be cleared via blunt dissection. With the lateral disc space clear of any remaining soft tissue the posterior blade can be deployed (▶ Fig. 50.12b). In cases of deformity, where competency of the

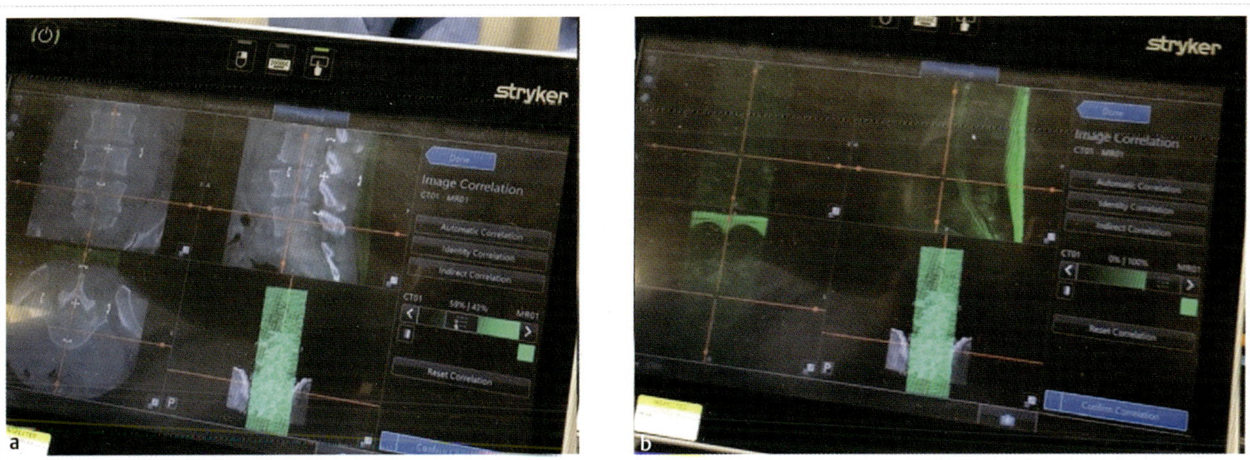

Fig. 50.10 (a, b) Use of navigation for lumbar spine surgery with the correlation of lumbar computed tomography (CT) and lumbar magnetic resonance imaging (MRI).

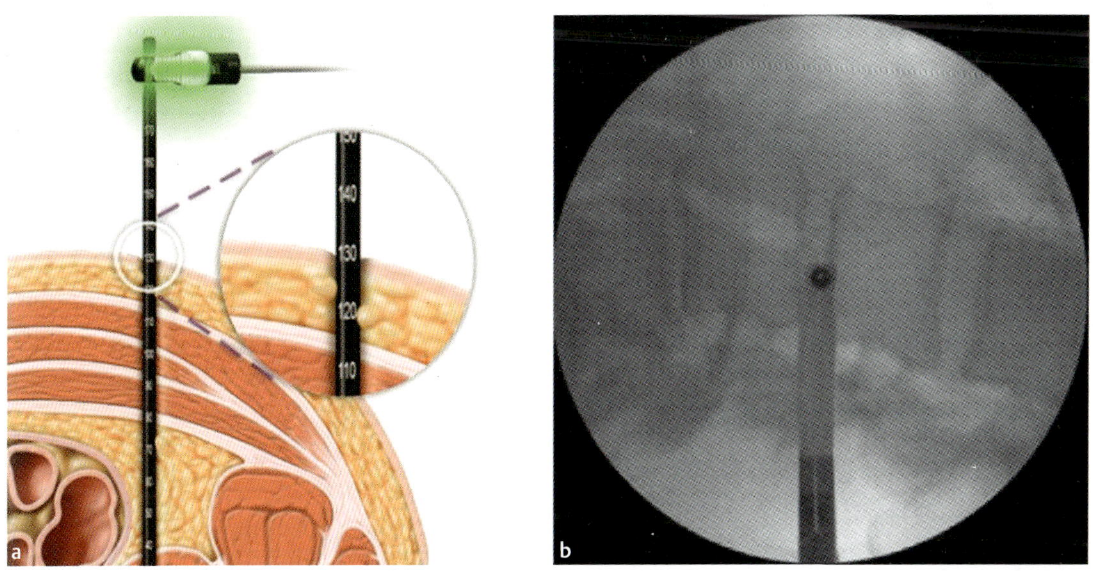

Fig. 50.11 (a) Dilator placement with neuromonitoring attachment. **(b)** Dilator positioning on the disc space. (Reprinted from NuVasive XLIF Guide. NuVasive, San Diego, CA. 2019; p. 10-11, Figs 21 and 23, with permission from NuVasive.)

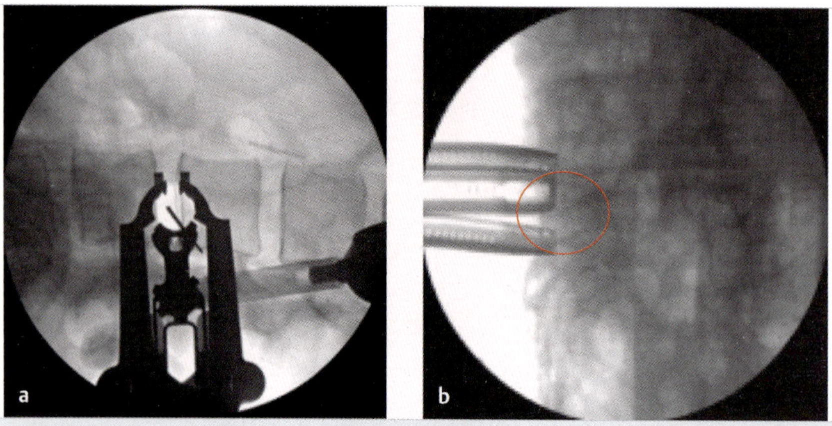

Fig. 50.12 **(a)** Placement of retractor system. **(b)** Posterior shim (circled) for retractor stability.

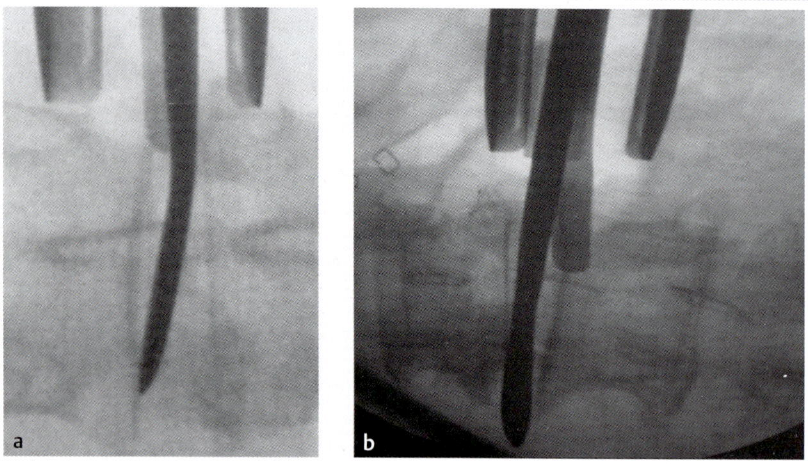

Fig. 50.13 **(a)** End plate preparation with Cobb elevator. **(b)** Contralateral annular release essential to restoration of coronal balance.

anterior longitudinal ligament (ALL) is important to allow for placement of lordotic cages while minimizing the risk of cage dislodgement, an optional retractor can be placed anteriorly to allow direct visualization of the ALL.

> Single-stage spinal surgery is rapidly evolving with the help of improved implants, instrumentation, and imaging/navigation technologies. Robotic navigation may have some advantages over freehand three-dimensional navigation in this setting and in our experience, the lateral position also allows direct tubular decompression if necessary.

50.8.4 Discectomy

With exposure to the lateral disc space obtained, an annulotomy is performed in a rectangular fashion and a pituitary is used to remove any remaining nucleus pulposus. A Cobb elevator is passed along the superior and inferior end plates (▶ Fig. 50.13a). In our experience, an angled Cobb is most useful to ensure the cartilaginous end plate is fully removed, specifically along the superior end plate. An AP radiograph is taken at this time to ensure the Cobb elevator has removed the end plates on the far-lateral side of the disc. A contralateral annular release is essential to correction of coronal deformity (▶ Fig. 50.13b). A combination of curettes and shavers are used to clean any remaining portions of the cartilaginous end plate with care taken to avoid bony end plate violation, which is a risk factor for graft subsidence.

50.8.5 Trialing and Graft Placement

Placement of the cage in the correct position is essential for deformity correction and to decrease the risk of subsidence. Sizing is performed via sizing trials. A reasonable amount of tension should be obtained on sizing trials. The alignment of the cage selected should be established when evaluating your indications for the procedure. In our case a hyperlordotic cage was used to obtain correction of lumbar lordosis and sagittal parameters. On the AP radiograph, the cage should extend to the lateral rim of the end plate on each side, which enables better correction of coronal plane deformity (▶ Fig. 50.14a). On the lateral radiograph, the cage should be centered to slightly anterior to allow for maximal fusion surface area, sagittal plane correction, and preventing end plate subsidence.[11] Once trialing is complete, the

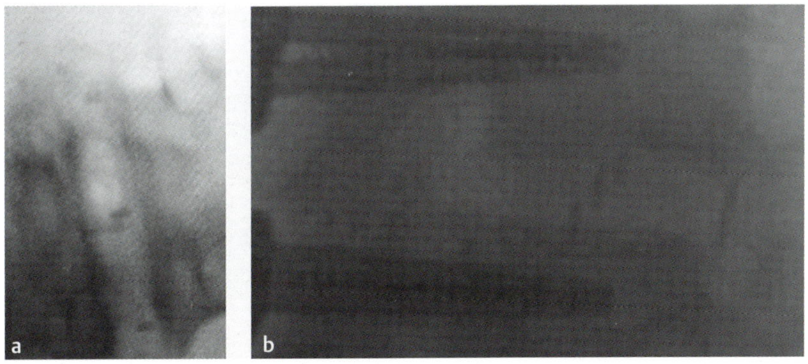

Fig. 50.14 **(a)** Placement of interbody cage should extend past the lateral rim of end plate. **(b)** Interbody cage should be slightly anterior/centered on lateral radiograph.

interbody cage with bone graft is placed in the interbody space (▶ Fig. 50.14b). A graft slider is used to prevent violations of the end plate with graft/cage insertion. These steps are then repeated for the remainder of the levels that will be addressed from the lateral position. Hemostasis is obtained prior to removal of the retractor and a layered closure is performed.

50.8.6 Addressing the L5–S1 Level

TLIF, ALIF, and OLIF can all be used to obtain interbody access to the L5–S1 level. Since most of lumbar lordosis comes from the L4–S1 level in the lumbar spine any approach to this level of the spine for deformity and loss or lordosis should be one that can reliably restore lumbar lordosis. Our preference is to perform an ALIF for this level due to the ability to place large hyperlordotic cages.

50.8.7 Lateral ALIF

Our preference is to perform an ALIF from the lateral position without the need to reposition the patient. The advantages of performing the ALIF from the lateral position are decreased operative time as the patient does not have to be repositioned and the effects of gravity assisting with exposure as the peritoneum can fall away from the surgical field. The main disadvantages to a laterally based ALIF are surgeon's disorientation as it is a novel approach with a learning curve and having an approach surgeon who is comfortable performing an ALIF approach. This novel technique requires an incision that overlies the L5–S1 disc space. A lateral radiograph is obtained with a marker over the L5–S1 disc space and an incision is marked out anterior to the iliac crest in line with the L5–S1 disc space (▶ Fig. 50.15a). Bedrail attachments should be placed—one that is distal and anterior to planned incision and one that is posterior and superior to planned incision (▶ Fig. 50.15b). An approach surgeon should be used. An incision is made anterior to the iliac crest and the external oblique, internal oblique, and transversalis are bluntly dissected until the peritoneum is reached. Blunt dissection is then carried out to the level of the sacral promontory (▶ Fig. 50.16). The left common iliac vein and artery are then palpated and the lateral blade is then inserted to retract these vessels (▶ Fig. 50.17a). The next step is insertion of a medial blade with a reverse tip on the contralateral side of disc space (▶ Fig. 50.17b). A cranial blade is then inserted for additional exposure (▶ Fig. 50.17c). All of these blades are then attached to a retractor ring called a C-frame (▶ Fig. 50.18a, b). Exposure to the L5–S1 disc space can be safely performed from the lateral position, which facilitates placement of a hyperlordotic interbody cage to restore LL. The obviation for the need to reposition the patient allows for increased OR efficiency and decreased anesthesia time, blood loss, and operative time. If this technology is not available, other alternatives for addressing the L5–S1 level are OLIF which can be performed in the lateral position and ALIF with the patient in a supine position.

50.8.8 Percutaneous Pedicle Screw Placement

Once all of the interbody cages are in place, the surgical wounds are closed and the patient is placed in a prone position. There are two separate techniques for pedicle screw placement. Our preference is for placement of pedicle screws based on navigation, but standard fluoroscopy can be used as well.

A second intraoperative fluoroscopic CT scan is taken with the patient in the lateral position because the first three-dimensional fluoro spin will no longer be accurate with the addition of the interbody cages. These images are then transferred to the navigation system to allow placement of pedicle screws based on the navigation software. This obviates the need for continuous fluoroscopy. Alternatively, if fluoroscopy is used properly aligned AP radiographs are obtained. Irrespective the method used, the steps for pedicle screw placement remain the same. The Jamshidi needle should be docked at the lateral margin of the pedicle and should be gently advanced while working toward the medial border of the pedicle (▶ Fig. 50.19a). If fluoroscopy is used, a lateral radiograph should be obtained at this time to ensure that the Jamshidi needle is ventral to the posterior border of the vertebral body prior to placement of a guidewire (▶ Fig. 50.19b). There should be a bony end point on insertion of the guidewire. This step is repeated for all instrumented levels. The pedicle of each level is tapped over a guidewire under radiographic guidance or with navigation. Screws are then placed over a guidewire, with the guidewire being removed after the screw has advanced past the posterior aspect of the vertebral body. Each screw should then be tested to ensure there is no evidence of pedicle breach. After all screws are in place, the length of the rod is measured with calipers.

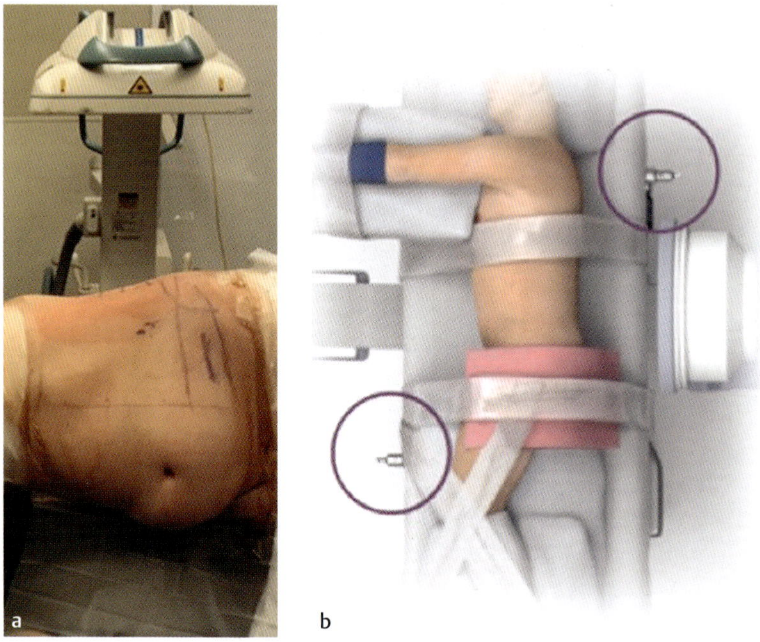

Fig. 50.15 (a) Marking incision between iliac crest and lateral portion of rectus. (b) Placement of bedrail attachments. (Reprinted from Lateral ALIF Guide. NuVasive, San Diego, CA. 2017; p. 4, Fig. 8, with permission from NuVasive.)

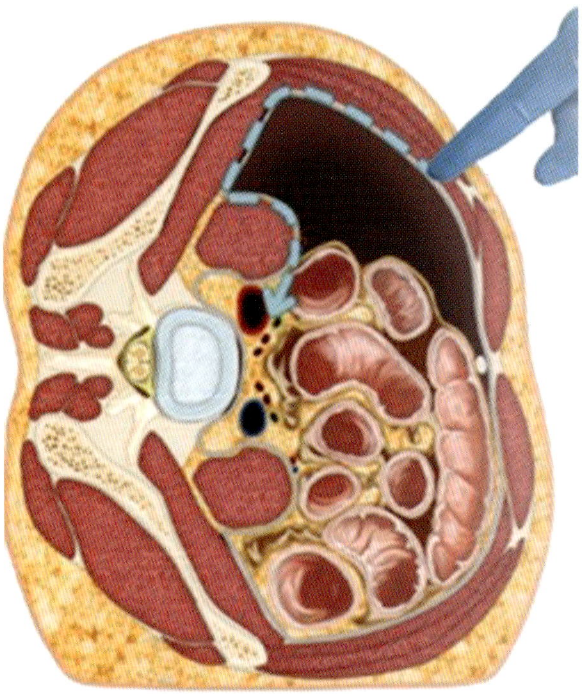

Fig. 50.16 Access to retroperitoneum to the level of sacral promontory. (Reprinted from Lateral ALIF Guide. NuVasive, San Diego, CA. 2017; p. 5, Fig. 9, with permission from NuVasive.)

The appropriate length rod is then placed under the fascia through the rod sleeves. This can be done with either a mini-open technique or percutaneously with a fixed angle rod inserter. Our preference is to use a fixed angle rod inserter to prevent further dissection through the muscle. Insertion of the rod will depend on the specific system used, but care must be taken to ensure the rod passes through the pedicle screw extender sleeve; some systems have a mechanism built in to check that the rod is inserted through each tulip correctly. Fluoroscopy should be used to check that the rod has extended far enough past the tulip head on either side. Our preference is to use precontoured rods that match the desired sagittal contour. Screws caps are then placed and the rod sleeves are removed. A layered closured is then performed.

50.9 Postoperative Course

Each of these patients are admitted for 2 to 3 days barring any complications in the postoperative course. We do not believe in the use of drains for this procedure. Adequate hemostasis should be obtained at the time of surgery and drains have been shown to increase patient's discomfort and increase operative time. Physical therapy is undertaken on hospital day 0 or day 1. We do not place any postoperative precautions on our patients. We also give a multimodality control regimen including Skelaxin, Tylenol, tramadol, and possibly Toradol if needed. We limit any stronger narcotics unless absolutely needed by the patient as we feel this will prolong hospital stays and prevent patients from participating in physical therapy as effectively. In the postoperative period,

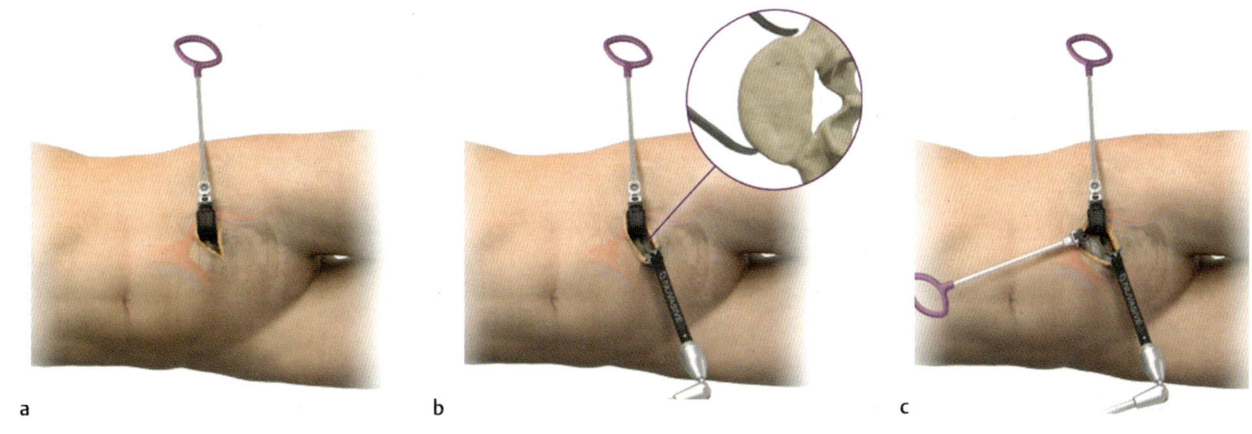

Fig. 50.17 (a) Lateral blade. (b) Medial blade with reverse tip (circled). (c) Cranial blade. (Reprinted from Lateral ALIF Guide. NuVasive, San Diego, CA. 2017; pp. 6–7, Figs 11–13; with permission from NuVasive.)

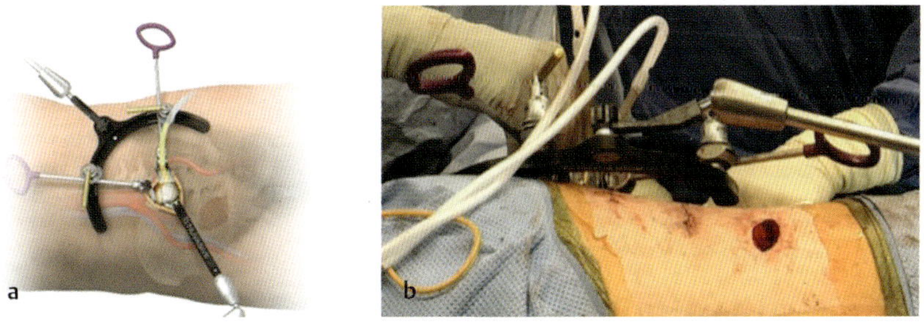

Fig. 50.18 (a) C-frame. (Reprinted from Lateral ALIF Guide. NuVasive, San Diego, CA. 2017; p. 8, Fig. 14, with permission from NuVasive.) (b) Setup for lateral anterior lumbar interbody fusion (ALIF) at L5–S1.

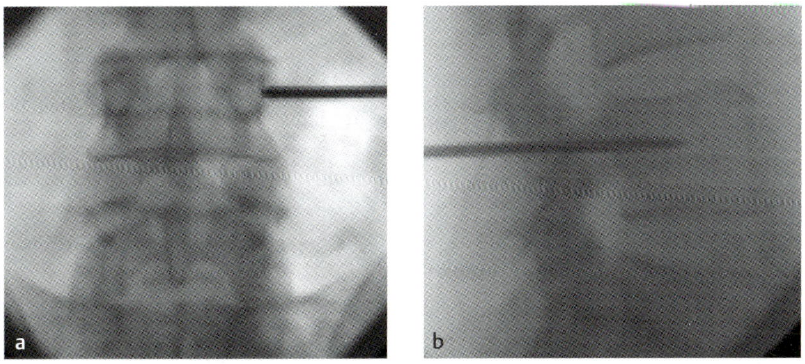

Fig. 50.19 (a) Jamshidi needle at lateral border of pedicle. (b) Placement of Jamshidi needle is ventral to posterior border of vertebral body.

it is common to have some hip flexion weakness on the ipsilateral side. This will commonly resolve by 6 months postoperatively. The patient is generally discharged home. We have patients follow-up at 2 weeks, 6 weeks, 3 months, 6 months, 1 year, and then yearly after that. We allow Dermabond to fall off naturally and do not use any nonabsorbable sutures. We allow showering after hospital discharge. We obtain EOS images at each postoperative visit to assess the change in pelvic parameters over time. If there is any clinical concern for a pseudoarthrosis we will obtain a CT scan between 6 months to 1 year to assess for fusion.

50.10 Back to Case

Our patient underwent an L1–S1 posterior spinal fusion (PSF) with L1–L5 LLIFs and L5–S1 lateral ALIF. She was able to be discharged from the hospital on postoperative day 5. She had iliopsoas (IP) weakness (3/5) on the ipsilateral side of surgical approach, which is slowly starting to resolve. She was informed that postoperative IP weakness was one of the most common risks of lateral lumbar surgery prior to surgery. She is currently able to ambulate without pain and has no complaints of radicular

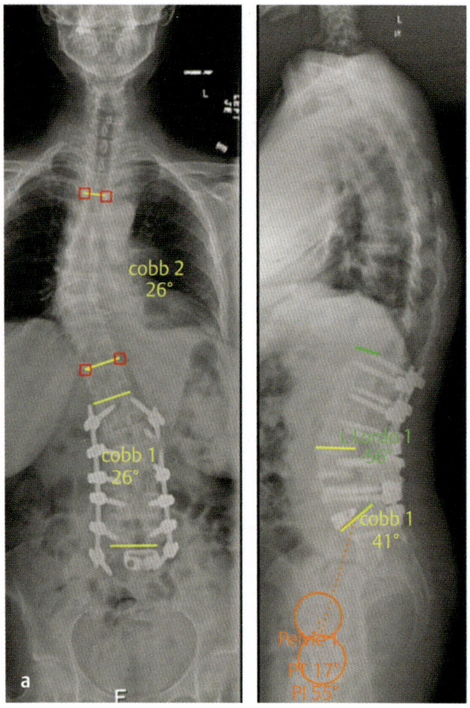

a

Parameter	Preoperative	Postoperative
Pelvic incidence	56	55
Pelvic tilt	25	17
Lumbar lordosis	28	56
L4-S1 Lordosis	29	41
SVA	4.5 cm	4.9 cm

b

Fig. 50.20 **(a)** Anteroposterior (AP) and lateral EOS images. **(b)** Preoperative versus postoperative pelvic parameters.

or claudicatory type pain. Her postoperative radiographs show a restoration of pelvic parameters and correction of coronal deformity (▶ Fig. 50.20a). Her pelvic parameters were improved to age-adjusted values compared to preoperatively (▶ Fig. 50.20b).

50.11 Tips and Pearls for Treating ADLS with Minimally Invasive Surgery

In going over the steps for successful minimally invasive spine surgery, we have identified different pearls that allow the surgery to be done successfully:

a) We used a Wilson frame on a Jackson table with the Wilson frame pieces placed maximally together. This allows for superior creation of separation between the vertebral bodies, allowing for easier access to the disc space. We feel this is superior to using a regular table in a jack-knife position. In addition, it also makes flipping the patient to the posterior position more streamlined as the Wilson frame is already in place.
b) When performing lateral surgery, many surgeons will manipulate the table (i.e., table positioned to the right or left) to obtain the perfect lateral radiograph. We feel that this step is time consuming. We opt to control and manipulate the C-arm to obtain the perfect lateral radiograph of the lumbar spine. This saves us time without increasing the danger of the operation. However, you must operate in the same plane as the C-arm to ensure proper trajectory.
c) The use of large hyperlordotic cages has enabled minimally invasive spine surgery to be used for deformity procedures. Previously, smaller cages were unreliable for correcting both segmental and overall lordosis.
d) For interbody lumbar surgery, it is imperative to obtain coverage of the hypophyseal ring to prevent subsidence of the graft/interbody.
e) For correction for coronal deformity, a contralateral annular release should be performed and the graft/cage should extend beyond the lateral end plate of the vertebral body on both the ipsilateral and contralateral sides.
f) The most important factor that allows successful implementation of minimally invasive surgery is to treat each surgery according to standard deformity principles. In both open and minimally invasive surgery, the goals of treatment should be the same. Restoration of most lumbar lordosis at L4–S1, correction of SVA, and balancing of coronal deformities are the goals of the operation. Minimally invasive techniques and technology are just tools to help achieve the application of these discussed principles.

References

[1] Cho K-J, Kim Y-T, Shin SH, Suk S-I. Surgical treatment of adult degenerative scoliosis. Asian Spine J. 2014; 8(3):371–381
[2] Wang G, Hu J, Liu X, Cao Y. Surgical treatments for degenerative lumbar scoliosis: a meta analysis. Eur Spine J. 2015; 24(8):1792–1799
[3] Kotwal S, Pumberger M, Hughes A, Girardi F. Degenerative scoliosis: a review. HSS J. 2011; 7(3):257–264

[4] Sebaaly A, Grobost P, Mallam L, Roussouly P. Description of the sagittal alignment of the degenerative human spine. Eur Spine J. 2018; 27(2):489–496
[5] Wiesel SW. Operative Techniques in Orthopaedic Surgery. Wolters Kluwer; 2016
[6] Mobbs RJ, Phan K, Malham G, Seex K, Rao PJ. Lumbar interbody fusion: techniques, indications and comparison of interbody fusion options including PLIF, TLIF, MI-TLIF, OLIF/ATP, LLIF and ALIF. J Spine Surg. 2015; 1(1):2–18
[7] Dangelmajer S, Zadnik PL, Rodriguez ST, Gokaslan ZL, Sciubba DM. Minimally invasive spine surgery for adult degenerative lumbar scoliosis. Neurosurg Focus. 2014; 36(5):E7
[8] Mummaneni PV, Shaffrey CI, Lenke LG, et al. Minimally Invasive Surgery Section of the International Spine Study Group. The minimally invasive spinal deformity surgery algorithm: a reproducible rational framework for decision making in minimally invasive spinal deformity surgery. Neurosurg Focus. 2014; 36(5):E6
[9] Moro T, Kikuchi S, Konno S, Yaginuma H. An anatomic study of the lumbar plexus with respect to retroperitoneal endoscopic surgery. Spine. 2003; 28 (5):423–428, discussion 427–428
[10] Epstein NE. Extreme lateral lumbar interbody fusion: do the cons outweigh the pros? Surg Neurol Int. 2016; 7 Suppl 25:S692–S700
[11] Anand N. How to create sagittal balance in MIS correction of adult spinal deformity. Spine. 2017; 42 Suppl 7:S17–S18

51 Strategies to Minimize Invasiveness and Optimize Success: T10-Pelvis

Neel Anand, Alisa Alayan, and Sheila Kahwaty

Summary
This chapter provides a step-by-step description of patient evaluation and surgical execution of degenerative spinal deformity correction with circumferentially minimally invasive approach.

Keywords: deformity correction, circumferential minimally invasive, MIS, ante-psoas, multilevel OLIF, LLIF

Case Example

51.1 Preoperative Presentation

A 71-year-old male—competitive tennis player—presented with progressive low back pain and leaning forward posture over the last several months prior to being seen. He had L5–S1 transforaminal interbody fusion (TLIF) 4 years prior and initially did well postoperatively, but slowly began developing low back pain. He did not have radicular symptoms on presentation. His pain limited his desired activities, especially within the last year prior to seeking consultation. He attempted conservative measures such as physical therapy, exercises, and massage. He had partial relief from nonsteroidal anti-inflammatory drugs (NSAIDs) such as Celebrex and Toradol. Past medical history included cardiac stent placement and prostate surgery, but no active problems. On examination, he had full strength in his lower extremities and no gait instability. Posture was observed to have positive sagittal balance and mid back kyphosis.

51.2 Imaging Studies

a) Standing 36-inch scoliosis X-rays to assess global alignment and spinopelvic parameters:
   1. In this patient, we observed degenerative lumbar dextroscoliosis, with apex at around L3. There was mild shift to the left, but overall balanced coronally. Prior L5–S1 hardware was noted. Significant multilevel disc collapse was observed: L4–L5 collapsed to right; T12–L1, L1–L2, L2–L3, and L3–L4 collapsed to left; T11–T12 collapsed to the right. On the lateral film, loss of lumbar lordosis (LL) is observed, with kyphosis at T12–L1. L1–L2 retrolisthesis is also noted (see ▶ Fig. 51.1).
   2. Pelvic incidence (PI) 70.8 degrees, pelvic tilt (PT) 37.7 degrees, LL 50.7 degrees, sagittal vertical axis (SVA) 114.5 mm, PI-LL mismatch 20.1 degrees.
b) Computed tomography (CT) thoracic and lumbar spine without contrast to assess bony anatomy and rule out spondylolysis or bony fusion of interbody segments or facet joints.
c) In this case, since the patient had previous surgery at L5–S1, we observed the bilateral L5 and S1 screws in appropriate position. We also noted an interbody graft with no evidence of bridging bone across the levels, suggesting pseudarthrosis at the L5–S1 level. The facets at L5–S1, as well as levels above, did not appear fused. We noted presence of gas in each lumbar disc space (see ▶ Fig. 51.2).
d) Magnetic resonance imaging (MRI) lumbar spine without contrast to assess stenosis, disc quality, spinal anomalies, and soft tissue anatomy. Most importantly, MRI allows the team to study the access corridor to the disc through the ante-psoas approach and evaluate the vascular anatomy:
   1. In this patient, we observed multilevel central and lateral recess stenosis at T10–T11, T11–T12, T12–L1, L1–L2, L2–L3, L3–L4, and L4–L5. No large central or far-lateral disc herniation was observed (see ▶ Fig. 51.3).
e) Bone density scan of the hips and spine to assess bone quality:
   1. The femoral neck T-score for this patient was −0.3. The T-score for the lumbar spine was 2.1.

51.3 Decision-Making for MIS

The patient appeared healthy enough to be a surgical candidate with realistic goals and significant impairment of his desired activities. He had exhausted conservative measures. He had progressive sagittal imbalance, measuring 114.5 mm. He had presence of gas in all the lumbar disc spaces on the CT scan, suggesting mobility of the discs. This reassured us that we would be able to elevate the disc spaces and achieve some degree of deformity correction, lordosis, and indirect decompression with interbody grafts at each level. These are the foundation of the corrective forces in this specific MIS technique. Finally, we looked on the MRI for open corridors between the psoas and the vessels, making sure we could place the interbody grafts safely in an ante-psoas MIS fashion.

51.4 Factors Favoring Open Surgery

a) Previous complex abdominal surgery preventing the ante-psoas and MIS L5–S1 oblique lateral interbody fusion (OLIF) approach.
b) High-risk medical comorbidities and osteoporosis (bone density scan T score of −3.0 or worse).
c) Multiple fused segments on CT/prior multilevel fusion surgery.
d) Aberrant vessels visualized on MRI which prevent safe access to the disc spaces safely.

51.5 Details of Surgery

Medtronic instrumentation is used for both stages by the senior author.

Somatosensory evoked potential (SSEP) monitoring not required for stage 1.

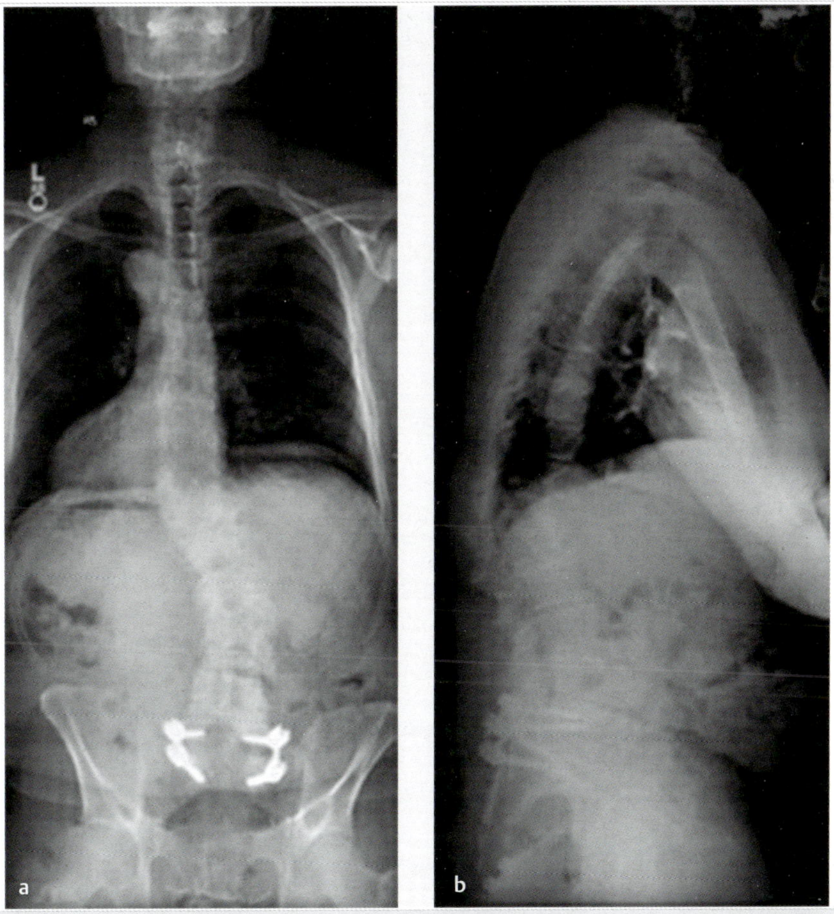

Fig. 51.1 (a) Anteroposterior AP) and (b) lateral standing scoliosis radiographs. Previous L5–S1 fusion hardware is noted. (b) Degenerative lumbar dextroscoliosis, with apex at around L3 is noted. (b) Loss of lumbar lordosis is observed, with kyphosis at T12–L1. Overall positive sagittal balance. The global deformity measurements include: Cobb angle 25, pelvic incidence (PI) 70.8, pelvic tilt (PT) 37.7, lumbar lordosis (LL) 50.7, sagittal vertical axis (SVA) 114.5 mm, PI-LL mismatch 20.1.

51.5.1 Stage 1

1. **Positioning**: Right lateral decubitus position (left side up) on a flat top Jackson table, with an axillary roll under the right axilla. A pillow is placed under the right knee to protect the peroneal nerve. The kidney rest is elevated to open the left flank. Tape is placed across the iliac crest, chest, greater trochanter, and legs. The C-arm is parked at the patient's back and the surgeon stands in front of the patient. The retractor system is attached on the table rail behind the patient at the level of the shoulder.
2. **Approach to L5–S1:**
   Mark the anterior and posterior margins of the disc space at L5–S1 with lateral view X-ray. Draw a diagonal line toward the pubis in line with the disc space. Draw a second line from the posterior aspect of the disc space extending perpendicular to the body. An oblique incision is made between these lines, approximately 2 finger breadths anterior to the anterior superior iliac spine (see ▶ Fig. 51.4).
   a) A vascular surgeon makes the incision in the left lower abdominal quadrant. The transversalis fascia is cut lateral to the rectus sheath, accessing the retroperitoneal space. The peritoneum and the ureter are carefully identified and mobilized as needed. The left iliac vessels and middle sacral vessels may need to be mobilized to gain access to the L5–S1 disc space.
   b) A table-mounted tubular retractor system is used to maintain the access. Three blades are positioned: one superiorly retracting the left common iliac vein and artery, one blade retracting the bifurcation cephalically, and one inferiorly by the right common iliac vein and artery.
   c) A lateral X-ray is taken to confirm the level and ascertain a clear view of the end plates is available. Some Ferguson tilt with the C-arm may be needed to achieve this. A linear incision is then made within the disc space and a straight, large, long-handled Cobb elevator is employed to enter the disc space all the way to the posterior margin.
   d) Discectomy continues with all long-handled instruments: large Cobb elevators, straight and angled curettes, rasps, pituitary rongeurs, and Kerrisons. X-ray is used to confirm depth.
   e) The posterior longitudinal ligament (PLL) is released using small straight and angled curettes under lateral fluoroscopy.
   f) The Medtronic DLIF Clydesdale trials are used next to dilate the disc space, starting with an 8-mm height trial, followed by 10- and 12-mm trials. Lateral X-ray is used to

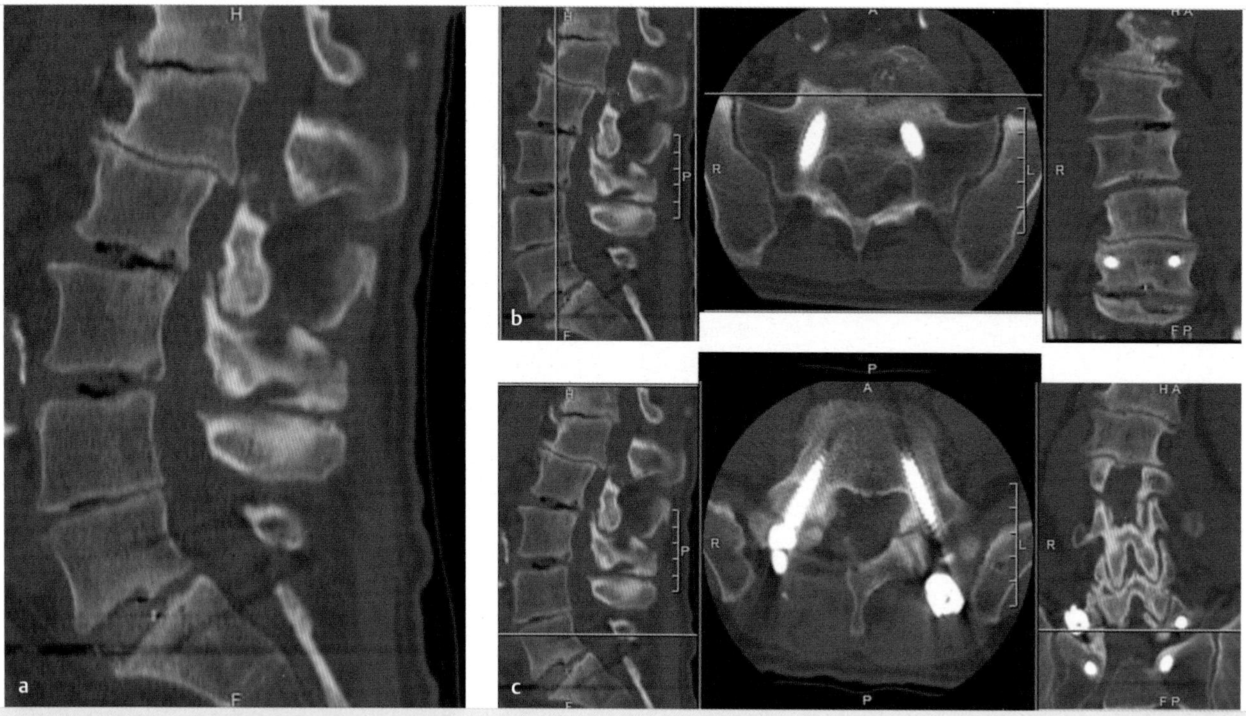

Fig. 51.2 **(a)** Sagittal view of the lumbar spine demonstrating the multilevel degeneration. Presence of gas is noted at L5–S1, L4–L5, L3–L4, L2–L3, and T12–L1 levels on this particular cut. **(b)** Sagittal, axial, and coronal cuts demonstrating the pseudarthrosis at L5–S1 with presence of interbody graft. **(c)** Sagittal, axial, and coronal cuts demonstrating open facet joints posteriorly at L5–S1.

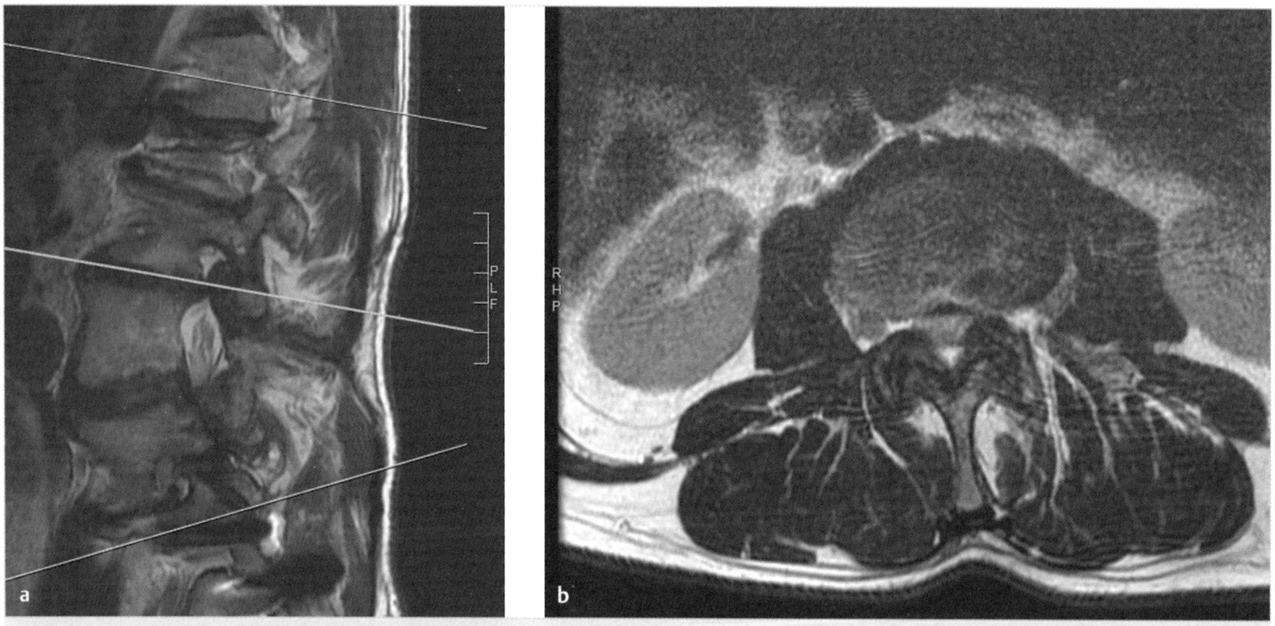

Fig. 51.3 **(a, b)** Sagittal and axial views of the lumbar spine at L3–L4 disc space, demonstrating clear ante-psoas access from the left side. The axial images also show no large central disc herniation. Each instrumented level is examined in this manner.

check the depth and angle of the trials and that the posterior height of the disc space is increasing appropriately (see ▶ Fig. 51.5).

g) Next, the Medtronic OLIF Divergence trials are used, beginning with a medium-sized trial with 10 mm of height and 12 degrees of lordosis. As the height is progressively increased, it is important to select a trial that provides at least 4 to 6 mm of posterior height. Anteroposterior (AP) X-ray is used to confirm the position of the trial and the chosen PEEK spacer is inserted with an anterior plate under lateral fluoroscopy.
1. The PEEK spacer is packed with approximately 4 mg rhBMP-2 and Grafton putty.

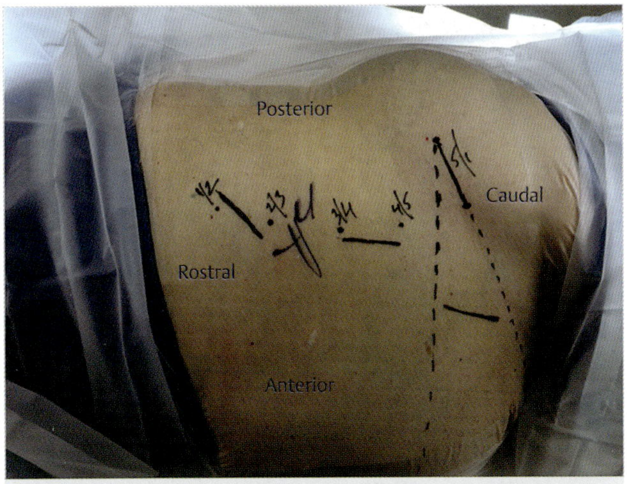

Fig. 51.4 Clinical photo of a patient in a right lateral decubitus position with incision markings for the multiple levels that are planned to be instrumented. Single incision is used for L1–L2 and L2–L3, another incision is used for L3–L4 and L4–L5. Finally, the most anterior incision, in between the hash marks, is used to approach L5–S1.

2. A long-handled screwdriver, with a guide for the screws, is mounted obliquely to the plate and spacer prior to insertion. This guide is a safe tool for lumbar and sacral screw placement across the anterior plate.
3. Grafton putty is packed on either side of the spacer.

h) In this particular case, the previously implanted TLIF graft at L5–S1 was found to be loose without any evidence of bony fusion. A Cobb elevator was used around the graft and then the graft was removed completely from the space. The steps above were then followed.

3. **Ante-psoas approach to levels above L5–S1:**

a) L4–L5 and L3–L4 can be accessed through one skin incision, while L2–L3 and L1–L2 through another (see ▶ Fig. 51.4). The external oblique muscle and the internal oblique muscle are split in line with their fibers. The transversalis fascia is entered with finger dissection. The finger dissection is used to sweep under the iliac crest and under the 12th rib. The peritoneum is swept anteriorly, while palpating for the psoas muscle.

b) With gentle superficial hand-held retraction and mobilization of the psoas muscles, the psoas minor tendon can be visualized and is often a landmark for the docking site at the anterior disc space.

c) A probe is placed onto the anterior one-third of the disc space under direct visualization. Once the position is confirmed on lateral X-ray, the probe is then advanced into the disc space, half the length of the disc space. Check this on AP view X-ray.

d) Sequential dilators are carefully passed over the initial probe and an appropriate size retractor is chosen. The final retractor blades are attached to the table-mounted post. The retractor blades are then opened in the cephalad-caudal direction and all the dilators, except for the initial probe, are removed. The initial probe acts as a guide for the anterior-posterior point of entrance into the disc space.

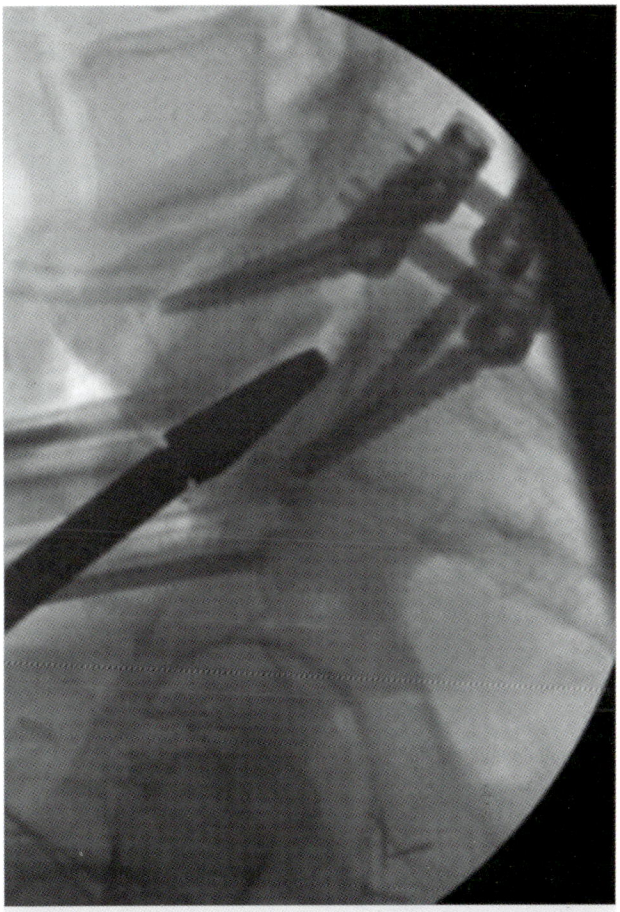

Fig. 51.5 Lateral X-ray demonstrating a trial being inserted into the L5–S1 discectomy site. Hardware from prior surgery is seen posteriorly as well.

e) Once the disc surface is cleared off with a Penfield #4 and the anterior longitudinal ligament (ALL) visualized, a linear incision is done with a long 15 blade scalpel just behind the ALL. The initial probe can be removed at this point.

f) A small long-handled Cobb elevator is inserted into the disc space all the way to the contralateral margin (but not through the contralateral annulus), under AP fluoroscopy. It is rotated gently to help open up the disc space. Same is repeated with a large Cobb elevator.

g) Discectomy continues with long-handled instruments: Uterine curette, straight double-sided rasp, pituitary and Kerrison rongeurs.

h) Medtronic DLIF Clydesdale trials are used next, starting with an 8-mm height, followed by a 10-mm trial. AP view fluoroscopy is used to check the trajectory of the trial (see ▶ Fig. 51.6).

i) Medtronic combo tool is used next to prepare the end plates. A 12-mm height trial is impacted into the disc space and the position checked with a lateral X-ray.

j) Usually, a 12-mm height × 50-mm length × 12 degrees lordosis spacer containing approximately 4 mg rhBMP-2 and Grafton putty is then inserted into the irrigated disc space

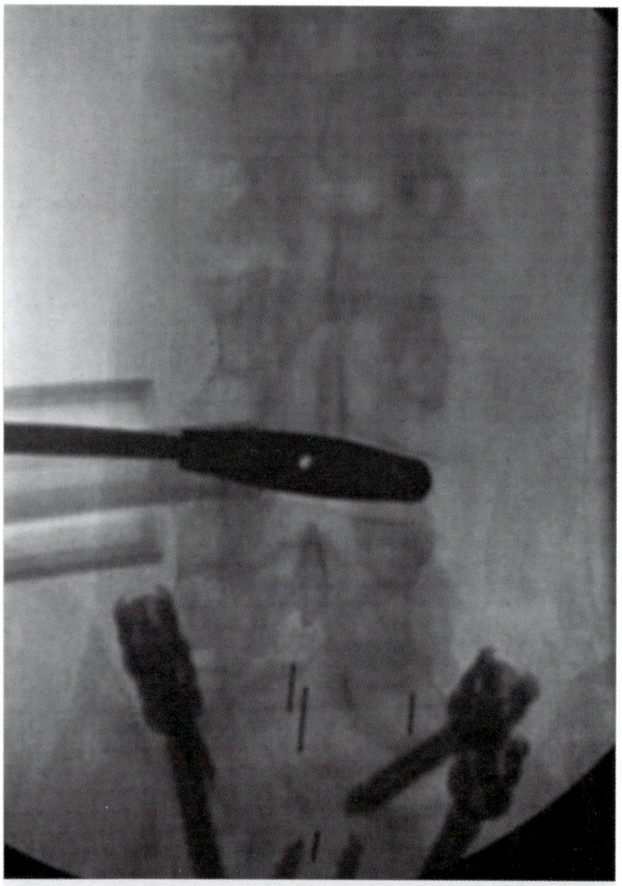

Fig. 51.6 Anteroposterior (AP) X-ray demonstrating a trial inserted all the way across the L3–L4 disc space, spanning from pedicle to pedicle.

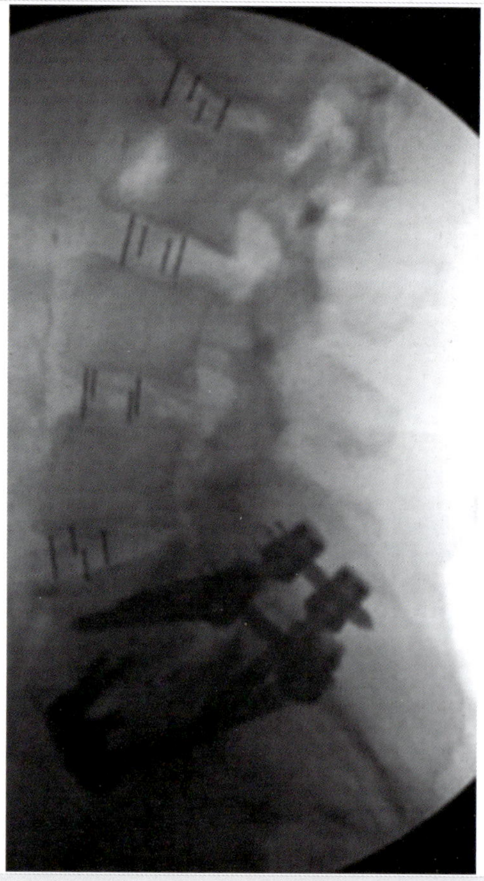

Fig. 51.7 Final lateral X-ray in stage 1 demonstrating all the instrumented levels. Previous posterior hardware with the screws and rods at L5–S1 is seen as on the preoperative imaging. L5–S1 graft with the anterior plate is visible, as well as interbody grafts at L4–L5, L3–L4, L2–L3, and L1–L2. Achievement of smooth lumbar lordotic curve is evident.

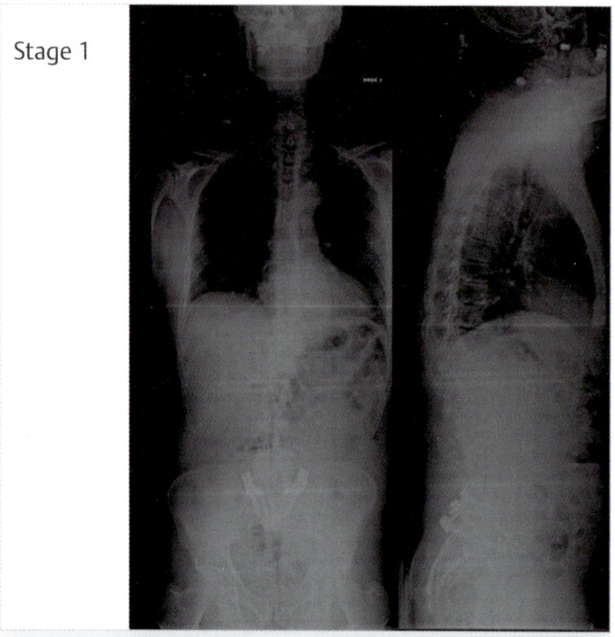

Fig. 51.8 Anteroposterior (AP) and lateral standing scoliosis films post stage 1 procedure. The global deformity measurements are as follows: Cobb angle 17.8, sagittal vertical axis (SVA) 86.8 mm, lumbar lordosis (LL) 61.2, PI-LL mismatch 7.4, pelvic incidence (PI) 68.6, pelvic tilt (PT) 24.4, sacral slope (SS) 44.1.

under AP fluoroscopy. Final X-rays are taken to confirm the position of the graft (see ▶ Fig. 51.7).

4. **Closure:**
   a) Running 1-PDS or 0-Vicryl for fascial layer. Interrupted 2-0 Vicryl for subcutaneous layer, and 3-0 Vicryl for the dermal layer.
   b) Steri-Strips and dry gauze dressing.
5. **Imaging:**
   a) Standing AP and lateral X-rays are obtained after patient ambulates post stage 1 (see ▶ Fig. 51.8).
   b) MRI or CT only indicated if patient has new radicular pain/ weakness or if the patient complains of persistent preoperative radicular symptoms.

51.5.2 Stage 2

1. **Positioning:** Patient is placed in a prone position on a Jackson table. All prominences are padded. Maximize lordosis with hip padding.
2. **Surgical steps:**
   a) A revision midline incision was made and extended from T10 to the pelvis. Bilateral skin flaps were created. Bilateral paraspinal fascial incisions were made medial to the iliac

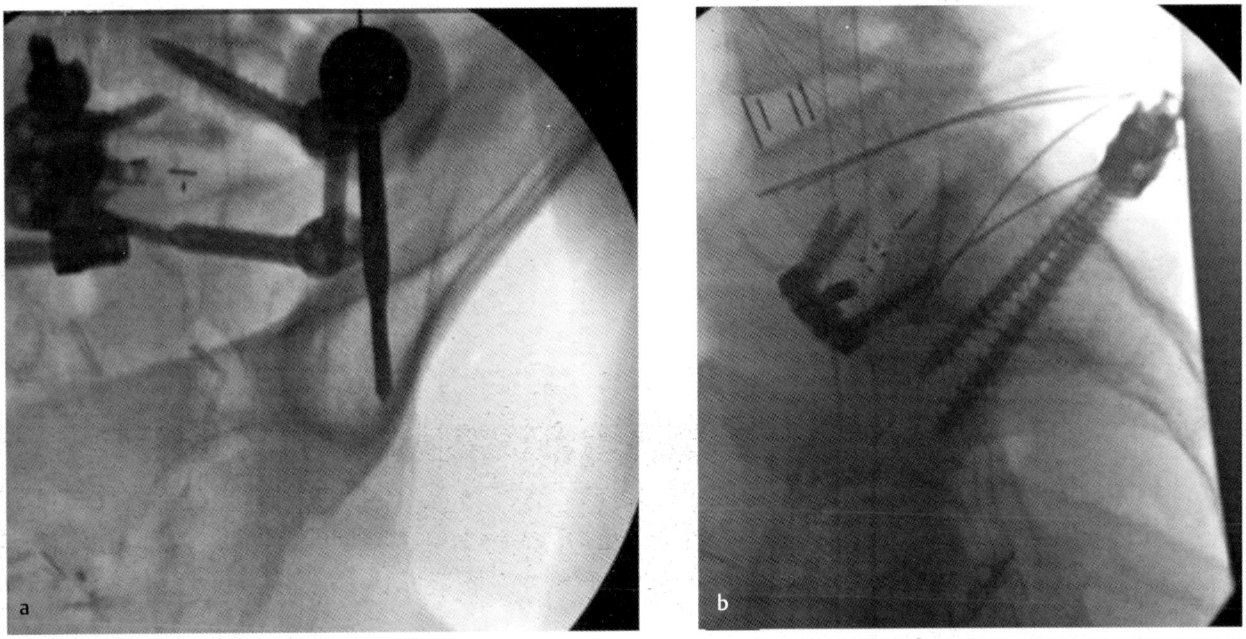

Fig. 51.9 **(a)** A teardrop view demonstrating the pedicle finder within the boundaries of the bony channel of the inner and outer margins of the ilium. **(b)** Lateral X-ray demonstrating placement of iliac screws, positioned superior to the sciatic notch.

crest for placement of iliac screws (8.5 × 90 mm). Pelvic outlet, inlet, and teardrop views were used to place the screws accurately (see ▶ Fig. 51.9). The start point of the iliac screw is on the deep and medial aspect of the superior one-third portion of the posterior inferior iliac spine (PIIS). This way, the head of the screw can be tucked in deep to PIIS and avoid prominence postoperatively. The other option is multiple paraspinal percutaneous incisions.

b) The previous hardware was exposed and removed. Guidewires were placed in the preexisting L4 and L5 screw paths bilaterally. Fluoroscopy was then used to cannulate the pedicles with Jamshidi cannulas, starting at T10 and working distally. Jamshidi cannulas were used to cannulate the pedicles at T10, T11, T12, L1, L2, L3, and L4 bilaterally (see ▶ Fig. 51.10). A guidewire was then placed down each of the Jamshidi cannulas. The Jamshidi cannulas were removed, followed by sequential dilation through the muscles, followed by tapping over the guidewire, followed by placement of a screw attached to a Medtronic Longitude extender over the guidewire. Screws were placed starting at S1 and moving rostrally in a sequential fashion. The screws were all checked on AP and lateral fluoroscopy, and all found to be satisfactory.

c) The rods were then appropriately measured and contoured, following which they were passed subfascially through the extenders within the slots of the extenders. Sequential reduction of the rods was then carried out into the tulips of the screws (see ▶ Fig. 51.11). The apex of lordosis was reduced first sequentially over several screws. Fluoroscopy was used to check the movement of the rod into the tulips. The apex of the lordosis was locked down with top-locking nuts, following which further nuts were used to lock down the rods to the screws.

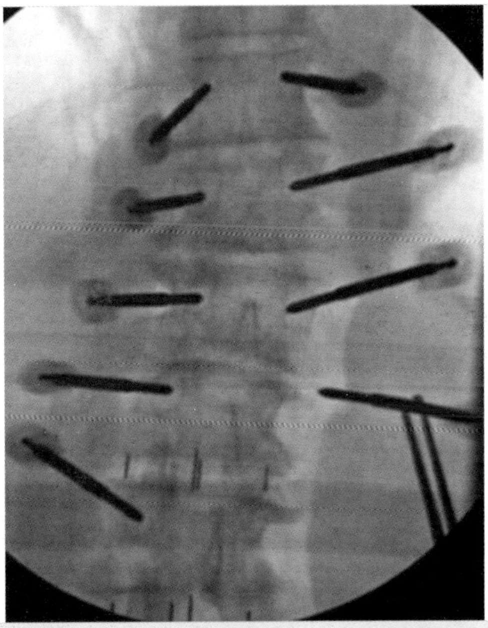

Fig. 51.10 Anteroposterior (AP) X-ray of the thoracolumbar spine demonstrating pedicle cannulation with Jamshidi cannulas, starting at T10 superiorly.

Good solid reduction and lordosis were obtained in this fashion and locked in place. Final X-rays, AP and lateral, were checked.

d) Posterior and posterolateral fusion was then carried out at T10–L1 level without the interbody spacers. The paraspinal muscles were carefully split. The pars-facet complex was satisfactorily exposed and decorticated. This was

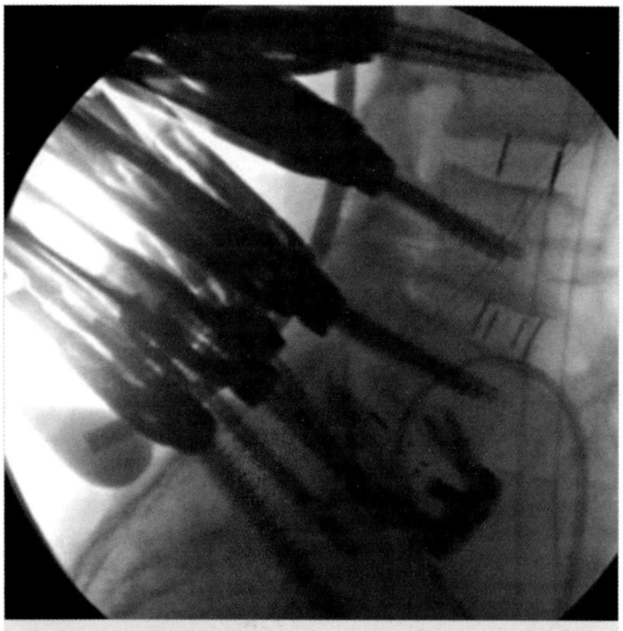

Fig. 51.11 Lateral X-ray demonstrating insertion and reduction of the rod through the extenders that are attached to the pedicle screw tulips. Interbody grafts at L5–S1, L4–L5, and L3–L4 from stage 1 are observed in this image.

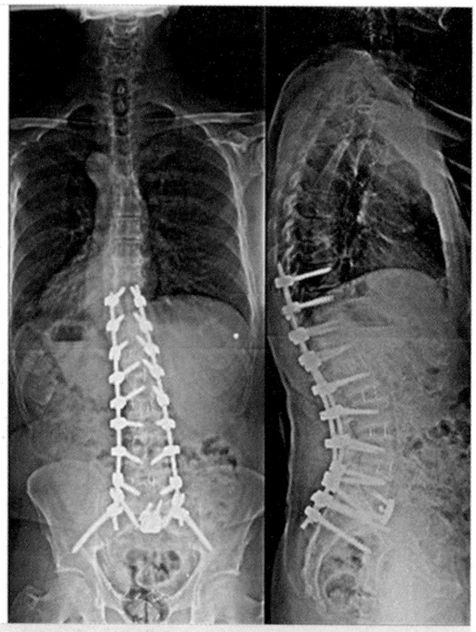

Fig. 51.12 Anteroposterior (AP) and lateral standing scoliosis X-rays 4 months post-op. T10-pelvis posterior instrumentation and L1–S1 interbody graft are in excellent position. Coronal and sagittal balance appears satisfactory and significant lumbar lordosis is noted.

followed by placement of rh-BMP2 that was divided from a large BMP kit with Grafton putty and local bone. Following grafting, the wound was thoroughly irrigated and washed out with antibiotic solution. Meticulous hemostasis was achieved.

e) Closure was obtained with 1 PDS to the fascia. Closure continued with 2–0 Vicryl to subcutaneous tissue, 3–0 Vicryl to subdermal tissues, and Steri-Strips to skin. Estimated blood loss was 200 mL.

3. **Postoperative care:** The patient is encouraged to ambulate as soon as tolerated, preferably on the same day, without a brace. Foley is removed usually on postoperative day 1. Prophylactic antibiotics are continued until Foley and drains (if any) are removed. Diet is advanced to clear once the patient has flatus and advanced to regular as tolerated from that point on. Aggressive bowel regimen is made available as needed, including stool softeners, laxatives, and enema. The dressings are changed on postoperative day 2. The posterior incision remains covered with a dry dressing while in the hospital. The lateral wounds may remain open to air. Steri-Strips are left until the first postoperative visit. Once the patient has mobilized and is medically/surgically stable, he/she is discharged to home or rehab facility.
4. **Follow-up:** The patient returns to the office in 2 weeks for a wound check and AP/lateral standing scoliosis X-rays (▸ Fig. 51.12 and ▸ Fig. 51.13). The subsequent visits are at 6 weeks, 3 months, 6 months, 9 months, 12 months, 18

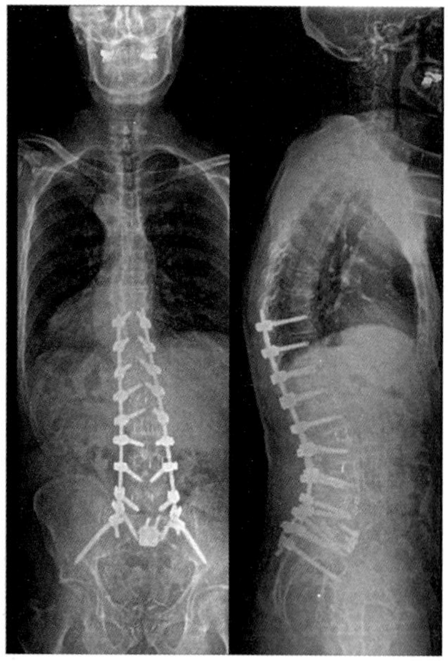

Fig. 51.13 Anteroposterior (AP) and lateral standing scoliosis X-rays 8 months post-op. T10-pelvis posterior instrumentation and L1–S1 interbody graft are in excellent position. Coronal and sagittal balance appears satisfactory and significant lumbar lordosis is noted. The global deformity measurements are as follows: Cobb angle 3.6, sagittal vertical axis (SVA) 27 mm, lumbar lordosis (LL) 59.3, PI-LL mismatch 10, pelvic incidence (PI) 68.6, pelvic tilt (PT) 29.8, SS 40.7.

months, 2 years, and then annually. Imaging studies at each visit include AP/lateral standing scoliosis films. CT scan is obtained at 18 months to 2 years to confirm fusion.

51.6 Trips and Tricks

a) Do not retract the psoas and find access planes to the disc pre-psoas between the bifurcation or lateral to the aorta.
b) Do not violate the end plates. This is imperative to prevent subsidence, get restoration of height, indirect decompression, and correct segmental deformity.
c) Take care not to damage surrounding soft tissues when impacting the PEEK graft into L5–S1 or the levels above.
d) Use AP fluoroscopy to confirm that you are in line with the disc space when using the Cobb or trials.
e) Hold handle firmly when inserting prosthesis to prevent rotation of the implant.
f) When inserting the trials at levels above L5–S1, first enter at an anterior angle underneath the psoas muscle and slowly straighten out handle to end up perpendicular to the body while impacting the trial in.
g) At L1–L2 and L2–L3, try to stay below the diaphragm. You can hold expiration or use right hand to hold diaphragm out of the way during placement of retractors.
h) L1–L2 and L2–L3 can be accessed on opposite sides of the rib.
i) At L1–L2, a 6-degree lordotic cage is used rather than 12-degree lordotic cage.

52 Lifestyle Medicine: Optimizing Recovery Following MIS of the Spine

Jaspal Ricky Singh and Kyle F. Worell

Summary

Lifestyle medicine is the use of evidence-based therapeutic approaches utilizing exercise, nutrition, and behavior science. In order to adequately address the burden of chronic disease and dysfunction, we must consider not only spine surgical treatments, but also preventative health measures to ensure optimal functional recovery. Through integrated exercise therapy, nutrition, health coaching, mindfulness, and sleep hygiene we have the potential to improve a patient's quality of life, as well as achieve greater outcomes following minimally invasive spine surgery.

Keywords: lifestyle medicine, exercise therapy, core stability, segmental stabilization, co-contraction, nutrition counseling, chronic inflammation, lifestyle modification, sleep hygiene, behavior change, coaching

52.1 Benefits of Minimally Invasive Spine Surgery

This chapter discusses the benefits of minimally invasive surgery (MIS) of the spine and provides a framework to optimizing functional recovery following the surgery. The primary goal of MIS of the spine is to reduce disability, pain and improve function during the postoperative setting. Technical advancements and MIS have led to increased safety and effectiveness by decreasing complications and tissue trauma. However, in order to fully optimize functional recovery, a comprehensive rehabilitation program along with lifestyle modifications must play a role in the postoperative treatment guidelines. An evidence-based comprehensive therapy program improves outcomes following MIS of the spine. These lifestyle modifications include, but are not limited to, optimal nutrition, sleep hygiene, smoking cessation as well as mindfulness/biofeedback. Together these modifications once applied synergistically to a postoperative program will not only achieve greater surgical outcome but may also improve the patient's overall quality of life.

MISS allows earlier mobilization and initialization of a comprehensive perioperative rehabilitation program than traditional open surgery. This approach of combining the benefits of MISS with an earlier rehabilitation program of lifestyle modifications can amplify the outcome from spinal surgery beyond the benefits provided by the technical aspects of MISS alone (▶ Table 52.1).

MIS of the spine has continued to evolve over the past several years and is now considered by many as the gold standard for spine surgery. With improved instrumentation and innovative buyout technological advances, the goal of MISS is to improve patient outcomes.[1] It has been estimated that approximately 60 to 80% of people will suffer from back pain at some point in their lives. The World Health Organization's statistics find that lower back pain is one of the leading causes of disability in both developed and developing countries.[2] Given a continued increase in spine-related disorders requiring surgical intervention, it is likely that MISS will also evolve and grow accordingly. MIS procedures and techniques evolve with the aim of improving clinical outcomes. MIS seeks to reduce surgical complications, reduce postoperative pain, improve recovery times, reduce blood loss, shorten hospital stays, and reduce the need for pain medication. MIS allows for preservation of posterior motion segments and paraspinal musculature that allows for a quicker recovery and optimizes postsurgical functioning.[3,4,5]

In this regard, MISS offers the great advantage over traditional spinal surgery of incorporating a comprehensive rehabilitation program much earlier and with potentially greater impact on patient recovery and health.

Table 52.1 Components of a comprehensive rehabilitation program
Exercise, therapy, and spine care
Nutrition/health eating
Smoking cessation
Sleep
Health and wellness coaching

52.2 Exercise and Spine Therapy

Adequate amounts of exercise and physical activity promotes a healthy back (▶ Fig. 52.1). Muscle makes up 40% of our body weight and healthy muscle is a key component for an active and pain free life. Conversely, as outlined in Chapter 5, there is an increased awareness that injured muscle itself can be a pain generator. Exercise and spine physical therapy are, therefore, critical during the postoperative phase. The purpose of physical therapy is to restore muscular conditioning and spinal structure in order to restore function and avoid reinjury.[6,7,8] Identifying the exercise objectives for each patient is critical to any spine program.[9]

For example, after a noncomplicated minimally invasive one-/two-level lumbar spinal fusion or decompression procedure we will progress rapidly with physical activity according to the following protocol:

- Start walking the same day.
- Upright bike, elliptical within 1 to 2 weeks after surgery, keep back straight.
- Pool exercises starting 2 weeks after surgery, when incision is healed.
- No bending, stretching, twisting for 6 weeks after surgery, abdominal quick draw binder optional and as per patient preference.
- Core exercise, stretching, and flexibility exercise starting 6 weeks after surgery.

52.2.1 Core Stability

One of the most fundamental concepts in the management of spine-related disorders, particularly cervical and lumbar pathologies, is the utilization and implementation of the upper

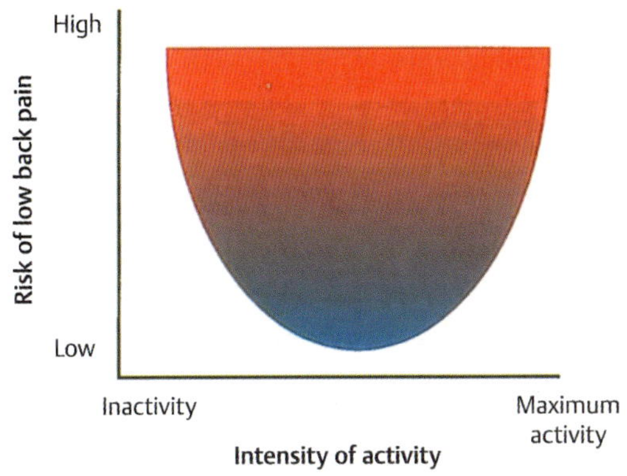

Fig. 52.1 Relationship between physical activity and low back pain. Adequate amounts of physical activity promotes a healthy back. However, a U-shaped relationship exists between physical activity and chronic low back pain, excessive activity may raise the risk of pain. Physical therapy and healthy exercise are a key treatment of muscle generated low back pain (see Chapter 5).[10] Minimally invasive surgery will allow patients to return to a healthy lifestyle and physical activity much faster than after traditional open surgery.

back and core stability exercises. It is important to note that the terms "core" and "core stability" have been misused not only in the public in media, and but often among health care professionals also. The core and muscles involved in truncal stability are more than just "sixpack muscles." Following MIS surgery of the spine, core strengthening exercises will vary depending on beginner, intermediate, or advanced levels. However, most central to the concept of core stability is facilitation and activation of the muscles involved with abdominal bracing (▶ Fig. 52.2).

***Abdominal bracing** is an activity targeting the deep transverse abdominis muscle and the multifidi group contracting together with the surrounding abdominal and back muscles.*[8] This concept is known as "co-contraction." The deep transverse abdominis is the muscle commonly called the "Corset of the Spine." This muscle has been recognized as integral to the bracing process.

52.2.2 The McGill Spine Exercises

Just as each individual's condition, diagnosis, and spinal dysfunction are unique, no two exercise programs will be the same. The following exercises have been chosen as general recommendations. These exercises are meant to serve as examples with the understanding that every individual and their specific needs vary. These exercises serve three main purposes: they spare the spine, they enhance the muscle challenge, and they ensure that spine stability is maintained.[8]

1. *Cat-camel*: The cat and camel, or spine flexion–extension cycle, is a motion exercise rather than a stretch (▶ Fig. 52.3). These motions reduce spine viscosity (internal resistance and friction) and "floss" the nerve roots as they outlet at each lumbar level, followed by hip and knee mobility exercises. As the cat-camel is a motion and not a stretch, emphasis should be taken on motion rather than "pushing" at the ranges of flexion and extension. Five to eight cycles are sufficient to reduce most viscous-frictional stresses.

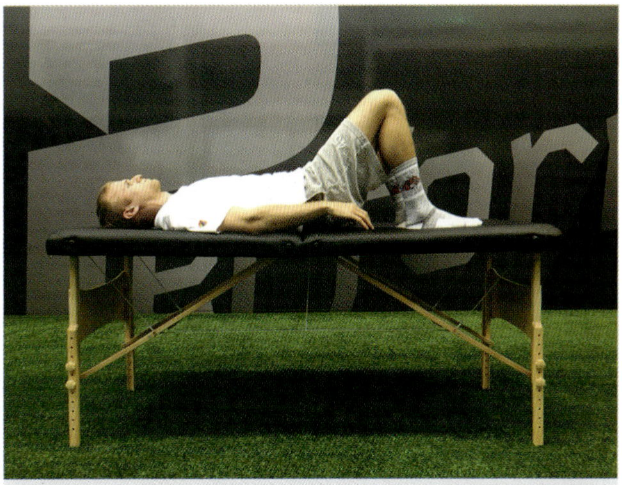

Fig. 52.2 Abdominal bracing.

2. *Bent knee curl-up*: The bent knee curl-up is an effective exercise to target the six-pack muscles, also known as the rectus abdominis (▶ Fig. 52.4). One can target these muscles by lying flat on the back while bending one leg up and keeping the foot flat on the floor. The other leg is left straight. Lifting the hands behind the head, raise the head and shoulders off the mat and contract the rectus abdominis muscles. Hold for 3 to 5 seconds. Slowly lower and repeat the exercise.
3. *Bird-dog*: The bird-dog exercise is critical in strengthening the lower back muscles. These include the lumbar paraspinal and the multifidus (▶ Fig. 52.5). These muscles are often strained and weakened from sitting at work or at home for long periods of time. Begin by placing one's hands and knees on a mat, keeping the elbows, wrists, and shoulders in alignment. Slowly string one leg behind the body. It is important to keep the pelvis level, as it is natural to rotate. A level pelvis will engage the multiphoton muscles. Hold this for 3 to 5 seconds and slowly lower it back to the mat.
4. *Side plank*: The side plank is the most advanced and difficult exercise that targets the deep abdominal muscles, particularly the obliques and the transverse abdominis muscle (▶ Fig. 52.6). These muscles are very important for keeping one's core stable and strong. To do this exercise, one must lie on the side, making sure that the elbow is aligned with the shoulder, and the knees are bent. Slowly straighten the top leg. Push off the elbow and knee, and raise the pelvis and hips off the ground. It's very important to ensure that one's bellybutton is pointed straight, as there is a tendency to either rotate upward or downward. However, make sure that the pelvis is level, and hold this for 10 to 30 seconds. Slowly release.

52.2.3 Segmental Stabilization

Another key benefit of MIS of the spine is the maintenance of spinal segmental stabilizers following surgery. In order to maximize segmental stability, the deep spinal extensor muscles are often spared during MIS and this can often lead to faster recovery.[11]

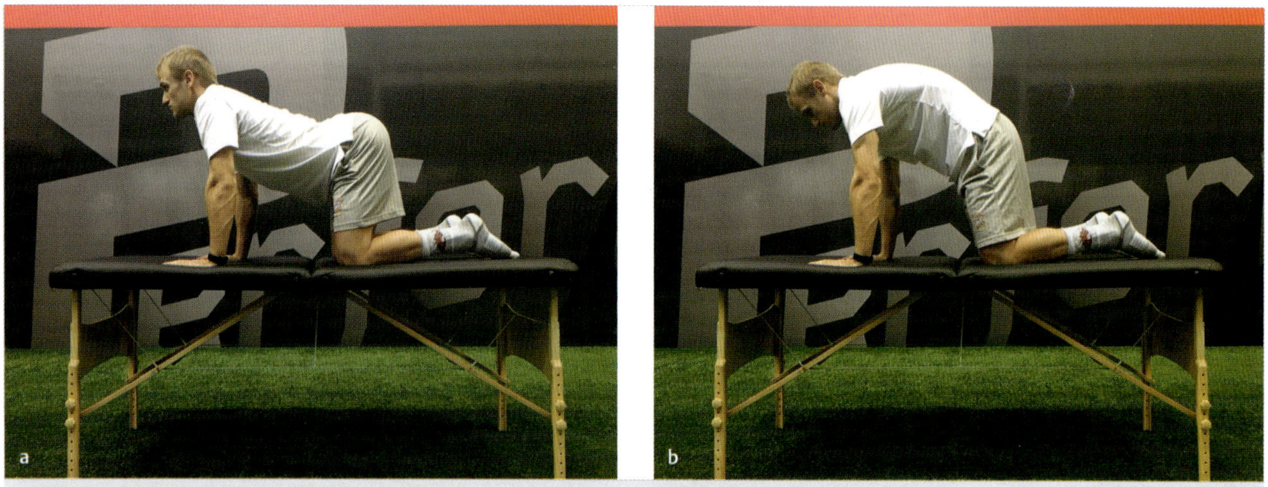

Fig. 52.3 (a, b) Cat–camel.

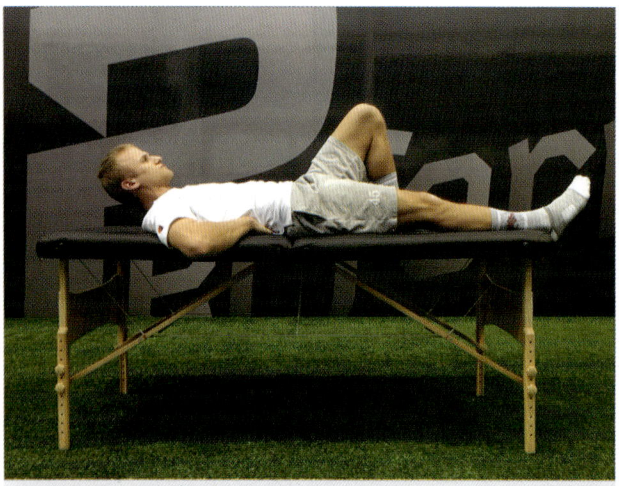

Fig. 52.4 Bent knee curl.

One of the major benefits of MISS is the reduction for potential spinal muscular injury to these structures.[11] The benefits for this include decreased muscular atrophy and a quicker return of neuromuscular facilitation. The targeting of specific muscular groups, namely the multifidi and the transverse abdominis, appear to be the focus in a large majority of spinal rehabilitation programs. Studies have shown the presence of atrophy in the multifidus group at the level of a known disc herniation. So while minimally invasive techniques may resolve the anatomic compression of nerves related to the disc herniation, surgical intervention on its own will not adequately resolve muscular weakness. Therefore, a graduated progressive exercise protocol for spinal stability should be emphasized.[12,13,14]

Nutrition

Diet changes can be made to improve overall health and wellness, specifically spine health. Current recommendations reflect that a diet consisting of whole foods, with avoidance of inflammatory foods is the key to success and recovery.[15] In addition, lean protein, an increase in key vitamins, and adequate hydration will promote tissue healing and bone health. It is important to note that following these diet recommendations helps to avoid chronic disease and pain as well as assists in recovery from MIS.[15]

Inflammation is the body's response to any threat that challenges homeostasis. The body responds to this threat by releasing inflammatory chemicals.[15] Assaults to the system such as lack of sleep, lack of or too much exercise, consumption of pro-inflammatory foods, illness, infection, or trauma eventually lead to a state of chronic inflammation (▶ Table 52.2). Chronic inflammation can damage tissues without the presence of swelling, pain, redness, or warmth.[15]

Research has now demonstrated that inflammation can also be triggered by psychological stress.[16] Acute inflammation plays a positive role in the immune responses as it acts to repair and restore the body after infection.[17] Inflammation is also a contributing factor to 8 out of the 10 leading causes of death in the United States.[18] An increase in inflammation can also increase the risk of a major depressive episode by 21%.[18] Chronic inflammation can lead to significant behavioral changes including depressed mood, anxiety, pain, disturbances in sleep, anhedonia, fatigue, irritability, social withdrawal, and psychomotor retardation.[19]

An anti-inflammatory diet reduces inflammation and moves the body toward a “deflamed” healthy state.[15] The average American diet consists of 40% of calories coming from refined carbohydrates.[15] These include refined sugars and refined grains. In total, a typical American diet consists of approximately 60% of calories derived from refined sugar, flour, and oils.[15] Although these products may help make food taste good, they lack nutritional value and lead to “dietary injury” which causes inflammation, pain, chronic disease, suffering, and a slowed healing process.[15] Foods made from these products also tend to trigger an addictive response in the body, creating an ongoing process.[20]

Diets that focus on anti-inflammatory foods reduce pain, suffering, and aid those with chronic illness (▶ Fig. 52.7). It is quite possible to eat an anti-inflammatory diet that allows one to lose weight, enjoy the food, and feel satisfied. One important concept that has gained more attention over the past few years is *Glycemic Index (GI)*. ***GI*** is a value assigned to a food based on

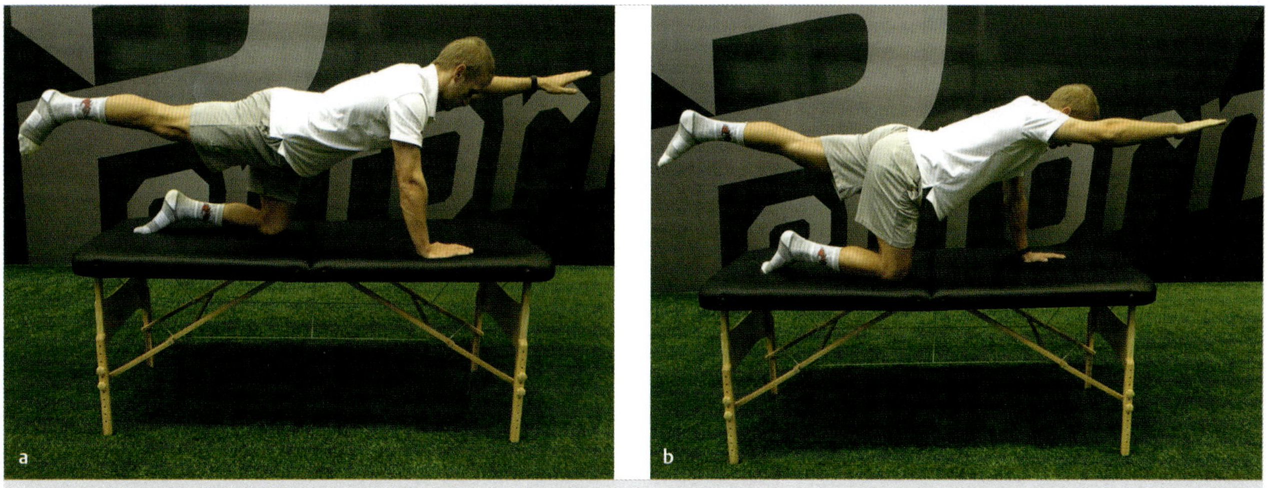

Fig. 52.5 **(a, b)** Bird-dog.

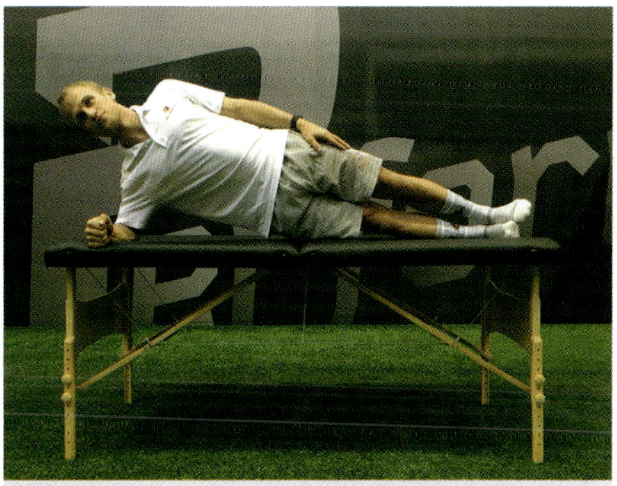

Fig. 52.6 Side plank.

how it affects one's blood sugar levels.[20] Foods with medium to high GI levels should be avoided as they tend to raise circulating glucose and insulin levels. Eventually, elevated circulating glucose and insulin levels lead to not only general pro-inflammation but metabolic syndrome.[20]

Diet and nutrition counseling lends itself to the greater aspect of coaching for health and wellness. Nutritional counseling and health and wellness coaching (HWC) is an area that requires ongoing behavioral modification that can be difficult to maintain.[21] A patient-centered collaborative approach inclusive of nutritional and lifestyle medicine counseling can provide realistic individualized change while including the necessary components of mindfulness, self-awareness, self-motivation, resilience, optimism, and self-efficacy.[21] Changes to diet and nutrition require both external and internal motivation. Research has shown that external motivation alone is not effective. A *coach* (health and wellness, nutrition, or other trained behavior change practitioner) functions as an educator, motivator, listener, and supporter as the patient incorporates a change in thinking, emotions, and behaviors.[21] Patients not only require the knowledge to make the necessary changes, but also the tools needed to intrinsically place a high value and vested interest in the outcome. The area of diet and nutrition works well with the technique of creating *SMART* goals.[21] The coaching professional, working in a collaborative partnership with the patient, looks to the future while breaking down goals using the SMART goal method. These have been described as S: smart, M: measurable, A: attainable, R: relevant, and T: timely (▶ Table 52.3).

Table 52.2 Pro-inflammatory foods

	Pro-inflammatory foods	
Refined sugar	Grain flour products	Refined omega-6 seed oils (corn, safflower, sunflower, canola, cottonseed, etc.)
Refined grains	Trans fats	
Coffee	Soda, carbonated beverages	Alcohol, beer
	Anti-inflammatory foods	
Grass-fed meat and wild game	Tubers/roots: potatoes, yams, sweet potato	Olive oil, coconut oil, avocado
Red wine and stout beer	Nuts (raw or dry roasted, walnut)	Omega-3 seeds: hemp, chia, flax
Wild caught fish	Fruit	
Berries	Vegetables	Tea (green tea is the best option)
Chicken (organic pasture raised)	Salads (leafy greens)	Ginger
Eggs (Omega 3)	Dark chocolate	Turmeric
Curcumin	Spices of all kinds	Cinnamon

Table 52.3 SMART goals

S	Specific
M	Measurable
A	Attainable
R	Relevant
T	Timely

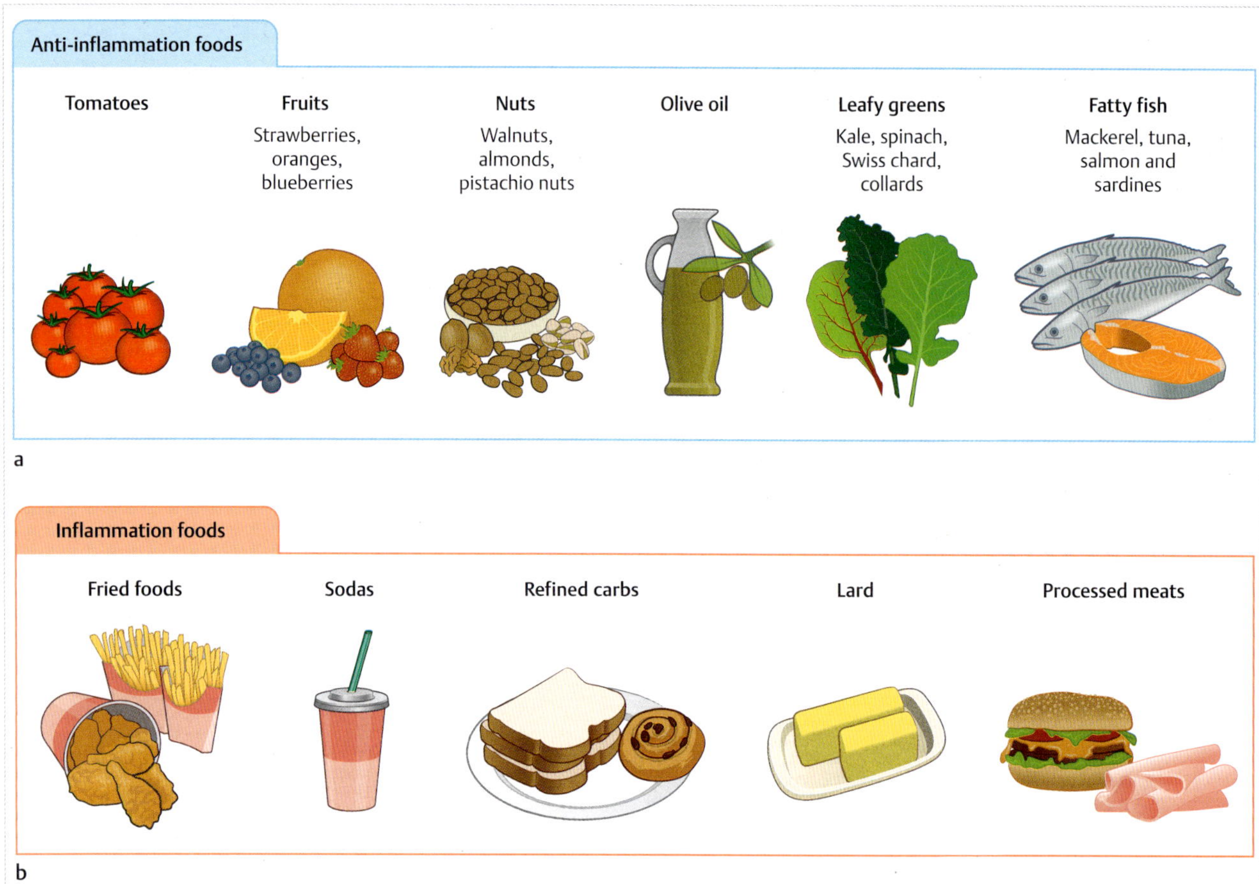

Fig. 52.7 (a, b) Foods that fight inflammation: anti-inflammatory foods versus foods linked to chronic inflammation, cancer, arthritis, and other nutrition-related disease processes.

52.3 Smoking Effects in Spine Surgery

Cigarette smoking has significant negative effects on the overall health of individuals including being causally related to malignancy, coronary and peripheral arterial disease, hypertension, hyperlipidemia, cerebrovascular accident, and chronic pulmonary disease.[22] In addition to general health, the effects of smoking on the musculoskeletal system comprise an increase of bone resorption and decrease in bone formation.[23] When it comes specifically to bone health, smoking increases cortisol which inhibits the proliferation of periosteal cells. Furthermore, smoking downregulates estrogen leading to decreased bone density and ultimately osteoporosis. Bone formation is decreased as smoking destroys osteoblasts and inhibits calcitonin and most importantly, smoking leads to decrease in oxygen supply to tissues.

MISS, including both decompression and fusions, are often indicated for various diagnoses, including disc degeneration, spinal stenosis, spondylolysis as well as traumatic spinal fractures. Tobacco smoking has been shown to affect all stages of healing including the inflammatory stage, repair stage, and late remodeling.[24] Particularly, smoking decreases the function of inflammatory cells and the mechanisms used to kill bacteria. As previously mentioned, smoking decreases oxygen supply which is essential to angiogenesis. Notable factors necessary for angiogenesis include bone morphogenetic proteins, transforming growth factor-beta, fibroblast growth factor, and vascular endothelial growth factor—all of which are affected by smoking. Without angiogenesis, the scaffolding of bone is impaired. In addition, smokers have been shown to have increased level of postoperative infections compared to nonsmokers.[25]

Patients who smoke report a greater rate of dissatisfaction after spinal fusion compared to nonsmokers.[26] This correlation may also relate to the increased incidence of depression in smokers as well as the increase in pain medication utilization in this group which is the most important factor when it comes to smoking and spine surgery in relation to the rate of successful fusion. Patients who smoke cigarettes are more likely to have nonunion during spinal fusion at the cervical and lumbar region. If a patient smokes more than 10 cigarettes a day, there is an 18.2% rate of nonunion compared to 9% of that of nonsmokers and those who smoked less than 10 cigarettes a day.[27] However, this study has shown that the amount of smoking also plays a role as those who smoke less than 10 cigarettes have the same rate of nonunion as nonsmokers. When it comes to comparing single-level fusion versus multilevel fusion procedures, smokers also have a significantly higher rate of nonunion (10.9 vs. 29.2%).[28]

Table 52.4 Recommended sleep position instructions postoperatively

Lay face up on the bed
Elevate the upper back/shoulder/head using supportive pillows or adjustable bed
Place a pillow or rolled up blanket under the back of the knees, so the hips and knees are slightly bent

The research also demonstrates the clinical benefits in patients who stop smoking prior to surgery. Carpenter et al noted that in 86 patients with a history of nonunion, smoking cessation improved pain, functional status, and postoperative satisfaction.[29] How long patients should stop smoking prior to surgery has also been studied, revealing that when patients manage to quit 4 weeks prior to the operation, there is a decreased risk of infection and respiratory complications.[30] If patients manage to quit for more than 6 months after surgery, the healing process is more efficient due to angiogenesis taking place during this time period.

52.3.1 Sleep

Adequate sleep is a critical component of recovery from spine surgery but often underemphasized as part and prescription to a healthy life. One of the inherent benefits of MIS of the spine is decreased postoperative pain which can result in better sleep hygiene than conventional open spine surgery. It has been proposed by numerous researchers across preventative and lifestyle medicine, of all health strategies, sleep is the most powerful.[31] Healthy sleep helps boost mood and intelligence quotient (IQ), improves memory, and improves concentration.[31] Plentiful, restful sleep has been shown to decrease the risk of heart disease, diabetes, depression, and even obesity.[32] The average number of sleep hours per day appears to be decreasing with increased busier lives and work demands.[33] The average of 8 to 9 hours has now dropped to 7 hours or less.[33] Sleep disturbances and a cumulative deprivation known as "sleep debt" is a chronic stressor that causes cognitive problems, possibly exacerbating pathways toward disease through inflammation.[34,35] Getting enough continuous, uninterrupted sleep helps the body to heal faster from spine surgery.[36] There may be recognizable limitations to sleep postoperatively especially following open large-incision spine surgery. A fundamental metric in favor of MISS over open spine surgery is the patient's ability to restore proper sleep hygiene due to their ability to sleep in a comfortable position. It is generally accepted after back surgery to sleep in a position that is most comfortable. Some prefer to sleep on their side with a pillow between their knees and/or behind them to support the back. General long-term sleep health suggests a lateral position could be most favorable (▶ Table 52.4).[37]

Proper pillow height is crucial for those who suffer from ongoing pain and especially those recovering post procedure.[38] Proper pillow selection and height is related to the sleeping position (▶ Fig. 52.8).[38] If the patient prefers to sleep on their back, choose pillows that support the natural curvature of the neck.[38] When lying down to sleep, the head and neck position should mimic the position that occurs when standing with proper posture. Side sleepers should consider a thicker pillow, if needed for this sleeping position.[38] The head position should be in the middle of the shoulders. Although sleeping on the stomach is generally not recommended, if the patient chooses this sleeping position, use an extra slim pillow or no pillow at all.[38]

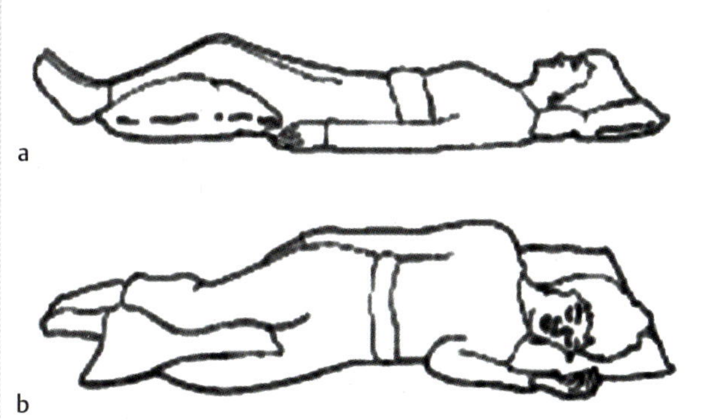

Fig. 52.8 (a) Place pillow under knees. A pillow with cervical support and a roll around waist are also helpful. **(b)** Place pillow between knees. Use cervical support under neck and a roll around waist as needed.

52.4 Health and Wellness Coaching

Coaching, and in particular HWC, is a new concept with relatively little scientific literature documented prior to 2005.[21] The roots of professional coaching in health care are firmly based in evidence-based psychological domains and theories on how to generate effective and durable behavior change. Health coaching is a technique designed to promote improvement in health behaviors of patients and clients, through self-actualization, using motivation and behavioral methods.[21] The primary goal of the patient is to have the best quality of life possible, by reducing spine-related pain and injuries. The primary goal of the health care system is to reduce the costs of health care by preventative measures and to improve the quality of life by promoting effective self-management and improve adherence of the individual receiving health coaching services. In a compendium of HWC literature conducted by Moore, HWC and patient outcomes were examined. The review examined 38 data-based articles looking at HWC and wellness. Moore found that the most consistent effects found while examining the effects of HWC on wellness outcomes were exercise behavior (92%), psychological outcomes (80%), nutrition behavior (88%), and smoking cessation (50%). Examining outcome results in this manner is valuable in that the profusion of positive patient outcomes cannot be overlooked.[39] Physicians are traditionally trained in an "expert approach," which is problem-focused and relies on the clinician's skills and knowledge to determine the correct diagnosis and treatment for each patient. This approach is most effective when handling acute problems and emergency situations. The patient-centered model focuses on the person as a whole while emphasizing overall health and the patient's role in the process. Following MIS of the spine, involving patients as an active participant in the postoperative care will promote lifestyle modifications that will be sustained long after the postoperative recovery period. Advances in MIS procedures with the integration of a lifestyle medicine approach when combined together provide greater opportunity for recovery and rehabilitation by working together synergistically.[40]

References

[1] Samartzis D, Shen FH, Perez-Cruet MJ, Anderson DG. Minimally invasive spine surgery: a historical perspective. Orthop Clin North Am. 2007; 38(3):305–326, abstract v

[2] Chang X, Chen B, Li HY, Han XB, Zhou Y, Li CQ. The safety and efficacy of minimally invasive discectomy: a meta-analysis of prospective randomised controlled trials. Int Orthop. 2014; 38(6):1225–1234

[3] Banczerowski P, Czigléczki G, Papp Z, Veres R, Rappaport HZ, Vajda J. Minimally invasive spine surgery: systematic review. Neurosurg Rev. 2015; 38 (1):11–26, discussion 26

[4] Telfeian AE, Veeravagu A, Oyelese AA, Gokaslan ZL. A brief history of endoscopic spine surgery. Neurosurg Focus. 2016; 40(2):E2

[5] Kim CW. Scientific basis of minimally invasive spine surgery: prevention of multifidus muscle injury during posterior lumbar surgery. Spine. 2010; 35 (26) Suppl:S281–S286

[6] Verkuilen P. Practical advice for recovering from back surgery. Veritas Health, LLC. https://www.spine-health.com/treatment/back-surgery/practical-advice-recovering-back-surgery. Published 2006. Accessed 2019

[7] Arnett J. Breaking down the exercises that break down your spine. National Spine Health Foundation. https://spinerf.org/breaking-down-the-exercises-that-break-down-your-spine/. Published 2015. Accessed 2019

[8] McGill SM. Low Back Disorders: Evidence-based Prevention and Rehabilitation. Human Kinetics; 2015

[9] McGill SM, Grenier S, Kavcic N, Cholewicki J. Coordination of muscle activity to assure stability of the lumbar spine. J Electromyogr Kinesiol. 2003; 13 (4):353–359

[10] Target MN. The muscle as a pain generator and key element to protect during MIS surgery. In: Hartl R, Navarro-Ramirez R, eds. Ten Step Techniques for Minimally Invasive Spine Surgery. New York, NY: Thieme; in press

[11] McFarland CM. Physical therapy after minimally invasive back surgery. Veritas Health, LLC. https://www.spine-health.com/treatment/physical-therapy/physical-therapy-after-minimally-invasive-back-surgery. Published 2007. Accessed 2019

[12] Balon J, Aker PD, Crowther ER, et al. A comparison of active and simulated chiropractic manipulation as adjunctive treatment for childhood asthma. N Engl J Med. 1998; 339(15):1013–1020

[13] Wallwork TL, Stanton WR, Freke M, Hides JA. The effect of chronic low back pain on size and contraction of the lumbar multifidus muscle. Man Ther. 2009; 14(5):496–500

[14] Yoshihara K, Shirai Y, Nakayama Y, Uesaka S. Histochemical changes in the multifidus muscle in patients with lumbar intervertebral disc herniation. Spine. 2001; 26(6):622–626

[15] Seaman DR. The Deflame Diet: Deflame Your Diet, Body, and Mind. Florida: Shadow Panther Press; 2016

[16] Slavich GM, Irwin MR. From stress to inflammation and major depressive disorder: a social signal transduction theory of depression. Psychol Bull. 2014; 140(3):774–815

[17] Couzin-Frankel J. Inflammation bares a dark side. Science. 2010; 330 (6011):1621

[18] Hoyert D, Xu J. Deaths: Preliminary Data for 2011. Natl Vital Stat Rep. 2012; 61(6)

[19] Slavich GM. Understanding inflammation, its regulation, and relevance for health: a top scientific and public priority. Brain Behav Immun. 2015; 45:13–14

[20] Egger G, Binns A, Rossner S, Sagner M. Lifestyle Medicine: Lifestyle, the Environment and Preventive Medicine in Health and Disease. London: Academic Press/Elsevier; 2017

[21] Frates EP, Moore MA, Lopez CN, McMahon GT. Coaching for behavior change in physiatry. Am J Phys Med Rehabil. 2011; 90(12):1074–1082

[22] Gandini S, Botteri E, Iodice S, et al. Tobacco smoking and cancer: a meta-analysis. Int J Cancer. 2008; 122(1):155–164

[23] Truntzer J, Vopat B, Feldstein M, Matityahu A. Smoking cessation and bone healing: optimal cessation timing. Eur J Orthop Surg Traumatol. 2015; 25 (2):211–215

[24] Berman D, Oren JH, Bendo J, Spivak J. The effect of smoking on spinal fusion. Int J Spine Surg. 2017; 11:29

[25] Olsen MA, Mayfield J, Lauryssen C, et al. Risk factors for surgical site infection in spinal surgery. J Neurosurg. 2003; 98(2) Suppl:149–155

[26] Jackson KL, II, Devine JG. The effects of smoking and smoking cessation on spine surgery: a systematic review of the literature. Global Spine J. 2016; 6 (7):695–701

[27] Andersen T, Christensen FB, Laursen M, Høy K, Hansen ES, Bünger C. Smoking as a predictor of negative outcome in lumbar spinal fusion. Spine. 2001; 26 (23):2623–2628

[28] Bydon M, De la Garza-Ramos R, Abt NB, et al. Impact of smoking on complication and pseudarthrosis rates after single- and 2-level posterolateral fusion of the lumbar spine. Spine. 2014; 39(21):1765–1770

[29] Carpenter CT, Dietz JW, Leung KY, Hanscom DA, Wagner TA. Repair of a pseudarthrosis of the lumbar spine. A functional outcome study. J Bone Joint Surg Am. 1996; 78(5):712–720

[30] Glassman SD, Anagnost SC, Parker A, Burke D, Johnson JR, Dimar JR. The effect of cigarette smoking and smoking cessation on spinal fusion. Spine. 2000; 25 (20):2608–2615

[31] Irish LA, Kline CE, Gunn HE, Buysse DJ, Hall MH. The role of sleep hygiene in promoting public health: A review of empirical evidence. Sleep Med Rev. 2015; 22:23–36

[32] West C, Egger G. To sleep, perchance to... get everything else right. In: Egger G, Binns AF, Rössner SR, Sagner M, eds. Lifestyle Medicine: Lifestyle, the Environment and Preventive Medicine in Health and Disease. Elsevier; 2017:291–308

[33] National Sleep Foundation-Sleep Research & Education. https://sleepfoundation.org. Accessed 2019

[34] Koren D, O'Sullivan KL, Mokhlesi B. Metabolic and glycemic sequelae of sleep disturbances in children and adults. Curr Diab Rep. 2015; 15(1):562

[35] Kryger MH, Roth T, Dement WC. Principles and Practice of Sleep Medicine. 6th ed. Elsevier; 2017

[36] Auvinen JP, Tammelin TH, Taimela SP, et al. Is insufficient quantity and quality of sleep a risk factor for neck, shoulder and low back pain? A longitudinal study among adolescents. Eur Spine J. 2010; 19(4):641–649

[37] Moeller A. 5 Little-known tips for sleeping with chronic pain. Veritas Health, LLC. https://www.spine-health.com/blog/5-little-known-tips-sleeping-chronic-pain. Published 2016. Accessed 2019

[38] Schubbe J. Best pillows for different sleeping positions. Veritas Health, LLC. https://www.spine-health.com/wellness/sleep/pillows-different-sleeping-positions. Published 2018. Accessed 2019

[39] Sforzo GA, Kaye MP, Todorova I, et al. Compendium of the Health and Wellness Coaching Literature. Am J Lifestyle Med. 2017; 12(6):436–447

[40] Rippe JM. Lifestyle Medicine. CRC Press; 2013

53 Three-Dimensional Navigation in MISS

Bernhard Meyer and Yu-Mi Ryang

Summary

No other field in spine surgery is expanding at such a pace as spinal navigation technologies. While 3D spinal navigation with or without robotic assistance has already become the standard/default procedure for many spine surgeons, especially for MIS spinal instrumentation, iCT might be the next step to total navigation. Other promising technologies such as videoexoscopy, augmented and mixed reality may help expand surgical indications and overcome surgical limitations. This chapter gives insight into future perspectives of next level spine surgery.

Keywords: spine, navigation, MISS

53.1 Introduction

Spinal navigation has greatly facilitated the use of minimally invasive spine surgery (MISS) worldwide. Numerous studies and meta-analyses were able to show the benefits of computer-assisted navigation (CAN) in spine surgery by improving accuracy and safety of open spine procedures[1] and by decreasing the rate of pedicle screw-related complications and revision surgeries.[2,3] Intraoperative assessment of pedicle screw accuracy and immediate revision during the same surgery made it possible to further reduce the rate of revision surgeries. Another major benefit is the significant reduction of radiation exposure to surgeon, operating room (OR) staff and patient.[4,5] These advantages of CAN are even more important in minimally invasive spine procedures where anatomical landmarks for additional visual orientation are missing, which may result in increased complication rates and increased fluoroscopy and OR time. The benefits of CAN in MISS are therefore obvious[5,6] and generally accepted among experienced spine surgeons around the globe.

53.2 State-of-the-Art—Where Are We Heading?

53.2.1 iCT NAV and Total Navigation

Evolving from two-dimensional image guidance through three-dimensional, fluoroscopy-guided spinal navigation, the best navigation systems available today in terms of image quality, field of view, and gantry size are intraoperative computed tomography (CT) navigation systems (iCT NAV).

These rapid technological advances made it possible to greatly expand the indications for CAN in MISS from mere pedicle screw placement to other MISS procedures such as navigated interbody fusions, vertebral column and tumor resections, and spinal reconstruction procedures.[7,8] Härtl and colleagues thus coined the term "total navigation." They used iCT NAV for skin incision and index level localization to verification of implant position and assessment of the extent of neural decompression. In this way, they were able to replace fluoroscopy in 75% of spinal procedures, of which the majority were MISS procedures, and to eliminate radiation exposure to the staff completely.[5]

53.3 Future Perspectives

53.3.1 Robotic Systems

Robot-assisted spine surgeries are being performed with increasing frequency and success to assist in pedicle screw placement. However, this technology is still in its infancy and far from what we would like it to be capable of in the future. Robotic arms are for the time being merely very expensive drill holders. Their functions are usually limited to executing one basic task. Indefatigability and the ability to perform repetitive monotonic tasks with constant precision already make robots a valuable asset for simple procedures such as assisting navigated facet joint injections.[9] In the near future, robots could advance from being able to execute one task to being able to perform a sequence of tasks. In the far future robots might be able to perform even complex surgical MISS procedures by means of machine learning. By providing robots with algorithms that enable them to learn, interact, predict, and even make decisions during surgery.[10]

Robotic arms are presumably only a first tiny step in the development of fully integrated robotic arms capable of executing surgical tasks ranging from simple tailored skin incisions and minimally invasive approaches to highly sophisticated MISS procedures through minimally invasive working portals. A remote surgeon, for example, might guide robots via sensor gloves which give the surgeon direct haptic feedback and can enhance his or her dexterity and maneuverability.[8] This also facilitates telesurgical procedures enabling surgeons to perform surgeries around the world without the need to travel.

53.3.2 Virtual Reality (VR) and Augmented Reality (AR)

VR and AR systems which are already indispensable in the flight and military industry, and greatly promoted by the entertainment industry, are yet to be implemented in the medical industry. In the surgical field these systems are still quite rare and mainly used for training purposes. These systems could be useful adjunct tools in navigating MISS procedures by displaying AR images into a head-mounted display projecting, for example, pedicle screw trajectories or target structures superimposed on the real-time images.[10] They have thus great potential especially for MISS, where the underlying anatomy is hidden.

53.3.3 Videoexoscopic Navigation

Recently videoexoscopes were introduced to neurosurgery. These surgical optical tools provide high-definition images, superior to microscopic images, which are visualized on a screen through a small camera mounted on a robotic platform

at the surgical site. These tools can be integrated into existing navigation systems providing the possibility of simultaneous visualizations of reconstructed navigation and surgical field images for real-time navigation and/or live image-guided surgery. The high-definition display allows for projections of the surgical field off-axis to the surgeon's inline loup or the microscopic view. This tool could also be a great adjunct in MISS navigation procedures facilitating procedures in a MISS fashion that usually need wide exposure of the surgical site such as pedicle subtraction osteotomies or vertebral column resections.[11]

53.4 Conclusion

CAN is the ideal tool to facilitate and expand the indications for MISS. Many technological innovations such as real-time navigation, live image-guided surgery, and spinal robotics are promising tools that can help to further augment MISS CAN in the future.[8] To be able to fully use the benefits of MISS CAN the learning curve needs to be overcome by fully integrating it into the OR workflow.[12]

We have no doubt that spinal navigation will someday become standard of care.[12,13] A major goal must be making these technologies affordable and widely available. Expanding applications is one way to achieve and improve cost-effectiveness. Among other advantages, CAN improves surgical accuracy and eliminates wrong-level and wrong-side surgery. We as surgeons should not forget that our main goal in using and developing these new technologies should be to improve patient outcomes and quality of life. We are convinced that an exciting future lies ahead of us. Books like this will help to propagate MISS techniques in the community of spine surgeons, especially those who are still reluctant to adopt these techniques.

References

[1] Mason A, Paulsen R, Babuska JM, et al. The accuracy of pedicle screw placement using intraoperative image guidance systems. J Neurosurg Spine. 2014; 20(2):196–203

[2] Shin BJ, James AR, Njoku IU, Härtl R. Pedicle screw navigation: a systematic review and meta-analysis of perforation risk for computer-navigated versus freehand insertion. J Neurosurg Spine. 2012; 17(2):113–122

[3] Fichtner J, Hofmann N, Rienmüller A, et al. Revision rate of misplaced pedicle screws of the thoracolumbar spine—comparison of three-dimensional fluoroscopy navigation with freehand placement: a systematic analysis and review of the literature. World Neurosurg. 2018; 109:e24–e32

[4] Villard J, Ryang Y-M, Demetriades AK, et al. Radiation exposure to the surgeon and the patient during posterior lumbar spinal instrumentation: a prospective randomized comparison of navigated versus non-navigated freehand techniques. Spine. 2014; 39(13):1004–1009

[5] Navarro-Ramirez R, Lang G, Lian X, et al. Total navigation in spine surgery; a concise guide to eliminate fluoroscopy using a portable intraoperative computed tomography 3-dimensional navigation system. World Neurosurg. 2017; 100:325–335

[6] Kim TT, Johnson JP, Pashman R, Drazin D. Minimally invasive spinal surgery with intraoperative image-guided navigation. BioMed Res Int. 2016; 2016:5716235

[7] Lian X, Navarro-Ramirez R, Berlin C, et al. Total 3D Airo® navigation for minimally invasive transforaminal lumbar interbody fusion. BioMed Res Int. 2016; 2016:5027340

[8] Overley SC, Cho SK, Mehta AI, Arnold PM. Navigation and robotics in spinal surgery: where are we now? Neurosurgery. 2017; 80 3S:S86–S99

[9] Zettinig O, Frisch B, Virga S, et al. 3D ultrasound registration-based visual servoing for neurosurgical navigation. Int J CARS. 2017; 12(9):1607–1619

[10] Madhavan K, Kolcun JPG, Chieng LO, Wang MY. Augmented-reality integrated robotics in neurosurgery: are we there yet? Neurosurg Focus. 2017; 42(5):E3

[11] Huang M, Barber SM, Steele WJ , III, et al. Videoexoscopic real-time intraoperative navigation for spinal neurosurgery: a novel co-adaptation of two existing technology platforms, technical note. J Robot Surg. 2018; 12(2):251–255

[12] Ryang Y-M, Villard J, Obermüller T, et al. Learning curve of 3D fluoroscopy image-guided pedicle screw placement in the thoracolumbar spine. Spine J. 2015; 15(3):467–476

[13] Meyer B, Ryang Y-M. Yes, we CAN! World Neurosurg. 2013; 79(1):85–86

Part V

Teaching and Training/Future

54 Surgical Training and Simulation in MISS 414

55 The Role of Biologics in Minimally Invasive Spine Surgery 420

56 Summary and Outlook—Future of Lumbar Minimally Invasive Surgery 423

57 Achieving MISS on a Global Level 427

V

54 Surgical Training and Simulation in MISS

Carolin Melcher, Thana Theofanis, Yusef Mosley, Geoffrey Stricsek, Sertac Kirnaz, and James S. Harrop

Summary
This chapter provides an overview of the integration of minimally invasive spine surgery into a trainee's surgical education and how simulation plays a vital role in making one proficient with the relevant tools and techniques.

Keywords: simulation, surgical education, cadaver, virtual reality

54.1 Introduction

The use of simulation in surgical training has become an essential part of education, particularly in the highly technical and complex fields of neurosurgical and orthopaedic spine procedures. Although nothing can replace time in the operating room alongside master surgeons, simulation allows for trainees to create a uniform foundation upon which they can build upon.[1] This is particularly true in minimally invasive spine surgery (MISS), wherein simulation can more closely mirror the actual procedure.

We recently published our procedural metrics for minimally invasive ULBD in combination with a realistic surgical simulator and demonstrated that "simulators" can be used to improve the skills and confidence of trainees. Surgical simulation may offer an important educational complement to traditional methods of skill acquisition and should be explored further with other MIS techniques.[2]

A basic example of the utility of simulation in spine is from Ghobrial et al, describing a simulated educational model for cerebrospinal fluid (CSF) leak repair for neurosurgery residents, showing this to be a valuable tool for training, synergistically building both a clinical knowledge base and operative technical skill set.[3] Chitale et al also demonstrated success with a minimally invasive simulation model for pedicle screw placement, showing improvement in trainees after completing the module.[4] Thus, simulation allows for effective learning and, most importantly, repetition—so the trainee can rehearse key steps of various clinical scenarios or operative procedures. Leaders in the field have already begun to describe curricula relying on simulation to master core competencies in neurosurgical training.[1,5]

Concurrently, external drivers of today's health care environment, such as patient satisfaction, quality improvement, and cost-effectiveness, have become leading priorities for hospital administration. Thus, the trend toward less invasive surgeries with faster recovery, particularly in spine, will continue due to improved patient satisfaction, deceased hospital length of stay, and other patient-centric outcomes.

Constructivist approaches to human learning have led to the development of a theory called cognitive apprenticeship. This theory holds that masters of a skill often fail to consider the implicit processes involved in carrying out complex skills when they are teaching novices. To ameliorate these tendencies, cognitive apprenticeships "…are designed to bring these tacit processes into the open, where students can observe, enact, and practice them with help from the teacher…"[6]

So how does one become an expert in MISS?

54.2 Methods

Historically, trainees have developed operative skills through the surgical apprenticeship model, following the adage "see one, do one, and teach one."[7] This saying oversimplifies the traditional method of teaching trainees. However, it accentuates the observation period of a particular procedure so that one is expected to be capable of performing that procedure. Further, teaching a colleague how to conduct that procedure is also reduced due to the lack of exposure and understanding of the procedure. Thus, trainees are presently expected to accomplish these tasks through exposure to a high volume of cases rather than specifically designed curricula.[7,8,9]

Meanwhile, opportunities for education through interacting with "real" patients diminish after residency due to issues with exposure, time, and resources. Therefore, developing formal education curricula has gained significant interest, specifically designed to teach new surgical skill sets to fully trained surgeons. These formal and defined curriculum are especially relevant for those adopting MISS techniques in their training or clinical practice[5,10] (▶ Table 54.1). The top three identified limitations to adopting MISS technology are: the technically challenging aspect of the procedures (both for the surgeon and operating rooom staff), lack of mentoring and tutored training opportunities, and the increased radiation exposure and its potential adverse effect on the patient and surgical team.[11]

54.2.1 Learn by Observing an Experienced MISS Surgeon

In spine surgery, particularly MISS procedures, managing and navigating the sequence of steps during an operative procedure require mastery of all the technically complex maneuvers in addition to understanding how to coordinate these numerous individual components such that they ultimately accomplish

Table 54.1 Table showing general skills. Material is available and can be integrated according to participant's knowledge

General skills
Using a microscope
Using an enoscope
Using a burr with an endoscope
Using a drill for MISS
Using 2D and 3D navigation and assistive technologies
Managing a dural tear
Bleeding control
Radiation reduction
Placing a tubular retractor (or retractor)
Abbreviation: MISS, minimally invasive spinal surgery.

the goals of the surgery. Education in the operating room is often an intimate, intense, and complex series of didactics and demonstrations. This includes advising, illustrative hand gestures, supportive physical actions, and repositioning of teaching instruments. Education research has shown that there are usually two general categories of teaching behaviors: surgical actions and teaching gestures.

Surgical actions assist the trainee in completing individual surgical steps of the procedure, which include: retracting, using instruments, and manipulating tissues. Gestures are expressed with the teacher's hands, fingers, and arms to point at an object, or to illustrate the shape of anatomy.[12]

54.2.2 Fellowships/Grants

There are numerous opportunities to expand one's knowledge base in MISS techniques since medical industry and spine educational foundation support these surgical procedures by offering fellowship or grants to support training for surgical programs affiliated to MISS. These postresidency experiences in surgical techniques for orthopaedic and neurological surgeons are designed to familiarize younger surgeons with the principles, indications, planning, techniques, and complications of the MISS procedures. Some noteworthy opportunities are listed below:

1. AO Fellowship Program.
2. Eurospine Observership Grant.
3. NASS Fellowship Connect/NASS International Visiting Surgeon Fellowship.
4. Industry-sponsored MISS Fellowships.

54.2.3 Courses

For established spinal surgeons in practice, there is no standard formula for learning and incorporating new surgical techniques into their practice. Currently available educational methods include: traditional continuing medical education (CME) symposia (1-day courses),[13] instructional videos, mentoring, and comprehensive courses that combine lectures and skills laboratories.

Cadaver

Development of MISS skills in cadaver models provides a valuable opportunity to exercise techniques in a controlled environment where the learning curve can be optimized to enhance proficiency.[14] The value of cadaveric dissection courses in imparting practical and essential knowledge of anatomic structural relationships in the spine has been clearly established. The human cadavers closely emulate intraoperative environments maximizing the technical aspects; but two limiting factors are the time the cadaver is available and the fact that surgical incidents, such as bleeding and CSF leak, cannot be experienced, minimizing the feedback from the model to the trainee.[9] Furthermore, human cadaveric models may be even less expensive than animal models and have the advantages of the native human anatomy releationships. The basic training techniques have been shown to be of high value not only for research and development but also for the surgeon's own clinical experience. Many of the scientific meetings and courses provide the opportunity for hands-on cadaveric teaching courses (▶ Fig. 54.1).

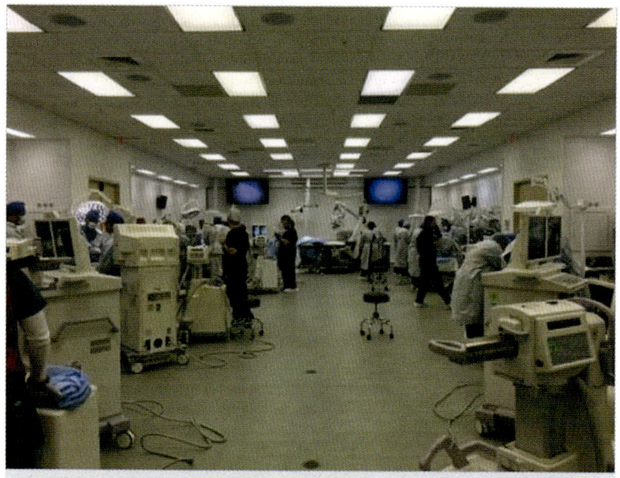

Fig. 54.1 Cadaver lab with two participants per table, with the same number of image intensifiers per station.

a) NASS (North American Spine Society), AANS (American Academy of Neurological Surgeons), CNS (Congress of Neurological Surgeons), AAOS (American Academy of Orthopaedic Surgeons):
   1. Specialty Education & Research Center.
b) NYCMISS
c) EUCMISS (European Course for Minimally Invasive Spine Surgery).
d) AO Foundation.
e) Eurospine.
f) National organizations.
g) Industry-sponsored.

Animal

Animal models provide high fidelity training with the ability to reproduce the entire operation procedure and associated techniques in order to prepare and avoid complications. However, the use of living animals is problematic due to ethical concerns, high costs, and the need for specialized facilities to perform the procedures. As large animals provide the most similarity to human anatomy, porcine models are commonly used in surgical training of spine procedures.[15,16,17]

Artificial Bone

There is a wide range of artificial bones available throughout industry, from single to multibone models, fractured, intact, or with foam coverings. In the past several years, these models have become more anatomically accurate, particularly in representing the relationship of the pedicles to the anterior and posterior bony elements of the spine. There have been recent advances in the models with the addition of soft tissue and skin on some models. Some examples include:

a) Sawbone.
b) Synbone:
   1. Ammolite.
   2. SpineStud.

Simulators

A simulator is a device or model used for training individuals by imitating situations and environments that they will encounter in uncontrolled situations.[18] Simulation devices have been used in military and aviation training for years, thus providing prospects to exercise technically demanding skills in a safe and controlled environment.[19,20] Advances in simulation training models have gone beyond a single procedural skill set to presently incorporating decision-making, problem solving, and judgment in a complex training environment.[21] Overall, simulation-based teaching can be divided into five components: Preparation, Exposure, Progression, Feedback, and Repetition.[22]

A critical aspect of a simulation model is the constant feedback accomplished through debriefing and reflection, which is a unique opportunity to reinforce the core assumptions of adult learning, providing external motivation, and stimulating guided reflection.[23,24] Understanding how the experience affects future practice is a crucial step to improve performance.[25]

Virtual Reality

Many of the general surgery disciplines have incorporated simulation through virtual reality (VR) training models into residency training curriculum, allowing trainees to safely develop surgical proficiency and to practice fine motor skills that are directly applicable in live procedures.[26,27] In recent years, the neurosugical and orthopaedic educational programs have have used this approach through MISS procedures. The MISS training has incorporated VR paradigms for simulation and teaching.[28,29,30,31,32]

RealSpine

RealSpine/Realists is one industry model that utilizes an artificial wetlab training system for lumbar spinal procedures such as discectomies and decompression. This lumbar spine simulator includes all relevant anatomical structures such as the vertebrae, ligamentum flavum, posterior ligamentous complex (PLC), epidural connective tissue, ligaments, intervertebral disc, and dura mater with spinal nerves (▶ Fig. 54.2 and ▶ Fig. 54.3). An impressive feature that differentiates it from other simulation models is the ensemble of different materials that closely mimic reality. The simulator can bleed in a controlled and quantifiable way by a two-point bleeding system for diffuse bleeding in the upper part of the simulator and intralaminar osseous bleeding; while drilling the bone and dissecting the tissues, the surgeon feels as if he or she is operating on a real patient. In addition, the model can serve to train on surgical complications management like CSF leaks, if required. The materials for all anatomical structures are made of specially designed synthetics (i.e., polyurethane, epoxy, silicone, gelatine, and latex). This simulator also includes sensors for the feedback of the pressure and the traction on the nerves in the dura and the CSF pressure.[28]

54.2.4 Societies

The following spine societies are dedicated to MISS education.

SMISS

The Society for Minimally Invasive Spine Surgery (SMISS) is an international community of orthopaedic and neurological surgeons who are dedicated to MISS. The society's overarching goal is to create knowledge and deliver standardized programs, tools, and techniques that raise the competencies and quality. SMISS features 10 informative video modules that address indications, techniques, and outcomes for current minimally invasive spine techniques. Participants who review the modules may take a brief online test for CME credits.

SMISS Core Curriculum

The purpose of the SMISS Core Curriculum is to educate orthopaedic and neurological surgeons in the nuances of care for the MISS patient. Each course of study champions the society's mission to improve patient care by advancing the practice of MISS through education, research, and advocacy:

1. Didactic lectures in video format.
2. Faculty-led hands-on cadaveric training at contemporary facilities.

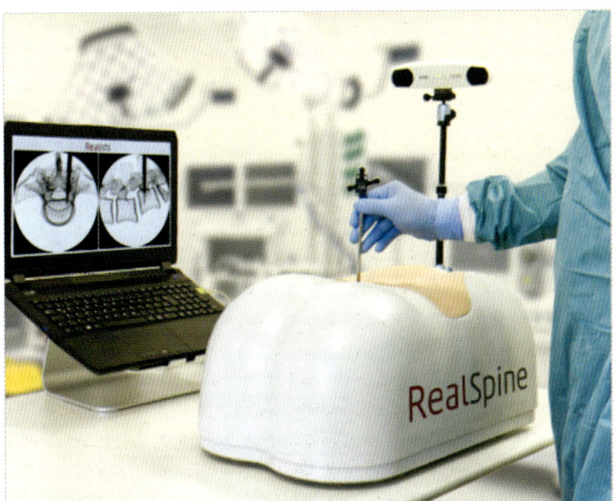

Fig. 54.2 RealSpine model. (Used with permission from RealSpine.)

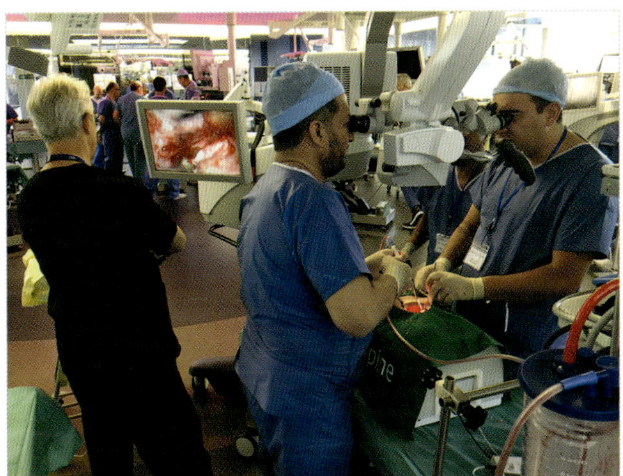

Fig. 54.3 The trainees operate on a RealSpine model under the supervision of a trainer.

3. Comprehensive and focused cadaveric lab opportunities are offered during the society's Spring Meeting and the annual SMISS Program each fall.

SMISS Continuing Professional Development (CPD) Program

The SMISS Continuing Professional Development (CPD) Program follows the principle of "Lifelong Learning," which is to impart a surgeon with education, tools, and support that will develop and maintain the surgeon's competence, proficiency, and expertise in MISS throughout his/her career.

The SMISS Syllabi consists of online assessment, workshop, and practice-based assessment modules to earn credits in four domains:

1. **Patient:** History, anatomy, diagnosis, selection.
2. **Imaging:** Systems, quality, interpretation, problems and controversies.
3. **Surgical technique:** Room setup, procedure, instrumentation, problems and controversies.
4. **Outcomes:** Best practices, complications, patient reported outcome measures (PROMs), rehabilitation.

ISMISS

The International Society for Minimal Intervention in Spinal Surgery (ISMISS) is an international nonprofit organization with members from Europe, the USA, and Asia. Over the last 30 years, members and participants have witnessed the evolution of percutaneous nucleotomy to endoscopic fragmentectomy, foraminoplasty, and segmental stabilization. In recent years, ISMISS has held several meetings and courses worldwide.

ISASS

The International Society for the Advancement of Spine Surgery (formerly The Spine Arthroplasty Society) (ISASS) is a special interest group of medical and associated specialists devoted to the field of clinical and structural restoration or replacement of spinal joints after normal function is lost by degenerative conditions. Its mission is to provide an independent, international, educational, and scientific venue to discuss and address the issues involved in all aspects of basic and clinical science of motion preservation, stabilization, innovative technologies, MISS procedures, biologics, and other fundamental topics.

AANS/CNS Spine Section (of Both the AANS and CNS)

The mission of the Spine Section is to advance spine and peripheral nerve patient care through education, research, and advocacy and foster the use of spinal neurosurgical methods for the treatment of diseases of the spinal neural elements, the spine, and the peripheral nerves.

54.2.5 Online Material

Literature/Webinars/Videos

With the growth of the electronic age, technology and education have evolved rapidly through the internet. Thus, searching the internet offers the latest literature published on the topic on Pubmed, Researchgate, Google Scholar as well as webinars and videos, either on journal and/or society websites (AO Spine, NASS, Spinesection, Global Spine Journal "MISS" special issue [https://journals.sagepub.com/toc/gsja/10/2_suppl], Eurospine). Furthermore, video-centric domains such as Youtube (https://www.youtube.com/user/AANSNeurosurgery), Vumedi (https://www.vumedi.com/term/spinelumbar-spine/), and Orthobullets (http://www.orthobullets.com/topic/dashboard?id=2&specialty=2&expandLeftMenu=true) might provide insight on the work of surgeons from all over the world implementing MISS into their daily routine using different devices for teaching purposes or to share a single surgeon's developed approaches and techniques.

Table 54.2 Procedures defined on the first MISS Task Force meeting

Procedure
Interlaminar microscopic tubular lumbar discectomy (IMTLD)
Posterior microscopic tubular cervical foraminotomy (PMTCF)
Extraforaminal microscopic tubular lumbar discectomy (EMTLD)
Interlaminar endoscopic lumbar discectomy (IELD)
Transforaminal endoscopic lumbar foraminotomy and discectomy (TELF/TELD)
Lumbar endoscopic unilateral laminotomy for bilateral decompression (endoscopic "over the top" decompression or endoscopic LE-ULBD)
Microscopic tubular unilateral laminotomy for bilateral decompression ("over the top" decomp, MT-ULBD)
Percutaneous screw and rod placement
MISS TLIF

Abbreviation: MISS TLIF, MISS transforaminal lumbar interbody fusion.

AO Spine Education

On the AO Spine website, an entire online-learning curriculum is offered including an MISS section. Here videos, surgical references, and step-by-step guides on procedures can be found (▶ Table 54.2). Furthermore, the education section contains the Case Base and many webinars and videos.

During the Global Spine Congress in Singapore in May 2018, a group of international leaders from Europe, Southern Africa, Middle East, Northern Africa, Asia Pacific, North America, and Latin America launched the Minimally Invasive Spine Surgery (MISS) curriculum. This task force defined MISS as "...a suite of technology-dependent techniques and procedures that reduces local operative tissue damage and systemic surgical stress enabling earlier return to function striving for better outcomes than traditional techniques."

The curriculum was geared toward educating surgeons who performed open surgery but had little or no MISS experience. This also included surgeons with some experience with the microscope and tubes but not with complex MISS, surgeons with experience in MISS who use the microscope (▶ Fig. 54.4) and burr even for complex cases, and surgeons of any level without any experience with the endoscope (▶ Fig. 54.5). In short, the curriculum is a guide on how to start MISS and is independent of a surgeon's background, training level, and location of practice and, therefore, applicable to all surgeons worldwide.[33] The task force created educational materials, including presentations, cases, exercises and guides, videos, and assessments.

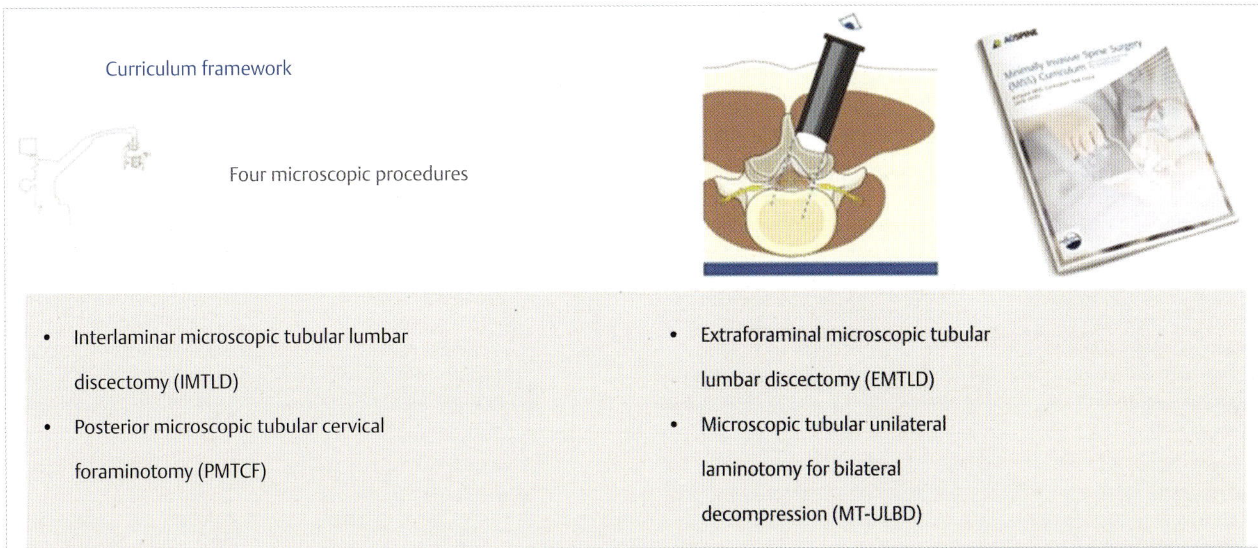

Fig. 54.4 Picture showing an example of educational material for microscopic procedures.

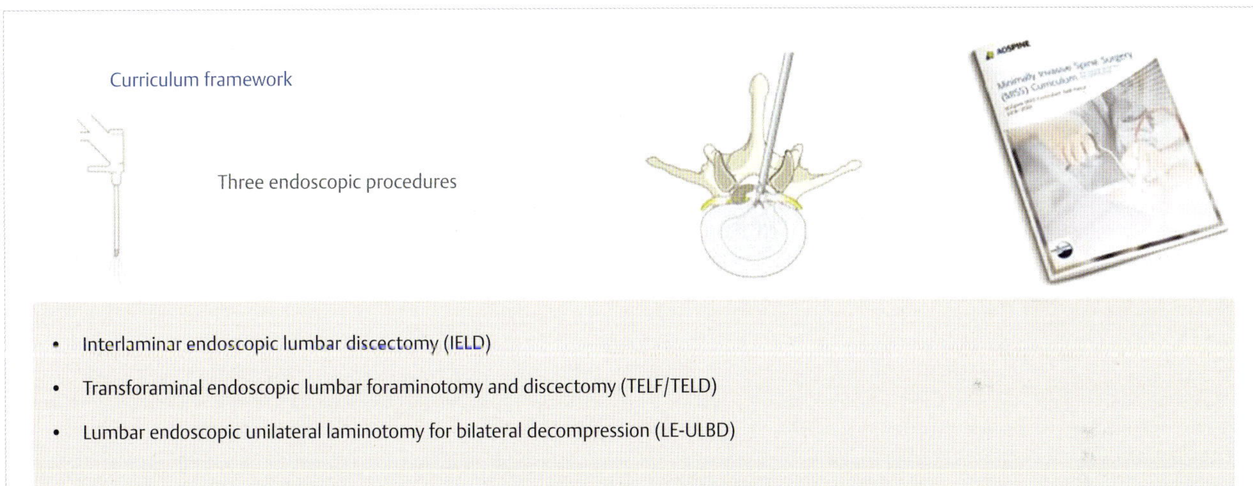

Fig. 54.5 Picture showing an example of educational material for endoscopic procedures.

NASS—Ask the Experts Videos and Podcasts

Online educational videos and podcasts are created in an effort to offer high-quality, evidence-based, spine-focused, electronic CME content.

EANS Academy

EANS is offering a comprehensive online library of neurosurgical material. Access is partly free, partly included in the membership fee.

eccElearning Spine Surgery Education Programme (Affiliated to European Spine Journal)

eccElearning is the world's first comprehensive *online* postgraduate education program in a medical subspeciality. The course is designed to meet the demands of today's spine surgeon trainee in terms of educational rigor, quality, and innovation. The program complements your practical training schedule, and typically the spine course takes 12 to 18 months to complete.

54.2.6 Textbooks

A multitude of books have been published on the topic of MISS by the experts in the field. Many of them offer a visual step-by-step guide to MISS procedures and instrument handling.[34]

54.2.7 Step-by-Step Transformation of Familiar Technique

As with any new technique, the first attempts at performing minimally invasive surgical approaches will involve learning the procedure itself, how to handle the instruments, and maybe new implants, if required. Even though aiming for a familiar technique, a steep learning curve and an extended time for surgery

must be taken into account. By taking a familiar technique using a microsurgical access with a larger incision and modifying it to a minimal invasive procedure by adopting an entirely different approach and philosophy, the novice can become an expert in spine surgery.

References

[1] Robison RA, Liu CY, Apuzzo ML. Man, mind, and machine: the past and future of virtual reality simulation in neurologic surgery. World Neurosurg. 2011; 76(5):419–430

[2] Melcher C, Hussain I, Kirnaz S, et al. Use of a high-fidelity training simulator for minimally invasive lumbar decompression increases working knowledge and technical skills among orthopedic and neurosurgical trainees. Global Spine Journal. 2022. doi:10.1177/21925682221076044

[3] Ghobrial GM, Anderson PA, Chitale R, Campbell PG, Lobel DA, Harrop J. Simulated spinal cerebrospinal fluid leak repair: an educational model with didactic and technical components. Neurosurgery. 2013; 73 Suppl 1:111–115

[4] Chitale R, Ghobrial GM, Lobel D, Harrop J. Simulated lumbar minimally invasive surgery educational model with didactic and technical components. Neurosurgery. 2013; 73 Suppl 1:107–110

[5] Harrop J, Lobel DA, Bendok B, Sharan A, Rezai AR. Developing a neurosurgical simulation-based educational curriculum: an overview. Neurosurgery. 2013; 73 Suppl 1:25–29

[6] Collins A, Brown JS, Newman SE. Cognitive Apprenticeship: Teaching the Craft of Reading, Writing and Mathematics. Centre for the Study of Reading, University of Illinois; 1987

[7] Kotsis SV, Chung KC. Application of the "see one, do one, teach one" concept in surgical training. Plast Reconstr Surg. 2013; 131(5):1194–1201

[8] Haluck RS, Krummel TM. Computers and virtual reality for surgical education in the 21st century. Arch Surg. 2000; 135(7):786–792

[9] Reznick RK, MacRae H. Teaching surgical skills—changes in the wind. N Engl J Med. 2006; 355(25):2664–2669

[10] Birch DW, Misra M, Farrokhyar F. The feasibility of introducing advanced minimally invasive surgery into surgical practice. Can J Surg. 2007; 50 (4):256–260

[11] Webb J, Gottschalk L, Lee YP, Garfin S, Kim C. Surgeon perceptions of minimally invasive spine surgery. SAS J. 2008; 2(3):145–149

[12] Sutkin G, Littleton EB, Kanter SL. How surgical mentors teach: a classification of in vivo teaching behaviors part 2: physical teaching guidance. J Surg Educ. 2015; 72(2):251–257

[13] Birch DW, Sample C, Gupta R. The impact of a comprehensive course in advanced minimal access surgery on surgeon practice. Can J Surg. 2007; 50 (1):9–12

[14] Krähenbühl SM, Čvančara P, Stieglitz T, et al. Return of the cadaver: key role of anatomic dissection for plastic surgery resident training. Medicine (Baltimore). 2017; 96(29):e7528

[15] Olinger A, Pistorius G, Lindemann W, Vollmar B, Hildebrandt U, Menger MD. Effectiveness of a hands-on training course for laparoscopic spine surgery in a porcine model. Surg Endosc. 1999; 13(2):118–122

[16] Hildebrandt U, Pistorius G, Olinger A, Menger MD. First experience with laparoscopic spine fusion in an experimental model in the pig. Surg Endosc. 1996; 10(2):143–146

[17] Mayer HM. A new microsurgical technique for minimally invasive anterior lumbar interbody fusion. Spine. 1997; 22(6):691–699, discussion 700

[18] Valentine R, Padhye V, Wormald PJ. Simulation training for vascular emergencies in endoscopic sinus and skull base surgery. Otolaryngol Clin North Am. 2016; 49(3):877–887

[19] Murray JS. Walter Reed National Military Medical Center: simulation on the cutting edge. Mil Med. 2010; 175(9):659–663

[20] Fletcher JD. Education and training technology in the military. Science. 2009; 323(5910):72–75

[21] Marcus H, Vakharia V, Kirkman MA, Murphy M, Nandi D. Practice makes perfect? The role of simulation-based deliberate practice and script-based mental rehearsal in the acquisition and maintenance of operative neurosurgical skills. Neurosurgery. 2013; 72 Suppl 1:124–130

[22] Taylor DC, Hamdy H. Adult learning theories: implications for learning and teaching in medical education: AMEE Guide No. 83. Med Teach. 2013; 35 (11):e1561–e1572

[23] Gallagher AG. Metric-based simulation training to proficiency in medical education:- what it is and how to do it. Ulster Med J. 2012; 81(3):107–113

[24] Pelargos PE, Nagasawa DT, Lagman C, et al. Utilizing virtual and augmented reality for educational and clinical enhancements in neurosurgery. J Clin Neurosci. 2017; 35:1–4

[25] Kaufman DM. Applying educational theory in practice. BMJ. 2003; 326 (7382):213–216

[26] Hassan I, Bin Dayne K, Kappus C, Gerdes B, Rothmund M, Hellwig D. Comparison of minimally invasive surgical skills of neurosurgeons versus general surgeons: is there a difference in the first exposure to a virtual reality simulator? Minim Invasive Neurosurg. 2007; 50(2):111–114

[27] Seymour NE, Gallagher AG, Roman SA, et al. Virtual reality training improves operating room performance: results of a randomized, double-blinded study. Ann Surg. 2002; 236(4):458–463, discussion 463–464

[28] Adermann J, Geissler N, Bernal LE, Kotzsch S, Korb W. Development and validation of an artificial wetlab training system for the lumbar discectomy. Eur Spine J. 2014; 23(9):1978–1983

[29] Alaraj A, Lemole MG, Finkle JH, et al. Virtual reality training in neurosurgery: review of current status and future applications. Surg Neurol Int. 2011; 2:52

[30] Jones F, Passos-Neto CE, Braghiroli OFM. Simulation in medical education: brief history and methodology. Principle and Practice of Clinical Research. 2015; 1(2):56–63

[31] Ray WZ, Ganju A, Harrop JS, Hoh DJ. Developing an anterior cervical discectomy and fusion simulator for neurosurgical resident training. Neurosurgery. 2013; 73 Suppl 1:100–106

[32] Kockro RA. Neurosurgery simulators—beyond the experiment. World Neurosurg. 2013; 80(5):e101–e102

[33] Schmidt FA, Wong T, Kirnaz S, et al. Development of a curriculum for minimally invasive spine surgery (MISS). Global Spine J. 2020; 10(2) Suppl:122S–125S

[34] Härtl R, Korge A. Minimally Invasive Spine Surgery: Techniques, Evidence, and Controversies. Thieme; 2012

55 The Role of Biologics in Minimally Invasive Spine Surgery

Howard An

Summary

In performing spinal fusion in MIS, proper selection of bone grafts and bone graft substitutes is paramount in achieving solid fusion. Proper surgical indications, meticulous preparation of the host endplates, and appropriate selection of interbody cage and biologics will lead to good surgical outcomes with fewer complications.

Keywords: biologics, intervertebral disc repair and regeneration, bone grafts and bone graft substitutes

55.1 Introduction

The narrower access corridors used in minimally invasive (MI) spine surgery has necessitated several technological advances. Although advances in instrumentation and technique have been critical, the success of MI spine surgery would be unthinkable without advances in biologic tools. On the one hand, technologies like novel bone graft extenders, bone morphogenetic protein (BMP), and bioactive materials are all critical to the success of modern MI techniques. On the other hand, bioregenerative interventions to treat degenerative disc disease have also been used with initially promising results. This chapter provides a brief overview of biologics in MI spine surgery and discusses exciting technologies that are currently in development.

55.2 Biologics for Spinal Arthrodesis

Spinal biologics enhance bone formation via osteoinductive, osteoconductive, osteogenic, or a combination of the three mechanisms.[1,2,3] Osteoinductive materials "induce" pluripotent stem cells to differentiate into osteoblastic, bone-forming phenotypes. Osteoconductive materials provide a scaffold for new bone formation. Osteogenesis refers to continued production of bone by pre-existing bone-forming cells.

Because MI approaches rely on narrow access corridors, surgeons often have access to a limited quantity of local autograft bone. Despite this fact, good results have been described when local bone shavings, excised facet bone, and iliac crest autograft[4,5,6] are used in MI transforaminal lumbar interbody fusions. Autograft bone remains a desirable graft choice when available because it is osteoinductive, osteoconductive, and osteogenic.

Allograft bone, in contrast, is primarily osteoconductive with only weak osteoinductive effects.[3] For this reason allograft bone is typically used in conjunction with osteoinductive agents (e.g., BMP).[7,8] Corticocancellous allografts provide mechanical support in addition to osteoconduction and are commonly used in the cervical spine.[9,10]

In addition to allograft bone, synthetic osteoconductive scaffolds and osteoinductive materials may be utilized. These products are referred to as bone graft extenders and include demineralized bone matrix (DBM), bone ceramics, and rhBMP. DBM is allograft bone that has been demineralized using a chemical process. DBM consists of an osteoconductive scaffold that also contains bone-forming proteins (e.g., BMP) to provide an osteoinductive effect, albeit weak due to low concentrations of BMPs in the products. Bone ceramics are comprised of a mix of hydroxyapatite (HA) and tricalcium phosphate (TCP). Their structure provides an osteoconductive scaffold for bone growth.[3,11,12] BMPs are proteins within the transforming growth factor beta (TGF-β) superfamily. They induce the differentiation of pluripotent mesenchymal stem cells toward osteogenic and chondrogenic phenotypes by stimulating angiogenesis and alkaline phosphatase activity.[13] Recombinant human BMP in the supraphysiologic concentration is widely utilized in MI surgeries via the anterior, lateral, or posterior approaches to assist with interbody fusion, but caution should be taken to avoid complications such as inflammation of surrounding structures, including nerves and ectopic ossification.[6,14]

55.2.1 Biomaterials in Spine Surgery

Using lessons learned from total joint arthroplasty, there have been several recent advances in spinal biomaterials to improve bony on-growth at the bone–implant interface. Traditional polyether ether ketone (PEEK) cages are widely used because of their radiolucency and desirable biomechanical properties. Although excellent results have been reported, there are concerns about the halo formation at the PEEK–bone interface.[15] Several surface modifications to PEEK have been proposed to improve osseointegration. These include the development of porous PEEK and surface treatments with titanium, HA, and various bone ceramics.[16,17,18,19] Although clinical data is limited,[20] there is promising animal and biomechanical data supporting these technologies. Novel ceramic materials such as silicon nitride with favorable biomechanical, osseointegrative, and antimicrobial properties have also been developed recently. Clinical trials studying this new material are currently underway.[21,22]

55.2.2 Biologic Approaches to Treating Degenerative Disc Disease

Given the immense burden of degenerative disc disease, strategies to repair and regenerate degenerative intervertebral discs (IVD) are an active area of investigation that are likely to represent the "next wave" in spine surgery. Strategies to repair discs include: injection of proteins (e.g., BMP7[23,24]), injection of growth factors (e.g., platelet-rich plasma, PRP[25,26]), gene therapy to reduce the expression of degradative molecules,[27,28,29] annular repair,[30] cell-based therapies,[31,32] and total disc transplantation[33,34] (▶ Fig. 55.1). There is strong in vitro and animal model data to support these strategies. Injection of BMP7 in a rabbit model of IVD degeneration, for example, has been shown to restore disc height and restore the biomechanical properties of degenerated intervertebral discs.[23,24] Similarly, injection of autologous or allogeneic chondrocytes into the IVD results in the production of disc matrix and decreased signs of

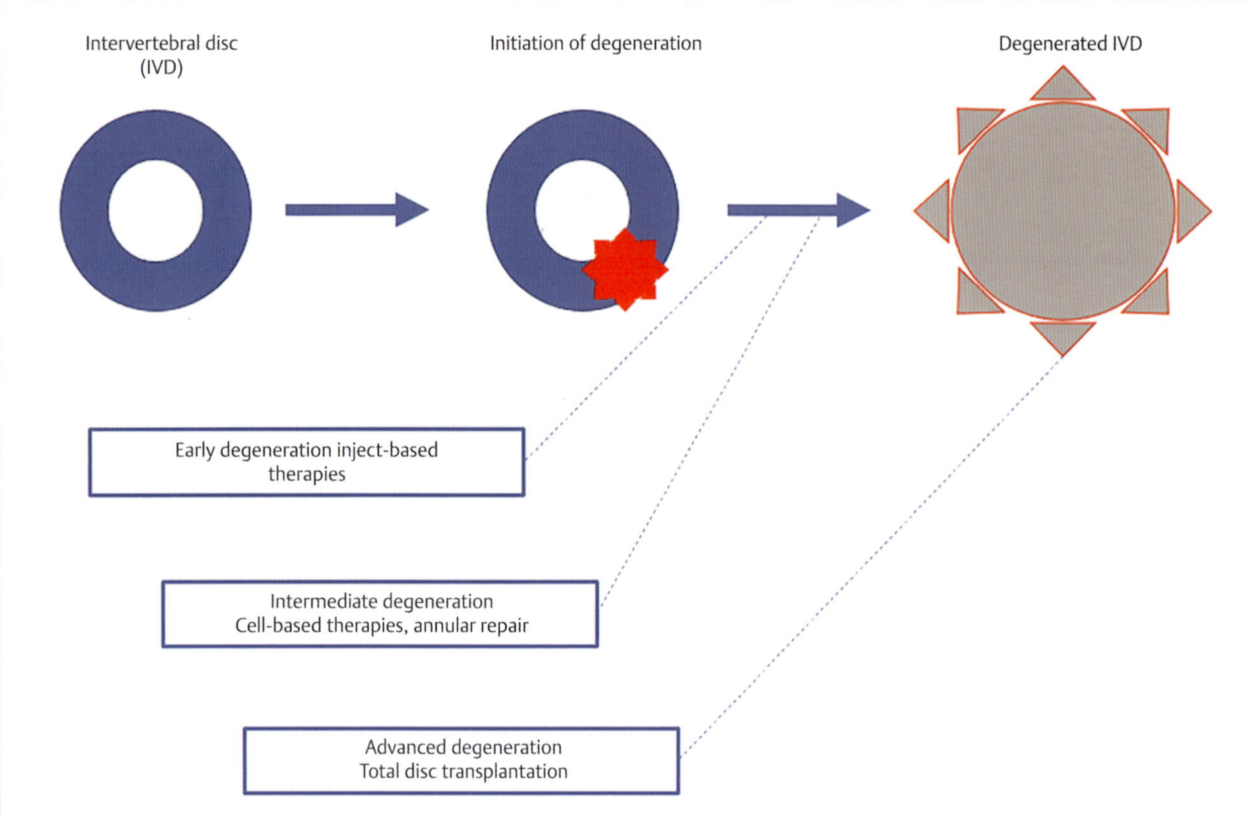

Fig. 55.1 Approaches to treat degenerated intervertebral discs based on the severity of degeneration. Although early degenerative changes may be treated with injection-based therapies, more advanced degeneration requires interventions such as tissue-engineered discs transplantation.

degeneration on magnetic resonance imaging (MRI).[32] Mesenchymal stem cells harvested from bone marrow or adipose tissue can differentiate into bone, cartilage, and other connective tissue. Implantation of these cells into the disc has also been shown to help regenerate disc matrix.[31] Although existing clinical data is limited, there are several clinical trials underway to determine the efficacy of these approaches to slow and potentially reverse disc degeneration.

Annular repair following microdiscectomy has often been considered an attractive strategy to prevent recurrent disc herniation. Strategies that have focused on material repair (i.e., suture repair of the annulus lesion or securing synthetic polymers to seal the defect) have yielded only limited success in *in vivo* studies.[30] Many biologically active strategies, however, have been successfully applied in large animal models. These include: injection of BMP13,[35] repair with an absorbable poly (glycolic acid) (PGA) material dipped in blood serum,[36] interstinal submucosa patch,[37] collagen patches,[38] hyaluronan-soaked sponges,[39] and fibrin tissue sealants.[40] Although these approaches were deployed in models of varying injury severity (annulus slit vs. box annulotomy, for example), they do show promising results with potential for future clinical translation.

Although annular repair and cell-based therapies might be promising for IVDs with intermediate degeneration, severely degenerated discs are unlikely to be managed with these methods. Tissue-engineered discs and disc transplantation might represent an attractive alternative in these patients. Ruan et al were the first to attempt transplantation of the whole intervertebral disc in the cervical spine.[41] They described promising results (mild disc degeneration but preserved motion and stability) at 5-year follow-up in a pilot study with five patients. Despite their positive results, their approach is limited by a lack of healthy donor discs and the possibility for disease transmission. These limitations have led investigators to pursue tissue-engineered approaches to disc transplantation. Moriguchi and colleagues recently described successfully implanting tissue-engineered discs in a canine cervical spine model.[33]

55.3 Conclusion

Biologically active materials are critical to the success of present-day MI spine surgery. Future advances in our understanding of graft technology, biomaterials, and disc biology will allow spine surgeons to successfully treat more varied pathology through less invasive methods.

References

[1] Grabowski G, Cornett CA. Bone graft and bone graft substitutes in spine surgery: current concepts and controversies. J Am Acad Orthop Surg. 2013; 21 (1):51–60

[2] Albrektsson T, Johansson C. Osteoinduction, osteoconduction and osseointegration. Eur Spine J. 2001; 10 Suppl 2:S96–S101

[3] Kannan A, Dodwad S-NM, Hsu WK. Biologics in spine arthrodesis. J Spinal Disord Tech. 2015; 28(5):163–170

[4] Lopez GD, Hijji FY, Narain AS, Yom KH, Singh K. Iliac crest bone graft: a minimally invasive harvesting technique. Clin Spine Surg. 2017; 30(10):439–441

[5] Kasliwal MK, Deutsch H. Clinical and radiographic outcomes using local bone shavings as autograft in minimally invasive transforaminal lumbar interbody fusion. World Neurosurg. 2012; 78(1–2):185–190

[6] Parajón A, Alimi M, Navarro-Ramirez R, et al. Minimally invasive transforaminal lumbar interbody fusion: meta-analysis of the fusion rates. what is the optimal graft material? Neurosurgery. 2017; 81(6):958–971

[7] Banwart JC, Asher MA, Hassanein RS. Iliac crest bone graft harvest donor site morbidity. A statistical evaluation. Spine. 1995; 20(9):1055–1060

[8] Summers BN, Eisenstein SM. Donor site pain from the ilium. A complication of lumbar spine fusion. J Bone Joint Surg Br. 1989; 71(4):677–680

[9] An HS, Simpson JM, Glover JM, Stephany J. Comparison between allograft plus demineralized bone matrix versus autograft in anterior cervical fusion. A prospective multicenter study. Spine. 1995; 20(20):2211–2216

[10] Chau AMT, Mobbs RJ. Bone graft substitutes in anterior cervical discectomy and fusion. Eur Spine J. 2009; 18(4):449–464

[11] Zadegan SA, Abedi A, Jazayeri SB, Bonaki HN, Vaccaro AR, Rahimi-Movaghar V. Clinical application of ceramics in anterior cervical discectomy and fusion: a review and update. Global Spine J. 2017; 7(4):343–349

[12] Nickoli MS, Hsu WK. Ceramic-based bone grafts as a bone grafts extender for lumbar spine arthrodesis: a systematic review. Global Spine J. 2014; 4 (3):211–216

[13] Campana V, Milano G, Pagano E, et al. Bone substitutes in orthopaedic surgery: from basic science to clinical practice. J Mater Sci Mater Med. 2014; 25 (10):2445–2461

[14] Hofstetter CP, Hofer AS, Levi AD. Exploratory meta-analysis on dose-related efficacy and morbidity of bone morphogenetic protein in spinal arthrodesis surgery. J Neurosurg Spine. 2016; 24(3):457–475

[15] Phan K, Hogan JA, Assem Y, Mobbs RJ. PEEK-Halo effect in interbody fusion. J Clin Neurosci. 2016; 24:138–140

[16] Hsu WK, Goldstein CL, Shamji MF, et al. Novel osteobiologics and biomaterials in the treatment of spinal disorders. Neurosurgery. 2017; 80 3S:S100–S107

[17] Lee JH, Jang HL, Lee KM, et al. In vitro and in vivo evaluation of the bioactivity of hydroxyapatite-coated polyetheretherketone biocomposites created by cold spray technology. Acta Biomater. 2013; 9(4):6177–6187

[18] Stübinger S, Drechsler A, Bürki A, Klein K, Kronen P, von Rechenberg B. Titanium and hydroxyapatite coating of polyetheretherketone and carbon fiber-reinforced polyetheretherketone: a pilot study in sheep. J Biomed Mater Res B Appl Biomater. 2016; 104(6):1182–1191

[19] Wang S, Deng Y, Yang L, Shi X, Yang W, Chen Z-G. Enhanced antibacterial property and osteo-differentiation activity on plasma treated porous polyetheretherketone with hierarchical micro/nano-topography. J Biomater Sci Polym Ed. 2018; 29(5):520–542

[20] Chong E, Mobbs RJ, Pelletier MH, Walsh WR. Titanium/polyetheretherketone cages for cervical arthrodesis with degenerative and traumatic pathologies: early clinical outcomes and fusion rates. Orthop Surg. 2016; 8(1):19–26

[21] Kersten RF, van Gaalen SM, Arts MP, et al. The SNAP trial: a double blind multi-center randomized controlled trial of a silicon nitride versus a PEEK cage in transforaminal lumbar interbody fusion in patients with symptomatic degenerative lumbar disc disorders: study protocol. BMC Musculoskelet Disord. 2014; 15(1):57

[22] Arts MP, Wolfs JFC, Corbin TP. The CASCADE trial: effectiveness of ceramic versus PEEK cages for anterior cervical discectomy with interbody fusion; protocol of a blinded randomized controlled trial. BMC Musculoskelet Disord. 2013; 14(1):244

[23] Ohara A, Miyamoto K, Naganawa T, Matsumoto K, Shimizu K. Reliabilities of and correlations among five standard methods of assessing the sagittal alignment of the cervical spine. Spine. 2006; 31(22):2585–2591, discussion 2592

[24] Miyamoto K, Masuda K, Kim JG, et al. Intradiscal injections of osteogenic protein-1 restore the viscoelastic properties of degenerated intervertebral discs. Spine J. 2006; 6(6):692–703

[25] Levi D, Horn S, Tyszko S, Levin J, Hecht-Leavitt C, Walko E. Intradiscal platelet-rich plasma injection for chronic discogenic low back pain: preliminary results from a prospective trial. Pain Med. 2016; 17(6):1010–1022

[26] Akeda K, Ohishi K, Masuda K, et al. Intradiscal injection of autologous platelet-rich plasma releasate to treat discogenic low back pain: a preliminary clinical trial. Asian Spine J. 2017; 11(3):380–389

[27] Paul R, Haydon RC, Cheng H, et al. Potential use of Sox9 gene therapy for intervertebral degenerative disc disease. Spine. 2003; 28(8):755–763

[28] Yoon ST, Park JS, Kim KS, et al. ISSLS prize winner: LMP-1 upregulates intervertebral disc cell production of proteoglycans and BMPs in vitro and in vivo. Spine. 2004; 29(23):2603–2611

[29] Nishida K, Kang JD, Gilbertson LG, et al. Modulation of the biologic activity of the rabbit intervertebral disc by gene therapy: an in vivo study of adenovirus-mediated transfer of the human transforming growth factor beta 1 encoding gene. Spine. 1999; 24(23):2419–2425

[30] Sloan SR , Jr, Lintz M, Hussain I, Hartl R, Bonassar LJ. Biologic annulus fibrosus repair: a review of preclinical in vivo investigations. Tissue Eng Part B Rev. 2018; 24(3):179–190

[31] Feng G, Zhao X, Liu H, et al. Transplantation of mesenchymal stem cells and nucleus pulposus cells in a degenerative disc model in rabbits: a comparison of 2 cell types as potential candidates for disc regeneration. J Neurosurg Spine. 2011; 14(3):322–329

[32] Ganey T, Libera J, Moos V, et al. Disc chondrocyte transplantation in a canine model: a treatment for degenerated or damaged intervertebral disc. Spine. 2003; 28(23):2609–2620

[33] Moriguchi Y, Mojica-Santiago J, Grunert P, et al. Total disc replacement using tissue-engineered intervertebral discs in the canine cervical spine. PLoS One. 2017; 12(10):e0185716

[34] Ruan D, He Q, Ding Y, Hou L, Li J, Luk KD. Intervertebral disc transplantation in the treatment of degenerative spine disease: a preliminary study. Lancet. 2007; 369(9566):993–999

[35] Wei A, Williams LA, Bhargav D, et al. BMP13 prevents the effects of annular injury in an ovine model. Int J Biol Sci. 2009; 5(5):388–396

[36] Hegewald AA, Medved F, Feng D, et al. Enhancing tissue repair in annulus fibrosus defects of the intervertebral disc: analysis of a bio-integrative annulus implant in an in-vivo ovine model. J Tissue Eng Regen Med. 2015; 9 (4):405–414

[37] Ledet EH, Jeshuran W, Glennon JC, et al. Small intestinal submucosa for anular defect closure: long-term response in an in vivo sheep model. Spine. 2009; 34(14):1457–1463

[38] Pennicooke B, Hussain I, Berlin C, et al. Annulus fibrosus repair using high-density collagen gel: an in vivo ovine model. Spine. 2018; 43(4):E208–E215

[39] Fuller ES, Shu C, Smith MM, Little CB, Melrose J. Hyaluronan oligosaccharides stimulate matrix metalloproteinase and anabolic gene expression in vitro by intervertebral disc cells and annular repair in vivo. J Tissue Eng Regen Med. 2018; 12(1):e216–e226

[40] Oehme D, Ghosh P, Shimmon S, et al. Mesenchymal progenitor cells combined with pentosan polysulfate mediating disc regeneration at the time of microdiscectomy: a preliminary study in an ovine model. J Neurosurg Spine. 2014; 20(6):657–669

[41] Ruan F, Zheng Q, Wang J. Mechanisms of bone anabolism regulated by statins. Biosci Rep. 2012; 32(6):511–519

56 Summary and Outlook—Future of Lumbar Minimally Invasive Surgery

Joel Martin, Laura Hein, Vincent Cheung, and William Taylor

Summary
Minimally invasive spine surgery continues to expand both procedurally and in interest to patients. We review possible future directions for this expanding field.

Keywords: minimally invasive surgery (MIS), lumbar minimally invasive surgery, transforaminal lumbar interbody fusion (TLIF), posterior lumbar interbody fusion (PLIF), diffusion of innovation

56.1 Adoption and Diffusion

Lumbar minimally invasive spine surgery has continued to evolve in the past decade, although not with the rapidity initially projected. In 2016, approximately one-third of all surgeries were done with the minimally invasive approach and it was estimated that by 2020, approximately half of all surgeries will be conducted using these methods.[1] Despite multiple positive studies and continued expansion of techniques, the adoption rate of minimally invasive spine surgery has not been as rapid as initially expected. This is often compared with the case of laparoscopic procedures, in which within a span of 1 to 2 years, abdominal surgeries done via laparoscopic technique almost completely supplanted open procedures, and rapidly became the standard of care. This certainly has not happened as quickly in the case of minimally invasive spine surgery despite multiple studies showing that minimally invasive approaches to spinal surgery offer decreases in blood loss, length of stay, infection rates, and have similar, if not improved, outcomes to open procedures. Leaders in minimally invasive surgery (MIS) have described a possible upper limit on MIS techniques and have postulated whether MIS has reached its maximum capability.[1]

Rate-limiting factors such as enhanced learning curves and uncertain applications in complex spinal disease have been suggested to impose a significant limitation in the adoption and diffusion of lumbar MIS techniques. In his classic writing on the diffusion of innovation topic published in 1983, Rodgers predicted an initial steep adoption curve as innovators and early adopters led the way to early adoption. Eventually, the market share of the innovation reaches saturation, much like the laparoscopic cholecystectomy and appendectomy have experienced, and what is currently being seen with robotic assisted prostatectomies.[2] Perhaps the reason why this trend is not being observed in lumbar MIS lies in the issue of technical complexity? The diffusion of medical techniques differs significantly from diffusion of new products and equipment. These features are described by Hinsch et al in 2014, which suggests that diffusion of technique also requires diffusion agents and interpersonal interaction, along with technical performance. Hinsch et al also purport that diffusion of technique is a prerequisite for diffusion of any related product or technology.[3] It can been suggested that minimally invasive lumbar spine surgery is more likely a diffusion of technique in which interaction between potential adopters and diffusion agents is the most important factor affecting adoption. For example, a classic diffusion of technique related to MIS of spine is akin to the diffusion of anterior, as opposed to standard lateral, hip replacement. The reasons are very similar, as the lateral approach is a well-respected technique in which many patients do very well, similar to open lumbar spine surgery. In addition, the latter technique is well established, and the anterior approach does not require new specific technology but rather the diffusion of training and technique.

56.2 Patient Care and Procedures

The question of standard of care for lumbar MIS still remains. Lumbar MIS has been defined as "one that by virtue of the extent and means of surgical technique will results in less collateral tissue damage, results in measurable decrease in morbidity and more rapid functional recovery than traditional exposures, without differentiation in the intended surgical goal."[4] Inclusive evidence has been reported on both nonfusion techniques, including MIS microdiscectomy, direct decompression (laminectomy/laminotomy), indirect decompression (interspinous process devices), as well as minimally invasive (MI) fusion techniques including percutaneous pedicle screw fixation, MIS transforaminal lumbar interbody fusion (TLIF), posterior lumbar interbody fusion (PLIF), and lateral lumbar interbody fusion (LLIF). Nonfusion techniques require a learning curve, and as expected, evidence suggests that clinical outcomes are similar in open and MIS cohorts.[5,6,7,8,9]

Despite similar clinical outcomes, decreased blood loss, shorter hospitalization, and cost savings seen in fusion lumbar MIS, the increased radiation exposure and learning curve may affect its overall use.[10,11,12,13] Evidence demonstrates that the use of MIS versus open surgery for lumbar disc herniation reaches clinical equipoise, but MIS can be inferior in regard to pain relief of the legs and lower back, quality-of-life, and rehospitalization rate.[14] For fusion cases, three randomized controlled trials have demonstrated that MIS-TLIF demonstrates advantages, most prominently in reduced hospitalization, cost, and time to return to work.[14,15,16,17] From this literature, it appears that more complicated procedures have a larger opportunity to gain from MIS. Simple discectomy, done with MIS, may serve best as a learning tool for more complicated procedures to follow, and therefore complicated deformity procedures should not be a surgeons' initial MIS and learning can occur progressively along a natural pathway. Clinical success with MIS appears more likely than with non-MIS fusions, but while these data are intriguing, they should be interpreted cautiously considering the level of heterogeneity of the studies available. Further, high-quality comparative studies are warranted to better understand the relative benefits of more complex interbody and MIS fusions for these conditions. Patient selection and matching the procedure to specific pathology remains key, along with appropriate technique.

In terms of minimally invasive approach (▶ Fig. 56.1), LLIF and oblique lumbar interbody fusion (OLIF) have changed practice patterns in lumbar MIS in an unprecedented way. Minimally invasive posterior approaches have evolved in an attempt to reduce approach related complications. Anterior/lateral approaches avoid the spinal canal, cauda equina, and nerve roots, along with muscular insertions using a unique natural tissue plane to the spine. With its high fusion rates, well-established complication profile, and ability for use in routine degenerative or complex deformities, the adoption and proliferation of minimally invasive fusion techniques have been rapid. A study by Watkins et al of 220 consecutive patients with 309 operative levels were compared by surgery type, namely, anterior lumbar interbody fusion or ALIF (184 levels), LLIF (86 levels), and TLIF (39 levels), with an average follow-up of 19.2 months. They concluded that improvement of lordosis was significant for both the ALIF and LLIF groups, but not the TLIF group. Intergroup analysis showed the ALIF group had significantly improved lordosis compared to both the other groups. The ALIF and LLIF groups had significantly increased disc height compared to the TLIF group. All the three groups showed significantly reduced spondylolisthesis, with no difference between the groups.[18] A recent review analyzed fusion, complications, and clinical success for lumbar fusion performed with various surgical technique, and found that PLIF-All, TLIF-All, and LLIF had significantly higher odds of fusion than instrumented posterior lateral fusion (▶ Table 56.1), most notable for PLIF with an odds ratio of 3.2. ALIF had a slightly lower odds of fusion compared to PLIF (odds ratio 0.47), and MIS procedures had significantly higher odds of fusion than non-MIS (OR 2.20). Lastly, consistent with previously reported studies, instrumented PLF had significantly higher fusion odds than uninstrumented PLF (OR 2.20).[19]

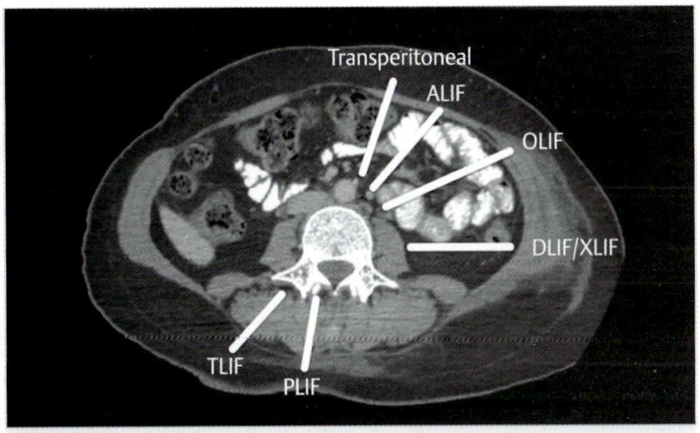

Fig. 56.1 Surgical approaches to the lumbar spine for interbody fusion techniques. The five primary interbody fusion approaches are shown here schematically: anterior lumbar interbody fusion (ALIF), lateral or extreme lateral interbody fusion (LLIF or XLIF), oblique lumbar interbody fusion/anterior to psoas (OLIF/ATP), transforaminal lumbar interbody fusion (TLIF or MI-TLIF), and posterior lumbar interbody fusion (PLIF). (Reproduced from Raheja A, Tandon V, Garg K et al. A Review of Minimally Invasive Techniques in Thoracolumbar Trauma. Indian Journal of Neurotrauma 2021; 18(01): 07-13.)

Adoption of the LLIF approach, in particular, despite its MIS advantages, may be related to the logistical hurdles of positioning the patient in lateral decubitus. The technique requires significant attention to initial positioning as well as intraoperative repositioning (to prone) for posterior fixation and direct decompression when required. Sagittal alignment is also of concern, as studies show only limited segmental and regional correction while in lateral decubitus.[22] Advancements in LLIF include the introduction of a technique to perform a transpsoas lateral approach to the interbody space with the patient in

Table 56.1 Odds ratio of fusion, complications, and clinical success between fusion techniques

Comparison	Fusion	Complications	Clinical success
ALIF-All vs. instrumented PLF	1.51 [1.15, 1.99]	0.89 [0.69, 1.15]	2.29* [1.86, 2.81]
PLIF-All vs. instrumented PLF	3.20* [2.53, 4.04]	0.65* [0.54, 0.79]	3.60* [3.03, 4.29]
TLIF-All vs. instrumented PLF	2.46* [1.90, 3.18]	0.54* [0.42, 0.70]	4.80* [3.95, 5.85]
LLIF vs. instrumented PLF	2.20* [1.55, 3.10]	1.66* [1.29, 2.14]	0.51* [0.40, 0.65]
Circumferential vs. instrumented PLF	1.49 [1.18, 1.89]	1.11 [1.09, 1.64]	1.19 [0.98, 1.44]
Instrumented vs. uninstrumented PLF	2.20* [1.74, 2.69]	1.00 [0.76, 1.42]	1.10 [0.86, 1.52]
ALIF vs. PLIF-All	0.47* [0.34, 0.66]	1.37 [1.02,1.79]	0.63* [0.50, 0.80]
ALIF vs. TLIF-All	0.62 [0.43, 0.87]	1.65 [1.10, 2.30]	0.48* [0.37, 0.61]
ALIF vs. LLIF	0.69 [0.45, 1.05]	0.54* [0.39, 0.74]	4.50* [3.38, 6.01]
PLIF-All vs. TLIF-All	1.30 [0.95, 1.79]	1.21 [0.91, 1.59]	0.75 [0.60, 0.94]
PLIF-All vs. LLIF	1.46 [0.98, 2.16]	0.39* [0.30, 0.52]	7.10* [5.44, 9.27]
TLIF-All vs. LLIF	1.12 [0.75, 1.68]	0.33* [0.24, 0.45]	9.47* [7.15, 12.5]
PLIF-MIS vs. PLIF non-MIS	1.01 [0.62, 1.64]	1.08 [0.75, 1.52]	18.6* [10.8, 32.1]
MIS-TLIF vs. TLIF non-MIS	0.95 [0.59, 1.58]	0.84 [0.48, 1.47]	12.3* [7.17, 21.1]
PLIF-MIS vs. MIS-TLIF	1.34 [0.76, 2.41]	1.45 [0.81, 2.58]	1.15 [0.56, 2.37]
MIS vs. non-MIS	1.59* [1.32, 1.90]	1.20 [1.03, 1.41]	2.44* [2.16, 2.75]
Biologic vs. no biologic	2.29* [1.75, 2.99]	1.28 [1.05, 1.55]	3.40* [2.82, 4.10]

Abbreviations: ALIF, anterior lumbar interbody fusion; LIF, lumber interbody fusion; LLIF, lateral lumbar interbody fusion; MIS, minimally invasive surgery; PLF, posterolateral fusion; PLIF, posterior lumbar interbody fusion; TLIF, transforaminal lumbar interbody fusion.
Source: Reproduced with permission from Makanji H, Schoenfeld AJ, Bhalla A, Bono, CM. Critical analysis of trends in lumbar fusion for degenerative disorders revisited: influence of technique on fusion rate and clinical outcomes. Eur Spine J. 2018;5.
Note: *Significant $p < 0.0025$.

prone position (e.g., prone transpsoas), maximizing positional lordosis and enabling concomitant posterior procedures such as direct decompression, posterior releases, and pedicular fixation, all without the need for patient repositioning. The prone transpsoas (PTP) technique was only described recently,[23] but initial results are promising.[20] The prone transpsoas procedure shown here can shorten or time with no need for repositioning and improve lordosis. Over 200 cases have been completed to date and this represents a new option for single position surgery using the lateral approach.

Technology continues to improve and change with the adoption of Enhancing Recovery After Surgery (ERAS) programs and endoscopic procedures.[24] These permeate other areas of medicine and surgery and have had a relatively stable adoption rate in minimally invasive lumbar spine surgery. New techniques that allow intracanal discectomy and decompressions allow the surgeon to perform a more recognizable procedure that may increase endoscopic use. Percutaneous, endoscopic or awake fusions coupled with ERAS are well documented.[24] Camera technology (chip on a tip) will provide improved visualization to endoscopically assisted procedures. This will allow a further decrease in approach-related tissue disruption which remains key for lumbar MIS. There are currently multiple investigational device exemption trials for the intradiscal treatment of degenerative disc disease. These include stem cells, small molecules, and device related ideas. The medical treatment of degenerative disc disease with injections into the disc space may eliminate and/or slow the need for fusion decompressions and discectomies from open and/or minimally invasive techniques.

The question remains if and when MIS will come to predominate lumbar spine surgery. Chronological studies have suggested that surgical complications can arise in the initial learning phase in lumbar MIS. Ancillary technology such as robotics and/or navigation can aid in reducing the learning curve and possibly ensure improved outcomes with MIS approaches. This concept fits well into the diffusion of innovation outline proposed by Rodgers. Diffusion of innovation states that technology itself is information, and a lack of awareness and exposure to this information can result in failure of diffusion. Rodgers reports the main types of innovation diffusion, including optional innovation-decision made by individual users or surgeons, and collective innovation and authority innovation made by authoritative bodies and hospitals. These factors, along with additional authority derived from the legal system or individuals who possess power or status within the field (key opinion leader [KOL] effect), can affect regional adoption. Thus, we should consider state laws that limit malpractice awards that have a direct effect on the adoption of new and often superior technologies. One study found that patients from states with malpractice caps were 70% more likely to receive minimally invasive radical prostatectomy than those without such caps.[25]

Overall, there remain several areas for continued lumbar MIS advancements including in new diagnostics and prognostics to aid in patient selection, the treatment of rigid and complex deformities, the expanded use of navigated technologies, and in the reduction of radiation exposure. Adoption of these new technologies and effective training programs in order to learn MIS effectively and safely may provide the impetus to continue to advance MIS past its current limitations.

References

[1] Phillips FM, Cheng I, Rampersaud YR, et al. Breaking through the "glass ceiling" of minimally invasive spine surgery. Spine. 2016; 41 Suppl 8:S39–S43

[2] Parsons JK, Messer K, Palazzi K, Stroup SP, Chang D. Diffusion of surgical innovations, patient safety, and minimally invasive radical prostatectomy. JAMA Surg. 2014; 149(8):845–851

[3] Hinsch ME, Stockstrom C, Luthje C. User innovation in techniques: a case study analysis in the field of medical devices. Creat Innov Manag. 2014; 23 (4):484–494

[4] McAfee PC, Garfin SR, Rodgers WB, Allen RT, Phillips F, Kim C. An attempt at clinically defining and assessing minimally invasive surgery compared with traditional "open" spinal surgery. SAS J. 2011; 5(4):125–130

[5] Skovrlj B, Gilligan J, Cutler HS, Qureshi SA. Minimally invasive procedures on the lumbar spine. World J Clin Cases. 2015; 3(1):1–9

[6] Kamper SJ, Ostelo RW, Rubinstein SM, et al. Minimally invasive surgery for lumbar disc herniation: a systematic review and meta-analysis. Eur Spine J. 2014; 23(5):1021–1043

[7] Anderson DG, Patel A, Maltenfort M, et al. Lumbar decompression using a traditional midline approach versus a tubular retractor system: comparison of patient-based clinical outcomes. Spine. 2011; 36(5):E320–E325

[8] Khoo LT, Fessler RG. Microendoscopic decompressive laminotomy for the treatment of lumbar stenosis. Neurosurgery. 2002; 51(5) Suppl:S146–S154

[9] O'Toole JE, Eichholz KM, Fessler RG. Surgical site infection rates after minimally invasive spinal surgery. J Neurosurg Spine. 2009; 11(4):471–476

[10] Seng C, Siddiqui MA, Wong KP, et al. Five-year outcomes of minimally invasive versus open transforaminal lumbar interbody fusion: a matched-pair comparison study. Spine. 2013; 38(23):2049–2055

[11] Parker SL, Mendenhall SK, Shau DN, et al. Minimally invasive versus open transforaminal lumbar interbody fusion for degenerative spondylolisthesis: comparative effectiveness and cost-utility analysis. World Neurosurg. 2014; 82(1–2):230–238

[12] Vertuani S, Nilsson J, Borgman B, et al. A cost-effectiveness analysis of minimally invasive versus open surgery techniques for lumbar spinal fusion in Italy and the United Kingdom. Value Health. 2015; 18(6):810–816

[13] Mobbs RJ, Sivabalan P, Li J. Technique, challenges and indications for percutaneous pedicle screw fixation. J Clin Neurosci. 2011; 18(6):741–749

[14] McClelland S , III, Goldstein JA. Minimally invasive versus open spine surgery: what does the best evidence tell us? J Neurosci Rural Pract. 2017; 8(2):194–198

[15] Wang HL, Lü FZ, Jiang JY, Ma X, Xia XL, Wang LX. Minimally invasive lumbar interbody fusion via MAST Quadrant retractor versus open surgery: a prospective randomized clinical trial. Chin Med J (Engl). 2011; 124(23):3868–3874

[16] Rodríguez-Vela J, Lobo-Escolar A, Joven E, Muñoz-Marín J, Herrera A, Velilla J. Clinical outcomes of minimally invasive versus open approach for one-level transforaminal lumbar interbody fusion at the 3- to 4-year follow-up. Eur Spine J. 2013; 22(12):2857–2863

[17] Wang J, Zhou Y, Zhang ZF, Li CQ, Zheng WJ, Liu J. Minimally invasive or open transforaminal lumbar interbody fusion as revision surgery for patients previously treated by open discectomy and decompression of the lumbar spine. Eur Spine J. 2011; 20(4):623–628

[18] Watkins RG , IV, Hanna R, Chang D, Watkins RG , III. Sagittal alignment after lumbar interbody fusion: comparing anterior, lateral, and transforaminal approaches. J Spinal Disord Tech. 2014; 27(5):253–256

[19] Makanji H, Schoenfeld AJ, Bhalla A, Bono CM. Critical analysis of trends in lumbar fusion for degenerative disorders revisited: influence of technique on fusion rate and clinical outcomes. Eur Spine J. 2018; 27(8):1868–1876

[20] Pimenta L, Amaral R, Taylor W, et al. The prone transpsoas technique: preliminary radiographic results of a multicenter experience. Eur Spine J. 2021; 30(1):108–113

[21] Mobbs RJ, Phan K, Malham G, Seex K, Rao PJ. Lumbar interbody fusion: techniques, indications and comparison of interbody fusion options including PLIF, TLIF, MI-TLIF, OLIF/ATP, LLIF and ALIF. J Spine Surg. 2015; 1(1):2–18

[22] Yson SC, Sembrano JN, Santos ER, Luna JT, Polly DW , Jr. Does prone repositioning before posterior fixation produce greater lordosis in lateral lumbar interbody fusion (LLIF)? J Spinal Disord Tech. 2014; 27(7):364–369

[23] Pimenta L, Taylor WR, Stone LE, Wali AR, Santiago-Dieppa DR. Prone transpsoas technique for simultaneous single-position access to the anterior and posterior lumbar spine. Operative Neurosurg (Hagerstown) 2020.; 20(1):E5–E12

[24] Wang MY, Chang PY, Grossman J. Development of an enhanced recovery after surgery (ERAS) approach for lumbar spinal fusion. J Neurosurg Spine. 2017; 26(4):411–418

[25] Hellinger FJ, Encinosa WE. The impact of state laws limiting malpractice damage awards on health care expenditures. Am J Public Health. 2006; 96 (8):1375–1381

57 Achieving MISS on a Global Level

Roger Härtl, Franziska Anna Schmidt, Taylor Wong, and Sertac Kirnaz

"The future is already here—it's just not very evenly distributed."
(William Gibson, 1993)

Summary

This chapter provides a succinct overview of the history, global prevalence, challenges, and economic impacts of MISS. Authors illustrate the concept of "leapfrogging" over the older techniques directly into MISS with the use of 2D and 3D navigation along with robotic surgery. This leads to the main challenges of training and equipment. Centers that received temporary spinal surgery assistance though MISS saw a great benefit to their outcomes, even if the assistance was temporary due to the emergency. A novel MISS curriculum has been developed by the AO Spine as a representation of the framework for providing access to MISS education globally. The global future looks to the organized spine societies to capture the initiative of implementing MISS education.

Keywords: global MISS, economic analysis, future directions

57.1 Introduction

Minimally invasive spine surgery (MISS) has rapidly evolved over the past decades in Europe, North America, and parts of Asia. Key events in the evolution of MISS included Yasargil's and Caspar's introduction of microscopic discectomy in 1977,[1,2] Böhler's odontoid screw in 1981,[3,4] Magerl's C1/2 transarticular screws[5] and his description of thoracic and lumbar percutaneous skeletal fixation in 1984,[6] computed tomography (CT)–guided navigation for pedicle screws in the early 2000s,[7,8] Foley's minimal invasive surgery (MIS) transforaminal lumbar interbody fusion (TLIF),[9] Pimenta's transpsoas fusion,[10] and more recently, the introduction of robotic surgery and augmented reality for pedicle screw placement.[11,12,13,14] An important publication that laid a lot of the groundwork for spinal MISS and microsurgery was Paul Young and John McCulloch's book *Essentials of Spinal Microsurgery* published in 1998.[15] Improvements in endoscopic systems and percutaneous implants have increased the range of applications for MIS in spinal surgery.[16] In addition, ongoing technological advancement in the field of MIS has led to improvements in surgical outcomes. The spectrum of MISS now includes the whole spectrum of spine, namely, spinal degenerative diseases, spinal trauma, spinal deformity, and spinal tumors.[17]

Promising current developments in MISS include the increased potential in outpatient surgery,[18] "single stage–single position" lateral decompression and fusion surgery,[19] three-dimensional printing technologies,[20] and MISS for metastatic and primary spinal tumors.[21] The frontiers for MISS are multilevel instrumentation of the cervical spine,[22] complex cervical and thoracolumbar deformity correction[23] as well as the potential for biological and tissue-engineered disc repair, regeneration, and replacement.[24,25,26]

As outlined in Chapter 1, Fig. 1.2, a large portion—we estimate up to 75%—of spinal procedures could be performed completely or partially using MISS, illustrating the potentially huge impact on spinal surgery worldwide.

Some of the MISS related strengths, weaknesses, opportunities, and threats based on the opinions of MISS leaders from around the globe are summarized in Chapter 2 (Table 2.2). In this final chapter, we address three aspects of MISS that are relevant in order to understand its significance for the global landscape of spinal surgery:

a) MISS can be performed with relatively modest investment in surgical equipment and resources while still having a big impact on patients' outcomes and overall costs savings.
b) Concept of leapfrogging; MISS accelerates the advancement of spinal surgery by skipping older techniques and "jumping" directly to advanced spinal procedures.
c) Economic impact of MISS on health care in health care systems worldwide.

Although some aspects of MISS require substantial investment by hospitals and/or surgical centers in infrastructure, equipment, and expensive implants, a lot of what MISS is about can be achieved with relatively inexpensive technology and techniques. This pertains especially to what has been covered under "Surgical Techniques" and "Training" in Chapter 1. A good example is the unilateral tubular or endoscopic laminotomy for bilateral decompression (ULBD); compared to open surgery this minimizes instability and avoids fusion surgery in a large proportion of patients[27] and therefore, it has a potentially big impact on cost reduction in spinal surgery. In addition, benefits like reduction of infection and blood loss as well as less postoperative pain and earlier return to normal activities with these surgical techniques provide big advantages for communities worldwide, especially in the settings with limited resources.

Good examples from personal experiences are places like Tanzania or Pakistan where surgeons are being trained in tubular surgery and can use this approach to perform lumbar decompression surgery effectively and with all above benefits including relatively low costs when compared to more traditional open surgery. This saves resources because less spinal instrumentation is needed. Although MISS avoids fusion surgery in patients who, if treated with open surgery, may need a stabilization, it allows for an expansion of the benefits of spinal stabilization to patient groups that were previously deemed too old or sick for traditional open fusion surgery. Together this can help retain elective patients who would have otherwise been sent elsewhere for expensive surgery abroad. In addition, this has a hugely positive impact on self-esteem and surgical growth in those countries.

The challenge then is adequate surgical training and education in tubular, endoscopic, and minimal access surgery. In large parts of the world, surgeons assume that decompression surgery automatically requires stabilization which consumes significant resources. Although this may be true with open surgery in certain scenarios, the need for fusion surgery can be significantly reduced by using tubular, specular, or endoscopic "over-the-top" decompression procedures. Therefore, the development of a curriculum for MISS and the dissemination of

teaching and training opportunities globally is key. This was recently started by AOSpine and the resulting curriculum and roll-out has been described.[28] Much more work needs to be done along these lines of course.

A recent neurosurgical survey was conducted in Africa that focused on the possibility of introducing MISS into the operating rooms of developing nations. One of the main takeaways from the study is the need for organization and structured training to implement MISS.[29] The lack of trained surgeons and overall poor infrastructure are contributing factors for the situation especially in Eastern Africa.[30]

57.2 MISS and Leapfrogging

The introduction of MISS can accelerate the advancement of spinal surgery by skipping older techniques and "jumping" directly to MISS and advanced spinal procedures. One example is the introduction of three-dimensional navigation and robotics that may lead to more procedures done percutaneously and pedicle screws being inserted without exposing anatomic landmarks. We witnessed this firsthand during a 2014 Hands-on Neurotrauma Course held in Dar-es-Salaam, Tanzania, where percutaneous screw fixation was performed in patients with spinal fractures using two-dimensional navigation.[31] A BrainLab Kick® (Brainlab Munich, Germany) two-dimensional portable navigation system with software was made available by the company and sent to Tanzania for the duration of the course and for a week after. Local spine surgeons without previous MISS experience or K-wire use were trained using two-dimensional navigated percutaneous pedicle screw placement and performed these procedures independently by the end of the week with excellent results in patients with spinal fractures.

After an earthquake struck Port au Prince, Haiti in 2010, a team of neurosurgeons from Miami successfully demonstrated the benefits of treating patients with spinal fractures using minimally invasive, percutaneous stabilization surgery.[32] A total of 15 trauma patients with fracture-dislocation at the thoracolumbar junction (ASIA grade B) were treated with MISS. Unfortunately, in both examples, the introduction of MISS could not be sustained by the local surgeons because the MISS equipment was only available for a limited time period.

Other more durable examples include the major advancements in endoscopic spine surgery, especially in some Asian regions where traditional open surgery seems to have been "skipped" and/or replaced in favor of MISS.

A concern related to this phenomenon of "skipping" more traditional surgical techniques is that trainees may not gain experience and confidence in older procedures and that their knowledge of anatomy may suffer as a consequence; this is especially a concern with modern three-dimensional navigation and robotics. Although this sounds like a reasonable concern, it should be remembered that similar concerns were voiced upon introduction of three-dimensional navigation in brain surgery in the 1990. More than 20 years later navigation has become a standard part of most cranial surgeries and the concerns regarding the quality of surgical training seem to have faded. One reason for this may be the tendency within surgery to subspecialize—surgeons tend to specialize and acquire expert knowledge in a particular field, while the concept of "general neurosurgeon or orthopedist" or even a "general spine surgeon" may slowly disappear.

57.3 Economic Impact of MISS on Health Care in Health Care Systems Worldwide

MISS can have a significantly beneficial impact on overall cost savings not only in North America[33,34] but also in Europe.[35]

The mechanisms by which costs are reduced are:

a) Lower infection rates requiring less revision surgery.
b) Greater implant accuracy with navigation/robotic surgery which avoids revision surgery.[7]
c) Less perioperative complications and earlier return to daily activities of living and normal function.[36]
d) Less postoperative pain.
e) Decreased need of fusion surgery because patients can be successfully decompressed without causing iatrogenic instability.[37]

The potential economic benefits of MISS have to be balanced against the initially higher costs associated with the MISS equipment and implants. Although several studies show the potential of MISS to be cost-effective, it is not clear how durable these results are over time. Longer follow-up and better outcome and cost data are needed compared to open or nonsurgical interventions.

In summary, MISS and the techniques and skills that it is associated with holds great benefits for spinal surgery worldwide. Approximately 75% of all spinal procedures can be performed partially or completely with MISS, and as MISS improves this percentage may increase.

Contrary to widespread belief, MISS can be performed with limited investment in expensive resources, especially MISS decompression procedures with low complication rates that avoid costly fusion surgery in many patients.

The introduction of MISS in regions that are surgically less developed than others is viable and may allow surgeons and health care systems to skip aspects of traditional open surgery which are associated with more complications, longer hospital stays, and slower return to normal function. Although MISS avoids fusion surgery in patients who, if treated with open surgery, may need a stabilization procedure, it allows us to expand the benefits of spinal stabilization to patient groups that were previously deemed too old or sick for traditional open fusion surgery.

Lastly, MISS has the potential to be of high economic value. More work on cost-effectiveness is needed to clarify this.

Only through a collaborative effort through research, teaching, and investment, accompanied by coordinated local and international action, can the vision of universal access to affordable minimally invasive surgery, particularly spinal surgery, be implemented in our global community. The recently developed curriculum for MISS by AOSpine, which has been used at courses worldwide, is an example of how MISS teaching can be disseminated around the globe.[28] These and other educational initiatives by organized spine societies need to be expanded and offer a promising opportunity for a new generation of spine surgeons.

References

[1] Caspar W. A new surgical procedure for lumbar disc herniation causing less tissue damage through a microsurgical approach. In: Wüllenweber R, Brock M, Hamer J, Klinger M, Spoerri O, eds. Lumbar Disc Adult Hydrocephalus. Springer; 1977:74–80

[2] Yasargil M. Microsurgical operation of herniated lumbar disc. In: Wüllenweber R, Brock M, Hamer J, Klinger M, Spoerri O, eds. Lumbar Disc Adult Hydrocephalus. Springer; 1977:81–81

[3] Böhler J. Anterior stabilization for acute fractures and non-unions of the dens. J Bone Joint Surg Am. 1982; 64(1):18–27

[4] Böhler J. [Screw-osteosynthesis of fractures of the dens axis (author's transl)]. Unfallheilkunde. 1981; 84(6):221–223

[5] Magerl F, Seemann P-S. Stable posterior fusion of the atlas and axis by transarticular screw fixation. In: Kehr P, Weidner A, eds. Cervical Spine I. Springer; 1987:322–327

[6] Magerl FP. Stabilization of the lower thoracic and lumbar spine with external skeletal fixation. Clin Orthop Relat Res. 1984(189):125–141

[7] Shin BJ, James AR, Njoku IU, Härtl R. Pedicle screw navigation: a systematic review and meta-analysis of perforation risk for computer-navigated versus freehand insertion. J Neurosurg Spine. 2012; 17(2):113–122

[8] Haberland N, Ebmeier K, Grunewald JP, Hliscs R, Kalff RL. Incorporation of intraoperative computerized tomography in a newly developed spinal navigation technique. Comput Aided Surg. 2000; 5(1):18–27

[9] Schwender JD, Holly LT, Rouben DP, Foley KT. Minimally invasive transforaminal lumbar interbody fusion (TLIF): technical feasibility and initial results. J Spinal Disord Tech. 2005; 18 Suppl:S1–S6

[10] Ozgur BM, Agarwal V, Nail E, Pimenta L. Two-year clinical and radiographic success of minimally invasive lateral transpsoas approach for the treatment of degenerative lumbar conditions. SAS J. 2010; 4(2):41–46

[11] Theodore N, Ahmed A, Karim B. The history of robotics in spine surgery. Spine. 2018; 43 7S:S23

[12] Theodore N, Arnold PM, Mehta AI. Introduction: the rise of the robots in spinal surgery. Neurosurg Focus. 2018; 45 VideoSuppl1:Intro

[13] Elmi-Terander A, Burström G, Nachabe R, et al. Pedicle screw placement using augmented reality surgical navigation with intraoperative 3D imaging: a first in-human prospective cohort study. Spine. 2019; 44(7):517–525

[14] Elmi-Terander A, Nachabe R, Skulason H, et al. Feasibility and accuracy of thoracolumbar minimally invasive pedicle screw placement with augmented reality navigation technology. Spine. 2018; 43(14):1018–1023

[15] Young PH, McCulloch JA. Essentials of Spinal Microsurgery. Lippincott-Raven; 1998

[16] Oppenheimer JH, DeCastro I, McDonnell DE. Minimally invasive spine technology and minimally invasive spine surgery: a historical review. Neurosurg Focus. 2009; 27(3):E9

[17] Snyder LA, O'Toole J, Eichholz KM, Perez-Cruet MJ, Fessler R. The technological development of minimally invasive spine surgery. BioMed Res Int. 2014; 2014:293582

[18] Basil GW, Wang MY. Trends in outpatient minimally invasive spine surgery. J Spine Surg. 2019; 5 Suppl 1:S108–S114

[19] Lamartina C, Berjano P. Prone single-position extreme lateral interbody fusion (Pro-XLIF): preliminary results. Eur Spine J. 2020; 29 Suppl 1:6–13

[20] Yamaguchi JT, Hsu WK. Three-dimensional printing in minimally invasive spine surgery. Curr Rev Musculoskelet Med. 2019; 12(4):425–435

[21] Barzilai O, Robin AM, O'Toole JE, Laufer I. Minimally invasive surgery strategies: changing the treatment of spine tumors. Neurosurg Clin N Am. 2020; 31(2):201–209

[22] Hussain I, Schmidt FA, Kirnaz S, Wipplinger C, Schwartz TH, Härtl R. MIS approaches in the cervical spine. J Spine Surg. 2019; 5 Suppl 1:S74–S83

[23] Mummaneni PV, Park P, Shaffrey CI, et al. International Spine Study Group (ISSG). The MISDEF2 algorithm: an updated algorithm for patient selection in minimally invasive deformity surgery. J Neurosurg Spine. 2019; 32(2):221–228

[24] Sloan SR , Jr, Wipplinger C, Kirnaz S, et al. Combined nucleus pulposus augmentation and annulus fibrosus repair prevents acute intervertebral disc degeneration after discectomy. Sci Transl Med. 2020; 12(534):eaay2380

[25] Moriguchi Y, Borde B, Berlin C, et al. In vivo annular repair using high-density collagen gel seeded with annulus fibrosus cells. Acta Biomater. 2018; 79:230–238

[26] Moriguchi Y, Mojica-Santiago J, Grunert P, et al. Total disc replacement using tissue-engineered intervertebral discs in the canine cervical spine. PLoS One. 2017; 12(10):e0185716

[27] Schöller K, Alimi M, Cong GT, Christos P, Härtl R. Lumbar spinal stenosis associated with degenerative lumbar spondylolisthesis: a systematic review and meta-analysis of secondary fusion rates following open vs minimally invasive decompression. Neurosurgery. 2017; 80(3):355–367

[28] Schmidt FA, Taboada N, Kirnaz S, Wong T, Hartl R. Development of MISS curriculum. Global Spine Journal. 2020; In print

[29] El Khamlichi A. African neurosurgery: current situation, priorities, and needs. Neurosurgery. 2001; 48(6):1344–1347

[30] Coburger J, Leng LZ, Rubin DG, et al. Multi-institutional neurosurgical training initiative at a tertiary referral center in Mwanza, Tanzania: where we are after 2 years. World Neurosurg. 2014; 82(1–2):e1–e8

[31] Njoku I, Wanin O, Assey A, et al. Minimally invasive 2D navigation-assisted treatment of thoracolumbar spinal fractures in East Africa: a case report. Cureus. 2016; 8(2):e507

[32] Wang MY. Devastation after the Haiti earthquake: a neurosurgeon's journal. World Neurosurg. 2010; 73(5):438–441

[33] Hopkins B, Mazmudar A, Kesavabhotla K, Patel AA. Economic value in minimally invasive spine surgery. Curr Rev Musculoskelet Med. 2019; 12(3):300–304

[34] Al-Khouja LT, Baron EM, Johnson JP, Kim TT, Drazin D. Cost-effectiveness analysis in minimally invasive spine surgery. Neurosurg Focus. 2014; 36(6):E4

[35] Vertuani S, Nilsson J, Borgman B, et al. A cost-effectiveness analysis of minimally invasive versus open surgery techniques for lumbar spinal fusion in Italy and the United Kingdom. Value Health. 2015; 18(6):810–816

[36] Kim CW. Scientific basis of minimally invasive spine surgery: prevention of multifidus muscle injury during posterior lumbar surgery. Spine. 2010; 35 (26) Suppl:S281–S286

[37] Boukebir MA, Berlin CD, Navarro-Ramirez R, et al. Ten-step minimally invasive spine lumbar decompression and dural repair through tubular retractors. Oper Neurosurg (Hagerstown). 2017; 13(2):232–245

Index

Note: Page numbers set **bold** or *italic* indicate headings or figures, respectively.

6

6 Ts *2*, 2, 4

A

abdominal bracing 404, *404*
ACDF, *see* anterior cervical discectomy and fusion (ACDF)
Adson test 28
alcohol, as pro-inflammatory food 406
ALIF, *see* anterior lumbar interbody fusion (ALIF)
ALL, *see* anterior longitudinal ligament (ALL)
allograft
– in cervical front/back surgery 371
– in oblique lumbar interbody fusion 311
– in occipitocervical fusion 363
– in spinal fusion 119, **119**
– in transforaminal lumbar interbody fusion 331
anesthesia
– in transforaminal lumbar interbody fusion 96
– in vertebroplasty/kyphoplasty, thoracic **198**
– intraoperative computed tomography and *69*
– optical tracking and 64
– outpatient 136
animal models, training by **415**
anterior cervical discectomy and fusion (ACDF), outpatient 138, **138**
anterior column release (ACR)
– accidental 291
– in cervical front/back surgery 291
– in extreme lateral interbody fusion 286
– traditional vs. minimally invasive 4
anterior longitudinal ligament (ALL)
– in extreme lateral interbody fusion 286–287
– in lateral lumbar interbody fusion 281
– release, in class 3 deformity 44
anterior lumbar interbody fusion (ALIF) 46
– in degenerative scoliosis surgery **390**, *391–392*
– in T10-pelvis fusion 398
– indirect decompression in 107
– posterior lumbar interbody fusion vs. 424
anterior psoas lateral interbody fusion (APLIF), indirect decompression in 107
anterior transcervical submandibular approach *362*
APLIF, *see* anterior psoas lateral interbody fusion (APLIF)
arthrodesis
– biologics in **420**
– facet joint **233**
Asia 14, **14**
atlantoaxial fixation and fusion
– closure in **187**
– complications in **187**, *189*
– contraindications for **183**
– incision in **184**
– indications for **182**
– navigation in *186*, **186**, *187–188*
– patient positioning in **183**, *184*
– postoperative care in **187**
– preoperative planning in *183*, **183**
– technique **184**, *185*
augmented reality (AR) **358**, **410**
Australia **15**

B

Babinski's sign 22
back pain, myofascial 33–34
bent knee curl-up 404, *405*
biologics
– in degenerative disc disease **420**, *421*
– in spinal arthrodesis **420**
biomechanics, of spinal fusion **118**
biopsy, in vertebroplasty/kyphoplasty, thoracic *200*, **200**
bird-dog exercise 404, *406*
bisphosphonates 123
blood loss minimization **128**, *130*
BMA, *see* bone marrow aspirate (BMA)
BMP, *see* bone morphogenic protein (BMP)
bone marrow aspirate (BMA), in spinal fusion *120*
bone morphogenic protein (BMP) **120**, 329
bone mounting platforms, with robotics *82*, **82**
bone scalpel **111**, *112*
bone stimulators, in transforaminal lumbar interbody fusion **123**
brachial plexopathy 26
brachial plexus anatomy *27*
bracing
– abdominal 404, *404*
– after transforaminal lumbar interbody fusion **123**

C

cadaver, training by **415**
cage placement
– among 4 surgeons 302–303
– bone morphogenic protein and 120
– expandable *232*, **232**
– facet, posterior cervical
–– complications in **162**
–– contraindications for **157**
–– indications for **157**
–– patient positioning for **157**
–– postoperative care in **161**, *162*
–– preoperative planning for **157**
–– technique **158**, *159–161*
– hyperlordotic
–– in class 3 deformity 44, 46, *46*
–– in extreme lateral lumbar interbody fusion 287
– in extreme lateral lumbar interbody fusion 287
– in transforaminal lumbar interbody fusion 122, *122*
– in transpedicular corpectomy **228**, *229*
– interbody
–– in indirect decompression 107
–– in transforaminal lumber interbody fusion 121
cat-camel exercise 404, *405*
CDR, *see* cervical disc arthroplasty (CDR)
central canal stenosis
– cervical 22, **149**, *150–155*
– lumbar 28
ceramics, in spinal fusion **119**
cerebral spinal fluid (CSF) leak repair
– instrumentation in *113*
– technique **112**, **114**, 115, *116*
cervical front/back surgery, for spinal deformity **367**, *369–371*
cervical segment
– as target **22**, *23*, *25–27*
– brachial plexopathy in 26
– central canal stenosis in 22
– facet joint arthropathy in 24, *25*
– neck pain in 25, *26*
– neural foraminal stenosis in 23, *24*
– shoulder pathology in, primary 25
cervical spondylotic myelopathy (CSM) 149
chicken, as anti-inflammatory food 406
China 14
clinical presentation
– of brachial plexopathy 26
– of central canal stenosis
–– cervical 22
–– lumbar 28
– of cervical radiculopathy 23
– of disc herniation, lumbar 30
– of facet joint arthropathy
–– cervical 24
–– lumbar 31
– of lateral recess stenosis 29
– of muscle pain **49**
– of neural foraminal stenosis
–– cervical 23
–– lumbar 30
–– thoracic 27
– of piriformis syndrome 32
– of sacroiliac joint pain 31
– of thoracic outlet syndrome 28
– of thoracic radiculopathy 27
closure
– among 4 surgeons 304–305
– in atlantoaxial fixation and fusion **187**
– in extreme lateral interbody fusion **291**
– in kyphoplasty, thoracic **201**, *202*
– in lateral lumbar interbody fusion **283**
– in muscle-sparing approaches *178*, **178**, *179*, **181**
– in oblique lumbar interbody fusion **311**
– in pedicle subtraction osteotomy **217**
– in percutaneous endoscopic interlaminar approach **258**, *259*
– in percutaneous pedicle screw placement *379*, **379**
– in posterior lumbar interbody fusion 317
– in T10-pelvis fusion 399
– in vertebroplasty, thoracic **201**
– with intradural extramedullary tumors 353, *354*
coaching, health and wellness **408**
coffee, as pro-inflammatory food 406
complications
– dural tears as 112
– in atlantoaxial fixation and fusion **187**, *189*
– in bone morphogenic protein **120**
– in computer assisted spine surgery 61
– in craniocervical junction endoscopy **167**
– in deformity correction 42, 46
– in endoscopic interlaminar lumbar laminectomy **278**
– in extreme lateral lumbar interbody fusion **291**
– in far-lateral lumbar discectomy **249**
– in iliac crest bone autograft 118
– in intradural extramedullary tumors **354**
– in lateral lumbar interbody fusion **283**
– in lateral retropleural thoracic discectomy and corpectomy **211**
– in oblique lumbar interbody fusion **312**
– in pedicle screw placement **346**
–– percutaneous **380**
– in pedicle subtraction osteotomy **218**
– in percutaneous endoscopic interlaminar approach **260**
– in posterior cervical facet cage **162**
– in posterior cervical foraminotomy **143**, *146–147*
– in posterior lumbar interbody fusion **318**
– in posterior paramedian endoscopic thoracic discectomy **224**
– in sacroiliac joint fusion **348**
– in thoracic discectomy **205**
– in three-dimensional cervical navigation **194**
– in transforaminal approach for endoscopic decompression **270**
– in transforaminal lumbar interbody fusion **329**
– in transpedicular corpectomy **229**
– in unilateral lumbar over-the-top bilateral decompression **243**
– in unilateral tubular over-the-top cervical laminectomy **154**
– in vertebroplasty/kyphoplasty, thoracic **201**
computed tomography (CT)
– cone beam, intraoperative *67*, 68

- in patient evaluation 126
- intraoperative *67*, **67**, 68, **68**, 69, *69–70*, **410**
-- in pedicle screw placement 61
- preoperative, in navigation **65**
computer assisted spine surgery (CAS), *see* navigation
- deformity correction and **231**
- in atlantoaxial fixation and fusion *186*, **186**, *187–188*
- in pedicle screw placement 61
- overview of 61
- technology **62**
contralateral decompression **103**, *104–106*
contralateral transforaminal approach 268
core stability, lifestyle medicine and **403**, *404*
corpectomy
- lateral retropleural thoracic discectomy and **207**, *208–212*
- transpedicular **226**, *227–229*
courses, training **415**
craniocervical junction (CCJ) endoscopy
- case examples *168*, **168**, *169*
- complications in **167**
- endonasal approach in **163**, *164–165*
- indications for **163**
- postoperative care in **168**
- techniques **163**
- transcervical approach in **163**, **166**, *167*
- transoral approach in **163–164**, *166*
CSF, *see* cerebral spinal fluid (CSF)
CSM, *see* cervical spondylotic myelopathy (CSM)
curriculum development 10, **10**

D

da Vinci Surgical System Robot 81
DBM, *see* demineralized bone matrix (DBM)
decompression, *see* unilateral laminotomy for bilateral decompression (ULBD)
- contralateral **103**, *104–106*
- endoscopic transforaminal *262*, **262**, *263–267*, *269*, *271*
- indirect *107*, **107**, *108*
- muscle sparing *175*, **175**, *176*
- over-the-top bilateral, unilateral lumbar approach for **238**, *239–242*
- robotics in 80
deep tendon reflexes (DTRs)
- in central canal stenosis
-- cervical 22
-- lumbar 28
- in cervical radiculopathy 23
- in neural foraminal stenosis, cervical 23
deformity, spinal
- anterior approach to thoracic **232**
- anterolateral approach to thoracic *232*, **232**
- cervical front/back surgery for **367**, *369–371*
- class 1 **43–44**, *45*
- class 2 **43**, *45*, **45**
- class 3 *46*, **46**
- class 4 **44**, **46**, *47*
- computer assisted navigation and **231**
- correction opportunity **41**
- examples **44**, *45–46*
- extreme lateral lumbar interbody fusion for 286
- minimally invasive spine surgery and *42*, *44–47*
- MISDEF algorithm for **43**, *44*
- patient selection with **43**
- percutaneous approach to thoracic **233**
- posterior approach to thoracic **233**, *234*
- posterolateral approach to thoracic **232**, *233*
- robotics and **231**
- transfascial approach to thoracic **233**

degenerative disc disease 45, *45*, *53*, 279, *279*, 286, **420**, *421*
degenerative spondylolisthesis 137, 172, 254
demineralized bone matrix (DBM) 119, 420
dermatomes *23*
diagnostic injections
- in brachial plexopathy 26
- in central canal stenosis
-- cervical 23
-- lumbar 29
- in cervical radiculopathy 24
- in disc herniation, lumbar 30
- in facet joint arthropathy
-- cervical 25
-- lumbar 31
- in lateral recess stenosis 30
- in neck pain 25
- in neural foraminal stenosis
-- cervical 24
-- lumbar 31
- in piriformis syndrome 33
- in sacroiliac joint pain 31
- in shoulder pathology, primary 25
- in thoracic outlet syndrome 28
disc herniation *142*
- endoscopy for 96
- lateral 245
- lumbar 30, *30*, 34
- percutaneous endoscopic interlaminar approach for 253
discectomy
- far-lateral lumbar **245**, *246–251*
- in degenerative scoliosis surgery *389*, **389**
- in laminoforaminotomy 136
- in transforaminal lumbar interbody fusion 122
- lateral retropleural thoracic, and corpectomy **207**, *208–212*
- mini-open lumbar **58**
- navigation in 65
- posterior paramedian endoscopic thoracic **220**, *222–224*
- specular retractor in 57, **58**
- thoracic, posterior transpedicular tubular approach in *203*, **203**, *205*
- tubular lumbar approach in **57**, *58*
- tubular retractor in 56
discectomy, among 4 surgeons 300–301
dorsal root ganglion (DRG)
- in L5radiculopathy *30*
- in lateral recess stenosis 29
- transforaminal ligaments and 262
dorsolateral approach 268
DRG, *see* dorsal root ganglion (DRG)
drills *112*
DTR, *see* deep tendon reflexes (DTRs)
dural tear
- in curriculum development 10
- in lateral retropleural thoracic discectomy and corpectomy 211
- in transforaminal approach for endoscopic decompression **270**
- in unilateral laminotomy for bilateral decompression 105
- in unilateral tubular over-the-top cervical laminectomy **155**
- mini-open procedures and risk of 58
- repair
-- instrumentation in *113*
-- technique **112**, **114**, 115, *116*

E

economic impacts **428**
eggs, as anti-inflammatory food 406
electromagnetic registration **64**
electromyography (EMG)
- in brachial plexopathy 26
- in central canal stenosis
-- cervical 23
-- lumbar 29
- in cervical radiculopathy 24
- in disc herniation, lumbar 30
- in lateral recess stenosis 30
- in neural foraminal stenosis
-- cervical 24
-- lumbar 31
-- thoracic 28
- in piriformis syndrome 33
- in thoracic radiculopathy 28
EMG, *see* electromyography (EMG)
endoscopic discectomy, posterior paramedian thoracic **220**, *222–224*
endoscopic interlaminar lumbar laminectomy **273**, *274–277*
endoscopic transforaminal decompression *262*, **262**, *263–267*, *269*, *271*
endoscopic transnasal odontoid resection *229*, 364, **364**
endoscopy
- channel sizes 96
- courses for learning **100**
- endonasal approach in **163**
- equipment purchase **100**
- expanding indications for **97**
- foraminal window and **95**
- in complex spine problems 96
- in craniocervical junction pathology **163**, *164–169*
- in facet cysts 96
- in foraminal stenosis 96
- in upper versus lower lumbar **96**
- instruments 96
- interlaminar lumbar approach **97**, *99*
- Kambin's triangle and *95*, **95**
- mentorship in **100**
- pathologies treated with **96**
- targeting and *95*, **95**
- teaching **100**
- training **100**
- transcervical approach in **163**
- transforaminal lumbar approach **96**, *97–99*
- transoral approach in **163**
Enhanced Recovery After Surgery (ERAS)
- basic principles of **132**, *133*
- exclusion criteria 133
- implementation of **134**
- inclusion criteria 133
- insulin resistance and 132
- intraoperative technique and **134**
- physiological principles of *133*
- postoperative management and **134**
- preoperative preparation and **132**
- protocol *133*
epidural hematoma
- in synovial cyst resection 129, *130*
- in unilateral lumbar over-the-top bilateral decompression 243
Europe **16**
ExcelsiusGPS *81*
exercise, lifestyle medicine and **403**, *404*, **404**
extraforaminal stenosis, lumbar 30
extreme lateral interbody fusion (XLIF)
- closure in **291**
- complications in **291**
- contraindications for **286**, *287*
- incision in **290**
- indications for **286**
- patient positioning in **287**, *288–289*
- postoperative care in **291**
- preoperative planning in **286**, 287

F

FABER maneuver 31
facet cysts, endoscopy in 96
facet joint arthrodesis **233**
facet joint arthropathy
- cervical 24, *25*
- lumbar 31
facet joint fusion **233**
FADIR test 32
far-lateral approach 268
fellowships **415**
fish, as pro-inflammatory food 406
fluoroscopy
- in navigation **65**, *66*, 68
- radiation exposure and **128**, *129*
foraminal window **95**
foraminotomy, muscle-sparing **180**
Fortin's finger test 31, 33, 34
fracture
- Jefferson 182
- lateral lumbar interbody fusion in 279, *280*
- odontoid 182
- vertebral compression 197
front/back surgery, cervical, for spinal deformity **367**, *369–371*
fruit, as anti-inflammatory food 406
fusion, *see* spinal fusion

G

Gaenslen's test 31
ginger, as anti-inflammatory food 406
global perspectives 14, **14**, 20, **427**
grains, as pro-inflammatory food 406
grants **415**

H

Hawkins test 25
health coaching **408**
hematoma
– epidural
–– in synovial cyst resection 129, *130*
–– in unilateral lumbar over-the-top bilateral decompression 243
– in transforaminal approach for endoscopic decompression **270**
hemostasis, in unilateral tubular over-the-top cervical laminectomy **155**
hip osteoarthritis 33–34
Hoffman's sign 22
Holmgren, Gunnar 88, *89*

I

iCBCT, *see* intraoperative cone beam computed tomography (iCBCT)
iCT, *see* intraoperative computed tomography (iCT)
IDEM, *see* intradural extramedullary (IDEM) tumors
iliac crest bone autograft (ICBG), in spinal fusion 118
imaging
– blood loss and 129
– evaluation 126
– in sacroiliac joint fusion **347**
– in vertebral compression fractures 197
– pain patterns and 5, *6*
incision
– among 4 surgeons 296–297
– for lumbar fusions **128**
– in atlantoaxial fixation and fusion **184**
– in extreme lateral lumbar interbody fusion **290**
– in far-lateral lumbar discectomy **247**
– in intradural extramedullary tumors 352
– in lateral lumbar interbody fusion **281**
– in lateral retropleural thoracic discectomy and corpectomy **208**, *210*
– in oblique lumbar interbody fusion **309**, *310*
– in pedicle screw placement, percutaneous **375**
– in pedicle subtraction osteotomy **216**
– in posterior lumbar interbody fusion 315
– in thoracic discectomy **204**
– in three-dimensional cervical navigation **192**
– in transforaminal lumbar interbody fusion 324
– in transpedicular corpectomy **226**, *227*
– in unilateral lumbar over-the-top bilateral decompression *240*, **240**
– in unilateral tubular over-the-top cervical laminectomy **150**, *151*
– tubular retractors and **127**
India 14
indirect decompression *107*, **107**, *108*
inflammation
– foods promoting 406
– myogenic vs. neurogenic **49**, *50*
injections, diagnostic, *see* diagnostic injections
instability minimization *106*, **106**
instrumentation
– bayoneted *110*, **110**, *111*
– bone scalpels **111**, *112*
– curved *110*, **110**, *111*
– drills **111**, *112*
– endoscopic *112*, **112**
– in cerebral spinal fluid leak repair **112**, *113*
– in percutaneous endoscopic interlaminar approach **254**, *255*, 256
– in unilateral tubular over-the-top cervical laminectomy **149**
– retractors
–– in unilateral laminotomy for bilateral decompression 104, *104*
–– specular **57**, *58*
––– advantages of 59
––– in lumbar microdiscectomy *58*
––– limitations of 59
–– tubular **56**, *57*, **110**, *111*
––– advantages of 59
––– blood loss and 129
––– in lumbar microdiscectomy **57**, *58*
––– in unilateral tubular over-the-top cervical laminectomy *151*, *153*
––– incision planning and **127**
––– limitations of 59
– visualization and **111**
insulin resistance, after surgery 132
International Society for Minimal Intervention in Spine Surgery (ISMISS) **417**
International Society for the Advancement of Spine Surgery (ISASS) **417**
interspinous process device (IPD), outpatient **137**
intracanal technique 266
intradural extramedullary (IDEM) tumors *71*
– closure with 353, *354*
– complications with **354**
– contraindications for **350**
– incision in 352
– indications for surgery **350**
– localization in 352
– navigation with **352**
– patient positioning with **352**
– patient selection with **350**
– postoperative care in **354**
– preoperative planning with *351*, **351**
intraoperative computed tomography (iCT) *67*, **67**, 68, **68**, 69, *69–70*, **410**
intraoperative cone beam computed tomography (iCBCT) *67*, 68
IPD, *see* interspinous process device (IPD)
ISASS, *see* International Society for the Advancement of Spine Surgery (ISASS)
ISMISS, *see* International Society for Minimal Intervention in Spine Surgery (ISMISS)

J

Japan 14
Jefferson fracture 182

K

K-line 171–172
K-wires, in atlantoaxial fixation and fusion 185–186, *187*
Kambin's triangle *95*, **95**, 246, 248, *249*, 250, 268, 270
Kemp's test 31, *32*, 34
Kerrison rongeurs *104*, 105, 107, *111*
Kraus-Weber test 50, *52*
Kurze, Theodore 88
kyphoplasty, thoracic
– balloon inflation in **200**
– biopsy in **200**
– cannula insertion in **199**
– closure in **201**, *202*
– complications in **201**
– contraindications for **197**
– image optimization in **198**
– indications for 197
– localization in **198**, *200*
– patient positioning in **198**, *199*
– postoperative care in **201**
– preoperative planning in **198**
– skin entry point in **199**
– trajectory planning in **199**
– unipedicular vs. bipedicular **198**

L

laminectomy
– endoscopic interlaminar lumbar **273**, *274–277*
– muscle-sparing **176**, *177–178*, **180**
– outpatient **137**
laminoforaminotomy, outpatient **136**
laminoplasty, muscle-sparing **176**, *177–178*, **180**
lateral interbody fusion (LIF), in class 1 deformity 43
lateral lumbar interbody fusion (LLIF) 46
– closure in **283**
– complications in **283**
– contraindications for **279**
– future of 424
– in thoracolumbar junction *279*, **279**, *280–282*, 283, *284*
– incision planning in 128, **281**
– indications for *279*, **279**, *280*
– operating room setup for 280, *281*
– outpatient **138**
– patient positioning for **280**, *281*
– postoperative care in **283**
– preoperative planning for **280**
– technique **281**, *282*, 283
lateral recess stenosis 29, 34
leap-frogging **428**
lifestyle medicine
– core stability and **403**, *404*
– exercise and **403**, *404*, **404**
– nutrition in **405**, 406, *407*
– segmental stabilization in **404**
– sleep in 408, *408*, **408**
– smoking in **407**
ligamentum flavum
– in central canal stenosis 28
– in contralateral decompression 104, *104*
– in endoscopic interlaminar approach 256–257, *257*, 258–259
– in far-lateral lumbar discectomy 245, 248, *249*, 250
– in mini-open lumbar discectomy 59
– in spinal stenosis 262, *262*
– in unilateral tubular over-the-top cervical laminectomy *150*, **152**, *153*
Littmann, Hans 87, *88*
LL, *see* lumbar lordosis (LL)
LLIF, *see* lateral lumbar interbody fusion (LLIF)
local grafting, in spinal fusion 118
loupes, microscopes vs. **91**
LSS, *see* lumbar spinal stenosis (LSS)
Lukens trap 118, *119*
lumbar lordosis (LL) 41, *42*
lumbar segment
– as target **28**, *29–30*, *32–33*, 34
– central canal stenosis in 28
– disc herniation in 30, *30*, 34
– facet joint arthropathy in 31
– hip osteoarthritis in 33–34
– lateral recess stenosis in 29, 34
– neural foraminal stenosis in 30, *32*
– piriformis syndrome in 32, 34
– zones *29*
lumbar spinal stenosis (LSS)
– percutaneous endoscopic interlaminar approach for 253
– transforaminal endoscopic decompression in 262, *262*

M

magnetic resonance imaging (MRI)
– disc herniation in *142*
– in degenerative disc disease *45*
– in endoscopy *98*
– in low back pain 34
– in pathology localization *71–72*
– in patient evaluation 126
– in registration 63
– in spinal stenosis *239*
– in spondylolisthesis *45*, *47*
– in stenosis *47*, *106*
Mazor X *81*, *83*
McGill spine exercises **404**
meat, as anti-inflammatory food 406
microdiscectomy, lumbar, tubular retractor in **57**, *58*
microscopy
– advantages of **88**, 89
– co-observation with 89
– coaxial lighting with 89
– costs of 89
– disadvantages of **89**, 91
– documentation with 89
– ergonomic workflow with 89, *90*
– fluorescence with 89
– future of *92*, **92**, *93*
– hand-eye coordination with 89
– history of **87**, *88*
– illumination with 89
– in thoracic spine **235**
– light intensity measurement with 90
– limited visual field with 89, *90*
– loupes vs. **91**
– magnification with 89–90
– operating room setup with **91**
– photometric analysis with 90
– radiometric analysis with 90
– three-dimensional imaging with 89
– tissue injury with 90
– training with **92**, *93*
– visual axis with 89

mini-open lumbar discectomy, retractor use in *58*, **58**
Minimally Invasive Spinal Deformity (MISDEF) algorithm **43**, *44*
minimally invasive spine surgery (MISS)
- defined *2*, **2**
- global 14, **14**, 20
- limitations of **42**
- potential of 3, *3*, **3**, *4*
MISS, *see* minimally invasive spine surgery (MISS)
MRI, *see* magnetic resonance imaging (MRI)
muscle(s)
- as target **49**, 50, *50*, *52–53*
- operative considerations with **51**, *52*
- pain
-- clinical presentation of **49**
-- myogenic vs. neurogenic inflammation in **49**, *50*
-- neuroanatomy of **49**, *50*
-- neurophysiology of **49**, *50*
-- spinal surgery and **51**
muscle-sparing approaches
- closure in *178*, **178**, *179*, **181**
- contraindications for **172**
- decompression *175*, **175**, *176*
- exposure in *174*, **174**, **180**
- foraminotomy in **180**
- in class 1 deformity 43
- indications for **171**
- laminectomy **176**, *177–178*, **180**
- laminoplasty **176**, *177–178*, **180**
- patient positioning in *173*, **173**, **180**
- postoperative care in **179**
- preoperative planning for **172**
myofascial back pain 33–34
myofascial neck pain 25, *26*
myogenic pain **49**, *50*

N

navigation **128**
- automated registration in **63**
- electromagnetic registration in **64**
- fluoroscopy in **65**, *66*, 68
- image acquisition in **63**
- in atlantoaxial fixation and fusion *186*, **186**, *187–188*
- in intradural extramedullary tumors **352**
- in pedicle screw placement **343**, *344*
- intraoperative image-based **65**
- learning curve with **76**
- O-arm *76–77*
- operative time and 61
- optical tracking in **63**
- pathology localization and **70**, *71–73*
- point-matching registration in **63**
- preoperative CT **65**
- registration system **63**
- robotic **67**, **81**, **410**
- surface-matching registration in **63**
- system types *64*, **64**, 68
- teaching **76**
- technology **62**
- three-dimensional 68
-- cervical
--- closure in **194**
--- complications in **194**
--- contraindications for **192**
--- in trauma 191
--- incision in **192**
--- indications for **191**
--- patient positioning in **192**, *193*
--- postoperative care in **194**
--- preoperative planning in *192*, **192**
--- screw insertion in **193**, *194*
--- screw trajectory confirmation in **193**
--- surgical steps *193–194*
-- lumbar
--- contraindications for **356**
--- indications for **356**
--- patient positioning for **356**
--- patient selection with **356**
--- pedicle screw insertion in **357**, *358*
--- preoperative planning for **356**
--- registration in *357*, **357**
--- table in **356**
- total **410**
- tracking system in **63**
- training **76**
- two-dimensional **65**, *66*, 68
- videoexoscopic **410**
NCS, *see* nerve conduction studies (NCS)
neck musculature *26*
neck pain, myofascial 25, *26*
Neer test 25
nerve conduction studies (NCS)
- in brachial plexopathy 26
- in central canal stenosis, lumbar 29
- in cervical radiculopathy 24
- in disc herniation, lumbar 30
- in lateral recess stenosis 30
- in neural foraminal stenosis
-- cervical 24
-- lumbar 31
- in piriformis syndrome 33
neural foraminal stenosis
- cervical 23, *24*
- endoscopy in 96
- indirect decompression in *107*, 108
- lumbar 30, *32*
- thoracic 27
neurogenic pain **49**, *50*
neurologic examination
- in central canal stenosis
-- cervical 22
-- lumbar 28
- in disc herniation, lumbar 30
- in facet joint arthropathy
-- cervical 24
-- lumbar 31
- in lateral recess stenosis 30
- in neural foraminal stenosis 23
-- cervical 23
-- lumbar 30
-- thoracic 28
- in piriformis syndrome 32
- in thoracic outlet syndrome 28
- in thoracic radiculopathy 28
neuromonitoring, in unilateral tubular over-the-top cervical laminectomy **154**
North America **18**
nutrition, in lifestyle medicine **405**, 406, *407*
nuts, as pro-inflammatory food 406
Nylén, Carl-Olof 87, *88*

O

O-arm *76–77*
Ober's test 34
oblique lumbar interbody fusion (OLIF)
- anatomical considerations **308**, *309*
- closure in **311**
- complications in **312**
- contraindications for **308**
- development of minimally invasive 14
- future of 424
- history of term 14
- incision in **309**, *310*
- indications for **308**
- patient positioning for **309**, *310*
- postoperative care in **312**
observation, training by **414**
occipitocervical fusion
- anterior transcervical submandibular approach in *362*
- case example **361**, *362–363*, **363**, *364–365*
- endoscopic transnasal odontoid resection in *229*, 364, **364**
- invasiveness reduction in *361*, **361**, *362*
- occipital plate in **362**
- outcomes with **360**
- risks of **360**
- screw fixation in **362**, *364*
odontoid fracture 182
OLIF, *see* oblique lumbar interbody fusion (OLIF)
OPG, *see* osteoprogenitor (OPG) cells
optical tracking (OT) **63**
osteoarthritis, hip 33–34
osteoprogenitor (OPG) cells 118
OT, *see* optical tracking (OT)
outpatient surgery
- anesthesia in 136
- anterior cervical discectomy and fusion 138, **138**
- in lumbar spine **136**
- interspinous process device **137**
- laminectomy **137**
- laminoforaminotomy **136**
- lateral lumbar interbody fusion **138**
- procedure choice and **136**
- transforaminal lumbar interbody fusion **137**, 138

P

pain
- back, lower 33–34
- clinical examination for 50, **50**
- muscle
-- clinical presentation of **49**
-- myogenic vs. neurogenic inflammation in **49**, *50*
-- neuroanatomy of **49**, *50*
-- neurophysiology of **49**, *50*
-- spinal surgery and **51**
- myogenic **49**, *50*
- neck 25, *26*
- neurogenic **49**, *50*
- sacroiliac joint 31, 34
- sources of spinal *53*
pain patterns 5, 6
patient positioning
- among 4 surgeons 294
- in atlantoaxial fixation and fusion **183**, *184*
- in degenerative scoliosis surgery *386*, **386**
- in extreme lateral lumbar interbody fusion **287**, *288*
- in far-lateral lumbar discectomy **246**, *247*
- in intradural extramedullary tumors **352**
- in kyphoplasty, thoracic **198**, *199*
- in lateral lumbar interbody fusion **280**, *281*
- in lateral retropleural thoracic discectomy and corpectomy **207**, *208*
- in muscle-sparing approaches *173*, **173**, **180**
- in oblique lumbar interbody fusion **309**, *310*
- in pedicle screw placement **343**
-- percutaneous **374**, *375*
- in pedicle subtraction osteotomy **216**
- in percutaneous endoscopic interlaminar approach *254*, **254**
- in posterior cervical facet cage **157**, *315*
- in posterior cervical foraminotomy **142**, *143*
- in posterior lumbar interbody fusion **314**
- in posterior paramedian endoscopic thoracic discectomy **221**, *222*
- in sacroiliac joint fusion **348**
- in T10-pelvis fusion 396
- in thoracic discectomy **204**
- in three-dimensional cervical navigation **192**, *193*
- in three-dimensional lumbar navigation **356**
- in transforaminal approach for endoscopic decompression *264*, **264**, *323*
- in transforaminal lumbar interbody fusion **323**
- in transpedicular corpectomy **226**
- in unilateral lumbar over-the-top bilateral decompression **239**, *240*
- in unilateral tubular over-the-top cervical laminectomy *150*, **150**
- in vertebroplasty, thoracic **198**, *199*
patient selection **126**
- in endoscopic interlaminar lumbar laminectomy **273**
- in posterior paramedian endoscopic thoracic discectomy **221**
- in three-dimensional lumbar navigation **356**
- in transforaminal lumbar interbody fusion **322**
- in transpedicular corpectomy **226**
- in unilateral tubular over-the-top cervical laminectomy **149**, *150*, **154**
- with spinal deformity **43**
Patrick's test 31
PCFo, *see* posterior cervical foraminotomy (PCFo)
pedicle screw placement
- biomechanics of 118
- complications in **346**
- computer assisted surgery in 61, *71*, **71**, *74–75*
- contraindications for **343**

– in atlantoaxial fixation and fusion 186
– in three-dimensional lumbar navigation **357**, *358*
– in transpedicular corpectomy **226**, *227*
– indications for **343**
– intraoperative computed tomography in 61
– localization in **343**, *344*
– patient positioning for **343**
– percutaneous **343**, *344–348*
–– closure in *379*, **379**
–– complications in **380**
–– contraindications for **374**
–– in degenerative scoliosis surgery **390**, *392*
–– incision in **375**
–– indications for **374**
–– navigation in *378*, **378**, *379*
–– patient positioning in **374**, *375*
–– postoperative care in **379**
–– preoperative planning for *374*, **374**
–– technique *375*, **375**, *376–377*
– preoperative planning for **343**
robotics in **79**
pedicle subtraction osteotomy (PSO)
– advantages of 215
– closure in **217**
– complications in **218**
– contraindications for **215**
– disadvantages of 215
– in class 3 deformity 44
– in class 4 deformity 46
– incision in **216**
– indications for **215**
– patient positioning in **216**
– postoperative care in **217**
– preoperative planning for **215**
technique **216**, *217–218*
pelvic incidence (PI) 41, *42*
pelvic tilt *42*
percutaneous approach
– in transforaminal lumbar interbody fusion, in trauma **123**
– to thoracic spinal deformity **233**
percutaneous endoscopic interlaminar approach
– closure in **258**, *259*
– complications in **260**
– contraindications for **254**
– indications for **253**
– instrumentation in **254**, *255*, 256
– operating room setup for **254**
– patient positioning in *254*, **254**
– postoperative care in **258**, *259*
– preoperative planning in **254**
percutaneous pedicle screw placement
– closure in *379*, **379**
– complications in **380**
– contraindications for **374**
– in degenerative scoliosis surgery **390**, *392*
– incision in **375**
– indications for **374**
– navigation in *378*, **378**, *379*
– patient positioning in **374**, *375*
– postoperative care in **379**
– preoperative planning for *374*, **374**
– technique *375*, **375**, *376–377*
physical examination
– in brachial plexopathy 26
– in central canal stenosis
–– cervical 22
–– lumbar 28
– in disc herniation, lumbar 30
– in facet joint arthropathy
–– cervical 24
–– lumbar 31
– in lateral recess stenosis 30
– in neural foraminal stenosis 23
–– cervical 23
–– lumbar 30
–– thoracic 28
– in piriformis syndrome 32
– in shoulder pathology, primary 25
– in thoracic outlet syndrome 28
– in thoracic radiculopathy 28
PI, *see* pelvic incidence (PI)
piriformis syndrome 32, 34
PLIF, *see* posterior lumbar interbody fusion (PLIF)
Ponte osteotomy 214, *214*
posterior cervical foraminotomy (PCFo)
– complications in **143**, *146–147*
– contraindications 141
– indications for 141, *142*
– labeling in **142**
– micro **142**, *144–146*
– operating room setup in *144*
– patient positioning in **142**, *143*
– patient selection for **141**
– postoperative care in **143**
– preoperative planning in **141**
– technique **142**, *144–146*
posterior lumbar interbody fusion (PLIF)
– anterior lumbar interbody fusion vs. 424
– bone morphogenic protein and 120
– closure in 317
– complications in **318**
– contraindications for **314**
– incision in 315
– indications for **314**
– lateral lumbar interbody fusion vs. 424
– maximum access **314**, *315–319*
– patient positioning for **314**, *315*
– postoperative care in **317**
– preoperative planning in **314**
– transforaminal lumbar interbody fusion and 121
posterolateral fusion
– bone marrow aspirate in 120
– with transforaminal lumbar interbody fusion **121**, *122*
postoperative considerations
– among 4 surgeons 307
– deformity correction and **134**
– Enhanced Recovery After Surgery and **134**
– in atlantoaxial fixation and fusion **187**
– in craniocervical junction endoscopy **168**
– in degenerative scoliosis surgery **391**
– in dural tear repair 115
– in extreme lateral lumbar interbody fusion **291**
– in far-lateral lumbar discectomy **249**
– in intradural extramedullary tumors **354**
– in lateral lumbar interbody fusion **283**
– in lateral retropleural thoracic discectomy and corpectomy **211**
– in muscle-sparing approaches **179**, **181**
– in oblique lumbar interbody fusion **312**
– in pedicle screw placement, percutaneous **379**
– in pedicle subtraction osteotomy **217**
– in percutaneous endoscopic interlaminar approach **258**, *259*
– in posterior cervical facet cage **161**, *162*
– in posterior cervical foraminotomy **143**
– in posterior lumbar interbody fusion **317**
– in posterior paramedian endoscopic thoracic discectomy **224**
– in T10-pelvis fusion 401
– in thoracic discectomy **205**
– in three-dimensional cervical navigation **194**
– in transforaminal approach for endoscopic decompression **270**
– in transforaminal lumbar interbody fusion **326**
– in transpedicular corpectomy **228**
– in unilateral lumbar over-the-top bilateral decompression **242**
– in unilateral tubular over-the-top cervical laminectomy **154**
– in vertebroplasty/kyphoplasty, thoracic **201**
– with bone morphogenic protein 120
preoperative planning **127**, **132**
– among 4 surgeons 294
– for vertebroplasty/kyphoplasty, thoracic **198**
– in atlantoaxial fixation and fusion *183*, **183**
– in extreme lateral lumbar interbody fusion **286**, 287
– in far-lateral lumbar discectomy *246*, **246**
– in intradural extramedullary tumors *351*, **351**
– in lateral lumbar interbody fusion **280**
– in lateral retropleural thoracic discectomy and corpectomy **207**
– in muscle-sparing approaches **172**
– in pedicle screw placement **343**
–– percutaneous *374*, **374**
– in pedicle subtraction osteotomy **215**
– in percutaneous endoscopic interlaminar approach **254**
– in posterior cervical facet cage **157**
– in posterior cervical foraminotomy **141**
– in posterior lumbar interbody fusion **314**
– in posterior paramedian endoscopic thoracic discectomy **221**
– in thoracic discectomy **203**
– in three-dimensional cervical navigation *192*, **192**
– in three-dimensional lumbar navigation **356**
– in transforaminal approach for endoscopic decompression **263**
– in transforaminal lumbar interbody fusion **322**
– in transpedicular corpectomy **226**
– in unilateral lumbar over-the-top bilateral decompression *239*, **239**
– in unilateral tubular over-the-top cervical laminectomy **149**
presentation, *see* clinical presentation
provocative maneuvers
– in central canal stenosis
–– cervical 23
–– lumbar 29
– in disc herniation, lumbar 30
– in facet joint arthropathy
–– cervical 25
–– lumbar 31
– in neural foraminal stenosis, lumbar 31
– in piriformis syndrome 32
– in sacroiliac joint pain 31
– in shoulder pathology, primary 25
– in thoracic outlet syndrome 28
PSO, *see* pedicle subtraction osteotomy (PSO)

R

radiation exposure **80**, **128**, *129*
RealSpine **415**, *416*
retractor
– among 4 surgeons, use of 299
– in unilateral laminotomy for bilateral decompression 104, *104*
– specular **57**, *58*
–– advantages of 59
–– in lumbar microdiscectomy *58*
–– limitations of 59
– tubular **56**, *57*, **110**, *111*
–– advantages of 59
–– blood loss and 129
–– in lumbar microdiscectomy *57*, *58*
–– in unilateral tubular over-the-top cervical laminectomy *151*, *153*
–– incision planning and **127**
–– limitations of 59
retropleural effusion, in lateral retropleural thoracic discectomy and corpectomy **213**
rheumatoid arthritis 182
robotic navigation **67**, **81**, **410**
robotics **128**
– benefits of **79**
– blood loss and **80**
– bone mounting platforms and *82*, **82**
– costs and **81**
– deformity correction and **231**
– early evolution of **81**
– future directions with **84**
– in bony decompression 80
– in pedicle screw placement **79**
– in three-dimensional lumbar navigation **358**
– learning curve with **83**
– limitations of **79**
– operating table with **82**
– operative times and **80**
– planning with **82**
– radiation exposure and **80**
– registration with **82**, *83–84*
– trajectory execution with **83**
– workflow with **82**
rongeurs, Kerrison *104*, 105, 107, *111*
Roos rest 28

S

sacral slope *42*
sacroiliac joint fusion **347**, *348*
sacroiliac joint pain 31, 34
sagittal balance 41
SAP, *see* superior articulating process (SAP)
scalpel *104*
– bone **111**, *112*
scoliosis, degenerative 44, *45*, 215, 238
– anterior lumber interbody fusion in **390**, *391–392*
– discectomy in *389*, **389**
– imaging in **382**
– indications for surgery **382**
– interbody devices in 383
– lateral approach in *386*
– patient positioning in *386*, **386**
– percutaneous pedicle screw placement in **390**, *392*
– postoperative care in **391**
– presentation of **382**, *383*, **383**, *384–385*
segmental stabilization, in lifestyle medicine **404**
shoulder pathology, primary 25
side plank 404, *406*
simulation, in training **416**
single-step pedicle screw system (SSPSS) **71**, *74–75*
sleep 408, *408*, **408**
SMISS, *see* Society for Minimally Invasive Spine Surgery (SMISS)
Smith-Peterson osteotomy 214, *214*
smoking **407**
Society for Minimally Invasive Spine Surgery (SMISS) 416, **416–417**
soda, as pro-inflammatory food 406
South America **19**
South Korea 14
specular retractor **57**, *58*
– advantages of 59
– in lumbar microdiscectomy *58*
– limitations of 59
spinal fusion, *see* anterior lumbar interbody fusion (ALIF), anterior psoas lateral interbody fusion (APLIF), lateral interbody fusion (LIF), lateral lumbar interbody fusion (LLIF), transforaminal lumbar interbody fusion (TLIF)
– allografts in 119, **119**
– biology of **118**
– biomechanics of **118**
– bone marrow aspirate in *120*
– bone morphogenic protein in **120**
– ceramics in **119**
– demineralized bone matrix in 119
– interbody **121**, *122*
spinal stenosis, *see* central canal stenosis, lumbar spinal stenosis (LSS), percutaneous endoscopic interlaminar approach for
spinopelvic parameters **41**, *42*
spondylolisthesis 44–45, *45*, 46, *47*, 137, 172, 254, 273
Spurling's maneuver 31
SSPSS, *see* single-step pedicle screw system (SSPSS)
stem cells, in spinal fusion 118
sugar, as pro-inflammatory food 406
superior articulating process (SAP), as target **96**

T

T10-pelvis fusion
– ante-psoas approach in 398
– closure in 399
– patient positioning in 396
– postoperative care in 401
Taiwan 14
talent, in 6 Ts 2, *2*, *11*, **11**
target
– cervical segment as **22**, *23*, *25–27*
– endoscopy and *95*, **95**
– foraminal window as **95**
– in 6 Ts 2, *2*, **4**, *5–8*
– in unilateral tubular over-the-top cervical laminectomy **149**
– Kambin's triangle as *95*, **95**
– muscle as **49**, 50, *50*, *52–53*
– superior articulating process as **96**
– thoracic segment as **27**
technique, in 6 Ts 2, *2*, **10**
technology, in 6 Ts 2, *2*, *9*, **9**
teriparatide 123
testing, in 6 Ts 2, *2*, **11**
textbooks **418**
thoracic kyphosis *42*
thoracic outlet syndrome (TOS) 28
thoracic segment
– as target **27**
– neural foraminal stenosis in 27
– radiculopathy in 27
thoracolumbar junction, lateral lumbar interbody fusion in *279*, **279**, *280–282*, 283, *284*
three-column osteotomies **232**
three-dimensional navigation
– cervical
–– closure in **194**
–– complications in **194**
–– contraindications for **192**
–– in trauma 191
–– incision in **192**
–– indications for **191**
–– patient positioning in **192**, *193*
–– postoperative care in **194**
–– preoperative planning in *192*, **192**
–– screw insertion in **193**, *194*
–– screw trajectory confirmation in **193**
–– surgical steps *193–194*
– lumbar
–– contraindications for **356**
–– indications for **356**
–– patient positioning for **356**
–– patient selection with **356**
–– pedicle screw insertion in **357**, *358*
–– preoperative planning for **356**
–– registration in *357*, **357**
–– table in **356**
TLIF, *see* transforaminal lumbar interbody fusion (TLIF)
TOS, *see* thoracic outlet syndrome (TOS)
tracking, optical **63**
training
– by animal model **415**
– by cadaver **415**
– by observation **414**
– by simulation **416**
– by virtual reality **416**
– courses **415**
– endoscopy **100**
– fellowships and **415**
– grants and **415**
– in 6 Ts 2, *2*, 10, **10**
– methods 414, **414**
– online materials for **417**
– textbooks for **418**
– with microscopy **92**, *93*
– with RealSpine **415**, *416*
trans iliac approach 269, *269*
transarticular screws
– in atlantoaxial fixation and fusion 182, 185
– in occipitocervical fusion 362, *364*
transforaminal endoscopic decompression *262*, **262**, *263–267*, *269*, *271*
transforaminal lumbar interbody fusion (TLIF) 46, 121, **121**
– bone morphogenic protein in 120, 329
– bone stimulators in **123**
– bracing after **123**
– complications in **329**
– contraindications for 322
– in class 1 deformity 43
– incision planning in 128, 324
– indications for 322
– medication augmentation in **123**
– outpatient **137**, 138
– patient positioning in *323*, **323**
– patient selection for **322**
– percutaneous, in trauma **123**
– posterior lumbar interbody fusion vs. 424
– posterolateral fusion with **121**, *122*
– postoperative care in **326**
– preoperative planning for **322**
– technique **121**, *122*
– traditional vs. minimally invasive 3
transpedicular approach 268
transpedicular corpectomy **226**, *227–229*
tubers, as pro-inflammatory food 406
tubular retractor **56**, *57*, **110**, *111*
– advantages of 59
– blood loss and 129
– in lumbar microdiscectomy **57**, *58*
– in unilateral tubular over-the-top cervical laminectomy *151*, *153*
– incision planning and **127**
– limitations of 59

U

ULBD, *see* unilateral laminectomy for bilateral decompression (ULBD), unilateral laminotomy for bilateral decompression (ULBD)
unilateral laminotomy for bilateral decompression (ULBD)
– contralateral decompression in **103**, *104–106*
– instability minimization in *106*, **106**
– outpatient **137**
– traditional vs. minimally invasive 3
unilateral lumbar over-the-top bilateral decompression **238**, *239–242*
unilateral tubular over-the-top cervical laminectomy 22, **149**, *150–155*

V

VATS, *see* video-assisted thoracoscopic surgery (VATS)
vegetables, as anti-inflammatory food 406
vertebral augmentation procedures (VAPs) 197
vertebral compression fractures (VCFs) 197
vertebroplasty, thoracic
– biopsy in **200**
– cannula insertion in **199**
– cement injection in **200**
– closure in **201**, *202*
– complications in **201**
– contraindications for **197**
– image optimization in **198**
– indications for 197
– localization in **198**, *200*
– patient positioning in **198**, *199*
– postoperative care in **201**
– preoperative planning for **198**
– skin entry point in **199**
– trajectory planning in **199**
– unipedicular vs. bipedicular **198**
video-assisted thoracoscopic surgery (VATS) **234**
videoexoscopic navigation **410**
virtual reality (VR) **410**, **416**
VR, *see* virtual reality (VR)

W

wellness coaching **408**
wine, as anti-inflammatory food 406

X

X-ray, in patient evaluation 127, *127*
XLIF, *see* extreme lateral interbody fusion (XLIF)

Y

yellow ligament
– in endoscopic interlaminar lumbar laminectomy 274, **275**
– in posterior cervical foraminotomy *146*
– in transforaminal approach for endoscopic decompression 264
– in unilateral lumbar approach for over-the-top bilateral decompression 239, 241

"

"Slalom" technique *155*, **155**